Vascular Surgery

Edited by

G. Heberer and R.J.A.M. van Dongen

With the Assistence of

K.W. Jauch and H. Stiegler

Foreword by

D.C. Sabiston

With Contributions by

K. Aigner, K. Balzer, M.G.M.H. Barwegen, R.G.H. Baumeister
H.M. Becker, D.P. van Berge Henegouwen, R.G.M. Biemans, E. Biemer
U. Brunner, G. Carstensen, H. Denck, H. Denecke, R.J.A.M. van Dongen
F.W. Eigler, F. Franke, F.P. Gall, K.H. Gänger, R. Giessler, J. Greebe
J.D. Gruss, B. Günther, G.W. Hagmüller, H. Hamann, R. Häring
G. Heberer, H. Hess, A. Hirner, A. von Hochstetter, F. Husemann
H. Ingrisch, H.D. Jakubowski, K.W. Jauch, W. Klinner, H. Kortmann
H. Kuppe, K.L. Lauterjung, H. Loeprecht, E. Martin, R. May
H.M. Mehdorn, H. Müller-Wiefel, L. Nieuborg, F. Piza, E. Pratschke
D. Raithel, B. Reichart, H. Rieger, D. Rühland, M. Schemper
F.W. Schildberg, W. Schoop, K. Schwemmle, E.-D. Schwilden, A. Senn
W.-J. Stelter, H. Stiegler, L. Sunder-Plassmann, O. Thetter, H.H. Thiele
M. Trede, A. Valesky, E. U. Voss, O. Wagner, A. Zehle

With 660 Figures, Mostly in Color in 1457 Separate Illustrations

Springer-Verlag Berlin Heidelberg New York
London Paris Tokyo Hong Kong

Professor Dr. G. Heberer
Klinikum Grosshadern, Chirurgische Klinik
und Poliklinik der Universität München
Marchioninistr. 15, D-8000 München 70

Professor Dr. R.J.A.M. van Dongen
Academisch Ziekenhuis bij de Universiteit van Amsterdam
Academisch Medisch Centrum, Vaatchirurgie
Meibergdreef 9, 1105 AZ Amsterdam Zuidoost
The Netherlands

Title of the German Edition: Gefäßchirurgie
(Volume XI of Kirschnersche allgemeine und spezielle Operationslehre,
edited by G. Heberer and R.J.A.M. van Dongen)

ISBN 3-540-18280-2 Springer-Verlag Berlin Heidelberg New York
ISBN 0-387-18280-2 Springer-Verlag New York Berlin Heidelberg

Library of Congress Cataloging-in-Publication Data. Gefässchirurgie. English. Vascular surgery. "Translated from Kirschnersche allgemeine und spezielle Operationslehre, Band XI: Gefässchirurgie" – T.p. verso. Includes bibliographies and index. 1. Blood-vessels – Surgery. I. Heberer, G. (Georg), 1920– . II. Dongen, R.J.A.M. van (Reinier Johannes Antonius Maria) III. Aigner, K. (Karl), 1947– . IV. Title. [DNLM: 1. Vascular Surgery. WG 170 G2987] RD598.5.G4413 1989 617.4′13 89-11274 ISBN 0-387-18280-2 (U.S.: alk. paper)

Illustrations: I. Daxwanger, K. Finch, C. Hengerer, R. Henkel, H. Konopatzki, J. Kühn, J. Pupp, A.A. van Horssen, B. Zimmermann

Reproduction of the Figures: Graphische Kunstanstalt G. Dreher, Stuttgart

Typesetting, Printing and Bookbinding: Universitätsdruckerei H. Stürtz AG, Würzburg

2122/3130-543210 – Printed on acid-free paper

List of Contributors

Aigner, K., Priv.-Doz. Dr., Chirurgische Abteilung des Kreiskrankenhauses, Siegertshöhe 1, D-8223 Trostberg

Balzer, K., Dr., Evangelisches Krankenhaus, Chirurgische Klinik, Teinerstr. 62, D-4330 Mülheim/Ruhr

Barwegen, M.G.M.H., Dr., Sint Maartens Gasthuis, Tegelseweg 210, 5912 BL Venlo, The Netherlands

Baumeister, R.G.H., Prof. Dr., Klinikum Grosshadern, Chirurgische Klinik und Poliklinik der Universität, Marchioninistr. 15, D-8000 München 70

Becker, H.M., Prof. Dr., Gefässchirurgische Abteilung des Städtischen Krankenhauses München-Neuperlach, Oskar-Maria-Graf-Ring 51, D-8000 München 83

van Berge Henegouwen, D.P., Dr., St. Elisabeth-Ziekenhuis, Hilvarenbeekseweg 60, 5000 LC Tilburg, The Netherlands

Biemans, R.G.M., Dr., Zilverstraat 12, B-2120 Schoten

Biemer, E., Prof. Dr., Klinikum rechts der Isar der Technischen Universität, Abteilung für Plastische Chirurgie, Ismaninger Str. 22, D-8000 München 80

Brunner, U. Prof. Dr., Departement Chirurgie, Klinik für Herzgefässchirurgie, Rämistr. 100, CH-8091 Zürich

Carstensen, G., Prof. Dr., Evangelisches Krankenhaus, Chirurgische Klinik, Teinerstr. 62, D-4330 Mülheim/Ruhr

Denck, H., Prof. Dr., Krankenhaus der Stadt Wien-Lainz, I. Chirurgische Abteilung, Wolkersbergenstr. 1, A-1130 Wien

Denecke, H., Prof. Dr., Klinikum Grosshadern, Chirurgische Klinik und Poliklinik der Universität, Marchioninistr. 15, D-8000 München 70

van Dongen, R.J.A.M., Prof. Dr., Academisch Ziekenhuis bij de Universiteit van Amsterdam, Academisch Medisch Centrum, Vaatchirurgie, Meibergdreef 9, 1105 AZ Amsterdam Zuidoost, The Netherlands

Eigler, F.W., Prof. Dr., Klinikum der Gesamthochschule, Chirurgische Klinik und Poliklinik der Universität, Abteilung für Allgemeine Chirurgie, Hufelandstr. 55, D-4300 Essen 1

Franke, F., Prof. Dr., Waldkrankenhaus St. Marien, Chirurgische Klinik, Rathsberger Str. 57, D-8520 Erlangen

Gall, F.P., Prof. Dr., Chirurgische Universitätsklinik, Maximiliansplatz 1, D-8520 Erlangen

Gänger, K.H., Dr., †, CH-Bern

Giessler, R., Dr., Aggertalklinik, Chirurgische Abteilung, Klinik für Gefässerkrankungen, D-5250- Engelskirchen

Greebe, J., Dr., Majella Ziekenhuis, Nieuwe Hilversumseweg 20, 1406 TE Bussum, The Netherlands

Gruss, J.D., Prof. Dr., Kurhessisches Diakonissenhaus, Gefässchirurgische Abteilung, Goethestr. 85, D-3500 Kassel

Günther, B., Prof. Dr., Städtisches Krankenhaus München-Neuperlach, 1. Chirurgische Abteilung, Oskar-Maria-Graf-Ring 51, D-8000 München 83

HAGMÜLLER, G.W., Doz. Dr., Wattmannsgasse 71, A-1130 Wien
HAMANN, H., Prof. Dr., Klinikum der Universität, Abteilung für Thorax- und Gefässchirurgie, Steinhövelstr. 9, D-7900 Ulm
HÄRING, R., Prof. Dr., Universitätsklinikum Steglitz, Chirurgische Klinik und Poliklinik, Hindenburgdamm 30, D-1000 Berlin 45
HEBERER, G., Prof. Dr., Klinikum Grosshadern, Chirurgische Klinik und Poliklinik der Universität, Marchioninistr. 15, D-8000 München 70
HESS, H., Prof. Dr., Thaddäus-Eck-Str. 3, D-8000 München 60
HIRNER, A., Priv.-Doz. Dr., Universitätsklinikum Steglitz, Chirurgische Klinik und Poliklinik, Hindenburgdamm 30, D-1000 Berlin 45
VON HOCHSTETTER, A., Prof. Dr., Kantonsspital, Universitätskliniken, Departement für Chirurgie, Abteilung für topographische und klinische Anatomie, CH-4031 Basel
HUSEMANN, F., Dr., Gynäkologische Klinik, Kreiskrankenhaus, Schwarzenmoorstr. 70, D-4900 Herford
INGRISCH, H., Prof. Dr., Abteilung für Strahlendiagnostik des Städtischen Krankenhauses München-Bogenhausen, Englschalkinger Str. 77, D-8000 München 81
JAKUBOWSKI, H.D., Prof. Dr., Schmölderstr. 78, D-4050 Mönchengladbach 2
JAUCH, K.W., Priv.-Doz. Dr., Klinikum Grosshadern, Chirurgische Klinik und Poliklinik der Universität, Marchioninistr. 15, D-8000 München 70
KLINNER, W., Prof. Dr., Klinikum Grosshadern, Herzchirurgische Klinik der Universität, Marchioninistr. 15, D-8000 München 70
KORTMANN, H., Prof. Dr., Klinikum Grosshadern, Chirurgische Klinik und Poliklinik der Universität, Marchioninistr. 15, D-8000 München 70
KUPPE, H., Dr., Deutsches Herzzentrum, Augustenburger Platz, D-1000 Berlin
LAUTERJUNG, K.L., Prof. Dr., Klinikum Grosshadern, Chirurgische Klinik und Poliklinik der Universität, Marchioninistr. 15, D-8000 München 70
LOEPRECHT, H., Prof. Dr., Krankenhauszweckverband Augsburg, Klinik für Gefäss- und Thoraxchirurgie, Chirurgische Klinik I, Stenglinstr., D-8900 Augsburg
MARTIN, E., Prof. Dr., Klinikum Nürnberg, Institut für Anästhesiologie, Flurstr. 17, D-8500 Nürnberg 91
MAY, R., Prof. Dr., †, A-Innsbruck
MEHDORN, H.M., Priv.-Doz. Dr., Universitätsklinikum der Gesamthochschule, Neurochirurgische Klinik, Hufelandstr. 55, D-4300 Essen 1
MÜLLER-WIEFEL, H., Prof. Dr., St. Johannes-Hospital Duisburg-Hamborn, Gefässchirurgische Klinik, An der Abtei 7-11, D-4100 Duisburg 11
NIEUBORG, L., Dr., Geerstraat 19, 6456 AK Bingelrade, The Netherlands
PIZA, F., Prof. Dr., Allgemeines Krankenhaus der Stadt Wien, I. Chirurgische Universitätsklinik, Alser Str. 4, A-1097 Wien IX
PRATSCHKE, E., Priv.-Doz. Dr., Klinikum Grosshadern, Chirurgische Klinik und Poliklinik der Universität, Marchioninistr. 15, D-8000 München 70
RAITHEL, D., Prof. Dr., Klinikum Nürnberg, Zentrum für Chirurgie, Fachabteilung für Gefässchirurgie, Flurstr. 17, D-8500 Nürnberg
REICHART, B., Prof. Dr., Department of Cardio-Thoracic Surgery, Groote Schuur Hospital, 7925 Cape Town, Republic of South Africa
RIEGER, H., Prof. Dr., Aggertalklinik, Spezialklinik für Gefässerkrankungen, D-5250 Engelskirchen
RÜHLAND, D., Prof. Dr., Städtisches Krankenhaus, Chirurgische Klinik, Virchowstr. 10, D-7700 Singen
SCHEMPER, M., Dr., Allgemeines Krankenhaus der Stadt Wien, I. Chirurgische Universitätsklinik, Alser Str. 4, A-1090 Wien IX

Schildberg, F.W., Prof. Dr., Klinikum Grosshadern, Chirurgische Klinik und Poliklinik der Universität, Marchioninistr. 15, D-8000 München 70

Schoop, W., Prof. Dr., Aggertalklinik, Spezialklinik für Gefässerkrankungen, D-5250 Engelskirchen

Schwemmle, K., Prof. Dr., Klinikum der Universität, Medizinisches Zentrum für Chirurgie, Anästhesiologie und Urologie, Klinik für Allgemeinchirurgie, Klinikstr. 29, D-6300 Giessen

Schwilden, E.-D., Dr., Städtische Krankenanstalten, Chirurgische Klinik, Abteilung Gefässchirurgie, Hirschlandstr. 97, D-7300 Esslingen

Senn, A., Prof. Dr., Holligenstr. 93, CH-3008 Bern

Stelter, W.-J., Prof. Dr., Städtisches Krankenhaus Frankfurt/Main-Höchst, Chirurgische Klinik, Gotenstr. 6–8, D-6230 Frankfurt/Main 80

Stiegler, H., Priv.-Doz. Dr., Klinikum Grosshadern, Chirurgische Klinik und Poliklinik der Universität, Marchioninistr. 15, D-8000 München 70

Sunder-Plassmann, L., Prof. Dr., Klinikum Grosshadern, Chirurgische Klinik und Poliklinik der Universität, Marchioninistr. 15, D-8000 München 70

Thetter, O., Prof. Dr., Chirurgische Klinik Innenstadt und Chirurgische Poliklinik der Universität, Nußbaumstr. 20, D-8000 München 2

Thiele, H.H., Dr., Krankenhaus Bruchsal, Chirurgische Klinik, Gutleutstr. 9/14, D-7520 Bruchsal

Trede, M., Prof. Dr., Klinikum der Stadt Mannheim, Chirurgische Klinik, Postfach 23, D-6800 Mannheim 1

Valesky, A., Prof. Dr., Stadtkrankenhaus, Chirurgische Klinik, Leinenstr. 20, D-6450 Hanau

Voss, E.-U., Priv.-Doz. Dr., Klinikum Karlsruhe, Gefässchirurgische Abteilung, Moltkestr. 14, D-7500 Karlsruhe

Wagner, O., Prof. Dr., Krankenhaus der Barmherzigen Brüder, Chirurgische Abteilung, Grosse Mohrengasse 9, A-1021 Wien

Zehle, A., Prof. Dr., Städtisches Krankenhaus, Chirurgische Klinik, Abteilung Allgemein-, Gefäss- und Thoraxchirurgie, Röntgenstr. 2, D-7900 Friedrichshafen 1

Foreword

In view of the extraordinary advances which have been made in the field of vascular surgery during the past 30 years, this English translation of Professors HEBERER and VAN DONGEN is a *monumental* achievement. In this unusually thorough, yet concise and superbly written monograph, the authors have brought the state of the art in this field to a new standard of *excellence*. In achieving this important task, they have sought the most outstanding vascular surgeons in Germany, the Netherlands, Austria, and Switzerland as contributors.

Quite appropriately, this remarkable text begins with a review of the pioneers in vascular surgery whose contributions later proved to be fundamental to both the initiation and development of vascular surgery. The contributions of CARREL and GUTHRIE in perfecting the technique of vascular anastomosis, and the work of LERICHE in developing clinical arterial surgery are engagingly reviewed. Appropriate attention is also given the fundamental contributions of GOYANES in his first successful use of the saphenous vein graft to restore circulatory continuity following resection of a popliteal aneurysm in 1906. Well deserved praise is given another pioneer whose contributions are seldom given the credit which they deserve, specifically those of JEGER, whose monograph published in 1913 entitled *"Die Chirurgie der Blutgefäße und des Herzens"* is one of the most impressive and visionary documentaries ever written in vascular surgery.

The editors next turn to an excellent chapter on anatomical aspects of vascular surgery. The illustrations in this chapter, as in all others in this text, are especially noteworthy for their clarity and the vivid impressions they make. Readers have come to regard this feature as a hallmark of Springer-Verlag publications. Following are well described accounts of the fundamentals of vascular hemodynamics and the general principles involved in the *techniques* of vascular surgery. In a very effective manner, the authors illustrate *poor* techniques often employed and contrast them with those which have been proven to be superior. This approach is particularly effective in emphasizing the importance of meticulous technique in determining the final clinical result. Very helpful, especially to young surgeons in training, are the sections on microsurgery and angiocardiography. The advances made during the past decade in *percutaneous transluminal angioplasty* are admirably described and convincingly illustrated with a summary of the current results obtained with this important technique.

The various disorders of the vascular system amenable to surgical correction are systematically reviewed by recognized authorities in the field with carefully detailed descriptions of the indications for operation, preparation of the patient, diagnostic techniques, and operative approach in appropriate detail. The potential complications of each of the procedures are presented as well as an updated discussion of modern management.

In the closing words of the Preface, the editors state: "Let us hope that this manual, the product of more than 30 years of personal experience, will become a useful source of sound advice in the field of vascular surgery." This reviewer is convinced beyond doubt that this has been achieved in this praiseworthy text. It can be confidently predicted that this monograph will become a worldwide standard by which *all* other similar works will be compared, and it is regarded as an essential text for all surgeons who practice vascular surgery.

DAVID C. SABISTON, Jr., M.D.

James B. Duke Professor of Surgery
and Chairman of the Department
Duke University Medical Center
Durham, North Carolina, USA

Preface

In recent decades surgical procedures for reconstruction of the aorta, arteries, veins, and lymph vessels have undergone extensive development. Advances were made possible through the improvement of instruments and suture material, through progress in biologic and synthetic grafts, and through developments in anesthesiology and surgical techniques as well. The initial result worldwide was the almost precipitate growth of the field of vascular surgery. For a time, opinions changed rapidly on fundamental matters such as operative procedures and techniques, choice of grafts for the various vascular areas, and clinical indications. Since that time, however, operative techniques have been standardized to a considerable degree, and a manual of vascular surgery therefore seems called for (exclusive of the coronary vessels, which are dealt with in the volume *"Heart Surgery"*). The present volume, the German edition of which is *Volume 11 of Kirschner's series of manuals,* consists of contributions by the editors and their colleagues and by numerous experts on vascular surgery from Germany, The Netherlands, Austria, and Switzerland.

In the *General Section* the preparation of the patient and indications for operation are discussed, as well as documentation and quality control. Surgical anatomy, instruments, and general operative techniques are clearly illustrated in comprehensive figures. Furthermore, general complications such as infection, bleeding, and reocclusion are outlined with particular emphasis on their prevention, early detection, and indication, as well as on the timing of reintervention.

In the *Special Section* the operative treatment of diseases of the aorta and arteries of all body regions, as well as of veins and of lymph vessels are discussed, also indications, operative approaches, and operative procedures. The various steps of the operations are presented dynamically using clear multicolored sequences of figures. Microsurgical techniques and rare operative procedures are also taken into consideration. Alternative techniques of vascular surgery and angiology to overcome unexpected difficulties are also mentioned.

We owe special thanks to our contributors for their much-appreciated collaboration. The procedures of the various operative phases are explained by figures and figure sequences, some of which cover an entire page. We are indebted to the artists, Mrs. I. DAXWANGER of Munich, Mr. J. KÜHN and colleagues of Heidelberg, and Mr. A.A. VAN HORSEN of Amsterdam. We would also like to thank the staff of Springer-Verlag, especially Dr. H. GÖTZE, Mr. W. BERGSTEDT, Mrs. I. LEGNER, and Mr. E. KIRCHNER, for the excellent preparation and appearance of the book. In addition, we would like to thank K.W. JAUCH, Munich, and H. STIEGLER, Munich, for their collaboration and their efforts in correcting the text. We are also indebted to Prof. Dr. H.H. LÖHR, Hamburg, for preparing the index.

Finally, we appreciate the translation into English by R. HATZ, Munich, R.K. TEICHMANN, Munich, and T. HAU, Wilhelmshaven, and thank Mr. W. POHL for the care he has taken in revising the text. We also thank Miss J. ESSLINGER and Miss C. DAEHNE for typing the manuscript.

Let us hope that this manual, the product of more than 30 years of personal experience, will become a useful source of sound advice in the field of vascular surgery.

Munich and Amsterdam

G. Heberer
R.J.A.M. van Dongen

Table of Contents

General Section

Special Section

General Section

1 History of Vascular Surgery

R.J.A.M. VAN DONGEN

CONTENTS

A. Introduction

Toward the end of the nineteenth century, experiments were performed in physiological and surgical laboratories all over the world in search of new vascular suture techniques (ECK 1877, JASSINOWSKY 1889, HEIDENHEIM 1895, VILLAR and BRACHET 1895, MURPHY 1897, DÖRFLER 1899, JENSEN 1903). Methods of vascular replacement were likewise sought [17]. Most of these investigations were carried out in Europe, where it was the French school which contributed most to the development of vascular surgery. Three men, all of them from Lyon, made decisive contributions: MATHIEU JABOULAY and his pupils, ALEXIS CARREL (Fig. 1.1) and RENÉ LERICHE (Fig. 1.2) [13]. JABOULAY was not as well known as the others, partly because his papers were published solely in the regional journal Lyon Medical, and partly because he died in a train accident at an early age. LERICHE made significant advances in the basic physiology and surgery of the sympathetic nervous system. CARREL was really the pioneer and founder of experimental vascular surgery [18, 21].

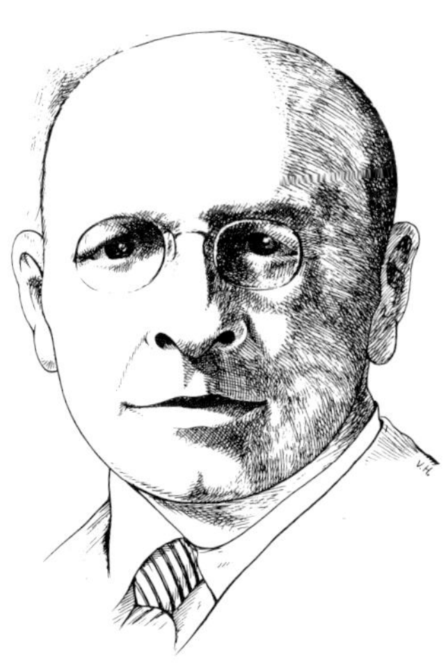

Fig. 1.1. ALEXIS CARREL (1873–1944)

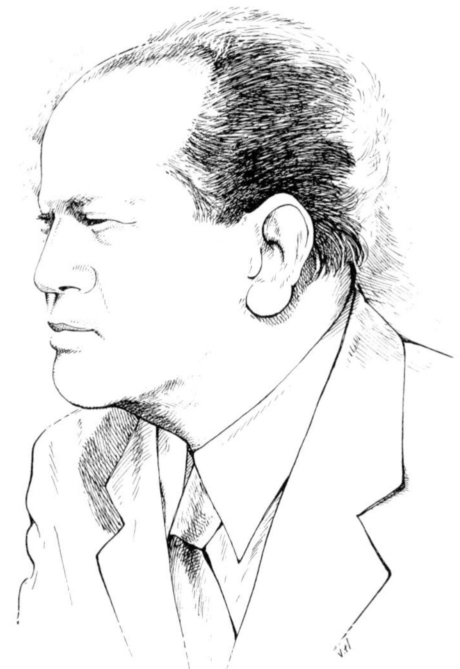

Fig. 1.2. RENÉ LERICHE (1879–1955)

In 1890, CARREL was admitted to the medical school of Lyon. As a student he was already greatly interested in the possibility of repairing blood vessels. This interest was precipitated by the assassination of the President of the French Republic,

MARIE FRANCOIS SADI CARNOT, by the Italian anarchist, SANTO CASERIO in 1894. The President underwent laparotomy immediately after the assault and injury of the portal vein was found. He bled to death because none of the surgeons was able to reconstruct the injured vessel. CARREL publicly discussed the inability of his teachers to repair a vascular injury and decided to devote himself to intensive research on the surgery of blood vessels. He had his first opportunity in the laboratory of SOULIER in Lyon where he worked together with MOREL.

However, CARREL did not receive much recognition in Lyon. In May 1904 he emigrated to Canada (Montreal and Toronto) where he was given the opportunity to continue his experiments. Only a short time later, in 1905, he received an appointment at the Hull Laboratory of Physiology at the University of Chicago, where he was able to continue his research in productive cooperation with GUTHRIE.

In August, 1906 GUTHRIE moved to St. Louis, where he worked at the Washington University, and CARREL changed to the Rockefeller Institute in New York; they kept in contact with each other through their common interest.

From the beginning, they recognized that vascular sutures and vascular anastomoses can only be successful if they are done with the utmost precision and care. In 1906, CARREL wrote the following which is still valid 80 years later: "The vessels must be handled very gently and the endothelium must be protected from drying by isotonic saline solution. The sutures must be impregnated and the vascular wall coated with vaseline. No dangerous metallic forceps are used. Great care is exercised to obtain accurate and smooth approximation of the endothelium of the vessels without invagination. Sutures should be made with very fine needles while the wall is somewhat stretched. Stenosis or occlusion only occurs as a result of faulty technique" [3].

All kinds of arterial and venous reconstructions were developed and tried out in experiments, including free arterial and venous grafts. CARREL's epoch-making work found recognition all over the world. In 1912 he received the Nobel Prize in Medicine "in recognition of his work on vascular suture and the transplantation of blood vessels and organs."

B. Homologous Vascular Replacement

CARREL understood that the availability of autologous grafts was limited and that they were not suited for the replacement of large arteries; therefore, he showed great interest in homologous grafts and in the creation of an experimental blood vessel bank.

The first clinical transplantation of a homologous artery from one human to another was performed by PIROVANO in 1910 and published in the Presse Médicale in 1911. However, it was not a success. The method was discredited and forgotten for many decades. Not until 1949 did the homologous transplant graft regain importance when ROBERT GROSS et al. successfully employed a homologous graft to bridge an aortic defect between the left subclavian and the left pulmonary artery during surgery of an aortic coarctation and a Blalock-Taussig operation. These first successful implantations led to the idea of preserving the arteries of persons who died in accidents and of storing them for clinical purposes in a blood vessel bank.

Over the years, various methods of preservation have been recommended. CARREL (1908) and GROSS (1949) worked with vessels that had been stored in a liquid medium at 4° C. However, such vessels were only preservable for 4–6 weeks. EASTCOTT and HUFNAGEL and also CHARLES ROB [11] employed a method of deep freezing at −20° C. These grafts could be preserved almost indefinitely. MARANGONI (1951), HEBERER and GIESSLER (1956), LINDNER (1955) and STAUDACHER (1974) recommended freeze-drying, and the method of lyophilization, which also preserved grafts indefinitely. In Tilburg MOEYS successfully preserved arteries of corpses in 4% formaldehyde and published his experimental results in Archivum Chirurgicum Neerlandicum in 1954.

RENÉ FONTAINE was enthusiastic about the possibility of using homologous arteries for vascular replacement and founded the first vessel bank of Europe in 1951.

Since 1950, homologous artery transplant grafts have been the method of choice for replacing blood vessels. Enormous advances in vascular surgery, especially at the aortoiliac level, were made possible by homeotransplant grafts. The first replacements of the aortic bifurcation were done using such grafts.

In 1923 RENÉ LERICHE predicted, that "ideal treatment of thrombosis of the terminal aorta should consist of a resection of the occluded segment and reestablishment of arterial continuity by a graft," but he never performed this operation himself. LERICHE and his younger colleague RENÉ FONTAINE were convinced that an occluded vessel provokes a vasoconstrictive response of the collaterals. Therefore they assumed that arterial resection was the therapy of choice in arterial occlusions. An occluded aortic bifurcation was resected without replacement, followed by bilateral sympathectomy. LERICHE did not trust vascular grafts. At the beginning of the century he tried to replace two thrombosed arteries by grafts, but could not find the correct site for anastomosis. It will be recalled that arteriography did not exist at that time. Angiography was developed 20 years later by EGAZ MONIZ and RAYNALDO DOS SANTOS, both in Lisbon.

In 1950, some 27 years after LERICHE had predicted it, the first replacement of the aortic bifurcation was performed by JACQUES OUDOT. A preserved bifurcation from an accident victim was transplanted. OUDOT was not only a good vascular surgeon, but also an enthusiastic mountain climber and automobile driver. In 1950 he participated in the first ascent of the Annapurna in Nepal which is over 8000 m high. His second hobby, driving, proved fatal: he died in a car accident in 1953 at the age of 40.

In 1951, the first resection of an aortic aneurysm with vascular replacement was performed by CHARLES DUBOST in Paris [19]. The infrarenal aneurysm was exposed by means of a left-sided thoracicoabdominal incision and resected. There was no aortic bifurcation graft available. Therefore, a 3-week-old homologous graft of a thoracic aorta was implanted between the infrarenal aorta and the right common iliac artery. The occluded left common iliac artery was endarterectomized and connected to the graft.

Until 1960, transplantation of homologous arteries was the method of choice for replacing diseased arterial segments. Unfortunately, the long-term results of homologous grafts were unsatisfactory. Progressive degenerative changes within these homologous grafts often led to reocclusion or caused serious complications, such as calcification, aneurysm formation, and rupture.

Meanwhile, it was found that synthetic arterial grafts were clearly superior to homologous arterial transplants in their biologic qualities. The homologous artery transplant was abandoned, and in large arteries alloplastic material, in small arteries autologous vein grafts were used instead.

More favorable results have been achieved in recent years using homologous vein grafts in the form of preserved umbilical veins. In 1973, HERBERT DARDIK published his experiences using such vein grafts in baboons. Some years later (1976) [5], he reported on his first clinical results. DARDIK first used Ringer's lactate solution at a temperature between 0° and 20° C to preserve these umbilical veins. However, they developed ectasias and aneurysms, inflammation, focal necroses and microabscesses. Later, he used dialdehydes to fix and eliminate antigenicity from the veins and after that changed to glutaraldehyde with reinforcement of the vessels using a polyester net to prevent aneurysms. The prostheses were stored in a 50% ethyl alcohol solution.

In contrast to Dardik's graft, the umbilical vein of Mindich is fixed by a different solution and has both umbilical arteries still present; the graft, furthermore, is not reinforced with alloplastic material.

C. Heterologous Vascular Replacement

Heterologous grafts have been employed much less frequently. The first experiments – also done by CARREL in 1906 [3] using these heterologous arterial grafts seemed very promising at first. But it soon became apparent that the complication rate was very high. Attempts by SAUTOT (1952) and KIMOTO (1954) to overcome the species-specific characteristics of such animal vessels were disappointing.

In 1956 NORMAN ROSENBERG et al. began to conduct experiments with bovine arteries treated with the proteolytic protein-splitting enzyme extracted from wild figs and kept in a buffered solution.

This eliminated all antigenic structures such as muscle tissue and elastic fibers. A nonantigenetic collagenous tube remains, which, however, is porous. These prostheses are made leak-proof by treating them with buffered dialdehyde starch solution. Since 1965, ROSENBERG has gained much clinical experience with his "artegrafts" in the United States. Other American surgeons, e.g., DALE, KESHISHIAN and JOHNSON, also reported satisfactory results. However, the clinical application of these modified bovine grafts remained limited.

In Europe artegrafts have been used much less frequently. Not until AMGWERD [1] and SEGE

(1975) reported on the first clinical experiences using modified heteroplastic arterial grafts from calf arteries, did the golden era of vascular replacement with such prostheses begin in Europe. However, the solcograft was soon abandoned because of the high rate of complications (thromboses, ruptures).

D. Alloplastic Vascular Replacement

As already mentioned, the homologous transplant in large arteries was replaced by the alloplastic prosthesis starting about 1960. The idea of replacing blood vessels with synthetic material is about 400 years old, but not until the beginning of this century did surgeons begin to investigate this problem experimentally. One of the pioneers in this field was ALEXIS CARREL [3]. His attempts to replace arteries with compact, rigid tubes made of glass and aluminum and covered with a layer of paraffin failed. Tubes made of ivory and rubber as well as the tubes developed by TUFFIER (1917), which were made of silver and covered with a layer of paraffin, were also unsuccessful. These silver tubes were used during the First World War, but only as temporary arterial shunts. BLAKEMORE tried vitallium prostheses during the Second World War, and DONOVAN experimented with polyethylene tubes later on (in 1949). But all these attempts were unsuccessful, as were the experiments with polyethylene prostheses by MOORE (1950).

Then, in 1952, came the surprising report by VOORHOEVE, JARETZKI, and BLAKEMORE [22] in the Annals of Surgery on the application of Vinyon-N tubes made of porous, biologically inert material that remained patent in animal experiments. This paper had an explosive effect in the field of vascular surgery and marked the beginning of further rapid advances in alloplastic vascular replacement, above all, after EDWARDS'S and TAPP'S introduction, in 1955, of crimping, which gave the synthetic prosthesis more elasticity in longitudinal and transverse directions and prevented kinking in curved vessels.

When Vinyon-N was no longer available, Ivalon was introduced commercially. Later, tubes consisting of Orlon were produced ready for use. In 1957 woven Nylon prostheses were introduced, in 1958 woven and knitted Teflon tubes. Finally, Dacron prostheses appeared. WESELOWSKI, SZILAGYI, HEBERER, COOLEY, SAUVAGE, and many others contributed greatly to the development and application of synthetic prostheses.

E. Autologous Vascular Replacement [2, 11]

For replacement of small vessels the arterial homologous transplant was abandoned in favor of the venous autograft. As early as 1903 HÖPFNER performed experiments with autologous vein grafts. Previously, CLEMENTI (1894), JABOULAY and BRIAN (1896), and EXNER (1903) had reported on unsuccessful attempts. The first successful application of this technique was in 1906, when CARREL and GUTHRIE replaced the carotid arteries of dogs with segments of the jugular vein. The fact that CARREL was successful where his colleagues had failed was undoubtedly due to his previous advances in the field of vascular anastomoses.

In 1906 the pioneer studies of CARREL and GUTHRIE were already well known throughout the entire surgical world. The Madrid surgeon, JOSE GOYANES, must have been well acquainted with them when, shortly before CARREL, he published two papers in the Spanish medical weekly journal El Siglo Med. (1 and 8 September 1906) on the successful replacement of the aorta by segments of the vena cava in dogs. These reports were read by very few outside of Spain.

Only much later was it reported that GOYANES had not only succeeded in experiments, he was also the first to use venous autografts clinically. In his first publication on 1 September 1906, he reported on a case in which he divided the iliac artery and sutured it to the proximally ligated iliac vein. He had divided the femoral vein above the knee joint and connected the proximal end to the distal femoral artery, thus bypassing an obstruction of the upper half of that artery. The result of this first bypass operation (strictly speaking it was an in situ bypass) was reported to be good, although no explicit details of the postoperative course are known.

The basic surgical principle of a bypass procedure using a free venous autograft was clearly described and studied in animal experiments for the first time by ERNST JEGER [14], a surgeon at the Berlin University Hospital who, in 1913 at the age of 29, wrote an impressive book with the daring title: The Surgery of Blood Vessels and the Heart – "dedicated to ALEXIS CARREL in gratitude and admiration." He not only described the vascular techniques developed by CARREL, but he also reviewed the entire field of vascular and heart surgery as it existed at that time. In addition, he wrote extensively about his own experiences as a vascular surgeon and predicted the future development of heart, vascular, and transplantation surgery.

GOYANES, in his second paper a week after the first one, reported on a 41-year-old patient with a luetic aneurysm of the popliteal artery. He had resected this aneurysm on 12 June 1906 and replaced it with a segment of the popliteal vein, which had remained in situ. Even though the wound became infected, the operation was a success. Blood circulation of the lower limb was maintained.

Some 6 months later ERICH LEXER from the University Hospital in Königsberg was confronted with a similar problem [15]. It concerned a 69-year-old man with a false aneurysm of the axillary artery. Primary anastomosis of the remaining vascular stumps following resection of the aneurysm was not possible. Therefore, he decided to restore continuity by using a segment of the great saphenous vein. Unfortunately, the patient died 5 days after the operation, of delirium tremens. But the autopsy, which LEXER himself performed, showed that the graft was patent. He reported on this operation at the 36th Congress of the German Surgical Society in April 1907 and published the case in Archiv für Klinische Chirurgie. This paper caused great interest in the Anglo-American countries, where renowned surgical centers had begun laboratory testing of vascular replacement by autografts. It did not take long for the first results to be published. In 1913 PRINGLE (Glasgow) reported in The Lancet on two patients in whom he had removed aneurysms of the popliteal artery and brachial artery and bridged the defects with autologous vein grafts. In the United States BERTRAM BERNHEIM, a colleague of WILLIAM S. HALSTED at John Hopkins Hospital, was the first to publish successful results.

The first experiments with the use of autologous vein grafts for treatment of arterial injuries and traumatic aneurysms were performed by SOUBBOTITCH, a surgeon from Belgrade who served as a military physician in the Serbian army during the Balkan War.

By 1917, according to WARTHMÜLLER a total of 51 patients had received autologous vein grafts, of whom 39 showed successful results. This led LEXER to conclude: "the replacement of arterial defects with autologous vein grafts is justly beginning to gain great importance in surgery."

However, interest in the venous autograft subsided for 30 years. During that time the entire field of vascular surgery seemed to have been forgotten. WEGLOWSKI was one of the very few surgeons who continued to amass experience. During the First World War he used autografts in 55 wounded soldiers. Patency of the graft could be shown in 40 of 47 survivors. His publications were hardly known in foreign countries, probably because they were published in Russian and Polish journals. Not until 1925 did his results receive recognition upon publication in the Zentralblatt für Chirurgie.

During this period of inactivity, two very important requirements for successful reconstructive vascular surgery were fulfilled: the possibility of diagnosing vascular disease with respect to its nature and extent, and the control of blood coagulation.

The first gap was closed by two Portugese investigators. Although HASCHEK and LINDENTHAL had already filled the arteries of corpses with contrast medium and had taken X-ray photographs of them in 1896, clinical angiography was not introduced until 1927–1929, when EGAZ MONIZ and REYNALDO DOS SANTOS employed it for the first time.

The introduction of anticoagulants, especially heparin (discovered in 1916 by JAY MACLEAN, animal experiments in 1918 by HOWELL and HOLT, chemical purification in 1933 by CHARLES and SCOTT, and first application by CRAWFORD in 1935) made it possible to control thrombosis. However, these discoveries were not applied generally and routinely until the last years of the Second World War. This represented the magic key to reconstructive vascular surgery, and the future success of artery replacement using vascular grafts was assured.

On 3 June 1948, JEAN KUNLIN (Fig. 1.3) performed his first bypass operation using a free autologous vein graft at the small Hopital Americain in Paris. The technique of this operation had been perfected beforehand by KUNLIN. His method of anastomosis has remained a standard technique to this day. KUNLIN, who had knowledge of JEGER's book [14], got the idea of bridging an obliterated arterial segment after JEAN CID DOS SANTOS had demonstrated his method of endarterectomy in the Hopital Americain. He perceived that an occlusion was limited to a particular arterial segment, and that the vessel was relatively normal

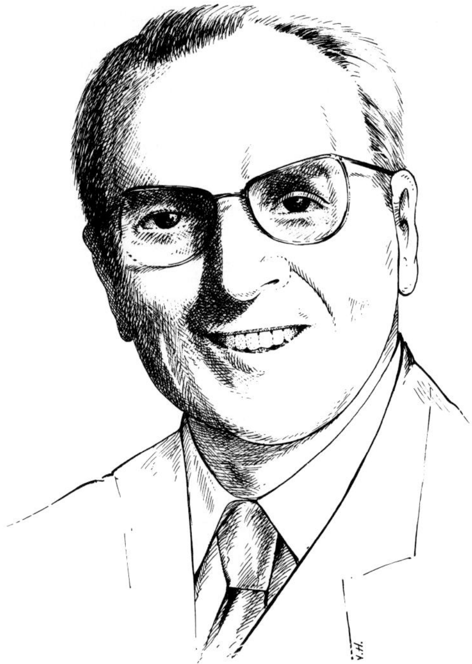

Fig. 1.3. JEAN KUNLIN (*1904)

distal to the occlusion and showed good patency in any case.

In the same year, KUNLIN performed 13 venous graft bypass operations. Encouraged by the excellent results, LERICHE soon became convinced that bypass surgery was the technique of the future.

Soon, this new method was being used all over the world. The great breakthrough came during the Korean War. The American surgical team which introduced reconstructive vascular surgery in the front lines in 1953 achieved good results. The publications of DYE et al. (1956), DALE (1974), as well as LINTON and DARLING (1962) made venous bypass grafting very popular [4].

F. Thromboendarterectomy

In the era before the discovery of heparin, open disobliteration of arteries had already been attempted, but without success. Not until heparin achieved clinical significance did new opportunities appear in this field.

JEAN CID DOS SANTOS (Fig. 1.4), the son of the famous inventor of angiography, utilized the antithrombotic effect of heparin when he performed his first successful disobliteration.

JEAN CID DOS SANTOS had studied with LERICHE in Strasbourg during the 1930s, repeating many of CARREL's experiments under the supervision of LERICHE, who had become director of the surgical department in 1924. During the war he served in the Azores. Following his return to Lisbon, where he directed the surgical department, he had the opportunity to apply his knowledge and skill in the practice of vascular surgery. In June 1946, he removed an acutely formed thrombus from the femoral artery. As he examined the specimen, he discovered that he had inadvertently removed the intima and a portion of the media. The artery remained patent for many months.

He concluded that, in order to keep an artery patent, an uninjured intima is not absolutely necessary if heparin is used for anticoagulation. As in many instances of medical progress, the discovery of thromboendarterectomy came by chance.

During the next few years, open disobliteration was performed mainly by French surgeons (BAZY, REBOUL, HUGUIER). Despite initial enthusiasm, it was shown that the long-term results were not satisfactory. The fervent discussions of thromboendarterectomy soon quieted down. However, this technique experienced a renaissance following the introduction of patch graft angioplasty and the

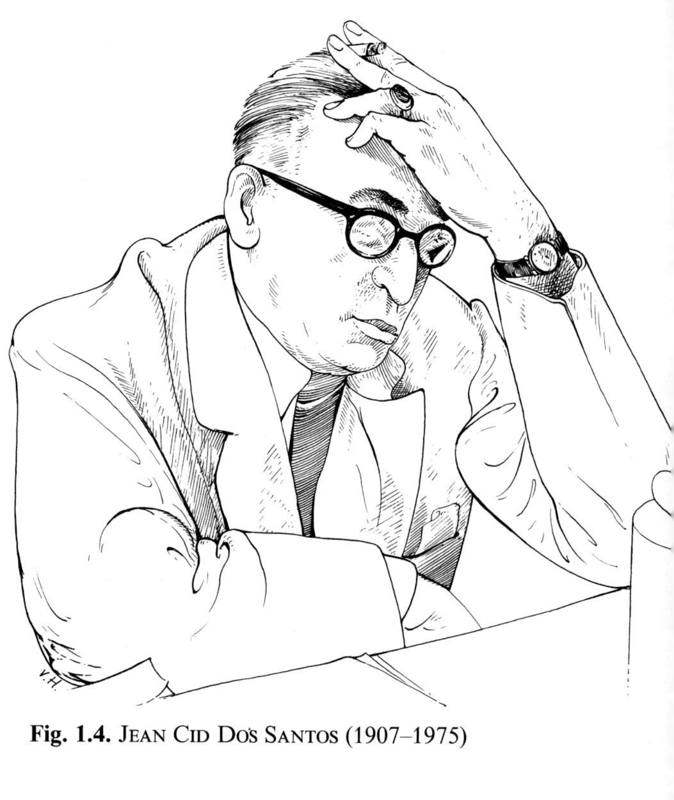

Fig. 1.4. JEAN CID DOS SANTOS (1907–1975)

extension of disobliteration beyond the occluded segment ("overpass", J.C. Dos Santos, 1963). Patch graft angioplasty had already been mentioned by Carrell and Guthrie in 1906. It was propagated especially by DeBakey [6] at the beginning of the 1950s.

In 1952, the American surgeons Cannon and Barker introduced ring stripping, a semiclosed method. However, this method lost its importance after 1960 in favor of the bypass technique, especially in the femoropopliteal region.

G. Other Applications of Vascular Surgical Techniques

Until 1952, all reported materials and methods were used exclusively in the aortoiliac region and the extremities. As reconstructive vascular surgery progressed, it was applied to other regions.

In 1951 Shimizu and Sano made the first attempt to disobliterate the internal carotid artery. They proceeded from the external carotid artery, which was sacrificed. A slight improvement was noticed. In a second patient the carotid bifurcation was resected and replaced by a venous homotransplant; here, too, the external carotid artery was sacrificed. Postoperatively, the patency of the graft could not be confirmed.

The first successful open thromboendarterectomy of the carotid bifurcation was performed by DeBakey on 7 August 1953. In the following years, it was Eastcott, Pikkering and Rob in London who contributed most to the development of carotid surgery [6]. Relatively soon, the basic principles of vascular reconstruction were applied to renal arteries. The first revascularization of a kidney was accomplished in 1952 by Thompson and Smithwick by means of a splenorenal anastomosis. Unfortunately, this operation was not a success, and the kidney had to be removed 17 days after surgery. A year later (1953), Freeman reconstructed a stenotic renal artery by endarterectomy. The first bilateral renal artery reconstruction was performed by Poutasse in 1956 using a homologous arterial graft.

Surgical treatment of chronic occlusive disease of the visceral arteries did not exist until 1958, when the first endarterectomy of the superior mesenteric artery was performed by Shaw and Maynard. A year later, Mikkelsen and Zaro became the first to transect and reimplant the superior mesenteric artery. DeBakey devised a new bypass procedure for reconstruction of the intestinal arteries in 1961.

H. Embolic Occlusions

The first embolectomy was attempted by Suabanejew in the year 1896. In 1911, Lahey in Paris was the first surgeon to successfully remove an embolus from the common femoral artery. The report of Key (1923) on a series of 10 embolectomies, of which 6 were successful, substantially contributed to the further widespread application of this new operative technique.

The technique of indirect embolectomy was also performed very early. The English surgeon Handley made an attempt to remove a blood clot by suction in 1907. Griffiths (1938) used a coiled corkscrew-like wire, Key (1936) used curets, and Seen (1963) pliers. Since Fogarty reported on his inflatable balloon catheter in 1963, his method has been preferred by most surgeons worldwide.

The first attempt to remove an embolus from the superior mesenteric artery was made by the Russian surgeon Ryvlin in 1943. However, he was not able to restore blood flow through the vessel. In 1951, Klass was more successful, but the patient died a few days after the operation. In 1955, a patient of Wise survived an embolectomy without additional bowel resection.

The history of vascular surgery is very extensive [21, 23]. It is not limited to the development of new techniques, methods, and materials. Many other advances in the most widely varying fields of medicine have made progress in vascular surgery possible. The most important advances have come in asepsis, anesthesiology, blood transfusion, blood coagulation, angiography, and microsurgery. Furthermore, one should not forget the refinements of diagnostic procedures, the simplification of flow and pressure measurement, the improvement of instruments, etc. Further development in these and many other fields will surely lead to great possibilities in the future [8, 10].

REFERENCES

1. Amgwerd R (1975) Unsere ersten klinischen Erfahrungen mit chemisch modifizierten heteroplastischen Arterientransplantaten aus Rinder- und Kalbskarotiden. Schweiz Med Wochenschr 105/17:522–527
2. Baird RN, Abbott WM (1977) Vein grafts: An historical perspective. Am J Surg 134:293–296
3. Carrel A (1906) The surgery of blood vessels. Bull Johns Hopk Hosp 19:18–27
4. Dale WA (1974) The beginnings of vascular surgery. Surgery 76:849–866
5. Dardik H, Dardik J (1976) Successful arterial substitution with modified human umbilical vein. Ann Surg 183/3:252–258
6. DeBakey ME (1979) The development of vascular surgery. Am J Surg 137:697–738
7. Dye WS, Grove WJ, Olwin JH, Julian OC (1956) 2- to 4-year behavior of vein growth in lower extremities. AMA Arch Surg 72:64–68
8. Edwards WS (1978) Arterial grafts: past, present, and future. Arch Surg 113:1225–1233
9. Goyanes J (1906) Nuevos trabajos de cirurgia vascular substitucion plastica de las venas e arterioplastica venosa, aplicada cuno nuevo metodo al tratamiento de los aneurismos. Siglo Med 53:543–561
10. Haimovici H (1963) History of arterial grafting. J Cardiovasc Surg (Torino) 4:152–174
11. Harrison LH Jr (1976) Historical aspects in the development of venous autografts. Ann Surg 183:101–106
12. Heberer G, Giessler G (1956) Bedeutung und Aufbau einer Arterienbank. Chirurg 27:289
13. Jarrett F (1979) René Leriche (1879–1955) father of vascular surgery. Surgery 86:736–741
14. Jeger E (1913) Die Chirurgie der Blutgefäße und des Herzens. Hirschwald, Berlin
15. Lexer E (1907) Die ideale Operation des arteriellen und arteriovenösen Aneurysmas. Arch Klin Chir 83:459–463
16. Linton RR, Darling RC (1962) Autogenous saphenous vein bypass grafts in femoro popliteal obliterative arterial disease. Surgery 51:62–73
17. Rob CG (1973) A history of arterial surgery. Arch Surg 105:821–823
18. Schmitt W (1983) Das chirurgische Erbe. Alexis Carrel. Zentralbl Chir 108:495–503
19. Shumacker HB Jr (1980) A history of modern treatment of aortic aneurysms. World J Surg 4:503–509
20. Staudacher M (1974) Die homologe Transplantation der gefriergetrockneten Vene – ein experimenteller Beitrag zum Problem: Gefäßersatz. Vasa [Suppl] 2:3–22
21. Thompson JE (1977) The founding fathers. Surgery 82:801–808
22. Voorhoeve AB, Jaretzki A, Blakemore AH (1952) Use of tubes constructed from vinyon "N" cloth in bridging arterial defects, preliminary report. Ann Surg 135:332–336
23. Wylie EJ (1981) Presidential address: vascular surgery; reflections of the past three decades. Surgery 88:743–747

2 Anatomy

This chapter presents a general overview of those anatomical features that are of fundamental importance in vascular surgery. Most of the ensuing chapters contain brief summaries of the special vascular anatomy encountered in each region. These descriptions, of course, are not intended as a substitute for textbooks and monographs on anatomy.

Rather, they try to present the most important topographic aspects of those body regions with which the vascular surgeon must be familiar. This being the case, the customary presentation of an anatomy of arteries and veins is not called for. There is only a very short chapter on the venous system of the lower extremity. The portal system is discussed together with the visceral vessels.

The number of anatomic variations in the blood vessels, in terms of their tributaries, varying diameters, positions, and collaterals is immense. The picture becomes even more complex if one takes into account variations due to age and sex. Using schematic drawings, we have tried to represent the most common variations. The corresponding monographs are referred to in the references. It was not possible to consider the numerous variations in the vasculature of individual organs, for example, the liver, which is very specific and should be reviewed in textbooks on liver surgery. Pathologico-anatomic details such as kinking and loop formation of the arteries, of the carotid artery, for example, or possible collaterals in an atypical aortic coarctation, are presented in the corresponding special chapters on these topics.

2.1 Surgical Anatomy of the Arteries

B. GÜNTHER and G. HEBERER

CONTENTS

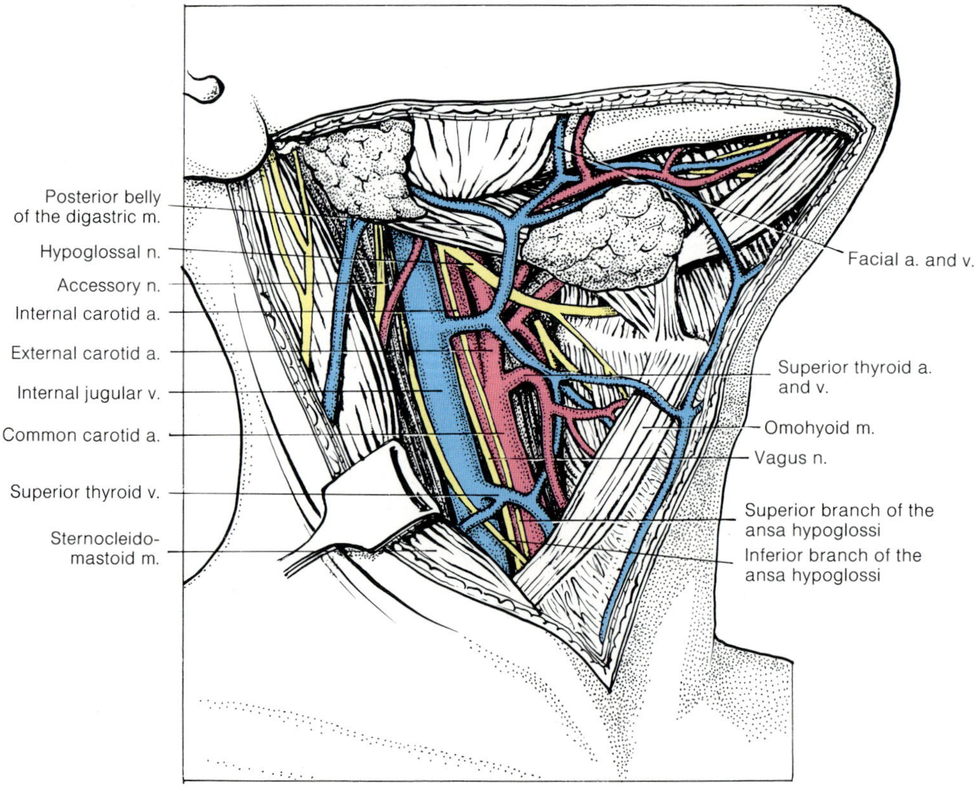

A. Common, Internal, and External Carotid Arteries

The cervical course of these vessels in the carotid triangle is shown (Fig. 2.1.1).

Following skin incision, dissection of the subcutaneous tissue, platysma, and anterior cervical fascia, the internal jugular vein is usually exposed first at the front margin of the sternocleidomastoid muscle. Its caudal portion lies ventral and lateral to the common carotid artery and its cranial portion at the same level as the artery. The medial branches of the jugular vein vary greatly. The main branches are the common facial vein, usually found at the level of the carotid bifurcation, and the caudally terminating superior thyroid vein, but a common thyrolinguofacial trunk is also possible.

The vagus nerve transverses dorsal to and between both large neck vessels. The arch of the hypoglossal nerve forms the cranial margin of surgical exposure of the carotid artery and its branches. The caudal margin of dissection is flanked by the omohyoid muscle, which runs obliquely to the lateral side of the neck. In the uppermost portion of the carotid triangle the accessory nerve crosses the internal jugular vein. Usually, it is not encountered during exposure of the carotid branches. The carotid body, a structure 5 to 6 mm long and 2 to 3 mm wide, lies in and behind the bifurcation of the common carotid artery. During dissection of this area, the carotid sinus nerve, a branch of the hypoglossal nerve, may be divided. One should watch out for the superior laryngeal nerve running dorsal to the carotid body.

The branching sequence of the external carotid artery varies greatly. Only the superior thyroid artery, which branches off medially, is of importance to the surgeon because it must be clamped before incising the carotid bifurcation. Rarely, the ascending pharyngeal artery, which branches off cranially at the carotid bifurcation, must be ligated.

Variations in the topographical position of the internal carotid and external carotid arteries relative to one another, e.g., the dorsomedial course of the internal carotid artery, do not play an important role in the surgical exposure of cervical vessels. The level at which the carotid bifurcation is located is much more important for dissection, because the higher the origin of the internal carotid artery, the more difficult its exposure is. In most cases, branching occurs at about the level of the fourth cervical vertebra and the upper margin of the thyroid cartilage.

◁ **Fig. 2.1.1.** Carotid triangle. View following resection of the platysma and anterior cervical fascia as well as lateral retraction of the sternocleidomastoid muscle

B. Subclavian Artery and Branches

The operative approach to the subclavian artery and its branches, which is especially important to the surgeon, is located in the caudal portion of the sternocleidomastoid region below the omohyoid muscle (Fig. 2.1.2a). The subclavian artery, as it passes through the scalene area, gives off the following branches along a 3-cm-long segment: the vertebral artery and the thyrocervical trunk upward toward the head, the internal mammary (thoracic) artery, and the costocervical trunk in a downward direction (Fig. 2.1.2b). On the left side of the neck, these arteries are very close to the junction of the thoracic duct at the venous angle, a fact of great significance (Fig. 2.1.2c). Because the aortic arch curves from the right front backward and to the left, the right subclavian artery lies anterior to the left one. The bifurcation of the brachiocephalic vein lies just behind the right sternoclavicular joint.

The phrenic nerve descends obliquely toward the midline, passing along the anterior surface of the anterior scalene muscle. Its middle portion runs lateral to the thyreocervical trunk, crosses over the subclavian and internal thoracic arteries, and then passes medially downward into the thorax. The sympathetic nerve usually forms a loop around the uppermost portion of the thyreocervical trunk and then enters the thorax with some of its branches running in front of and some behind the clavicular portion of the subclavian artery (ansa subclavia). The middle cervical sympathetic ganglion usually lies just above the thyreocervical trunk, and the inferior cervical sympathetic ganglion just above the crossing point between the sympathetic trunk and the subclavian artery (Fig. 2.1.2b).

The thoracic duct curves upward on the left side behind the internal carotid artery and internal jugular vein, but in front of the vertebral artery and vein and the thyreocervical trunk. It joins the venous angle from behind, branching delta-like into several tributaries (Fig. 2.1.2c and special lymphatic vessel anatomy).

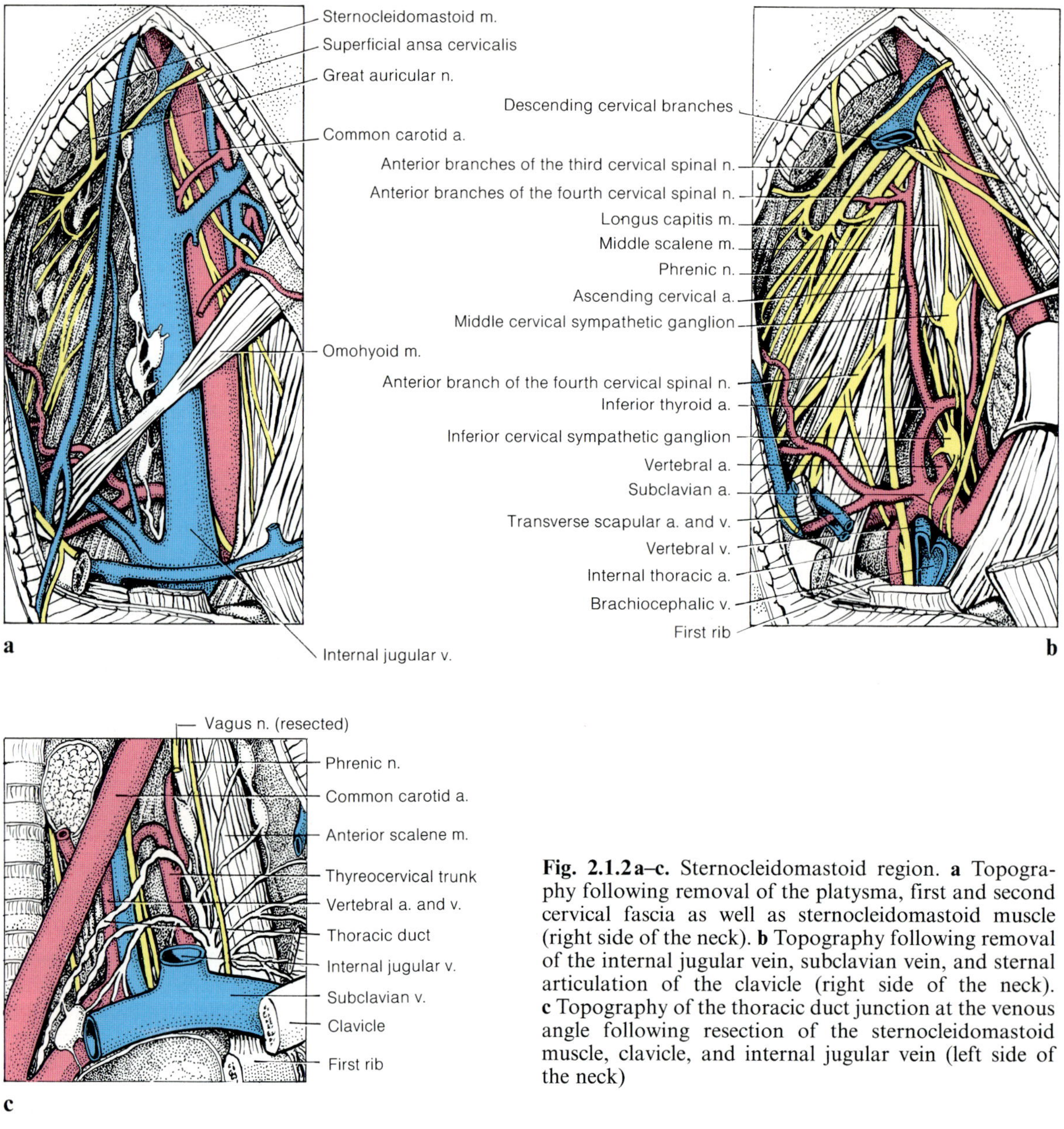

Fig. 2.1.2a–c. Sternocleidomastoid region. **a** Topography following removal of the platysma, first and second cervical fascia as well as sternocleidomastoid muscle (right side of the neck). **b** Topography following removal of the internal jugular vein, subclavian vein, and sternal articulation of the clavicle (right side of the neck). **c** Topography of the thoracic duct junction at the venous angle following resection of the sternocleidomastoid muscle, clavicle, and internal jugular vein (left side of the neck)

C. Intrathoracic Vessels

I. Vessels of the Left Hemithorax

The descending aorta extends from the fourth thoracic vertebra downward directly in front of the vertebrae (Fig. 2.1.3a). In the middle portion of the descending aorta, the segmental posterior intercostal arteries, emerging in corresponding pairs, run horizontally and in the superior portion climb steeply upward until they reach the corresponding intercostal spaces. The left subclavian artery, the last branch of the aortic arch, originates at the distal end of the latter and ascends steeply upward.

The left longitudinal thoracic vein, which receives the posterior intercostal veins, crosses the posterior intercostal arteries on the lateral surfaces of the vertebrae. At a lower level, this vein becomes larger. It is then called the inferior hemiazygos vein. It crosses to the other side behind the aorta at the level of the seventh to the ninth thoracic vertebra, joining the azygos vein on the right side.

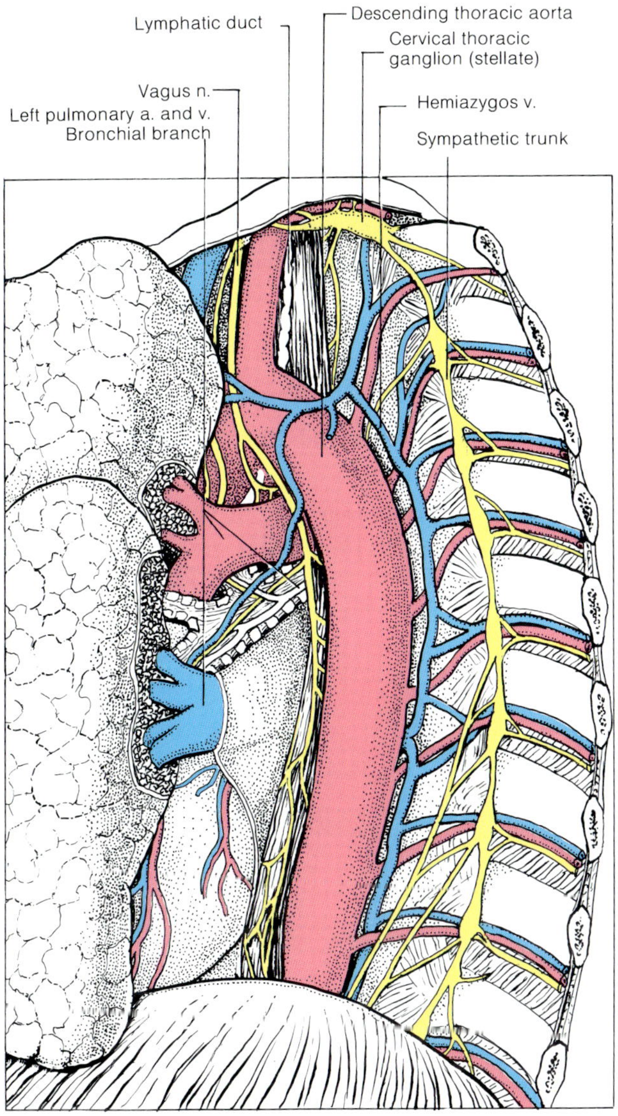

a

The sympathetic chain lies farthest laterally, on the heads or joints of the ribs in front of the posterior intercostal arteries and veins. At the level of each rib, it forms a thoracic ganglion. The first thoracic ganglion often joins the inferior cervical ganglion to form the cervical thoracic ganglion or stellate.

The vagus nerve runs downward next to or on the ventral aspect of the left subclavian artery, crossing the aorta laterally at the origin of the subclavian artery. This is where the vagus nerve gives off the recurrent nerve posteriorly. The thoracic duct also lies behind the left subclavian artery.

Fig. 2.1.3a–c. Schematic representation of the large intrathoracic vessels and nerves. **a** Left hemithorax. **b** Upper third of the right hemithorax. **c** Upper mediastinum

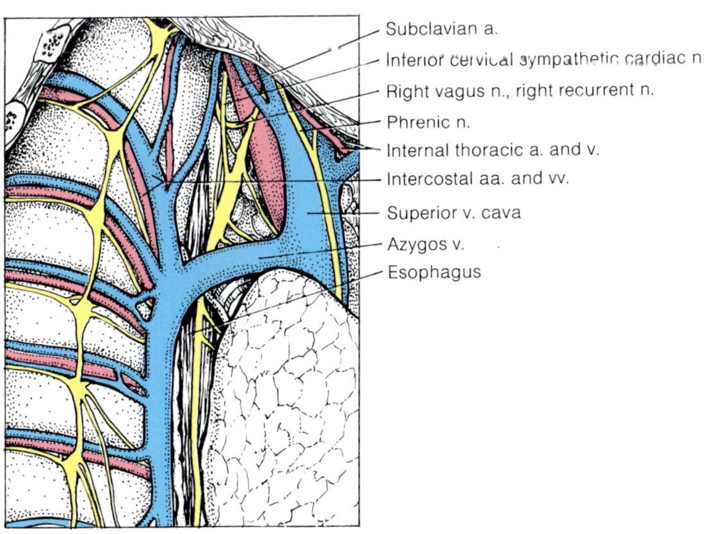

b

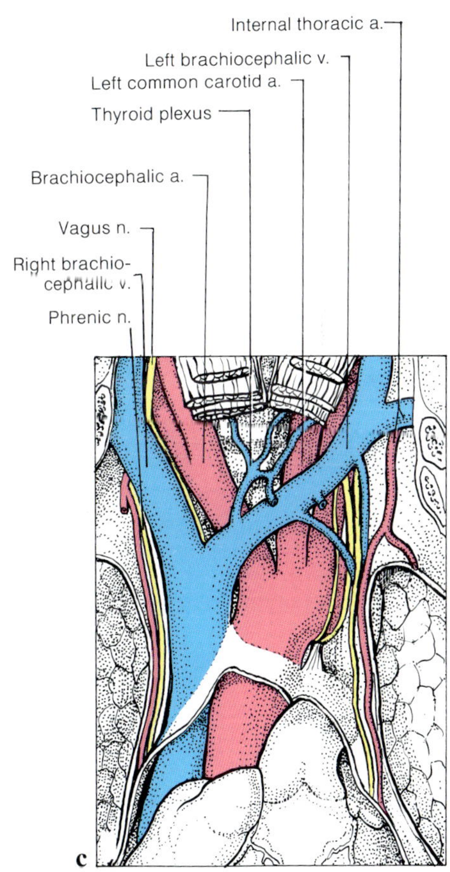

c

II. Vessels of the Right Hemithorax

The topography of the middle and lower third of the right hemithorax is similar to the left side. In the upper third, the azygos vein enters into the superior vena cava just above the hilus of the right lung, lateral and anterior to the esophagus and trachea (Fig. 2.1.3b). The right vagus nerve passes behind the azygos vein to the lateral aspect of the esophagus. The phrenic nerve descends directly on or lateral to the superior vena cava.

The thoracic duct ascends between the esophagus and the azygos vein. At the level of the azygos arch, it passes over to the left side behind the esophagus.

III. Aortic Arch and Branches

The aortic arch and its branches are exposed transsternally through the upper anterior mediastinum (Fig. 2.1.3c). They are covered in front by the left brachiocephalic vein. During dissection, one must pay attention to the lower thyroid veins coming from above and the superior hemiazygos vein entering laterally from below.

The origins of the supra-aortal branches show numerous variations. Between 1 and 5 different origins of the branches of the aortic arch and up to 25 combinations of different anomalies have been classified [16, 20].

D. Visceral Arteries and Portal System

Knowledge of the topography of visceral vessels is equally important in vascular and abdominal surgery. Because of its connections with the inferior vena cava, the portal system has a special position.

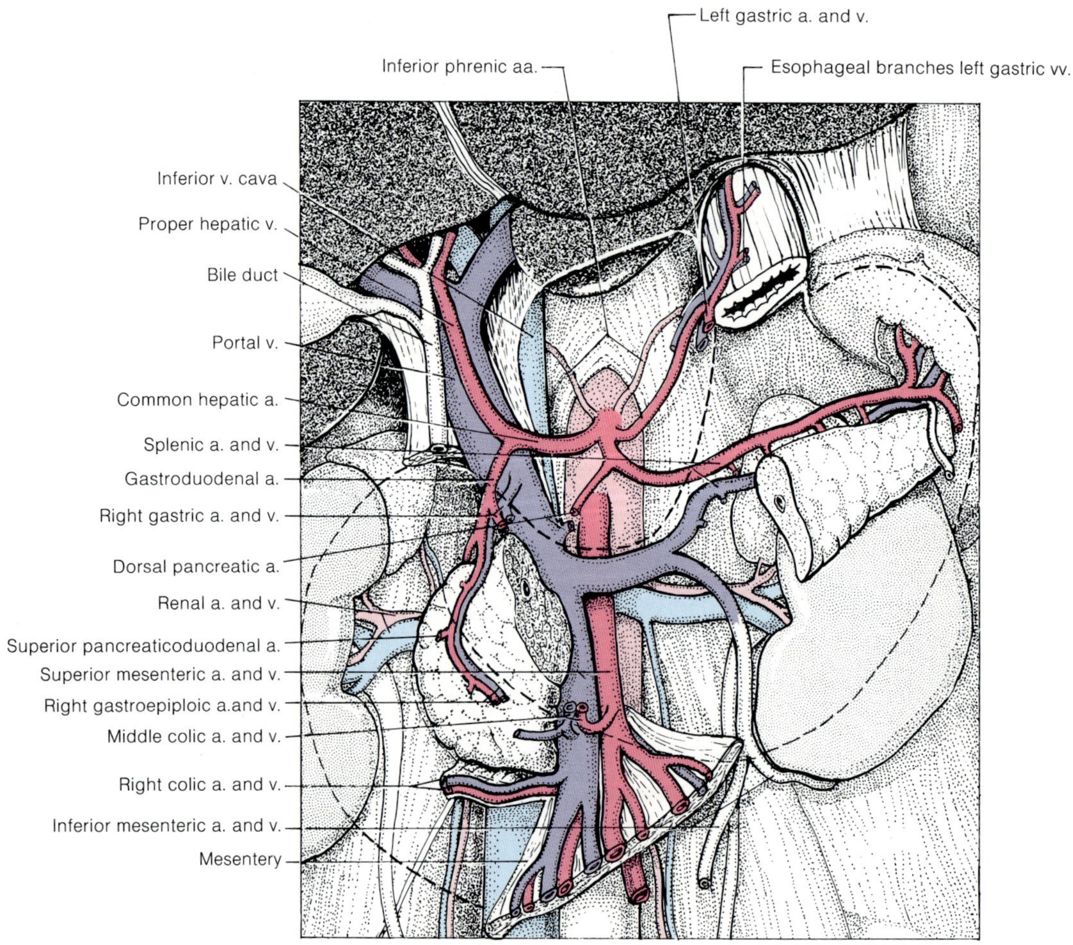

I. Visceral Arteries

The celiac trunk arises from the aorta just below the aortic hiatus (Fig. 2.1.4). Usually, it divides into three branches: the thin left gastric artery, the splenic artery, and the common hepatic artery. The latter two are about equal in diameter. The splenic artery runs along the upper margin of the pancreas to the splenic hilus, giving off numerous pancreatic branches. Before entering the splenic hilus, it also gives off the short gastric arteries and the left gastroepiploic artery to the greater gastric curvature.

Just before entering the hepatoduodenal ligament at the posterior upper margin of the duodenum, the common hepatic artery separates into the gastroduodenal artery, which descends behind the duodenum, and the proper hepatic artery, which enters the ligament. The superior mesenteric artery arises from the descending aorta 5–10 mm below the celiac artery and runs behind the pancreas and under the splenic vein, but anterior to the renal vein. Before separating into 5–20 visceral branches at the base of the mesentery, it gives off the inferior pancreaticoduodenal artery at the lower pancreatic margin. The inferior mesenteric artery arises from the abdominal aorta as the last visceral vessel below the duodenojejunal flexure at the level of the third lumbar vertebra.

MICHELS classifies six different variations of the origins and branches of both of these arteries (Fig. 2.1.5a). He calls the standard anatomic situa-

◁ **Fig. 2.1.4.** Schematic presentation of the visceral arteries, portal, and retroperitoneal vessels following resection of the stomach, duodenum, and body of the pancreas

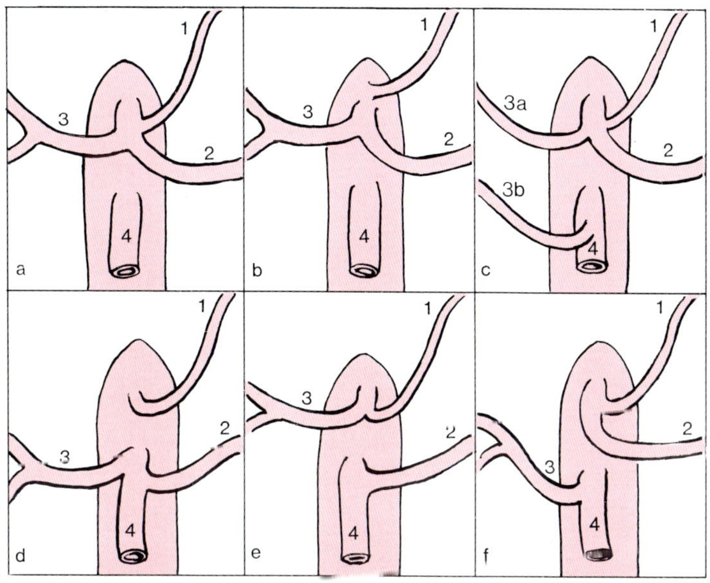

a

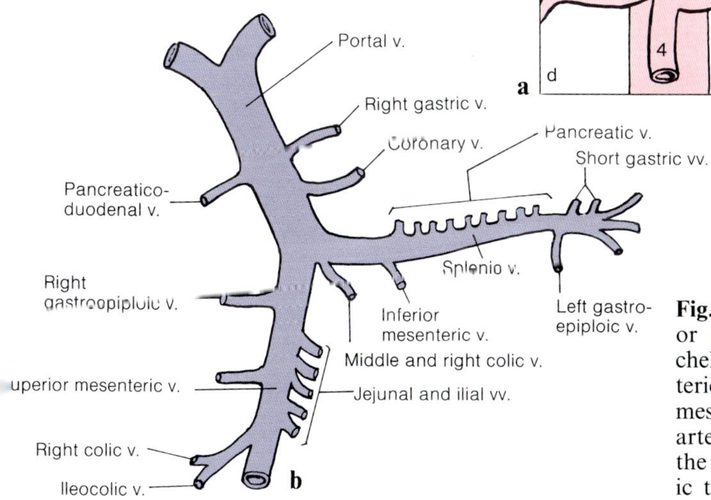

b

Fig. 2.1.5. a Variations of the celiac artery and the superior mesenteric artery (classification according to Michels). *a*, Hepatogastrosplenic trunk and superior mesenteric artery: type I; *b*, hepatosplenic trunk and superior mesenteric artery: type II; *c*, origin of the left hepatic artery at the celiac artery, the right hepatic artery at the superior mesenteric artery; *d*, hepatosplenomesenteric trunk: type III; *e*, hepatogastric trunk: type IV, *f*, splenogastric trunk: type V; *1*, left gastric artery; *2*, splenic artery; *3*, common hepatic artery; *3a*, left hepatic artery; *3b*, right hepatic artery; *4*, superior mesenteric artery. **b** Schematic representation of the most important branches of the portal system (modified according to PAPADOPOULOS [18]) tion as described above, with a normal hepatogastrosplenic trunk and an independent superior mesenteric artery, the Type I variation [12]. A frequently occurring Type I variation consists of a separate left hepatic artery arising from the celiac artery, while the right hepatic artery arises from the superior mesenteric artery (11.5%). Type II is encountered in 3.5%, Type III in 0.5%, Type IV in 1.5%, and Type V in 15.5%. Type VI, having one single trunk for all visceral arteries and Type VII, with the middle colic artery and/or left colic artery arising from the celiac artery, are very rare.

The variability of arterial supply to different organs, especially the liver, is more important in liver surgery. For example, an accessory hepatic artery is found in over 20%, two additional hepatic arteries in almost 10%, three in 7%, and four in 3% of patients.

II. Portal System

Lateral to and below the origin of the superior mesenteric artery, the superior mesenteric vein and splenic vein join behind the pancreas to form the portal vein. This vessel lies posterior to the proper hepatic artery in the hepatoduodenal ligament, following a diagonal course laterally to the hepatic porta, where it lies just medial and anterior to the inferior vena cava. The splenic vein ascends in a posterior direction to the spleen, starting about the middle of the pancreatic body. The infe-

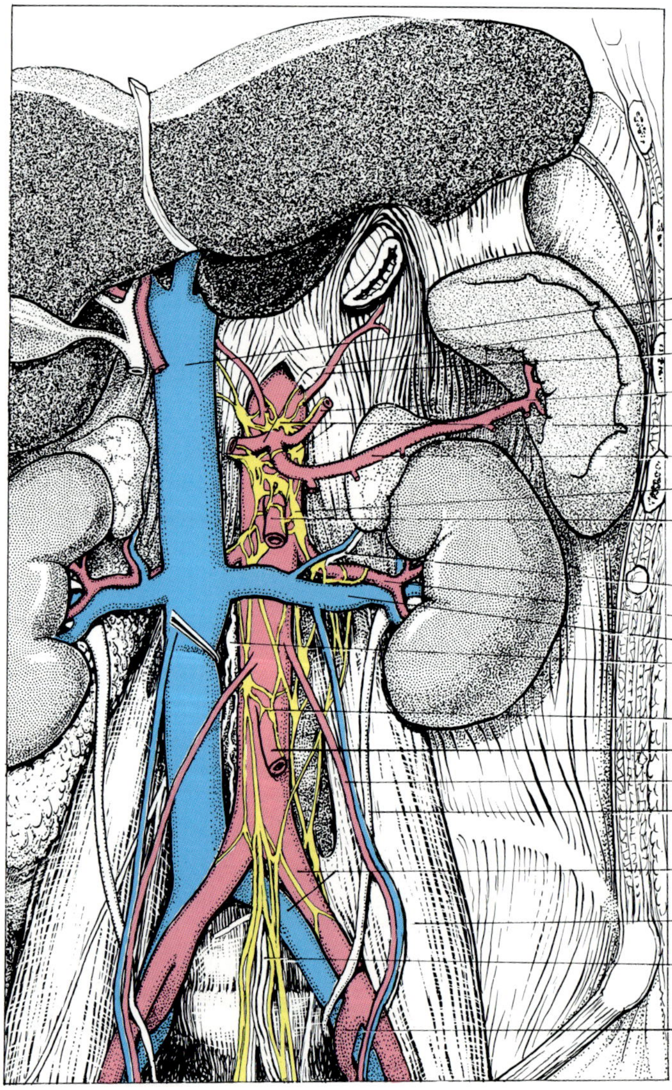

rior mesenteric vein enters the splenic vein about 2 cm to the left of the confluence.

The individual branches of the portal vein vary greatly. Not only the junction of these tributaries with the superior mesenteric and portal veins is of great importance for dissection in this region, but their stereotactic arrangement as well, i.e., whether they enter from behind, below, or from the front [18]. Figure 2.1.5b is a schematic representation of the most important branches. Particular attention should be paid to the posterior tributaries entering along the 4.5-cm-long segment leading to the confluence. The splenic vein should only be mobilized dorsally because of the danger of injuring the numerous ventral branches from the pancreas. Before the portal vein separates at the hepatic porta, a 1.5-cm-long segment of this main vessel is usually entirely free of tributaries.

E. Abdominal Aorta, Inferior Vena Cava, Renal Artery and Vein, Other Retroperitoneal Vessels

The abdominal aorta usually gives off two renal arteries just below the origin of the superior mesenteric artery (Fig. 2.1.6). In addition, four pairs of lumbar arteries arise from the abdominal aorta. The vena cava is formed by the junction of both common iliac veins to the right and behind the aortic bifurcation at the level of the fourth lumbar vertebra. In the mesogastric region, it lies posterior to the duodenum and pancreas and farther up between the right suprarenal gland and the portal vein within the hepatoduodenal ligament. The left renal vein crosses the aorta on its way to the inferior vena cava. Both renal arteries arise at the same level in most humans, in younger persons at the center of L1, in older persons at the lower quarter of L1 or at the level of the intervertebral disk L1/L2. The sympathetic chain lies farthest back and toward the side and is covered to some extent by the lateral border of the vena cava.

The arteries of both kidneys and also the veins of the left kidney show especially numerous variations. In 20%–25% of patients one finds aberrant and accessory renal arteries, sometimes originating at the common iliac and spermatic arteries.

◁ **Fig. 2.1.6.** Schematic representation of retroperitoneal vessels

Multiple renal veins are encountered in 25%. Other variations of the renal vein, such as crossing behind the aorta or duplication, with one part in front and one part in back of the aorta, are usually combined with anomalies of the inferior vena cava. The frequency of duplication of the inferior vena cava is reported to be 1%–3%, crossing of the left renal vein behind the aorta 1.8%, and loop formation around the aorta 1.5% of patients.

F. Vessels of the Upper Extremity

I. Axillary Artery

The axillary artery lies posteriorly and laterally to the axillary vein in the axilla (Fig. 2.1.7a). There is a very close topographical relationship between the axillary artery, the brachial plexus, and the peripheral nerves. In the upper portion of the axillary artery, extending from the infraclavicular region to the upper border of the pectoralis minor muscle, the brachial plexus lies above and behind the artery.

In the lower portion, as it runs down to the lower border of the pectoralis minor muscle, it is surrounded by the fascicles of the brachial plexus. Distal to this muscle, the median nerve lies on the artery, with the ulnar nerve medial and the musculocutaneous nerve lateral to it. The radial nerve, which lies behind the artery, arises from the posterior fascicle. The arterial branches of the axillary artery, running downward to the posterior structures of this area and accompanying the various nerves, are not of any importance for surgical dissection.

The cephalic vein penetrates the clavipectoral fascia below the clavicle in the deltoideo pectoral triangle (Mohrenheim's fossa) and terminates in the subclavian vein (Fig. 2.1.7b). Posterior to the cephalic vein, the thoracico-acromial artery runs in a lateral direction, and multiple anteriorly pectoral nerves descend for motor innervation of the pectoralis major muscle.

II. Brachial Artery

The brachial artery is the extension of the axillary artery. It continues downward, usually accompanied by two concomitant veins, reaching the cubital fossa beneath the bicipital aponeurosis

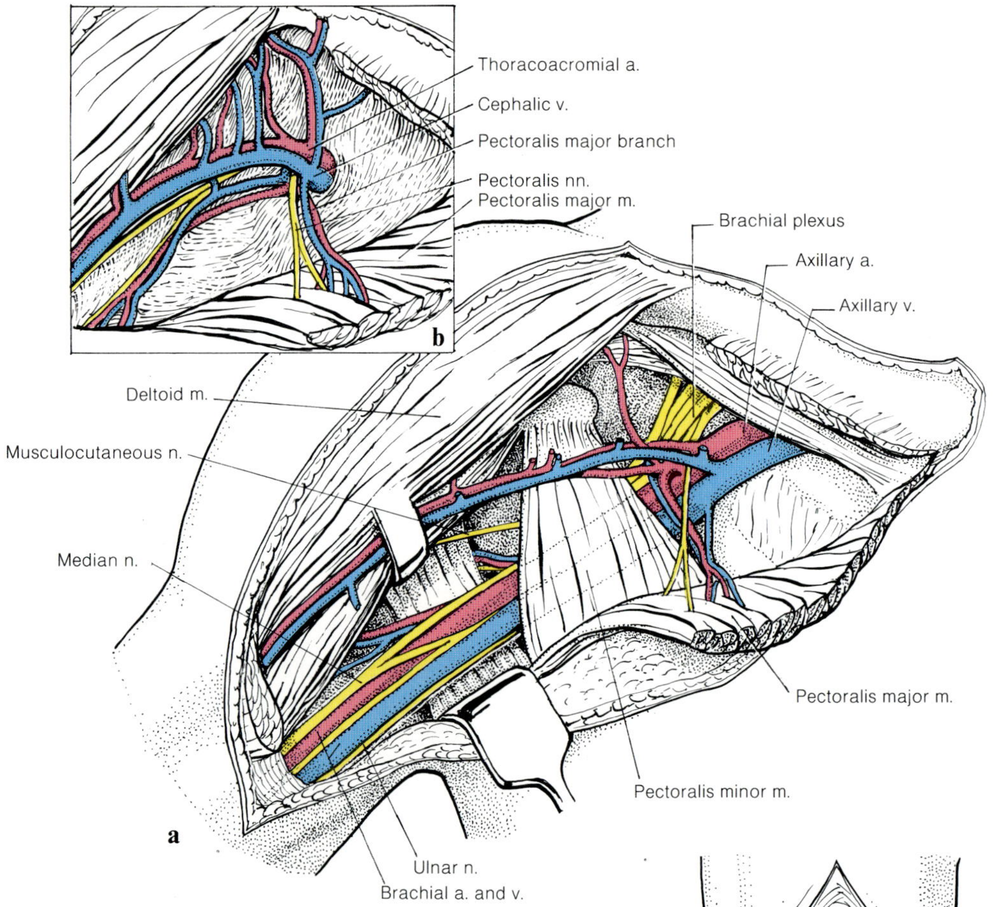

Fig. 2.1.7. a Infraclavicular and axillary region following resection of the pectoralis major muscle and the fasciae. **b** Deltoideopectoral triangle

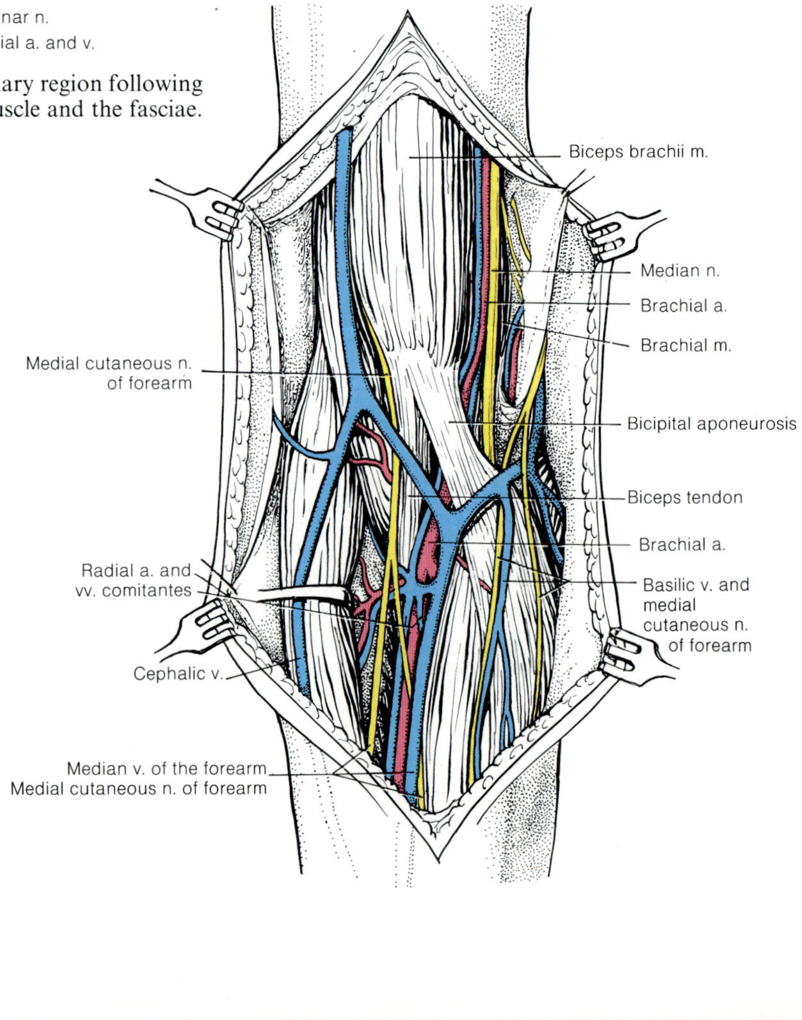

Fig. 2.1.8. Superficial and deep vessels of the cubital fossa

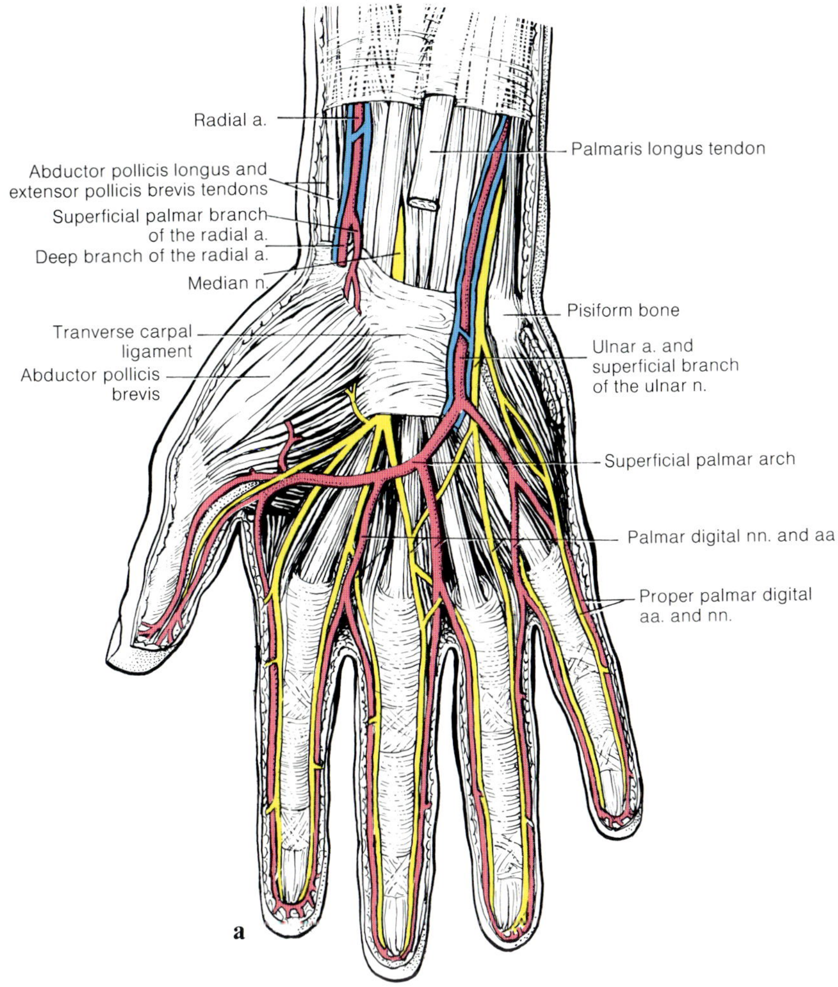

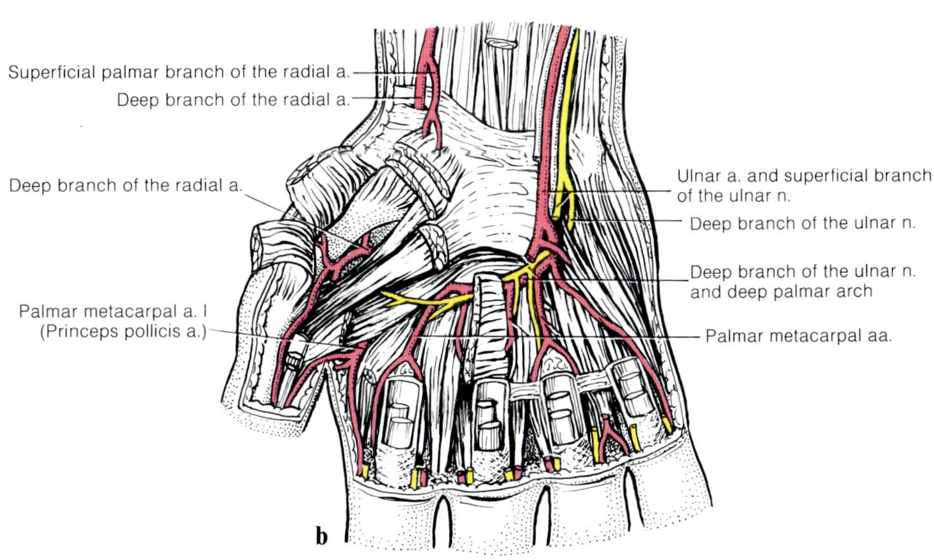

Fig. 2.1.9. Superficial (**a**) and deep (**b**) dissection of the palm

(Fig. 2.1.8). It extends into the forearm as the radial artery, while the ulnar artery branches off medially. The cranial collateral as well as the distal recurrent arteries form the arterial network of the elbow joint, a natural system of anastomosis between the upper and lower arm vessels.

The brachial artery is accompanied on its ulnar side by the median nerve, which crosses in front of it. The radial nerve with its deep and superficial branches on the lateral side of the arm comes in close contact with the radial artery at the cubital fossa.

III. Vessels of Wrist and Hand

The ulnar artery enters the palm of the hand radial to the pisiform bone in front of the transverse carpal ligament, covered only by the palmar fascia (Fig. 2.1.9a). At the pisiform bone it gives off the deep palmar branch to the deep palmar arch (Fig. 2.1.9b). Its course distal to the transverse carpal ligament has about the same direction as the linea vitalis on the palm of the hand, continuing under the superficial palmar arch, making a distally convex half circle to the radial side of the hand. Three or four common palmar digital arteries arise from this arch.

The radial artery turns toward the radial side of the hand as soon as it reaches the wrist, crossing within the tabatière formed by the abductor pollicis longus and extensor pollicis brevis muscles to the dorsum of the hand. Anteriorly, it gives off the superficial palmar branch which continues ulnar to the thenar muscles under the tendons of the digital flexor muscles and, together with the ulnar artery, forms the deep palmar arch just above the base of the metacarpal bones (Fig. 2.1.9b).

The ulnar artery runs lateral to the ulnar nerve, which splits up into several branches as it reaches the pisiform bone. The median nerve enters the palm radially, together with the long digital flexor tendons, and divides at the distal edge of the transverse carpal ligament into three common palmar digital nerves which spread out to the fingers just beneath the superficial palmar arch.

The superficial and deep palmar arches show numerous variations. For example, a complete superficial palmar arch is present in only 50%. For further study of these variations consult the references at the end of this chapter [6, 8].

G. Vessels of the Pelvic Region and the Lower Extremity

I. Iliac Arteries

Distal to the iliac bifurcation the common iliac artery subsequently divides, giving rise to the external and internal iliac arteries. Just below the inguinal ligament the former of these gives off the deep inferior epigastric artery medially upward and the deep circumflex ileal artery laterally (Fig. 2.1.10).

At the iliac bifurcation the ilac vein crosses beneath the artery, running downward toward the inguinal ligament on the medial side of the external iliac artery.

At about the same level, the ureter crosses in front of the common iliac artery or the iliac bifurcation.

II. Femoral Artery

The main vessel of the anterior femoral region is the femoral artery. Relative to the sartorius muscle, it can be divided into three segments: The first – and surgically the most important – segment proximal to the sartorius muscle; the second, beneath the sartorius muscle; and the third, covered by the vastoadductor membrane (Fig. 2.1.10).

At the inguinal ligament the femoral artery usually gives off two smaller branches, the superficial epigastric artery and the superficial circumflex ileal artery (Figs. 2.1.10 and 2.1.11a), which deserve attention when dissecting around the common femoral artery. Smaller external pudendal arteries branch off further distally at variable distances. The origin of the profunda femoris artery usually lies 2 cm below the inguinal ligament on the lateral and posterior side of the femoral artery. It extends only a short distance and gives off the lateral circumflex artery and the medial circumflex artery. The latter passes beneath the femoral vein and superficial femoral artery.

At first the femoral vein lies medial to the artery, however, along its middle and lower course it runs more and more behind the artery. The greater saphenous vein enters into the femoral vein from the medial side at about the same level as the origin of the profunda femoris artery. Just before entry it takes up numerous subcutaneous veins (venous star) which are very variable in their

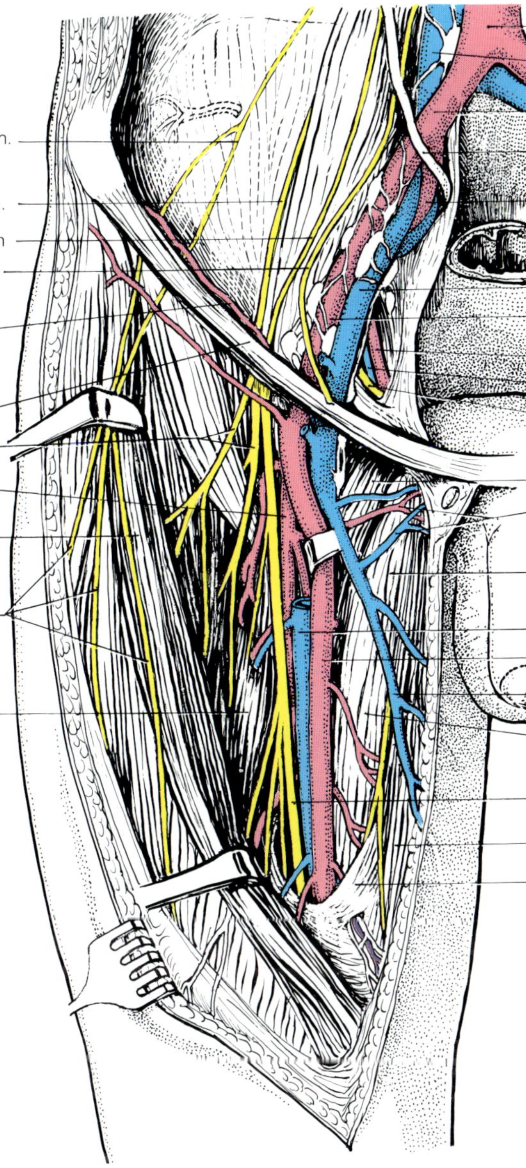

Fig. 2.1.10. Schematic representation of vessels in the pelvic and thigh regions

course and site of entry. When dissecting around the profunda femoris artery one should pay special attention to the crossing lateral circumflex vein. It is often accompanied by two additional venae comitantes (Fig. 2.1.11b).

The branches of the femoral nerve lie lateral to the artery and usually cross the tributaries of the profunda femoris artery on their course to the lateral side of the leg. At the uppermost part of the anterior femoral region, the saphenous nerve comes in close contact with the superficial femoral artery, running laterally next to or on this vessel downward to the adductor canal.

The division of the common femoral artery shows numerous variations, not only in the number of tributaries, but also in the level of their origin and in their topographic relationship to the corresponding veins [8, 26].

The standard anatomical situation is encountered in only 50%: lateral origin of a perfect profundocircumflex trunk (Fig. 2.1.11c). The commonest variations, especially in the origin of the circumflex arteries, are shown as described by VAAS in order of their frequency from left to right (Fig. 2.1.11d–g).

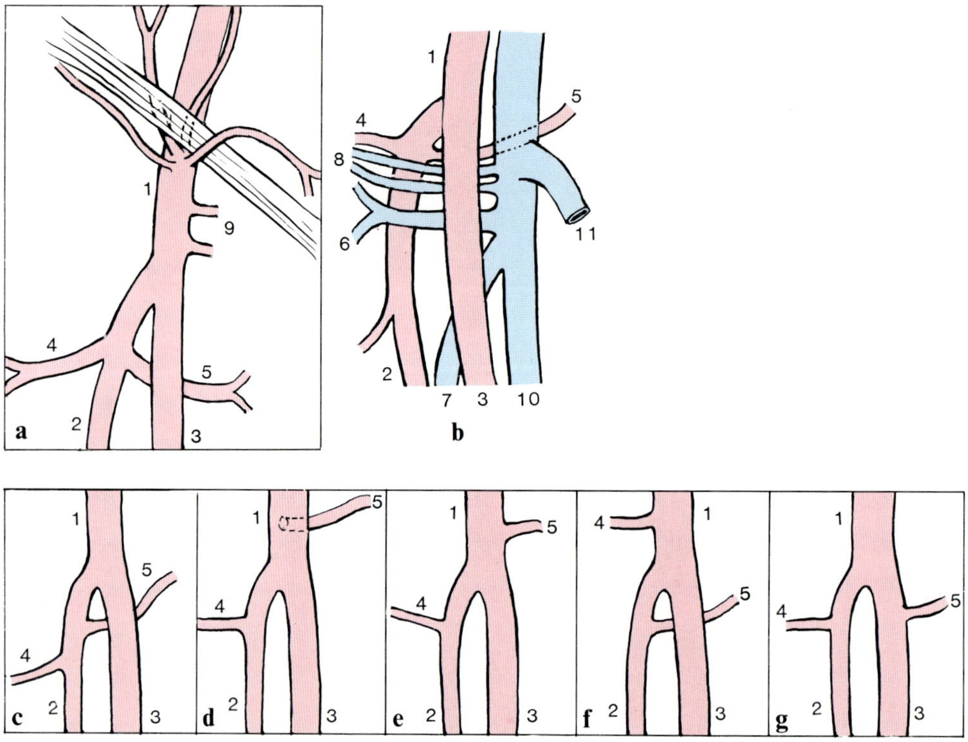

Fig. 2.1.11 a–g. Schematic representation of the branches of the femoral artery and vein with important variations and topographical relationships between arteries and veins. **a** Branches of the common femoral artery. **b** Vessels at the femoral bifurcation. **c–g** Variations in the order of vessels arising from the femoral bifurcation according to their frequency (as described by F. Vaas [26]). *1*, Common femoral artery; *2*, profunda femoris artery; *3*, superficial femoral artery; *4*, lateral circumflex artery; *5*, medial circumflex artery; *6*, lateral circumflex vein; *7*, profunda femoris vein; *8*, venae comitantes; *9*, pudendal arteries; *10*, femoral vein; *11*, greater saphenous vein

III. Popliteal Artery (Middle Segment)

The sciatic nerve and its branches, the tibial nerve, and the common peroneal nerve run superficially within the popliteal fossa (Fig. 2.1.12) above the popliteal vein and artery. In the upper and middle portions of the popliteal fossa, the sciatic nerve and tibial nerve lie lateral to the vascular bundle and in the lower portion directly in front. The vascular bundle is separate from the nerve, which makes dissection and exposure of both structures easy.

When dissecting around the popliteal artery one must carefully note the origins of the small branches of the arterial network of the knee which arise from the popliteal artery on the medial and lateral sides (superior, medial, and inferior genicular arteries).

The lesser saphenous vein enters the popliteal fossa between both heads of the gastrocnemius muscle and joins the popliteal vein.

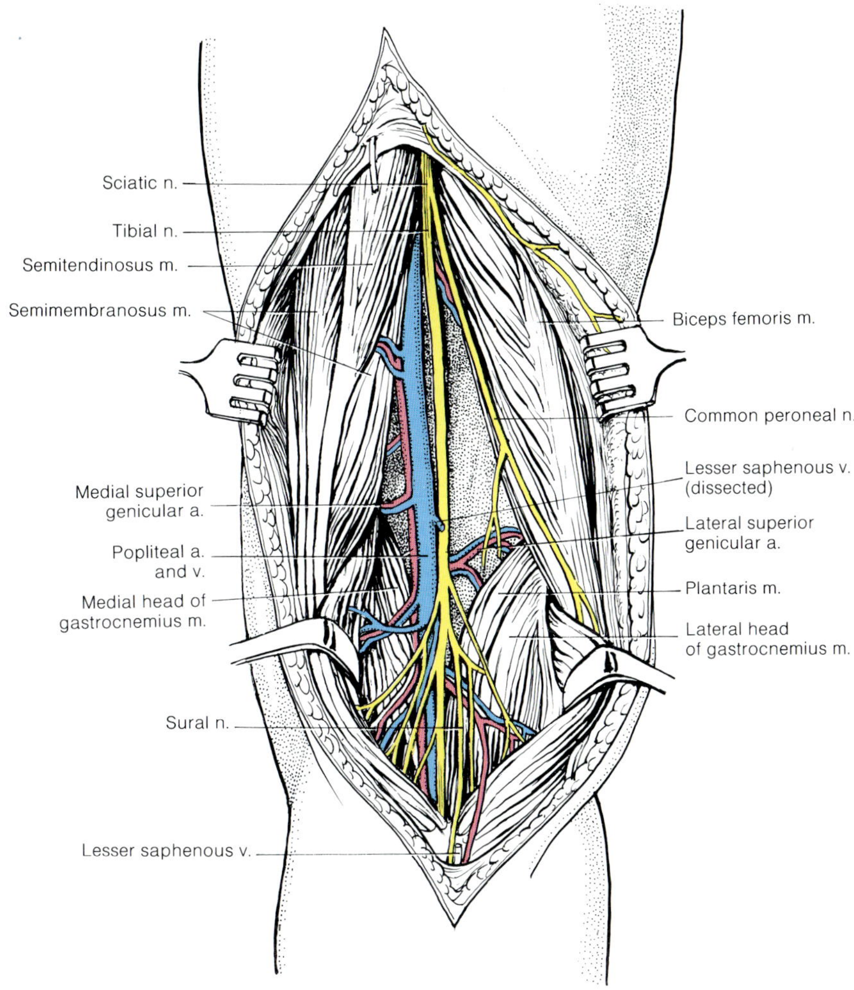

Fig. 2.1.12. Popliteal fossa following resection of the popliteal fascia

IV. Popliteal Artery (Distal Segment) and Posterior Tibial Artery

On the tibial side (medial side of the lower limb) the distal popliteal segment and the topography of the posterior tibial artery are of special interest (Fig. 2.1.13).

The space containing the distal segment of the popliteal artery is bordered by the medial head of the gastrocnemius muscle cranially and posteriorly, by the hamstring muscles in front and above, as well as by the soleus arcade distally. Just above the soleus arcade, the popliteal artery gives off the anterior tibial artery in front and the tibioperoneal trunk which passes downward under the soleus arcade. At this point, in some cases, the popliteal vein is already separated into two venae comitantes, and the tibial nerve lies dorsal and lateral to the vessels.

In the middle portion of the crural segment, the posterior tibial artery lies between the posterior tibial muscle covering the dorsal surface of the tibia and interosseous membrane and the soleus muscle. Thus, the posterior tibial artery can be exposed through a medial incision at the tibial edge following dorsal retraction of the medial head of the gastrocnemius muscle as well as division of the soleus muscle.

In the upper region, the tibial nerve lies medial to the posterior tibial artery, in the middle and lower segments it lies posterior and medial to the vascular bundle. One should note carefully the paired veins and numerous arterial muscle branches. The division of the popliteal artery and the caliber of its branches vary, and therefore the importance of each branch for blood circulation in the lower limb also varies. For further details see reference [8].

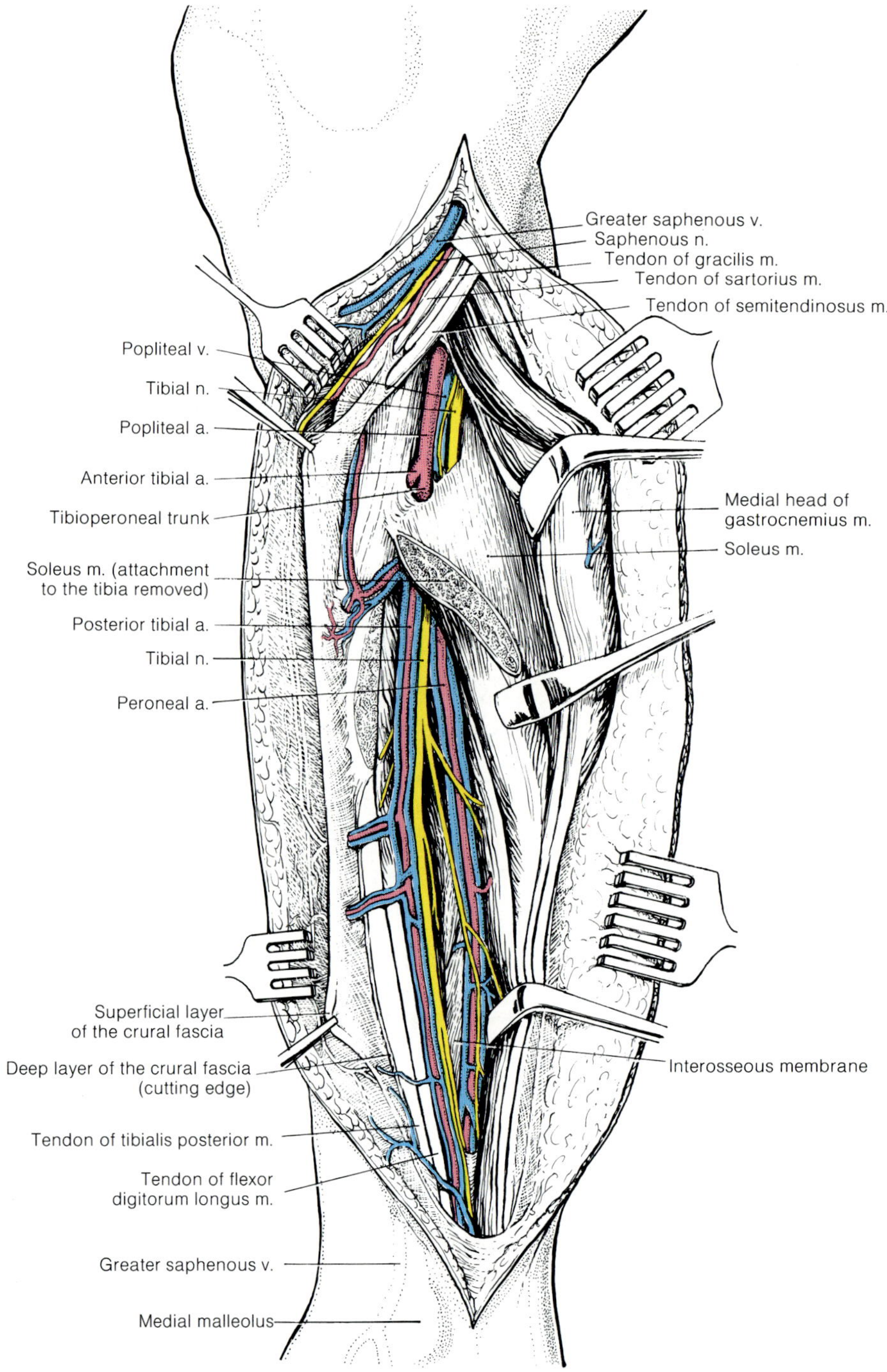

Fig. 2.1.13. Medial view of lower leg – distal third of the popliteal artery

V. Anterior Tibial Artery

On the lateral side of the lower leg (Fig. 2.1.14) nerves and vessels lie on the interosseous membrane posterior to the tibialis anterior muscle and lateral to the fibular surface of the tibia. Nerves and vessels lie between the tibialis anterior muscle

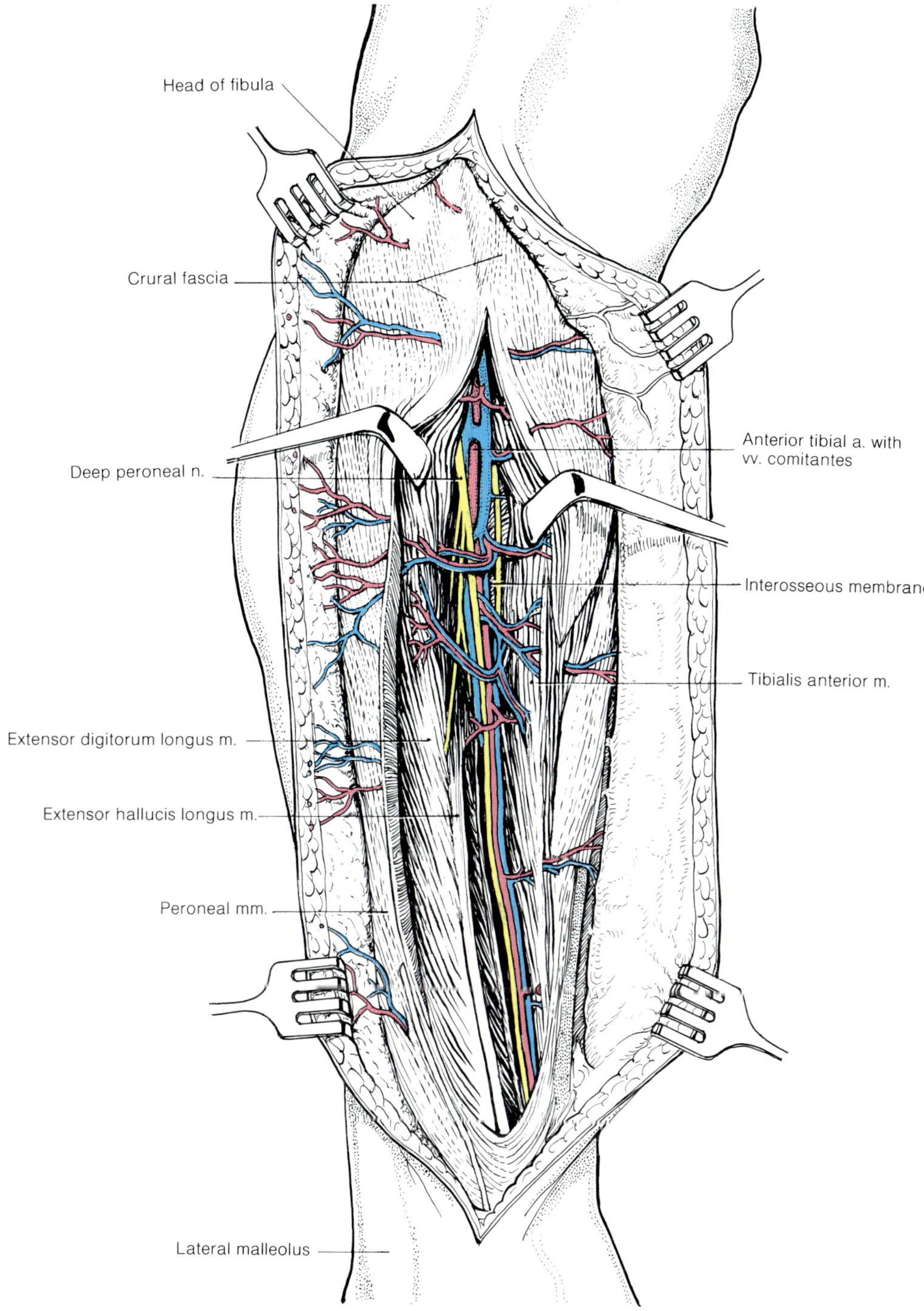

Fig. 2.1.14. Lateral view of the lower leg

and the extensor digitorum muscle. The venae comitantes exist in pairs and show numerous connections. The deep peroneal nerve runs laterally and superficially in the space between both extensor muscles, comes in close contact with the anterior tibial artery in the middle portion of the thigh, and crosses in front of it in the lower portion.

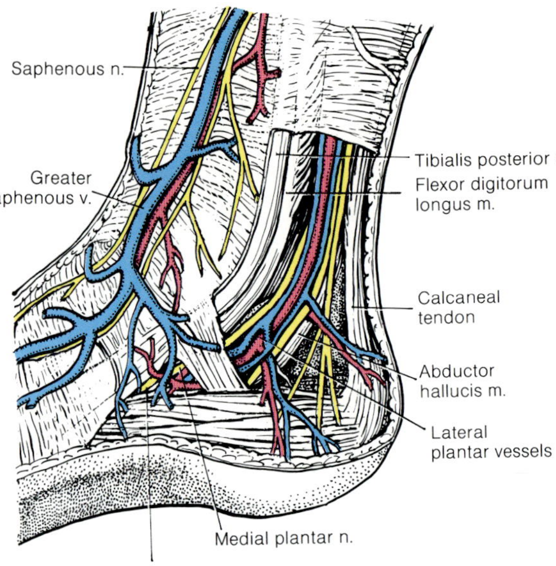

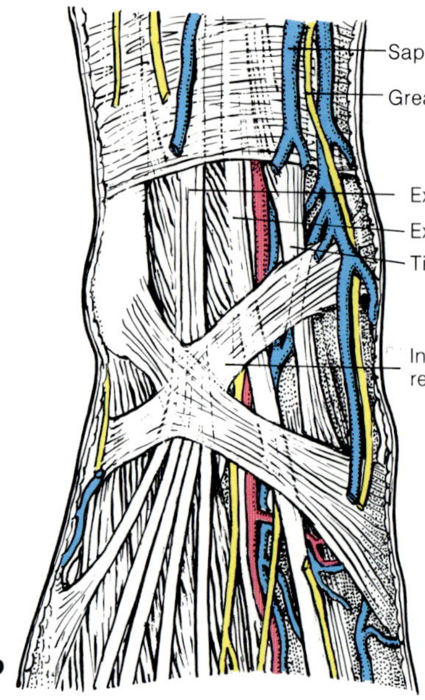

Fig. 2.1.15 a, b. Vessels of the dorsum of the foot and ankle region. **a** Medial malleolar region following resection of the superficial layer of the crural fascia and abductor hallucis muscle. **b** Dorsum of the foot after removal of the fasciae

VI. Vessels of the Ankle and Foot Region

The neurovascular bundle can be found between the medial malleolus and the calcaneal tendon (Fig. 2.1.15 a). It can be exposed by dissecting the superficial layer of the crural fascia. The nerve lies lateral to the artery and its venae comitantes.

The posterior tibial artery, covered by the abductor hallucis muscle, separates into a medial and lateral plantar branch about 1–2 cm distal to the medial malleolus. The tibial nerve also gives off a medial and lateral branch at the level of the malleolus. Just after its division, the nerve lies medial to the vascular bundle.

As soon as the anterior tibial artery reaches the malleolar axis, it passes beneath the tendon of the extensor hallucis longus muscle, remaining on its lateral side as it continues downward (Fig. 2.1.15 b). Thus, the artery lies superficially between the lateral attachment of the extensor hallucis brevis muscle and the tendon of the extensor hallucis longus muscle.

The deep peroneal nerve and the tendon of the extensor hallucis longus muscle cross in front of the vascular bundle, remaining anterior and medial to the vessels.

REFERENCES

1. Adachi B (1928) Das Arteriensystem der Japaner, Druckerei der Universität Kyoto, Kyoto
2. Babaian RJ, Johnson DE (1979) Major venous anomalies complicating retroperitoneal surgery. South Med J 72:1254–1258
3. Buurman R, Bücheler E (1976) Die Mißbildungen der unteren Hohlvene. ROFO 125:337–345
4. Ehringer H, Fischer H, Netzer C, Schmutzler R, Zeitler E (1979) Venöse Abflußstörungen. Enke, Stuttgart
5. Grewe H-E, Kremer K (1977) Chirurgische Operationen, Bd 1. Thieme, Stuttgart
6. Hafferl A (1957) Lehrbuch der topographischen Anatomie. Springer, Berlin Göttingen Heidelberg
7. Heberer G, Rau G, Löhr H-H (1966) Aorta und große Arterien. Springer, Berlin Heidelberg New York
8. Von Lanz T, Wachsmuth W Praktische Anatomie, Band 1/4. Teil: Bein und Statik 1972 (Lang J, Wachsmuth W), 2. Teil: Hals 1955, 3. Teil: Arm 1959, Springer, Berlin Heidelberg Göttingen
9. Loose KE, van Dongen RJAM (1976) Atlas of angiography. Thieme, Stuttgart
10. Martin R (1962) Lehrbuch der Anthropologie, Band III. Fischer, Stuttgart
11. May R (1973) Die Chirurgie der Bein- und Beckenvenen. Thieme, Stuttgart
12. Michels NA (1955) Blood supply and anatomy of the upper abdominal organs. Lippincott, Philadelphia
13. Mitty HA (1975) Circumaortic renal coller, a potentially hazardous anomaly of the left renal vein. Am J Roentgenol Radium Ther Nucl Med 125:307–310
14. Molz G (1976) Abnormer Abgang der Arteriae subclaviae. Basic Res Cardiol 71:420–427

15. Nadjati AS, Vollmar J (1976) Die klinische Bedeutung und die chirurgische Behandlung der Knickstenosen der A. carotis interna. Med Welt 27:2420–2422
16. Nizankowski C, Raichel Z, Zirlkowski M (1975) Abnormal origin of arteries from the aortic arch in man. Folia Morphol (Warsz) 34:109–116
17. Noczynski L (1976) Vascular anomalies of the hepatic arteries and their practical importance. Folia Morphol (Warsz) XXXV:85–93
18. Papadopoulos NJ (1981) Stereotactic patterns of the extrahepatic portal venous system. Anat Clin 3:143–148
19. Pick JW, Johnson B (1940) The renal vascular pedicle: an anatomical study of 430 body-halves. J Urol 44:411
20. Platzer W (1982) Atlas der topographischen Anatomie. Thieme, Stuttgart
21. Schmidt GP (1975) Über eine besondere Form der doppelseitigen V. cava inferior. Anat Anz 137:200–206
22. Schwemmle K (1980) Die allgemein-chirurgischen Operationen am Halse. Springer, Berlin Heidelberg New York (Allgemeine und spezielle Operationslehre, vol 5, part 4)
23. Strandness DE Jr (1969) Collateral circulation in clinical surgery. Saunders, Philadelphia
24. Testut L, Latarjet A (1949) Traité d'anatomie humaine, tome deuxième et quatrième. Doin, Paris
25. Töndury G (1981) Angewandte und topographische Anatomie. Thieme, Stuttgart
24. Vaas F (1975) Some considerations concerning the deep femoral artery. Arch Chir Neerl 271:25–34
27. Van Limborgh J (1961) L'Anatomie du système veineux de l'extrémité inférieure en relation avec la pathologie vanqueuse. Folia Angiol (Pisa) VIII:3
28. Wicke L, Spängler HP, Dimopoulos J, Fibras W, Olbert F (1974) Zur Dignität der Variationen der Nierenarterienabgänge im Angiogramm. Anat Anz 135:140–150

2.2 Surgical Anatomy of the Veins

B. GÜNTHER and G. HEBERER

As stated earlier, we have chosen to present those topographic aspects of the vascular system that are of greatest importance for the surgeon, rather than a systematic anatomy with a division into arteries and veins. The veins that have been discussed, together with their corresponding regions, are: internal jugular vein, carotid triangle (p. 13); subclavian vein, sternocleidomastoid region (p. 13); axillary vein, axillary region (p. 19); inferior vena cava, renal veins, and variations, discussed in the section on the retroperitoneum (p. 19); iliac veins, femoral veins, saphenous vein junction and variations in the sections on pelvic and lower limb vessels (p. 22).

A. The Greater Saphenous Vein with Its Most Important Branches and Communicating Veins

Because of its special importance in vascular surgery, the greater saphenous vein, with its most important branches and communicating veins, is discussed separately.

The greater saphenous vein collects the entire epifascial venous blood of the leg. The perforating and communicating veins connect the greater saphenous vein system to the deep system of the femoral vein (Fig. 2.2.1).

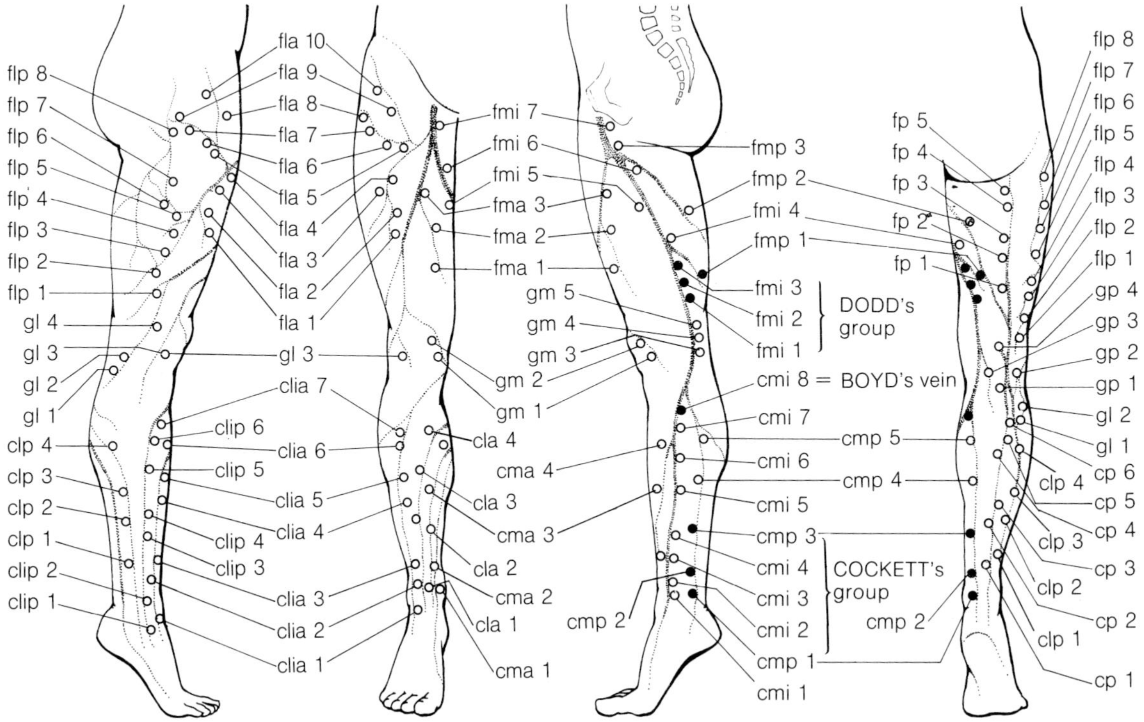

Fig. 2.2.1. Schematic representation of the superficial venous system of the lower extremity with the location of communicating veins (perforating) as described by VAN LIMBORGH [1]

The 100 or more perforating veins of the lower extremity are classified either as direct connections, which run between the muscles, or as indirect connections, which link the superficial and deep system through veins belonging to the muscle itself. Only the direct connections, such as Cockett's, Boyd's and Dodd's veins are of particular importance in vascular surgery. Usually, the communicating veins of Cockett's group are located 6, 12 and 15 cm above the plantar surface of the foot and Boyd's veins 25 cm above. Dodd's or Hunter's group is situated at the level of the vastoadductor membrane.

REFERENCE

1. Limborgh J van (1961) L'Anatomie du système veineux de l'extrèmitè inférieure en relation avec la pathologie variqueuse. Folia Angiol (Pisa) VIII: 3

2.3 Surgical Anatomy of the Lymphatic System

R.G.H. Baumeister

CONTENTS

A. General Remarks

The anatomy of the lymphatic system is of interest mainly because of its function as a drainage network.

The blind precapillaries are the beginning of the lymphatic system in the tissue. They have slits in their sides which can open and close. They are fixed to the surrounding tissue by specific fibers, so that as the tissue becomes saturated with body fluid, the tension on the fibers increases leading to dilatation of the precapillaries and opening of the slits [1, 2].

Near the skin, precollectors drain limited small regions, so-called lymphatic skin regions. Several precollectors, connected to one another in series, drain the lymph into the superficial skin collector. The skin regions drained in this manner together comprise a strip, called a lymphatic skin zone. The skin regions and skin zones overlap so that for every point on the skin there are several lymphatic drainage possibilities (Fig. 2.3.1), all in close proximity to one another.

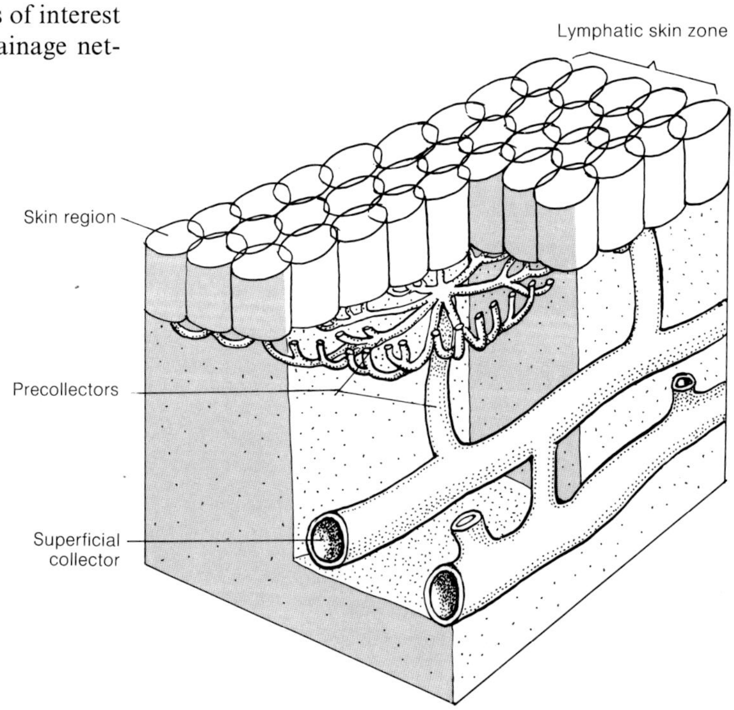

Fig. 2.3.1. Lymphatic drainage of the skin

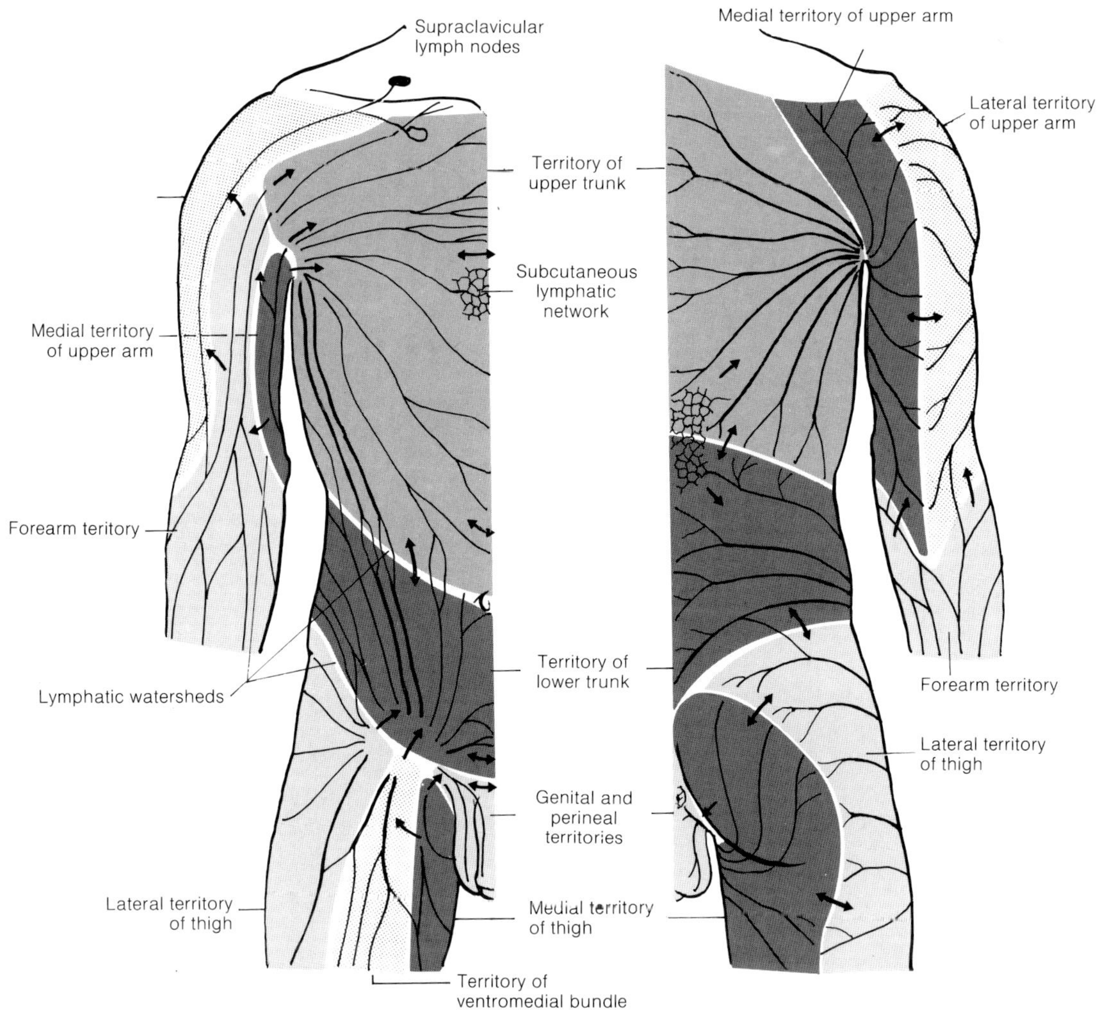

Fig. 2.3.2. Superficial lymphatic drainage territories of the trunk and proximal areas of the upper and lower extremities (afferent and efferent collaterals)

Finally, several collectors form bundles or groups of collectors. The corresponding drainage areas are then named territories. Between these skin territories there are lymphatic watersheds which can be transgressed only by interterritorial anastomoses within the cutaneous network. Knowledge of these territories is of great importance in the understanding and possible correction of lymphedema (Fig. 2.3.2) [3, 4, 5, 6].

B. Anatomy

I. Lymph Vessels of the Lower Extremity

The lymph vessels vary greatly with respect to their course. Therefore, a schematic representation of the different types of lymph vessel distribution may be misleading. In serial examinations Kubik described lymph vessel variations in the lower limb which play an important role in the development of iatrogenically induced lymphedema. Two principal types of lymphatic vessel distribution can be distinguished in the region of the anteromedial bundle: those with a very abundant, dense vasculature, and others with fewer lymphatic vessels (Fig. 2.3.3a) [3].

Schematically, the lymph vessels of the lower limb can be subdivided into superficial and deep lymphatic networks.

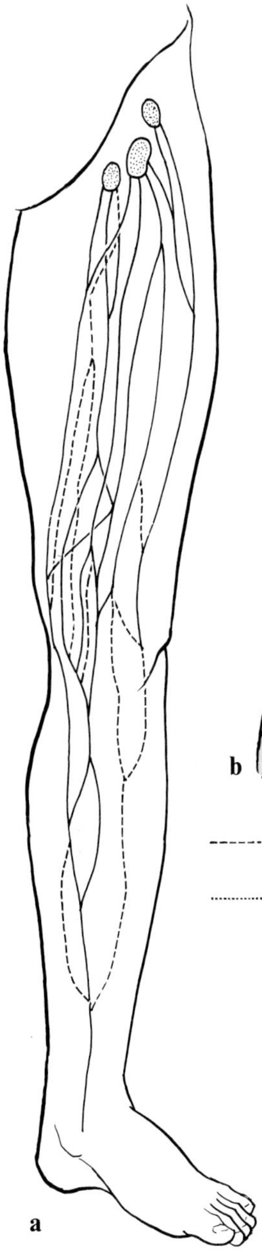
a

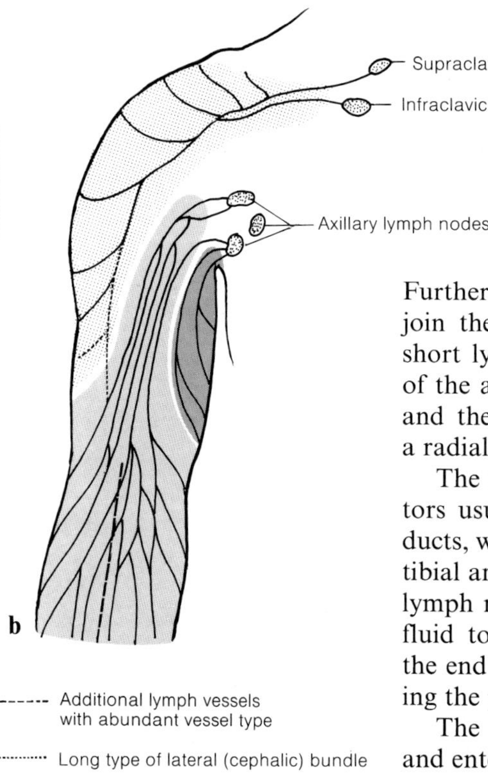

Fig. 2.3.3. a Main variations of lymphatic vessels of the anteromedial bundle in the lower extremity. **b** Types of distribution of lymphatic vessels of the cephalic bundle in the upper extremity

The superficial lymphatic vessels form three large collector groups:

a) The medial collectors. They follow the course of the greater saphenous vein and enter into the superficial inguinal lymph nodes in the region of the inferior group.
b) The anterolateral collectors. They ascend on the anterior aspect of the lower leg and on the anterolateral side of the thigh.
c) The dorsal collectors. They follow the course of the lesser saphenous vein and enter into the lymph nodes near the popliteal vein.

Furthermore, the collectors of the gluteal region join the superficial inguinal lymph nodes. Also, short lymph vessels originating at the distal wall of the abdomen, the genital and perineal regions, and the anus enter the inguinal lymph nodes in a radial arrangement.

The larger lymphatic ducts of the deep collectors usually run alongside the large vessels. The ducts, which follow the same course as the anterior tibial artery and vein, enter into the anterior tibial lymph nodes and from there transport the lymph fluid to the popliteal lymph nodes. This is also the end point of lymphatic collectors accompanying the posterior tibial and peroneal vessels.

The efferent ducts follow the femoral vessels and enter into the deep inguinal lymph nodes. Additional drainage of the lower extremities is possible through the obturator canal to the obturator lymph node and by lymphatic vessels along the sciatic nerve. These join the upper group of internal iliac lymph nodes [7, 8, 9].

II. Lymph Vessels of the Upper Extremity

In the region of the upper extremity, one can also distinguish between a superficial and a deep lymphatic system.

Commencing from the lymphatic network of the fingers and the hand, three lymphatic collector groups form at the level of the wrist:

a) Medial collectors. They follow the basilic vein. Together with the vein, they penetrate the fascia and join the deep lymphatic ducts of the upper arm. The lymph fluid of this region is transported to the lateral axillary lymph node group.

b) Lateral collectors. They follow the cephalic vein, penetrating the infraclavicular fascia. They transport lymph fluid to the infraclavicular lymph nodes. Often additional lymph nodes may be found in the deltopectoral fascia. There are two types of cephalic bundles (Fig. 2.3.3b). In the long type the lymphatic fluid can flow from the radial side of the forearm to the cephalic bundle. In the short type, only the lateral portion of the upper arm is drained.

If the lymphatic drainage is blocked at the axilla, the ultimate size of the areas drained in the arm by bypassing the axillary lymph nodes will vary according to drainage type [5].

c) Lymph collectors which do not run parallel to the previously mentioned groups perforate the axillary fascia at the lower edge of the pectoralis major muscle. The lymph fluid drains into the lateral axillary lymph nodes.

Principally, the deep lymphatic ducts also follow the large vessels in the upper extremity. They form collectors at the elbow which are in close contact with the brachial artery and vein. The lymph flows into the lateral axillary lymph nodes, where a connection to the superficial lymphatic network exists.

III. Lymph Vessels of the Pelvic Region

The lymph vessels of the pelvic region are interrupted by the large lymph node groups which surround the large vessels. The external iliac lymph nodes form a lateral, medial, and intermediate chain. They are followed by the common iliac lymph nodes. Most of the lymph flows from the left medial group of these lymph nodes to the right medial group and, unlike the remaining lymphatic fluid, directly into the aortocaval lymph nodes which surround the abdominal aorta and inferior vena cava. They form lateral, pre-, and retrovascular chains or groups.

IV. Lymph Vessels of the Thorax

In the thorax, one may distinguish between mural and visceral lymph node groups and their efferent ducts.

a) Mural nodes and efferent ducts. Intercostal lymph nodes lie next to the spine and form two rows of nodes parallel to the thoracic duct. These function as collaterals if the thoracic duct is obstructed. Efferent ducts of the uppermost nodes ascend to the right and left junction between the brachiocephalic vein and subclavian vein (venous angle). The efferent ducts of the middle nodes enter directly into the thoracic duct. The lowest nodes form efferent ducts which run downward through the diaphragm.

Parasternal nodes have efferent vessels which also ascend to both venous angles.

The efferent ducts of the diaphragmatic lymph nodes lead to the anterior mediastinal, juxtaesophageal, and parasternal nodes.

b) Visceral nodes and efferent ducts. The efferent ducts of all visceral lymph node groups, the regional nodes of the lung, the nodes of the hilus and bifurcation, the bilateral tracheobronchial chains, as well as the anterior and posterior mediastinal nodes ascend to the upper aperture of the thorax. They form the bronchomediastinal vessels which extend to the right and left venous angle.

V. Lymph Vessels of the Head and Neck

The lymph of the head and neck is collected in two large drainage systems: the jugular lymph node chain, located near the internal jugular vein, and the juxta-accessory and supraclavicular lymph node chains. Together they form one main jugular duct at the base of the neck which, being joined by the infraclavicular and bronchomediastinal ducts, may form the right lymphatic duct or enter directly into the venous system at the venous angle. On the left side, the jugular trunk may join the thoracic duct or enter directly at the left venous angle.

VI. Thoracic Duct

The thoracic duct collects the lymphatic fluid of almost the whole body. Only the right arm, the right side of the head and neck, and the right side of the thorax are drained through the right lymphatic duct.

The course of the thoracic duct, from its origin beneath the diaphragm to its entry into the venous system, may vary considerably [7].

1. Normal Course

The thoracic duct begins at the cisterna chyli at the level of the second to the third lumbar vertebra behind the aorta and between the crura of the diaphragm. The cisterna chyli has the shape of a pea, bean, or pear. The thoracic duct passes through

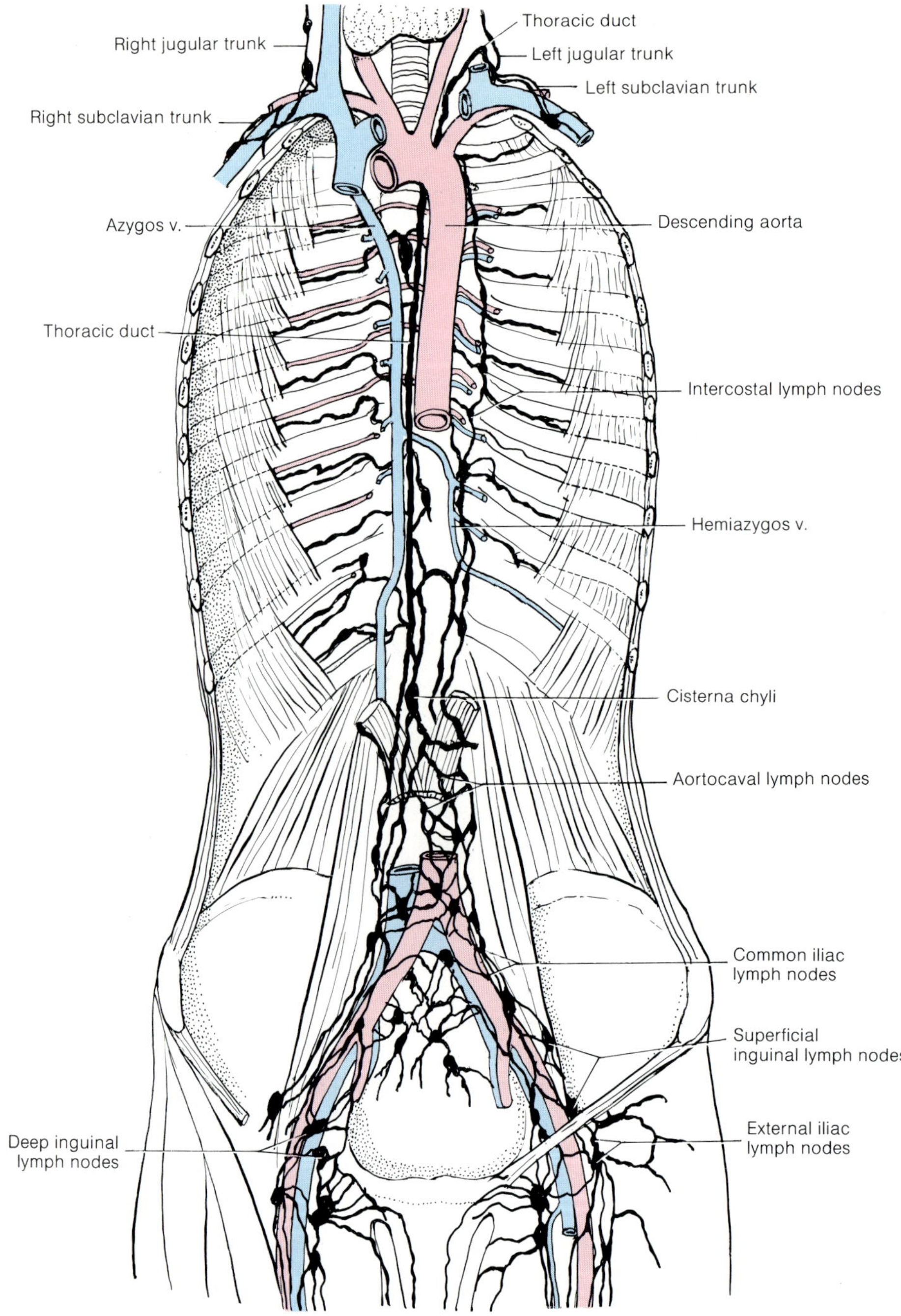

Fig. 2.3.4. The central lymphatic drainage system

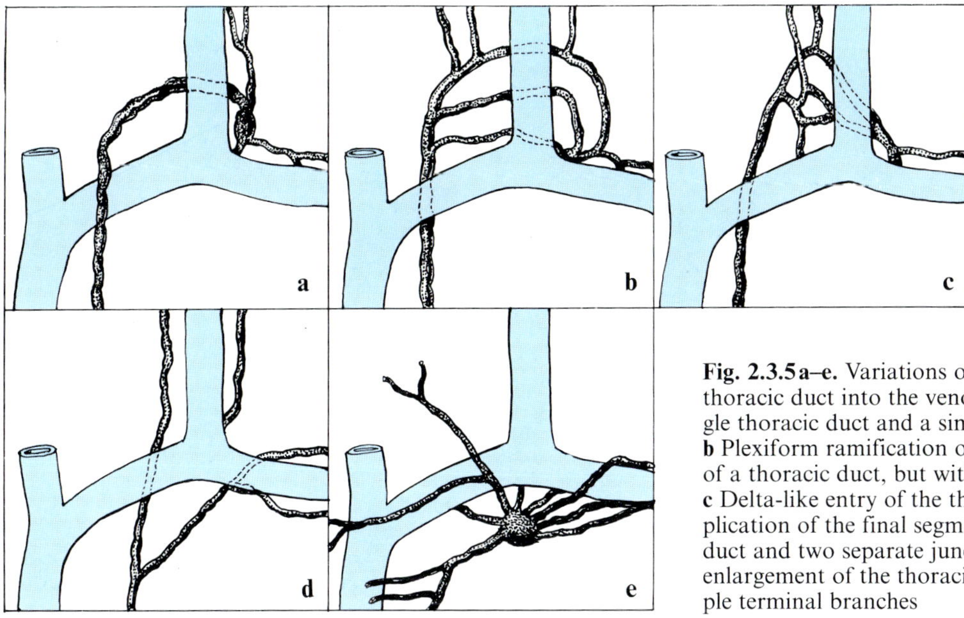

Fig. 2.3.5a–e. Variations of the entry of the thoracic duct into the venous system. **a** A single thoracic duct and a simple junction. **b** Plexiform ramification of the final segment of a thoracic duct, but with a simple junction. **c** Delta-like entry of the thoracic duct. **d** Duplication of the final segment of the thoracic duct and two separate junctions. **e** Ampullary enlargement of the thoracic duct with multiple terminal branches

the diaphragm together with the aorta and continues in the posterior mediastinum to the right side of the spine. It lies in front of the intercostal vessels in the prevertebral tissue.

The thoracic duct changes its direction at the level at which it crosses the hemiazygos vein and passes behind the esophagus and the aorta. Sometimes, it may ascend together with the vagus nerve. It joins the left subclavian artery above the aortic arch reaching at that site the upper aperture of the thorax. Sometimes, lymph nodes may be found. In the neck the thoracic duct curves to the front at the level of the seventh cervical vertebra and enters at the venous angle, the junction between the internal jugular vein and the left subclavian vein. In this region the left bronchomediastinal trunk and the left subclavian collectors join the thoracic duct. After receiving these vessels the thoracic duct widens to form an ampulla. Valves are often found at this site (Fig. 2.3.4).

2. Variations

The following variations are often found: a division of the cisterna chyli into two or three parts or a plexiform construction of the first segment of the thoracic duct.

In some cases, the thoracic duct may exist as two vessels. The duct often separates into two channels when it reaches the thoracic region. These run either apart from one another, or they have interconnections. These branches may then resemble a plexiform ramification of the thoracic duct. However, there is usually only one vessel present above the aortic arch. As it curves toward the venous angle, the thoracic duct may separate into several channels which in part may cross each other, but they can reunite shortly before entering into the venous angle or enter separately in the vicinity of the venous angle. The curve may be missing, and the thoracic duct may enter into the veins alone or together with other vessels from below (Fig. 2.3.5).

VII. Right Lymphatic Duct

The right lymphatic duct lies on the right side deep in the neck, between the jugular vein and the subclavian vein. It collects all lymphatic vessels which do not enter the thoracic duct. These are chiefly the subclavicular, jugular, and bronchomediastinal trunks on the right side. The length of the right lymphatic duct measures about 8–15 mm. Numerous variations are also found at its venous junction. Its tributaries can also enter directly into the subclavian vein, jugular vein, or brachiocephalic vein (Fig. 2.3.6a–c).

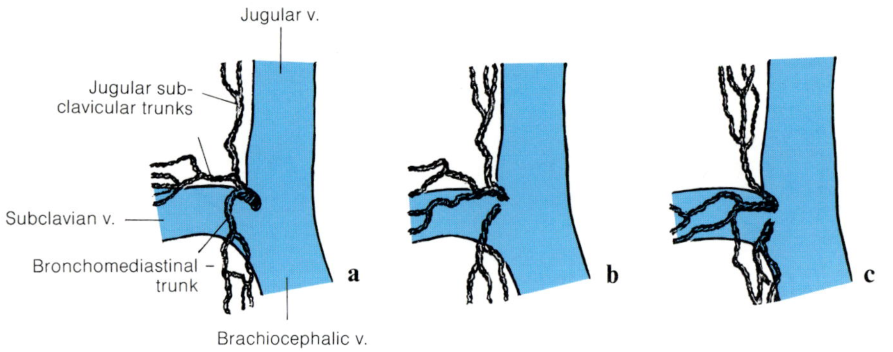

Fig. 2.3.6a–c. Variations of the lymphatic junctions at the right venous angle. **a** Entry of the tributaries into the right lymphatic duct. **b** Partial entry into the right lymphatic duct. **c** Separate entry of the tributaries near the right venous angle

REFERENCES

1. Casley-Smith JR (1977) The structural basis for the conservative treatment of lymphedema. In: Clodius L (ed) Lymphedema. Thieme, Stuttgart
2. Casley-Smith JR (1982) The fine structure and fine functioning of initial lymphatics. In: Bartos V, Davidson W (eds) Advances in lymphology. Avicenum, Prag
3. Kubik S (1969) Die normale Anatomie des Lymphsystems unter besonderer Berücksichtigung der Sammelgebiete der Lymphknoten der unteren Körperhälfte. Strahlentherapie 69:8–17
4. Kubik S (1974) The anatomy of the lymphatic system. Recent Results Cancer Res 46:5–17
5. Kubik S (1980) The role of the lateral upper arm bundle and the lymphatic watersheds in the formation of collateral pathways in lymphedema. Acta Biol Acad Sci Hung 31:191–200
6. Kubik S (1980) Drainagemöglichkeiten der Lymphterritorien nach Verletzungen peripherer Kollektoren und nach Lymphadenektomie. Folia Angiologica 28:228–237
7. Testut L, Latarjet A (1948) Canaux cellecteurs lymphatiques, In: Traitè d'anatomie humaine. Doin, Paris
8. Testut L, Latarjet A (1948) Lymphatiques et groupes ganglionnaires, In: Traitè d'anatomie humaine. Doin, Paris
9. Toldt C, Hochstetter F (1979) Anatomischer Atlas. Urban & Schwarzenberg, München

3 Hemodynamic Aspects in Vascular Surgery

L. SUNDER-PLASSMANN

CONTENTS

A. Introduction

Occlusive arterial disease is primarily a disease of the large transporting and distributive arteries. Essential for the development of clinical symptoms, however, are the effects of this disease on the microcirculation, which must function with only a small fraction of normal perfusion pressure. All surgical measures of revascularization, whether by thromboendarterectomy or bypass grafting, aim at reestablishing normal perfusion pressure at the level of the arterioles [6, 12].

It is of crucial importance for tissues in the resting state and during exercise that the blood be distributed to those regions within the microcirculation in accordance with the demand. "Demand-orientated blood distribution" means that the controlling mechanisms of the arterioles do not guide blood to those regions with the greatest conductivity – the widest and shortest capillaries – but to all those areas where an increased oxygen supply is actually needed, e.g., in the longer, thinner capillaries. Thus, the arterioles function as inlet or distributive valves of nutritive blood flow: Just like a valve they regulate the flow of blood under high pressure from the arteries to the capillaries. Therefore, it is most important for the correct function of blood supply distribution that the blood actually has enough energy, i.e., circulatory pressure, at the level of the arterioles [5, 10].

B. Energy Losses of Circulating Blood in Occlusive Arterial Disease

The loss of energy of the blood from the ascending aorta to the arterioles may be demonstrated objectively by direct measurement of the fall in pressure. Flow resistance was introduced as a measure of energy loss within the entire circulatory system in analogy to Ohm's law.

$$P_1 - P_2 - R \times Q$$

$$P_1 - P_2 = \text{Pressure gradient before and after the perfusion} \quad (1)$$

Q = flow; R = flow resistance

The decline in pressure from central to peripheral areas has two principal causes:

I. Frictional Resistance to Blood Flow in Tubular Vessels

This is defined by the Hagen – Poiseuille law:

$$R = \frac{8\eta \times L}{\pi \times r_4} \quad (2)$$

η = blood viscosity; L = length of vessel, r = radius of vessel

II. Loss of Kinetic Energy

The second reason for a drop in pressure is kinetic energy loss caused by inertia, turbulence, and velocity changes in blood flow at stenoses, bifurcations, and curves. The drop in pressure is proportional to the density of blood p and the square of the difference between both velocities $v_1 - v_2$.

$$\Delta P = k \times \frac{p}{2} \times (v_1 - v_2)^2. \tag{3}$$

Figure 3.1 shows that the pressure loss, the sum of friction, turbulence, inertia, pulse reflection, and flow diversion from the aorta to the arterioles is very low. Flow resistance of the aorta together with the large transporting and distributive arteries and their terminal branches, is less than 20% of the entire resistance. In contrast, the short arterioles, as inlet and distributive valves, constitute over 40% of the entire vascular resistance [5]. In healthy arteries, the main drop in pressure within the circulatory system happens at the arterioles. Thus, normally

$$R_{art} \ll R_{per} \tag{4}$$

R_{art} = partial resistance of the aorta and large arteries

R_{per} = resistance in the arterioles

In occlusive arterial disease the conditions are reversed: multiple narrowings and segmental vascular occlusions increase resistance within stenotic or occluded transporting arteries to such an extent that the main pressure drop within the circulatory system occurs before the arterioles (Fig. 3.1). The arterioles react, dilating completely to cause a reduction of resistance. Therefore, R_{art} may become much greater than the peripheral resistance R_{per}. In occlusive arterial disease, the following condition is present:

$$R_{art} \gg R_{per}. \tag{5}$$

The reason for the enormous drop in pressure along an occluded vascular segment is the difficulty of forming collaterals, which may take months or years to develop. Because of this dilatation, the arterioles cease functioning as distributors or valves for the microcirculation. Blood distribution is not oriented toward oxygen and nutritive demands, but is subject only to the laws of hydrodynamics. Blood flows to the shortest and widest capillaries. Local distribution within the microcirculation is disturbed, leading to local tissue hypoxia.

Figure 3.2 schematically illustrates these pathogenetic mechanisms in the lower limb: in a totally obstructed segment (superficial femoral artery) the blood flows exclusively through the collaterals, which take months or years to develop completely. The goal of all conservative measures is to accelerate the growth of collaterals and reduce collateral flow resistance. Surgical therapy is much more effective because blood flow is completely restored

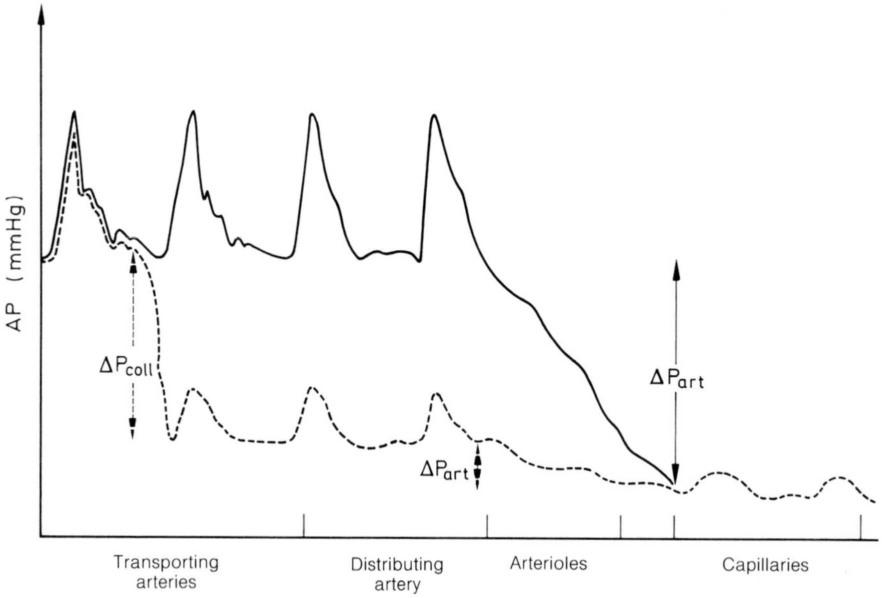

Fig. 3.1. Pressure distribution within the circulatory system, starting at its central portion (transporting arteries) continuing to its peripheral portions all the way down to the capillaries in the case of undiseased vessels (*solid line*), and in occlusive arterial disease (*broken line*). In healthy individuals, the reduction of pressure (ΔP_{art}) and kinetic energy of the blood occurs at the level of the arterioles, which function as inlet valves to the microcirculation. In occlusive arterial disease, this pressure drop and energy loss happens along the course of the transporting arteries or collaterals (ΔP_{coll}) so that flow pressure at the arterial level is not adequate for microcirculatory regulation

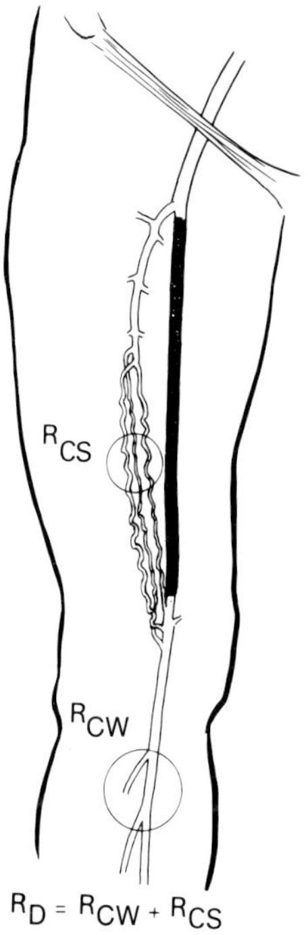

Fig. 3.2. Changes of flow resistances within the lower extremity due to obstruction of the superficial femoral artery. The total resistance (R_D) which the blood must overcome to reach the calf muscles is the sum of the collateral resistance (R_{CS}) and peripheral calf resistance (R_{CW}). If the formation of collaterals is poor, R_{CS} may become the most important obstacle ($R_{CS} \gg R_{CW}$), so that the flow energy is insufficient in peripheral regions of the calf muscle

following endarterectomy or bypass grafting of the previously occluded segments. The technique and possible applications of endarterectomy and bypass grafting are described on p. 78ff. Hemodynamically, they both aim at reducing resistance (R_{art}) to such an extent that an almost normal perfusion pressure is restored peripheral to the reconstruction, and this is usually achieved in single-level occlusions. In multiple-level occlusions of the pelvic – thigh type, it must borne in mind be that the resistances of pelvic arteries (R_I), collateral circulation ($R_F + R_C$), and calf (R_W) add up to a total resistance, because they are connected in series

$$R_{total} = R_I + R_F + R_C + R_W. \qquad (6)$$

The Hagen – Poiseuille law can also be applied using the frictional resistance of a stenosis. This resistance is directly proportional to the viscosity of the fluid, the length of the stenosis, and above all indirectly proportional to the fourth power of the radius of the stenosis:

$$R_{sten} = \frac{8\eta \times L}{\pi \times r_4} \qquad \text{(see reference 2).}$$

From a hemodynamic point of view in multiple-level occlusions, the stenosis with the smallest diameter must be removed in every case [11]. For example, if only R_I is reduced by thromboendarterectomy and R_F remains unchanged (e.g., high grade stenoses at the origin of the profunda femoris artery), the mere reconstruction of pelvic arteries will not lead to improved blood flow in the calf. Conversely, a peripheral reconstruction will fail if a hemodynamically effective stenosis remains in the proximal vascular segment. It has been proved experimentally as well as clinically that an autologous vein bypass constructed distal to a vascular stenosis shows a higher degree of thrombosis, owing to the absence of pulsatile flow and to turbulence [7, 12].

Therefore, in multiple-level occlusions the proximal stenosis is always corrected first.

C. Hemodynamics of Surgical Reconstruction

I. Thromboendarterectomy

Thromboendarterectomy is performed at the carotid bifurcation, in pelvic arteries as well as in the profunda femoris artery, and mainly in short occlusions or solitary stenoses (see p. 73ff). Bilateral long occlusions and multiple stenoses are more an indication for bypass grafting. A remaining distal intimal flap must always be fixed by an adequate additional suture. A longitudinal arteriotomy should not be sutured directly, but instead closed with a patch graft. Besides preventing narrowing at the suture site, the greater diameter of the vessel following patch angioplasty raises transmural pressure and increases the pressure against the intimal flap. Because of excessive neointima formation with subsequent recurrent stenosis, occlusions of the superficial femoral artery are seldom corrected nowadays by thromboendarterectomy, but almost always by bypass grafting.

II. Bypass Grafting

Autologous saphenous veins as well as synthetic Dacron and Teflon materials are used in bypass grafts. Two basic principles should be kept in mind: (1) All bypass grafts show a higher flow resistance than undiseased arterial segments of the same length and caliber. (2) Independent of all technical details concerning anastomosis, anastomotic angle, and dimensions of the graft, blood flow ultimately depends on the run-off in the vascular bed distal to the graft. Even a technically superb graft construction will develop thrombosis quickly if the run-off is obstructed by peripheral occlusions [7]. The only way to preserve patency in such a case is to construct a distal arteriovenous fistula (see p. 415).

This does not increase the peripheral nutritive circulation in muscle or skin: however, it does cause a considerable increase in flow velocity within the graft, thus preventing early thrombotic obliteration.

The entire energy loss of the blood during its passage through the bypass graft results from a combination of the following forces:

1. Frictional resistance

$$R_{\text{sten}} = \frac{8\eta \times L}{\pi \times r_4} \qquad \text{(see reference 2)}$$

2. Kinetic energy loss due to inertia caused by curvature of the vessel, turbulence, changes in flow velocity during in- and outflow from the prosthesis, as well as disturbance of streamline flow at the anastomotic angle ($\Delta P = K \times \frac{1}{2} \times v^2$).

Depending upon the graft's position within the circulatory system (supra-aortic, pelvic, lower leg region) as well as its dimensions, the frictional resistance may increase considerably (e.g., in prostheses below the knee joint with diameters less than 4 mm). Also, the loss of kinetic energy may be greater for abrupt changes of diameter in the pelvic arteries. In every case, the energy loss through friction, as calculated by Poiseuille's law, is considered to be minimal because these kinetic energy losses are not taken into account in practice. Therefore, the prosthesis is chosen on the one hand according to mathematical considerations and on the other according to instantaneous conditions within the circulatory system. Besides certain qualities of wall structure, the practical requirements which a bypass graft must fulfill are highly contradictory from a physical point of view [2, 3, 4, 7, 8, 9]. On the one hand, frictional resistance should be as low as possible so that the pressure does not drop too much, but on the other hand, flow velocity should not be too low (danger of thrombosis). Kinetic energy losses through inflow and outflow phenomena such as turbulence should be avoided. The anastomotic angle between the bypass graft and its parent artery should be as acute as possible in relation to the radius of the prosthesis. An additional difficulty consists in the different functional behavior of a prosthesis at rest and during exercise. For example, in the pelvic region, where blood flow varies substantially according to physical activity, a prosthesis might function superbly at rest, but lead to severe obstruction of blood flow during hyperemia under exercising conditions. The correct choice of the prosthetic diameter must always be the best compromise between mathematical considerations and practical requirements.

Thus, theoretically, the widest possible lumen should be used, since frictional resistance increases inversely with the fourth power of the radius (see Eq. 1). Furthermore, formation of pseudo- and neointima inside Dacron prostheses causes the initial diameter to the reduced by about 1–1.5 mm; calculation shows that in an 8-mm prosthesis this degree of narrowing would produce a 216% increase in frictional resistance. On the other hand, if the diameter is too large, flow velocity, which is directly proportional to the second power of the radius, is significantly reduced [2].

$$v_1 v_2 = (r_2/r_1)^2. \qquad (7)$$

Calculations reveal that a 7-mm prosthesis has a flow velocity almost three times as high as that in a 12-mm prosthesis. On the other hand, with increased flow velocity the effects of outflow phenomena at the distal anastomosis are intensified when the bloodstream emerges from the narrow prosthesis into the wider artery. The energy loss (P) is proportional to the square of the difference in velocity ($v_1 - v_2$)

$$\Delta P = \frac{K}{2} \times p \times (v_1 - v_2)^2 \qquad \text{(see reference 3).}$$

If the kinetic energy loss due to inflow and outflow phenomena is to be kept low, the prosthetic lumen at the upper anastomosis should be smaller than the lumen of the parent artery and the lumen at the distal anastomosis should be larger, because with such an arrangement there is less turbulence and less disturbance of the blood flow [2].

Therefore, an 8–10-mm Dacron bypass graft in occluded pelvic arteries is the best compromise between frictional resistance, flow velocity, and turbulence. Even if the whole internal surface of the prosthesis is narrowed by 1–1.5 mm through the formation of neointima, the frictional resistance in these arteries will not be too great.

By contrast, resistance can be a very critical problem in femoropopliteal vein bypass grafts. The saphenous vein is 4–6 mm in diameter. According to Poiseuille's equation [1] a graft 30 cm long will cause a drop in pressure under resting conditions (100 ml/min) and during active hyperemia (500 ml/min) of about 9 and 14 mmHg, respectively. A decrease in diameter of 3 mm produces a fall in pressure at rest of 14 mmHg and during hyperemia a drop of as much as 44 mmHg. This means that the frictional resistance of a narrow graft in the femoropopliteal segment can be just as high as in existing collaterals. Early graft thrombosis is inevitable. Therefore, the diameter of a femoropopliteal graft should never be smaller than 4 mm [12].

D. Technique of Anastomosis

I. Angle in End-to-side Anastomoses

In contrast to an end-to-end anastomosis, an end-to-side anastomosis causes energy losses due to kinetic and frictional forces which are proportional to the anastomotic angle (α) between bypass graft and parent artery, and the quotient of the radius of curvature (r_k) and the prosthetic diameter (r_p).

$$\Delta P \sim \alpha \times r_k / r_p \qquad (8)$$

Although the energy loss at the anastomotic angle is low, one may conclude that in practice an end-to-end anastomosis should be performed whenever possible, and in cases where an end-to-side anastomosis must be constructed the anastomotic angle should be as small as possible, e.g., less than 45°.

II. Configuration of the Anastomoses

When attached obliquely by end-to-side anastomosis, a graft will be elliptical in cross-section. Such elliptical distortion of a cylinder whose longitudinal radius (r_a) remains constant causes frictional resistance to increase as the transverse radius (r_b) decreases.

$$Q = \Delta p \times \frac{\pi}{4L} \times \frac{r_a^3 \times r_b^3}{r_a^2 \times r_b^2}. \qquad (9)$$

The smallest frictional resistance is achieved when the transverse diameter of the elliptical anastomosis and the diameter of the cylindrical prosthesis are equal. Therefore, slanting the prosthesis, which is necessary to achieve an acute angle, should not be extended so far that narrowing of the transverse diameter takes place (Fig. 3.3).

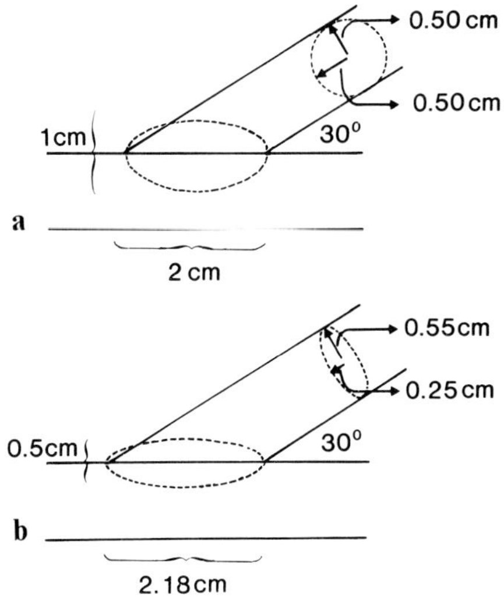

Fig. 3.3a, b. The obliquely cut end-to-side anastomosis. Proper oblique tailoring changes the circular shape of the prosthetic orifice (diameter 1 cm) to an elliptical shape with a longitudinal diameter of 2 cm and a transverse diameter of 1 cm at the anastomosis (**a**). Such an elliptical orifice has the same flow resistance as a circular prosthesis. However, if the anastomosis is too oblique, (**b**) and narrowing of the orifice changes the transverse radius from 1 cm to 0.5 cm, flow resistance increases by a factor of 4.4 (after STRANDNESS and SUMNER [12])

III. Special Characteristics of a Bifurcation Prosthesis

In a bifurcation graft, an energy loss is produced either through friction or inertia. If an energy loss through frictional resistance is to be kept as low as possible, according to Poiseuille's law (see Eq. 2), the quotient of the radii $r_2/r_1 = 0.884$, and then the quotient of the diameters is $2\ A_2/A_1 = 1.414$.

If, on the other hand, a change in velocity along the prosthetic segment must be avoided, then the relationship between both diameters must be ($2\ A_2 = A_1$), i.e., the ratio $r_2/r_1 = 0.707$. Finally, if maximal transmission of pulsatile energy is necessary, so that reflection of pulsatile waves is avoided, the inflow impedance (Z_0) should be equal to the impedance of both tubes (Z_1); but this is only achieved if the ratio of both radii $r_2/r_1 = 0.758$ (Fig. 3.4).

The customary bifurcation prostheses with $r_2/r_1 = 0.5$ and $2\ A_2/A_1 = 0.5$ are unfavorable because: frictional resistance at the bifurcation is increased by a factor of 8, flow velocity is doubled,

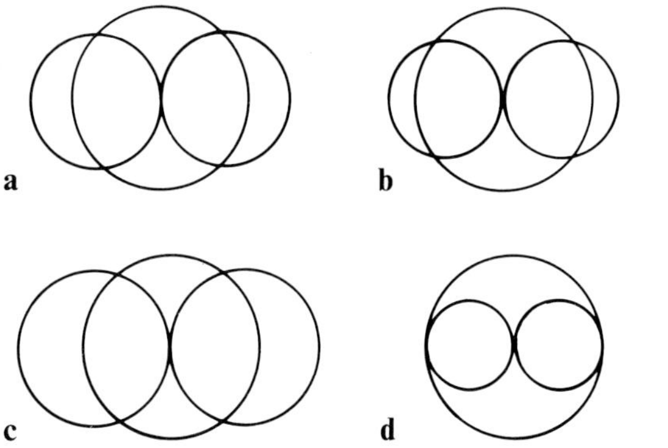

Fig. 3.4a–d. Dimensions of bifurcation prostheses. The ratio of the radii of both limbs of the prosthesis to the proximal radius of the prosthesis may be designed from different points of view: If a change in velocity is to be avoided, the diameter of the prosthesis A_1 and both diameters of the legs of the prosthesis A_2 must be equal ($A_1 = 2\,A_2$). In such a case the ratio $r_2/r_1 = 0.707$ (**b**). If a drop in pressure caused by frictional resistance along the bifurcation must be prevented, then, according to the Hagen-Poiseuille law (see Eq. 2), the following dimensions are necessary: $r_2/r_1 = 0{,}884$ and $2\,A_2/A_1 = 1.414$. **b** If the inflow impedances Z_0/Z_1 are equal, the ratio $r_2/r_1 = 0.758$ (**a**). Thus, the dimensions of the prostheses commonly available (**d**), with the arbitrarily chosen ratio $r_2/r_1 = 0.5$, are not suited to the creation of acceptable hemodynamic conditions. Prostheses with wider branches (e.g., 16/12 mm instead of 16/8) would be much more favorable (**c**)

and about 50% of the pulsatile energy is reflected upward, generating a higher amplitude of pulsatile waves above the terminal aorta and thereby producing an additional strain on the upper row of sutures (see below). In terms of physics, the common bifurcation prosthesis with $r_2/r_1 = 0.5$ is therefore not ideal. A ratio of 0.7 to 0.75 is much more desirable (e.g., 16/12 mm instead of 16/8 mm). The main problem is not the increased frictional resistance, since flow in the pelvic area is very high, but rather the reflection of pulsatile energy upward, which might be a common cause of the frequent anastomotic aneurysms in this region [1, 4, 8, 9].

E. Significance of the Run-off

The blood volume which flows through a bypass graft during a given time interval depends on the resistance of the graft (R_T) as well as the resistance of the calf (R_W)

$$(R_{ges} = R_T + R_W). \tag{10}$$

The resistance of the calf consists not only of the peripheral resistance of the arterioles and capillaries, but also the resistance of run-off vessels, such as the popliteal artery and crural arteries; for example, if the run-off consists of only one single lower leg artery which may also have multiple stenoses along its course, run-off resistance will become the most decisive factor influencing the function of the entire graft. It has already been shown quite often that the patency rate of a femoropopliteal or crural bypass is strongly dependent on blood flow at rest and during dilatation with Papaverine [13]. This blood flow is again directly dependent on the patency of the lower leg arteries as demonstrated angiographically. The differences in flow through a graft are, however, always more distinct during hyperemia than under resting conditions.

Thus, bypass grafting is only indicated if there is angiographic evidence that at least one lower leg artery is patent and the patient's clinical symptoms are severe (stage III–IV).

All other previously discussed aspects of graft resistance, – diameter, anastomotic angle, anastomotic diameter, etc. – are less important than the initial anatomic situation of the grafted artery.

F. Conclusions

Each surgical revascularization aims at normalizing perfusion pressure and blood distribution at the level of the microcirculation. Each bypass graft has a higher resistance and therefore causes a higher loss in energy than undiseased arterial segments. This resistance is the sum of different factors: frictional resistance (graft radius and graft length) and kinetic energy loss through curvature of the graft, the anastomotic angle, the transverse radius of the anastomosis, turbulence due to abrupt caliber changes from the parent artery to the prosthesis and vice versa. Thus, a compromise must always be made when looking for the right prosthesis. At the upper anastomosis, the diameter of the prosthesis should be equal to or somewhat smaller than that of the parent artery, and at the lower anastomosis it should be equal to or greater than that of the parent artery. The anastomotic angle should be as small as possible, which means that the bypass prosthesis should branch off from and reenter the parent artery at the most acute angle possible. However, the slant of the orifice should not be too great since, in an elliptical anastomosis, the transverse diameter should be equal to the diameter of the prosthesis. Nevertheless, all of the factors listed above concern only technical details. Ultimately, the decisive parameter of blood flow through a prosthesis is the patency of the run-off vessels which must be assessed preoperatively by angiography.

REFERENCES

1. Boughner DR, Roach MR (1971) Effect of low frequency vibration on the arterial wall. Circ Res 29:136
2. Daugherty HJ, Franzini JB (1965) Steady flow of incompressible fluids in pipes. In: Fluid mechanics with engineering applications, 6th edn. McGraw-Hill, New York, p 191
3. Deweg F (1979) Fluid mechanics of arterial flow. Exp Med Biol 115:55
4. Ferguson GG, Roach MR (1972) Flow conditions at bifurcations as determined in glass models with reference to the focal distribution of vascular lesions. In: Bergel DH (ed) Cardiovascular fluid dynamics, vol 2. Academic Press, London, p 141
5. Green H, Rapela CE, Conrad MC (1963) Resistance and capacitance phenomena in terminal vascular beds. In: Hamilton WF, Dow Ph (eds) Handbook of physiology. Circulation, vol 2. Washington, DC, p 935
6. Heberer G, Rau G, Löhr HH (1966) Aorta und große Arterien. Springer, Berlin Heidelberg New York, p 56ff
7. Kaminski DL, Barner HB, Dorighi JA, Kaiser GC, Willman VL (1972) Femoropopliteal bypass grafting. Arch Surg 104:527
8. Newman DL, Bowden LR, Gosling RG, Wille SD (1972) Impedance of aortic bifurcation grafts. J Cardiovasc Surg 13:175
9. Newman DL, Gosling RG, Bowden NLR, King DH (1973) Pressure amplitude increase on unmatching the aortopunction of the dog. Cardiovasc Res 7:6
10. Spencer MP, Denison AB (1963) Pulsatile blood flow in the vascular system. In: Hamilton WF, Dow Ph (eds) Handbook of physiology. Circulation, vol 2, Washington, p 839
11. Strandness DE, Sumner DS (1977) The effect of geometry on arterial blood flow. In: Strandness, Sumner (eds) Hemodynamics for surgeons. Grune & Stratton, New York, p 96
12. Strandness DE, Sumner DS (1977) Grafts and grafting. In: Strandness, Sumner (eds) Hemodynamics for surgeons. Grune & Stratton, New York, p 342
13. Terry HJ (1972) The electromagnetic measurement of blood flow during arterial surgery. Biomed Eng 7:466

4 Technique of Vascular Surgery

E.-D. SCHWILDEN and R.J.A.M. VAN DONGEN

CONTENTS

A. Preparation of Patients for Vascular Surgery

The majority of patients are older and have multiple risk factors especially because of arteriosclerosis. Therefore, the diagnosis and treatment of possible risk factors and concomitant diseases is an essential aspect of *routine preoperative preparation* (see p. 99, 191). Coagulation parameters have to be checked and, if necessary, therapeutic measures initiated preoperatively, intraoperatively, and/or postoperatively (see p. 104). Preoperatively, one should also discuss any necessary prophylaxis against infection. In case of a previously existing infection, the aim of preoperative preparation should be to determine the optimal time for vascular reconstruction (see p. 166).

The number of blood units requested usually depends on the experience of the surgeon. They may consist of donor blood or the patient's own blood prepared by isovolemic hemodilution.

The *local preparation of the operative area* should include a very much wider area than the operative field itself. The preparation of a possible site for the harvest of an autologous vein graft is also important. In cases of curved incisions or incisions across skinfolds, especially in the area of the groin, the incision should be marked, but not by scratching with a knife or a needle. For prophylaxis against infections in peripheral vascular surgery, the leg, including the groin, should be wrapped in an antiseptic dressing with polyvinylpyrrolidone-iodine solution the evening before the operation.

Preparation on the table should provide positioning for an optimal operative approach (head-down position, semithoracotomy position). Care must be taken to prevent decubital ulcers in patients with arteriosclerosis, especially in those with poor soft-tissue condition. The first critical area is the sacral region, especially in the presence of stenosis of iliac arteries or when the arterial blood supply to the pelvis is occluded for a significant time during the operation. Prophylaxis against decubitus may be achieved by placing a soft pillow underneath the patient or by means of a vacuum pillow. Use of an electric cushion may lead to burning of the skin because of the insufficient heat transport which can accompany interruption of the blood supply. Thermoregulated heating cushions or switching off the heating cushion during the time of occluded blood flow reduces these risks. The second critical point for intraoperative pressure sores is the heel. It should be protected routinely by a soft cushion or a cotton wool dressing. For intraoperative inspection of the foot, the operating table should be equipped with a suitable cushion at the site of the heel.

Continuous draining of the bladder is necessary during longer operations and in all cases where a full bladder might possibly impede the surgical procedures. Drainage of the bladder should be through a suprapubic catheter because of the well known postoperative complications from transurethral catheters. A suprapubic catheter, however, is contraindicated whenever a possible complication from the puncture might involve the area of vascular reconstruction.

Draping of the operative field should include adjacent regions in case the operative procedure has to be extended. In other words, if complications arise, exposure of adjacent regions should be possible without any further manipulation. For all reconstructions possibly requiring a vein graft, the region chosen for removal of the graft should also be draped. A vein patch should only be removed from the region of the ankle. Total vein segments for short interposition or bypass are best removed from the inguinal region. When performing an inguinal incision, special care must be taken in draping the genital area. In case of a unilateral inguinal approach, the scrotum and penis should be fixed at the contralateral thigh using a sterile double gauze pad with an adhesive. Whenever it is expected that the drapes might become soaked with fluid or blood, a water-resistant adhesive plastic material should be placed beneath the drapes. This adhesive plastic also protects the operative field from skin pockets due to fat or kinking. The gauze pads, which should always be double, will be fixed either by clamps or by the adhesive plastic used for skin draping. During the operation it may be wise to palpate the distal arteries for immediate recognition of thromboembolic complications. Figure 4.1 a, b illustrates two possibilities for intraoperative control of circulation in the lower extremity.

a

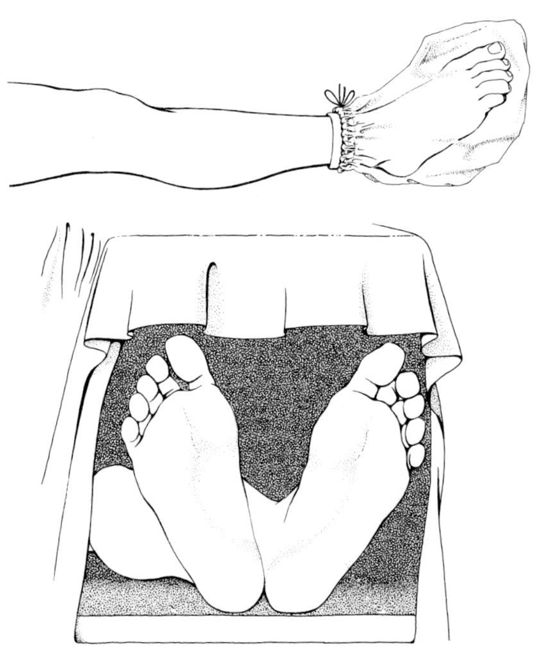

b

Fig. 4.1 a, b. Possibilities for intraoperative control of the circulation by wrapping the foot with a transparent sterile plastic sac (**a**) or by inspection from the end of the operative table (**b**)

B. Standard Vascular Instruments and Technical Aids

During vascular reconstruction, the risk of damage by unsuitable instruments or by their inappropriate use is especially high. Therefore, special instruments for vascular surgery are indispensable. There are two requirements which must be fullfilled by the instruments: function and optimal safety.

One of the first requirements for sound technique in vascular surgery is wide exposure of the operative field, allowing quick and precise reconstruction. For good exposure there are numerous

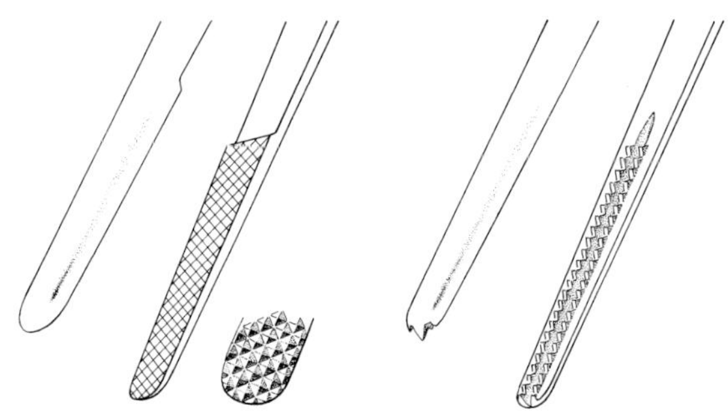

Fig. 4.2. Atraumatic jaw profiles of vascular forceps

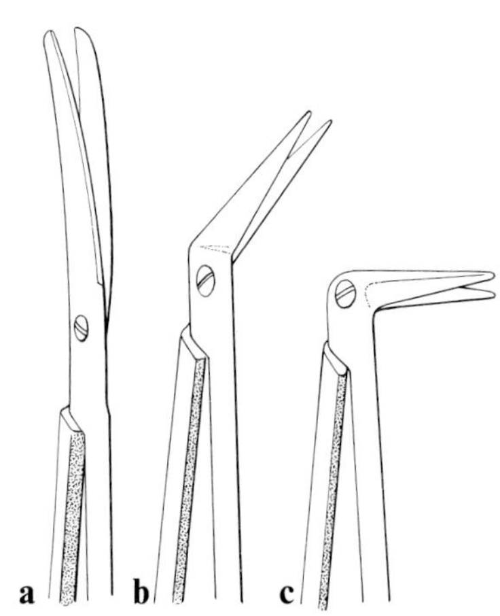

Fig. 4.3 a–c. Scissors for vascular dissection (**a**) and for arteriotomy (**b**, **c**)

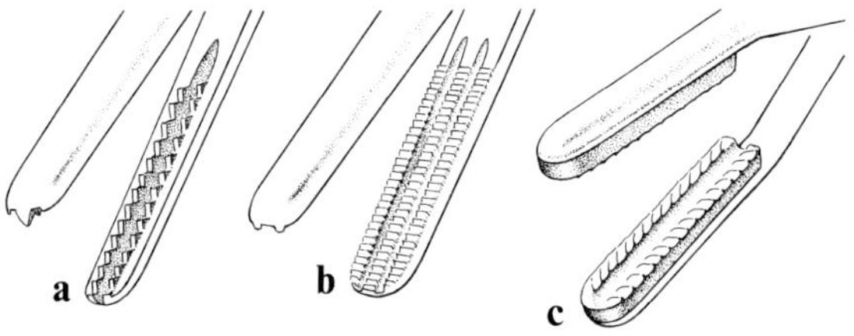

Fig. 4.4a–c. Jaw profiles of atraumatic vascular clamps

and multiform retractors on the market. A suitable assortment of various models, properly used, can greatly facilitate both the operative approach and the intraoperative manipulations.

The forceps for dissection of vessels should have different lengths because of the different depths of the operative field. The jaws should not traumatize the tissue, but they should grip it firmly and not let it slip. These features are best guaranteed by the jaw profiles shown in Fig. 4.2.

Vascular scissors should also be available in different lengths. The scissors should allow the surgeon to palpate the quality of the dissected tissue as with an extended finger. This may be achieved by rounded, slightly curved, and smoothly sliding blades (Fig. 4.3a). A model with a counter curve may be of advantage in a deep operative field. Scissors with various angles (Fig. 4.3b, c) are used for extension of arteriotomies and for partial incision of vessel walls.

Putting a band around a vessel is best performed with a moistened rubber catheter or silastic loops, the latter being available commercially.

Vascular clamps for temporary occlusion of blood flow should fulfill the following requirements: First, that they grip the vessel with absolute safety and with minimal trauma. Longitudinal and transverse rows of fine serrations, or teeth, on the inside (Fig. 4.4a) usually guarantee a firm grip and prevent slipping and the possibly disastrous consequences. The model devised by DARDIK is especially atraumatic because the serration is extremely flat and a firm grip is assured by an additional row of teeth (Fig. 4.4b). Clamps with a soft removable jaw profile (Fig. 4.4c) may be of great value for clamping extremely arteriosclerotic vessels.

The second requirement is a sufficiently long lock, allowing soft closure of the clamp and a stepwise, pressure-adapted release of the blood flow.

The third requirement, finally, is variety in the form and length of the handle and branches of the clamps. Such an assortment (Fig. 4.5) allows the surgeon to choose a clamp specifically suited to the particular operative approach and situs.

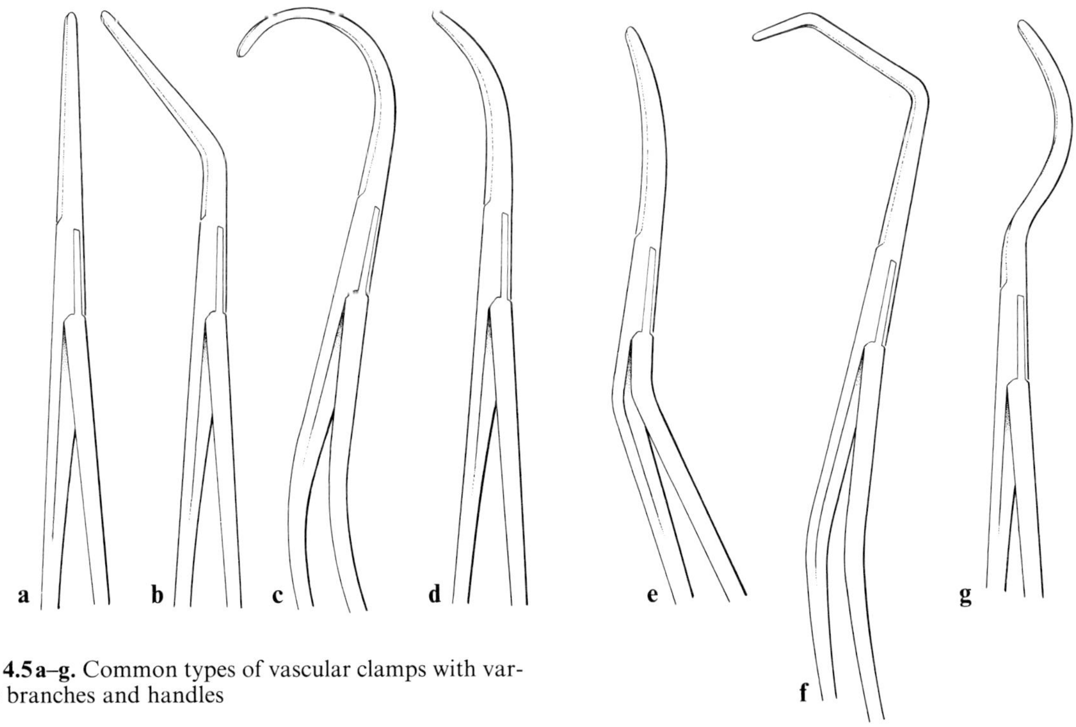

Fig. 4.5a–g. Common types of vascular clamps with various branches and handles

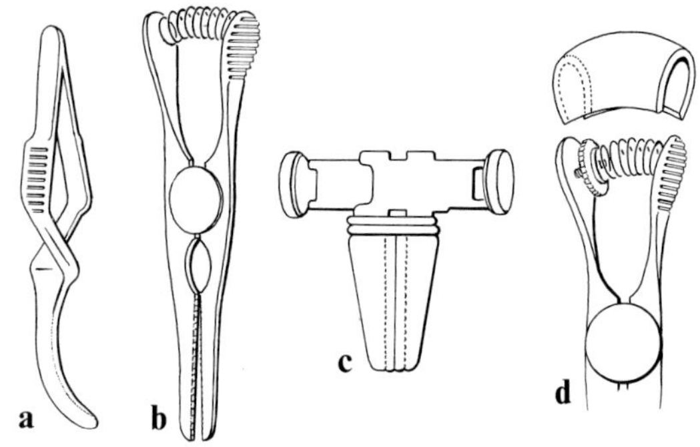

Fig. 4.6a–d. Atraumatic bulldog clamps with various clamping mechanisms

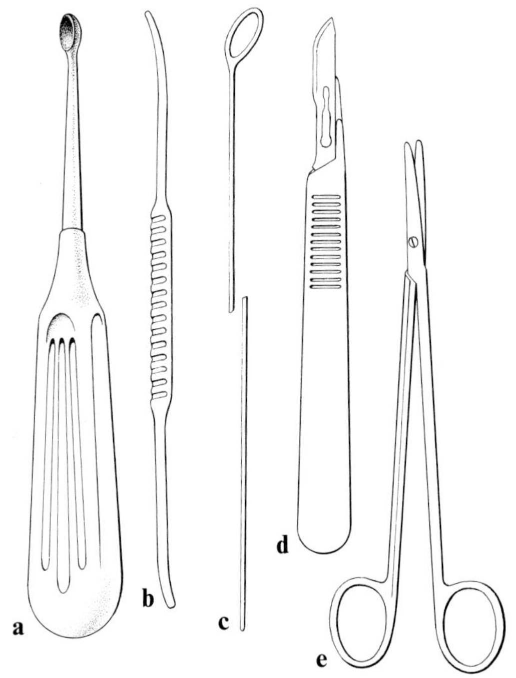

Fig. 4.7a–e. Instruments for open and semiclosed thromboendarterectomy

For cross-clamping smaller vessels, straight or curved so-called bulldog clamps of various sizes are preferred (Fig. 4.6). The clamping pressure is imparted by the elasticity of the metal (Fig. 4.6a), by a coil spring (Fig. 4.6b), or by a circular rubber band (Fig. 4.6c), depending on the model.

Those with adjustable springs are especially atraumatic (Fig. 4.6d). The pressure of the clamp should be chosen so that compression is extremely soft, just enough to occlude the vessel. In order to prevent a suture from being caught in the spring, the latter can be covered by a plastic cap made out of an infusion line (Fig. 4.6d).

The instruments shown in Fig. 4.7 are used for open and semiclosed thromboendarterectomy; e.g., scalpel, scissors, sharp spoon, spatula, and a set of ring strippers of various sizes. A stripper with an oval-shaped ring facilitates the dissection.

Vascular olives of various sizes (Fig. 4.8a) may be used as dilators (Fig. 4.8b), for intraoperative intraluminal control of anastomoses (Fig. 4.8c) or as a guide when suturing a small defect in a vessel wall or a graft (Fig. 4.8d). They may also be used for intraluminal occlusion (see p. 55).

Balloon-tipped catheters (Fig. 4.9a) of various sizes are important instruments for indirect thrombectomy and embolectomy. Older or partially adherent material may well be removed with an urologic Dormia catheter (Fig. 4.9b). Balloon-tipped catheters equipped with a lock may also be used for intraluminal occlusion (see p. 175, 241).

The requirements of a vascular needle holder are, first, not to damage the curve of the very fine vascular needles and, second, to avoid twisting of the needle in the jaws of the needle holder. A very finely profiled short jaw made of hard metal (Fig. 4.10) best guarantees these features.

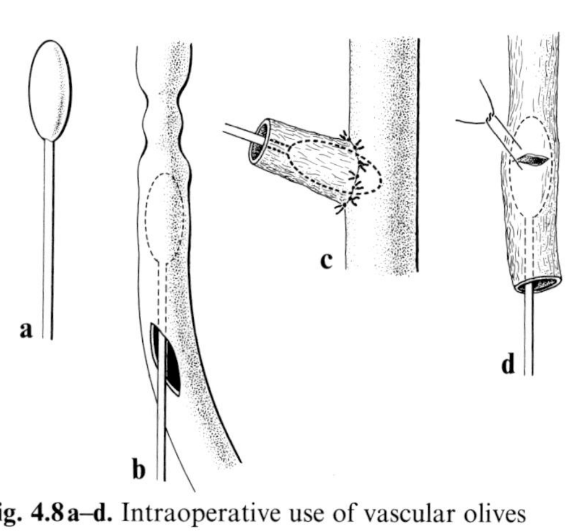

Fig. 4.8a–d. Intraoperative use of vascular olives

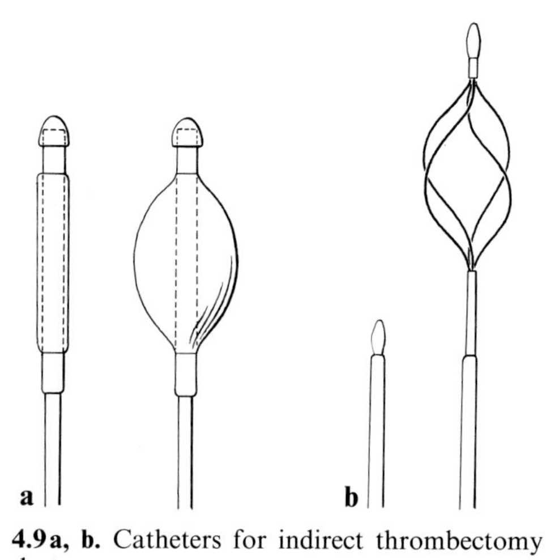

Fig. 4.9a, b. Catheters for indirect thrombectomy and embolectomy

Among the technical aids not usually found among the standard vascular instruments, but of great importance under certain circumstances, are the so-called temporary bypasses. They are used for the reconstruction of vessels for which the circulatory area tolerates only a brief interruption of the blood flow (e.g., carotid artery). In traumatic vascular surgery such bypasses are used for temporary restoration of the circulation whenever reconstruction takes longer or another procedure has priority, or to avoid possible severe ischemic damage during the transport of a patient to a specialized center.

In emergency cases, a plastic tube of appropriate size made out of an infusion line may be used as an intraluminal shunt for the carotid artery or for arteries of the extremities. Commercially available shunts of various lengths and diameters lie either completely within the lumen, as so-called inlying shunts (Fig. 4.11 a), or partially outside the vessel, forming a circle (Fig. 4.11 b) or an omega loop (Fig. 4.11 c), so-called outlying shunts. They facilitate intraluminal manipulations at the site of the arteriotomy. Kinking of shunt loops is avoided by spirals within the shunt wall. The shunt ends are rounded and thickened.

The sealing and the shunt fixation within the vessel is performed either by a tourniquet (Fig. 4.12a, b) or by a special clamp (Fig. 4.12c). Newer shunts are equipped with inflatable balloons or cuffs at the tip, which will interrupt the blood flow and simultaneously fix the shunt within the vessel (Fig. 4.13). This obviates the need for a clamp or a tourniquet, which may traumatize the vessel wall. To avoid intraoperative thromboembolic complications the shunts may be rinsed or perfused continuously via an additional line.

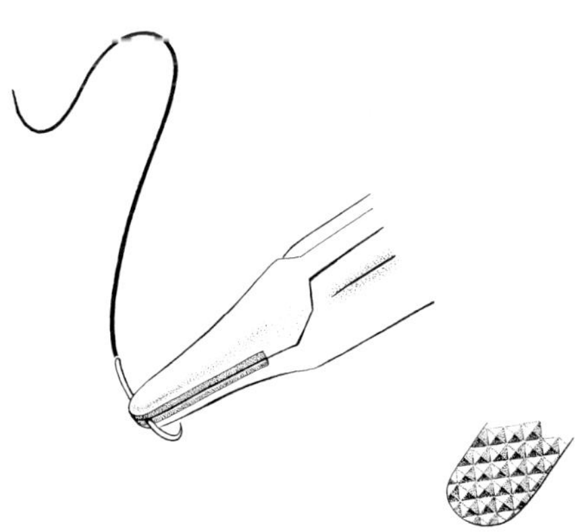

Fig. 4.10. Form and jaw profile of a vascular needle holder

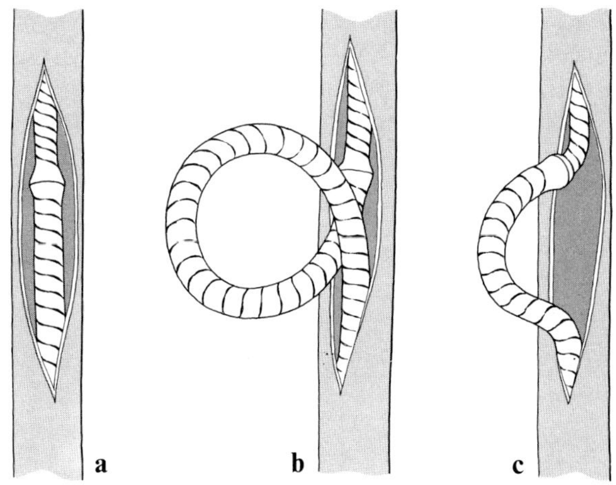

Fig. 4.11 a–c. Intraluminal shunts

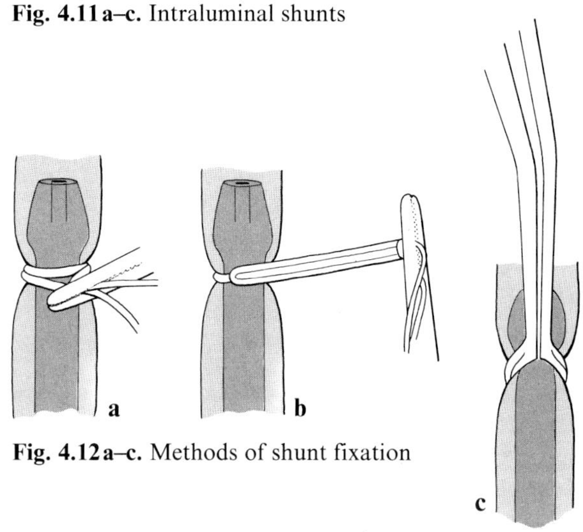

Fig. 4.12 a–c. Methods of shunt fixation

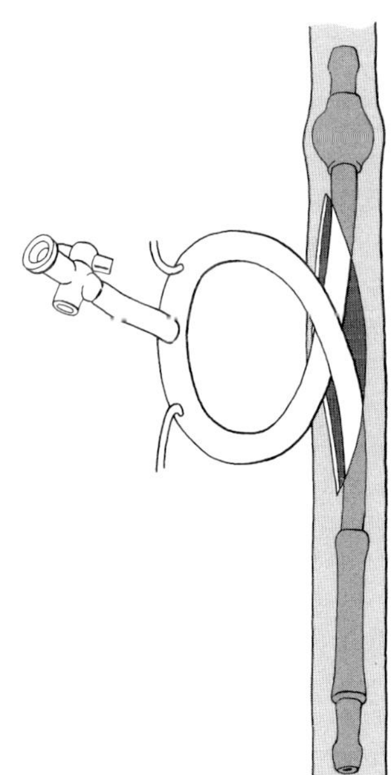

Fig. 4.13. Shunt with intraluminal balloon fixation

This also allows application of drugs and perhaps injection of contrast medium for angiography.

In emergencies or elective operations at the descending aorta or at the innominate artery (trauma, aneurysm) a so-called Gott shunt in the form of an aortoaortic, aortofemoral, or aortobrachiocephalic shunt may be used as an alternative to simple cross-clamping or extracorporeal circulation. The material is PVC. Its inner surface is coated with a heparin complex, providing an antithrombogenic surface. The shunt is inserted into the vessel through an arteriotomy.

C. Vascular Suture Material

The suture material for vascular surgery has to withstand the same hemodynamic forces as the reconstructed vessel itself. It should be inert to avoid infections. A high tensile strength and elasticity should be guaranteed. Simultaneously, the suture must glide well, and the knot must stay tight. The quality of the suture is dependent upon the material, the structure, and the size of the suture material.

The use of *absorbable suture material*, so-called temporary sutures, is still in its experimental phase. Absorbable material may only be used for suturing autogenous material, as only the suture of living vessels will heal without support by permanent sutures.

The basic material of absorbable sutures is hydrolyzable and consists of polyglycolic acid or polyglactin in the case of braided material. These materials are not suitable for vascular surgery because of their rapid absorption and consequent rapid loss of tensile strength and their braided structure. With the development in 1981 of the aliphatic polyester, polydioxanon, a synthetic monofilament absorbable material became available which, because of its significantly lower absorption rate and the smaller resulting loss of tensile strength, opens up new prospects for the future. These prospects include an increase of vascular anastomosis in children and the possibility of more favorable results in cases of sepsis.

In the majority of vascular reconstructions, the long-term safety of the suture depends on the strength of the suture material. Therefore, nonabsorbable suture is the material of choice. The major development among the so-called permanent suture materials is the monofilament polypropylene or polybutylene suture. Its ease of penetration and its high tensile strength enables smooth penetration through each tissue and therefore significantly reduces suture hole bleeding. Furthermore, this material allows one to tighten an already loose running suture, the so-called distance suture technique, without difficulty (see p. 61). This technique may be used, for instance, for difficult posterior wall sutures or after removal of intraluminal shunts. Its biologic inertness and extremely minimal foreign body reaction as well as the fact that it does not act as a wick, provide some resistance to bacterial contamination. One drawback is its low resistance to mechanical damage, for instance, by forceps or clamps, with the risk of suture disruption. Another disadvantage is its elasticity, often resulting in loops and kinking. The knot is relatively unsafe because of the ease of gliding. Security may be ensured by a sufficient number of knots (5–7) and an exact technique of knotting.

The braided nonabsorbable suture mostly consists of polyester made of high quality Dacron. The disadvantage of this suture is that it does not penetrate smoothly through the tissue. This "sawing" effect is intensified by dried blood. Furthermore, its ability to act as a wick may favor infections. An additional outer coating of the thread significantly reduces these disadvantages.

The size of the suture to be used is dependent on the size of the vessel and the condition of the vessel wall. The scheme in Table 4.1 may give a frame of reference for choosing the size of suture for the various vascular regions. The sutures are

Table 4.1. Suture size designations commonly used in various vascular regions according to the old conventional classification of the United States Pharmacopoeia (USP) and according to the classification of the new European Pharmacopoeia (Ph. Eur.). The latter is metric and gives the suture diameter as $^{1}/_{10}$ mm

Vascular region	Suture diameter	
	USP	Ph. Eur.
Thoracic aorta	3–0	2
Abdominal aorta, aortic branches	4–0	1.5
Iliac artery	5–0	1
Femoral artery, brachial artery	6–0	0.7
Carotid bifurcation, renal artery, visceral artery, lower extremity artery, forearm artery	7–0	0.5

swaged onto atraumatic, usually circular needles. Different sizes may facilitate the suture technique in various situations. A special configuration or serration of the body of the needle and a trocarlike piercing tip guarantee a secure seating for the needle holder and atraumatic penetration of the needle through the vascular wall, especially in vessels with extreme calcification or scars. Sometimes double-armed sutures may be advantageous.

D. Vascular Exposure

The exposure of a vessel requires exact anatomic knowledge and a subtile operative technique. First, an incision of the vascular sheet is performed over the anterior wall of the artery, which usually has no branches.

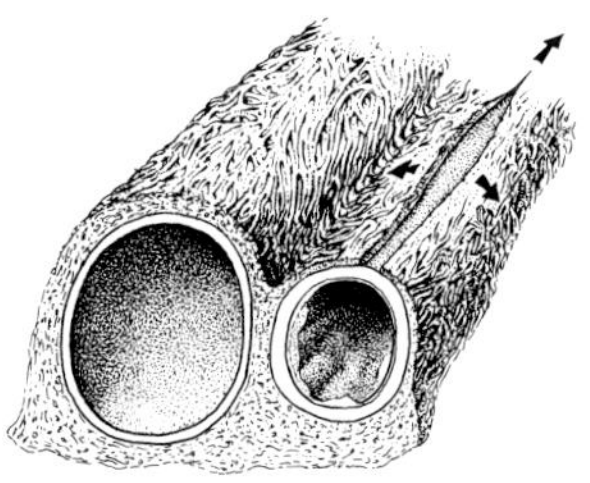

Fig. 4.14. Beginning the exposure of the vessel by longitudinal incision of the periadventitial tissue and subsequent isolation of the vessel in all directions

Dissection continues by removing the periadventitial tissue, staying close to the arterial wall and proceeding proximally and distally on both sides (Fig. 4.14). The dissection is easier if both the surrounding tissue and the adventitia of the vessel are picked up and traction is applied gently to each. The vessel wall itself has to be handled with maximal care, and squeezing by forceps has to be avoided. This dissection may be difficult whenever endangitis has caused inflammatory reactions, when hematomas following angiography, old trauma, or previous operations have caused fibrotic reactions, and also in the case of aneurysms, which usually adhere to the surrounding structures, especially the vein.

When dissecting the artery, especially laterally, each string should be considered as a possible branch of the artery and should be preserved. Temporary occlusion of such small branches is performed by so-called tourniquets (Fig. 4.15) and controlled by the weight of a hemostat. If there is a branch at the posterior wall of the vessel and exposure is difficult the technique of "blind double-encircling at a distance" (Fig. 4.16) is useful. This will avoid damage to the branch. Following sufficient dissection of the artery at both sides, the dissection clamp is passed underneath the vessel and a tape is placed around it. When using

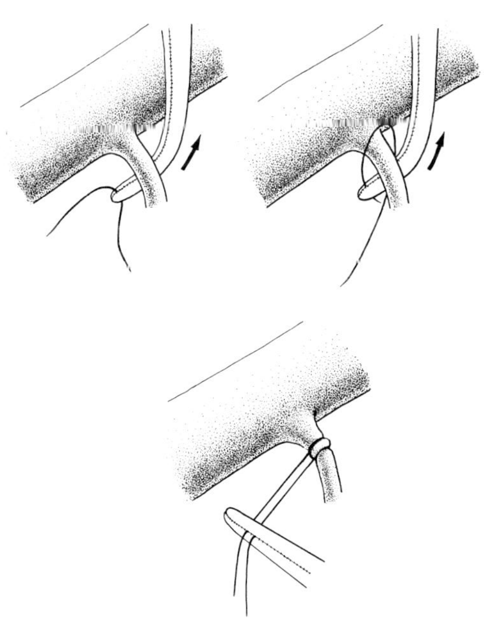

Fig. 4.15. Technique of temporary occlusion of branches by a tourniquet

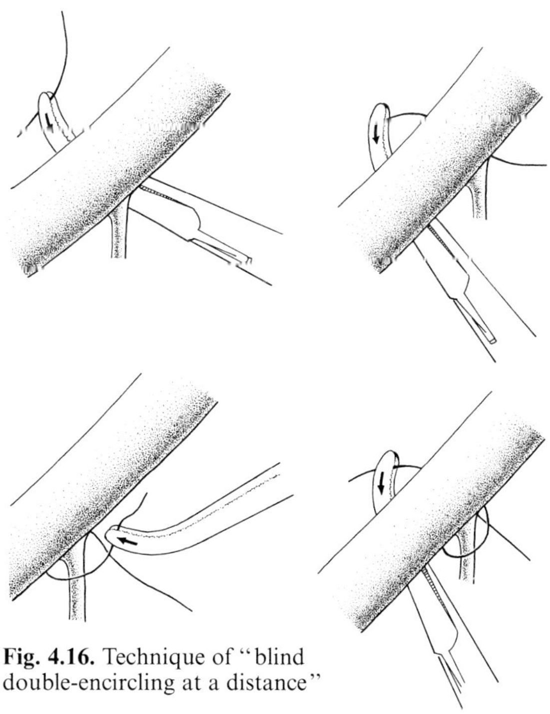

Fig. 4.16. Technique of "blind double-encircling at a distance"

this procedure, special attention must be paid to the posterior collaterals, and the approach should always be from the side next to the vein (Fig. 4.17).

In this way, inadvertent injury to a posterior branch or to the major vein can be avoided. Passing the tape around the vessel is best performed by using a moistened rubber catheter or the so-called vessel loops that are commercially available. Simple sutures or textile tapes are not recommended because of the danger of cutting into the vessel wall or the possibility of twisting the vessel and possibly causing fracture of a plaque. The first dissection of a major vessel should be performed proximally in the area of intended vessel occlusion. This area, as well as the distal tape around the major artery, should be sufficiently far from the segment to be reconstructed or from the site of the anastomosis to insure that the later occlusion will not impair the reconstruction. In case of bleeding during the distal dissection, blood loss is diminished by traction on the proximal tape or by clamping with a hemostat. As in the case of major arteries a tape is also put around larger branches or bifurcations, and they are prepared for cross-clamping. During this procedure, the proximal and distal tapes around the major artery may be carefully drawn upward, allowing one to encircle the branch much more easily (Fig. 4.18). If the exposure of a branch is difficult, the tape may be passed around "blind at a distance."

In case of inadvertent injury to a small arterial branch or to small veins, a ligation, or suture ligation, is called for. Care should be taken not to cause a purse-string effect or to leave a stump that might lead to local thrombosis (Fig. 4.19).

When a tributary is torn out of the major vessel, the lesion is closed by interrupted sutures (Fig. 4.20a) or by an atraumatic suture ligature (Fig. 4.20b). Lesions of the major artery or larger branches, as well as lesions of the concomitant major vein, must be corrected by vascular suture under good visibility. One should beware of blind suture or blind clamping. The bleeding site should be occluded with the finger or a cotton applicator; efferent and afferent arteries should then be isolated and clamped; finally, after complete hemostasis, the lesion of the vessel wall should be properly sutured. In case of injuries to the vein, compression of the vein distally and proximally by means of a cotton applicator will usually stop the bleeding and provide sufficient exposure.

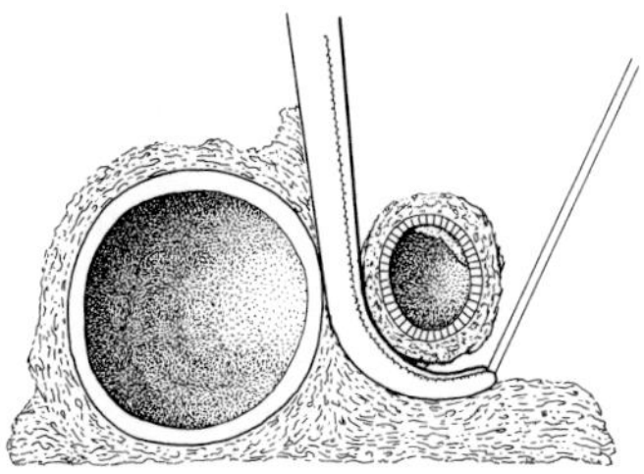

Fig. 4.17. Technique of passing a tape around the major artery, approaching from the venous side with a dissecting clamp

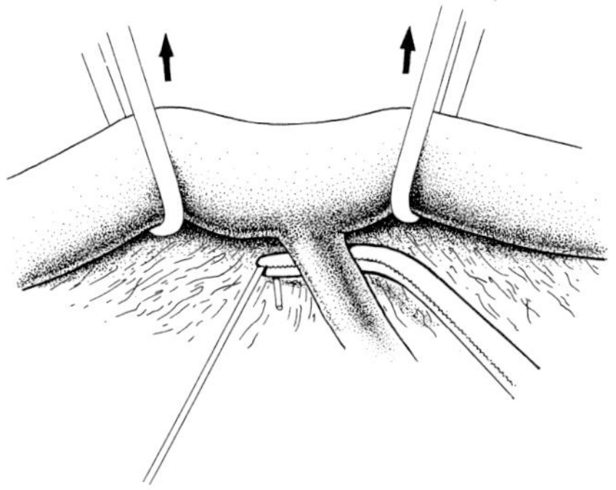

Fig. 4.18. Technique of passing a tape around major arterial branches or bifurcations

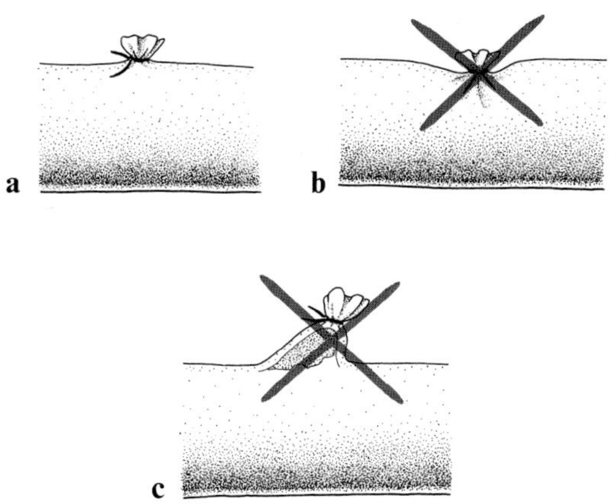

Fig. 4.19a–c. Correct (**a**) and wrong (**b, c**) suture ligation of arterial branches

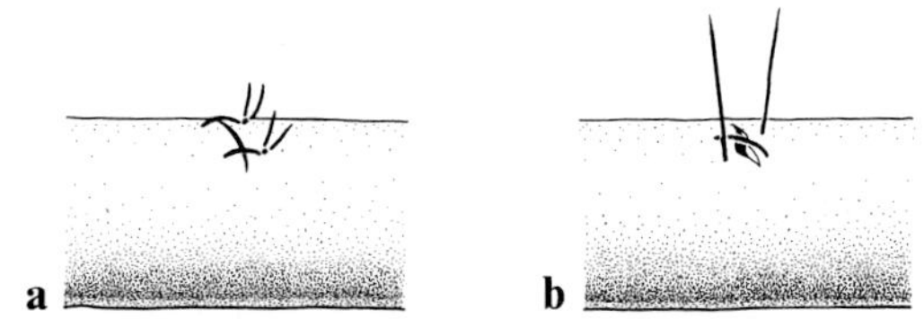

Fig. 4.20a, b. Techniques of hemostasis of arterial branches after lesions or evulsions

E. Vascular Clamping

A requirement for an optimal vascular suture is complete hemostasis by temporary occlusion of the blood flow. Of utmost importance is the avoidance of additional lesions, i.e., lesions of the intima that might result from repeated or otherwise unnecessary manipulation. Occlusion of the blood flow can be achieved by various techniques:

1. Partial tangential clamping (Fig. 4.21). This is done using appropriate vascular clamps. Except for anastomoses of the ascending aorta, the aortic arch, and perhaps the descending aorta, there is hardly a situation where a complete occlusion of the blood flow will not be tolerated for the period of reconstruction. Tangential clamping is still frequently performed for an end-to-side anastomosis at the abdominal aorta and carries the risk that the often significantly sclerotic intima will be injured and dissected by the clamp. Another disadvantage is the difficulty of exposing the vessel lumen owing to the compressed vessel walls. This may complicate a correct suture technique, especially as regards the spacing of the stitches. Furthermore, there is the danger that the clamp may slip.

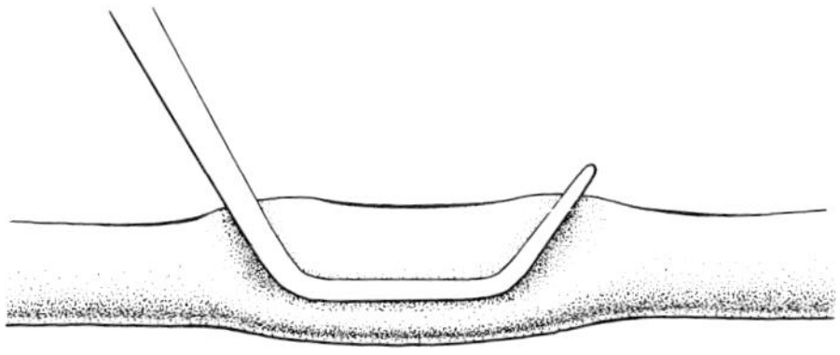

Fig. 4.21. Partial tangential clamping of the vessel by a Satinsky clamp

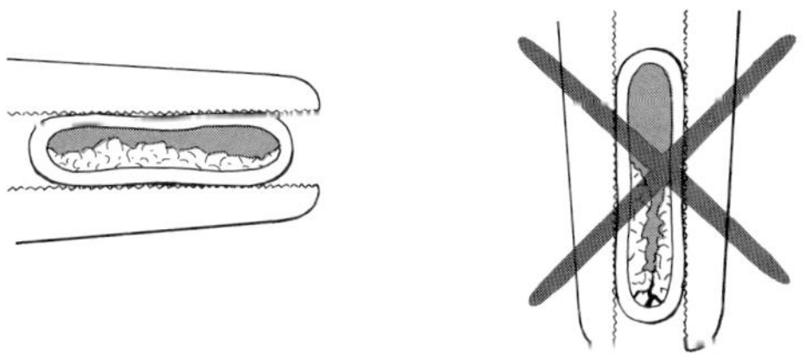

Fig. 4.22. Correct and wrong technique for cross-clamping a partially arteriosclerotic vessel

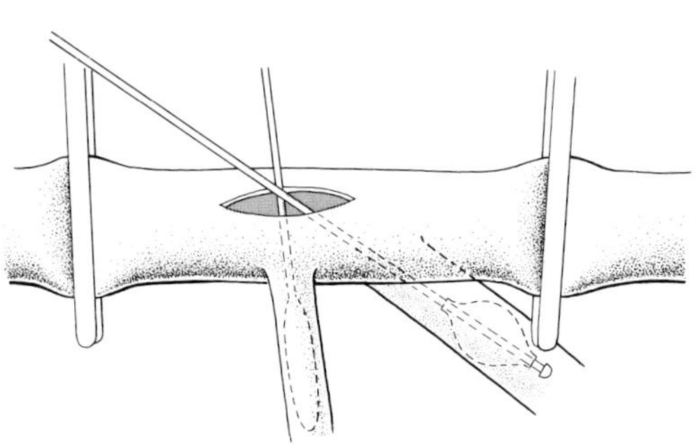

Fig. 4.23. Technique of occluding the blood flow by a combination of cross-clamping and intraluminal balloon or olive occlusion

2. Cross-clamping. The advantage of this technique is that it can be used at each site and provides a sufficient exposure of the vascular segment to be reconstructed. The risk of injury to the vessel wall is less when the clamp is placed at a site free of arteriosclerosis. But since this is seldom the case, placement of the clamp must be appropriate to the pathology of the arterial wall. This means that the soft part of the arterial wall should be pressed against the arteriosclerotic part so that the plaque will not be fractured (Fig. 4.22).

3. Intraluminal occlusion (Fig. 4.23). This may be performed by balloon-tipped catheters or olives of appropriate sizes. In emergency cases, a simple Foley urinary catheter may also be used. Intraluminal occlusion is recommended: (1) for thin vessel walls which may easily be injured by clamps, for instance following open endarterectomy, (2) in case of difficult and time-consuming or risky dissection for cross-clamping, for instance in repeat operations or inflammatory conditions, (3) in the case of unexpected bleeding, when dissection for cross-clamping requires a cost significant amount of time and would therefore cause great blood loss.

F. Arterial Ligature

Because of the severe consequences of a slipped ligature, the ligation should be done in such a way that slipping is virtually impossible. Furthermore, because of the danger of cutting through the artery, the ligature should not be placed in the groove left by a clamp and should be tied slowly and carefully.

Because of these risks, smaller arteries should be tied by suture ligature. Middle-sized arteries are ligated twice; here the central ligature, which is a suture ligature, secures the peripheral ligation (Fig. 4.24a).

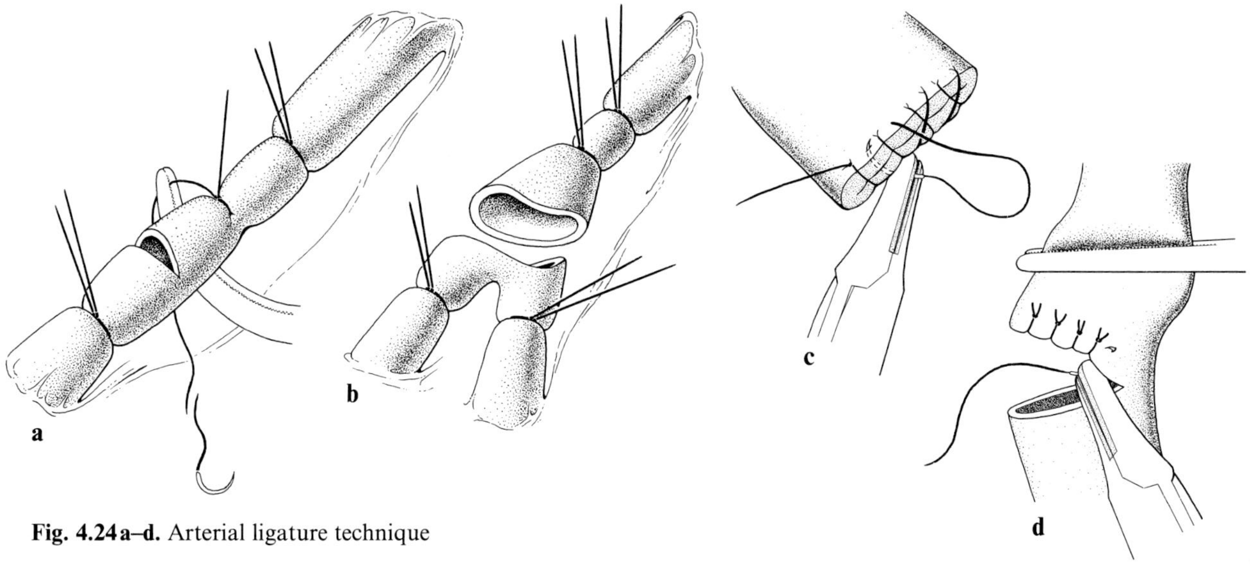

Fig. 4.24 a–d. Arterial ligature technique

When ligating a bifurcation, a small remaining bridge of the bifurcation will prevent the ligature from slipping off (Fig. 4.24b). If the lumen of the artery is wide, both ends are closed by a two-layer continuous suture (Fig. 4.24c) or by a two-layer horizontal mattress suture (see p. 338). If the stump is rather short, or if there is a danger that the clamp may slip off, this risk can be met by stepwise division and suture (Fig. 4.24d).

G. Arteriotomy

Arteriotomy may be performed longitudinally or transversely. A longitudinal arteriotomy can always be employed. The indication for a transverse incision, however, is restricted mainly to indirect embolectomies in healthy vessels. Its advantage is that it can be closed by direct suture, without a time-consuming patch graft. But it can also lead to problems: for one thing, exposure of the lumen, particularly in small vessels, is difficult; furthermore, in case of local complications, e.g., dissection of the intima or loosening of a plaque, considerable difficulties can result from the need to extend the incision for an endarterectomy or a bypass. The area of the arteriotomy itself should be free of adventitia, as it may cause difficulties for exact placement of the stitches or incisions. The arteriotomy is facilitated if the vascular segment is filled with blood.

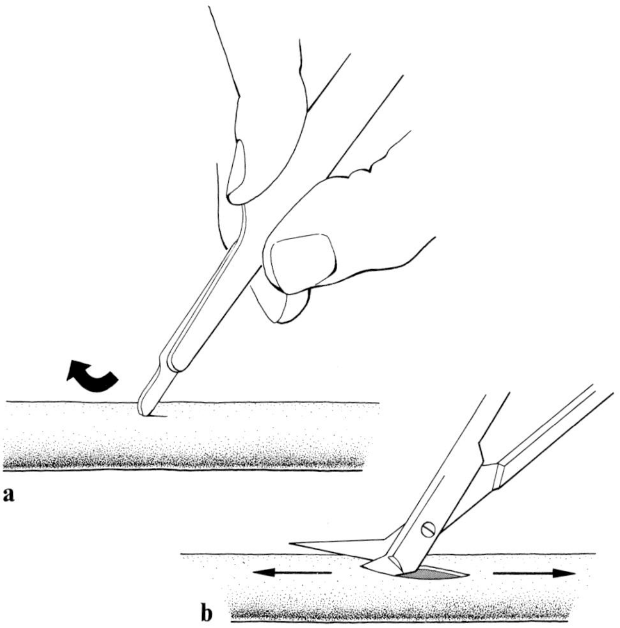

Fig. 4.25 a, b. Technique of stitch incision of the vessel by scalpel and its extension with angled vascular scissors

When the blood flow has been interrupted, the segment may be filled by transmural injection of heparinized saline solution.

The arteriotomy is initiated by an incision using a scalpel with the blade upward. The direction of the incision should be away from the surgeon (Fig. 4.25a). In this way, injury to the posterior wall of the vessel may be avoided. It is important to know that the incision should be performed at right angles through all layers to prevent dissection. The extension of the incision is made by angled scissors. The blade of the scissors inside the vessel (especially arteriosclerotic vessels) should not leave the lumen throughout the entire length of the incision in order to avoid dissection (Fig. 4.25b).

H. Suture Techniques

I. Common Suture Techniques

The basic principle of every functional intact suture should be that both vessel ends are exactly approximated in such a way that no leakage occurs and the patency of the lumen is guaranteed. This is achieved by eversion of the vessel wall with intima-to-intima approximation. The following techniques may be used:

1. The continuous over-and-over suture (Fig. 4.26a). This is the standard method and may be used for any reconstruction.
2. The interrupted suture (Fig. 4.26b). This is indicated for circular end-to-end anastomosis of smaller vessels and for arterial sutures in young patients, as it allows the anastomosis to grow. Disadvantages are possible bleeding between stitches and time-consuming knotting.
3. The interrupted horizontal mattress suture (Fig. 4.26c). Advantages are strength and absence of leakage owing to the broad intima-to-intima approximation. This suture is therefore recommended for great arteries near the heart. One disadvantage is the danger of a purse-string effect, especially in the case of a circular anastomosis of smaller vessels.
4. The continuous horizontal mattress suture (Fig. 4.26d). This has the same advantages and disadvantages as the interrupted horizontal mattress suture. If the suture line is not secure, a second anastomotic layer may be called for. The second layer will be a simple continuous suture, grasping only the everted rim of the first layer (Fig. 4.26e).
5. Noneverting, transluminal suture (Fig. 4.27). This is used mainly if the operative field is rather deep and the exposure of the posterior wall for an end-to-end or end-to-side anastomosis is difficult.

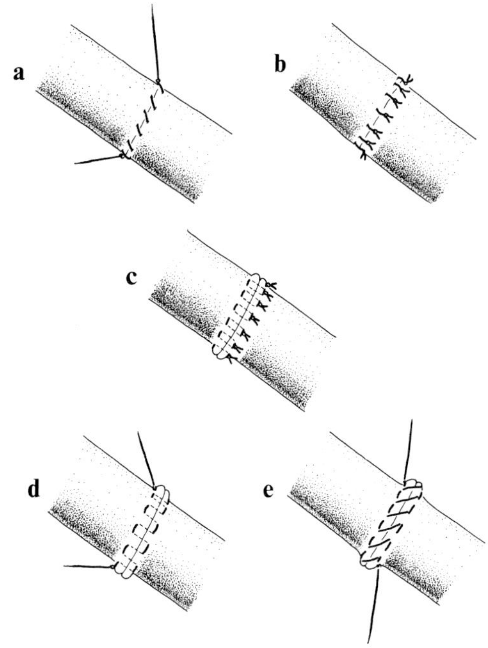

Fig. 4.26a–e. Suture techniques in vascular surgery

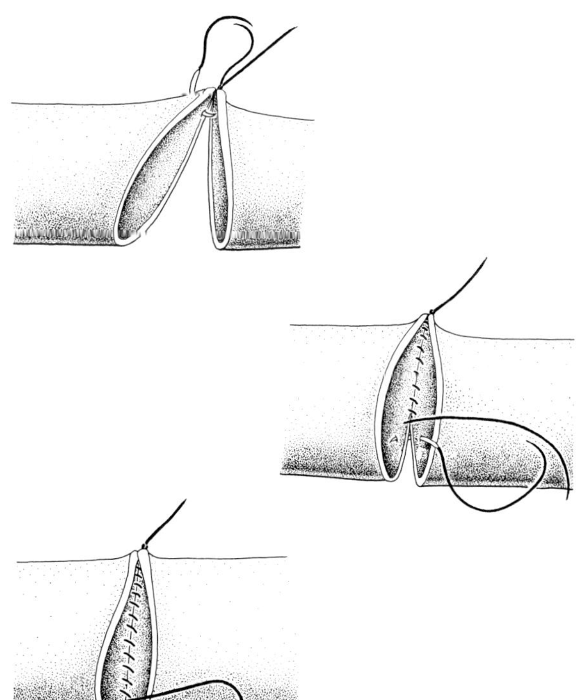

Fig. 4.27. Noneverting transluminal suture technique

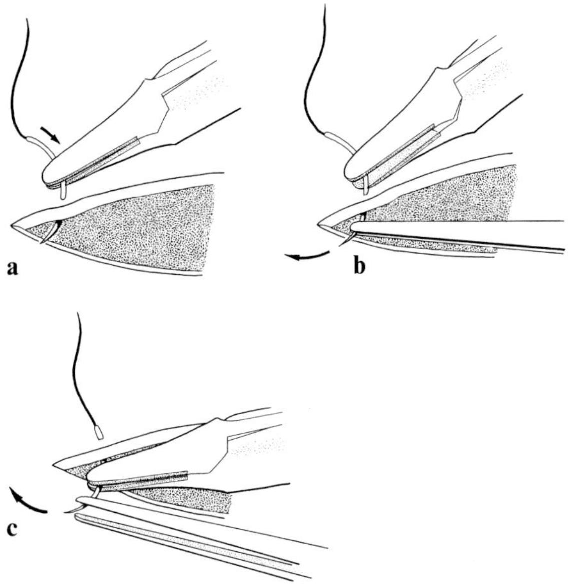

Fig. 4.28a–c. Technique for passing a suture through the vessel wall using a needle holder and forceps (**a**) the needle is grasped and partially pulled through by a forceps (**b**), and correct positioning of the needle holder for the next suture (**c**)

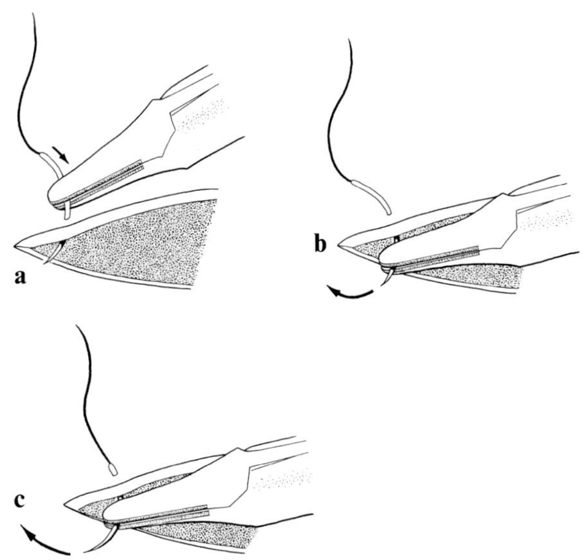

Fig. 4.29a–c. Technique for passing a suture through the vessel wall using a needle holder alone (**a**), the needle is grasped and partially pulled through by the repositioned needle holder (**b**), and correct positioning of the needle holder for the following suture (**c**)

For any vascular suture, the following technical details have to be considered, as they may decide the success or failure of a vascular reconstruction. As instruments for vascular suture, only a needle holder and a forceps should be used. Unnecessary corrections of the needle within the needle holder or grasping the needle by the finger should be avoided. The technique with needle holder and forceps is demonstrated in Fig. 4.28. The use of the needle holder by itself is shown in Fig. 4.29.

The *direction of the needle* through the vascular wall should be performed in accordance with its curvature. Any other manipulations significantly enlarge the stitch hole. An exact right-angled passage through all layers and without distortion of the needle is best performed when the tip of the needle holder is placed in the middle of the needle. Passage may be facilitated by traction on or pressing against the appropriate wall. Traction should only be applied to the adventitia (Fig. 4.30a). Grasping the whole wall may cause lesions of the endothelium, dissection of plaques, or rupture of the intima (Fig. 4.30b). Pressure against the wall should only be applied with a closed forceps against the direction of the stitch (Fig. 4.30c).

The *direction of the suture* is dependent upon the condition of the arterial wall, the reconstruction, and the suture material. The following facts should be taken into consideration: In arteriosclerotic vessels penetration from the outside into the lumen may cause dissection of plaques or intima (Fig. 4.31a).

When using autologous venous material the adventitia of the vein may be dragged into the suture hole (Fig. 4.31b). This is even more likely to result where braided suture material is used. With an eye toward this phenomenon, the following technique, adapted to local pathology, is recommended:

1. When suturing alloplastic material and artery, the direction of the suture should always be from the prosthesis toward the artery and consequently from the inside of the artery out.
2. When suturing vein and artery, the suture direction should be from the artery to the vein, which usually presents no problems following endarterectomy. If the risk of possible dissection of the intima or plaque seems too high, even when applying pressure from inside with closed forceps, then the direction of the stitch should be the reverse, from the vein to the artery. In such cases only a monofilament smooth suture should be used, so as to reduce the risk of dragging adventitial tissue into the anastomosis.

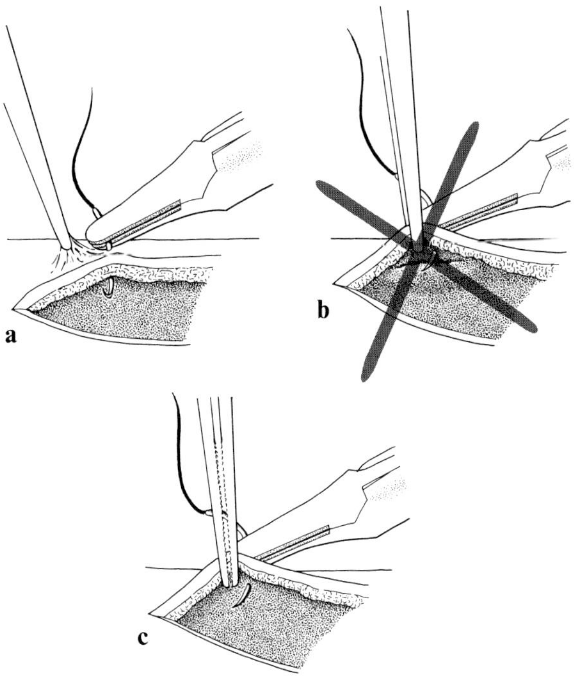

Fig. 4.30 a–c. Correct (**a**, **c**) and incorrect (**b**) ways of passing a suture through the vessel wall

The suture should not be grasped by instruments, but by the fingers, and should be kept at a right angle to the vascular wall (Fig. 4.32a). In this way, one avoids enlarging the stitch hole or even tearing the wall (Fig. 4.32b). The suture itself is kept under elastic tension. If it is too loose, bleeding between the sutures may occur. On the other hand, too much tension may cause tears or stenoses. The exact placement of the suture loop during a running suture is performed by a closed forceps (Fig. 4.33a). If a loop is placed incorrectly, it can be loosened with the back of a needle and replaced correctly again using the closed forceps (Fig. 4.33b). If the suture is grasped by a forceps, it may be damaged, leading to a break in the suture and bleeding from the anastomosis (Fig. 4.33c).

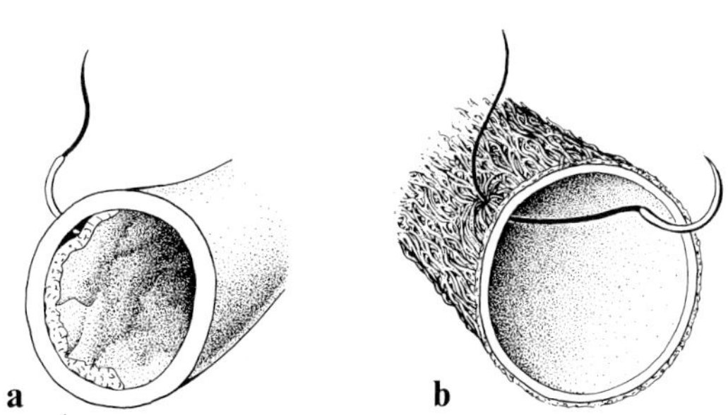

Fig. 4.31 a, b. Potential hazard to (**a**) artery and (**b**) vein placing a suture from the outside in

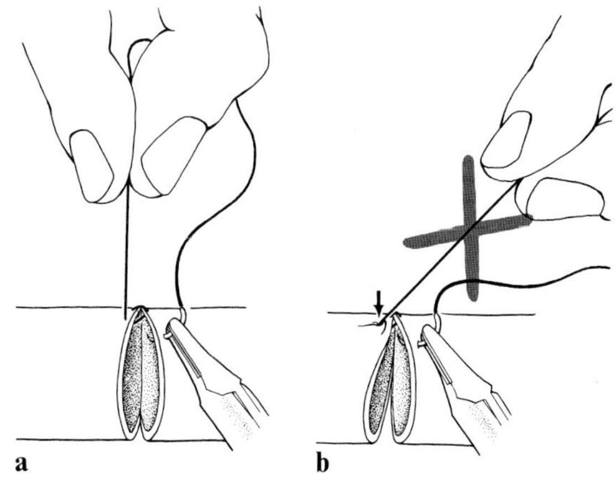

Fig. 4.32 a, b. Correct (**a**) and incorrect (**b**) direction of the suture

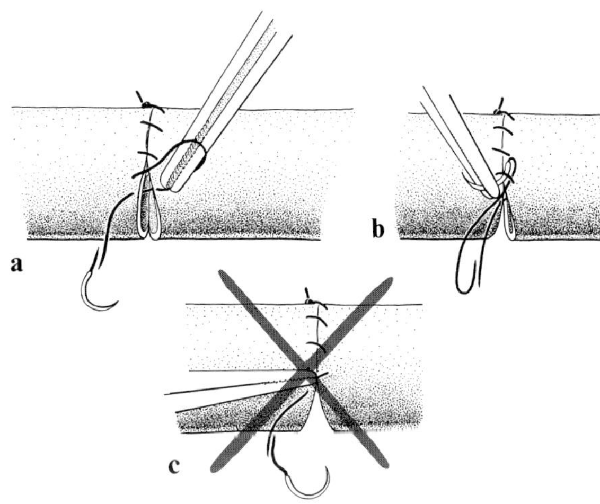

Fig. 4.33 a–c. Right and wrong technique for placement and correction of a suture loop

II. Suture Techniques Without Graft Material

The direct suture of the vessel may be used for closure of an arteriotomy; it can also be employed following tangential resection of aneurysms and for certain types of injuries, as well as for numerous anastomotic techniques. All of the different suture techniques may be applied, depending upon the size of the vessel and the local condition of the arterial wall.

1. Direct Closure of the Arteriotomy

Closure of a *transverse arteriotomy* is carried out using either a row of interrupted sutures

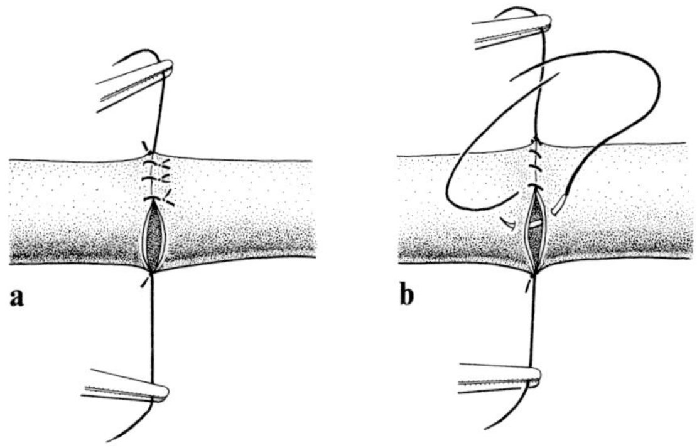

Fig. 4.34a, b. Suture techniques for closure of a transverse arteriotomy

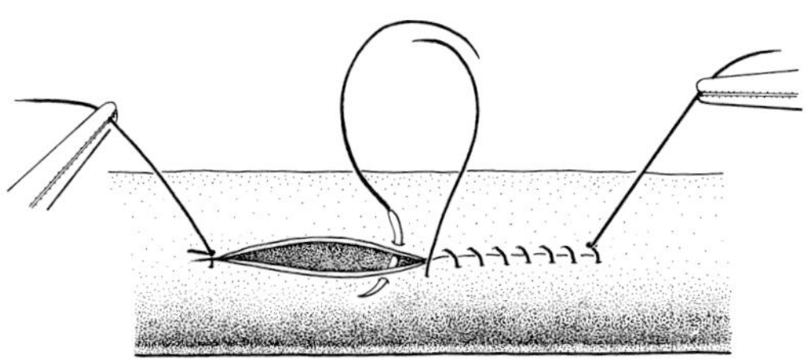

Fig. 4.35. Technique of closure of a longitudinal arteriotomy

(Fig. 4.34a) or an everting continuous suture (Fig. 4.34b). If the continuous suture is pulled too tightly, a purse-string effect, narrowing the lumen, may occur. Therefore, gentle tension should be applied to the sutures by pulling each strand of the suture in opposite directions. In order to avoid kinking at the closure, the edges should be grasped as little as possible, especially those of smaller vessels. This may often be impossible because of pathologically altered vessel walls. In this case, a transverse arteriotomy and suture of the small vessels should be avoided. Everting mattress sutures aggravate such stenoses and therefore should only be used for closure of transverse arteriotomies of great vessels close to the heart.

Direct closure of a *longitudinal arteriotomy* is usually performed with a continuous over-and-over suture. But first a suture must be placed at each corner and gentle traction should be applied (Fig. 4.35). An "hourglass constriction" created by this suture line is unavoidable, even in healthy vessels and with subtile technique. The resulting hemodynamic properties are directly related to the size of the vessel. This risk is even greater where, in the presence of arteriosclerosis or following endarterectomy, bigger "bites" of the vessel wall have to be taken, and it is not reduced significantly when the suture is performed using an olive or a temporary inlying shunt. Therefore, the closure of the arteriotomy of small and middle-sized vessels should usually be done using a patch graft (see p. 62). In view of its disadvantages, a direct suture should be used only if there is a high risk of infection, a necessarily short operation time, or the likelihood of impaired healing of the graft.

2. Direct Anastomotic Techniques

a) *End-to-end Anastomosis.* A direct end-to-end anastomosis is indicated for traumatic or complete iatrogenic vascular transsection, resections of a short stenosis or of elongated vessels, and possibly for some types of dialysis shunts. The end-to-end anastomosis of large arteries is done using a circumferential suture. The two ends are cut transversely (Fig. 4.36a). The anastomosis of small or middle-sized vessels should be S-shaped (Fig. 4.36b) to achieve a larger diameter and to avoid a stenosis.

The diameter of the anastomosis will be the greater the more obliquely the vessel is cut and the suture placed. If the lumina of the segments are not equal, adaptation may be achieved by beveling the segments differently, by leaving larger intervals between sutures on the larger vessel (Fig. 4.36c), or by making a wedge-shaped incision at the end of the smaller segment (Fig. 4.36d).

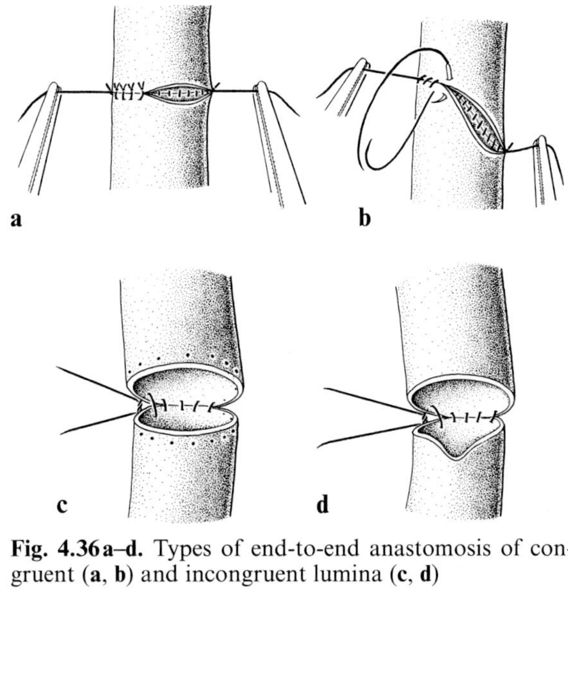

Fig. 4.36a–d. Types of end-to-end anastomosis of congruent (**a**, **b**) and incongruent lumina (**c**, **d**)

Interrupted, continuous, or mattress sutures are the common techniques for anastomosis. In accordance with the principles of direct vascular suture, interrupted sutures should be used in small vessels and running sutures only in greater vessels. Where interrupted sutures are used, pressure may cause the anastomosis to dilate. However, the diameter of an anastomosis completed using a running suture is related to the length of the suture. When both vascular segments are mobile, the anastomotic technique is the so-called rotation method. Using the method of "suture rotation", two tied corner sutures are inserted at corresponding sites on the circumference. When a circumferential anastomosis is performed and both ends are sufficiently mobile, these two corner sutures should be placed on the lateral side of the circumference. When the anastomosis is oblique or following wedge-shaped incision, the corner sutures are usually placed in the middle of the anterior and posterior wall. Rotating the vessel ends by turning the corner sutures through 180° or 90°, respectively, rotates the posterior wall of the artery around to the front, thereby affording optimal direct vision for either continuous or interrupted sutures (Fig. 4.37). When the posterior wall has been sutured, the stays are released, and the vessel rotates back to its normal position. The anterior wall is then sutured.

When it is not possible to move the vessel ends because they may be torn, the vessel end can be rotated in either direction, using clamps ("clamp rotation"). In this way, the posterior wall can be brought around to the front one half at a time and thus sutured in two stages (Fig. 4.38).

If the two segments to be anastomosed are not mobile, suture of the posterior wall can be done by means of a noneverting, transluminal suture (see p. 57). Alternatively, the suture at a distance (Fig. 4.39), with a continous over-and-over suture for small vessels and a horizontal mattress suture for larger vessels, may be used. For this type of technique an optimally gliding monofilament suture should always be chosen. When the suture is tied later, the two segments should be brought together by approximating the clamps.

b) *End-to-side Anastomosis.* The end-to-side or side-to-end anastomosis is seldom done by direct suturing. Typical indications are reinsertions of branches, portosystemic anastomoses, and sometimes dialysis shunts. The advantage of this technique is that luminal incongruities are not impor-

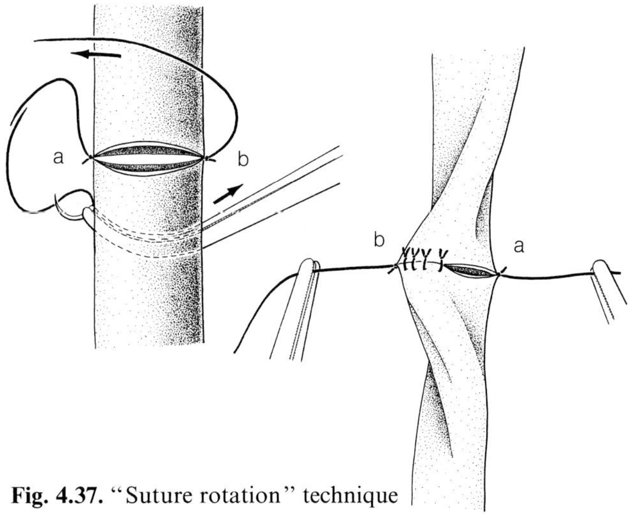

Fig. 4.37. "Suture rotation" technique

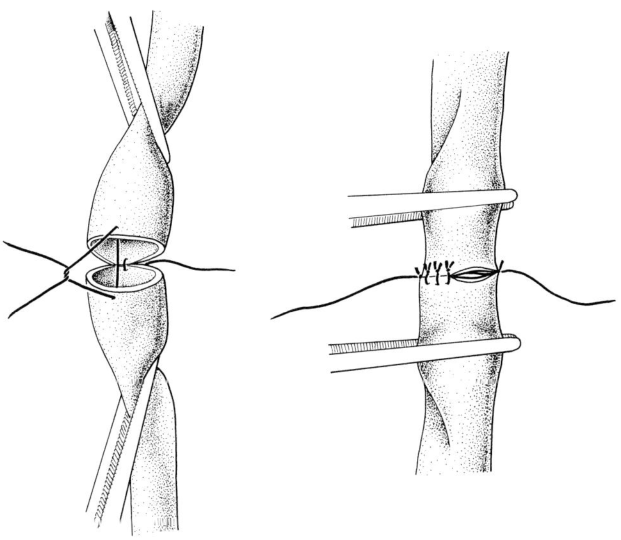

Fig. 4.38. "Clamp rotation" technique

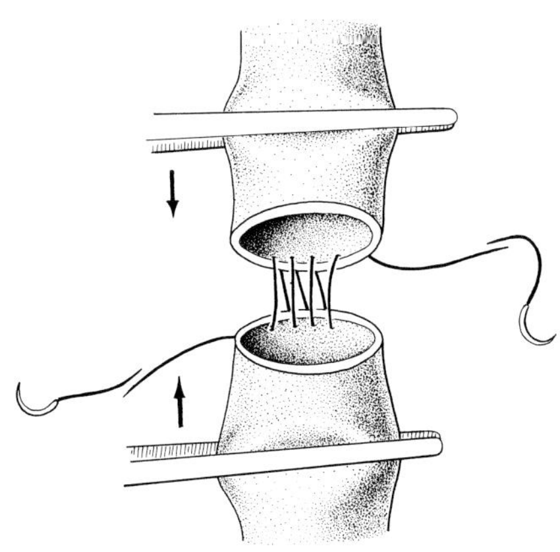

Fig. 4.39. Technique of "suture at a distance"

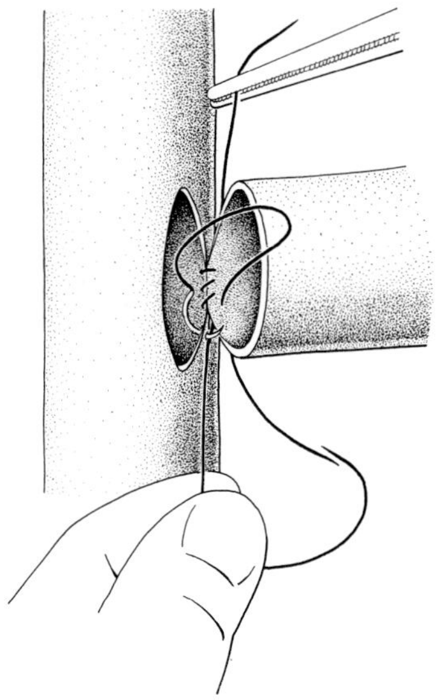

◁ **Fig. 4.40.** Technique of end-to-side anastomosis with everting continuous over-and-over suture of the posterior wall

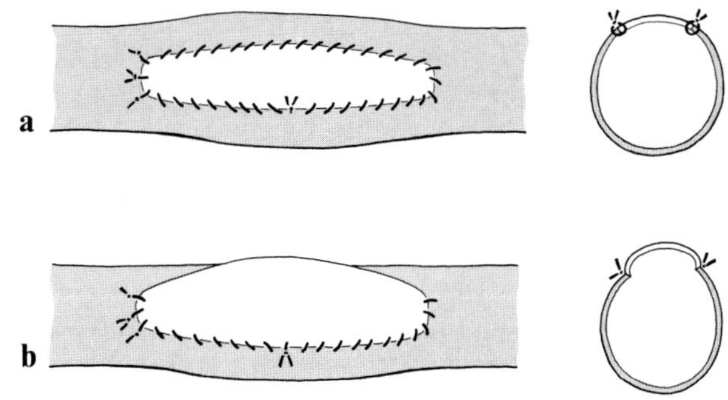

Fig. 4.41 a, b. Correct (**a**) and incorrect (**b**) patch width

tant, and the diameter of the anastomosis can be varied by beveling the end of the segment to be implanted. The anastomosis is usually performed using a continuous suture. The suture row begins with either a double-threaded suture or two separate ones in the middle of the posterior wall and continues, by means of everting sutures, around to the front, where it is tied in the middle of the anterior wall. The suture should be kept under tension and parallel to the longitudinal axis of the main artery. This allows exact placement of the suture and eversion of the posterior wall (Fig. 4.40). If the operative field is deep and the approach difficult, then the so-called "suture at a distance" or the "noneverting transluminal suture" may be used.

c) *Side-to-side Anastomosis.* The only indications for this anastomosis as a direct suture are portosystemic anastomoses or dialysis shunts. The technique is not different from the end-to-side anastomosis. This means that if there is good exposure, the everting continuous suture is performed. If the operative approach is difficult, the "suture at a distance" or the "noneverting transluminal suture" should be employed.

III. Suture Techniques with Graft Material

1. Closure of Arteriotomy with Patch Angioplasty

The aim of closing an arteriotomy by patch angioplasty is to avoid stenosis of a longitudinal incision by enlarging the lumen. A direct longitudinal suture may create a stenosis, especially in small vessels with pathologic changes. In such cases, therefore, a patch graft should always be employed. The patch will compensate for shrinking of the lumen as a result of excessive healing processes following thromboendarterectomy.

Where the vessel is already stenosed, a direct enlargement of the stenosis is effected by the patch. The patch can consist of: alloplastic material, an already obliterated vessel segment secondarily reopened by thromboendarterectomy (obliterated superficial femoral artery), an arterial segment replaceable by a graft (external iliac artery), autologous vein. The patch has to be of such a size that the artery will regain its original diameter or become slightly greater (Fig. 4.41 a) following release of the clamps. If the patch is too small, the same disadvantages will be encountered as after a direct suture. If it is too wide, there will be an nonphysiological bulging, causing turbulence, thrombus formation, and the risk of an aneurysm (Fig. 4.41 b). The shape of the patch should be longitudinal – oval with the ends either bluntly rounded (Fig. 4.42a) or angled (Fig. 4.42b). If the end of the patch is pointed, the purse-string effect may

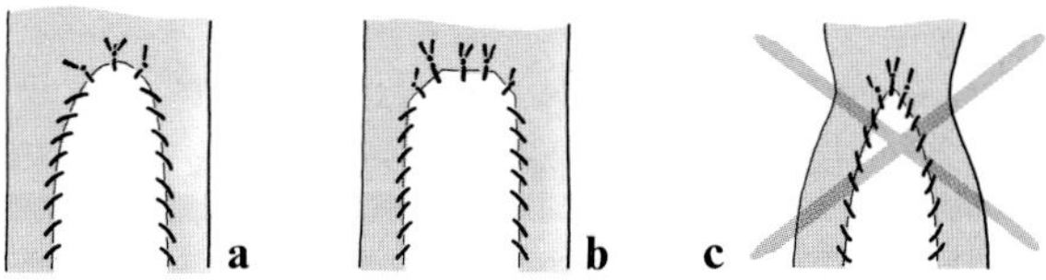

Fig. 4.42 a–c. Correct (**a**, **b**) and incorrect (**c**) preparation of the end of the patch

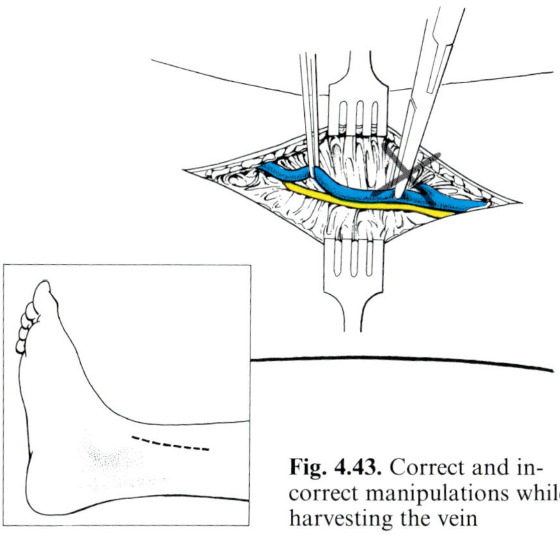

Fig. 4.43. Correct and incorrect manipulations while harvesting the vein

cause constriction of the vessel (Fig. 4.42c). A patch with four right angles is usually not satisfactory.

a) *Harvest and Preparation of Autogenous Vein Graft.* The graft of choice is the greater saphenous vein. But it should be obtained from the distal segment, above the inner malleolus, (Fig. 4.43a) rather than from the femoral site. The latter segment of the vein should be saved for other purposes. Caution is in order, however, where significant arterial occlusive disease of the leg is present which might impair proper healing of the surgical wound at the distal harvest site. In such cases it may be possible to use a proximal tributary of the greater saphenous vein, the smaller saphenous vein, or the cephalic vein.

The harvesting of a segment of the greater saphenous vein should be performed as atraumatically as possible. One should be especially careful not to harm the endothelium. After exposure of the vein, a dissecting clamp is passed under it, thus allowing placement of a "vessel loop." During the following sharp dissection of the surrounding tissue, the venous segment is moved only by means of this loop and must not be grasped by forceps or clamps (Fig. 4.43b), as this would cause fractures of the endothelium – the most common site of thrombus formation – and might also cause late stenosis as a result of fibrotic shrinking.

After harvest of the venous segment, which should be somewhat longer than the arteriotomy, a round-tipped cannula is introduced in the distal end and the vein flushed with heparinized blood. Next, the segment is carefully dilated; this overcomes the spasm of the venous wall that usually occurs and also identifies open tributaries, which are either ligated or excised when the vein is cut longitudinally. A surplus of periadventitial tissue is removed when the vessel is filled. Following longitudinal incision and any necessary resection of valves, the patch is trimmed to the appropriate width, but for the time being only one end is tailored (see p. 62).

b) *Technique of Patch Graft Angioplasty.* A patch graft angioplasty begins with fixation of the patch using two or three interrupted sutures at the most critical point, usually the distal corner of the arteriotomy. The other end of the patch, which is at first excessively long and will later be cut away and disposed of, is held by means of a hemostat. This keeps the patch under gentle traction and allows it to be moved without damaging the endothelium by forceps (Fig. 4.44a). Then the patch is fixed by continuous suture beginning on the side opposite the surgeon and continuing almost to the proximal corner of the anastomosis. The proximal end of the patch is then cut and the surplus material and the clamp removed (Fig. 4.44b). The con-

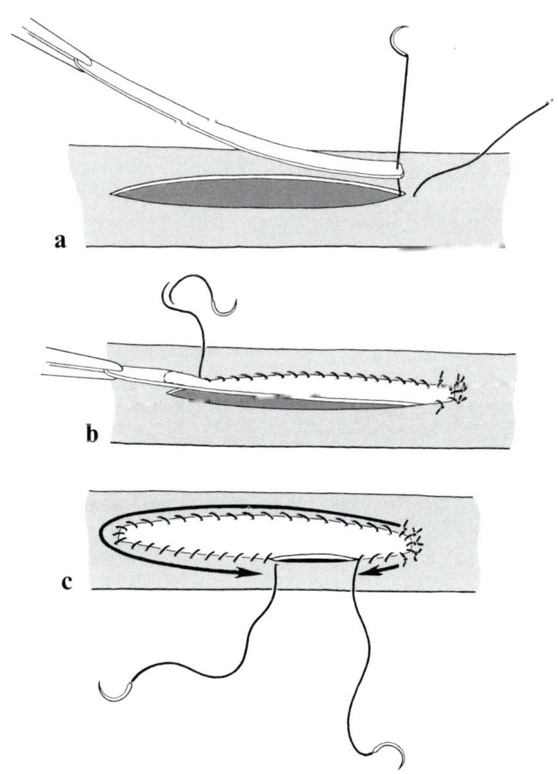

Fig. 4.44a–c. Venous patch graft technique

tinuous suture is brought around the proximal corner to the middle of the arteriotomy on the surgeon's side. A second continuous suture starts from the distal corner and completes the patch graft (Fig. 4.44c). Before placing the last stitches, the remaining gap allows control, and eventual dilation of the end of the patch or the corner of the arteriotomy by instruments. Furthermore, the area of run-in and run-off can be checked and cleaned by flushing.

2. Anastomotic Techniques with Graft Material

a) *End-to-end Anastomoses.* Graft material is typically used for bypass operations with proximal or distal exclusion and graft interpositions. They can be performed using the direct anastomotic techniques detailed earlier (see p. 60) and also by employing the following technical modifications:

1. Partially circumferential anastomosis with a dilatation patch in the anterior wall. The major artery to be anastomosed and an appropriate prepared transplant are incised longitudinally in the middle of the anterior wall for about 1.5–2 cm.

The opposing corners are approximated by interrupted sutures (Fig. 4.45a). If there is a great difference between the diameters of the two vessels, an appropriate wedge-shaped resection is performed on the vessel with the larger diameter

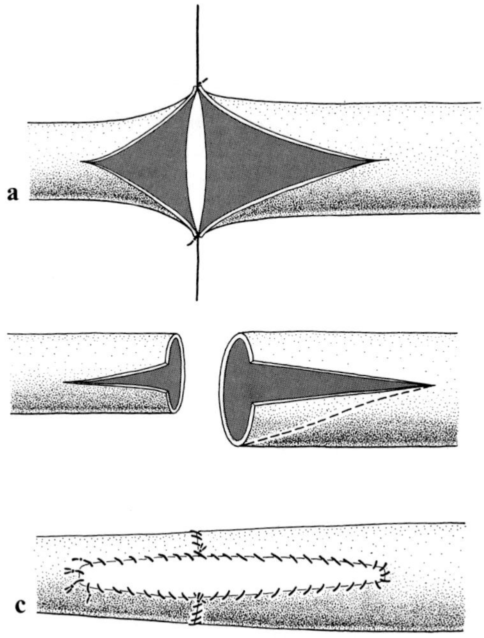

Fig. 4.45a–c. Technique of partially circumferential end-to-end anastomosis with patch graft of the anterior wall

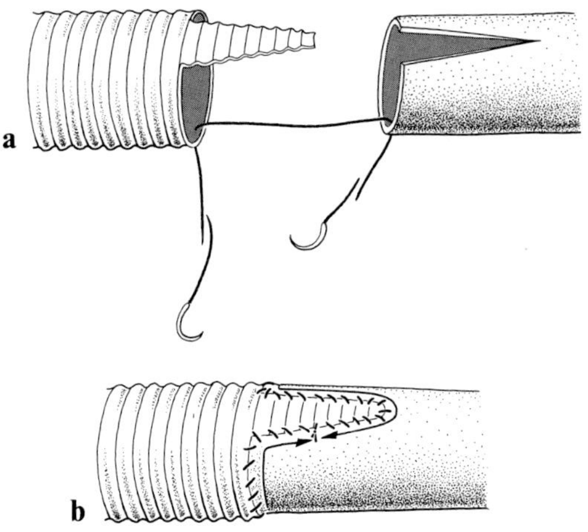

Fig. 4.46a, b. Technique of a partially circumferential end-to-end anastomosis with wedge-shaped patch graft of the anterior wall

(Fig. 4.45b). After rotating both vessels according to the method earlier described (see p. 61), the posterior wall of greater vessels is anastomosed by a running suture, that of small and middle-sized vessels by interrupted sutures. The vessels are then rotated back, and the anastomosis of the anterior wall is completed by the patch graft (Fig. 4.45c). When the diameters of the lumina are different, the patch should be tapered, resulting in a smooth funnel-shaped anastomotic area.

2. The partially circumferential anastomosis with a wedge-shaped patch graft in the anterior wall. This form is used for end-to-end anastomoses of prostheses to smaller arteries. A longitudinal incision about 1.5–2 cm long is made in the anterior wall of the arterial stump. The opposing end of the prosthesis is trimmed to create a wedge configuration (Fig. 4.46a). The size of the wedge depends on the luminal discrepancy. The row of sutures begins with two interrupted sutures or one double-armed suture in the middle of the posterior wall and runs around the anastomosis, as indicated in Fig. 4.46b. If the prosthesis is mobile, the posterior wall is sutured, drawing the transplant up. If the prosthesis is already fixed, the anastomosis is performed using corner sutures or clamp rotation. An end-to-end anastomosis of grafts to large arteries (for instance infrarenal aorta) may be secured additionally by a sheath of graft material (Fig. 4.47). This sheath favors hemostasis at the anastomosis and prevents bulging of the aorta due to the pulsating blood flow with possible secondary development of an anastomotic aneurysm.

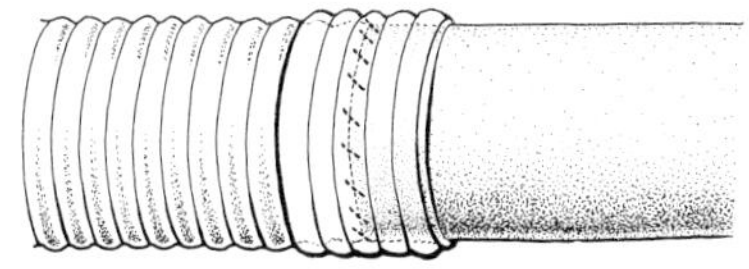

Fig. 4.47. Securing an end-to-end anastomosis by a sheath of prosthetic material

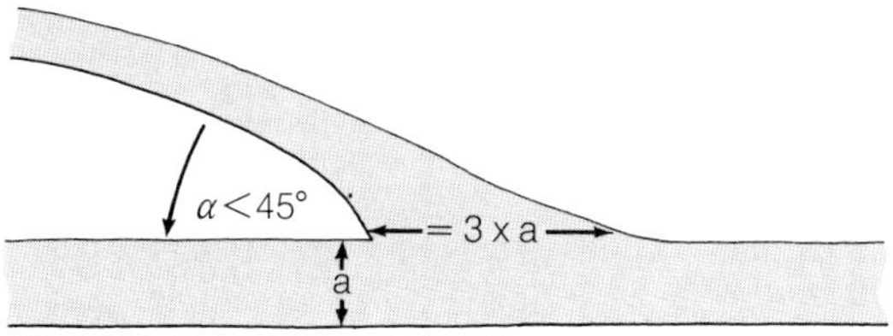

Fig. 4.48. Parameters for hemodynamiclly favorable end-to-side anastomosis

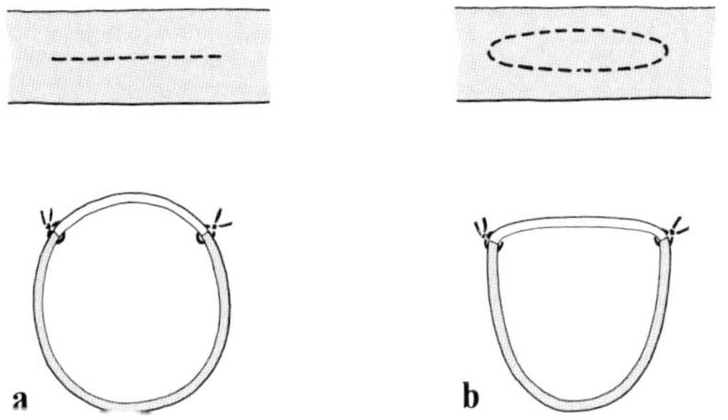

Fig. 4.49 a, b. Correct (**a**) and incorrect (**b**) preparation at the site of graft insertion

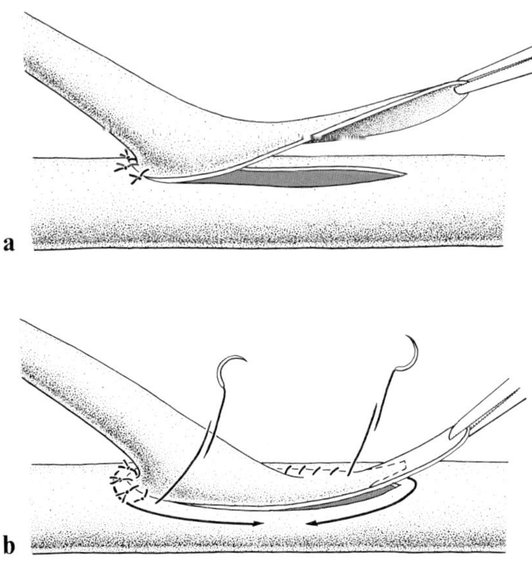

Fig. 4.50 a, b. Technique of end-to-side anastomosis

b) *End-to-side Anastomosis.* Today, the end-to-side anastomosis is the most frequently used reconstruction method in vascular surgery, owing to the increasing use of grafts for bypass procedures. The advantage is that luminal discrepancies do not pose a problem and the cross-section of the anastomosis can be selected optimally by appropriate beveling of the graft end. Blood-flow properties at an anastomosis bypassing larger vessels are better the more acute the angle of entry in relation to the run-off segment. The angle of entry should never be greater than 45°. It is determined by the length of the incision anastomosed to the graft. This incision should be at least three times the diameter of the segment of the recipient artery. The incision should be longer, especially in smaller arteries, to achieve a cone-shaped anastomosis and, consequently, favorable hemodynamics (Fig. 4.48).

An oval excision of the recipient artery makes no sense, because it diminishes the enlarging effect achieved by the graft (Fig. 4.49). The suture begins at the most critical point of the anastomosis, at the "heel", with two or three interrupted sutures (Fig. 4.50 a). The suture continues to the end of the arteriotomy on the side away from the surgeon. The end of the transplant is then cut and the suture continued around to the middle of the anastomosis on the surgeon's side. A second continuous suture completes the anastomosis (Fig. 4.50 b). If the end of the graft is too pointed, or if too much of the arterial wall is grasped, or if the suture is pulled too tight, constriction of the vessel at the end of the graft may occur (Fig. 4.51 a). These hemodynamically adverse effects can be avoided by appropriate preparation of the graft and by the use of interrupted sutures instead of a running suture at this critical point (Fig. 4.51 b).

The second drawback to such beveled end-to-side anastomoses is a possible constricting of the graft at the angle of the entry or exit, caused by the suture line (Fig. 4.51 a). Often simple dissection of the strangulating adventitia is sufficient to free the stenosis. Otherwise, a patch angioplasty has to be performed (Fig. 4.51 b).

When using a vein graft, the diameter of the graft may be extended at this critical point by creating a small "collar" out of a tributary (Fig. 4.52).

When anastomosing a bypass to major branches (organ arteries), the technique is essentially the same as described under the direct suture

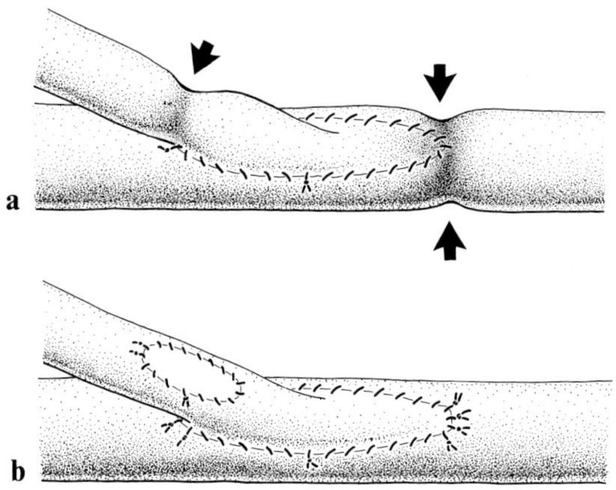

Fig. 4.51 a, b. Stenosis of the anastomosis by constriction of the artery or the graft (**a**) and prophylaxis or correction by correct preparation of the graft or by a patch plasty (**b**), respectively

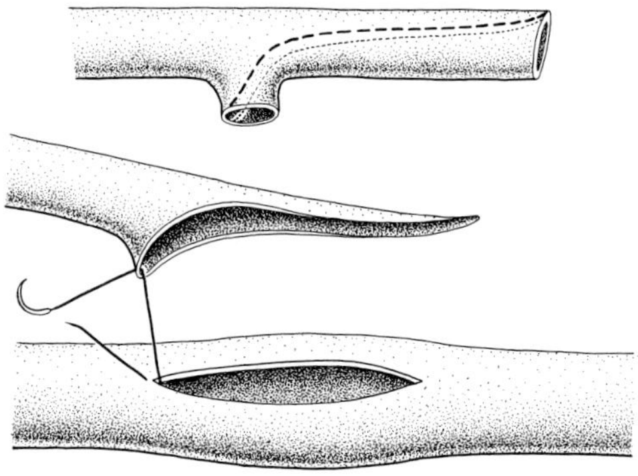

Fig. 4.52. Technique of extending the orifice of a graft by creating a "collar" out of a tributary ("boot-shaped anastomosis")

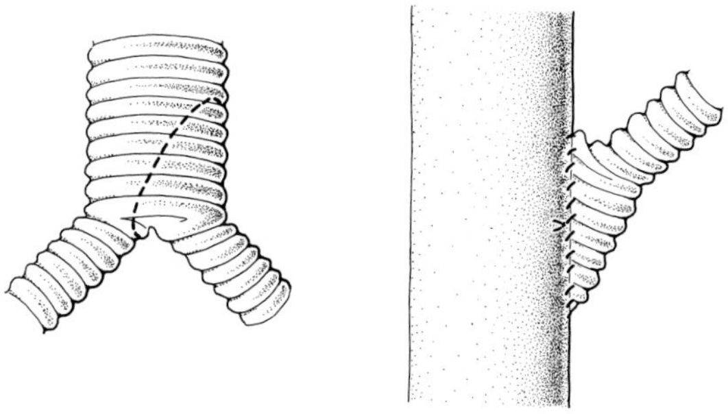

Fig. 4.53. Extension of the graft orifice with a small bifurcation prosthesis

Fig. 4.54a–g. Technique of extension of the orifice by means of various vein configurations (**a–d**), by excision of the greater saphenous vein providing a collar of femoral vein (**e**), or by a partially circumferential anastomosis using a patch graft (**f, g**)

▽

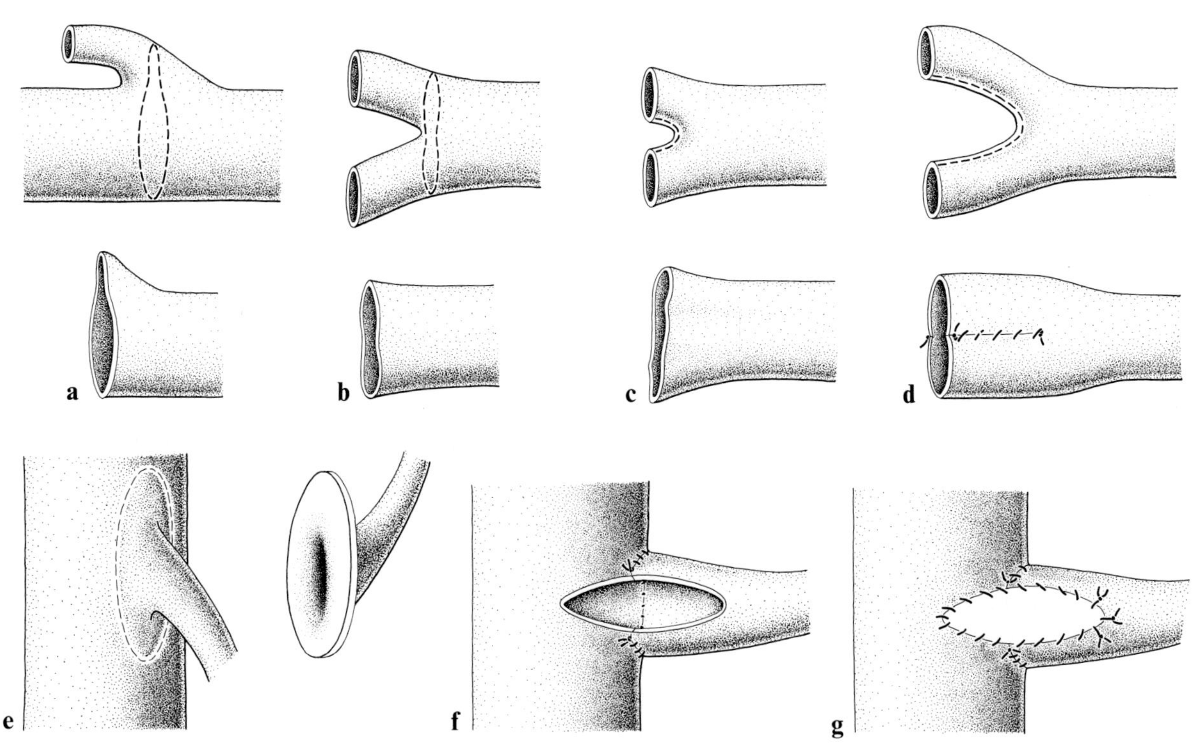

techniques (see p. 60). The suture of the posterior wall is usually even easier because of the mobility of the graft. From the perspective of hemodynamics the disadvantage of this type of reconstruction is the right-angle exit of the graft from the artery; it is usually unavoidable and causes a sudden change of direction in the blood flow. Maximizing the diameter of the anastomosis may diminish this negative effect.

The orifice of the graft may be extended by appropriate tailoring of a bifurcation prosthesis (Fig. 4.53). Figure 4.54 illustrates ways of extending vein graft orifices by making use of variations in vein anatomy.

c) *Side-to-side Anastomoses*. Side-to-side anastomoses with grafts are only indicated under certain circumstances, e.g., double bridging grafts for reconstructions of both renal and/or visceral arteries or for long aorto- or iliopopliteal bypasses with simultaneous revascularization of the hypogastric artery or profunda femoris artery by means of a side-to-side anastomosis. The technique used is essentially the same as the direct suture techniques.

I. Tissue Glues in Vascular Surgery

Tissue glues have been used experimentally and clinically in vascular surgery since early in the 1960s. A tissue glue must fulfill numerous requirements. Important characteristics are: sterilizability, storage stability, ease of handling, rapid hardening, and low heat production during polymerization. In regard to long-term effects, there should be a sufficient adhesive capacity and durability combined with complete absorption. There should be no toxicity, no major local reaction, and above all no carcinogenesis. Three types of tissue glues have been developed which fulfill the requirements in varying degrees and have been used clinically in vascular surgery.

1. Polymerizing Cyanoacrylic Acid Ester [6, 8,10, 12, 13, 22]

First synthesized in 1949, the extraordinary adhesive capacity of this compound was discovered only by chance 10 years later [6]. Structurally speaking, it is an alkyl ester of 2-cyanoacrylic acid. The substance comes in plastic ampules in a watery monomer form. It polymerizes to become a hard substance, most rapidly in the presence of anions, especially hydroxyl ions, and also in the presence of water or tissue fluid. The polymerization time may be altered and regulated by the addition of inhibitors. Thin layers of glue are completely absorbed within a short time. The absorption of massive deposits, however, may take a long time. Cyanoacrylic acid esters were of experimental and, sporadically, also of clinical significance for the performance of microvascular anastomoses until the beginning of the 1970s. The technique was very difficult and did not always allow a sufficiently rapid approximation of the vascular segments. Numerous instruments served to facilitate the manipulations; however, tissue glues never became fully established. There were experiments with outer splints of Dacron patches coated with glue, slit polyethylene tubes and adhesive rings, inner splints using polyethylene tubes and soluble hollow cylinders, and finally various gluing devices.

2. Gelatin – Resorcin – Formaldehyde [3, 27]

This glue, consisting of a mixture of gelatin, resorcinol, and formaldehyde was developed in 1965 [3]. The condensation of resorcinol and formaldehyde forms a matrix for the gelatin, resulting in tight adhesions. A final verdict on this glue cannot be given because of too little experience.

3. Fibrin Glue [1, 11, 16, 17, 20, 29]

This substance currently has the greatest clinical importance. Fibrin glue was first used in 1972 [20]. It consists of a biologic double-component glue, one component being highly purified, highly concentrated human fibrinogen and the second component being a solution of aprotinin – CaCl – thrombin. The gluing process completes the end phase of the coagulation. The effective principle is the coagulation of fibrinogen by thrombin at the tissue surface. This process is enhanced by CaCl. The high content of factor XIII induces optimal crosslinking and stability of the fibrin produced and guarantees appropriate mechanical stability and adhesive power of the fibrin meshwork. Fibrinolytic processes will be blocked by the addition of the inhibitor aprotinin.

Areas of indication for the use of fibrin glues include:

a) *Sealing of Fabric Prostheses*. Sealing may become necessary as an emergency measure following release of the clamps if there is rebleeding from an adequately preclotted prosthesis owing to the so-called "defibrination syndrome," to local fibrinolysis, or to manufacturing defects. As a primary prophylactic sealant for non-preclotted prosthesis, fibrin glue may be used in cases involving extracorporeal circulation and also in cases of blood loss resulting from coagulation defects, e.g., following perforation of an aortic aneurysm, or from other causes. This primary sealing allows the use of biologically superior, porous prostheses in areas where usually only prostheses of greater density are used because of the expected blood loss (aortic arch, thoracic aorta).

Advantages are: reduced blood loss, especially where transfusion blood is in short supply; reduced risk of rebleeding; shorter operation time, especially in patients at risk; and shorter clamping time. The technique is to apply both glue components to the prosthesis continuously, one after the other, and to rub them in with the prosthesis straightened. Afterward, the prosthesis is flushed with saline solution, thereby eliminating the increased thrombogenicity of its inner surface. The cost of fibrin glue is about half that of the prosthesis itself.

b) *Local Control of Hemorrhage*. Local control of hemorrhage by fibrin glues may be used for bleeding from suture holes or from the anastomosis, especially when the bleeding site is either difficult to expose for surgical suture or not suitable for suture owing to fragility of the vessel wall. The glue is not placed directly onto the bleeding site, but a carrier such as collagen fleece or collagen fascia is used. The drier the site of application, the more effective sealing is. One must avoid contact with the intima; otherwise local thromboembolic complications are likely to occur.

c) *Microvascular Anastomosis*. Fibrin glue may be used either as an adjuvant for the suture in a combined suture – glue technique or as a complete suture replacement in a sutureless microvascular anastomosis.

These techniques are still quite difficult; once they are perfected, however, one can expect the following beneficial results: a simplification of anastomotic technique; a shortening of operating and clamping time; improvement of implanted suture material; and avoidance of cicatricial stenosis.

d) *Graft Fixation*. This is indicated when the length of the graft has been incorrectly calculated owing to changes in organ position during graft implantation, with resultant kinking of the prosthesis. Thus, for example, fixation at an appropriate site may prevent kinking of an aortocoronary bypass.

Besides their significant costs, fibrin glues also involve certain risks. The risk of transmitting hepatitis cannot yet be excluded, despite the fact that donor selection and supervision insure a high level of safety for the currently available operations. Incidental penetration of the glue into the vascular lumen causes lesions of the endothelium and local thromboembolic complications. Doubts still remain regarding healing and other long-term effects of the glued graft.

In summary, tissue glues are of value and are in some cases vital aids to vascular surgery. The techniques of gluing, however, have not yet been perfected, and therefore one cannot completely delineate their possibilities.

K. Vascular Staplers

[2, 5, 9, 14, 15, 18, 21, 23, 25, 26]

The purpose of vascular staplers is to simplify and speed up a technically very difficult and time-consuming hand anastomosis, especially where smaller vessels are involved.

The first experiments with sutureless vascular anastomosis were carried out by PAYR [23]. His method of end-to-end anastomosis of vessels was to pull one end of the vessel through a ring or cylinder of absorbable magnesium and to evert it. The other end of the vessel was pulled over it, providing broad contact of both intima surfaces. Both vessel segments were fixed by sutures tied to the prosthesis. The unavoidable step effect produced at the anastomosis was compensated for by continuing proliferation of the intima.

The method of Payr was subsequently modified in many ways, especially in the mid-1950s, using other materials (vitallium, tantalum, silastic, Teflon, fibrin) and removable slit-ring prostheses [25]. Despite the improvements brought about using this method, sutureless vascular anastomoses are still in the experimental stage and so far have not been used clinically because of the high local complication rate (thrombosis, cicatricial stenosis, arrosion).

The first vascular stapler was developed by a group of Russian engineers and physicists between

1945 and 1950. ANDROSOV [2] experimentally and clinically tested vascular staplers in vascular traumatology. The stapler was developed especially for the anastomosis of smaller vessels with a diameter down to 1.5 mm. The operative principle is that the ends of the two vessels are freed of surrounding tissue, grasped by a holder, and everted. With the aid of the holder, the everted vascular stumps are then precisely adapted to one another and then joined together by a ring of U-shaped staples of tantalum. Technically simplified and improved versions of the Russian model have been developed in America and Japan, but these improved versions, like the basic Russian prototype, have failed to achieve clinical significance [5, 14, 15, 18, 26].

A somewhat different basic concept is embodied in Nakayama's model, which is considerably easier to handle. With this stapler, too, eversion of both vessel stumps is necessary. Each stump is pulled through a tantalum ring equipped with six ultra-fine spikes and holes. Then the rings are pressed together and secured with special clamps. The spikes of the one ring are automatically pressed into the holes of the opposite ring and fixed by turning them back (Fig. 4.55). If these fine spikes have been previously distorted, the anastomosis fails. The rings remain in situ and lie loose within the tissue after approximately 1 month.

On the whole, there has been relatively little interest in vascular stapling devices since their development. Except for certain special indications in the traumatology of small vessels, their use is restricted to the experimental laboratory. The development of modern microsurgery is chiefly responsible for this. Another limiting factor is the complicated handling and time-consuming servicing of vascular staplers and the local difficulties in cases of deep, limited operative approach. Finally, the necessary eversion of the vessel wall precludes the use of vascular staplers for reconstructive surgery in arteriosclerosis, because in an arteriosclerotic vessel eversion is either impossible or would be likely to cause lesions of the intima.

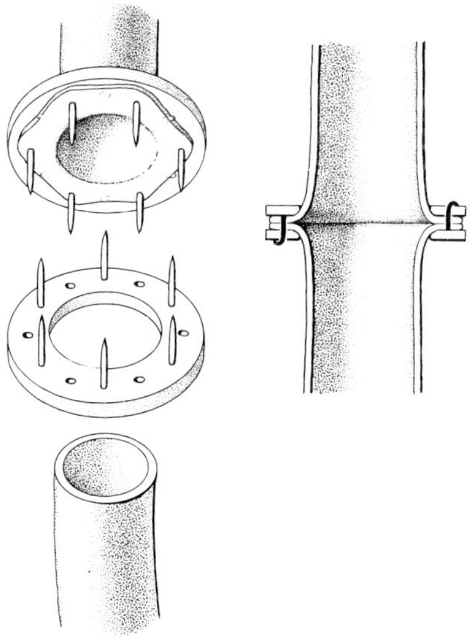

Fig. 4.55. Basic concept of the stapler model of Nakayama

REFERENCES

1. Akrami R, Kalmar P, Pokar H, Tilsner V (1978) Abdichtung von Kunststoffprothesen beim Ersatz der Aorta im thorakalen Bereich. Thoraxchirurgie 26:144
2. Androsov PI (1956) New method of surgical treatment of blood vessel lesions. Arch Surg 73:902
3. Braunwald NS, Gay W, Tatooles CJ (1966) Evaluation of cross linked gelatin as a tissue adhesive and hemostatic agent. Surgery 59:1024
4. Cooley DA, Wukasch DC (1980) Gefäßchirurgie – Indikation und Technik. Schattauer, Stuttgart
5. Cooper P, Christie SG (1963) Development of the surgical stapler with emphasis on vascular anastomosis Trans NY Acad Sci 25:365
6. Coover HW, Joyner FB, Shearer NH, Wicker TH (1959) Chemistry and performance of cyanoacrylate adhesives. J Soc Plast Eng 15:413
7. van Dongen RJAM (1970) Photographic atlas of reconstructive arterial surgery. Stenfert Kroese NV, Leiden
8. Gottlob R, Blümel G (1965) Gefäßanastomosen mit klebenden Ringen. Langenbecks Arch Klin Chir 313:708
9. Gudov VF (1950) Technique in mechanical application of vascular suture. Khirurgia 12:58
10. Hafner CD, Fogarty TJ, Cranley JJ (1963) Nonsuture anastomosis of small arteries using a tissue adhesive. Surg Gynecol Obstet 116:1
11. Haverich A, Walterbusch G, Borst HG (1983) Abdichtung poröser Gefäßprothesen unter Teil-Heparinisierung und extrakorporaler Zirkulation. Angio 5:215
12. Healey JE Jr, Moore EB, Brooks BF, Sheena KS (1962) A vascular clamp for circumferential repair of blood vessels. Surgery 51:452
13. Heiss WH (1968) Gewebeklebstoff – Applikationen, Eigenschaften und Anwendungsmöglichkeiten. Med Mitt 42:11
14. Holt GP, Lewis FJ (1961) A new technique for end-to-end-anastomosis of small arteries. S Forum 11:242
15. Indokuchi K (1958) A new type of vessel-suturing apparatus. Arch Surg 77:954

16. Kletter G, Matras H, Dinges HP (1978) Zur partiellen Klebung von Mikrogefäßanastomosen im intracraniellen Bereich. Wien Klin Wochenschr 90:1
17. Köveker G (1982) Clinical application of fibrin glue in cardiovascular surgery. Thorac Cardiovasc Surg 30:228
18. Levy MJ, Gifford PJ, Lillehei CW (1965) Stapler for cardiovascular surgery. J Cardiovasc Surg (Torino) 6:547
19. Linton RR (1973) Atlas of vascular surgery. Saunders, Philadelphia
20. Matras H, Dinges HP, Lassmann H, Mamoli B (1972) Zur nahtlosen interfaszikulären Nerventransplantation im Tierexperiment. Wien Med Wochenschr 517:523
21. Nakayama K, Tamiya T, Yamamoto K, Akimoto S (1962) A simple new apparatus for small vessel anastomosis (free autograft of the sigmoid included). Surgery 52:918
22. Ota K, Mori S (1965) Nonsuture anastomosis of vascular prosthesis utilising plastic adhesives. Angiology 16:521
23. Payr E (1904) Zur Frage der zirkulären Vereinigung von Blutgefäßen mit resorbierbaren Prothesen. Arch Klin Chir 72:32
24. Rutherford RB (1977) Vascular surgery. Saunders, Philadelphia
25. Schüttemeyer W (1952/53) Gefäßanastomosen mit Metallprothesen. Langenbecks Arch Klin Chir 723:893
26. Takaro T (1964) The American and the Russian vascular staplers. Arch Surg 89:536
27. Tatooles CJ, Braunwald NS (1966) The use of crosslinked gelatin as a tissue adhesive to control hemorrhage from liver and kidney. Surgery 60:857
28. Vollmar J (1982) Rekonstruktive Chirurgie der Arterien, 3rd edn. Thieme, Stuttgart
29. Walterbusch G, Haverich A, Borst HG (1982) Clinical experience with fibrin glue for local bleeding control and sealing of vascular prosthesis. Thorac Cardiovasc Surg 30:234
30. Wylie JE, Stoney RJ, Ehrenfeld WK (1980) Manual of vascular surgery, vol I. Springer, Berlin Heidelberg New York

5 Vascular Reconstruction

R. GIESSLER

CONTENTS

A. Basic Principles

The most outstanding *characteristic of vascular reconstruction* is its very *low tolerance of errors*. In general, it can be said that surgical risk is increased by shortcomings in the following areas: choice of the optimal time for surgery; choice of the most appropriate procedure; and correct execution. This is especially true in vascular surgery, particularly where vascular substitutes [trans- or implants] are involved. In such cases, failure and life-threatening complications are not limited to the early postoperative phase, but often continue to cast a shadow over the later postoperative period as well. Knowledge of this *fateful relationship between the quality of reconstruction and long-term success* has led to a search for new methods of *quality control*.

In the analysis of the *risk factors in vascular reconstructions* the surgeon ranks highest, followed by shortcomings in the observance of empirically established, approved principles. As a consequence, the specialized training of vascular surgeons has been strictly regulated, and its quality continuously improved. The vascular surgeon guaranties the *quality of the procedure*: he is expected to put scientific knowledge into practice and to guarantee the quality of his work. These expectations can only be fulfilled if the surgeon is well acquainted with the results of epidemiologic studies concerning the natural course of certain vascular diseases, with pathophysiology including hemodynamics, and with the interpretation and assessment of diagnostic findings, especially those based on noninvasive methods. In addition, the surgeon must perform self-critical quality control, using documentation and biostatistics. Surgeons should be fully competent to perform standard as well as low-risk alternative surgical procedures, including ancillary measures for improving and maintaining surgical results. They should be acquainted with the prophylaxis and treatment of infection. Finally, they should be able to prevent and treat perioperative complications.

Based on our own personal experience, the most important *guidelines for surgical technique* are the following:

1. The *priority of function over exact anatomic correction*
2. The strict observance of *hemodynamic principles*
3. The lowering of surgical risk by applying an *atraumatic and meticulous technique*

The first guideline is confirmed by extra-anatomic bypasses. Anastomotic techniques and other possibilities of improving blood flow must be mastered theoretically before they are applied practically. To *think in terms of collateral systems* means to eliminate all possibility of complications: a carefully planned clamping technique avoids stagnation of blood flow with the resulting increased risk of thromboembolism. At the same time, preservation of collateral blood flow is an effective protective measure against peripheral ischemia.

Careful handling of tissue prevents *local complications* such as compression or injury of neighboring structures, intimal dissection or fracture, thermal or osmotic disturbances, compression of bypass grafts due to faulty graft alignment, and local as well as distant thromboembolic episodes.

The surgeon's familiarity with a particular vascular substitute is of great importance during and after its implantation. Knowledge of specific instructions by the manufacturer guards against failure and complications [23]. This is an extremely important point, especially with new products. For, to ignore a manufacturer's instructions is in effect to disregard the technical progress embodied in such products.

The *structural quality* that a vascular surgery department should deliver cannot be defined exactly. At the very least, there should be well-functioning working units with appropriate personnel and equipment as well as an extensive number of cases involving a wide range of vascular diseases, thereby offering an optimal situation for teaching and for the enhancement of professional skill. Close contact and cooperation with colleagues in other specialties – e.g., angiology and angioradiology, internal medicine, cardiology, neurology, ophthalmology, otolaryngology, and orthopedic surgery – guarantees not only the best preoperative management but also excellent postoperative follow-up control.

High *quality of result* in vascular surgery can be achieved only if organization and quality of treatment are constantly improved [21]. The extension of reconstructive surgery far into the peripheral dimension has brought with it problems of inadequate blood flow in cases of high resistance and in long bypass grafts passing over joints. Added to these are new problems arising from the surgical management of elderly or multimorbid patients previously outside the range of such therapy. All of these new problems require the creative application of rigorous principles in individual cases.

B. Reconstructive Procedures

Vascular reconstructions *aim* at restoring the acutely or chronically impaired or completely interrupted function of the circulatory system within various tissues of the body, or preventing these pathologic states. Accordingly, the procedures can be classified as:

1. Operations which remove obstructions with or without the resection of wall segments (disobliteration)
2. Maneuvers which by angioplasty correct pathologic conditions by preserving or utilizing layers of the vascular wall
3. Procedures which use grafts to fortify, widen, substitute, or bypass diseased arterial segments

This chapter outlines the basic elements with respect to their practical application.

I. Disobliteration

1. Thromboembolectomy (see also p. 364)

Embolism is one of the most common indications for an emergency operation, the others being vascular injury and ruptured aneurysms. The logical strategy and quick success of a correctly performed embolectomy should not lead one to underestimate the dangers and possibilities for error which this procedure entails. This is also true of acute thrombotic occlusions, e.g., following vascular injury. However, these situations as well as complications following a reconstructive procedure, should be managed primarily by a vascular instead of a general surgeon.

The importance of percutaneous aspiration thromboembolectomy cannot be judged at the present time [28].

Today, basic *instruments for vascular procedures*, such as atraumatic clamps, forceps, balloon catheters of different sizes, and ultrafine suture material, are available everywhere. Dilating balloon catheters made of latex or PVC make extraction possible from any site to which access is easily gained if the obstruction site cannot be precisely localized according to clinical criteria.

As an example, let us take the lower extremity, which is the most frequent site of occlusions. Access to the femoral bifurcation is easily achieved and suturing in this area can be done without difficulty. Adequate, but not too extensive *exposure* makes a safe and quick operation possible. The lateral approach preserves the lymph nodes, and careful dissection leaves nerves (femoral saphenous nerves) and veins (common femoral, saphenous veins) untouched. Initial *clamping* is only necessary if inspection and delicate palpation indicate residual blood flow within the vessel. Thus, fragmentation of a fresh thrombus, which could be extracted easily as a whole, is avoided. A transverse *arteriotomy* of the anterior wall 0.5–1 cm above the origin of the profunda femoris artery can be sutured more quickly than a longitudinal incision in which patch angioplasty may also be necessary. However, in a transverse incision, more care must be taken to prevent dissection or tearing. Following incision, one should check the age, structure, and adherence of the thrombus by careful dilatation and flushing with heparinized solution. A fresh, coherent clot can often be "milked" by a careful, uniform pull with several forceps, making sure that branches of the thrombus are also removed from the tributaries of the outflow tract. Back-bleeding generally indicates successful removal of the thrombus. Then, the run-off may be tested by flushing with heparinized saline solution. Suction should merely ensure clear vision, not remove the detritus. The whole or fragmented thrombus is spread out on gauze covering the thrombectomized segment and should only be discarded after its beginning and end have been identified completetly.

If extraction is not accomplished by this simple method, a *balloon catheter* is inserted carefully. Obstructions along its way can be localized by markings on the catheter. As soon as the catheter penetrates the thrombus, the balloon is dilated by instilling the correct amount of fluid according to its size. Bursting by overdilating the balloon may lead to embolism of the remaining fragments. Advancement, filling, and retrieval must be performed without scraping defects and dissection. At the introduction site, the catheter is always moved parallel to the axis of the vessel in order to prevent mechanical injury and tearing at the corners of the wound. The thrombi pulled out by the catheter are arranged in a row, as described above, to make sure that the thrombotic material has been removed completely.

The number of passages of the catheter through the vessel depends on the extent and amount of thrombotic material. For peripheral segments thinner catheters are introduced. Following each passage, heparinized solution is slowly injected to prevent embolism.

Older, partially or totally adherent thrombi cannot be extracted by a balloon catheter alone. In such cases a *ring stripper* made of flexible wire, which is slipped over the thrombus, if possible under direct vision, has a much greater scraping effect. To prevent embolism of stripped particles, the outflow tract can be blocked by introducing a balloon catheter and advancing it through the ring stripper. This is called the "Rififi method."

Observing the sequence of peripheral thrombectomy followed by disobliteration of the proximal segment has the advantage that the former procedure can usually be performed without interference from a clamp on the inflow tract.

Extraction of the thrombus from proximal segments is done in the same manner. However, one can utilize the increased retrograde blood flow to flush out the thrombus. If a balloon catheter or a ring stripper is employed, the necessary length is estimated by measuring it alongside the course of the vessel before insertion (aortic bifurcation is located at the level of the umbilicus) and the pulse of the contralateral femoral artery is checked to identify disruption and distal migration of the thrombus.

The *suture* must include all layers. This not only guarantees secure closure, but also saves time. Before placing the last stitch one should allow bleeding to remove possible residues of the thrombus, which can be identified by holding gauze over the bleeding site. When the surgeon has checked the suture, blood flow can slowly be restored under continuous monitoring of blood pressure. This prevents sudden drops in blood pressure due to fluid loss into the maximally dilated ischemic peripheral vascular bed, which are especially dangerous in patients with cardiac risk factors. Steady digital pressure and, if necessary, a supplementary suture of the adventitia can prevent needless blood loss. A suction drain does not replace careful hemostasis.

The most common *causes of failure* to restore adequate blood flow are an impaired run-off due to thrombi or dissection of vascular wall structures. These failures can be prevented only by consistency in surgical technique and by the continuous control and documentation of results, beginning intraoperatively with palpation and inspection and continuing postoperatively in follow-up examinations using Doppler techniques for pressure measurement.

Today, the indication for arterial embolectomy within the extremities is no longer dependent on the *interval of time* since the manifestation of symptoms (6 h limit), but on the *reversibility of ischemia*. In delayed embolectomy, one may encounter extensive obstruction of peripheral vessels and branches following proximal and distal extension of the thrombus. Therefore, one should always be prepared to perform an additional incision at a crural artery. Whether or not local thrombolysis, by means of an intraoperatively introduced catheter, shows better results in such cases, remains uncertain at the moment.

Where preoperative *differentiation between an embolism and the acute thrombosis* of a preexisting arteriosclerotic lesion was uncertain, or where, during embolectomy, complete thrombosis of a high grade arteriosclerotic obstruction may be found, disobliteration or bypass grafting must be performed in every case, even in emergencies. One should not wait until further diagnostic measures are performed. This also applies to acute thrombotic occlusions in *aneurysmal disease*. This pathologic condition must be considered if an extraordinarily large amount of thrombotic material is extruded and the thrombi are not of the same age.

2. Endarterectomy and Thromboendarterectomy

Flow obstruction due to an intimal lesion or thrombus formation may be relieved by excision and removal of the obliterating material, leaving the outer layers of the vascular wall intact. Morphologically, the structure of the vascular wall in arteriosclerotic disease exhibits two regions with different physical characteristics, a sclerotic inner core and an undiseased elastic outer cover. In advanced arteriosclerosis ("mature", flaky atheromatous debris) a *preformed dissection plane* exists, making subintimal and subadventitial dissection with an elevator or a fine mosquito (Halsted) clamp easy. Because most atheromatous plaques extend into the media, dissection should preferably be performed near the adventitia.

Treatment by *disobliteration depends* on the type of vascular wall, the dimensions of the artery, and its pathomorphology. Unsuitable for this procedure are inflammatory and immature arteriosclerotic lesions, aneurysmal changes, the popliteal artery, and the delicate crural arteries. Calcified incrustations do not usually pose insoluble problems as long as the remaining outer layer is unaffected and it is possible to dissect the calcified inner core without injuring the outer layer. Even in seemingly hypoplastic, occluded, or nonpulsating narrow vessels, a normal diameter may be regained as the outer layer expands following removal of the obstruction.

Unfortunately, transmural vascular scars following previous diagnostic or radiologic punctures may often limit disobliteration or even make it completely impossible. The latter is the case at the site of a previous reconstruction.

Disobliteration may be *open* or *semiclosed*, depending on the length of the obstruction.

However, certain *errors and hazards* are common with all methods of endarterectomy. It is often difficult to find the ideal dissection plane and to stay in the plane once dissection is commenced. This leads to the formation of flaps and debris which are left behind with the possibility of obstructing blood flow and causing early occlusion. Ascertaining that the arterial sclerotic plaque has been removed completely and flushing with saline in the direction of blood flow may help to avoid these errors. To date, arterioscopy has not been widely used. At the distal and proximal boundaries of the endarterectomized segment, changes in caliber may act as valves, causing turbulence or narrowing. In such a case, disobliteration is continued beyond the plaque, or the remaining thickened layer is flattened with fine curved scissors. Cleavage too close to the adventitia may cause intraoperative hemorrhage, making a time consuming correction necessary. Even after a correctly performed endarterectomy, a relative dilatation of the disobliterated segment in comparison with the neighboring nonendarterectomized segments results. This generates a thrombogenic hemodynamic situation imitating aneurysmal changes. Finally, the disobliterating instruments are always moved along the boundary between hard core and tender outer layer. The surgeon needs a more sensitive and delicate touch and a more perfect control of the dissecting instruments during manipulations of the vascular wall than during implantation of a vascular prosthesis. This should be considered when choosing the method for vascular reconstruction.

a) Direct Endarterectomy with Direct Suture. Ideal locations for direct disobliteration are the commonest sites of arteriosclerotic plaques at the origins of branches of the internal carotid artery, celiac, superior mesentric, and renal arteries, and at the femoral bifurcation. The advantage at these sites is that they afford a good view of the distal end of the incision and also good exposure of bifurcations. The arteriotomy is extended beyond the palpable or visible edge of the plaque so that the distal protruding margin of the intima is exposed. Ideally, the plaque extends gradually and without abrupt interruptions onto the normal intimal surface. If an intimal flap or protrusion remains, many supplementary maneuvers are recommended, such as applying steady pressure until natural fixation prevents protrusion of the intima into the lumen. Transfixation by suturing the flaps to the vessel wall may cause additional injury to the vessel and is helpful only if the measures previously mentioned fail. The proximal intimal flap does not cause many problems because its edge is held down by the flow, in a manner reminiscent of a roofing shingle.

If the lumen is wide enough following removal of the inner core, the continuity of the artery can be restored by direct suture. Suturing should begin at the distal end of the incision. The flushing maneuver can be performed when the suture reaches the central portion of the incision, where the wall is not likely to tear easily.

An *alternative* method is the *eversion technique*. Today, it is helpful in only a few situations. When kinking of the carotid artery is present with simultaneous stenosis at its origin, one transects the internal carotid artery at its origin. Its outer layers are everted and peeled back until the whole diseased inner core with the arteriosclerotic plaque can be removed without an intimal flap remaining. The internal carotid artery is then anastomosed to the distal end of the common carotid artery. In a variant method of *profundaplasty*, the occluded superficial femoral artery is transected several centimeters distal to its origin and disobliterated according to the eversion technique. It is anastomosed distal to the stenotic origin of the profunda femoris artery instead of performing a time-consuming patch graft angioplasty.

b) Direct Disobliteration with Patch Angioplasty. Originally, a patch was used only to prevent possible narrowing and stricture of a longitudinal suture or to replace a damaged region of the vascular wall. Today, it is a prophylactic measure to prevent stricture during healing of a vascular suture [13]. Its advantages are that it overpasses incongruities and bridges abrupt changes in caliber. Disadvantages are, on the one hand, the amount of time needed to complete it, when compared with the simple direct suture, and on the other, the negative features of the material used for the patch: with synthetic material, an increased susceptibility to infection, and with autogenous vein patches, progressive dilatation or shrinking as a result of intima hyperplasia.

Technically, one starts with an everting horizontal mattress suture at the distal end of the arteriotomy so that the narrowest site of the reconstruction can always be inspected from the inside. The stitch is directed away from the patch to the internal surface of the vascular wall; the patch is attached in such a way that it acts as a washer to prevent these sutures from tearing out.

Complications may occur if the patch is too large, which may lead to an iatrogenic aneurysm. The correct width of an autogenous vein patch is difficult to determine because of its elasticity. This can only be learned through practice and experience. Compensating by taking larger bites during suturing may lead to narrowing of the patch.

Available patch materials include superficial autogenous veins (at the ankle) and various specially developed synthetic graft materials (see p. 78).

c) Indirect Semiclosed Endarterectomy. Indication: Open disobliteration with patch angioplasty in long occluded segments of the femoral artery was abandoned in favor of the semiclosed technique of disobliteration, which today is only rarely indicated. Isolated or extensive aortoiliac obstructions are the primary indications for disobliteration with a ring stripper.

The advantage of the procedure is that it can be performed by an experienced surgeon quickly and without the potential risks associated with synthetic vascular prostheses. There is no leakage as in the case of porous vascular prostheses. There is as a drawback, however, a certain dependence on the morphological structure as well as the vulnerability of the remaining outer wall layers.

Technique: A standard aortoiliac disobliteration can usually be performed without patch angioplasty. Adequate exposure is achieved by a transverse vessel incision. The correct plane of cleavage is then determined. Following circumferential dissection, the ring of the stripper, which should only be slightly larger than the inner core, is passed over the core and advanced by a combination of rotary and gentle pushing movements. Through a second incision above the distal bifurcation, the inner core can be carefully divided and extracted. Intimal flaps are handled in the same way as described above. Continuous suture of the incisions should be done while applying slight traction on the stay sutures so that no stricture can form after blood flow is restored.

Common errors and complications: Loose fragments of the vascular wall, atheromatous debris, clots, intimal flaps, and unrecognized thinning of the vascular wall are the main causes of complications. A meticulous operative technique, constant control by palpation, and thorough irrigation of the disobliterated segment are the best preventive measures.

Special applications of indirect disobliteration *are retrograde* transfemoral disobliteration of the external iliac artery and endarterectomy of the abdominal aorta. The former is performed only in exceptional cases. It is an alternate method with a lower surgical risk. There are no objections to the latter as a blind method since the obstructive plug is quickly and smoothly removed under direct vision with the help of the Vollmar disobliterotome.

d) Complications and Modifications. Numerous anatomic and instrumental variations of disobliteration, such as anterograde endarterectomy of the superficial femoral artery and common carotid arteries, the application of pneumatic or hydraulic methods, or the use of an oscillotome have been abandoned. The first results of using a laser for the disobliteration of peripheral arteries have been reported [7]. The combination of disobliteration with bypass grafting is still the most commonly used reconstruction. Local endarterectomy is performed at the site of anastomosis between graft and host artery. Disobliteration of the host artery is less commonly performed in a sequential bypass. Sometimes, it is used to salvage reconstructions in which the length of the venous graft is not adequate.

II. Angioplasty

This term comprehends all surgical procedures which correct pathologic changes in caliber in the vessel wall while preserving the original wall components and the topography of the artery. Their importance varies, but knowledge of these methods may be helpful in some special situations.

1. Plication

The restoration of a normal caliber by reducing the transverse diameter of the vessel was one of the first reconstructive procedures ever performed. Today, aneurysmorrhaphy according to MATAS is done only in localized saccular aneurysms, where replacement by a synthetic prosthesis must be avoided, e.g., in cases of an increased risk of infection or in lateral suture of the dilated central portion of a chronic arteriovenous fistula. Lateral aneurysmorrhaphy of saccular thoracic aneurysms is now a thing of the past.

2. Straightening

A still widely applied technique is the correction of congenital or degenerative elongations, most commonly seen in the internal carotid and vertebral arteries, and less often in the common iliac artery.

Leaving aside muscle flaps and arteriopexy to eliminate kinking, which are merely palliative measures, three *surgical techniques* are available for straightening. A loop of the internal carotid artery can be straightened by means of several adjacent longitudinal *plications*. The advocates of this method state that such a technique leads to only limited shortening without impairment of blood flow. The second preferred method is to divide the vessel at its origin and *reinsert* it proximal to the initial origin end-to-side. This technique not only straightens the vessel accurately, but also allows for the simultaneous removal of stenoses at the origin under direct vision. The third possibility is shortening of the artery by *resecting* the portion which is most severely diseased and reanastomosing both stumps end-to-end.

3. Transposition, Transposition Flap

Stenoses near the origins of organ arteries may be relieved by transposition. This is a very elegant method of correction in obstructions situated at the origins of the renal and superior mesenteric arteries. Transposition of the subclavian artery to the common carotid artery, following disobliteration if necessary, has long been our procedure of choice.

The stenosis in a coarctation of the aorta may be relieved by creating a transposition flap out of the left subclavian artery. The end-to-side insertion of a disobliterated superficial femoral artery has already been pointed out as a possible variation in profundaplasty.

Reimplantation of a short vascular stump may cause *technical difficulties*. As a rule, one should always suture first those portions of the wall which are most difficult to approximate. In the *open suture technique*, smooth, monofilament sutures are used to complete adaptation following suture of the back wall.

4. External Reinforcement

Recently, wrapping of aortic abdominal aneurysms has been suggested again, but has not been accepted as a method of reducing surgical risk. However, today the use of a sleeve, which may consist of different materials, is still common to reinforce the suture line. For example, porous vascular prostheses are put around the anastomosis. If only a portion of the vascular wall shows potential weakness, a small strip of Teflon felt sutured to this site may be adequate (see p. 338). Strips of fascia are obsolete. Woven prostheses inhibit migration and incorporation of fibroblasts. Doppler sonographic controls are recommended after such repairs.

5. Reentry Technique

This form of treatment tries to convert the double lumen of a dissecting aneurysm into a single one. The blood flow through the false lumen is conducted into the main aortic lumen by excising a small window of tissue out of the dividing membrane. Further dissection is prevented by suturing both walls directly to one another or connecting them with fibrin glue (see p. 358).

6. Decompression

The removal of external obstructions has increased with better knowledge of their pathophysiology. Originally, the phenomenon of poststenotic dilatation caused by external compression was known only in patients with an accessory cervical rib and occlusions beneath the adductor tendons. Today, we know the most frequent *sites* of intermittent or chronic narrowing of the vascular lumen that can lead to hemodynamic disorders, thromboembolic complications, or aneurysmal dilatation. These are at the origins of the celiac trunk, renal artery, and especially the popliteal artery (see p. 575). Compression following healing of a bone fracture is relatively uncommon.

The *operative techniques* employed in these disorders are discussed in the appropriate chapters. It is necessary to dissect sharply, owing to periarterial fibrosis, and to perform vascular reconstruction if arteriolysis is impossible or unsatisfactory. Alternatives other than operative decompression are not known, except in the treatment of cystic adventitial degeneration, in which percutaneous aspiration is performed by radiologic intervention.

7. Fixation

After blood flow has been restored, vascular reconstructions may have a tendency to kink. This may occur if the reconstructed arterial segment, for example, becomes redundant after removal of the supporting arteriosclerotic plug at the carotid bifurcation or after implantation of a graft that is too long. Small errors may be corrected by adapting the neighboring tissue firmly around the vessel. This gives enough support in most cases. Direct fixation of the vessel to its surrounding tissues with supplementary sutures should be done only in exceptional cases, as the vessel wall tears easily in these situations.

8. Dilatation

Dilatation of the outflow tract following reconstructive procedures has been done routinely for a long time. Bougienage of inaccessible portions of an artery, e.g., fibromuscular dysplasia of the subcranial internal carotid artery is a standard technique today. Advances in *interventional radiology* have not only changed the indications for treatment in different diseases, but have also brought about a new surgical strategy in obliterative arteriopathies. Only the simultaneous application of intraoperative transluminal dilatation during reconstructions of the arterial system will be discussed at this point.

Intraoperative transluminal dilatation (ITA) is applied in stenoses of the inflow or outflow tract in which removal is not absolutely indicated, is too time consuming, or correction is unsuitable for technical reasons.

Angioradiologic principles are applied in these maneuvers. A metal guide is not obligatory. There are two types of catheters available for dilatation, the Grüntzig and Olbert catheters. Fogarty catheters are not suited because the balloons expand uncontrollably in all directions.

In intraoperative dilatation of fibromuscular stenoses of the carotid artery the disruption and migration of thrombi do not occur. This danger cannot be excluded if the procedure is done percutaneously with the direction of blood flow.

Postoperative percutaneous dilatation of remaining and recurrent stenoses is possible in selected cases. When such a procedure is planned, we consider close cooperation with a vascular surgeon mandatory. The surgeon's knowledge of pathogenesis, pathomorphology, and their risks is a valuable aid.

9. Methods of Vascular Obliteration

These aim at achieving permanent, secure occlusion of a particular vascular segment or vascular stump.

The *induction of thrombosis* had been performed long before the resection of abdominal aortic aneurysms. It was reintroduced for treatment of high risk patients without resection under the protection of an extra-anatomic bypass. In smaller and peripheral arteries, *percutaneous therapeutic embolization* replaces surgical ligation. Fluids, such as fibrin or acrylic glues or particles such as microspheres or spirals, are used, e.g., in congenital angiodysplasia, acquired arteriovenous fistula (see p. 223), aneurysms, including false aneurysms, and cancer.

As a last resort reliable obliteration of large *vascular stumps* still causes problems, especially in the abdominal aorta, when insecure anastomotic conditions are present or an infection makes removal of the prosthesis necessary. The absorbable synthetic suture material used today keeps its tensile strength for a prolonged period of time and then deteriorates slowly. This is a significant improvement over materials used in the past which were readily absorbed or acted as foreign bodies. Covering with vital periaortal tissue or an omentum flap improves the prognosis. However, this cannot be guaranteed.

10. Adjuvant Flow Augmentation

The construction of additional peripheral anastomoses ultimately leads to a *reduction of run-off resistance*. Multiple anastomoses of long bypass grafts with several peripheral arteries, as in a sequential bypass, or *shunts* between arteries and the venous low pressure system, belong to this category. The thromboprotective effect of an increased blood flow in venous reconstructions and long arterial bypass grafts is evident. However, the peripheral circulatory effect of artificial arteriovenous fistulae has not yet been completely clarified.

III. Reconstruction by Vascular Replacement

Vascular replacement has become the main component in vascular surgery. Its applications are numerous, and its requirements differ greatly. First, the following *review* outlines the practically essential surgical and technical concepts. Then the biology and problems of vascular replacement are discussed.

1. Enlargement of the Lumen, Partial Replacement

The most common *purpose* of patch grafts is to increase the size of a vascular lumen *prophylactically* following any longitudinal suture. These grafts are also used in repairing *local vascular wall defects* following vessel injury, intraoperative mishaps, or after abandoning a bypass procedure. Furthermore, partial replacement allows vital, *growing sectors* of a congenitally hypoplastic segment to develop, e.g., in the correction of juvenile aortic coarctation. The *harmonization of an anastomosis* to overcome a disparity by the incorporation of a small, well-fitting patch, as described by VAN DONGEN, has already been discussed elsewhere (see p. 63).

2. Interposition and Substitution

Today, *total resection* and substitution are obligatory only in pathologic changes that affect the outer layers of the vascular wall, such as cancer, vascular tears of various origin, and high grade thinning of the vascular wall due to chronic hypervolemic circulatory conditions in long-standing arteriovenous fistula. In the abdominal aorta, substitution presents hemodynamic and anatomic advantages as an alternative to bypass grafting.

Partial resection and substitution are indicated when sections of the vascular wall in which tributaries branch off must be preserved by any means. For instance, during the resection of thoracic aortic aneurysms it may be employed to prevent spinal ischemia. It is also indicated in the resection of aneurysms of the aortic arch and thoracoabdominal aorta with preservation of visceral of supra-aortal branches (see p. 318). This technique is further applicable in the reimplantation of the interior mesenteric artery or the origin of the deep femoral artery.

A second variation of partial resection is partial aneurysmectomy. Thrombus and atheromatous material is scooped out from within the aneurysm, and the continuity of the artery is reestablished by the interposition of a straight tube prosthesis. Quick dissection within the preformed plane of cleavage, preservation of the outer wall layers, as well as avoiding an extra anastomosis are the main advantages of the "minimal dissection method."

A third variation is the *inlay graft technique* applied in emergency, life-threatening situations, where time and the amount of blood loss play a crucial role (see p. 344). In dissecting aneurysms of the thoracic or abdominal aorta as well as in typical abdominal aortic aneurysms, a prosthesis with reduced porosity is positioned within the original lumen and anchored without sutures by a ligature placed around cloth-covered stainless steel rings [6, 9]. Making a prosthesis fit the actual anatomic conditions by moving the distal ring into the right position is usually no problem. However, the attachment to the iliac arteries may cause difficulties.

Another concept of internal stabilization is the *percutaneous transluminal implantation of metal spirals* which may be attached by controlled elastic expansion [18]. Until now, there are only a few reports on the application of this very interesting percutaneous inlay technique.

3. Bypass Grafting Techniques

Vascular replacement makes it possible to imitate natural principles of collateral systems. Bypass grafting was originally conceived by JEGER in 1913 [14] as a functional way of bridging anatomic flow obstructions and was realized by KUNIN in 1948 [15] with a venous graft in an orthotopic position. Later on, bypassing of problematic zones, e.g., sites of infection following vascular reconstruction, with extra-anatomic grafts was developed.

Meanwhile, the technique of extra-anatomic bypass has established itself as a sound alternative with acceptable results. It is employed in patients in whom direct reconstruction is combined with high risk, e.g., elimination of aortoiliac occlusions or aneurysms in patients of poor general condition, in extrathoracic bypass of a symptomatic occlusion of the subclavian artery, or in the bridging of a popliteal aneurysm.

Technically, the principle of bypass has numerous advantages. Exposure is limited to the area of the anastomoses. Alignment of the graft and its course to the distal anastomosis can be constructed by subcutaneous tunneling. There should be no tension on the graft as it passes through the tissue. Collaterals are preserved. An end-to-side anastomosis makes it possible to connect lumina with differing calibers. Finally, because of its simplicity, bypass grafting can be applied everywhere.

The technique of implantation, positioning of the bypass, and secondary changes of the graft and its host artery may lead to *complications.* Correct construction of the anastomotic angle and diameter is necessary. Otherwise, narrowing at the take-off of the graft or an aneurysmal sac with the danger of tearing at the suture line will develop. While placing the graft in the subcutaneous tunnel, twisting, kinking and external compression by neighboring tendons, fascia, or scars must be avoided. The graft must not be too long, and tension should be absent as well. A good knowledge of hemodynamics (no competitive flow, no steal constellation, no situations causing turbulent flow) and a good visual estimation in order to make the grafts of different elasticity fit are necessary.

4. Combinations and Alternatives

Competing anatomic and pathomorphological requirements often make it necessary to combine techniques of vascular disobliteration and grafting. The situations requiring combined methods are discussed in the section on special topics.

5. Vascular Access

A specific application of vascular reconstructive techniques is the extra-anatomic end-to-side interposition of shunts between arteries and veins for chronic intermittent hemodialysis. The vein graft or prosthesis must withstand increased blood flow and is mechanically impaired by frequent punctures with large cannulas. It also carries an increased risk of infection (see Chap. 25, p. 659).

C. Vascular Replacement

I. General Remarks

Vascular replacement is almost as old as the circumferential arterial suture. Its principles – harvesting technique, preservation, morphological and functional fate – had already been systematically investigated during the first decade of this century. For decades, only autogenous veins were used clinically. The successful replacement of aortic and arterial segments with homologous transplants and the creation of blood vessel banks to provide a supply of such transplants have come about only since 1948.

At the beginning of the era of reconstructive vascular surgery *two basic discoveries* were made:

1. The maintenance of the graft's *function* as a blood conduit was not dependent upon its vitality, which prior to that time had been the main goal of transplantation.
2. The replacement of *small arteries* and *veins* posed problems.

Meanwhile, advances in the manufacturing of *synthetic prostheses* made it possible to produce grafts fulfilling specific anatomic and technical requirements in large arteries. With some limitations, these are also suited to medium-sized arteries as well as veins.

The systematic search for *biologic grafts* with the same characteristics as medium and small arteries was not very successful. Because the manufacture of non-autogenic grafts makes devitalization of tissue necessary, they were called bio*prostheses* or *im*plants.

Present efforts are concentrated on gaining a better understanding of hemostasis and resistance to thrombosis and their influence on the vessel wall (endothelium). These efforts are a result of experience with the inhibition of platelet aggregation to secure long-term postoperative patency.

The *requirements which grafts must fulfill* are multiple. Generally, they should be reliable, well tolerated by the surrounding tissues, not easily deformable, immunologically inert, and non-carcinogenic. Furthermore, they must fulfill the microbiologic requirements and must be available in the sizes required. They should be easy to handle and should incorporate themselves permanently into the surrounding tissues. They should prevent thrombus formation and be insensitive to degeneration and degradation by their environment. The different behavior of each material within the body led to the introduction of the term "scale of *biologic acceptance.*" In addition to long-term results, however, other aspects frequently take *clinical priority*. Short life expectancy or limited general operability of the patient may change the indication for certain vascular reconstructions. In such cases, lowering surgical risk ranks highest [9].

II. Autogenous Grafts

1. Arterial Grafts

The body's own arterial segments with their *preserved viability* and mechanical endurance are at the top of the list of grafts having the best biologic acceptance and tolerance. However, only short or small arterial segments can be transplanted freely. They can either be removed without replacement (internal iliac, splenic, internal thoracic [10], radial, epigastric arteries), or in very special cases exchanged with a vascular prosthesis (external iliac artery). *Indications* for transplantation exist during the period of growth, in potentially infected vascular injuries [25], and in the extracorporal correction of stenoses of the renal arteries.

2. Venous Grafts

a) Basic Principles. Practically speaking, the *most important* biologic graft is the greater saphenous vein which can be used in many situations because of its length and range of diameters [3, 11].

Its use is *limited* in aortic, renal, and iliac positions because of its delicate wall structure. It is commonly (20%–30%) unavailable for primary interposition or bypass owing to varicosis, previous phlebitis, or previous treatment of varices. If further operations are necessary following reconstruction with a greater saphenous vein graft, alternative veins must be found such as the greater saphenous vein of the other leg, the basilic, cephalic, and smaller saphenous veins, and even the femoral vein [1, 24]. Various techniques of lengthening or widening vein grafts, e.g., for the replacement of large veins, have been described. These are done in emergency situations if no other alternatives are available.

Often, extension by means of a synthetic prosthesis (*composite graft*) or connection to a disobliterated superficial femoral artery are possible. Patch grafts can also be harvested from tributaries of the saphenous vein or by resecting only a short malleolar saphenous vein segment.

b) Incorporation. The *morphologic changes* within grafts which influence their clinical and functional performance can be classified into six groups:

1. Proliferation of the intima with concentric narrowing at the anastomosis or along the whole length of the prosthesis
2. Arteriosclerosis
3. Fibrosis of the venous valves
4. Fibrotic scars following a traumatic operating technique
5. Stenosis at the origin of a tributary as a result of a ligature or suture at that point
6. Aneurysmal degeneration

Although LEXER claimed in 1907 [16] that the resection of an aneurysm and replacement with an autogenous vein graft was the *ideal* operation, today biopathologic research has led to a more realistic assessment. However, the autogenous saphenous vein graft is still unsurpassed, and its effectiveness constitutes the standard for determining the suitability of the newly developed prostheses.

c) Technique of Transplantation. Whether or not a vein can be used for grafting is judged intraoperatively. Its gross macroscopic appearance is evaluated, but always with the awareness that touching the vein may lead to contraction. *Harvesting* must be performed using a meticulous technique. To prevent injury of the endothelium the graft must not be pulled too tightly or squeezed. The graft should only be picked up by the adventitia [17]. Flushing of the graft overcomes spasms and detects leakage. However, normal physiologic pressure should never be exceeded during this maneuver [4]. To prevent osmotic injury, buffered heparinized saline solutions are recommended. The graft should stay in contact with the wound as long as possible. This minimizes warm ischemic time.

d) Errors and Complications. Insufficiently restrictive *patient selection* for the implantation of a great saphenous vein graft is one of the first errors which can be made. Examples are: uneconomic harvesting, uncertainty of results, usage instead of another equivalent prosthesis (dialysis shunt), and implantation in an unsuitable position which may jeopardize the graft's function.

During resection, any injury may lead to an anastomotic stricture later on. Therefore, small branches of the graft should be ligated far enough away from the main stem. During *implantation*, twisting of the vessel must be avoided. Pulling the graft through a tunneler with a smooth inside surface is preferred to positioning the graft using a long clamp.

3. Semiautogenous Grafts

The theoretically very interesting *concept of autogenous arteriogenesis* by SPARKS 1973 [27] deserves to be mentioned at this point, even though this method has proved impractical without further development. Likewise, the attempt to induce arteriogenesis over a prosthetic frame consisting of *absorbable* synthetic fibers has as yet found no clinical application.

III. Allogenic Grafts

1. Arterial Allografts

The implantation of allografts following resection of long isthmic stenoses (1948), aortic occlusions, and abdominal aortic aneurysms (1950/51) initiated the first period of progress in modern vascular surgery. However, because of aneurysmal complications, these arterial allograft techniques were soon abandoned in favor of the newly developed synthetic prostheses.

2. Venous Allografts

Hopes that allogenic transplantation of veins would lead to a never-ending supply of biologic grafts with the same advantages as a saphenous vein graft have not been fulfilled. The grafts were harvested during stripping and were implanted in a fresh or preserved state [2]. In contrast to arterial allografts, they show little antigenicity. They may possibly find application in secondary operations or as arteriovenous shunts and may also be able to offset shortages in the supply of synthetic prostheses.

3. Umbilical Vein Allografts

Of the allogenic biologic grafts, the human umbilical vein is still widely used clinically. By tanning with glutaraldehyde as described by DARDIK, it is changed into an immunologically inactive blood conduit which is supported by a net made of Dacron. Thus, the wall is thick and sensitive to incorrect handling. A scalpel is used to trim the prosthesis as needed. Because it is stored in alcohol, careful irrigation prior to its implantation is mandatory. Routine follow-up examinations at intervals are recommended for early detection of aneurysms.

IV. Xenogenic Bioprostheses

1. Arterial Xenografts

The immunologic barrier to the transplantation of *viable* arteries from slaughtered animals to humans proved insurmountable. However, by applying complicated techniques, some investigators did succeed in converting carotid arteries of calves and cows into *bovine bioprostheses*, which were manufactured and offered in standard sizes. Although early results and suitability of the graft for easy implantation were good, aneurysms commonly developed. This led to rejection of the grafts and discontinuation of their production.

2. Semixenogenic Grafts

New types of *biosynthetic* prostheses are bovine, glutaraldehyde fixed blood conduits, reinforced with a net of polyester, which are grown in situ on the backs of sheep using the mandril method, as described initially by SPARKS (see p. 81). The internal surface of the graft is covered by a cellular layer of neointima, which makes it suitable for the grafting of smaller arteries. Even though final assessment of the clinical results presently available is not yet possible, bovine grafts probably are of historical interest only.

V. Synthetic Prostheses

1. Special Requirements

In practical terms, synthetic prostheses are the most important conduits now being used in vascular reconstruction. This is due to their wide spectrum and frequency of clinical application [29, 30,

33, 34]. The *requirements* which an ideal prosthesis must fulfill have been defined many times:

- Unlimited production of a wide variety of *standard* qualities, dimensions, and configurations
- Easy and long-term *storage* and *reliable sterilizability* in routine surgical management
- *Mechanical durability* in everyday life
- *Biologic compatibility* thanks to biochemically inert and non-blastogenic materials, without induction of a foreign body reaction during the healing process
- Resistance to thrombosis, even under conditions of poor flow and low pressure
- *Secure and uncomplicated surgical implantation* owing to easy penetration of the material during suture, flexibility, good anchorage of suture materials, impermeability, twisting and kinking stability, and easy replacement in reoperations
- *Economical aspects:* it should at least be resterilizable and capable of being tailored with minimal waste of material

Surprisingly enough, these conditions have been fulfilled to a large extent. Yet, some tasks for the future are specified in this *negative list:*

- *Absence of thrombogenicity* on the basis of endothelialization rather than physical characteristics and capability of being implanted in important vessels of small size
- *Permanent flexibility* instead of fibrotic rigidity
- *Resistance to infection*, and finally – although impractical at the moment
- A *growing* prosthesis

2. Concept and Categories

The evolution of synthetic prostheses is not only the history of numerous unsuccessful attempts at replacing vessels, but also the maturation of the concept of arteriogenesis which converts porous flexible tubes consisting of suitable synthetic fibers into functioning blood conduits by capsulation with soft tissue components. Materials and manufacturing techniques make numerous combinations possible which differ with respect to permeability of blood during implantation.

3. Material, Structure, and Modifications

It is surprising that despite extensive testing with very different substances, the material of modern prostheses has remained the same for more than 30 years, namely, Dacron and – following the solution of several problems in textile manufacturing and advances in the production of synthetics – Teflon [22]. The mechanical, electrophysical, chemical, and biochemical properties of polymers meet most of the basic and specific requirements for synthetic prostheses. Physical bonding of both substances by the polymerization of Teflon onto microporous woven Dacron microfiber prostheses (*plasma TFE*) presents a possible improvement in the future, but at the moment it cannot be assessed clinically. The same is true for the interesting development of transluminally implanted metal prostheses, as described by MAAS et al. [18].

Proper *structure* should not be thought of merely as a key factor in the implantation procedure; structure also plays a crucial role – equal to that of the material – in promoting the *incorporation*, and therefore the longevity, of the prosthesis. Today's generation of prostheses consists of *knitted* or *woven* Dacron or Teflon and of microporous extruded PTFE (Teflon). Easier and more rapid fibroblast invasion, facilitated by using highly porous prostheses (*healing porosity*), is preferred to higher impermeability of the prosthesis during implantation (*implantation porosity*).

Modifications: The *implantation porosity* of a prosthesis can be modified either by structure or by application. Tightly woven prostheses prevent blood loss during operations with the heart-lung machine. ePTFE prostheses are initially impermeable. Sealing grafts with fibrin, albumin, or gelatine reduces blood loss during implantation and exposes the prosthetic frame following absorption. Parts of the trimmed grafts remaining after the operation, however, cannot be resterilized.

The firm *anchorage* of sutures is attained by coating the outer and inner surfaces of the prosthesis or both with velour. A modified method of textile processing is employed for this purpose. *Stability against kinking and collapse*, achieved by crimping the prosthesis, makes implantation easier. As in the cartilage structure of the trachea, externally attached rings or spirals consisting of radiopaque polypropylene fabric support joint-spanning prostheses. They are sometimes a hindrance in reintervention. To *avoid twisting*, marking lines are drawn on the external surface of the prosthesis.

The improvement of prosthesis *resistance to thrombosis* is of crucial importance in the reconstruction of medium and small arteries. The results of many attempts to influence the interaction between the inner surface of the prosthesis and the blood components (electrophysically, heparin bonding, hydrophobic polymers, etc.) show that endothelial seeding is the most promising method. However, this technique has not yet found widespread clinical applications, so that drug therapy is still the only way of preventing thrombosis.

Similar developments are seen in the improvement of prosthesis *resistance to infection*. Antibiotic bonding techniques have not replaced perioperative antibiotic therapy. The smallest bacterial adherence is seen in ePTFE prostheses.

Further improvements aim at the structural stability of the prostheses by elaborate knitting techniques to prevent dilatation after implantation. Also, the hemodynamic properties have been perfected and surgical implantation simplified.

4. Incorporation

The incorporation of a synthetic prosthesis within the human body is a very *complex process*. Only some practically important findings shall be discussed here.

The idealized conception of former experimental investigators that the synthetic frame is penetrated and covered by connective tissue, leading to an *outer* and an *inner* intimalike *capsule* cannot be applied to humans. Except for the fixation of the outer velour surface to the surrounding tissues, active incorporation, including endothelialization, is only present to some degree at the site of the anastomosis. The large surfaces of the prosthetic body are lined with a layer of fibrin of varying thickness. This is attached to the velour fibers. In contrast to animals, in which such coating with fibrin represents a transitional stage in the formation of neointima, in humans this fibrin film remains in a state of equilibrium between flowing blood and the prosthetic surface without progressive thickening. This explains the maintenance of function, despite incomplete incorporation on the one hand and the fine vulnerable balance between external and hematogenous complications on the other.

5. Specific Prosthetic Complications

The *pathology of prostheses*, a risk inherent in scientific progress, begins with the *worsening of common vascular complications* as they are found in all types of reconstruction. Besides the risk of thromboembolic occlusion following intimal dissection, *susceptibility to infection* poses a great problem. Though the modern generation of prostheses allows for a differentiated treatment, depending on the location of the infection close to or for away from the anastomosis, the foreign body character of the prosthesis itself decides the final outcome. *Late infections* may not only occur as a consequence of arrosion into neighboring bacteria-containing structures such as intestines, bronchi, ureter, but also by hematogenic spread, leading to septic symptoms in patients with prostheses. Such a complication is extremely severe and needs very special intensive treatment. Another difficulty is the *explantation* of an infected velour prosthesis which is very firmly embedded in connective tissue.

At the anastomosis, partial and total disruption at the suture line (pulsating hematoma or avulsion) caused by technical errors is usually limited to the early postoperative period. On the other hand, a *false aneurysm* is a typical late complication [8]. Its pathogenesis, diagnosis, and treatment are discussed elsewhere (see p. 173). A common cause of early reocclusions is *intimal hyperplasia* which, however, may also occur in patients without synthetic prostheses solely on the basis of hemodynamic disorders, e.g., following carotid disobliteration or autogenous vein bypass.

Other specific complications in synthetic prostheses are *structural defects*. These can be caused either by dilatation of the synthetic texture or by the more dangerous *disintegration* following fragmentation and disruption of synthetic fibers. Such defects are usually attributable to errors made during manufacture or handling; they seldom result from the simple wearing out of the prosthetic material itself [20].

Within the prosthetic bed, disorders of *incorporation* are: *incomplete attachment* to the surrounding connective tissue and *diapedetic hemorrhage* due to an unabsorbed hematoma and periprosthetic seroma or *"incompatibility."* A true immunologic reaction is less probable. Prolonged infections were not seen in such cases. Incorporation was achieved by exchanging the prosthesis with a synthetic graft of a different material. *Periprosthetic fibrosis* can lead to rigidity and compression, e.g., of the ureter. *Arrosions* of structures immediately surrounding the suture line usually lead to septic complications. They can also occur at a distance from the anastomosis. Finally, because neoplasms have been reported in the vicinity of synthetic prostheses, the question has once again been raised as to whether synthetic grafts *induce tumor growth* [32]. This discussion, however, has had no effect on the use of synthetic prostheses in vascular surgery.

6. Technique of Implantation

The most relevant practical questions concerning implantation of the prosthesis are summarized in the *checklist* below:

1. Is the *assortment* complete?
   - Standard sizes, standard variations?
   - Has the demand been calculated? Is it economical?
2. *Storage:*
   - Have the prostheses been stored correctly (temperature, humidity, exposure to light, etc.)?
   - Inventory, order list?
   - Are the resterilized prostheses appropriately marked?
3. *Sterilization:*
   - Have the manufacturer's instructions been observed?
   - How should the prosthesis be packaged?
   - Steam sterilization?
   - Maximum storage time?
   - Correct labeling: type of prosthesis, number, length, diameter, date of sterilization?
4. *Operating nurse:*
   - Has the prosthesis been removed from the package under strict aseptic conditions?
   - Have the data been checked? Tracer label?
   - Keep the prostheses covered until they are implanted!
   - Present the prostheses only on a clean, sterile cloth!
   - Touch and tailor it only with clean instruments!
   - Save unused parts of the prosthesis for resterilization or use them for training purposes following disinfection.
5. *Surgeon:*
   - Check the indication for surgery: Is there no alternative?
   - Choice of prosthesis: type, diameter to fit the host artery, porosity?
   - Suture material: "Standard" or a special needle – suture combination?
   - Has the prosthesis been measured for correct length?
   - Has a safety centimeter been added? In an ePTFE prosthesis high precision is necessary!
   - Is the angle of take-off appropriate?
   - Has the prosthesis been trimmed exactly? Has it been checked for any damage?
   - Should preclotting be performed according to the standard method or an alternative technique [12]?
   - Are the distances between the stitches adequate to prevent fraying of the prosthesis and tearing of the edge of the host vessel?
   - Are the edges of the anastomosis everted and approximated enough to guarantee tight closure?
   - Is the suture technique adapted to the type of suture material used?
   - Are supplementary sutures practical and necessary?
   - Are the vessels clamped carefully, is undue strain impossible?
   - Have the flushing maneuvers prior to restoration of blood flow been done carefully and without large blood loss?
   - Has complete hemostasis been obtained in the operative field?
   - Are the prostheses surrounded by living tissue?
   - Is drainage necessary?
   - Have the results of the reconstruction been checked?
   - Is a correction necessary?
   - Has the particular procedure been explained to the resident in training?
   - Was a sketch made of the operative situs for purposes of documentation?
   - Were notes made on the course of the operation?
   - Were the results and potential complications written down?
6. *Ward physician:*
   - Inform and *instruct* the patient!

7. Postoperative Care

a) Postoperative Treatment. The *basic principles* of postoperative treatment are *modified* according to the specific regional and pathologic situation of the reconstructed vessel in each patient. *Early mobilization* is preferred. However, in joint-spanning procedures, in difficult anastomoses, and in high-risk patients it may be postponed for 1–2 days, depending on the patient's condition. *Antibiotics* in single-shot or short-term administration [31] and *anticoagulants* or *antiaggregants*, respectively [5], are administered following the usual guidelines. *Adjuvant measures* such as the improvement of microcirculation during the immediate postoperative period are not generally accepted.

b) Basic Prophylactic Measures in Vascular Disease. These measures are an absolute necessity in preventing the progression of the underlying arterial disease as well as secondary pathologic changes within the reconstructed segment.

c) Guidelines for the Patient with a Prosthetic Graft. The patient should be *instructed* to protect the reconstructed segment from mechanical overstretching, compression, or kinking without limiting normal everyday activities. Furthermore, the patient should avoid positions which cause stasis and should conscientiously *check the pulse*. The patient should be informed that in the event of weakening of the pulse or other signs of reduced blood circulation, a *service operation* (see p. 460) can avoid extensive surgical reintervention. If the patient consults a physician because of any symptoms, the patient should *inform the physician of the implanted prosthesis*. The patient should *avoid injections* in the area of the inguinal lymph nodes (insulin injections), to prevent possible bacterial contamination of the graft. If a *puncture of the prosthesis* for diagnostic or therapeutic reasons is ever planned, the patient should insist on alternatives having a lower risk. Such punctures are by no means harmless, as is often asserted by some authors [23], who seem to ignore the potential hazards of prosthetic graft pathology.

d) The Physician's Duties in Caring for the Patient with a Vascular Prosthesis. Patients with vascular reconstructions, especially vascular replacement, need lifetime follow-up care. This starts with the passing on of *information* to the patient and to the family physician. *Follow-up examinations* should be planned at regular intervals. During clinical examination, attention must be paid to the region of the anastomosis and the course of the prosthesis by checking for expansive pulsation, condition of the skin above the suture site, etc. In addition, noninvasive imaging techniques should be used more often, especially sonography, and, if necessary, computerized tomography. Further diagnostic procedures such as intravenous pyelography, X-rays of the gastrointestinal tract, gastroscopy, etc., should be considered if symptoms following aortoiliac reconstructions lead one to suspect a complication. *If symptoms are obscure and the clinical course is atypical*, one should always think first of a possible complication and try to exclude it. A good example is recurrent gastrointestinal hemorrhage as a manifestation of either a late infection or a gastroenteric fistula at the aortic anastomosis (see p. 177).

REFERENCES

1. Auer AI, Hurley JJ, Binnington HB, Nunnelee JD, Hershey FB (1983) Distal tibial vein grafts for limb salvage. Arch Surg 118:597–601
2. Beaudoin G, Guidoin R, Gosselin C, Marois M, Roy PE, Gagnon D (1985) Characteristiques physiques des veines de stripping conservees a 4 degres C et susceptibles d'etre utilisees comme substituts arteriels. J Mal Vasc 10:147–151
3. Böhmig HJ, Polterauer P, Euler-Rolle J (1977) Orthograder, freier femoro-popliteo-cruraler Venenbypass. Chirurg 48:671–674
4. Boerboom LE, Olinger GN, Bonchek LI, Gunay II, Kissebah AH, Rodriguez ER, Ferrans VJ (1985) The relative influence of arterial pressure versus intraoperative distention on lipid accumulation in primate vein bypass grafts. J Thorac Cardiovasc Surg 90:756–764
5. Bollinger A, Brunner U (1985) Antiplatelet drugs improve the patency rates after femoro-popliteal endarterectomy. Vasa 14:272–279
6. Cave-Bigley DJ, Harris PL (1985) Use of a ringed intraluminal graft in the operative management of abdominal aortic aneurysms. Br J Surg 72:825–827
7. Geschwind H, Teisseire B, Boussignac G, Benhaiem N, Vieilledent C, Laurent D (1985) Desobstructions arterielles par laser. Arch Mal Coeur 78:961–966
8. Giessler R (1980) Anastomosen-Aneurysmen nach synthetischem Gefäßersatz. Chirurg 51:14–18
9. Goddard MB, Lucas AR, Curletti EL, Cohn MS, Sadighi PJ (1985) Sutureless intraluminal graft for repair of abdominal aortic aneurysm. Arch Surg 120:791–793
10. Grondin CM, Campeau L, Lesperance J, Enjalbert M, Bourassa MG (1984) Comparison of late changes in internal mammary artery and saphenous vein grafts in two consecutive series of patients 10 years after operation. Circulation [Suppl I]: 70:208–212
11. Gruss JD, Vargas-Montano H, Bartels D, Fietze-Fischer B (1985) 10 Jahre Erfahrung mit dem in situ-Bypass. Langenbecks Arch Chir 366:317–318
12. Hagmüller G, El Nashef B, Müller HM, Denck H (1984) Zur Abdichtung von gestrickten Gefäßprothesen: Alternativverfahren zum herkömmlichen Preclotting. Angio Archiv 6:167–171
13. Hamann H, Badmann A, Vollmar JF (1985) Rezidivstenosen nach Carotis-TEA. Langenbecks Arch Chir 366:323–326
14. Jeger E (1913) Die Chirurgie der Blutgefäße und des Herzens. Hirschwald, Berlin

15. Kunlin J (1949) Le traitment de l'arterite obliterant par le greffe veineuse. Arch Mal Coeur 42:371
16. Lexer E (1907) Die ideale Operation des arteriellen und arteriovenösen Aneurysma. Langenbecks Arch Chir 83:459
17. LoGerfo FW, Haudenschild CC, Quist WC (1984) A clinical technique for prevention of spasm and preservation of endothelium in saphenous vein grafts. Arch Surg 119:1212–1214
18. Maas D, Zollikofer CL, Largiader F, Senning A (1984) Radiological follow-up of transluminally inserted vascular endoprostheses: an experimental study using expanding spirals. Radiology 152:659–663
19. Müller-Wiefel H (1986) Gefäßprothesen. Chirurg 57:64–71
20. Pinkerton JA (1979) Erosion of Dacron graft by atherosclerotic plaque. J Cardiovasc Surg 20:385–387
21. Prenner K, Rendl KH, Wagner O, Hagmüller G, Maurer PC (eds) (1983) Qualitätssicherung in der Gefäßchirurgie. Angio Archiv 5 Demeter Gräfelfing
22. Sandmann W, Kremer K (1983) Materialprobleme in der Gefäßchirurgie. Chirurg 54:433–443
23. Sauvage LR (1984) Opportunities and responsibilities in the use of arterial grafts. Surg Annu 16:91–117
24. Schulman ML, Badhey MR (1981) Deep veins of the leg as femoropopliteal bypass grafts. Arch Surg 116:1141–1145
25. Seeger JM, Wheeler JR, Gregory RT, Snyder SO, Gayle RG (1983) Autogenous graft replacement of infected prosthetic grafts in the femoral position. Surgery 93:39–45
26. Smith DC (1984) Catheterization of prosthetic vascular grafts: acceptable technique. AJR 143:1117–1118
27. Sparks CH (1973) Silicone mandril method for growing reinforced autogenous femoro-popliteal artery grafts in situ. Ann Surg 177:293–300
28. Starck E, McDermott J, Crummy A, Holzman P, Herzer M, Kollath J (1986) Die perkutane Aspirations-Thromboembolektomie: eine weitere transluminale Angioplastiemethode. Dtsch Med Wochenschr 111:167–172
29. Tilanus HW, Obertop H, Van Urk H (1985) Saphenous vein or PTFE for femoropopliteal bypass. A prospective randomized trial. Ann Surg 202:780–782
30. Veith FJ (1985) Progress in limb salvage arterial surgery: components and results of an aggressive approach. Thorac Cardiovasc Surg 33:374–376
31. Vollmar J, Voss EU (1984) Antibioticaprophylaxe in der Gefäßchirurgie. Chirurg 55:227–231
32. Weinberg DS, Maini BS (1980) Primary sarcoma of the aorta associated with a vascular prosthesis: A case report. Cancer 46:398–402
33. Wright CB, Hobson RW, Hiratzka LF, Lynch TG (1983) Vascular grafting. Clinical applications and techniques. Wright, Boston Bristol London
34. Ziomek S, Quinones-Baldrich WJ, Busuttil RW, Baker JD, Machleder HI, Moore WS (1986) The superiority of synthetic arterial grafts over autologous veins in carotid-subclavian bypass. J Vasc Surg 3:140–145

6 Microvascular Surgery

E. BIEMER

CONTENTS

A. Development of Microvascular Surgery

With modern techniques of vascular surgery, very good results can be achieved in large vessels. However, these methods have not been successful in vessels smaller than 3 mm in diameter. Here, totally new surgical techniques had to be developed. Magnifying instruments were needed because careful manipulation of the very fine structures was not possible with the naked eye. Magnifying glasses, and especially the operating microscope, led to the breakthrough. At the same time, fine instruments and suture materials were developed.

Following the first attempts to anastomose such small vessels successfully [18], the rapid further development of these methods during the last two decades has led to their application in many different fields of clinical medicine. BUNCKE et al. were the first to report [10] on reimplantations of body parts in animal experiments. The first reimplantation in humans was done by TAMAI [19] in 1965. The first to report on vascularized free flaps were DANIEL and TAYLOR [13], after HARII [16] had already done such transplantations in humans.

Today these techniques are found in two main clinical fields: the reimplantation of peripheral-body segments and tissue transplantation.

Beyond this, the technique of microvascular surgery has spread into almost all surgical disciplines because of the possibility of operating on anatomic structures with the finest atraumatic methods. This has led to refined surgical techniques such as recanalization operations of the fallopian tubes, spermatic ducts, etc.

B. Equipment

I. Operating Microscope

The simplest instrument for magnification is the magnifying glass which can be used up to a magnification of $\times 6$. Beyond this, an operating microscope is needed. Following its introduction by NYLEN (1935) in the field of otolaryngology, it was used in ophthalmology. Further development, always in close contact with clinical needs, has made operating microscopes available today which can be put together in a modular fashion so that they can be adjusted to each and every situation. In microvascular surgery, the OPMI 2 and the OPMI 7D of the Zeiss Company have proved especially reliable. The most important features of an operating microscope are:

1. Good mobility and an adequate distance from the operating area
2. Binocular steroscopic vision for surgeon and assistant

3. A well-illuminated operating area
4. Continuous adjustment of magnification, as well as focusing by foot pedals
5. Photographic or video facilities

Further information can be obtained from the manufacturers.

II. Operating Chair (Fig. 6.1)

Special operating chairs have been developed in order to guarantee steady handling of microsurgical instruments without fatigue. Their main advantages are that they have adjustable armrests. These support the forearm from the elbow to the wrist, allowing the surgeon to handle the instruments in a very secure and steady manner. Furthermore, one can smoothly adjust the height of the chair in a vertical direction, which is especially important when operating with a microscope.

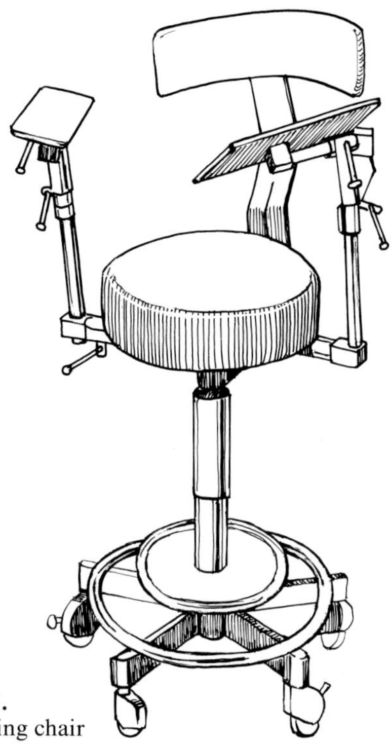

Fig. 6.1. Operating chair

III. Instruments (Fig. 6.2a–j)

On the one hand the basic instruments in microvascular surgery are very simple, while on the other hand they are of very high precision.

Mainly, two straight and one curved watchmaker's forceps (jeweler's forceps) of about 12 cm in length are used. The microsurgical needle holder cannot be locked. Only very little pressure should be needed to close the holder. Its form should be round so that delicate handling of the needle with the fingertips is possible without turning the hand.

Furthermore, one needs straight and curved bulldog scissors. Of great importance are the vessel clamps which are needed for temporary occlusion of the vessel stumps. The pressure on the vessel wall should be as light as possible in order to avoid vessel wall injury. However, the clamp has to occlude the vessel securely and have a good grip so that it does not slip off when touched, owing to the extraordinary flexibility of the vessel wall. Beyond this, its outer surface should be smooth and compact and also closed so that no suture material becomes entangled.

Experimental studies have shown that a closing pressure of 20 g/mm^2 is a good compromise among all of the requirements listed above.

Some surgeons use a vessel adapter. Such an adapter serves to stabilize the ends of both vessels and to approximate them so that a tensionless suture is possible. The great tension between the distal and proximal ends is usually overcome by a slight twisting of the vessel stumps during approximation. This allows the suturing to be done; however, after removing the instrument, the tension on the anastomosis is too great. According to our experience this usually leads to thrombosis. Because many adapters do not have a device for fine regulation of clamping pressure, we only use such adapters in experiments or for training, and never in routine procedures.

For exact cutting of very small vessels and nerve endings, special scissors with a guillotine-like cutting edge have proven very useful. Unlike normal scissors, which keep pushing the tissue forward, these totally encircle the small structures. When using these scissors, fixation with forceps is not needed. In very thin-walled veins, it is often very difficult to obtain a full view of the lumen because the front and back walls stick together. A special spreading instrument has proven very useful in overcoming these difficulties.

Bipolar coagulation is extremely important in microvascular surgery as it is the only method of effecting a precision hemostasis of the very delicate vessels.

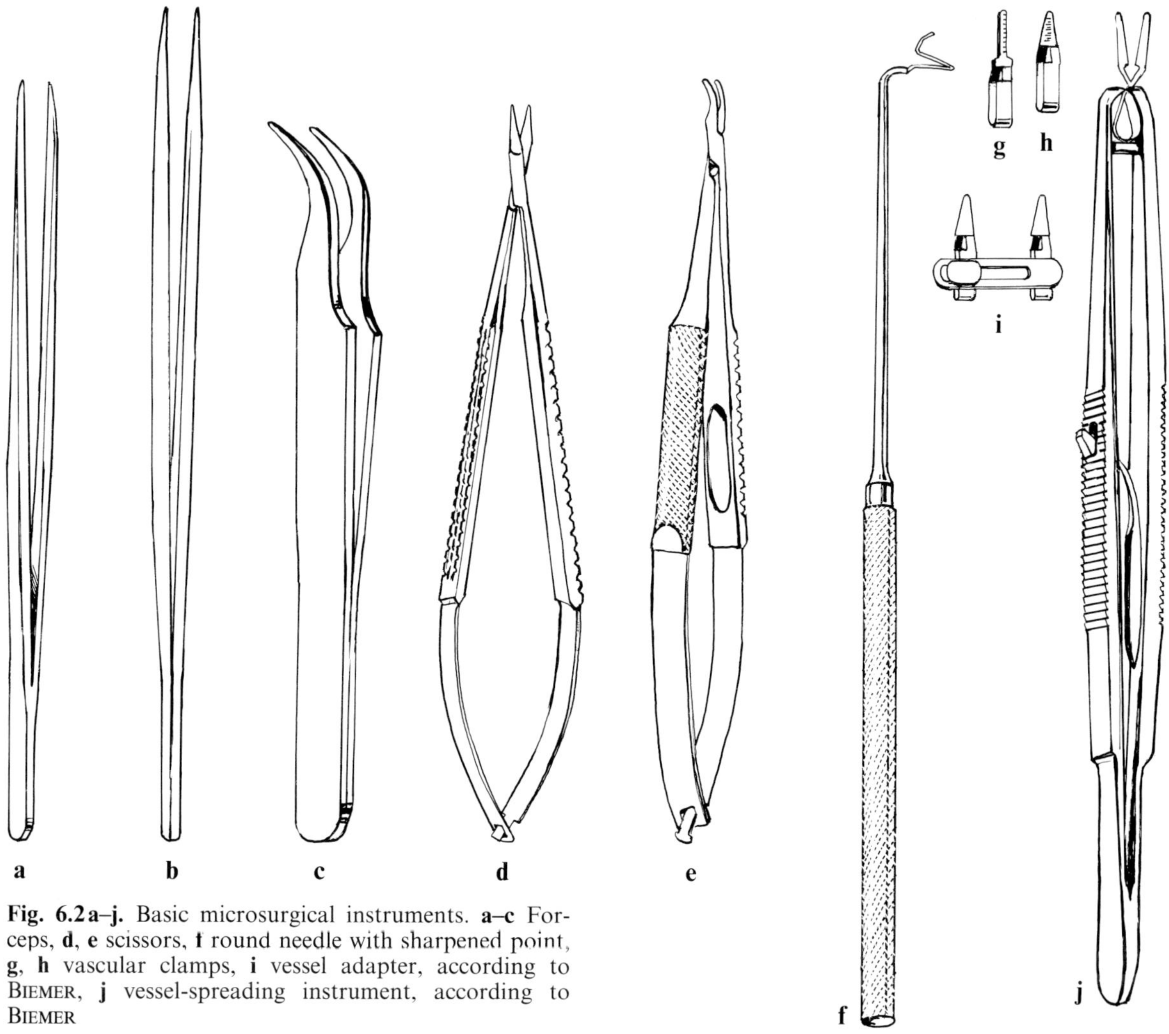

Fig. 6.2a–j. Basic microsurgical instruments. **a–c** Forceps, **d**, **e** scissors, **f** round needle with sharpened point, **g**, **h** vascular clamps, **i** vessel adapter, according to BIEMER, **j** vessel-spreading instrument, according to BIEMER

IV. Suture Materials

In microvascular surgery, the suture materials used are monofilament polyamide or nylon sutures in sizes 10 × 0 or 11 × 0 (25 or 15 μm thick). Sutures 12 × 0 in size (about 10 μm thick with metal-coated points; O'BRIEN 1973) are not usually used in routine procedures. They are sometimes employed in lymphatic – venous anastomoses or in experiments on very small laboratory animals.

Recently, absorbable polyglycol sutures in these sizes have become available. Their clinical use still has to be tested. First investigations show that when used for nerve sutures they are not absorbed soon enough and are therefore an obstacle to growing axons.

These suture materials come with swaged-on round needles that have a 3/8 circle (BV4-, BV6-needles from the Ethicon Company). For a better grasp by the needle holder, modern needles are flattened over their posterior third. Some surgeons prefer sharpened needle points.

C. Microsuture Techniques

I. General Remarks

Experimental training on a model or an animal is always necessary before practicing and learning microvascular surgical techniques. Working under the microscope requires special training if one is to be able to manipulate the microsurgical instruments blindly and confidently in the small magnified operating field. Even the assistant must have great precision and manual skill in these procedures as it is possible to jeopardize or destroy the success of the whole operation by one clumsy movement or through false handling of the vessels.

The small vessels are always picked up by the adventitia, using jeweler's forceps. Touching the intima should always be avoided. The knots are tied only instrumentally. The knots are always tied under direct vision, that is, until both edges of the vessel are adapted well. One can use the long sutures (about 20–25 cm) available commercially or short ones 5–7 cm in length. When using long sutures the needle must be released and put down after every stitch and the whole length of the suture pulled through the tissue. For the next stitch, the needle must again be picked up and grasped by the needle holder. In our experience, this technique is very time-consuming and leads to entanglement and fixation of the suture. This is why we cut the suture down to 5–7 cm. This allows for the needle to be held at all times and for a complete exposure of the whole suture during the sewing process. It is a basic principle to avoid tension at the anastomosis. We do this by incorporating the weakest point of the suture into the tying process which at the same time provides a good indication of the tension at the anastomosis. This weakest point is the segment where the needle is fixed to the suture material. If during the tying process both vessel edges cannot be adapted far enough and the suture tears at its weakest point, then the tension is too great. Under such circumstances the vessel stumps have to be approximated by further preparation, or a venous graft has to be interposed.

Anastomoses near vascular bifurcations or curves have to be avoided (turbulence). Furthermore, a small vessel should never be connected to a larger vessel as considerable turbulence may occur here as well. Although in the early days of microvascular surgery only end-to-end anastomoses were performed, today the end-to-side anastomosis is preferred, especially in tissue transplantations. The view during suturing is improved by putting a colored rubber or plastic strip under the vessel.

II. End-to-end Anastomosis (Fig. 6.3a–i)

In an end-to-end anastomosis of small arteries, a right-angled dissection plane is chosen instead of an oblique one as with larger vessels (Fig. 6.3a). The vascular stumps are occluded with clamps and stabilized (some surgeons achieve stabilization by using a double-clamp adapter.) To complete the suture, both vascular edges have to lie next to each other without tension. The periadventitial tissue and the adventitia are retracted in order to prevent them from falling into the lumen. The vascular lumen is carefully dilated with a jeweler's forceps (Fig. 6.3b). This gives a better view and eliminates spastic narrowing of the vessel. With this technique, one can compensate some differences in the diameter of the two vessel ends. Afterward, the lumina are flushed with a warm heparinized normal saline (10 units/ml; Fig. 6.3c). The anastomosis is completed with interrupted sutures tied instrumentally in the order 2, 1, 1, always using square knots. The needle holder is held like a pen. The suture should not be longer than 5–6 cm so that its whole length is visible within the operating field. The needle is inserted tangentially, not vertically, and, as with a skin suture, from the outside inward through all layers of the vessel wall, including the intima (Fig. 6.3d). Inserting the needle tangentially almost completely eliminates the danger of catching the back wall of the vessel. The distance of the suture from the vascular edges should be about twice the wall thickness.

When pushing the needle through, one has to be very careful to avoid catching the posterior wall. The stitch is completed by inserting the suture through the wall of the opposite stump from the inside to the outside. The needle is picked up by a microforceps, and the suture is pulled through until its end is clearly visible and has reached an accessible position.

When the needle is raised toward the lens of the microscope and then returned to the operating area, a loop is created which is directed toward the needle holder (Fig. 6.3e). This makes it easier to tie the knot. The vessel edges are approximated until they touch each other. One end of the suture is kept long in order to use it as a stay suture later on.

The second suture is placed at a distance of about 120° (COBBETT [11] asymmetric biangulation; Fig. 6.3f). Now, when traction is placed on both stay sutures, the posterior walls are pulled apart so that the surgeon has a better view of the anastomosis and can avoid accidentally catching the anterior wall when suturing the posterior wall.

The suture of the front wall is now completed (Fig. 6.3g). The vessel is then rotated by turning the double clamp or both vascular clamps

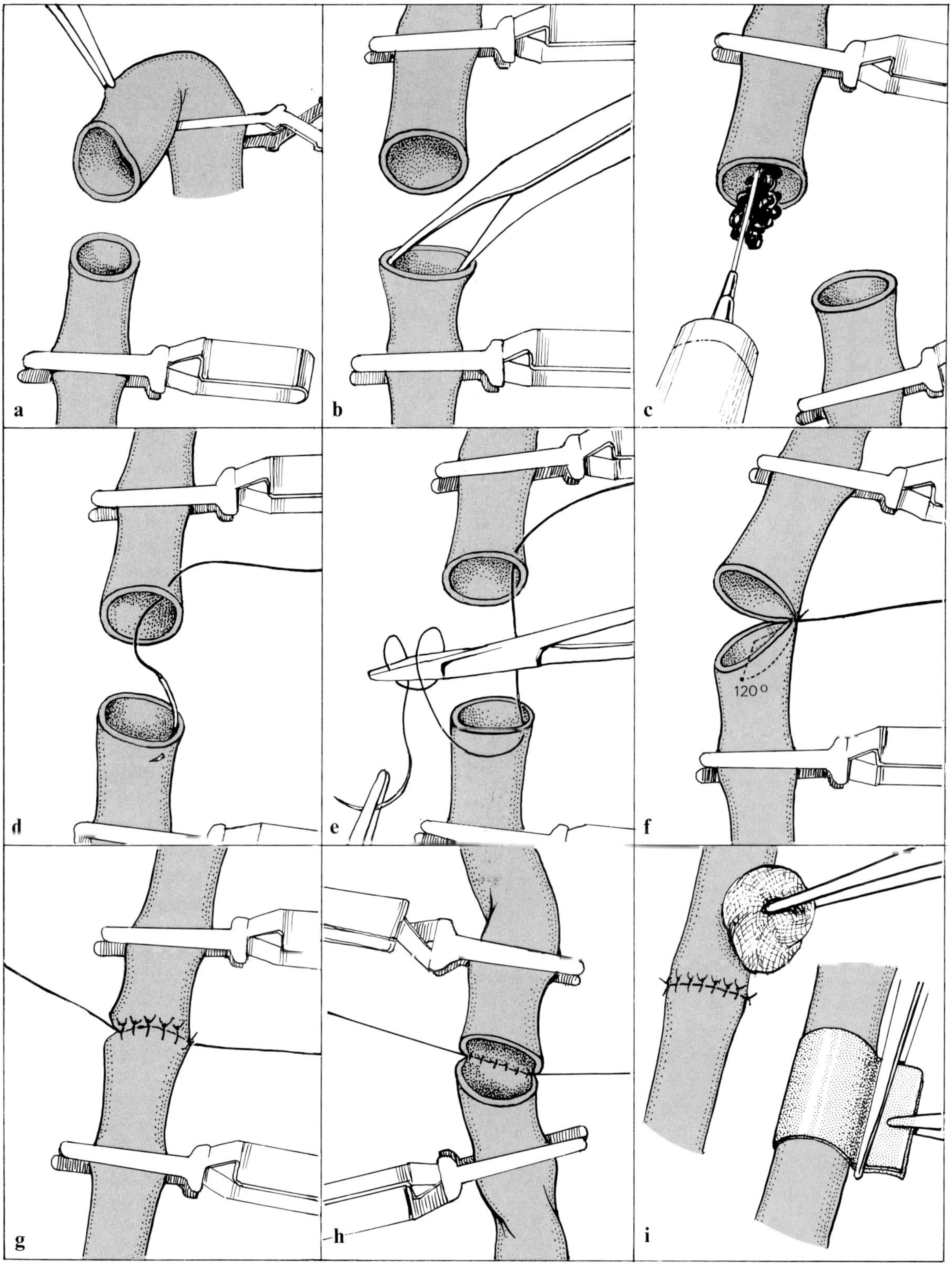

Fig. 6.3a–i. Microsurgical end-to-end anastomosis

(Fig. 6.3h). If rotation is not possible for spatial or anatomic reasons, the posterior wall may be sutured by means of a climbing technique in which each previously tied suture is left long and used for traction.

Basically, arteries and veins are sutured in the same fashion. Because the pressure in a vein is much lower than in an artery, only 4–6 stitches are needed to complete the anastomosis of a vein 1 mm in diameter. In an artery of the same size, 8–10 stiches are required.

After completion of the anastomosis, first the distal and then the proximal clamps are removed. For a few minutes the anastomosis is covered with gauze in order to achieve hemostasis. Final closure is achieved later by means of a platelet thrombus (Fig. 6.3i).

III. End-to-side Anastomosis (Fig. 6.4a, b)

Experiments show that angulation at the anastomosis between the vessel and the lumen being sutured to it is not of great importance. This is why the right-angled anastomosis technique is preferred.

An oval patch large enough for the anastomosis is cut out of the wall of the host vessel. Some authors recommend only a transverse incision which becomes a round hole under the tension of the vascular wall (Fig. 6.4a).

First, two sutures are placed 180° from each other at both corners of the incision (Fig. 6.4b). If the vessel cannot be rotated for direct visualization of the back wall, the back wall should be sutured first, followed by the front wall. It is advisable to place the last 2–3 sutures without tying them immediately. This makes it possible to maintain a better view during completion of the anastomosis.

The end-to-side anastomosis has the advantage that differences in diameter no longer matter and main vessels do not have to be transected during anastomoses of grafts.

IV. Telescopic Anastomosis (Fig. 6.5a–c)

As microsurgical techniques were being developed, there were many attempts to simplify suture techniques so as to speed up the anastomosis and achieve hemostasis sooner, thereby minimizing blood loss. For example the attempt was made to stabilize the anastomosis with 2–3 stay sutures and prevent leakage by filling the spaces in between with fibrin glue [21]. To facilitate hemostasis, plastic strips were wrapped around the anastomosis for a few minutes, or sometimes even a vein segment was slipped over the anastomosis. However, these techniques were never of any clinical value. The best solution seems to be the telescopic anastomosis which is performed by pulling a section of the vessel into the opposite lumen in the direction of blood flow (see Fig. 6.5a). Stabilization is established by two corner sutures placed

Fig. 6.4a, b. Microsurgical end-to-side anastomosis

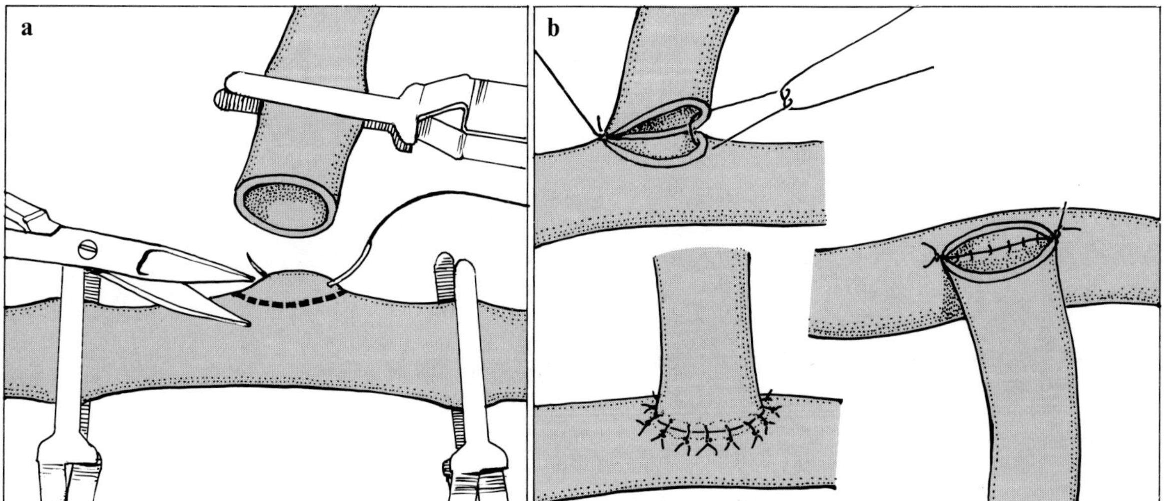

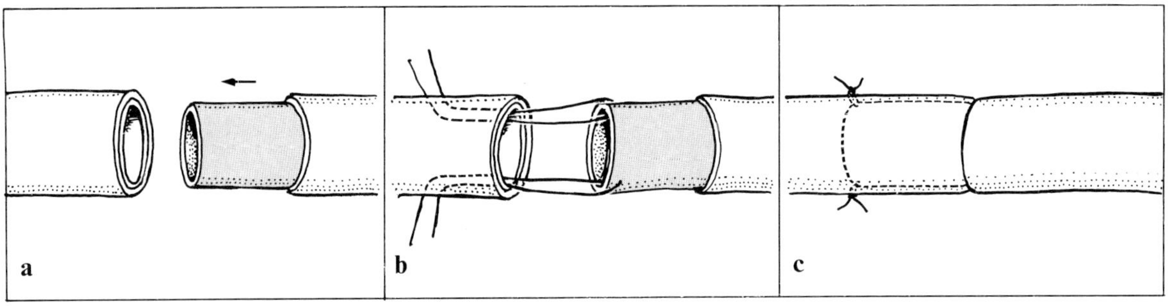

Fig. 6.5a–c. Telescopic anastomosis

exactly opposite to one another (Fig. 6.5b, c). The telescopic anastomosis is suited to situations in which the distal vessel is of greater diameter than the proximal one. Otherwise, kinking and distortion of the invaginated vessel is possible. Furthermore, this suture technique is successful only if completed in the direction of blood flow. Because in tissue transplantation and reimplantation the distal vessel is usually smaller than the proximal one, the telescopic anastomosis has limited indications. Beyond that, the end-to-side anastomosis is preferred because it preserves the continuity of the larger vessel.

V. Anastomosis of Vessels with Different Diameters (Fig. 6.6a–d)

Whenever possible, only vessels of the same or nearly the same diameter should anastomosed to one another. If this is not possible for anatomic reasons and if a direct end-to-end anastomosis seems too risky, one of the following techniques should be applied:

a) Dilatation (Fig. 6.6a)
b) Fishmouth incision (Fig. 6.6b)
c) Oblique transection (Fig. 6.6c)
d) Venous graft interposition (Fig. 6.6d)

When using the fishmouth method it is often very difficult to achieve an exact adaptation of both vessel ends.

If the edge of the smaller vessel is cut obliquely, the anastomosis may develop kinking later on, which can lead to thrombosis.

Therefore, we recommend the interposition of a venous graft. Because of the great elasticity of the walls of the vein, one end of the graft can be dilated to about three times the size of the other end. This ensures nonturbulent continuous blood flow at the anastomosis.

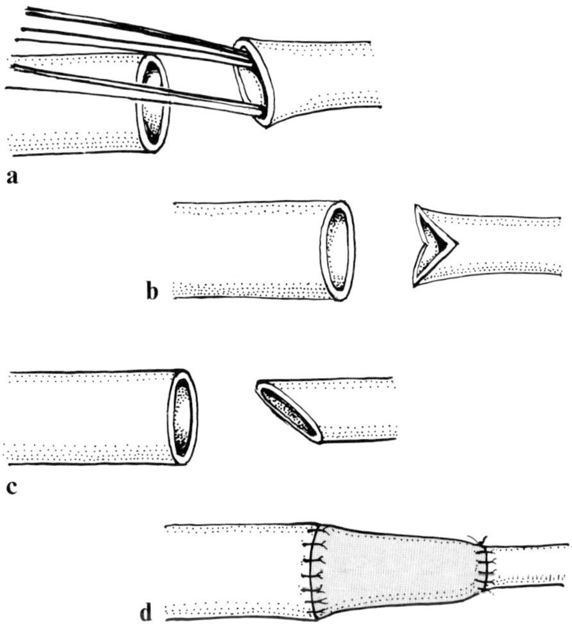

Fig. 6.6a–d. Anastomosis of vessels with different diameters. **a** Variable dilatation, **b** fishmouth incision, **c** oblique transection, **d** interposition of a venous graft after its ends have been dilated to fit the different calibers of the host vessel

VI. Venous Graft Interposition

Venous graft interposition plays an important role in microvascular surgery for such clinical applications as reimplantation and tissue transplantation.

Indications for microvenous graft interpositions are as follows:

1. Vascular defects
2. Tension at the anastomosis
3. Vascular shunts

4. Anastomosis of vessels with different diameters
5. Difficult anastomoses of very short vessels located deep in the wound (difficult to achieve good suture of the back walls by turning the vessel over because rotation is not possible)

Donor sites for small vein grafts: The best areas for obtaining microvenous grafts are the volar side of the wrist or the dorsum of the foot. There, one finds a clearly visible and easily dissectable venous network with vessels in suitable sizes, about 1–3 mm in diameter. They protrude when only slightly obstructed.

Technique of small vein graft interposition: Before implantation of the grafts, exact ligation of all tributaries must be carried out carefully; otherwise, clots will form at these sites.

Careful ligation is best performed under the microscope using 10×0 nylon purse-string ligatures. The graft must not be damaged, and the surrounding tissue must be removed. It should be kept moist with normal saline to prevent drying out. Where venous grafts are used between arteries, the veins must be reversed before insertion because of their valves.

Rules for venous graft interpositions:
1. Equivalent diameter
2. Correct length of graft
3. Removal of periadventitial tissue
4. Exact ligation of tributaries
5. No angulation of arterialized vein grafts

Before harvesting a vein graft, one should carefully estimate its diameter since spastic contraction often occurs following dissection. In such cases, pseudoaneurysmal dilatation may result after the spasm has subsided, often revealing a graft too great in diameter.

In oblique arteriovenous – arterial connections, distortion of the arterial stump must be avoided. Otherwise, pulsation causes straightening of the arteries, followed by twisting and narrowing of the vein graft. In conjunction with the acute angle at the anastomosis, thrombosis may occur at this site.

VII. Lymphatic Vessels

After accomplishing the successful anastomosis of small blood vessels, the next logical step was to try to connect lymphatic vessels using the same microscopic techniques. Indications for such operations were congenital and secondary lymphedema, such as lymphedema of the arm following radical mastectomy or axillary irradiation.

In the former group, the application of microsurgery is limited by agenesis of the lymphatic vasculature, especially of the collecting vessel. In the latter group, interrupted lymphatic vessel must be reconstructed or bypassed. Basically, there are two ways of accomplishing this:

1. Drainage of the lymph into the venous system (lymphatic – venous anastomosis)
2. Bypass of the interrupted lymphatic vessel by autogenous lymphatic or venous graft (see p. 798).

D. Functional Tests for Anastomoses
(Fig. 6.7a–c)

After completing a small vessel anastomosis, it is often very difficult to decide if there is blood flow through the vascular connection. Peripheral arterial and venous return may fill the vessel on both

Fig. 6.7a–c. Functional test of the anastomosis using two jeweler's forceps

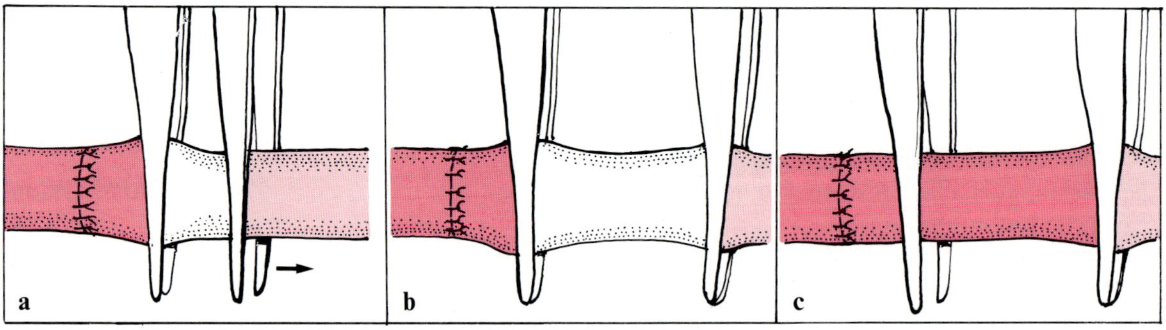

sides of the anastomosis, making this assessment even more difficult. Furthermore, a transmitted arterial pulse wave may simulate arterial pulsation distal to the suture line. The best proof of good flow at the anastomosis is, of course, visible perfusion of a reimplanted finger or of a transplanted tissue block. However, because this process is often delayed, a method of immediate assessment is needed.

The simplest technique is to express a portion of the vessel in the direction of the blood flow using a microsurgical forceps while at the same time occluding the vessel just distal to the anastomosis with a second forceps (Fig. 6.7a). Then, with pressure still on the first forceps, so as to maintain occlusion and prevent possible reflux, the pressure on the second forceps is released; if the anastomosis is intact, the vessel segment will be filled. The time needed for complete filling can be used for assessing a free or obstructed blood flow (Fig. 6.7b, c). One can distinguish between a localized or a transmitted pulsation by exerting tension on the pulsating vessel part in the direction of the segment to be examined. Such tension interrupts the transmission, and the tension release intensifies autonomous localized pulsation.

E. Thrombosis and Thrombectomy

Naturally, the severest complication in microvascular surgery is thrombosis at the suture line.

Expressing thrombotic material in the direction of blood flow is usually not successful because the cause of thrombosis is not eliminated. Therefore, recurrence is frequent.

Causes of thrombosis:
1. Unrepaired vascular wall damage, especially to the intima
2. Traumatic suture technique
3. Catching the back wall
4. Inverted adventitia
5. Anastomosis under tension
6. Connection of a vein to an artery
7. Unintended suturing and fixation of valves in the veins
8. A nearby tributary (formation of turbulence)

Therefore, it is necessary to resect the anastomotic site together with a small portion of the vessel containing the thrombus. A venous graft is then usually needed in most cases to bridge the defect.

Total occlusion of the anastomosis should always be detected as early as possible and should be corrected immediately. Stasis very quickly leads to enlargement of the thrombus which may spread into the capillary bed and become irreversible. In such a case, the smallest Fogarty catheter or flushing with heparinized normal saline may help.

If there is only an obstruction of the venous outflow and this cannot be eliminated, it is possible to prevent dangerous stasis in replants and transplants by other methods:

1. By exsanguination
2. By applying leeches

The blood which cannot flow through the venous system can be drained into the wound dressing through evenly distributed skin incisions. The measure is supported by systemic heparinization of the patient. It must be taken into account that this procedure may provoke severe bleeding which must be under constant observation by measuring hemoglobin and hematocrit levels. If necessary, blood transfusions must be given. A more elegant method is the application of leeches at regular intervals. By sucking the blood they facilitate good drainage of the venous congestion. These manipulations must be carried out until the 6th to 8th postoperative day, after which the necessary vascular connections have developed by spontaneous capillary growth. Because large amounts of blood are usually lost and transfusions are necessary, these methods should be applied only under special conditions with a strict indication.

F. Drug Therapy

All pharmacologic alternatives are used in the prevention of thrombosis.

Today, heparin is applied intraoperatively only as a local flushing agent, or it is given for a limited time (5000 units per 60 kg body weight). It is given postoperatively only in some instances where special indications in reimplantation surgery make it necessary (Chap. 14). Coumarin preparations have been given mainly as long-term preparations following reimplantations in China.

Dipyridamole and acetylsalicylic acid are given to block platelet aggregation. We give 20 mg dipyridamole intraoperatively and postoperatively as a compound preparation orally for 6 days (Asasantin, Thomae). Low molecular weight dextran

(Rheomacrodex, Knoll) has proven very efficient in improving microcirculation. This is also administered before reestablishing blood flow. During the postoperative period, 500 ml is given daily for 6 days in adults. Today, Promit (Knoll) must be given prior to dextran because of possible allergic reactions.

However, drug therapy has lost its importance in microvascular surgery. Today, most operations are done without any adjuvant drugs. Refined technique provides better results than any medication could ever achieve.

G. Clinical Application

I. Replantation of Peripheral Body Segments (Micro- or Small Replantation)

In addition to the now relatively common reattachment of amputated hands, microsurgical replantation has also been employed with remarkable success in dealing with other, less common injuries, such as scalping, avulsion inuries to the face, and amputations of the penis or the foot (Chap. 14).

II. Vascularized Free Flaps

Until now, defects of soft tissue or larger tissue parts such as bones, muscles, joints, thumbs, and long fingers could not be replaced at all. It is in this field that microvascular surgery has made an essential breakthrough and created new possibilities that surgeons for centuries could only dream of. The basic principle is to resect tissue or a tissue block together with its vascular supply and connect it to vessels at the site of the defect. The intensive study of the anatomy of peripheral nerve and vascular systems form the anatomic basis of this technique. Today, almost every loss can be replaced using the right flap. We distinguish:

Vascularized free flaps:

a) Simple flaps, consisting of skin and subcutaneous tissue
b) Combined flaps:
   1. Myocutaneous flaps, consisting of muscles, skin, and subcutaneous tissue
   2. Osteocutaneus flaps, consisting of bone, skin, and subcutaneous tissue
   3. So-called sensitive flaps, consisting of simple flaps together with their nerve supply
   4. Tendinocutaneous flaps, consisting of simple flaps with the corresponding tendons attached to them

Single Tissues: The following tissues may be transplanted: Muscles, epiphyses, thumbs, omentum, bones, parts of the gastrointestinal tract.

Complex Transplants: Toes, two toes en bloc, or a combination of simple flaps with different single tissues as needed. Such transplants have replaced other methods such as pediculated flaps which were formerly used to cover defects.

III. Surgery of the Lymphatic Vessels

Today, there are many procedures which can be applied in this field (see p. 791 ff., 796 ff.).

REFERENCES

1. Baumeister RGH, Seifert J, Wiebecke B, Hahn D (1981) Experimental basis and first application of clinical lymph-vessel transplantation of secondary lymphedema. World J Surg 5:401–407
2. Biemer E (1977) Microvenous grafts in microvascular surgery. Br J Plast Surg 30:197
3. Biemer E (1981) Salvage operations for complications following replantation and free tissue transfer. Int Surg 66:37
4. Biemer E (1984) Handrekonstruktion. Münchner Med Wochenschr 126:394
5. Biemer E, Duspiva W (1979) Rekonstruktive Mikrogefäßchirurgie. Springer, Berlin Heidelberg New York
6. Biemer E, Schmidt-Tintemann U (1983) Anatomische und funktionelle Grundlagen für die Wahl von Nahtmaterialien und Nahttechniken in der klinischen Mikrochirurgie. In: Thiede A, Hamelmann H (eds) Moderne Nahtmaterialien und Nahttechniken in der Chirurgie. Springer, Berlin, Heidelberg New York
7. Buck-Gramcko D (1984) Mikrochirurgie peripherer Gefäße. Experimentelle Untersuchungen und klinische Anwendung. Handchirurgie 6:101
8. Buncke HJ, Schulz WP (1966) Total ear reimplantation in the rabbit utilizing microminiature vascular anastomoses. Br J Plast Surg 10:15
9. Buncke HJ, Buncke CM, Schulz WB (1965) Experimental digital amputation and reimplantation. Plast Reconstr Surg 36:62
10. Buncke HJ, Buncke CM, Schulz WP (1966) Immediate Nicoladoni procedure in the rhesus monkey, or hallux-to-hand transplantation, utilizing microminiature vascular anastomoses. Br J Plast Surg 19:332
11. Cobbett JR (1969) Small vessel surgery in hand. Hand 1:57

12. Cobbett JR (1976) Small vessel anastomosis. Br J Plast Surg 20:16
13. Daniel RK, Taylor GI (1973) Distant transfer of an island flap by microvascular anastomoses. Plast Reconstr Surg 52:111
14. Daniel RK, Terzis JK (1977) Reconstructive microsurgery. Little, Brown and Co., Boston
15. Duspiva W, Biemer E (1976) Technik der Mikrogefäßchirugie. Med Welt 17:852
16. Harii K (1970) Mündliche Mitteilung
17. Ingianni G, Holzmann T (1983) Klinische Erfahrungen in der Anwendung von lymphovenösen Anastomosen beim sekundären Lymphödem. Handchirurgie 15:215–218
18. Jacobsen JH, Suarez EI 61960) Microsurgery in small vessel anastomosis. Surg Forum 11:243
19. Komatsu S, Tamai S (1968) Successful replantation of a completely cut-off thumb. Plast Reconstr Surg 42:374
20. Mandel H (1981) Experimentelle Untersuchungen zur mikrochirurgischen Rekonstruktion von Lymphgefäßdefekten. Plast Chir 5/2:70–92
21. Matras H, Chiari FM, Kletter G, Dinges HP (1977) Zur Klebung kleinster Gefäße im Tierversuch. Dtsch Z Mund Kiefer Gesichts Chir 1:19
22. O'Brien B McC (1977) Microvascular reconstructive surgery. Churchill Livingstone, Edinburgh
23. O'Brien B McC, Shafiroff BB (1979) Microlymphatic-venous and resectional surgery in obstructive lymphedema. World J Surg 3:3–15

7 Conservative and Radiologic Measures

7.1 General Procedures in the Management of the Vascular Surgical Patient

H. RIEGER and W. SCHOOP

CONTENTS

A. Introduction

Most patients who need vascular surgery have several risk factors and other diseases which raise the risk of anesthesia and surgery considerably [1]. The patient's preoperative condition is a very important parameter of surgical risk as shown by the American Society of Anesthesiologists in over 34000 patients (general overview in [11]).

Especially in the group of vascular surgical patients, preoperative risk is about two to three times higher than in general surgical patients [1]. Of course, this influences the surgeon's judgement of the patient's operability.

In elective vascular surgery, it is possible to treat the patient preoperatively in cooperation with the internist and anesthesiologist. This is not the case if vascular operations have to be performed under urgent or emergency conditions, which naturally have a much higher general risk. In elective vascular surgery, the patient's individual status must be considered. Besides preoperative reduction of local and general risk factors, a very important part of treatment as a whole is the postoperative therapy and follow-up. The latter, just as much as the former, are essential factors in successful therapy.

B. Preoperative Management

I. Improvement of Local Operating Conditions

1. Weight Reduction

Overweight raises the chance of local wound complications, especially deep wound infections with considerable risk to the extremity, or even to life. It also causes operative difficulties, thereby prolonging the duration of surgery. If elective surgery is planned, there is usually enough time for the reduction of body weight. There are different ways of reducing weight which are mentioned on p. 103. Success depends on the patient's motivation, mentality, and compliance; however, the physician has great influence on all of these.

2. Prophylaxis Against Infections (see p. 166)

The implantation of vascular prostheses must always be approached as a highly aseptic procedure. That it usually is explains why wound and prosthesis infections are very rare (1%–16%). General pre- and perioperative prophylaxis with antibiotics is not indicated [5].

However, deep infection of a surgical wound, usually in the inguinal region and orginating from an infection of a graft or anastomosis, is one of the most dangerous complications of any vascular reconstruction. Its consequences are dehiscence, anastomotic aneurysm (pseudoaneurysm), and life-threatening septic thrombosis. The following measures may be undertaken to prevent such complications:

- Hygiene of the inguinal region. If necessary local antibiotic, antimycotic, or antiseptic treatment
- Preoperative antibiotic treatment (determination of antimicrobial sensitivity!) of infected distal necroses (danger of lymphatic spread of bacteria from the groin)
- No preoperative angiograms within the designated operating area (arterial puncture, if possible, on the opposite side)
- Preoperative percutaneous transluminal angioplasty attempts using, if possible, a cross-over technique from the contralateral side to preserve the operating area
- Treatment of defects of host defense (immune defects) and bacteremia of different etiology and, if necessary, antibiotic prophylaxis
- Preoperative weight reduction (see p. 103)

3. Treatment of Edema in Chronic Venous Insufficiency

If a patient needing vascular surgery has chronic venous insufficiency, with or without visible edema, it is important to eliminate congestion preoperatively as such patients have a higher risk of developing deep vein thrombosis postoperatively. Raising the foot of the bed (20–30 cm) and compression (elastic bandages, intermittent mechanical pressure treatment with the Jobst apparatus) are the most important therapeutic measures. The principle of mechanical intermittent compression according to Jobst is that a boot surrounding the leg generates a certain pressure for a preselected length of time. Initially, treatment should commence with high compression to transport the interstitial fluid and inflammatory substances back into the vascular system (reabsorption pressure > filtration pressure). This goal is achieved best by a well-fitting nonstretchable pressure bandage.

The situation becomes more difficult if the congested leg presents with occlusive arterial disease reducing arterial pressure. In such a case, there is danger of intensifying ischemia by additional compression. However, above a systolic arterial ankle pressure of 70/80 mmHg, the arterial perfusion of the leg will not be affected in a negative way. At lower arterial pressures, the degree of compression must be carefully chosen, and the patient must be watched closely. Special care must be taken if the patient has reduced sensitivity (e.g., polyneuropathy) as ischemic pain is not noticed in such cases.

Mobilizing venous edema with diuretics should not be done (see p. 102).

If operative procedures on the venous system are planned (vein stripping, etc.) the preoperative measures for eliminating congestion mentioned above are indispensable. Inflammations in the area of the superficial venous systems (superficial thrombophlebitis) must be eliminated by drainage procedures without ordering bed rest(!). If necessary, local and systemic antiphlogistic treatment should be applied.

II. Improvement of General Operating Conditions

1. Concomitant Diseases in Other Vascular Regions

a) Coronary Arteries (see p. 191). In 3%–6% of all larger vascular operations, death is due to primary cardiac causes [13]. This is primarily a result of coronary heart disease, which occurs with high frequency in patients with peripheral circulatory disorders. Reports on the incidence of coronary artery disease in patients with peripheral vascular disease vary, depending on the severity of occlusive arterial disease and the diagnostic criteria for coronary artery disease. Of all patients who are candidates for aortoiliac reconstruction, 35% have coronary artery disease as diagnosed by coronary arteriogram [12].

The internist's main concern should be to estimate cardiac risk preoperatively. The cardiac risk index [8] given in Tables 7.1.1 and 7.1.2 may help in this evaluation. A subtle and discriminating inquiry into the patient's history of illness as well as resting and exercise electrocardiograms are necessary diagnostic procedures. However, sufficient interpretation of the exercise electrocardiogram on a bicycle ergometer is not always possible at the maximum exercising level because the patient's performance is limited by the occlusive arterial disease. If necessary, the ejection fraction must be determined by radionuclide ventriculography as a parameter for myocardial pumping capacity, and preoperative coronary angiograms must be performed. Especially prior to elective surgery, it must be judged whether cardiac function can be improved preoperatively (e.g., drug therapy). In

Table 7.1.1. Scoring system for the preoperative estimation of cardiac risk. (From [8])

Criteria	Points
Case history	
Older than 70	5
Myocardial infarction within the last 6 months	10
Medical examination	
Gallop rhythm, prominent jugular veins	12
Stenosis of the aortic valve	3
Electrocardiogram	
All types of rhythm except sinus rhythm	7
5 or more premature beats per minute	7
General condition	
PO_2 60 mmHg or PCO_2 50 mm Hg	3
K^+ 3 mmol/l or HCO_3^- 20 mmol/l	
Urea nitrogen 50 mg % or creatinine 3 mg %	
SGOT increase or liver diseases	
Vascular surgery planned	
Intraperitoneal, intrathoracic, aortic	3
Emergency operation	4

Table 7.1.2. According to the point catalogue in Table 7.1.1 the following risk groups can be classified. (From [8])

Group	Points	Complications (%)	Deaths (%)
1	0–5	0.7	0.2
2	6–12	5	2
3	13–25	11	2
4	26	22	56

emergency situations, these considerations are secondary. However, together with the internist, one should ask if the patient's cardiac situation may be improved within 12 h (this time interval is dependent on the acuteness of the vascular situation.

b) Cerebral Arteries (see also p. 193). Flow obstruction within the supra-aortal cerebral arteries can be diagnosed by history, auscultation, palpation, Doppler sonography, B-scan sonography, and angiographically by digital subtraction angiography or conventional techniques. The incidence of hemodynamically effective supra-aortal flow obstructions together with simultaneous peripheral obstructive arterial disease is 30%–35% in patients over 60–65 years old [17].

There is still great controversy as to what extent a concomitant arterial narrowing, especially within the internal carotid artery, is an anesthesiologic or surgical risk and whether such a lesion should be corrected prior to elective vascular surgery. The decision should be made after careful consideration of the clinical stage of cerebral arterial insufficiency.

Stage I. Generally, the spontaneous outcome of an asymptomatic stenosis of the internal carotid artery is not exactly known. The studies published covered too small a population and do not differentiate between localization and degree of stenosis, so that a general indication for a (prophylactic) operation cannot be concluded. Computer-tomographically positive stage 1 patients and those with high grade stenoses, where the remaining diameter is less than 1.5–2 mm, are possibly at risk for transient ischemic attack (TIA) or cerebrovascular accident (CVA). Such patients should undergo endarterectomy if the operative mortality is not greater than 2% [4].

At the moment there are no figures [2, 18] which show how many patients undergoing elective vascular surgery have a concomitant asymptomatic stenosis of the internal carotid artery and therefore a higher risk of having a TIA or CVA. The incidence of TIAs or CVAs within a surgical patient group for which there is no data on the carotid arteries is no greater than in a group of patients with repaired carotid arteries. This fact raises doubts as to the general necessity of operative correction of the carotid artery prior to vascular surgery for other reasons [20]. Here, too, high grade and double-sided asymptomatic stenosis have to be judged differently.

Stage II. Although many studies and reports emphasize the benefit of carotid surgery in TIAs for the prevention of repeated attacks or complete CVAs, the only controlled multicenter clinical study did not obtain clear results (general review in [15]). On the other hand, TIAs are obvious and impressive precursors of a neurologic deficit which may become manifest later on. Since the presence of TIAs implies greater likelihood of a CVA, the presumed stenosis of the carotid artery should be eliminated before other vascular procedures are performed.

Stages III and IV. Patients with a CVA or a progressive reversible ischemic neurologic defect (PRIND) should, of course, not undergo vascular surgery if the 8-h mark has been passed. Later, the possibility of an extra-intracranial bypass may be discussed in each case (see p. 488).

2. Further Important Diseases and Risk Factors

a) Arterial Hypertension (see also p. 192). Preoperative control of arterial hypertension should only be done after full consideration of total circulatory homeostasis. Naturally, the rare secondary forms of hypertension should receive causal treatment, or, if this is not possible, then at least normal blood pressure values should be reached by drug therapy. Essential hypertension is treated according to the usual guidelines of medical antihypertensive therapy. It is difficult to devise a special preoperative treatment scheme because sudden critical rises in blood pressure may occur intraoperatively (clamping syndrome, sympathetic hyperactivity, stimulation of the renin – angiotensin system), with the danger of acute left heart failure, a coronary infarct, intracerebral hemorrhage, or an anastomotic aneurysm as well as life-threatening drops in blood pressure (declamping syndrome, blood loss, vasovagal syndrome) with the danger of ischemic encephalomalacia. Compared with general surgical patients, patients having vascular surgery react more often intraoperatively with sudden critical hypertensive episodes (17.7% compared with 5%) or a sudden drop in blood pressure (31.4% compared with 9.9% [1]).

Basically, one can say that, preoperatively, hypertension should not be treated too rigorously because if hypertensive episodes occur during surgery, these can be brought under control more easily (clonidine, sodium nitroprusside, calcium antagonists) than a sudden drop in blood pressure, possibly with life-threatening shock symptoms. Less rigorously treated patients have a more stable blood pressure during the operation than untreated patients. Preoperative antihypertensive therapy should be chosen in such a way that reductions of the extracellular space and electrolyte shifts (for example, potassium loss) are avoided. Diuretic therapy should be discontinued or changed 24–48 h before the operation [6]. Monoamino oxidase inhibitors are contraindicated perioperatively because they block necessary sympathetic counterregulation. They reinforce the effect of barbiturates, morphine, atropine, ganglion blockers, and anesthetics [9]. Accordingly, reserpine, guanethidine, and methyldopa have more advantages because sympathetic activity is only partially suppressed. Beta-blockers, vasodilators (dihydralazine, prazosin, and others) and calcium antagonists may be considered more appropriate preoperatively, especially since they have a cardioprotective effect.

b) Diabetes Mellitus. In diabetes treated orally (type II diabetes) therapy is discontinued on the day of the operation and glucose levels are constantly monitored. Corrections may be achieved by 5% glucose solutions given intravenously or by an adequate dose of regular insulin (levels >250 mg %). In insulin dependent patients (especially in type I diabetes) total discontinuation of insulin substitution is not advisable because a basic requirement of about 1 unit/h insulin is needed, even though the patients have no food intake. It is advisable to reduce the morning dose on the day of the operation to about one half or one third of the patient's usual dose, administering it in 500 ml of a 5% levulose or 5% glucose solution.

c) Congestive Heart Failure. Preoperative treatment of myocardial insufficiency is the same as in internal medicine [3]. In clinically manifest cardiac insufficiency (stage III and IV CNYHA) – other than tachyarrhythmia absoluta – the indication for digitalis treatment is unquestionable [7]. Digitalization in stage II (signs of cardiac insufficiency only under great exertion, free of symptoms under normal conditions) is controversial. However, in view of the preoperative situation of a vascular surgical patient and the above-average incidence of hypertensive episodes (see p. 193) with sudden left heart failure and an abrupt increase of cardiac workload, preoperative digitalization cannot be rejected in general. On the other hand, routine preoperative (prophylactic) digitalization cannot be advocated today (overall review in [19]).

d) COPD. A clinical and pathologic – anatomic explanation of the term COPD will not be given at this point. Pulmonary emphysema, chronic bronchitis, and bronchial asthma show etiologic and pathogenetic similarities and interconnections which are most difficult to distinguish. These diseases may manifest themselves in chronic respiratory insufficiency, with or without right ventricular strain, and this fact is of decisive importance for the preoperative situation. Respiratory insufficiency is defined as a disorder of external breathing (ventilation) which is documented by pathologic pulmonary function values.

Some 60%–70% of surgical patients show pathologic spirometric and blood gas measurements. Obstructive ventilatory disorders are more common than restrictive ones. This is especially the case in vascular surgical patients because, naturally, the pulmonary risk factor nicotine is predominant in this group. The necessity of postoperative artificial respiration, primarily due to pulmonary causes, is 9.1% in the vascular surgery group, compared with 2.5% in the general surgery group [1].

Preoperative measures should be to quit smoking (elimination of mucous membrane irritants allowing for generation of the cilia), breathing exercises, aerosol administration (mucolytics and/or bronchodilators) and, in cases of infected sputum, antibiotic treatment. High grade obstructions (asthmatic or spastic bronchitis) make systemic bronchial dilatation necessary. Selected patients should acquaint themselves preoperatively with the method of intermittent positive pressure breathing ([14] see p. 313).

e) Obesity. Besides diminishing local complications (see p. 99), weight reduction in cases of obesity also improves general operating conditions. It has a positive influence on preexisting arterial hypertension or on diabetes mellitus. Experience shows that a reduction of body weight leads to a decrease in blood pressure and a better control of diabetic metabolism. Furthermore, diabetes mellitus may be converted to a less serious stage which may make insulin substitution unnecessary. All in all, one can obtain a drastic decrease of typical intraoperative and postoperative risks, which are present in vascular surgical patients at a much higher rate.

The most efficient form of treatment is the so-called zero diet, with certain precautions and adjuvant therapeutic measures (intake of the daily minimal requirement of calorie free fluids up to 3l, potassium substitution, uric acid reduction, etc.). One can achieve a daily reduction in body fat of about 400 g, depending on initial body weight. The undesirable protein catabolism may be compensated by daily administration of a protein mixture (Ulmer drink).

For a patient prior to vascular surgery, a calorie-reduced diet is preferable. Daily weight reduction on a 300 kcal diet is only about 10%–15% less on average than with the zero diet (about 350 g/day). Important advantages are the very low risk and the fact that the patient may remain under outpatient surveillance.

f) Defects of Hemostasis. Vascular surgery is complicated by intraoperative or postoperative bleeding two to three times more frequently than general surgery. Technical errors, wound infections, and clotting disorders are the main causes. Therefore, prior to every vascular operation, the function of hemostasis should be checked.

- Thromboplastin time (prothrombin time, Quick's value) for testing the exogenous coagulation system (factors VII, X, V, II, I)
- The partial thromboplastin time to evaluate the function of the endogenous coagulation system (factors XII, XI, IX, VIII, X, V, II, I)
- Plasma thrombin time (plasma thrombin coagulation time, thrombin time). This test evaluates the last phase of the coagulation cascade. Clotting disorders which are associated with a prolongation of the thrombin time are as follows:
  1. Antithrombinemia with an increase in the products of fibrinogen-fibrin lysis (hyperfibrinolysis)
  2. Dysfibrinogenemia
  3. Lack of fibrinogen
  4. Prolongation of the thrombin time under heparin

In the event of pathologic results of one of the above groups of tests, a single factor analysis must be performed for further evaluation.

The number (and if necessary also the function) of the platelets should be checked routinely as a control of the cellular hemostatic system. This is especially necessary in patients who have had treatment with antiplatelet drugs. A prolonged bleeding time must be expected for up to 7 days after their discontinuation (see part IV "Prophylaxis of Pneumonia and Thrombosis").

C. Postoperative Management

I. Postoperative Mobilization

Many operations on the vascular system are extensive procedures. Nevertheless, it is important to mobilize the patient as early as possible since this is a very effective means of preventing pulmonary and thromboembolic complications.

Following surgery on the peripheral venous system, the patient may usually get up out of bed in the evening of the day of surgery.

II. Positioning

Following operations on the carotid artery, or where there are symptoms of cardiac insufficiency at rest (dyspnea and/or congestion of the jugular veins), the patient should be lying in bed with the upper part of the body raised above the horizontal. After venous operations it is advisable to raise the foot of the bed on the day of the operation.

In the case of a severe disorder of the arterial circulation (after incomplete or unsuccessful recanalization), positioning the legs at a lower level, 10–20 cm below the horizontal, provides for the best possible perfusion.

Severe edema must be avoided because it impairs circulation. In case of edema of the lower legs one should elevate the legs if no symptoms of insufficient acral circulation are present (rest pain, increased pallor of the toes).

To prevent decubital ulcer, the vulnerable parts (especially the heels) should be padded and relieved of pressure. In a poorly perfused foot one must prevent the development of necrosis by cushioning the leg below the knee. The danger of decubitus over the sacrum is increased in patients with occlusion of the pelvic arteries.

Patients with postoperative paresis of the extremities should be positioned as prescribed by BOBATH and mobilized early.

III. Treatment of Necrosis

Local treatment of acral necrosis due to arterial circulatory disorders must be done with the utmost care postoperatively. In case of impaired compensation, pain is only a consequence of insufficient blood circulation. After successful surgery, it is usually due to bacterial infection.

To combat infection, which is almost always present at the margin of the necrosis, elimination of purulent retentions must be achieved first. If abscesses are present, they should be incised. The vital tissue should be freed of any debris (incrustations, necroses, parts of fingernails) that can be removed without injury and pain. If possible, checks should be made every day.

Secretions from lesions must be collected. This is best done with the help of a strip of linen, so that the tissue which is still intact is not macerated (especially interdigitally). If the secretion is strong, the wound dressings should be changed frequently, several times a day if necessary.

Local edema prevents or delays healing of lesions and dictates proper positioning (see above). If severe edema prevents a lesion from healing and the patient cannot tolerate horizontal positioning of the leg because of great pain, appropriate pain elimination is indicated. This is best done by peridural anesthesia, using a catheter.

IV. Prophylaxis of Pneumonia and Thrombosis

Prophylaxis of pneumonia is indicated after all more extensive vascular operations, especially in patients with chronic disease of the respiratory system (almost all heavy smokers): moistening of the air passages with an ultrasound atomizer, administration of secretolytic drugs in chronic bronchitis (for example with Mucosolvan i.v.). To improve pulmonary ventilation (prophylaxis of atelectasis), breathing exercises with an increase of dead space should be carried out three times daily in uncomplicated cases without pulmonary insufficiency. This should be done only if the number of breaths per minute does not increase during exercise. Obese patients should be instructed to use intermittent positive pressure breathing to deepen their inspirations [14]. Patients with asthmatic bronchitis may sometimes need an antibiotic and/or a corticosteroid besides bronchiolytic and secretolytic drugs (prophylaxis of thrombosis, p. 725).

V. Rehabilitation

Following reconstructive procedures on the arterial system, muscle atrophy and limitations of joint function are not infrequent. Directed physical therapy can be started prior to the operation and continued postoperatively for a few days. If arterial circulatory disorders are still present (e.g., occlusion of the femoral artery after reconstruction of the pelvic arteries), systematic walk training should commence, depending on compensation. Prior to or after operations on the peripheral venous system, measures are sometimes needed to strengthen the skin and muscle pump. These are especially important in persons with stiff ankle joints and muscle atrophy following chronic inflammations and ulcerations.

In patients who have undergone vein surgery, the leg operated on should be wrapped with an elastic bandage until the inflammatory irritations subside. If a disturbance of venous return remains, this treatment should be continued.

REFERENCES

1. Ahnefeld FW, Heinrich H (1983) Die Analyse und Bedeutung von Risikofaktoren sowie Möglichkeiten einer Vorbehandlung bei angiologischen Patienten aus der Sicht der Anästhesie. In: Nobbe F, Rudofsky G (eds) Probleme der Vor- und Nachsorge und der Narkoseführung bei invasiver angiologischer Diagnostik und Therapie. Pflaum, München, p 21
2. Barnes RW, Marszalak PB (1981) Asymptomatic carotid disease in the cardiovascular surgical patient: is prophylactic endarterectomy necessary? Stroke 12:497
3. Bleifeld W (1984) Strategien der Langzeittherapie bei der fortgeschrittenen chronischen Herzinsuffizienz. Internist 25:404
4. Busuttil RW, Baker JD, Davidson RK, Machleder HJ (1981) Carotid artery stenosis – hemodynamic significance and clinical course. JAMA 245:1438
5. Daschner F (1981) Antibiotikaprophylaxe – sinnvoll oder sinnlos? Dtsch Med Wochenschr 106:1150
6. Davison KJ (1978) Anesthesia for peripheral vascular disease. Int Anesthesiol Clin 17:129
7. Erdmann E (1984) Deutsche Gesellschaft für Innere Medizin, Wiesbaden, Mai 1984. Selecta 28:2394
8. Hallet JW, Brewster DC, Darling RC (1982) Manual of patient care in vascular surgery. Little, Brown and Co., Boston, p 72
9. Hallet JW, Brewster DC, Darling RC (1982) Manual of patient care in vascular surgery. Little, Brown and Co., Boston, p 75
10. Hartmann HG, Jutzler GA (1984) Medikamentöse Hochdrucktherapie: bewährtes Schema individuell modifizieren. Klinikarzt 13:611
11. Heinrich H, Ahnefeld FW, Kilian J, Seeling W, Sigel H, Spilker ED (1982) Der kardiozirkulatorische Risikopatient in der Anästhesie. Herz Kreislauf 14:429
12. Hertzer NR (1979) Routine coronary angiography prior to elective aortic reconstruction. Arch Surg 114:1336
13. Hertzer NR (1981) Fatal myocardial infarction following lower extremity revascularization. Ann Surg 193:492
14. Kilian J, Schwinn W (1984) Postoperative Atemtherapie. Dtsch Med Wochenschr 109:1084
15. Kistler JP, Röpper AH, Heros RC (1984) Therapy of ischemic cerebral vascular disease due to atherothrombosis. N Engl J Med 311:100
16. Lode H (1983) Antibiotikaprophylaxe bei Implantation von Gefäßprothesen. In: Nobbe F, Rudofsky G (eds) Probleme der Vor- und Nachsorge und der Narkoseführung bei invasiver angiologischer Diagnostik und Therapie. Pflaum, München, p 11
17. Neuerburg-Heusler D, Böke R, Gaentzsch A, Roth FJ (1980) Häufigkeit von haemodynamisch wirksamen Karotisobliterationen bei Patienten mit peripherer arterieller Verschlußkrankheit. In: Nobbe F, Rudofsky G (eds) Probleme der Vor- und Nachsorge und der Narkoseführung bei invasiver angiologischer Diagnostik und Therapie. Pflaum, München, p 390
18. Ropper AH, Wechsler LR, Wilson LS (1982) Carotid bruit and the risk of stroke in elective surgery. N Engl J Med 307:1388
19. Seipel L, Haasis R, Breithardt G, Borggrefe M (1983) „Prophylaktische" praeoperative Digitalisierung. In: Rietbrock N, Schnieders B, Schuster J (eds) Wandlungen in der Therapie der Herzinsuffizienz. Vieweg, p 255
20. Witschger PM, Nachbur BH (1984) Häufigkeit des zerebrovaskulären Insults nach gefäßchirurgischen Eingriffen. Präliminäre Sanierung des „asymptomatic bruit"? In: Mahler F, Nachbur B (eds) Zerebrale Ischämie. Hans Huber, Bern Stuttgart, Wien, p 26

7.2 Local Thrombolysis

H. HESS

CONTENTS

A. Fundamentals

The material of an occlusion of a large artery is always a blood clot if the obstruction did not originate traumatically. It is either an embolus from somewhere else or a locally formed thrombus. As long as the fibrin of such clots is not organized, it can be totally dissolved by thrombolytic treatment. Thus, an embolus or a thrombus can be changed back into its initial blood components [3, 4]. The organization of a clot occurs faster in narrow and healthy arteries than in wide and arteriosclerotic arteries. Beside these criteria there are radiologic criteria for determining the indication of thrombolytic treatment (Table 7.2.1) [5, 9, 10].

Today streptokinase and urokinase are available for thrombolytic treatment. Streptokinase acts faster and more intensively than urokinase. Both actually change inactive plasminogen into proteolytically active plasmin. Treatment is systemic, that is, by intravenous infusion, or localized by direct infiltration of the obstruction with either thrombolytic substance [6].

Table 7.2.1. Criteria for assessing the possibility of lysis of intra-arterial clots

Localization	Maximum time limit
Time criteria	
Finger	A few days (weeks)
Lower leg, forearm	A few weeks
Knee, thigh, upper arm	2–4 months
Pelvis	6 months and older
Abdominal aorta	Years
Radiologic criteria	
Parts of the thrombus surrounded by contrast medium	
Blurred, cloudy contours	

Systemic thrombolysis immediately activates the total circulating plasminogen, which attacks the thrombus from the outside (exogenous lysis), and at the same time acts proteolytically on the coagulation system. A very small portion of the intravenously given dose of about 2 million units streptokinase or urokinase penetrates the clot and activates the plasminogen accumulated within it, leading to endogenous lysis. This represents the main mechanism of thrombolysis [4]. Depending on the extent of the thrombus, systemic application of streptokinase may dissolve the clot within 0.5–5 days. Urokinase takes twice as long. By infiltrating an arterial clot with streptokinase directly, one can dissolve it with only a few thousand units within several hours, even if it is very extensive.

The advantages of systemic thrombolytic treatment are simultaneous lysis of all existing soluble thrombi and prevention of vascular lesions. The disadvantages are the higher risk of hemorrhage, provocation of systemic emboli, a large number of contraindications (Table 7.2.2), and a long time for successful thrombolysis to be accomplished [6]. The advantage of local low-dosage thrombolytic therapy is the lower risk of provoking bleeding or emboli in the arterial system, which in turn significantly reduces the number of contraindications

Table 7.2.2. Contraindications of thrombolytic therapy

Systemic thrombolysis	Local low dose thrombolysis
Increased risk of hemorrhage	
Coagulopathies	Coagulopathies
All stomach and intestinal ulcers	Bleeding stomach and intestinal ulcers
Bleeding hemorrhoids kidney stones	
Fresh wounds or operation	Polytrauma
Hypertension	Malignant hypertension
Intramuscular injection (recent)	
Endocarditis lenta (mycotic aneurysm)	
Old age (more than 70 years)	
CVA	Recent recovery from CVA
Embolic risk	
Mitral valve disease	
Dilatation of the heart + arrhythmia	
Dilating arteriosclerosis	Aneurysm as the cause of the occlusion

(Table 7.2.2). Furthermore, this therapy restores blood flow as fast as an operative procedure could. The disadvantage of local thrombolysis is an unavoidable trauma to the vessel, which may lead to further extension of the occlusion. In segmental occlusions, the risk of local macroemboli is present [6].

Indications for systemic thrombolic therapy which will not be discussed at this point are: acute and subacute acral ischemic syndrome, peripheral arterial (multiple) stenoses, or thrombotic occlusions, which fulfill the time and/or radiologic criteria for thrombolysis and, after careful consideration of the risks and positive outcome, do not present any contraindications.

B. Indications for Local Thrombolysis

1. All acute, subacute, and chronic thrombotic femoropopliteal occlusions, including the trifurcation, up to 8 months following obstruction.
2. Embolic femoropopliteal occlusions, including trifurcation, for a period of 4–6 weeks if the surgeon refused embolectomy.
3. Segmental femoropopliteal occlusions with a length >4 cm and poor compensation (stage IIb–IV) if systemic lysis is contraindicated and/or the obstruction is older than 4 months.
4. Embolic or thrombotic complications during or after primary transluminal angioplasty.
5. Acute embolic or thrombotic occlusions of the renal artery, also as a complication of catheter dilatation. Rare cases of successful local lysis of acute mesenteric artery occlusions have been reported. The decision to perform such a procedure must be made with great caution because of the danger of severe hemorrhage. Attempts at local lysis of cerebral occlusions involve a high risk of embolism or hemorrhage and should be considered only in very desperate situations (acute basilar artery occlusion).

Following local thrombolysis, older stenoses which remain can be dilated with a catheter during the same procedure. Extensive segmental femoropopliteal occlusions have an unfavorable long-term prognosis if they are treated by percutaneous transluminal angioplasty alone. Therefore, we start with local thrombolysis if the obstructions are longer than 4 cm. This regimen has several advantages:

1. It makes it easier to pass the guide wire through the thrombus by softening it.
2. It removes the soluble portion of the clot, which in some cases may make catheter dilatation unnecessary. However, in many cases it will reduce the size of the occlusion down to a residual stenosis of much smaller size, which may then be eliminated by dilatation. A shorter dilatation segment means less trauma to the vessel and thus a lower risk of repeated clot formation.
3. The lytic effect persists for some hours after the procedure, thus preventing reformation of the clot.

Local lysis causes local hyperemia for more than 1 day, which also counteracts clotting.

C. Preparation

For the prophylaxis of early recurrent clot formation the patient receives 1.0–1.5 g acetylsalicylic acid daily starting 1 day prior to the procedure and continuing for 3 days thereafter. It should not be given in combination with dipyridamole as dangerous drops in blood pressure have been observed following streptokinase treatment, which are probably due to an enhancement of the vasodilating effects of thrombolytic treatment. Further premedication is not necessary. Prior to the procedure an intravenous infusion is started so that necessary injections can be given immediately; if resting pain is present, 30 mg pentazocin is given.

D. Positioning

The procedure is best performed on an angiographic table, but it can be done with any intensifying unit. It is important to place a soft foam rubber pad on the table because the patient may have to lie in a certain position for several hours.

The patient should be placed in a supine position and the pelvis raised by placing a radiolucent roll about 10 cm in diameter under the sacrum. This makes it much easier to puncture the common femoral artery for lysis within the lower extremity. The roll can be removed following introduction of the catheter.

E. Technique of Local Thrombolysis

For treatment of a femoropopliteal occlusion the arterial cannula is introduced above the upper margin of the inguinal ligament by the Seldinger technique under local anesthesia. The pulsating common femoral artery is fixed between two fingers of one hand (Chap. 7.3). The needle is then inserted into the common femoral artery in the direction of the obstruction below the inguinal ligament. One should try not to injure the back wall of the vessel in order to prevent the formation of an extensive local hematoma later on. As soon as the needle lies completely within the artery, the flexible metal guide is carefully inserted. We prefer a straight wire (35×10^{-3} in) to a curved wire because it provides more sensitivity. If the wire cannot be introduced without resistance and a brief fluoroscopic check shows it to be in the profunda femoris artery, it is pulled back, and the needle location is controlled by injecting 1–2 ml diluted contrast medium. This maneuver often allows the needle to be directed in such a way that the wire can be inserted into the superficial femoral artery. If this cannot be accomplished, a new puncture is tried somewhat beneath or above the first site, depending upon the situation. An important word of caution: following its insertion, the flexible metal guide must not be advanced so far that it reaches or even penetrates the obstruction site. (An exception can be made only if the thrombus is located within the superficial femoral artery only a few millimeters below the origin of the profunda femoris.) After withdrawal of the needle a Teflon French catheter with only terminal opening is threaded over the wire. If a Y-piece is connected to the catheter, one can, without removing the metal guide, inject 1 ml of diluted contrast medium in order to verify the intraluminal position of the catheter. At the same time, both ends of the obstruction can be localized and marked with a radiopaque item (injection needle, ampule file). (If a Y-piece is not available, the metal guide must be removed before injection.)

Now the guide and the catheter are carefully advanced until they reach a position a few millimeters in front of the obstruction. The position of the catheter is again checked with a small amount of contrast medium. The tip of the catheter is placed close to the beginning of the obstruction without the guide.

Then, the thrombolytic substance is injected: 1000 units of streptokinase in a solution of 500 units/ml normal saline solution two to three times at intervals of 3 min to soften the presenting portion of the thrombus and thereby make it easier to advance the catheter a few millimeters into the thrombus. Then, the clot is infiltrated with 1000 units streptokinase. The catheter is advanced small distances of 0.5–1 cm, with or without the metal guide, at 3 to 5-min intervals, 1000 units streptokinase being injected at each step. The shorter the obstructed segment is, the longer the time intervals must be. Advancement must be possible without resistance. As soon as resistance is encountered, there is a danger of leaving the intraluminal path. In most cases, an old stenosis is the cause. Such stenotic segments can be infiltrated repeatedly without advancing the catheter any further. Usually one manages to manipulate the metal guide through such stenoses without any resistance. The catheter can be advanced over the guide, and infiltration can be continued until a connection is established with the open vessel on the distal side of the obstruction. Then the metal guide is placed distal to the former obstruction and the catheter is pulled back proximal to it, and 2–3 ml contrast medium is injected to control patency. It is advisable to take at least 1 h for the whole lytic process, the obstruction material must be totally infiltrated with streptokinase before blood flow is restored. This prevents persisting macroemboli and incomplete dissolution of the thrombotic material. As soon as blood flow is restored, thrombotic material must not be further infiltrated with streptokinase. Blood clots which still remain after streptokinase application are usually totally dissolved within the next few hours. As soon as good blood flow is present for 15 minutes, local lysis can be stopped. However, if flow velocity decreases after some time, the cause is usually a remaining high grade stenosis which cannot be lysed. Such a lesion should be documented by angiography and marked so that it can be dilated during the same session after changing to a Grüntzig catheter. It is important to limit the dilatation to such residual stenoses and not to extend it over the entire length of the previously occluded segment, even if remaining clots still obstruct flow within it. The larger the segment which has been dilated is, the higher the risk of recurrent thrombosis (Chap. 7.3).

At the end of the procedure, a last control angiogram is made. We never use more than 10 ml diluted contrast medium for this. Afterward 1000–2000 units streptokinase is given through the catheter, which is then removed.

We do not give heparin at the end of the procedure because if more than 30000 units streptokinase are applied during local thrombolysis, there is always a heparin-like effect lasting a few hours, owing to the cleared products of fibrinogen. Additional heparin would raise the risk of local hemorrhage.

The right approach to the prevention of early recurrent thrombosis is blockage of platelet function and not anticoagulation. Compression of the puncture site is done by hand and continued for 10 min after the bleeding has stopped. Then, an elastic bandage is wrapped around the leg and pelvis and the patient is instructed to remain in a horizontal position for 20 h. Sandbags or other means of mechanical compression should not be used because they tend to promote local hematoma rather than prevent it.

In the past we used total streptokinase dosages of 70000–120000 units. Now we try to use as little as possible (30000 units) in order to decrease the risk of hemorrhage in the system or of mobilization of emboli. Control evaluations of the clotting system and thrombolysis are not necessary in low dose local streptokinase treatment [7, 8]. Local thrombolysis can also be done successfully with urokinase; however, a higher dose is needed – reportedly 3–10 times higher than the streptokinase dose. Not all clinicians perform local thrombolysis in the way described in this chapter. Even in long occluded segments, some try to overcome the obstructed area with a flexible metal guide and catheter, just as in normal transluminal angioplasty, before applying streptokinase. Using the technique of normal transluminal angioplasty, for example, some try – even when the occluded segment is long – to pass a flexible metal guide and catheter beyond the obstruction before any streptokinase is administered. If this attempt succeeds, the catheter is pulled back into the thrombus, and only then is streptokinase administered. The main advantage of this technique is that one can be sure prior to infiltrating the thrombus that the catheter does not lie within the vessel wall. And in fact the result is a reduction in the number of failed attempts in cases where streptokinase is used. At the same time, however, the total number of patients helped by local thrombolysis is also reduced – by at least the number of cases in which a failed attempt, i.e., intramural passage of the catheter, could have been prevented by the prior initiation of local lysis. A further consideration is that previous canalization of the occluded segment makes it more difficult to achieve adequate infiltration of the entire thrombus.

In another version of local lysis a catheter with sideholes is placed within the thrombus, and an infusion pump is connected to it. Different doses of streptokinase are infused every hour (1000–100000 units), and the patients are kept in the intensive care unit. After 12–24 h control angiography is performed and, if the infusion therapy seems successful, it is sometimes continued for days [1, 2]. This method of treatment overlooks the fact that small doses of streptokinase, if given over a longer period of time, pose a greater danger to the clotting system, owing to persistent plasminemia, than high doses given over the same period of time, and therefore increase the chances of hemorrhage.

F. Causes of Failure

Penetration of the catheter into the wall is the most common cause of failure and always leads to termination of the procedure. The severity of the circulatory disorder increases only if this complication causes an extension of the obliterating process. Luckily, this happens only in a very small number of cases.

Penetration of the wall can begin at the site of puncture, the metal guide being thrust into the wall just after its insertion through the needle. Once in such an intramural position, it can often be advanced a long distance without perceivable resistance, just as if it were within the lumen of the vessel. This can happen even with an experienced surgeon. However, one becomes suspicious as soon as resistance is encountered at a site that was inconspicuous in a previous angiogram, or if the guide suddenly develops a long loop. In such a case, the wire should be pulled back immediately. A subsequent attempt to place the guide correctly, after changing the needle's position, or after new puncture, may be successful. However, if the situation is not recognized, and if the catheter is put in place and a control injection shows a pulsating stasis of the contrast medium, the procedure must be interrupted at once and no further injections given. Dissection can, but does not necessarily, lead to total obliteration of the vessel segment.

Shortly after introduction, the metal guide may lie intraluminally and may, during its advancement, penetrate the wall at a small plaque or a curve before reaching the occlusion. A catheter which is threaded over the guide may follow the same path without perceptible resistance, sometimes even reaching the obstructed lumen. At this point, the obligatory injection of contrast medium shows the intramural position of the catheter, recognizable by the pulsating stasis and impaired flow of the medium. In such a case, the procedure must be abandoned immediately.

The beginning of an obliterated vascular segment is a very critical site where the metal guide and the catheter can easily take an intramural path without any hint of trouble. At such a point, the thrombus and the endothelium often stick together very tightly. The latter may even be pulled off the intima by retraction of the clot. If the thrombus is very hard, the guide and/or the catheter will be easily deflected into the wall. Under certain circumstances they may even be advanced without much resistance down to the popliteal artery and even farther. This is why it is advisable to apply some thousand units of streptokinase at intervals at the point where the clot begins and then after 10–15 min to try to penetrate the softened thrombus. Thereafter, the catheter can still take the intramural path, especially if the stenosis has been present for a longer period of time. Such stenoses can often be made visible, and can therefore be more easily passed, by patient and repeated infiltration at the spot of the obstacle and by small injections of contrast medium.

Signs of an intramural catheter position are:

1. The metal guide develops a long loop or obviously changes its direction.
2. The contrast medium stands still for a longer period of time and pulsates.
3. Local pain is felt during injection of streptokinase or contrast medium.

In view of all of these possibilities for positioning the catheter intramurally, it is not surprising that in a series of 322 treatments it occurred in 19% of the patients. In 7% of the same series, the obliterating material was not soluble (Table 7.2.3). The cause of the occlusion may be an unknown aneurysm. If it is recognized during local lysis, the procedure must be abandoned because of the danger of provoking an embolus which would worsen the circulatory situation considerably. Examination of the occluded segment using ultrasonic tomography before the procedure may sometimes detect an aneurysm and should therefore be performed in all suspected cases. In an acute occlusion of the popliteal artery due to compression, one is usually able to dissolve the fresh thrombus and pass the obstruction with the catheter. However, during withdrawal of the catheter compression almost always occludes the segment again. In this case, a timely corrective operation is necessary [6, 8].

Table 7.2.3. Failures in 322 attempts of local lysis (%)

Causes	
Intramural path	19
Thrombus too old	7
Puncture technically impossible	3
Compartment syndrome	1
Aneurysm as the cause of occlusion	0.6

G. Complications

Complications which occurred at the Medizinischen Poliklinik in Munich are listed in Table 7.2.4. Local macroemboli are the most common complication and lead to further circulatory impairment in 1% of patients. They may be completely avoided by slow advance of the catheter, especially in short occlusions. One should try to follow the macroembolus with the catheter in every case and infiltrate it with streptokinase.
Some 3% of patients experienced a second thrombosis. In these cases, either a long intramural passage of the catheter was recognized too late or, more frequently, a long arterial segment was dilated. Keeping dilatation limited to the smallest segment possible is the best way of preventing recurrent thrombosis.

Bleeding into the parenchyma (brain, kidney) is rare. It cannot be totally prevented, and therefore the smallest dose possible should be given over a short time interval. The provocation of multiple emboli from a preexisting embolic source may be prevented in the same way. Mortality was 0.8% in 500 treatments. Two patients died of cerebral hemorrhage, one of a questionable dissection of the abdominal aorta, one 4 weeks after an above-knee amputation necessitated by recurrent extensive thromboses [6].

Table 7.2.4. Complications in 500 local lyses (%)

Macroemboli (local)	4
Macroemboli with circulatory impairment	1
Extensive thrombosis	3
Spasm of the femoral artery	0.2
Large local hematoma	1.5
Deep vein thrombosis of the treated limb	0.2
Injury of the femoral nerve	0.2
Cerebral hemorrhage	0.4
Renal hemorrhage	0.2
Cerebral embolism	0.2
Dissection of the abdominal aorta(?)	0.2
Amputation because of complications	0.4
Death	0.8

H. Results

According to our experience in 500 treatments over a period of $3^1/_2$ years, primary success, that is, recanalization, can be achieved in 70% of cases, including emergencies. However, one quarter of these reoccluded within the first 2 weeks. A repeat attempt achieved lasting success in about half of the cases. The reasons for early occlusion were remaining high grade stenoses which were relieved during the second procedure or insufficiently effective premedication with antiplatelet drugs. The most common cause of failure during a repeated catheterization was wall dissection during the first treatment. These dissections developed into non-thrombotic blood flow obstructions and therefore could not be eliminated by lysis.

The cumulative patency rate or number of successful recanalizations beyond a period of 2 weeks was satisfactory: 50% after 3 years.

I. Long-term Treatment

In thrombotic occlusions due to obliterating arteriopathy, the elimination or at least the reduction of risk factors is the basic therapy. In drug prophylaxis of recurrent thrombosis, and against the progression of angiopathic lesions, anticoagulants and anti-platelet drugs compete with one another. We have found both to be effective. Results of clinical studies are not available at the moment. Presently, we prefer anti-platelet drugs in a combination of acetylsalicylic acid (0.33 g) and dipyridamole (75 mg) known as Asasantin, in a dose of 3 × 1 capsule daily, instead of acetylsalicylic acid alone. With this combination we were able to show in our own study that an obliterating arteriopathy progressed significantly more slowly during a 2-year follow-up period.

For long-term treatment of embolic occlusions, anticoagulation with coumarin preparations is the treatment of choice if total elimination of the embolic source is not possible. The Quick value should be held constant at 15%–25% of the normal level. It is advisable to give acetylsalicylic acid in a dose of 2 × 0.5 g daily for 2 weeks after the procedure and to start coumarin therapy immediately after successful recanalization. We do not give heparin during the early postoperative period.

REFERENCES

1. Dembski IC, Zeitler E (1978) Selective arterial clot lysis with angiography catheter. In: Zeitler E, Grüntzig A, Schoop W (eds) Percutaneous vascular recanalization. Springer, Berlin Heidelberg New York, p 157
2. Dotter CD, Rösch I, Seaman AJ (1974) Selective clot lysis with low-dose streptokinase. Radiology 111:31
3. Gottlob R, Blümel G, Piza F, Brücke P, Böhmig HJ (1968) Die Lysierbarkeit operativ gewonnener menschlicher Thromben verschiedenen Alters in Streptokinase. Wien Med Wochenschr 118:1
4. Gross R (1964) Blutgerinnung und Fibrinolyse. Behringwerk-Mitteilungen 44:1
5. Heinrich F (1975) Streptokinase-Therapie bei chronischer arterieller Verschlußkrankheit. Medizinische Verlagsgesellschaft Marburg
6. Hess H (1982) Systemische und selektive Streptokinase-Therapie bei arteriellen Verschlüssen. Internist 23:405–409
7. Hess H, Mietaschk A, Ingrisch H (1980) Niedrig dosierte thrombolytische Therapie zur Wiederherstellung der Strombahn bei arteriellen Verschlüssen. Dtsch Med Wochenschr 105:787
8. Hess H, Ingrisch H, Mietaschk A, Rath H (1982) Local low-dose thrombolytic therapy of peripheral arterial occlusions. N Engl J Med 307:1627–1630
9. Schoop W, Martin M, Zeitler E (1968) Beseitigung von Stenosen in Extremitätenarterien durch intravenöse Streptokinase-Therapie. Dtsch Med Wochenschr 93:1629
10. Schopp W, Martin M, Zeitler E (1968) Beseitigung alter Arterienverschlüsse durch intravenöse Streptokinase-Infusion. Dtsch Med Wochenschr 93:2312

7.3 Percutaneous Transluminal Angioplasty

H. INGRISCH

CONTENTS

Percutaneous transluminal angioplasty (PTA) is the elimination of arterial stenoses and occlusions by means of a dilating catheter placed percutaneously into the lumen of a vessel. Today, the dilating catheter of GRÜNTZIG and HOPFF [5] is preferred to the coaxial catheter systems formerly used because of several disadvantages with the latter (remnant stenoses, frequent hemorrhages at the puncture site, rigid catheter system). This method may be applied in every arterial region into which the dilating catheter can be introduced: the coronary arteries, the supra-aortal branches, the visceral and renal arteries, and the arteries of the lower extremities, including the distal part of the abdominal aorta.

A. Introduction

The obliterating material, which consists of atheromatous thickenings and thrombotic deposits, may remain unorganized for months or years. Thus, it can be penetrated with a catheter and pressed against the vascular wall with a balloon. In their original report, DOTTER and JUDKINS [3] thought that the occluding material was compressed and the diameter of the vessel remained the same. According to recent studies of CASTANEDA-ZUNIGA et al. [2], the obliterating material is pressed, as a whole or in parts, toward the media which itself is stretched or even overstretched, depending on the strength of the dilatation. Tearing of the intima and the media occurs and the outer diameter of the vessel increases. The enlarged outer diameter remains constant after dilatation. It is therefore concluded that the media is irreversibly stretched and loses its elasticity (Fig. 7.3.1). In nonarterial sclerotic lesions, as in fibromuscular dysplasia, postanastomotic stenoses of graft arteries, recurrent postoperative stenosis, dilatation, and tearing of fibrous components play a greater

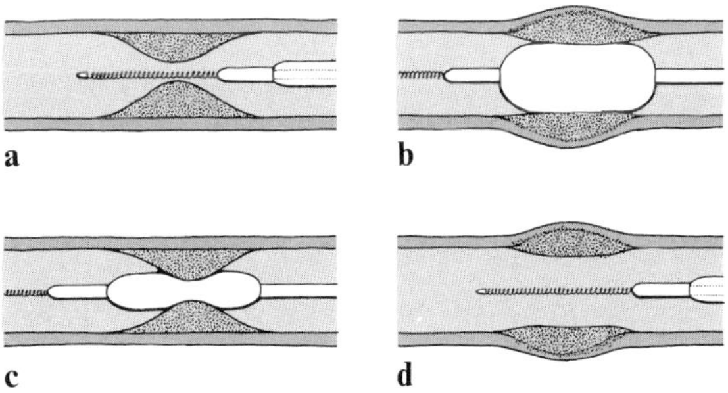

Fig. 7.3.1 a–d. Diagram of transluminal angioplasty. After passing the concentric stenosis with the straight guide wire (**a**), the dilatation catheter is threaded over the guide until the balloon lies within the stenosis (**b**). The non-compressible occluding material is pressed into the vascular wall, the wall is dilated, and the outer diameter increases (**c**). After withdrawal of the dilating catheter, a control angiogram is obtained with the guide wire (**d**) still in place

role. There is no explanation as to why a stenosis or a thrombus does not develop at the injured site of the vessel. There are probably a number of factors which are responsible for keeping the vessel patent: blood flow, which is immediately restored after dilatation, exerts pressure against the vascular wall, antiplatelet drug administration before, during, and after the procedure, and endothelialization which leads to smoothing of the injured site within weeks.

B. General Management

Percutaneous transluminal angioplasty involves the following steps:

- Informing the patient
- Preparation of the patient
- Procedure
- Follow-up treatment

I. Informing the Patient

A few days before PTA, the patient is informed about the indication, the procedure itself (dilatation is painless or only slightly painful; it takes about 1–3 h depending on the vascular region; following the procedure, bed rest is necessary for 24 h), and its possible complications (allergic reactions to contrast medium, percutaneous advancement of the catheter, and specific PTA complications, depending upon the vascular region) (see p. 119).

II. Preparation of the Patient

Independent of the vascular region being treated, the following applies to all patients:

- Preparation for a hospital stay of only a few days
- Medical examination with special attention to risk factors which might lead to further progression of occlusive disease
- Initiation of measures to eliminate risk factors
- Close contact with the vascular surgeon in cases where same-day surgery might become necessary as a result of complications (for example, PTA for stenosis of a transplant artery or for a stenosis of the profunda femoral artery with occlusion of the superficial femoral artery, PTA for a stenosis of a vertebral artery, and so on). Assessment of operability in these patients
- Administration of platelet aggregation inhibitors, starting 1–2 days before the procedure dosage: e.g., 1 tablet Asasantin (330 mg acetylsalicylic acid and 75 mg dipyramidamole) t.i.d.
- On the day of the procedure the patient must fast and receive a peripheral intravenous line
- In all patients at risk (history of allergy, hypertension, or older than 65 years, and others), dimethindenemaleate (1 ml/10 kg body weight, i.v.) and cimetidine (2 ml, i.v.) are administered as an additional allergy prophylaxis

Additional measures in certain vascular regions are listed in Sect. C.

III. Procedure

1. Necessary Equipment, Instruments, and Contrast Medium

Ideal equipment for this procedure is an angiographic unit with a high capacity generator within a radiology department. An image intensifier with video transmission, a below-table X-ray tube, an automatic cassette changer for 35×35 cm films, and a sliding table with an automatic table-shifting device are adequate for PTA procedures on the subclavian artery, renal artery, aorta, iliac artery, femoral artery, and popliteal artery.

However, for PTA procedures on the carotid, mesenteric, and coronary arteries, image intensification video transmission system in C-arch arrangement or with biplane exposure are necessary. Additional apparatus such as standard format cameras for 10×10 cm films attached to the image intensifier, an analog video recording system, and the digital subtraction technique for digital subtraction angiography (DSA) may be helpful in PTA, but are not absolutely necessary. However, an automatic contrast medium injector and a pressure-measuring instrument (Statham element), useful for intra-arterial pressure registration, are needed.

2. Instruments

Independent of the vascular region, the following basic instruments should be available:

1. A 20-ml syringe with 1% lidocaine for local anesthesia
2. A 10-ml syringe with a Luer-lock attachment for contrast medium
3. A 5-ml syringe with a Luer-lock attachment for filling the balloon (filled with 2 ml normal saline solution and 2 ml contrast medium)
4. A 25-ml syringe with a Luer-lock attachment for emptying the balloon
5. 1–2 50-ml syringes for flushing by the perfusor
6. Perfusor
7. 2 bowls of normal saline solution with heparin added (5000 units/l)
8. Seldinger needle
9. An 8-French introducer sheath with a hemostatic valve (Fig. 7.3.3)
10. A Y-piece attachment with stopcock (contrast medium can be injected with guide wire still in place; Fig. 7.3.4)
11. Guide wires, an angiographic catheter for exploration, and a dilating catheter (see Sect. C)

3. Contrast Media

The new, nonionic contrast media (Jopamidol or Johexol) cause less heat sensation and have less toxicity than the traditional ionic contrast media. As a rule, children should not receive more than 1 ml per kilogram body weight and adults not more than 2 ml per kilogram body weight per day. In exceptional cases, up to 250 ml can be given to adults with normal renal function. By applying DSA for control of superselective positioning and final assessment of morphology, the amount of contrast medium may be reduced considerably.

4. Positioning of the Patient

The supine position is suited for transfemoral, transaxillary, or transbrachial catheterization. For anterograde puncture in the region of the femoral artery, a cushion about 10 cm high should be placed under the pelvis, especially in obese patients. It can be removed after introduction of the catheter. In such a position, it must be ensured that the vascular region and its distal outflow can be reached with the image intensification fluoroscopy unit.

5. Introduction of the Catheter

The catheter can be introduced percutaneously or following exposure of the artery (e.g., intraoperatively). The transfemoral approach is used most often. The transaxillary or transbrachial approaches are very rarely chosen. For transfemoral and transaxillary catheterization, the percutaneous technique of SELDINGER is most often used (Fig. 7.3.2). In the transbrachial approach the catheter is usually inserted after operative exposure of the brachial artery in the cubital region. If the catheter needs to be changed very often, one should use an introducer sheath with a hemostatic valve through which catheters of different sizes may be inserted (Fig. 7.3.3).

In stenoses located within branches of the aorta (e.g., stenosis of the renal artery, subclavian artery, vertebral artery, and so on) an angiographic catheter is first introduced to locate the stenosed artery and then replaced by a dilating catheter over a guide wire. The dilatating catheter can be inserted directly into stenoses that are near the puncture site (for example: iliac stenoses, stenoses of the superficial femoral artery or popliteal artery).

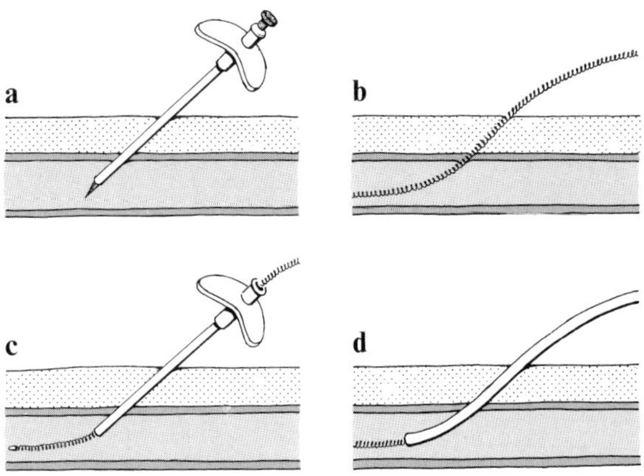

Fig. 7.3.2a–d. Diagram of percutaneous catheter introduction according to SELDINGER

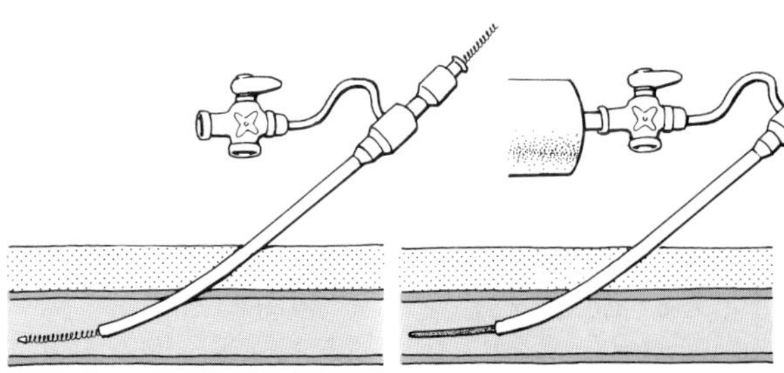

Fig. 7.3.3. Diagram of the catheter sheath introducer system. Catheters of different sizes can be changed as often as necessary. The sheath is constantly flushed by a perfusor connected to the system

A description of anterograde puncture of the femoral artery in stenoses of distal vessels is given in the section on catheterization of special vascular areas, p. 123.

6. Passage of a Stenosis

The passage of a stenosis or an occlusion with a guide or an angiographic catheter is the most important step in angioplasty. Morphologic details of the stenosis can be seen in a conventional angiogram. If only i.v. angiography with subtraction (DSA) or angiotomography has been performed prior to the procedure, a conventional angiogram must be obtained before passage of the narrowed vascular segment. The stenosis must be localized by fluoroscopy during a test injection and marked on the skin with a piece of metal. In stenoses of the renal arteries, one should note the position of these stenoses with reference to the edge of the vertebra or, in stenoses of the subclavian artery, with reference to the clavicle. It is a rule in all techniques that the passage of the stenosis with a guide wire and/or catheter must always be done under fluoroscopic control employing test injections of contrast medium to assure their intraluminal position. If a guide lies within the catheter, injection of contrast medium is only possible using a special Y-piece attachment (Fig. 7.3.4). If passage of the stenosis is achieved, it is usually very easy to advance the dilating catheter over the guide through the stenosis. Then dilatation can be performed without difficulty. Sometimes, however, passage is difficult owing to the location and morphology of the stenosis. Also, the guide wire and catheter may be advanced intramurally; or, loosening of thrombotic material may lead to embolization or conversion of the stenosis into a total occlusion. This is why different techniques must be employed, depending upon the location and structure of the stenoses. These techniques are described below.

a) Guide Wire Technique. The basic principle is to advance a catheter (angiographic or dilating catheter) until the stenosis is reached and to insert a guide wire through it. This guide passes the stenosis first. Afterward, the dilating catheter is advanced over the guide through the stenosis. The following possibilities may result:

Straight Catheter – Straight Guide (Fig. 7.3.5a). This method is suited for all concentric stenoses in straight vessel segments. Example: stenoses of the superficial femoral artery and popliteal artery, common iliac artery, and infrarenal abdominal aorta.

Preshaped Catheter – Straight Guide (Fig. 7.3.5c). By preshaping the catheter, the guide is given a different direction so that a stenosis can be passed which might not be passable using a straight catheter. Preshaped catheters are the "cobra," "side-winder," and "head-hunter" catheters. These catheters are necessary in eccentric stenoses with or without pockets, within straight or curved vascular segments, and in concentric stenoses within curved vascular segments (Fig. 7.3.5c). Example: eccentric stenoses within the elongated external or common iliac artery, concentric stenoses in the renal artery, the mesenteric artery, or the subclavian artery, among others.

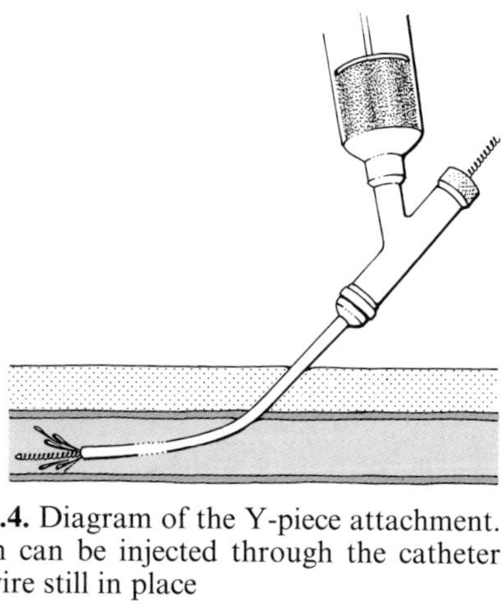

Fig. 7.3.4. Diagram of the Y-piece attachment. Contrast medium can be injected through the catheter with the guide wire still in place

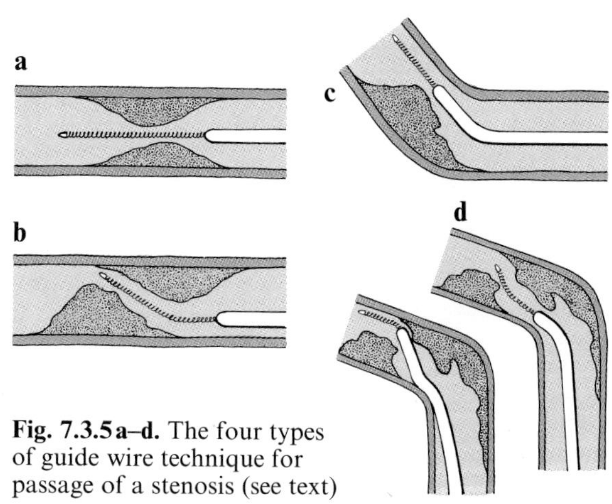

Fig. 7.3.5a–d. The four types of guide wire technique for passage of a stenosis (see text)

Straight Catheter – Preshaped and Steerable Guide (Fig. 7.3.5b). By a special manufacturing process the posterior portion of the guide is stabilized, allowing the front curved end to be rotated in any possible direction. This method is suited to eccentric stenoses in straight vascular segments. Example: eccentric stenoses in the superficial femoral artery and the popliteal artery, also in segments of the common iliac artery.

Preshaped Catheter – Preshaped and Steerable Guide (Fig. 7.3.5d). Guide and catheter can be used in stenoses that change direction. This method is suited to double eccentric stenoses in straight or curved vascular segments. Example: multieccentric stenoses in the iliac and renal arteries or in stenoses of segmental arteries of the renal artery.

b) Guide Catheter Method (Fig. 7.3.6). The basic principle of this method is to place a rigid preshaped guide catheter in front of the stenosis. A miniaturized balloon catheter is inserted through it and advanced through the stenosis with a guide wire. This method is used in coronary stenoses and also rarely in stenoses of the renal arteries.

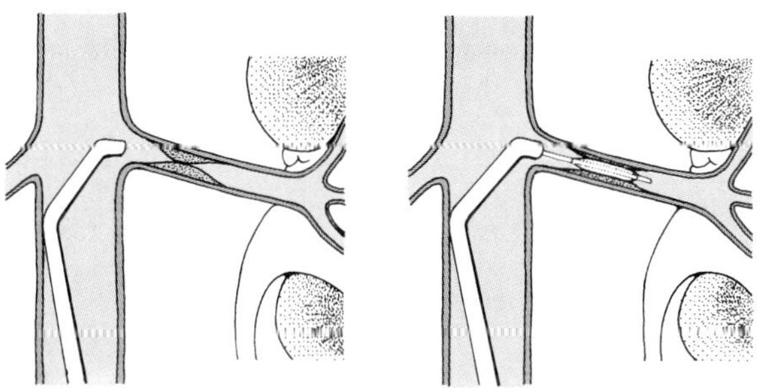

Fig. 7.3.6. Guide catheter technique

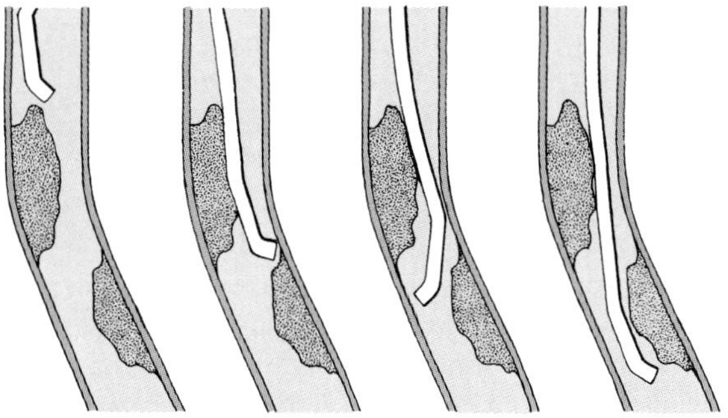

Fig. 7.3.7. Jet technique for passage of a stenosis without a guide wire

c) Jet Method (Fig. 7.3.7). A straight or preshaped catheter without a guide wire is advanced through the stenosis during constant administration of small test injections. The rebound at the tip of the catheter gives it the right direction. Once passage of the stenosis has been accomplished, the guide is advanced into the distal part of the vessel, and the passage catheter is exchanged for a dilating catheter. This method is used in eccentric stenoses in straight or curved vascular segments.

7. Passage of an Occlusion

The atheromatous fibrous portion of the obliterating material greatly obstructs the passage of the catheter. However, the thrombotic portion is easily traversed by a guide wire and/or catheter with relatively little resistance. We pass occlusions up to 4 cm without local streptokinase injection, and longer occluded segments with the injection (Chap. 7.2).

There are three ways of passing an obstruction. All three of them have about the same success rate. The author recommends maintaining the following sequence: First use the straight guide wire. If the occlusion cannot be passed, reinforce the guide wire by passing a catheter over it. It is best to use a curved guide, placing its end beyond the tip of the catheter and advancing both together through the occlusion. Penetration of the vascular wall with the catheter is less likely than with the guide wire alone because the former has a greater diameter. Thus, the risk of intramural advancement is greatly reduced. The beginning and end of the occlusion are marked on the skin. After passing the occlusion, the intraluminal position of the catheter must be checked by an injection of contrast medium.

8. Dilatation

Dilatation aims at the following:

- To enlarge the diameter of the narrowed vascular segment
- To create a smooth internal surface
- To injure the vascular wall as little as possible, especially proximal and distal to the stenosis
- To avoid microemboli

For the achievement of these goals, selection of the right dilating catheter is just as important as a sound knowledge of the dilatation procedure.

We prefer a polyethylene catheter. Its balloon, when filled, shows little compliance (increase of outer diameter when the pressure is raised). This guarantees that the application of maximum pressure is totally transmitted to the occluding material and does not lead to overdilatation of neighboring vessel segments. It is important to understand that less pressure is necessary to fill a balloon with a larger diameter (force A) than a balloon with a smaller diameter because A is a function of pressure X. The dilating force of the balloon at the stenosis is greater, the greater the narrowing at the stenosis. This is why a high grade stenosis can be eliminated with only one dilatation, whereas low grade stenoses or remnant stenoses cannot be removed, even if great pressure and repeated dilatations are employed.

Form of a Dilating Catheter. Length and diameter of the balloon must be chosen according to the individual situation. Usually, a straight dilating catheter is used. In renal or mesenteric arteries branching off at an acute angle in a caudal direction, a preshaped dilating catheter (e.g., the Side-Winder) may also be applied (Fig. 7.3.8). The diameter of the balloon depends on the supposed diameter of the treated vascular segment without poststenotic dilatation. It is sufficient to dilate the stenotic arterial segment until its lumen is as large as undiseased portions of the inflow and outflow tract. Overstretching can lead to mechanical injury. The length of the balloon depends on the length of the treated vessel segment, whereas in short stenoses a balloon length of 2–3 cm and in stenoses or occlusions up to 4 cm a balloon length of about 4 cm are needed. Longer occlusions require a longer balloon (up to 10 cm) if they cannot be treated by local lysis.

The *process of dilatation* is carried out as follows:

After advancing the catheter through the stenosis (see Sect. B.III.6) and making sure that the guide wire has an intraluminal position, the dilating catheter is passed over the guide (Fig. 7.3.1).

A lead marker placed distal and proximal to the balloon of the dilating catheter helps to position the dilating segment of the catheter exactly at the site of the stenosis. As mentioned earlier, the exact site of the stenosis must be marked by radiopaque material on the skin surface. When it is certain that the balloon is exactly within the stenotic segment, the balloon is filled with diluted contrast medium (1.5 ml contrast medium + 1.5 ml normal saline solution in a 5 to 10 ml syringe) under fluoroscopic control. Dilatation lasts about 20–30 s. It can be repeated several times. After the balloon has relieved the stenosis, the pressure remains constant. At this point, one should consider that a small syringe with a small piston (5 ml syringe) may build up more pressure faster, but on the other hand a large syringe (20–50 ml) speeds up pressure reduction and emptying of the balloon [1]. If the balloon is longer than the stenotic vessel segment (that is the way it should be), the catheter does not have to be advanced for a second dilatation. However, if the balloon is shorter, the dilating catheter is pushed forward until the distal end of the balloon lies 1 cm distal to the stenotic area. After the first dilatation, the balloon is withdrawn about three quarters of its length, and the proximal portion of the vessel is dilated. This procedure is repeated until the proximal end of the stenosis or the occlusion is reached. In such a way, multiple stenoses are dilated with a short balloon, starting at the distal end. Following dilatation, the dilating catheter is withdrawn, and the guide wire is left in place. A control angiogram is obtained (Fig. 7.3.9). If, after dilatation, a distinct stenosis remains, the catheter can be advanced again, and a second dilatation using the same or a larger balloon diameter may be attempted. A second dilating procedure is not necessary in smaller remnant stenoses because wall irregularities caused by thrombotic de-

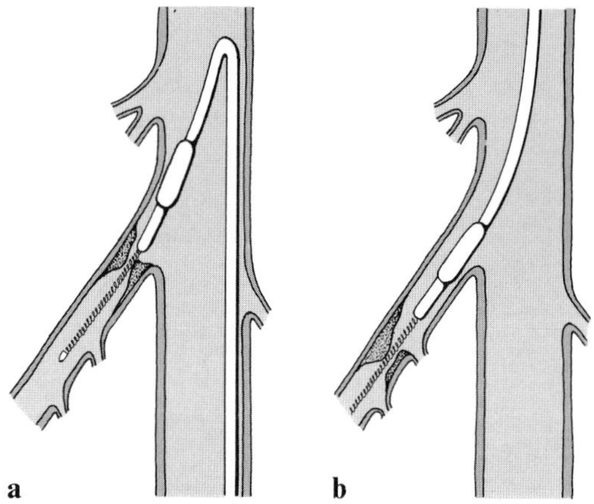

a b

Fig. 7.3.8a, b. PTA in a stenosis of the superior mesenteric artery. On the left (**a**) PTA is performed transfemorally with a preshaped dilating catheter (Side-Winder); on the right a transaxillary approach with a straight dilating catheter (**b**). In **b**, the stenosis is situated further distally. Basically, these methods can also be applied in renal arteries which branch off caudally at a very acute angle

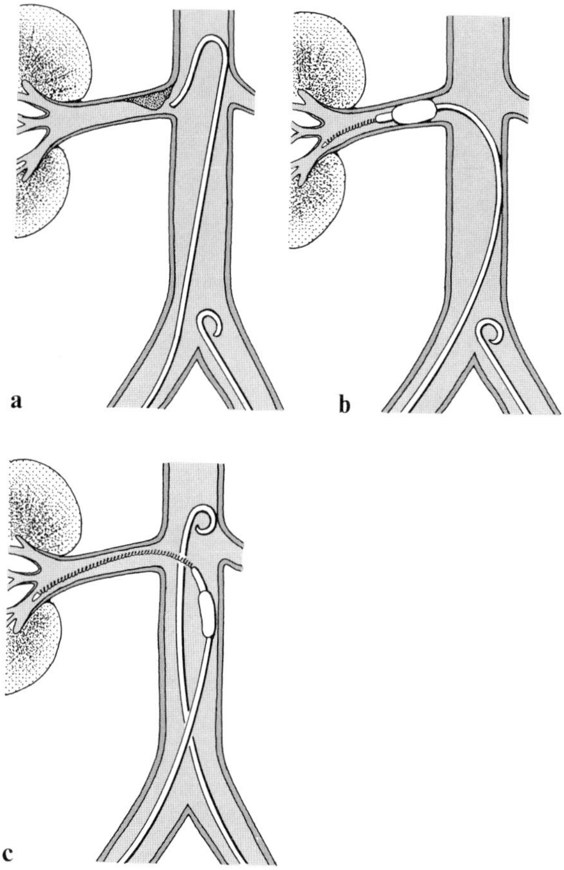

Fig. 7.3.9 a–c. PTA in stenosis of the right renal artery. The right renal artery is entered with a Side-Winder catheter since its tip can be advanced on the caudal side of the plaque (**a**). A catheter for orientation lies in the contralateral pelvic artery, which can be advanced upward for morphologic control at any time (**c**). Catheters for passage of the stenosis and dilating catheters should be inserted ipsilaterally through the femoral artery. This is the only way the dilating catheter can be easily introduced into the renal arteries (**b**). Following PTA, the guide wire remains in the right renal artery and the dilating catheter only is pulled back (**c**). A control aortogram is obtained

posits vanish, owing to autogenous lysis and smoothing (endothelialization).

9. Control Angiography

Control angiography should document the success of treatment and expose complications. Therefore, the vessels distal to the dilated segment should always be included. In small arteries, contrast medium can be injected through the catheter after it has been withdrawn about 10 cm proximally from the dilated vascular segment (the guide wire remaining distal to it (Fig. 7.3.4)).

In stenoses at the origin of the renal and mesenteric arteries an additional catheter is necessary for orientation in order to achieve the necessary concentration of contrast medium in the aorta (Fig. 7.3.9).

IV. Follow-up Treatment

- Pressure bandage over the puncture site.
- Bed rest until the next morning.
- Drug treatment: platelet aggregation inhibitors dose, for example Asasantin (330 mg acetylsalicylic acid and 75 mg dipyramidamole) t.i.d. for a period of at least 6 weeks. In arteriosclerotic patients, long-term treatment may be necessary.
- Noninvasive diagnostic procedures to control the results of treatment: e.g., auscultation and palpation, blood pressure measurement, Doppler sonography and Doppler pressure measurement, measurement of walking range, ^{131}I-hippuric-acid clearance on each side, DSA, and others according to the vascular region. When findings have normalized, the patient may be discharged after 1–2 days and should be seen again, on an outpatient basis, about 14 days after PTA.

C. Indications, Contraindications, Technique, and Complications of PTA in Particular Vascular Areas

I. Subclavian Artery, Axillary Artery, and Brachiocephalic Artery

Today PTA of stenoses of the subclavian artery has developed into a routine procedure. If done on the left side, it is relatively simple. PTA of the very rare right-side stenosis is more difficult. Occlusions of the subclavian artery should be treated by PTA only in exceptional cases.

Indications for PTA

- Cerebral symptoms as in vertebrobasilar insufficiency during arm exercise (vertigo, speech and visual disturbances, headaches, pareses, short episodes of unconsciousness, etc.)

- Brachial symptoms (arm weakness, pain at rest, gangrene caused by emboli, coldness, numbness
- Combination of cerebral and brachial symptoms

Preconditions for PTA

- Stenoses proximal to the origin of the vertebral artery with retrograde flow within the vertebral artery
- Stenoses distal to the origin of the vertebral artery and extending into the region of the axillary and brachial artery
- Stenoses of the brachiocephalic artery with total occlusion of the internal carotid artery and retrograde flow in the vertebral artery, both on the right side

Contraindications

- Asymptomatic stenosis of the subclavian artery
- Symptomatic proximal stenosis of the subclavian artery with anterograde flow in the vertebral artery
- Stenosis of the subclavian artery with an arterial thoracic outlet syndrome
- Stenosis of the brachiocephalic artery with an open internal carotid artery and/or anterograde flow in the vertebral artery
- Stenosis just at the origin of the right subclavian artery (danger of embolization into the right common carotid artery)

Technical Particulars

- Transfemoral approach in stenoses of the left side and transaxillary approach in stenoses and occlusions on the right
- Passage of the stenosis: preshaped angiographic catheters, e.g., "head-hunter"; guide wire 250 cm long, dilating catheter 100–120 cm long

Following deflation of the balloon, results can be checked by measuring blood pressure. Sometimes dilatation must be repeated until blood pressure is the same as in the opposite arm. A second passage of the stenosis with the guide wire and catheter must always be avoided as thrombotic material may be loosened and embolize into the vertebral artery, which already shows anterograde perfusion following the first dilatation.

Results. This treatment produced positive hemodynamic as well as angiographic results in 81 of 85 patients without neurologic complications (review of the literature [15]). The only complication which occurred was an embolization into the arteries of the arm. Our own results show primary success in 11 of 13 cases (a stenosis of the right subclavian artery and a stenosis of the peripheral brachial artery could not be passed). Out of these 11 cases we had one recurrence.

II. Carotid Artery

If the internal carotid artery is patent, PTA of an arterial sclerotic stenosis within the brachiocephalic artery or the common carotid or internal carotid arteries should not be attempted on either side, save in exceptional cases, owing to the danger of cerebral embolization [8]. An arteriosclerotic stenosis of the carotid bifurcation, the typical site, is treated only by vascular surgery. Fibromuscular dysplasia of the internal carotid artery, when situated near the base of the skull, and arteriosclerotic stenosis of the external carotid artery with simultaneous occlusion of the ipsilateral internal carotid artery are indications for PTA. In both cases, the risk of embolization into the brain is very low. The aim of treating a stenosis of the external carotid artery is to improve collateral circulation to the internal carotid artery which is of importance if an ipsilateral extra-intracranial bypass is planned. The technique is the same as in a stenosis of the subclavian artery described above (straight guide wire, 250 cm long; dilating catheter, 120 cm long, with a balloon diameter of 3–5 mm). Angiography of all cerebral arteries should be performed. A vascular surgeon should be on standby.

Results. Successful treatment of fibromuscular dysplasia of the internal carotid artery near the base of the skull [8] as well as of stenosis of the external carotid artery with simultaneous occlusion of the internal carotid artery [14, 15] has been reported. There were no complications in these cases.

III. Vertebral and Basilar Artery

These stenoses should be treated only in centers with a great deal of PTA experience. Stenoses of the vertebral artery are usually located at its origin and do not show ulcerating plaques.

Indications and Preconditions. Prior to PTA, a panangiographic survey of the cerebrovascular system should be performed. Carotid stenoses must be relieved by surgery before the procedure is attempted. If this correction does not change the clinical symptoms of vertebrobasilar insufficiency and the contralateral vertebral artery is occluded or shows a high grade stenosis, PTA is indicated. Again, it should be attempted only with a vascular surgeon on standby. The technique is similar to that used in stenoses of the subclavian artery (straight guide wire, 250 cm long; dilating catheter, 120 cm long, with a balloon diameter of 3–4 mm).

Results. MOTARJEME et al. [9] reported on 13 successful PTAs of stenoses at the origin of the vertebral artery. In three cases the catheter could not be passed through the narrowed segment of the artery. We do not have any experiences of our own to report.

PTA in a stenosis of the basilar artery is justified if the prognosis is unfavorable. Passage of the stenosis may be possible following operative exposure of the vertebral artery at the arch of the atlas (intraoperative PTA).

IV. Celiac Artery, Superior, and Inferior Mesenteric Arteries

Abdominal angina may be suspected when all three visceral arteries (celiac artery and both mesenteric arteries) are partially stenosed or occluded and other reasons for these symptoms have been excluded. Stenoses of these arteries near their origins may be treated by PTA with a vascular surgeon on standby. Biplanar fluoroscopy must be available. As in renal arteries, passage and dilatation of preshaped catheters is necessary (Fig. 7.3.8).

V. Renal Artery

In most cases, renal vascular hypertension is caused by arteriosclerotic stenoses of the renal arteries or fibromuscular dysplasia of one or more layers of the arterial wall. With only a few exceptions, both forms of stenosis are suitable for PTA. It is also the method of choice in stenoses of transplanted arteries, in stenoses which develop within venous interposition grafts postoperatively, and in recurrences following previous PTA.

Indication

- Renovascular hypertension in which the age of the patient and the pathogenesis of the stenosis is not important (arteriosclerosis, fibromuscular dysplasia, stenosis of transplant arteries, Takayasu arteritis)
- Renal insufficiency: stenoses of both sides and unilateral stenoses if the contralateral kidney is without function or only one kidney is present

Preconditions for PTA

- Correction of existing carotid stenoses
- Possibility of intensive care in high risk patients following PTA (history of myocardial infarction, coronary stenosis, cerebral insult, older than 65)
- Discontinuation of antihypertensive medication in the evening of the day before the procedure. Clonidine treatment is discontinued by slowly reducing the dose as abrupt withdrawl may lead to a rebound effect causing a hypertensive crisis
- Notification of the vascular surgeon

Contraindications

- Stenoses without hemodynamic effect (negative renin quotient, ^{131}I-hippurate clearance equal on both sides, no measurable pressure gradient across the stenosis)
- Stenoses with beadlike multisegmental fibromuscular dysplasia
- Stenoses caused by dissecting aortic aneurysms
- Large plaques in the aorta at the ostium of the renal artery which are easily dislodged
- Kinking stenoses (especially in graft arteries)
- High grade stenoses with a large amount of occlusive material

Technique. For passage and dilatation of a renal artery stenosis, the guide wire method (Fig. 7.3.5) and the guide catheter method are suitable (Fig. 7.3.6 in Sect. B.III.6). The guide wire method with very flexible, preshaped dilating catheters is usually successful; as a result the guide catheter method is rarely used. The transfemoral approach should always be ipsilateral; this allows the catheter to be advanced easily along a curve of large radius into the renal artery. A catheter for orientation can be inserted transfemorally on the contralateral side. This facilitates control angiography during each phase of the passing and dilating procedure without withdrawing the guide wire, the passage catheter, or the dilating catheter from the renal artery (Fig. 7.3.9). If control angiography shows a second dilating procedure to be necessary, the dilating catheter is advanced over the guide wire a second time. A further advantage of using a second catheter is that in the event of perforation or rupture of the renal artery, the artery can be occluded simply by advancing the dilating catheter over the guide wire into the ostium of the renal artery.

Complications. In addition to local complications at the puncture site (thrombosis, leakage, large hematoma, and others), complications occurring at the renal artery are also of great importance. Total occlusion of the main renal artery (2%) must be corrected operatively, even though this is not the case in obstructions of the segmental arteries. Before surgery, one can try to eliminate the occlusion by local streptokinase injection. Smaller dissections and intimal tears, spasms of the renal artery, and perforation with the guide wire are without consequences. However, perforation with the catheter must be monitored intensively (sonography and computed tomography, control angiography), and an operation may be necessary. In cases of rupture of the renal artery (selection of a too large balloon), one should attempt to occlude the orifice of the renal artery with the balloon catheter (see above). Immediate surgery is necessary. In patients with limited renal function, too much contrast medium may lead to reversible or even irreversible renal insufficiency. Therefore, nonionic contrast medium is recommended. Cumulative statistics show the complication rate to be 22.6% in 561 patients [7]. Most complications (70%) had no long-term sequelae for the patient. Surgical intervention at the puncture site was necessary in 1.2% following PTA. The renal arteries needed reconstruction in 2.1% of cases and the pelvic and leg arteries in 0.7%. In another 1.2% irreversible renal insufficiency made dialysis necessary. Mortality was 1%, whereas catheter manipulation caused only one death directly (mesenteric infarct). Myocardial infarctions ($n = 4$) and one cerebral insult in the days following PTA were the main causes of death.

Results. According to the literature, PTA treatment (primary success) is possible in 82%–94% of patients. Follow-up controls up to 4 years show an average success rate of 73% in 438 treated patients [7]. Patients with fibromuscular dysplasia have a higher cure rate than patients with arteriosclerotic stenoses. Systematic angiographic control 6 months after PTA showed not one occlusion of the renal artery or formation of an aneurysm in our patients. No stenosis was observed in the majority of renal arteries investigated (24/33). The vasculature was inconspicuous, and poststenotic dilatation had regressed.

The other patients had remnant stenoses without hemodynamic effects or recurrent stenoses (5/33). The recurrent stenoses were dilated a second time. According to the literature the average recurrence rate is about 11% (5%–25%). Repetition of PTA in a recurrent stenosis is possible without higher risk. The chances that a second PTA procedure will be successful are about equal to those for the first PTA.

VI. Infrarenal Abdominal Aorta

A single stenosis of the infrarenal aorta is very rare. It may be a preliminary stage of a total obstruction of the aortic bifurcation. It can be treated by PTA (Fig. 7.3.10).

Indication for PTA

- Intermittent claudication on both sides with pain in the gluteal and thigh muscles
- Impotentia coeundi (rare)

Preconditions for PTA

- Single stenosis
- Site of the stenosis between the renal artery and the aortic bifurcation
- Both pelvic arteries patent

Contraindications

- Long segments of the abdominal aorta showing arteriosclerotic lesions with loose plaques and ulcerations
- Additional occlusions and stenoses in the region of the iliac arteries (such patients should receive a bifurcation prothesis)

Technique. Depending on the diameter of the aorta, dilating catheters with balloon diameters of 8,

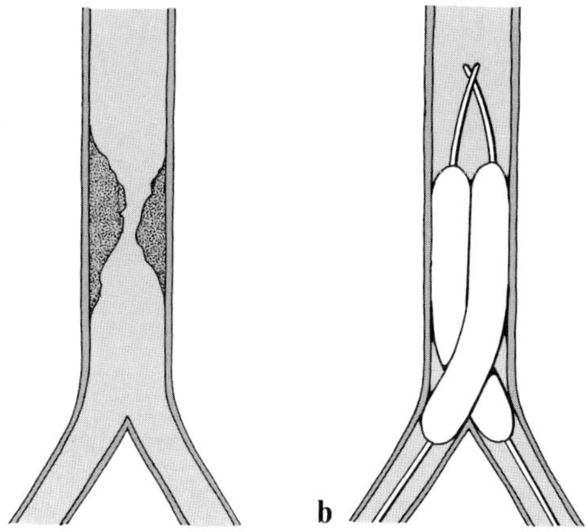

Fig. 7.3.10 a, b. Diagram of PTA in a distal aortic stenosis. The high grade stenosis just above the bifurcation is treated by the kissing balloon technique (**b**). This is the only way to achieve a dilatation wide enough for successful restoration of normal blood flow

10, or 12 mm can be used. If a large cross-section is to be achieved, or if the stenosis lies just above the aortic bifurcation (Fig. 7.3.10), the kissing balloon technique [6] with two dilating catheters should be employed. The two balloons are inflated simultaneously. If one balloon reaches down to the common iliac artery, the diameter of the common iliac artery will determine the diameter of the balloon.

Results. Besides reports on successful PTA treatments of concentric aortic stenoses in a few cases [11, 13], we have results for 19 of our own patients. During an average follow-up period of 48 months treatment was successful in 17 of the 19 cases.

Three complications without sequelae occurred: one aortic wall dissection, one embolization, and one hematoma at the puncture site [6].

VII. Pelvic and Femoral Arteries

The common occurrence of occlusive arterial disease in the lower half of the body explains why PTA is most often done in this vascular region. The procedure is easy to perform in this area because the arterial puncture site is in the vicinity of the vascular segments requiring dilatation.

Indication

- Any accessible stenosis situated anywhere between the common iliac artery and the distal tibioperoneal vessels, including stenoses in the distal profunda femoris artery. Clinical symptoms range from stages IIa to IV according to Fontaine's systems of classification
- Occlusions up to a length of 4 cm in the region of the superficial femoral and popliteal arteries and a length of 2 cm in the region of the common or external iliac arteries; occlusions causing stage IIb–IV symptoms, and especially in cases in which stage IIb cannot be improved by conservative therapy (e.g., walking exercise). Occlusions over 5 cm in length should be treated by a combination of local lysis and PTA and only in exceptional cases by PTA alone (Chap. 7.2)
- Any stenosis of the internal iliac artery if it is a possible cause of impotence
- Any recurrence following PTA treatment of these lesions

Contraindications

- Acute embolism and thrombosis
- Transfemoral approach not possible because of infection or considerable scar formation after surgery
- All stenoses at the origin of the profunda femoris artery that are indications for operative grafting procedures

Technique

1. Stenoses far away from the puncture site (at least 5–6 cm distal or proximal to the inguinal region).
   - Ipsilateral transfemoral approach, retrograde or anterograde puncture (for anterograde puncture see below)
   - A passage catheter is rarely necessary to overcome the stenosis. This is why a straight dilating catheter is inserted
   - Selective control angiography
2. Stenoses near the puncture site: cross-over technique.
   - Approach: contralateral transfemoral, retrograde puncture
   - Preshaped catheter for aortic bifurcations ("cobra," "side-winder")
   - Dilating catheter: straight, 65 cm long
   - Selective control angiography

In stenoses of the superficial femoral artery and the popliteal artery anterograde puncture of the ipsilateral common femoral artery is essential. The arterial puncture site lies at the upper margin of the palpable inguinal ligament. The needle is ad-

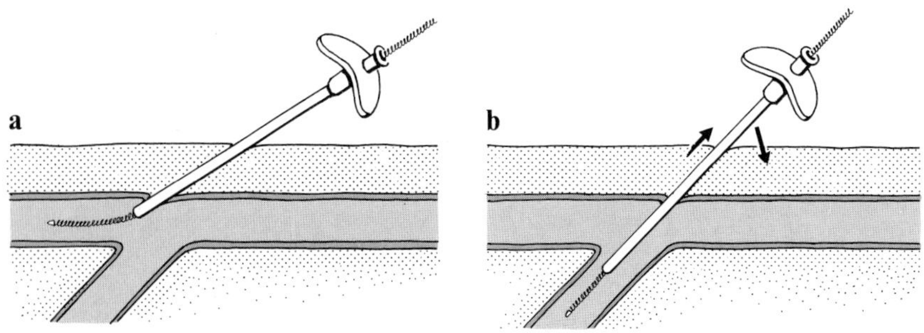

Fig. 7.3.11 a, b. Diagram of the anterograde puncture of the femoral artery. Needle and guide wire are often wrongly advanced into the deep femoral artery owing to the anatomy in this region (**a**). After partially withdrawing the needle and holding it in a more tangential direction towards the surface of the skin, the guide wire can be manipulated into the superficial femoral artery (**b**)

vanced at a 45° angle. In most cases localization and passage of the superficial femoral artery do not present any problems. However, owing to certain anatomic features of this region, the guide wire may slip off into the profunda femoris artery. Withdrawal and lowering of the needle (Fig. 7.3.11) may lead the guide wire into the correct artery. Using the Tuohy cannula makes anterograde passage of the superficial femoral artery easier [12].

Results. Review of the literature [4] shows a primary success rate of 93% in iliac stenoses (1600 patients), 96% in femoral stenoses (751 patients), and 68% in femoral occlusions (518 patients). The patency rate after 3 years in successfully treated patients in the same group was 85% in iliac stenoses, 75% in femoral stenoses, and 68% in femoral occlusions. The same cumulative statistics show a complication rate of 2.8% in iliac and 7.6% in femoropopliteal stenoses.

In iliac stenoses, local complications at the puncture site occured in 1.7%, systemic complications (e.g., pulmonary embolism, myocardial infarction, congestive heart failure, CVA, etc. during the first 10 days after the procedure) in 0.3%, and complications requiring surgical intervention (macroembolism, pseudoaneurysm formation, thrombosis at the puncture site, etc.) in 0.8%. In femoropopliteal stenoses the complication rate at the puncture site was 3.2%, the rate of systemic complications was 2.4%, and surgery was necessary in 2%.

D. Intraoperative Transluminal Angioplasty

This technique represents the application of transluminal angioplasty during vascular surgery for dilatation of remote proximal or distal stenoses or occlusions. Its purpose is to improve inflow and outflow in these regions. This technique limits the extent of surgery and lowers the operative risk. Intraoperative transluminal angioplasty is often used in long stenoses of the superficial femoral artery with simultaneous stenosis of the pelvic arteries or distal popliteal artery.

Stenoses lying within inaccessible vessel segments may be dilated by intraoperative transluminal angioplasty (e.g., stenosis of the basilar artery after operative exposure of the vertebral loop, peripheral stenosis of the renal artery after operative exposure of the main renal artery, fibromuscular dysplasia of the carotid artery near the base of the skull following operative exposure of the carotid bifurcation).

The essential equipment in the operating room (radiolucent operating table, devices for fluoroscopy and pressure registration, etc.) is just as important as cooperation between the surgeon and the radiologist. An arteriotomy is performed on the exposed vessel, or the Seldinger technique is applied. Passage and dilatation are done using the same technique as described in Sect. B.

More extensive studies have not yet been carried out. The results are probably equivalent to those achieved using the percutaneous technique in the corresponding vascular areas.

REFERENCES

1. Abele JE (1980) Balloon catheters and transluminal dilatation: technical considerations. AJR 135:901–906
2. Castaneda-Zuniga WR, Formanek A, Tadavarthy M, Vlodaver L, Edwards JE, Zollikofer C, Amplatz K (1980) The mechanism of balloon angioplasty. Radiology 135:565
3. Dotter CT, Judkins MP (1964) Transluminal treatment of arteriosclerotic obstruction. Circulation 30:654–670
4. Gailer H, Grüntzig A, Zeitler E (1983) Late results after percutaneous transluminal angioplasty of iliac and femoropopliteal obstructive lesions – a cooperative study. In: Dotter CT, Grüntzig A, Schopp W, Zeitler E (eds) Percutaneous transluminal angioplasty. Springer, Berlin Heidelberg New York, pp 215–218
5. Grüntzig A, Hopff H (1974) Perkutane Rekanalisation chronischer arterieller Verschlüsse mit einem neuen Dilatationskatheter. Dtsch Med Wochenschr 99:2502
6. Ingrisch H, Stiegler H, Rath M (1983) Nichtoperative Behandlung von infrarenalen Aortenstenosen durch Katheterdilatation. Röntgenpraxis 11/36:363–367
7. Ingrisch H (1984) Radiologische Therapie der Nierenarterienstenose durch perkutane transluminale Angioplastik. In: Arlart JP, Ingrisch H (eds) Renovaskuläre Hypertonie, Radiologische Diagnostik und Therapie. Thieme, Stuttgart New York
8. Mathias K, Bockenheimer St, von Reutern G, Weiss H-W, Ostheim-Dzerowycz W (1983) Katheterdilatation hirnversorgender Arterien. Radiologe 23:208–214
9. Motarjeme A, Keifer JW, Zuska AJ, Nabavi P (1983) Percutaneous transluminal angioplasty of the vertebral arteries. In: Dotter CT, Grüntzig A, Schoop W, Zeitler E (eds) Percutaneous transluminal angioplasty. Springer, Berlin Heidelberg New York, pp 241–244
10. Mullan S, Duda EE, Patronas NJ (1980) Some examples of balloon technology in neurosurgery. J Neurosurg 52:321–329
11. Olbert F, Kasprzak P, Muzika N, Schlegl A (1982) Perkutane transluminale Dilatation und Rekanalisation: Langzeitergebnisse und Erfahrungsbericht mit einem neuen Kathetersystem. VASA 11/4:327–331
12. Sepehr M-H, Altmann C (1984) Erleichterte Sondierbarkeit der Arteria Femoralis superficialis bei der PTA durch Anwendung der Tuohy-Kanüle. ROFO 140/2:212–214
13. Velasquez G, Castaneda-Zuniga W, Formanek A, Zollikofer Ch, Barreto A, Nicoloff D, Amplatz K, Sullivan A (1980) Nonsurgical aortoplasty in Leriche syndrome. Radiology 134:359–360
14. Vitek JJ, Morawetz RB (1982) Percutaneous transluminal angioplasty of the external carotid artery: preliminary. AJNR 3:541–546
15. Zeitler E, Berger G, Schmitt-Rüth R (1983) Percutaneous transluminal angioplasty of the supra-aortic arteries. In: Dotter CT, Grüntzig A, Schoop W, Zeitler E (eds) Percutaneous transluminal angioplasty. Springer, Berlin Heidelberg New York, pp 245–261

8 Intraoperative und Postoperative Assessment

G.W. HAGMÜLLER

CONTENTS

A. Introduction

In reconstructive vascular surgery, immediate assessment of therapeutic success by certain intraoperative procedures (evaluation of morphological and hemodynamic criteria) is of the utmost importance for preserving high standards. In reconstructive vascular surgery the quality of the operative procedure largely determines both the early and the late results. Long-term results can be improved through intraoperative control of vessel reconstruction. The discovery and elimination of technical errors within a reconstructed vascular segment is the ultimate goal of all intraoperative control measures.

Postoperative assessment should evaluate the immediate outcome of the operation. This is compared with preoperative diagnostic measures and the previous angiomorphological situation of the specific reconstructed arterial segment.

From the perspective of quality control, long-term follow-up at fixed time intervals makes it possible to keep track of patients and to evaluate the effectiveness of individual operations within larger patient groups.

B. Intraoperative Assessment

I. General

Intraoperative control is performed immediately after vascular reconstruction, so that any errors discovered can be immediately corrected. Morphological conditions are almost always judged by intraoperative angiography [11, 14, 17]. Vascular endoscopy as developed by VOLLMAR represents an important supplement to morphological judgement. However, this procedure can only be performed in a few medical centers since special equipment is needed [27].

Functional tests are a second means of immediate intraoperative control. Intravascular pressure registration and electromagnetic flow measurement have proven to be very reliable. Qualitative as well as quantitative blood flow parameters can be registered and compared [9]. In addition to these basic intraoperative methods, the literature discusses many highly specialized control techniques for specific vascular regions. However, since they usually involve very expensive equipment and are subject to constant modification, most of them cannot be recommended as standard methods of intraoperative assessment [26] (Table 8.1).

Table 8.1. Intraoperative assessment

I. Morphology:
1. Intraoperative angiography
2. Intraoperative vascular endoscopy
3. Other measures

II. Function:
1. Pressure registration
2. Electromagnetic flow measurement
3. Other measures

1. Angiography

The aim of intraoperative angiography is the radiomorphological display of an entire reconstructed vascular segment. The contrast medium is injected by hand either through a needle inserted proximal to the reconstruction or through a thin polyvinyl catheter that is fixed between two sutures during completion of the uninterrupted vessel suture with its tip lying proximal to the reconstruction. Following control angiography the needle or the catheter is removed, and the puncture site or the small anastomotic flap is compressed with the fingers. We prefer the catheter method because it is less traumatic than needle puncture. Detailed morphological pictures may be expected after arterial as well as after venous reconstructions.

Visual documentation is processed by an image-intensification fluoroscopy unit or an X-ray cassette of variable format which is exposed by standard X-ray apparatus. The advantage of a fluoroscopy unit to which a video recorder can be connected is that it allows precise observation of contrast medium run-off during injection. This allows the surgeon to judge the functional value of the reconstruction. The exposure of X-ray cassettes using a standard X-ray unit has the disadvantage of permitting only one exposure per injection. On the other hand, it is the better method of documentation. The quality of the X-ray picture is certainly higher than that of pictures obtained using fluoroscopy. During intraoperative angiography the dose of radiation can be estimated at 200–600 mR per X-ray using the conventional X-ray technique, and this is not insignificant. The radiation dose incurred during a fluoroscopic examination depends upon the length of the examination and may often be much higher than in conventional X-ray examinations. Intraoperative angiography is mainly applied in arterial and venous reconstructions of the extremities.

2. Vascular Endoscopy

According to VOLLMAR, endoscopic control of arterial and venous lumina depends upon three conditions:

1. Temporary interruption of blood flow
2. Establishment of a transparent environment by pressure-control perfusion through the inserted endoscope
3. Availability of an appropriate flexible or rigid endoscope

VOLLMAR lists the following main indications [27, 28]:

1. Semiclosed stripping of the pelvic and femoral artery
2. Venous thrombectomy within the ileofemoral segment

We have no experience of our own with this method. It should be seen as a complement to intraoperative angiography and as an aid in the identification of otherwise undetected vascular wall lesions within the inflow and outflow tract. One advantage is that the endoscopist has a three-dimensional view of the vessel and not merely a two-dimensional view as in angiography.

3. Intraoperative Pressure Registration

Historically, intravascular pressure registration is the oldest method of quantitative, intraoperative assessment. Here, too, technological progress has been dramatic – from a very complicated pressure gauge system to disposable pressure transducers. A pressure measuring system mainly consists of the following elements:

1. A conduction system to transmit the pressure from the vessel to the transducer
2. Pressure transducer
3. Amplifier
4. Registering instrument

A conduction system consists of transparent polyvinyl catheters with an average diameter of 1 mm. These are connected to the heart of the pressure measuring system, the transducer, and are filled with normal saline solution, making sure that no air bubbles are in the system. This is very important because gas bubbles are compressible and would falsify the measurements by influencing the volume-elasticity index. Continuous flushing of the whole pressure registration system is mandatory during intraoperative pressure measurement. The pressure chamber forms one unit with the actual pressure receptor (Fig. 8.1a, b).

The pressure transmitted from the vessel to the transducer by means of the conducting system acts upon an integrated strain gauge within the transducer through an elastic membrane. This gauge is part of an electrical resistance bridge. Responding to a change in electrical resistance, caused by

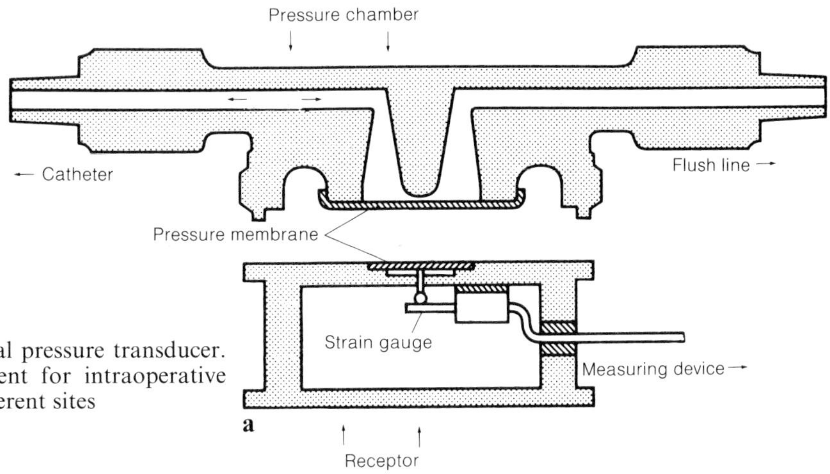

a

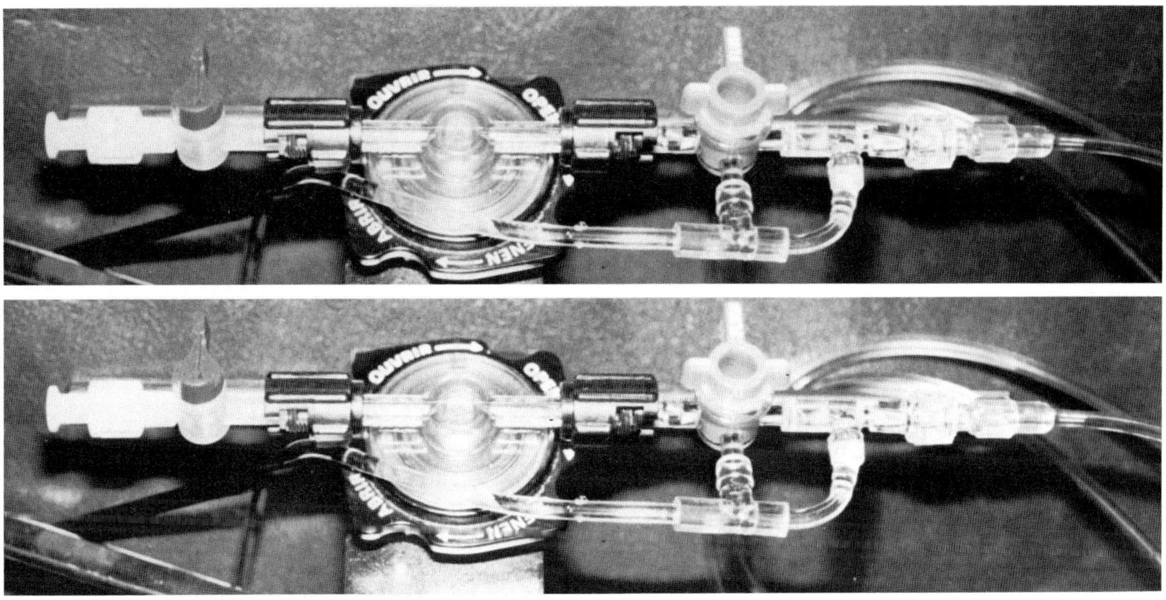

b

Fig. 8.1. **a** Diagram of an external pressure transducer. **b** Pressure transducer arrangement for intraoperative pressure measurement at two different sites

deformation of the strain gauge, a potential signal is produced in the measuring device, proportional to the changes in pressure. These electric impulses are amplified and recorded on a registering instrument. Information gained by intraoperative pressure registration is quantitative, i.e., it records the pressure in mmHg within the vessel segment being investigated. Pressure measurement should be performed in two different vessel segments simultaneously: one in the diseased vessel undergoing reconstruction and another in a segment with unaltered hemodynamic conditions, to serve as a reference (Fig. 8.2). This method is especially suited for intraoperative control of hemodynamically effective short stenoses and occlusions of arteries that are reconstructed by disobliterative endarter-

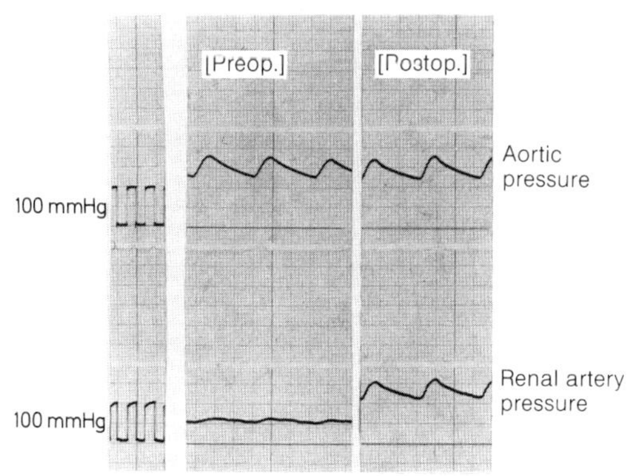

Fig. 8.2. Pressure curves before and after aortorenal vein bypass in subtotal renal artery stenosis. The calibration peak is equivalent to 100 mmHg. Postoperatively, renal artery pressure increased, equaling aortic pressure

ectomy or bypass (renal arteries, unpaired visceral arteries). A comparison of the preoperative and postoperative pressure differences between the reference pressure (e.g., aorta) and the pressure in the occluded vessel segment demonstrates the immediate effect of intraoperative reconstruction.

When puncturing the vessel for pressure measurement, one must be sure that the needle tip lies within the vessel, if possible against the direction of blood flow. The inside diameter of the needle should not be too small; otherwise, it damps the pressure curves. At least a 20-gauge needle should be used. The edge of the needle point should be blunt and steep. These details are extremely important for accurate pressure measurement. Bleeding at the puncture sites can be stopped by digital compression. They should not be oversewn; this might jeopardize the success of the operation.

4. Electromagnetic Blood Flow Measurement

This is the only method which can be applied intraoperatively to determine the functional state of the reconstructed vessel segment. The basic principle of electromagnetic flow measurement in a closed vessel is the practical application of Faraday's law of induction. Within the electrolyte fluid of the blood, an electric potential is induced across the two poles of the flowmeter by means of a magnetic field outside the vessel. This potential is registered by a pair of electrodes integrated into the flowmeter on the outside of the vessel. This so-called signal potential is proportional to the flow velocity averaged over the vessel diameter and therefore also proportional to the flow rate. The measuring device records the flow rate digitally. This method of flow measurement was described separately by KOLIN (1936) and WETTERER (1937) [13, 30]. Modern recording devices employ alternating magnetic fields, especially of the square wave form (square wave flowmeter), since there is no polarization at the electrodes and a constant zero level can be achieved. In combination with a recording machine, peak flow and mean flow should be registered as a flow curve during each measurement [9, 31].

The accuracy of electromagnetic measuring devices depends upon several factors: vessel wall thickness, vessel diameter, blood flow velocity, and hematocrit. The margin of error is about 10%–20%. The influence of hematocrit upon flow measurement can be eliminated in modern, programmable registration devices. However, in everyday practice, it can be disregarded because a reduction in hematocrit of 40%–20% lowers the relative measuring sensitivity of the devices by only about 1%. The registration electrodes must be in close contact with the vessel wall, and they should narrow the vessel lumen about 10%–20%. Interfering electrical potentials in the vicinity of the measuring site must be eliminated. Besides the recommended single ground electrode located in the subcutis near the measuring site, an additional surface ground electrode should be fixed to the patient (Fig. 8.3).

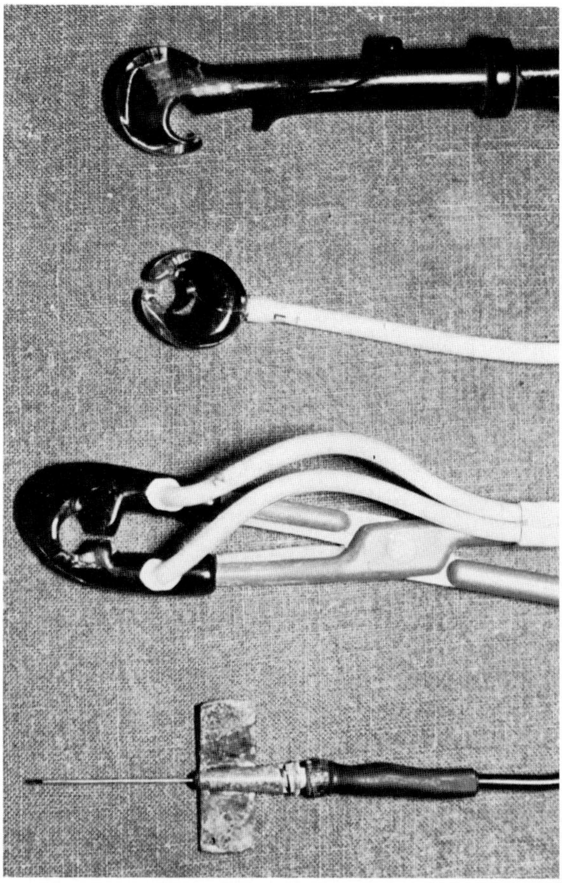

Fig. 8.3. Different models of flow probes for intraoperative electromagnetic flow measurement. Needle for subcutaneous grounding of the monitoring device

The functional value of electromagnetic flow measurement is demonstrated in a femoropopliteal vein bypass (Figs. 8.4, 8.5, 8.6). Of course, these results may be applied to other vascular regions.

1. The analysis of the registered curves shows the functional state of inflow and outflow. Pharmacodynamically induced hyperemia (papaverine

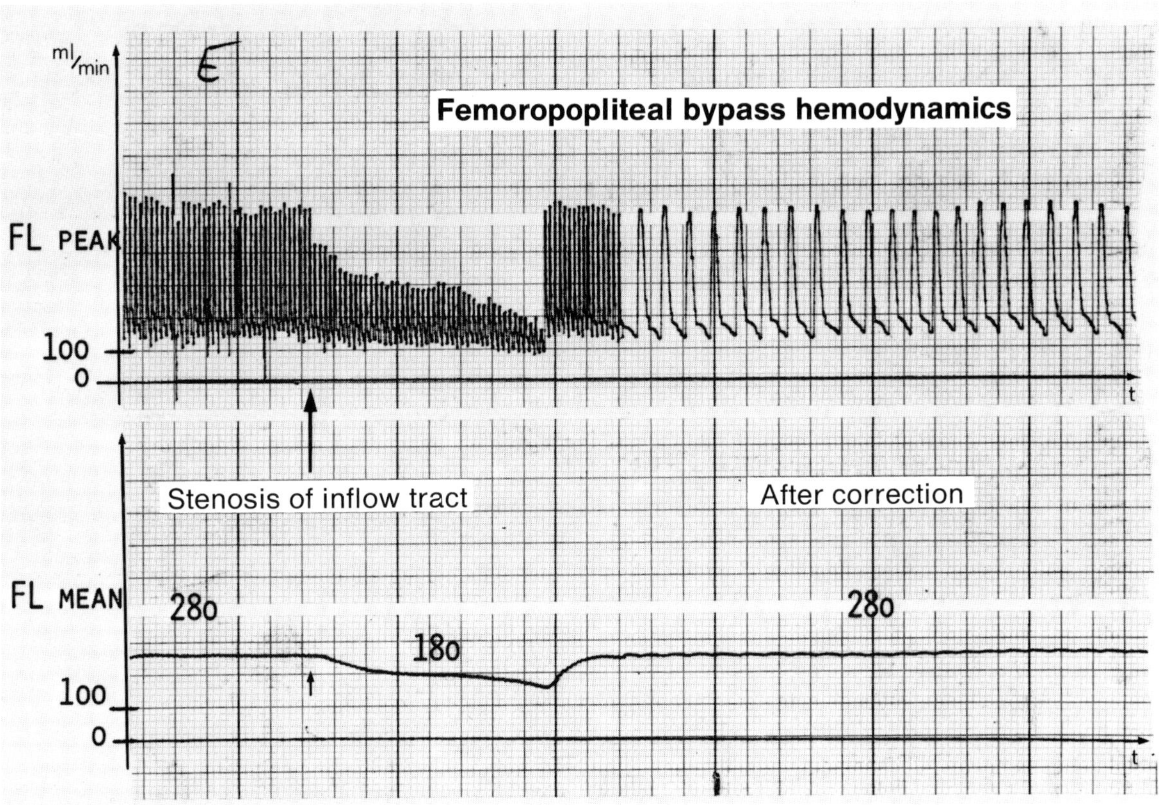

Fig. 8.4. Peak and mean flow registration during progressive narrowing of the inflow tract of a femoropopliteal vein bypass. Significant decrease of peak systolic flow at a 50% stenosis within the inflow tract of the vein bypass without detectable change of diastolic flow (*left portion of the upper flow curve*). The drop in mean flow from 280 to 180 ml is due to the decrease in peak systolic flow (*lower flow curve*). Conclusion: a stenosis of the inflow tract of a vessel reconstruction can be identified only by the decreased peak systolic flow rates during pulsatile curve registration. The cause of a decrease in blood flow cannot be determined from the mean flow rate curve

0.5 mg per kilogram body weight, naphtydrofuryl 1 mg/kg etc., are injected into the vascular segment) leads to an increase in blood flow parameters that are monitored by mean flow measurement. This increase of blood flow is caused by a rise in peak diastolic flow, which is due to a decrease in peripheral vascular resistance developing after vasodilatation. This increased take-up capacity of the periphery leads to a secondary rise in systolic flow. These changes during registration of flow curves give a limited evaluation of the functional value of a reconstruction.

2. If the registered flow measurements do not coincide with values normally obtained after different reconstructive procedures, a technical error must be sought. Intraoperative angiography should help find the error in order to perform immediate correction.

In analyzing the registered flow curves, the peak systolic and diastolic amplitudes in relation to the zero line are of great importance. A small systolic amplitude with round and angled peaks is an indication of a stenosis within the inflow tract (Fig. 8.4). The peak diastolic flow gives information on peripheral resistance. The higher it is, due to an impaired outflow tract, the lower is diastolic flow (Fig. 8.5). Functional behavior of a femoropopliteal vein bypass during electromagnetic flow measurement is depicted in Fig. 8.6. All criteria needed for intraoperative measurement are described here. Blood flow is measured as mean (lower curve) as well as peak flow (upper curve). A calibrating spike of 100 ml/min is present at the beginning of each curve registration. Flow behav-

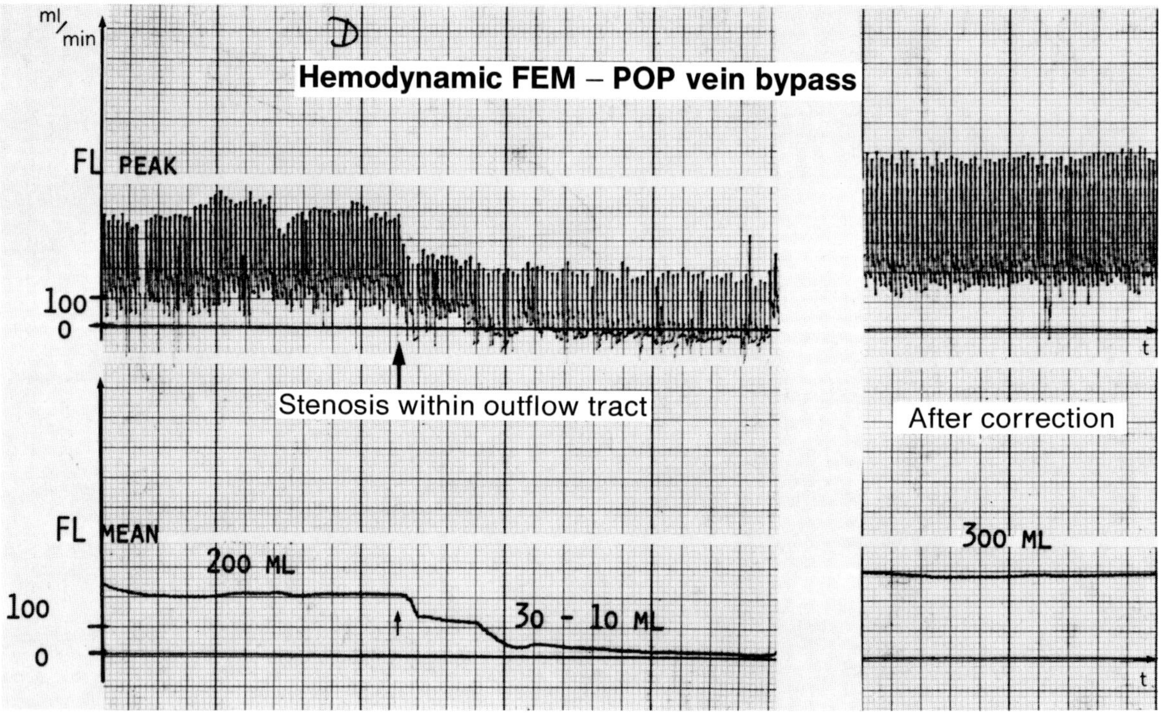

△

Fig. 8.5. Flow measurement in progressive narrowing of the outflow tract of a femoropopliteal vein bypass. Increase of resistance peripheral to the measuring site lowers diastolic flow below the zero line. The flow amplitude between diastolic and systolic flow does not change during an increase of peripheral resistance (*upper curve*). The fall in mean blood flow from 200 ml to 30–10 ml is due to the decrease in peak diastolic flow (*lower curve*). Results: During pulsatile curve registration, peak diastolic flow values near the zero line indicate increased peripheral resistance due to an angiomorphologically impaired outflow tract

Fig. 8.6. Typical blood flow curve of a femoropopliteal vein bypass at rest and after pharmacodynamically induced hyperemia (naphtydrofuryl 1 mg/kg); increase from 260 to 480 ml; this rise is achieved with three patent lower leg arteries (group 1). By converting the distal bypass anastomosis from an end-to-side (*ES*) to an end-to-end (*EE*) anastomosis the flow drops here to an average flow of 200 ml owing to the decrease in peak diastolic flow. The latter drops because the exclusion of the retrograde perfused proximal popliteal segment above the distal anastomosis leads to an increase of peripheral resistance for the bypass

▽

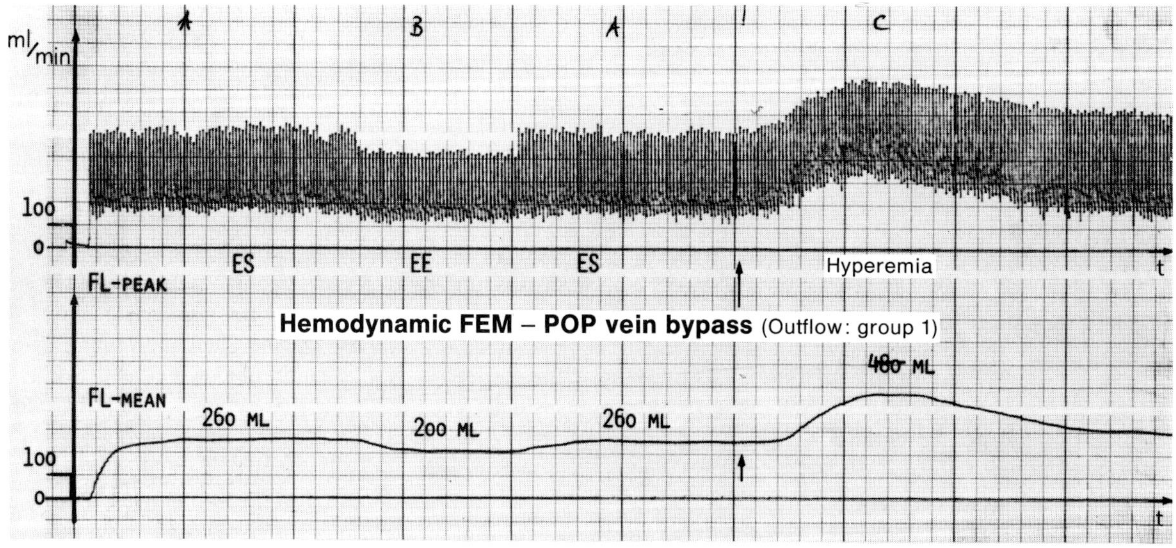

ior after changing peripheral resistance by converting an end-to-side into an end-to-end anastomosis within the region of the distal bypass anastomosis is clearly shown. Flow measurement following pharmacodynamically induced hyperemia is always performed at the end of the procedure. As mentioned earlier, an increase of flow during hyperemia is due to a rise in diastolic flow, which is caused by a reduction of vascular resistance during peripheral vasodilatation. Besides registering absolute values of mean blood flow at rest and during hyperemia, intraoperative flow measurement also helps analyze inflow and outflow conditions.

II. Special

1. Carotid Artery

Various techniques for measuring blood pressure in the carotid artery have been developed (direct intravascular pressure measurement, indirect pressure measurement of the orbital arteries using ophthalmodynamography and oculopneumoplethysmography) and also various control methods using Doppler sonography (registration of supratrochlear flow signals, direct ultrasound of the internal carotid artery, quantitative determination of local flow disturbance with measurement of the perturbation index, Doppler ultrasonic techniques with frequency analysis) [12, 20, 21, 24].

a) Pressure Measurement. Pressure registration following direct needle puncture of the common carotid artery and internal carotid artery distal to the reconstructed vessel segment allows one to evaluate the elimination of a preoperative pressure gradient (Fig. 8.7). However, an estimation of local flow conditions at the carotid bifurcation cannot be achieved by intravascular pressure measurements, which allow only a rough assessment of successful intraoperative reconstruction. Indirect pressure measurement by continuous ophthalmodynamography or oculopneumoplethysmography evaluates the function of the collateral circulation

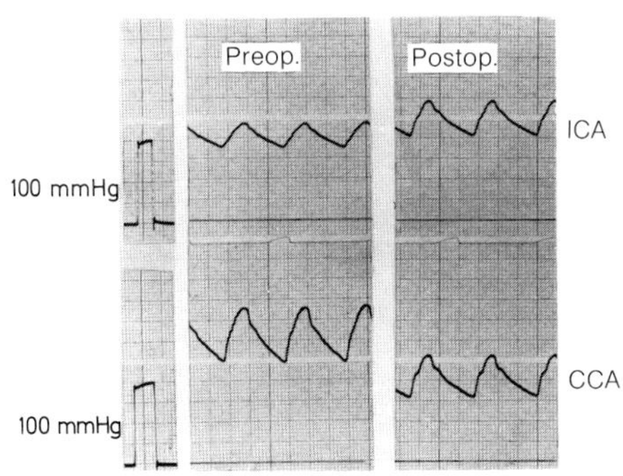

Fig. 8.7. Intraoperative pressure measurement before and after endarterectomy of the internal carotid artery. Registration of pressure gradient elimination between the common carotid artery (*CCA*) and internal carotid artery (*ICA*)

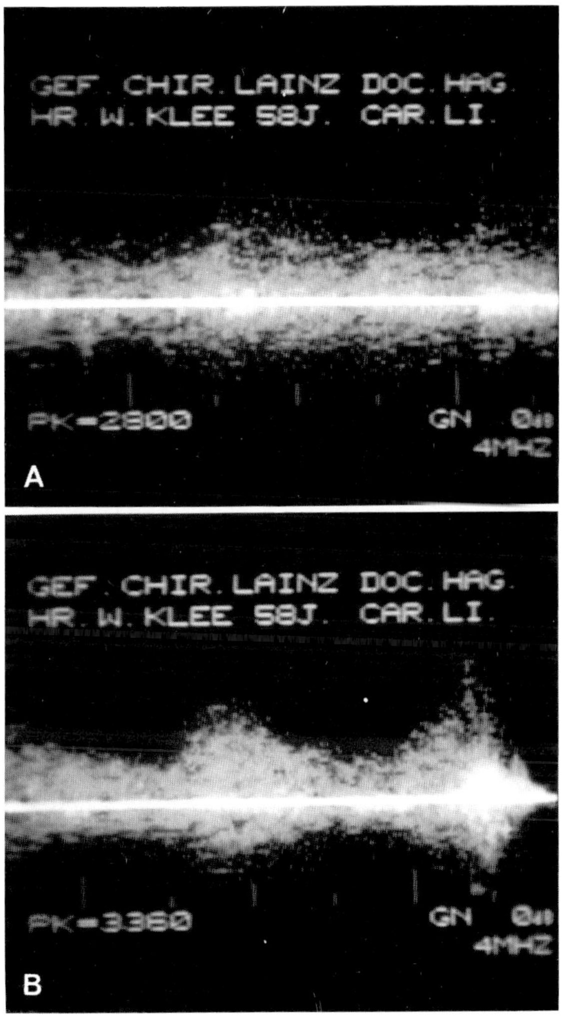

Fig. 8.8 A, B. Intraoperative echoflow frequency analysis at the internal carotid artery before (**A**) and after (**B**) endarterectomy (Polaroid photo). **A** Echoflow with a wide uniform frequency band and low flow velocity characterize the stenosis with turbulent flow. **B** Following endarterectomy distinct pulse waves with a uniform color spectrum and peak amplitude of 3360 Hz clearly demonstrate a decrease of turbulent flow with reconstitution of laminar flow

of the external carotid artery and correct position of internal shunts and documents pressure changes achieved by surgery of the internal carotid artery.

b) Indirect and Direct Ultrasonic Doppler Sonography. The indirect registration of flow signals from the supratrochlear artery demonstrates a change in flow direction from retrograde to anterograde following successful carotid artery reconstruction. Nevertheless, a quantification of blood flow is not possible. Direct ultrasound of the carotid artery with sterile Doppler probes affords the opportunity to judge conditions by analyzing the registered curves [12, 24].

c) Doppler Ultrasonic Frequency Analysis. A localized flow disturbance may be determined quantitatively with the Doppler ultrasonic method. The calculation of the so-called perturbation index is a new technique developed by SANDMANN et al. during the last few years for clinical use [20, 21]. It can detect deviations in laminar flow. If serious turbulence occurs within the operating field, the situation is monitored immediately. Such a direct assessment of localized flow turbulences at the carotid bifurcation may also be done with an echoflow scanner (Fig. 8.8). Its clinical application has not yet been fully developed.

The intraoperative use of high-precision Doppler ultrasonic frequency analyses can lead to a significant reduction in intraoperative and postoperative neurologic complications. Therefore, it is absolutely essential that these control methods for intraoperative assessment of the success of carotid reconstructions be further developed and applied.

2. Subclavian Artery

The main indications for reconstruction of the subclavian artery are central subclavian occlusions with evidence of a clinical and angiographic subclavian steal syndrome. Intraoperative surgical success (carotid – subclavian bypass, subclavian transposition, subclavio-subclavian bypass) is recognizable by the postoperative reverse of vertebral blood flow. This can be easily detected at the vertebral artery by electromagnetic flow measurements. According to our own investigations of central occlusions of the subclavian artery, retrograde flow in the vertebral artery is 100–200 ml/min. Following successful reconstruction, antegrade flow should reach physiologic values of 80–120 ml/min.

3. Arteries of the Arm

After reconstructive procedures within the arteries of the arm (embolectomies, traumas), surgical success is checked intraoperatively by judging the quality of the peripheral pulse and by angiography. It is especially important to make sure that the palmar arch system is patent as most recurrent occlusions are caused by obstruction of peripheral arterial segments, leading to a maximum increase of peripheral resistance.

4. Visceral Arteries

Functional assessment after procedures on visceral arteries is most accurately performed by intraoperative intravascular pressure measurement. A prerequisite for assessing success is preoperative pressure measurement prior to reconstruction. Preoperative and postreconstructive pressure registration should be performed on the same vessel segments (aortic pressure measurement as a reference). It is not the comparison between the absolute pressure values that is important, but the removal or reduction of the pressure gradient between aorta and postreconstructive arterial segment. If synthetic material is used for reconstruction, a puncture of the synthetic material for pressure measurement should be avoided. Its wall elasticity influences the registered pressure curves, and needle puncture may cause unpleasant hemorrhage.

5. Renal Arteries

In quality control after renal artery reconstruction, the same requirements apply as in visceral arteries. Here, change of the pressure gradient before and after reconstruction is the most important intraoperative check (see Fig. 8.2). According to our own experience, electromagnetic flow measurement is not indicated in intestinal and renal arteries since no comparative values on normal blood flow through these arteries are available in the literature. Furthermore, the adjustment and fixation of the small flow probes to these fine arteries could jeopardize the reconstruction.

6. Aortic and Pelvic Arteries

Instrumental measurement for quality control following reconstruction of the abdominal aorta (endarterectomy, aortic bifurcation prosthesis) and reconstruction of the pelvic arteries is not employed routinely since clinical pulse control alone suffices. Intraoperative measurements of flow rate through the pelvic arteries show values between 600 and 800 ml/min in one leg of the bifurcation prosthesis when the femoral artery is patent. The results of aortoiliac reconstructions can be measured only at the superficial femoral artery and the profunda femoris artery. This will be described in the following section.

7. Femoropopliteocrural Artery Axis

Methods of intraoperative control for the many reconstructive procedures within the lower extremity can be summarized as follows:

1. Angiography
2. Electromagnetic flow measurement
3. Pressure measurement
4. Continuous registration of skin temperature
5. Ultrasonic Doppler pressure measurement
6. Vascular endoscopy

Two main methods are employed: angiography for morphological control and electromagnetic flow measurement for functional control.

a) Intraoperative Angiography. Intraoperative angiography is probably the oldest method of intraoperative functional control following reconstructions within the lower extremity. References on this subject are numerous. The technique of intraoperative angiography has been described earlier. The great advantage of angiography is that technical errors can be found immediately and corrected during the same operation. According to KRETSCHMER et al., the commonest errors requiring correction are found after thromboendarterectomy of the femoral artery, followed by femoropopliteal vein bypass and synthetic graft bypass. In the literature, the intraoperative correction rate following angiography of femoral artery reconstructions is between 9% and 27%. After thromboendarterectomy the lesions most often encountered are more or less extensive intimal residues necessitating a correction.

Control angiography after bypass operations should give information on the proximal and distal anastomosis, where intraoperative errors are most often discovered. Surgically induced peripheral embolisms are easily found by means of image intensification, using the preoperative angiogram for reference.

b) Electromagnetic Flow Measurement. The technique of intraoperative electromagnetic flow measurement has been described earlier. Its value in assessing the success or failure of reconstructive procedures in different vascular regions will be reemphasized here [9, 19].

The flow rate following profunda patch angioplasty in an inoperable femoral artery occlusion is 130 ml/min on average, according to our own investigations. The benefit of additional lumbar sympathectomy is evident from a 30% increase in blood flow (Fig. 8.9). The augmentation of blood flow starts immediately after resection of the sympathetic chain, as the figure shows. This increase is a result of a rise in peak diastolic flow, initiated by a drop in peripheral resistance within the profunda femoris circulation as a result of sympathectomy. The measurement of flow through the profunda femoris artery is especially important after iliac reconstruction in multiple two-level occlusions [1]. Mandatory measurement of the hyperemic reaction of the profunda femoris artery tests the response of the outflow tract. From an increase in peak and mean flow during hyperemia, it is possible to predict the likely effect of lumbar sympathectomy. Circulatory improvement in an aortoprofundal synthetic bypass graft following lumbar sympathectomy is shown in Fig. 8.10. Maximum hyperemia after sympathetic chain resection reaches 130 ml, with a steady level of 90 ml. This is an increase of about 50% with respect to a control value of 60 ml before sympathectomy.

The importance of electromagnetic flow measurement in a vein graft and its typical functional characteristics have already been described earlier (see Fig. 8.6). We present here, calculated from our own data, the absolute values of the necessary minimum flow rates. These rates depend upon outflow tract morphology as demonstrated in angiograms (Table 8.2). A predictive value for long-term patency of a vein bypass is 300 ml/min in three patent lower leg arteries, 250 ml/min in two open arteries, and 150 ml/min in one open artery.

The increase of flow during hyperemia (papaverine, naphtydrofuryl, etc.) should be 200 ml in three arteries, 150 ml in two, and 100 ml in one artery. If these values are not reached during hyperemia, early thrombosis of the reconstruction must be expected. In such a case intraoperative angiography might help discover technical errors at the anastomosis or outflow obstructions (intraoperative embolism). The absolute values listed

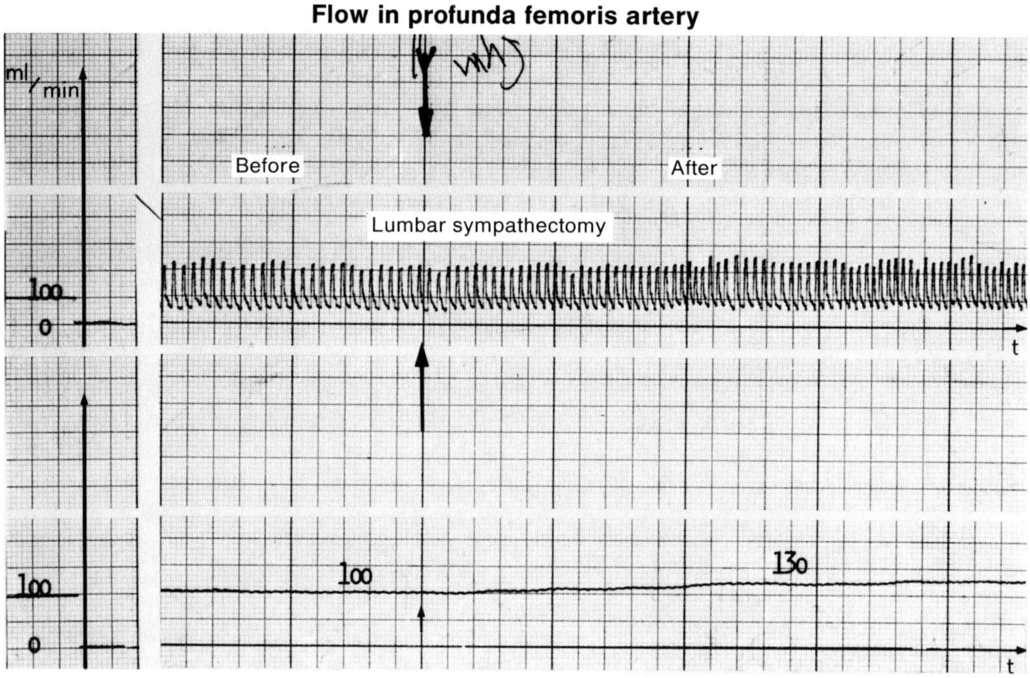

Fig. 8.9. Intraoperative flow measurement following extensive profunda patch angioplasty before and during lumbar sympathectomy. After sympathetic trunk resection (see *arrow*) a slow increase of mean flow from 100 to 130 ml is registered. Vasodilatation due to sympathectomy is indicated by the rise in diastolic flow during pulsatile curve registration (*upper curve, right-hand portion*). A fall in peripheral resistance due to sympathectomy is observed

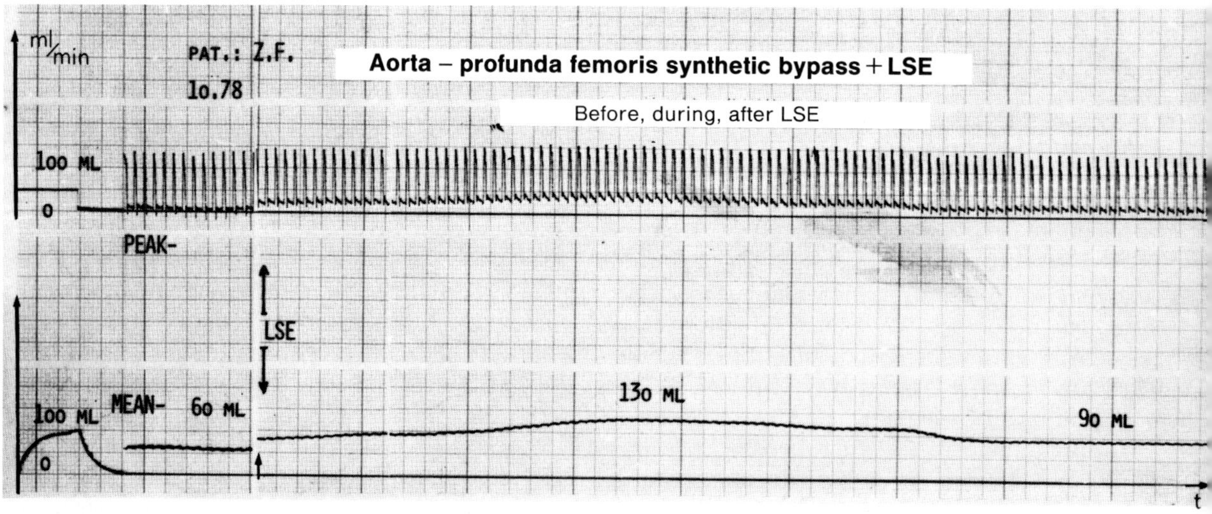

Fig. 8.10. Intraoperative flow measurement following aortoprofunda synthetic bypass. Registration of increased flow within the profunda femoris circulation from 60 to over 130 to 90 ml, caused by peripheral vasodilatation after lumbar sympathectomy (LSE)

Table 8.2. Flow values at rest (Fl_r) and during hyperemia (Fl_{hyp}) in a femoropopliteal vein bypass with respect to the patency of the outflow tract

	Patent lower leg arteries		
	Three	Two	One
Fl_r $x \pm SD$	306.7 ± 168.6	246.5 ± 102.6	148.4 ± 113.3
Fl_{hyp} $x \pm SD$	500.8 ± 203.4	407.0 ± 149.9	252.0 ± 154.3

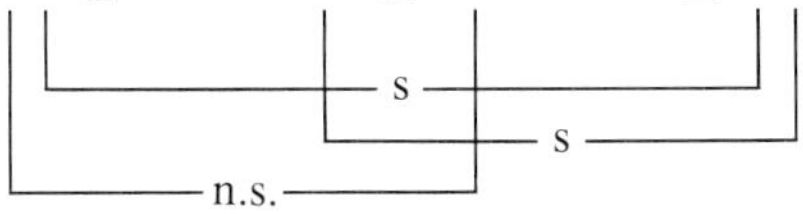

s = significant ($p < 0.05$); n.s. = not significant (Student's test)

also depend on the circulatory situation as a whole, the method of anesthesia, and intraoperative volume substitution. A critical bypass flow rate, which is always mentioned in the literature, cannot be generally defined without classifying the outflow tract in terms of patent lower leg arteries, as in Table 8.2 [2, 19].

Further methods of intraoperative control such as measurement of skin temperature, percutaneous oxygen measurement, and intraoperative ultrasonic pressure measurement may also help estimate surgical success, especially during operations on the extremities. However, these controls cannot be used as absolute indicators of successful reconstruction since comparable quantitative values do not exist in the literature.

C. Postoperative Assessment

The aim of immediate postoperative control is to evaluate the anticipated circulatory improvement using clinical and technical methods. Preoperative findings with the same methods must be present for adequate judgement. According to KRIESSMANN we differentiate between stage-dependent and stage-independent parameters [5]. In the extremities, dynamic stages (i.e., postoperative conversion of clinical symptoms, stages II–IV according to the classification of FONTAINE) are a very simple and important check.

Immediately after surgery the most impressive change in symptoms is the conversion from stage III to the painless stage II. A similar effect may be seen following operations on the extracranial carotid artery. In these cases, initial quality control may be performed by a simple clinical neurologic examination.

Stage-independent parameters are hemodynamic dimensions such as:

1. Pressure
2. Flow
3. Volume

These parameters are obtainable by noninvasive measuring techniques.

Some arterial regions cannot be judged by noninvasive methods (visceral arteries, renal arteries, and in some instances the carotid artery). If there is clinical doubt that reconstruction has been successful, postoperative morphological control (angiography) must be performed [5].

I. General

Qualitative diagnostic measures:
- Oscillometry
- Rheography
- Doppler ultrasonography

Quantitative diagnostic measures:
- Plethysmography (Doppler flow measurement)

Morphological diagnostic measures:
- Angiography
- Ultrasonic imaging

1. Doppler Ultrasonography

The most widely applicable method of qualitative control, one that can be employed in virtually every region of the arterial system, is based on the Doppler ultrasonic technique [22, 25]. This is a special form of echo technology, involving the evaluation of echo signals whose frequency differs from that of the transmitter signals. The underlying principle is illustrated in Fig. 8.11.

From a stationary transmitter, a strong ultrasound beam is directed toward the solid blood components flowing within the blood vessel. The ultrasound waves traverse the vascular lumen with the velocity of sound c. The speed of the blood particles in the direction of the ultrasound waves is equivalent to $v_i \cos \alpha$. The ultrasound waves are dispersed by the blood particles. When the receiver, located in the Doppler probe, registers this dispersion, the receiving frequency of the backscat-

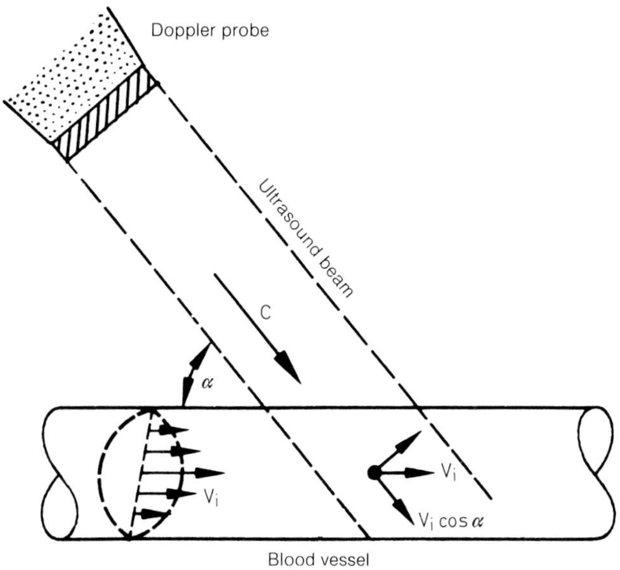

Fig. 8.11. Doppler ultrasonography

tered ultrasound wave demonstrates the characteristic Doppler shift. The sum of the intensities of all blood components within the ultrasound wave area result in a broad frequency spectrum, the Doppler signal. The Doppler effect with ultrasound was used for the first time by SATOMURA to determine the direction of blood flow. The first clinical studies were reported by SUMMER, BAKER, and STRANDNESS. Since then, Doppler ultrasonography has become indispensable as a diagnostic tool in vascular disease. The Doppler instruments used for qualitative determination of blood flow operate at frequencies of 5–10 MHz. The measuring sensitivity of these devices is rather small because the dispersion at the blood particles is limited. This is why they can only be used in peripheral vessels and have only a short depth of penetration. The directional Doppler devices register the direction of blood flow and display it as a trace on an oscilliscope or recording device. One of the most important applications is the measurement of systolic blood pressure in the extremities by the cuff method. A blood pressure cuff proximal to the site of measurement is inflated above the level of systolic pressure. The systolic pressure value reached at the point where pulsatile blood flow recommences during slow reduction of cuff pressure can be detected by the Doppler probe, even after the audible pulse signals have vanished. Distal to an arterial obliteration (e.g., femoral artery occlusion) systolic pressure is lowered significantly. The quotient between the registered Doppler pressure value and systemic arterial blood pressure is a good estimate of the severity of flow obstruction. The comparison between preoperative and postoperative quotients (Doppler index) is best suited to postoperative functional control following arterial reconstructions within extremities. However,,for assessment of existing circulatory insufficiency in an extremity, it is certainly better to consider the absolute pressure values [15, 18, 29].

Further detailed information on the use of Doppler ultrasonography in blood flow measurements, such as the pulsed Doppler flowmeter for determination of flow profiles and blood volume, and Doppler angiography, may be found in the literature.

2. Plethysmography

Venous outflow plethysmography consists of quantitative determination of flow parameters in extremities. Today strain-gauge plethysmography is mostly applied. Flow is measured quantitively in ml per 100 g tissue per minute. This flow measurement is performed at rest and under standard exercising conditions. Resting blood flow is influenced regionally by different factors and is therefore not the decisive parameter in evaluating circulation. Instead, exercise flow, which is not measured as reactive hyperemia, but under standardized exercising conditions up to 280 W/s, is better suited to this purpose. We have abandoned the measurement of reactive hyperemia because the occluding cuff necessary to provoke reactive hyperemia increases the risk of recurrent obliteration of the reconstructed femoral artery. Provocation is achieved by exercise with a pedal ergometer. An important point in using plethysmography as a method of postoperative quality control is that an individual reference value is obtained preoperatively. According to our own investigations, a mean value of 25 ± 5 ml can be measured in the leg during exercise at 280 W/s [8, 10, 29]. Oscillography and rheography cannot be discussed any further in this chapter.

3. Control Angiography

Presently, three methods are at our disposal:

1. Conventional transarterial angiography [5, 6]
2. Digital video subtraction angiography (DSA, DVI) [3, 23]
3. Transvenous xeroarteriography [7]

Table 8.3. Indications for postoperative control angiography (as proposed by VAN DONGEN)

Early postoperative period:
Reocclusion
Suspected malfunction of the reconstruction
Suspected change of the outflow tract
Suspected false aneurysm (postoperative bleeding, infection)
Late postoperative period:
Extension of a reocclusion
Localization of a recurrent stenosis
Obliteration of a parallel or dependent arterial segment
Anastomotic aneurysm
Aortoenteric fistula

The technical bases of these diagnostic methods is given in more detail in the literature.

The indications for postoperative control angiography following arterial reconstructions are shown in Table 8.3, as proposed by VAN DONGEN [6]. Early postoperative angiography should be performed if clinical findings and noninvasive control methods indicate signs of reocclusion or raise doubt as to the patency of the reconstructed vascular segment. Control angiography during the late postoperative period should be performed if, following initial symptomatic relief, ischemic complications within the reconstructed area reoccur. Also, if during long-term follow-up with noninvasive measuring techniques functional impairment is detected, control angiography is essential to determine the extent of a recurrent occlusion, on the one hand, and to localize recurrent stenosis, on the other.

Although there are numerous noninvasive control methods for the evaluation of the postoperative hemodynamic situation in the extremities, possibilities for control following reconstructions of the visceral or renal arteries are limited. These should be inspected by angiography. The same should be done after reconstructions of the carotid artery if morphological changes at the site of endarterectomy are suspected.

Thus, control angiography is indispensable in many postoperative situations. In many cases, it is very useful in finding errors which have been overlooked during surgery. Besides being an important tool in the diagnosis and treatment of complications, it can be used to examine the morphological and functional state of a reconstruction. Angiography is also a well-established method of exact documentation and control during the follow-up period (VAN DONGEN).

II. Special

1. Carotid Artery – Vertebral Artery

Ultrasound imaging as well as angiography are of equal importance in the postoperative control of extracranial cerebral arteries [4, 7]. They should always be performed if intraoperative control is not possible and there is doubt that the reconstruction is functioning properly.

2. Supra-aortic Arterial Segments – Subclavian Artery

Aortic angiography is essential for control of supra-aortic arterial segments. It should always be performed for postoperative documentation [6]. Reconstructions of the subclavian artery can be inspected by control angiography or ultrasonic imaging.

3. Arteries of the Arm

For routine control of the arteries of the upper extremity, the following are sufficient: separate pulse examinations on each side, blood pressure measurement according to Riva-Rocci, and Doppler ultrasonic pressure measurements in the forearm arteries. Of course, if there are factors which make control angiography necessary, this procedure should be performed prior to a second operation.

4. Visceral and Renal Arteries

Following reconstructions within both arterial systems, postoperative control angiography is indispensable [6]. Although one can detect absent or reduced blood flow of the kidney with noninvasive techniques, such as renography and scintigraphy, true assessment of success or failure of a renal artery reconstruction is possible only by angiography. The same is true after reconstructions of visceral arteries. A constriction at the anastomosis of an aortomesenteric vein bypass graft can lead to thrombosis of the graft, which would not only endanger vital organs, but also the life of the patient. Control angiography is always indicated after operations on the abdominal aorta in which visceral and renal arteries are also reconstructed.

5. Aorta and Pelvic Arteries

Quality control in these regions is not problematic and can easily be performed in the lower extremity. Noninvasive techniques, especially Doppler ultrasonography and plethysmography, are available.

6. Aortofemoral Occlusion

a) Total Correction of the Aortofemoral Occlusion. Total correction of a two-level occlusion, using an aortofemoral synthetic bypass graft for the obliterated upper segment and a femoropopliteal venous bypass graft for the lower arterial segment, shows excellent clinical and hemodynamic results during the early postoperative period (Fig. 8.12).

The Doppler indices increase to 0.88 ± 0.11 in the posterior tibial artery and to 0.80 ± 0.10 in the dorsalis pedis artery. Exercise flow values measured plethysmographically during pedalergometry increase to subnormal values of 18.6 ± 2.4 ml/min. The values demonstrated here are representative of patient groups that have undergone such operations.

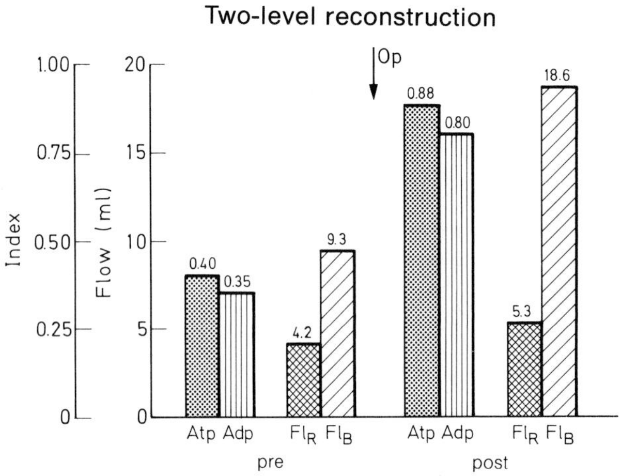

Fig. 8.12. Early hemodynamic results after total correction of an ileofemoral occlusion. The Doppler index of the posterior tibial artery (*Atp*) and dorsalis pedis artery (*Adp*) and the plethysmographically measured resting flow (Fl_R) and exercise flow (Fl_B) are shown. Postoperative indices: Atp, 0.88; Adp, 0.80; resting flow, 5.3; exercise flow, 18.6

b) Aortoprofunda Reconstruction Excluding a Long Segment of the Profunda Femoris Artery. In 18 patients with stage II and III symptoms, the following values were obtained (Fig. 8.13). The postoperative Doppler indices show an increase of more than 80% over preoperative values, to 0.48 and 0.46 ± 0.16, respectively. Exercise flow rises about 11% to 9.7 ± 3.0 ml/min. Symptomatic improvement from stage III to II may be expected.

c) Aortoprofunda Synthetic Bypass Including a Long Segment of the Profunda Femoris Artery. In 22 patients with stage III and IV symptoms, the following values were obtained (Fig. 8.14). (Direct comparison between both groups is not legitimate because the morphology of the outflow tract differs in each case.) The relative increase of blood flow after simple and extended profunda recon-

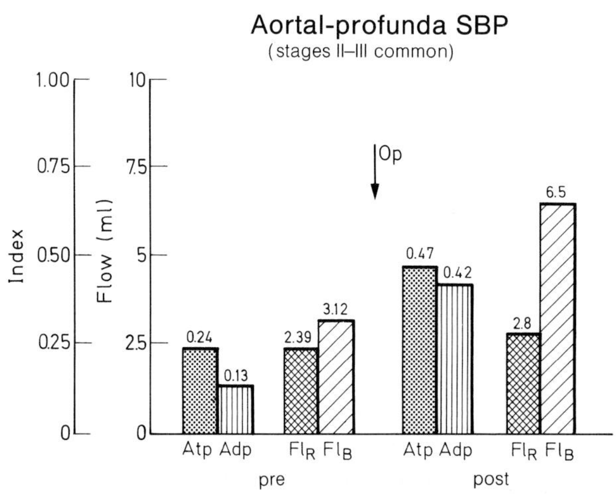

Fig. 8.13. Early hemodynamic results of postoperative quality control following common aortoprofunda synthetic bypass (for explanation of abbreviations see Fig. 8.12)

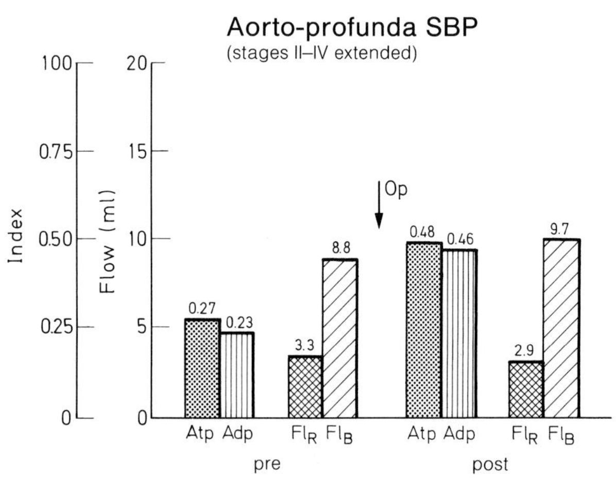

Fig. 8.14. Early hemodynamic results of postoperative assessment following aortoprofunda synthetic bypass with extended long angioplasty at the profunda femoris artery. Significant increase of Doppler indices and plethysmographic exercise flows, in contrast to Fig. 8.13

struction is of special interest. The Doppler indices increase more than 100% to 0.47 and 0.42±0.16; exercise flow rises 108% to 6.5±2.56 ml/min. Statistically, the aortoprofunda synthetic bypass with extended profunda revascularization clearly shows better results [8, 9].

If clinical stage improvement is not achieved and intraoperative control measures are not possible or inconclusive, control angiography of the whole reconstructed segment is necessary.

7. Femoropopliteocrural Reconstruction

Noninvasive control methods are mainly employed after procedures on the femoral artery. The results of Doppler ultrasound pressure measurement and plethysmographic flow measurement after long femoropopliteal vein bypass grafting are shown in Fig. 8.15 and correspond to the values reported in the literature. The postoperative Doppler indices are 0.88 and 0.87±0.16. Exercise flow increases to 16.6±2.2 ml/min. These hemodynamic parameters demonstrate the subnormalization of blood flow in successful femoropopliteal vein bypass grafting.

If during the early postoperative period the expected pressure values in the foot arteries are not reached, even though a positive pulse can be palpated over the open graft, a control angiogram is indicated. The morphology of the lower leg arteries enables the examiner to predict the prognosis of each individual reconstruction, provided that the anastomosis is correct. The most important control measure after crural bypass operations is Doppler ultrasound pressure measurement. According to our experience and reports in the literature, the morphological state of lower leg arteries following crural reconstruction differs so much from case to case that no collective values representative of postoperative hemodynamic function can be determined. Each case must be evaluated separately. Nevertheless, angiography is indicated whenever there is doubt. The fate of the extremity depends on the quality of the reconstruction.

Methods of intraoperative and postoperative control are summarized in Table 8.4.

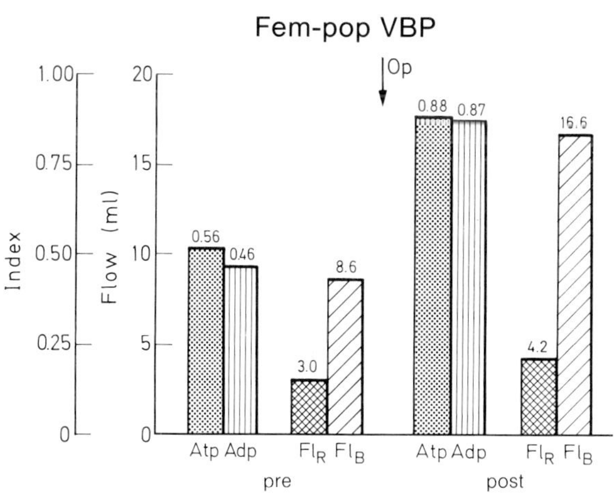

Fig. 8.15. Early hemodynamic results of postoperative assessment following long femoropoliteal venous bypass grafting. Improvement of postoperative Doppler indices and plethysmographic exercise flows to subnormal values

Table 8.4. Diagnosis and control measures in patients with occlusive arterial disease

Preoperative measurement:
- Clinical symptoms, stages II–IV
- ↓
- Functional assessment (Doppler ultrasonography, plethysmography, others)
- ↓
- Morphological assessment (angiography)

Intraoperative measurements:
- Functional assessment (pressure measurement, electromagnetic flow measurement, Doppler ultrasonography, others)
- ↓
- Morphological assessment (intraoperative angiography, Doppler ultrasound frequency analysis)

Postoperative measurements:
- Clinical symptoms (change in stage)
- ↓
- Functional assessment (change of preoperative parameters)
- ↓
- Control angiography (if anticipated functional improvement is not achieved)

REFERENCES

1. Berguer R, Higgins RF, Cotton LT (1975) Geometry, blood flow and reconstruction of the deep femoral artery. Am J Surg 130:68
2. Capellen C, Hall K (1967) Electromagnetic blood flowmetry in clinical surgery. Acta Chir Scand [Suppl] 368:3
3. Chilcote WA, Modic MT, Pavlicek W (1981) Digital subtraction angiography of the carotid arteries: a comparative study in 100 patients. Radiology 139:287
4. Comerota AJ, Cranley JJ, Cook SE (1981) Real-time-B-mode carotid imaging in diagnosis of cerebrovascular disease. Surgery 89:718

5. van Dongen RJAM (1970) Photographic atlas of reconstructive arterial surgery. HE Stenfert Kroese NV, Leiden
6. van Dongen RJAM (1983) Postoperative Kontrollangiographie. Angio Archiv 5:53
7. Dörrler J, Kramann M, Maurer PC, Schleicher P, Wiesmeier R (1983) Optimierung der Carotischirurgie-Nachsorge unter besonderer Berücksichtigung der transvenösen Xeroradiographie. Angio Archiv 5:156
8. Hagmüller GW, Weidinger P (1979) Die Bedeutung und Erfassung der prae-, intra- und postoperativen Hämodynamik für das Therapiekonzept beim Zweietagenverschluß. Angio 1:25
9. Hagmüller GW (1981) Klinisch-experimentelle Studie der Durchflußänderungen bei rekonstruktiven Eingriffen an der femoropoplitealen Arterienachse. Angio Archiv, vol 2. Demeter, Gräfelfing
10. Hallböök T (1971) Blood flow measurement with strain-gauge plethysmography in the early postoperative course after reconstructive arterial surgery in lower limbs. Acta Chir Scand 137:233
11. Heiss JM, Roder J, Lange J, Dörrler J, Maurer PC (1983) Angiographie mit Videosystem – wirkungsvolle und einfache intraoperative Diagnosesicherung und Therapiekontrolle. Angio Archiv 5:46
12. Keller HM, Turina M (1983) Die peroperative Beurteilung der Carotisperfusion mittels Doppler-Ultraschall. Angio Archiv 5:86
13. Kolin A (1936) An electromagnetic flowmeter. Principle of the method and its application to blood flow measurement. Proc Soc Exp Biol Med 35:53
14. Kretschmer G, Polterauer P, Wagner O, Winter M, Piza F (1981) Zur Wertigkeit der intraoperativen Kontrollangiographie im femoro-popliteo-cruralen Bereich. Langenbecks Arch Chir 354:89
15. Kriessmann A (1979) Welche Meßmethoden sind in der Langzeitbeobachtung gefäßchirurgischer Patienten sinnvoll. Angio 1:67
16. Piza F (1979) Die intraoperative Diagnostik in der Gefäßchirurgie. Wien Klin Wochenschr 91:403
17. Plecha FR, Pories WJ (1972) Intraoperative angiography in the immediate assessment of arterial reconstruction. Arch Surg 105:902
18. Rückert U, Burckhardt H (1975) Ultraschall-Druckmessung zur Erfolgsbeurteilung arterieller Rekonstruktionen. Dtsch Med Wochenschr 100:1473
19. Sandmann W, Kremer K, Wüst H, Florack G, Ruf S (1977) Funktionskontrolle von rekonstruierten Arterien durch postoperative elektromagnetische Strömungsmessung. Thoraxchirurgie 25:427
20. Sandmann W, Peronneau P, Kremer K (1980) Carotischirurgie und Pertubationsmessung. Angio 4:277
21. Sandmann W, Hennerici M, Klüsener K, Peronneau P (1981) Vergleich der Empfindlichkeit von Pertubationsmessung und Druckmessung zum Auffinden technischer Mängel in der Carotischirurgie. Vasa [Suppl] 8:70
22. Satomura S (1959) Study of the flow patterns in peripheral arteries by ultrasonics. J Acoust Soc Jap 15:75
23. Seyfert W, Marhoff P, Zeitler E (1982) Transvenöse und arterielle Videosubtraktionsangiographie (DVSA). ROFO 136:301
24. Sigel B, Coelho JCU, Flanigan DP, Schuler JJ, Spigos DG (1982) Ultrasonic imaging during vascular surgery. Arch Surg 117:764
25. Sumner DS, Baker DW, Strandness DE (1968) The ultrasonic velocity detector in a clinical study of venous disease. Arch Surg 97:75
26. Trusheim H (1983) Die intra- und postoperative Überwachung der Extremitätendurchblutung mit kontinuierlicher Temperaturmessung. Angio Archiv 5:93
27. Vollmar J, Storz LW (1974) Vascular endoscopy. Surg Clin North Am 54:111
28. Vollmar J (1982) Rekonstruktive Chirurgie der Arterien, 3rd edn. Thieme, Stuttgart New York
29. Weidinger P, Denck H, Olbert F (1977) Durchblutungsmessungen vor und nach Eingriffen wegen arterieller Durchblutungsstörungen in den oberen Extremitäten. Vasa 6:157
30. Wetterer E (1937) Eine neue Methode zur Registrierung der Blutgeschwindigkeit am uneröffneten Gefäß. Z Biol 98:26
31. Wyatt DG (1977) Theory, design and use of electromagnetic flowmeters. In: Hwang NHC, Norman NA (eds) Cardiovascular flow dynamics and measurement. University Park Press, Baltimore London Tokyo, p 89

9 Documentation and Statistics

O. WAGNER and M. SCHEMPER

CONTENTS

Vascular surgery is a specialty mainly based on clinical experience. Except for basic innovations like new vascular replacements development and progress rely on observations gained in everyday clinical practice. This information is then transmitted by surgeons' reports on their own therapeutic procedures and the results achieved through publications in medical journals and presentation of papers at meetings and congresses. Such retrospective reports depend on personal impressions and recollections and are seldom reflections on a broad base of facts. To avoid these pitfalls many medical investigaters have turned to prospective studies, this process was enhanced by the development of new statistical methods and improvement of computerized documentations systems.

For the correct assessment of therapeutic procedures and their results, the following factors must be taken into account: indication, preoperative pathomorphological situation, composition of patient groups, and the effects of these factors on immediate and long-term therapeutic results. In order to make comparisons between different institutions, the data must be comparable, and this means that all concepts and definitions must correspond, that patient groups must be classified in an analogous manner, and that analysis must be consistent and statistically correct.

Quality control has gained enormous importance as a result of increasing public interest in the efficiency and effectiveness of medical treatment. But quality cannot be ensured without the careful collection and interpretation of data. Therefore, modern techniques of comprehensive documentation, complemented by appropriate statistical analysis, are absolutely indispensable if the ever-growing demand for optimal health care is to be met.

A. Methods of Documentation

I. Historical Development

The basis of documentation is the patient's case history, together with the medical findings. Especially important in vascular surgery is the pictorial documentation of morphological changes (X-rays, computed tomography); this provides the most accurate description of the patient's preoperative condition and the postoperative results. While a small number of cases can be reviewed by case histories and pictures alone, other methods have to be used for continuous follow up and control of larger patient groups.

For better access to case histories, card-index systems have been devised which display diagnoses, operations, complications, and other details. In some instances, they are still a useful method for monitoring special patient groups.

Since the introduction of electronic data processing systems and the simplification of their usage in everyday life, medical documentation has changed considerably. Owing to the complexity of scientific problems and clinical research, even small patient groups necessitate the use of electronic data processing systems and adequate computer programs for statistical analysis. This presupposes, of course, that the importance of modern data processing within the field of clinical medicine is recognized and the proper equipment and personnel are available. It was in response to this rapidly developing need that a data processing center was founded at the medical school in Vienna in 1967.

The difficulties of systematization, definition, and quantification of medical data, as well as differences in technology and program languages have thus far prevented the broad-based standardization of medical documentation, despite the development of internationally accepted diagnostic and therapeutic codes (SNOMED, ICD) and surgery codes (VESKA in Switzerland, CHIDOS in Austria, the surgical therapeutic code according to Scheibe in the Federal Republic of Germany).

II. Methods of Documentation for the Systematic Study of Therapeutic Techniques and Their Effectiveness

To a large extent, scientific progress in vascular surgery has come through observation alone following the application of new techniques and materials. For this reason retrospective studies have accounted for most of the literature in this field. However, the data were not always adequately analyzed; important information on the description of patient groups was often missing, and correct statistical analysis was not employed. Only patients with nearly identical anatomic and functional forms of occlusive arterial disease and, for each such group, only similar reconstructive procedures are comparable. It is well known that vascular reconstructions above and below the knee, and within the lower leg region, using autogenous vein grafts, are quite different and dependent on the clinical stage and the outflow tract conditions. In such cases, explicit detailed information on each patient is needed. One reason why the results reported by different authors on the same reconstructive procedure are so different may be that these facts have not been taken into consideration. In retrospective studies, there have been some attempts to achieve group comparability by stratification on the basis of risk factors.

In the last years midterm follow-up documentation (for about 1–5 years) has been increasingly applied for prospective studies in systematic observation and control of the results of surgical and/or conservative therapy.

The first step that physicians and statisticians must take is to develop forms suitable for standardized data processing and containing the desired variable information. The quality of data collection is important for successful analysis and processing later on. The input of data should not be time-consuming and can be done, in part, by nonmedical personnel. The forms should contain coded facts (e.g., type of operation), quantitative details (e.g. distal perfusion pressure), or standardized alphanumeric input spaces (e.g., patient's name and address).

It is especially useful in the documentation of chronic diseases to divide the data into two groups: base-line and follow-up documentation. There are three ways of accomplishing the follow-up documentation:

- Only the last follow-up data is kept and considered during analysis.
- Each time the patient is seen, an additional follow-up data form is stored as part of a continuous series.
- At certain fixed time intervals (e.g., 3-month intervals), notes are made in specified spaces at each follow-up examination.

The first alternative is usually chosen because of its practicality and simplicity. Sometimes the investigator is interested only in assessing the patient's condition within a certain time interval (e.g., the function of a vascular reconstruction). The second method of data registration gives additional information on the patient's changes during the follow-up period, even if the patient is not seen at fixed time intervals. Precise and detailed follow-up analysis is necessary when using the third alternative.

An administrative system is necessary to make sure that the patients are seen at regular intervals and are reminded to come to the follow-up examinations [35]. The software package SAS [31–34] is an integrated data processing system [38] for clinical studies or special documentation. Several functions are available: printing of tables and graphic presentations, lists of patients who did not come to the follow-up examinations, number of expected follow-up examinations within a month, printing of address labels or standardized letters, and on-line information may be obtained on each patient. Such processing of information in connection with a study actually enhances the motivation of everyone involved. It is a continuous control and guarantees instantaneous statistical assessment of the patient groups. Besides SAS [38] there are other software packages available (e.g., SIR). With SAS and SIR, data analysis can be carried out using the high quality statistics packages BMDP [8] and SAS [31, 33]. Locally developed programs should be avoided in favor of internationally available and recognized software packages.

The term "documentation" is inseparably linked to the concept of a rigorously organized data registration process.

III. Computerized Documentation for Continuous Patient Observation

The computerized registration of data on vascular surgery patients must meet some special requirements. Since it is difficult to foresee what kind of information will be needed or what kinds of analyses will be carried out, the data must be extensive, precise, and continuous. Such a store of data increases our ability to answer the basic question: which method of treating a certain vascular disease shows the best long-term results? The amount of work required to gather such vast amounts of data can be discouraging; this is offset, however, by the advantages of having continuous, reliable information for purposes of quality control and scientific research.

Continuous data registration of vascular operations by electronic data processing systems can be organized in various ways, depending upon the particular mode of data entry, storage, and retrieval. All details which might eventually constitute relevant information must be registered, but without creating an intolerable workload.

There are many difficulties in defining pathologic vascular processes. The same is true for a particular operation because it usually consists of a great number of combined surgical procedures. Early and late results can be defined according to objective (measurement data) and subjective (symptoms) criteria. A special feature of treatment in vascular surgery is that the same patient may have surgery on different parts of the body. The patient may also be treated several times at the same site, which makes data analysis rather confusing and separate assessment of differently applied methods of treatment impossible. Trials with continuous computerized documentation of vascular operations and their late results have been initiated in only a few cases, e.g., the computerized vascular registry of the Cleveland Vascular Society [26] in which the frequencies and early results of operations performed by 26 vascular surgeons are being evaluated. Another group [15] has described a program for micro- and minicomputers. In the last few years several vascular registries have been established for continuous patient monitoring [14, 17, 44]. The Austrian Society of Vascular Surgery has maintained a computerized registry on vascular surgery at the Department of Surgery of the University of Vienna since 1970 [46].

1. The Electronic Data Processing System of the Austrian Society of Vascular Surgery

In 1968, at the first Annual Convention of the newly founded Austrian Society of Vascular Surgery the creation of a joint registry for all vascular surgery centers in Austria was suggested. The aim was to find analogue criteria and definitions for the assessment of morphological changes, of vascular operations as well as their results. As a consequence the present system was developed in the years 1968–1970 and the joint registry started in 1970 [46].

The system has been in use, almost unchanged, ever since. It focuses primarily on the operation itself and only secondarily on the patient. A four-page form is used in every vascular operation which contains information on the preoperative morphological situation, detailed surgical technique, preoperative clinical assessment, and immediate postoperative results. A second form is used to evaluate the late results of each operation with regard to function and preservation of the extremity. In the past, these data were entered into the computer by punched cards, since the end of 1984 have been directly entered by visual display units.

Until recently, many kinds of data were stored on magnetic tape in the form of BMDP files [8]. Since 1984, these data have been organized in an SAS file [31]. Each investigator has direct access to the data on each patient and each operative procedure on screen by using SAS-FSP software. The patient groups are analyzed statistically using BMDP [8] and SAS [31] commands. The SAS system makes it easier to analyze very complex data structures (e.g., follow-up periods). Beside these very well-known and widely used statistical program packages, Fortran programs [36] have been developed for special problems. Color graphics of statistical results are available in the graphics package, SAS Graph [32].

To analyze an individual patient throughout the entire course of treatment, the same patient number is assigned to the patient in all follow-up operations. The data forms are filled out by the surgeon while dictating the operation report. This usually takes only a few minutes. Information on the COD is added to the form by the ward physician. Follow-up forms are filled out during the patient's visits to the outpatient department. Computerized patient notification of routine follow-up medical examinations is an essential part of the clinical follow-up system Nasok [35]. When this information is stored, it is carefully examined to determine whether the entered data is complete, correct, and coherent for each case. If these requirements are not met, the forms are disregarded. A list of errors and a list of data within the file are printed. Finally, all the functions mentioned above are available to the data processing system. Information on deaths, together with the ICD-coded causes of death are sent annually from the Federal Data Center of Austria to the general medical data bank of the hospital and from there to the vascular registry. This not only helps in the statistical analysis of posttreatment survival rates, but also avoids sending notification of follow-up examinations to deceased patients.

The vascular archives contain information on 7047 operations performed on 4308 patients at the Surgical Depart I of the University of Vienna between 1965 and 1987. The tables and figures from this chapter are derived from this data.

B. Evaluation of Results of Vascular Operations

The assessment of the effectiveness of vascular reconstructions has led to the development of graft-patency function curves, similar to survival curves, [43], which permit a statistical comparison between different patient groups. Unlike prospective studies, comparability in retrospective studies is limited because the patient groups are not identical with respect to their disease and preoperative morphological situation. They have been deliberately selected and intentionally treated in different ways, according to their preoperative condition. Therefore, all publications should contain an exact definition of the preoperative state of disease, a description of therapeutic measures, and an assessment of surgical success.

I. Influence of Preoperative Clinical Status

1. Morphology

The morphology of the outflow tract is a very important factor influencing the effectiveness of a vascular reconstruction. Nevertheless, a uniform classification for the outflow tract has not been found. The classification according to the number of open or obliterated lower leg arteries (0/1/2/3) is often incorrect because the occlusions may be located within different portions of the distal part of the extremity, and high grade stenoses may have the same effect as an occlusion. In view of these problems, a criterion which may be used to differentiate between different patient groups is the percentage of sudden, unmanageable occlusions. The morphology in the area of the reconstruction itself (good or bad vein, endarterectomies in the right or wrong layer) is also of prognostic value, but it is very difficult to classify.

2. Preoperative Stage

Like morphology, the clinical stage is an indication of the extent of arteriosclerotic disease and therefore a very important factor in the prognosis. The clinical stage has considerable influence on all reconstructive procedures, less in operations within the pelvic area than for those in the periphery distal to the inguinal ligament [47]. The patient's clinical stage is especially important when comparing different vascular procedures as the indications for the various surgical procedures differ greatly (Table 9.1).

Table 9.1. Percentage of patients with stage III–IV disease and a typical reconstruction within a segment of the femoral artery (1966–1987)

Endarterectomy	$n=1280$	41%
Short vein graft	$n=413$	41%
Long vein graft	$n=375$	55%
Umbilical vein graft	$n=163$	58%
Profundaplasty	$n=596$	66%
Distal vein graft	$n=266$	74%

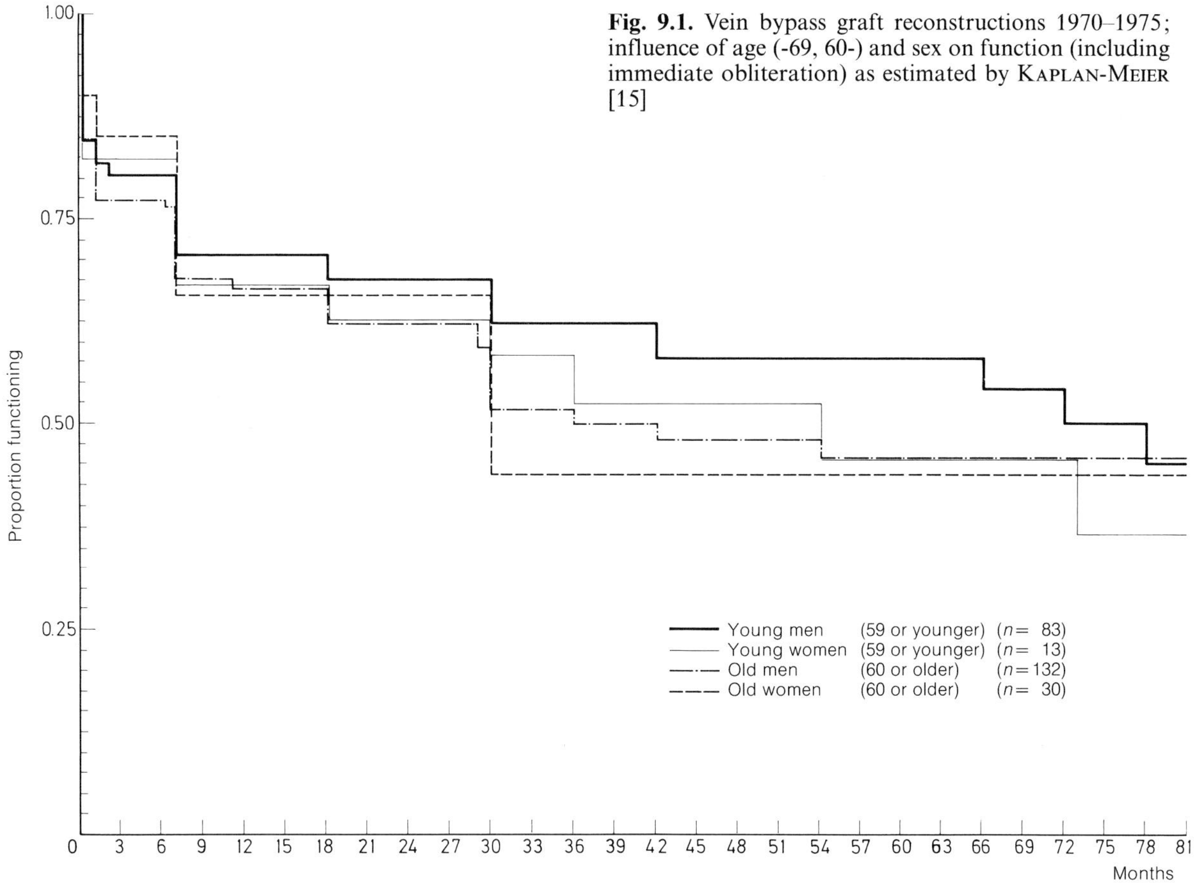

Fig. 9.1. Vein bypass graft reconstructions 1970–1975; influence of age (-69, 60-) and sex on function (including immediate obliteration) as estimated by KAPLAN-MEIER [15]

3. Surgical Risk – Influence of Concomitant Illness, Age, and Sex

The evaluation of individual surgical risk is difficult. Schematization of degree of dysfunction of different organs has not yet been achieved, satisfactorally. Risk factors often remain unknown until early results on complication rate and lethality are evaluated. In an individual case, the patient's age may not play an important role. However, patients of seventy and older have higher operative mortality and morbidity rates, due especially to cardiac and pulmonary complications. This is only true for general medical complications. Age does not have an influence on the frequency of local complications within the reconstructed area of the vessel during the early or late postoperative period [49, 50]. Likewise, there is no correlation between a patient's sex and late results of reconstruction (Fig. 9.1). Finally, the amputation rate must be included in the surgical risk.

II. Early and Late Results

1. Immediate Reocclusion

Immediate reocclusion is a common complication in vascular surgery, having great influence on the results. However, the rate of immediate reocclusion is not an absolute criterion of the quality of surgery at a vascular surgery center because it is largely dependent on the indication for surgery. This is why it is so important that reports on surgical results give exact information on the immediate reocclusion rate.

In some cases, successful correction of an immediate reocclusion is possible by reoperation. Patients who experienced immediate reocclusion of their vessels and whose patency was successfully reestablished by a second operation do not have as good a prognosis as patients without these early complications. One can either put them into the group of primary successful reconstructions or keep them separated. This should always be specified. For better comparability it is advisable to put the primary successful reconstructions into a separate group and at the same time provide information on the outcome of patients with immediate reocclusions.

2. Clinical Stage Conversion Due to Operation

The aim of surgery is to relieve symptoms, and the establishment of a functional reconstruction usually produces such relief. In some cases, however, improvement is not sufficient. Even if the reconstruction functions properly, sometimes the extremity must be amputated. This aspect must also be considered when assessing the effectiveness of an operation.

3. Objective Assessment by Angiologic Measurements

The only objective criteria of circulatory improvement are blood flow measurements; it is not enough merely to indicate whether a reconstruction is patent or occluded. Registration of distal perfusion pressure or other methods of peripheral circulation measurement may be employed. It is important to be able to assess to what extent peripheral circulation has been improved, and whether the occlusion itself has been relieved or not.

4. Change of Clinical Stage Following Reocclusion – Possibilities of Reoperation

A rather large number of patients must expect to experience a reocclusion in the long run. This occurs in about one third of all patients following femoropopliteal reconstructions. This means that in long-term follow-up assessment of reconstructive techniques, a change in clinical stage following reocclusion and the possibility of repair must be considered. Among our patients, many who underwent femoral artery reconstruction followed by late reocclusion regressed to their preoperative clinical stage. However, in some cases, the symptoms were slightly improved in comparison with the situation before the first vascular operation and some were in a worse clinical stage. If a reocclusion can be relieved by a second reconstructive procedure, the overall function of all reconstructions is important for the fate of the extremity and is an essential criterion for evaluating surgical therapy.

5. Completeness of Follow-up Examinations

Many authors deliberately refrain from reporting on the percentage of patients who have had follow-up examinations. Usually 10%–15% are not regularly assessed. Disregarding the missing information on patients who die long after vascular surgery (the mortality rate in vascular patients over a period of several years is between 30% and 50%), the important question arises: are the results more favorable or less favorable in patients who are not followed up? Are they:

a) Patients who are without symptoms and for this reason do not go to the follow-up examinations, or
b) Patients with recurrent occlusions who are not doing well, who are not interested in reoperation, or who have undergone amputation in another hospital and are therefore reluctant to reestablish contact with the original surgeon.

A sample audit of these aspects would be necessary to clarify the situation.

6. Walking Ability, Rehabilitation, Late Amputation

Since vascular surgery is actually a form of symptomatic treatment, preference should therefore be given to the assessment of the improvement of symptoms such as the prolongation of walking distance and disappearance of resting pain. The operation should not generate any residual symptoms such as swelling, pain, and ulcers which could counteract the benefit of increased circulation. The percentage of amputated patients who have been rehabilitated and are able to walk using a prosthetic device following lower leg or upper leg amputations should be specified.

7. Additional Problems in Assessment

The results reported by various authors for the same therapeutic procedure seem to differ considerably. Surely one reason for this is that the patient groups analyzed are much too small. Beyond this, it is to be expected that favorable results are more readily published than unfavorable ones. This leads to an overly optimistic view of results in the literature, especially in reports where new methods of treatment are compared. However, there are still additional explanations:

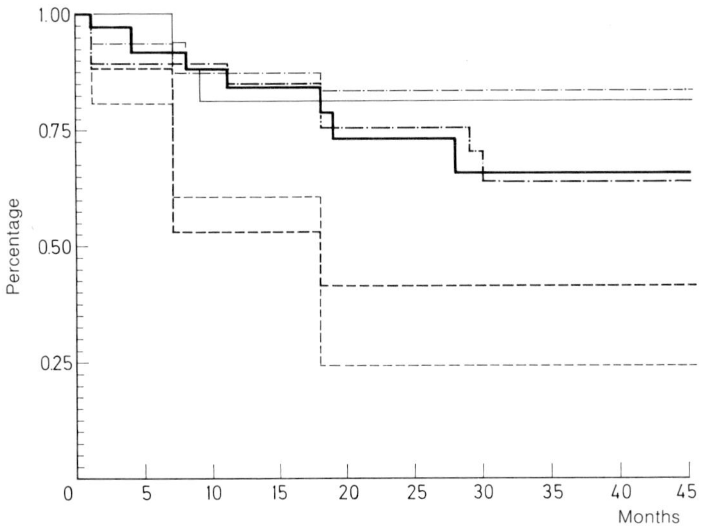

Fig. 9.2. Femoropopliteal vein bypass graft reconstruction; influence of stage (I, II or III, IV) and time periods of surgery (up to 1970, 1971–1978, 1979–1987) on function without immediate reocclusion, as estimated by KAPLAN-MEIER [16]

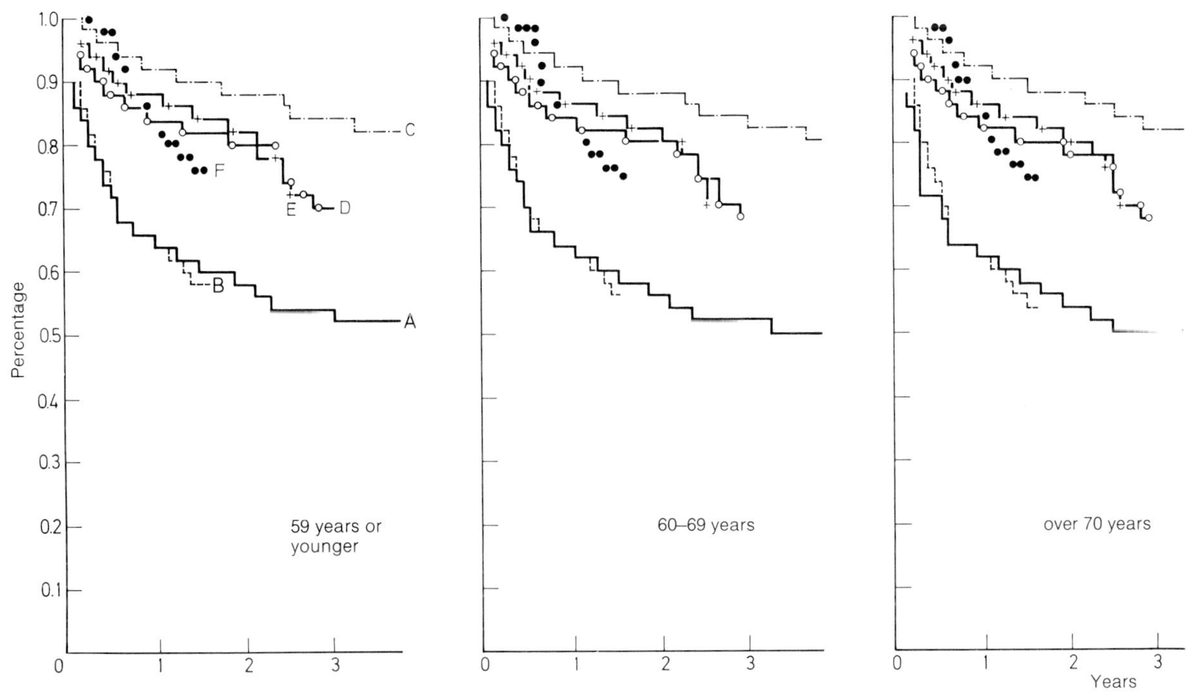

Fig. 9.3. Graft-patency function curves of femoropopliteal vein bypass grafts ($n = 240$) without immediate reocclusion, rearranged according to time intervals and clinical stages for three different age groups (59 or younger, 60–69, 70 or older). *A*, up to 1970, stage II; *B*, –1970, stage III–IV; *C*, 1971–1978, stage II; *D*, 1971–1978, stages III to IV; *E*, 1979–1987, stage II; *F*, 1979–1987, stages III to IV

a) Differences are only apparent, owing to different indications for surgery, different time intervals in which surgical technique has improved, and a change in the composition of patient groups over different evaluation periods (Fig. 9.2). We were able to show for our own patients that, over the years, a considerable shift in the composition of the patient groups has taken place [49, 50]. More and more patients belonged to clinical stages III–IV and were older than 70 (currently 34%). Therefore, it is essential to consider the composition of the patient groups and to correct it by stratification (Fig. 9.3).

b) On the other hand, results may actually differ. This may be due to qualitative differences in either operative technique or medical opinion. This happens even though most vascular operations have been standardized and technical competence at different vascular surgery centers is at the same level. Greater objectivity could be achieved by the increasing use of angiologic and radiologic assessment criteria.

C. Statistical Evaluation

I. Fundamentals

Statistical reasoning is always supported by a model [42] which tries to describe reality by means of different elements and their relationships to one another. Whether or not a statistical description is adequate depends upon the model on which it is based.

Furthermore, the extent of generalization of results obtained by clinical and statistical analysis may be limited by preselection of patient groups according to either known or unknown factors [29].

Meaningful statistical statements are only possible if correct and continuous data registration is guaranteed.

The main objective of descriptive statistics is to reduce observation data to a few relevant variables, tables, or graphs. In contrast, inductive statistics tries to draw out inferences about incompletely assessed and related hypothetical background populations on the basis of random samples. Induction can be performed in two ways:

1. By deriving an interval which covers a "true" parameter of the base population with a probability of, e.g., 95%
2. By employing statistical tests to judge whether or not a given null hypothesis (e.g., of no treatment effect) is compatible with a set of data

If the probability (usually represented by the letter *p*) is very small and large deviations from the null hypothesis are detected, the alternative hypothesis is accepted in exchange for the null hypothesis. The alpha error is the probability *p* (or alpha) of falsely rejecting the null hypothesis. The beta error is the probability, beta, of falsely keeping the null hypothesis. Differences in effectiveness of treatment regimens are confirmed by very small alpha values. Equal effectiveness or ineffectiveness of treatment regimens is confirmed by very small beta values.

Statistical analyses can be used to confirm a preconceived idea, such as the testing of the main hypothesis in a therapy study, or they may be employed in an exploratory way, which means that new hypotheses are postulated in the presence of small *p* values or recently discovered phenomena.

A brief survey of inductive statistical methods follows. The methods are useful in confirmatory and exploratory analysis.

II. Statistical Methods

1. Assessment of Dichotomous Variables

The relationship between two dichotomous qualitative variables (e.g., immediate occlusion, sex) may be examined by the χ^2 test for contingency tables. Simultaneous testing of a relationship between more than two variables requires long-linear models. To test the dependence of a dichotomous variable on an ordinal variable (e.g., age, pain intensity, laboratory parameters) the U test is adequate. To describe the dependence of a dichotomous variable as a function of several factors, logistic regression is available. Relationships to dichotomous criteria are evaluated by percentages, medians, quantiles, and by pie, bar or block diagrams (Fig. 9.4–9.6).

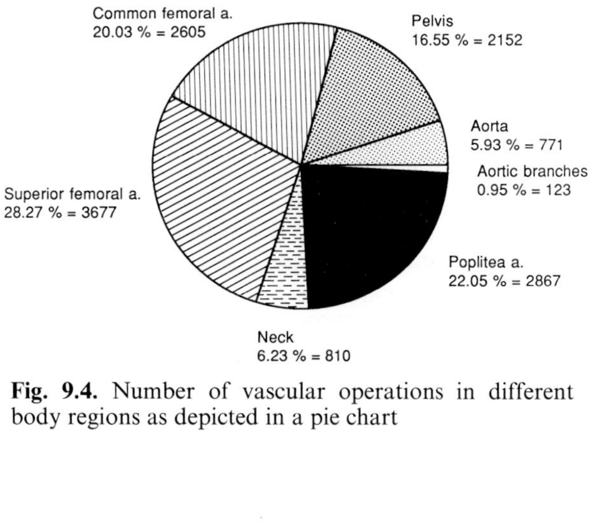

Fig. 9.4. Number of vascular operations in different body regions as depicted in a pie chart

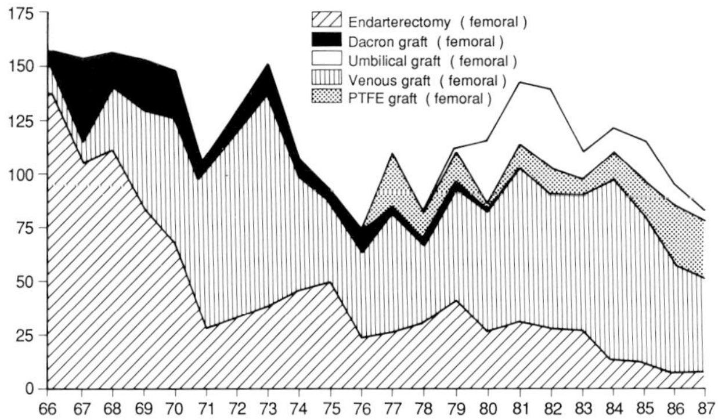

Fig. 9.5. Frequencies of typical procedures in the femoral artery region

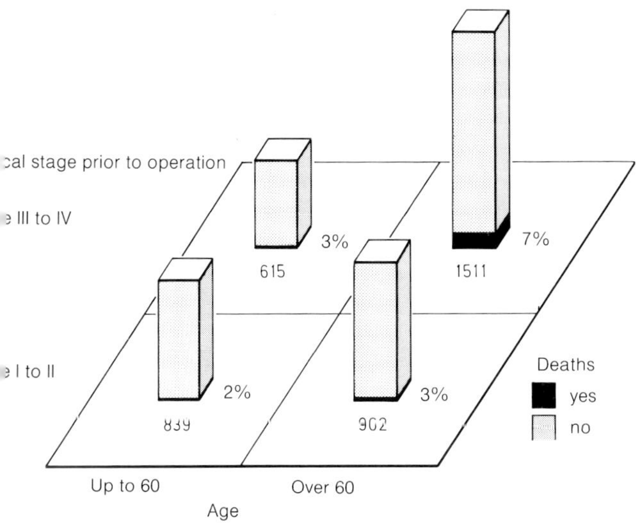

Fig. 9.6. Dependence of lethality on age and clinical stage at the time of vascular reconstructions (bar diagram)

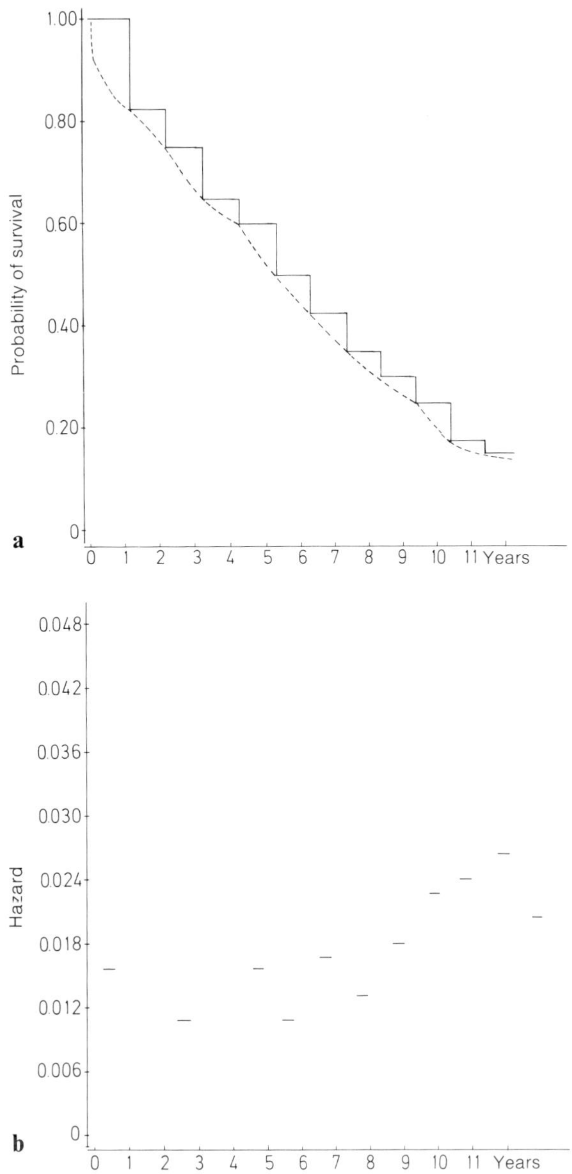

Fig. 9.7. Characterization of patient survival following vascular reconstructions within the pelvic region using (**a**) Kaplan-Meier estimation (----), life table (——), (**b**) hazard function. The age distribution of these patients is described by the following quantiles: $\chi_{0.1}=47.4$; $\chi_{0.25}=56.8$; $\chi_{0.5}=64.6$; $\chi_{0.75}=70.7$; $\chi_{0.9}=75.9$. (A quantile χ_p gives the value at which p percent o/a a distribution is equal or below)

2. The Assessment of Functional Longevity of Vascular Reconstructions

At the time of analysis of a patient group, there are still patients alive with properly functioning vascular reconstructions. Therefore, special methods [18, 38] must be employed to evaluate "censored" (that is, not fully observable) variables. Survival and the distribution of possibly censored graft functions are described by life tables as suggested by STOKES et al. as early as 1960, or, more accurately, by Kaplan-Meier estimations [16].

In both cases the probability of survival and of patency of the revascularized vessel is described by means of a table or a graph as a function of time which had passed since treatment or diagnosis. The patient's risk of death or of occlusion of the reconstructed vessel in the years following surgery is described by hazard functions (Fig. 9.7). To examine differences between groups, several

Table 9.2. Relative survival functions (standardization of mortality in a study group according to a control population)

Interval	(1)	(2)	(3)	(4)	(5)	(6)	(7)	(8)	(9)	(10)	(11)
Mortality table:											
Year											
1	1003	62	972.0	163	0.17	0.04	4.56	1.00	1.00	1.00	35.75
2	778	48	754.0	61	0.08	0.04	2.01	0.83	0.97	0.86	30.40
3	669	40	649.0	61	0.09	0.04	2.14	0.76	0.93	0.82	28.57
4	568	40	548.0	37	0.07	0.05	1.40	0.69	0.90	0.77	26.39
5	491	27	477.5	50	0.10	0.05	1.99	0.65	0.86	0.75	25.11
6	414	15	406.5	26	0.06	0.06	1.11	0.58	0.82	0.70	23.33
7	373	16	365.0	33	0.09	0.06	1.45	0.54	0.79	0.69	22.78
8	324	23	312.5	21	0.07	0.07	0.99	0.49	0.75	0.66	21.15
9	280	24	268.0	23	0.09	0.07	1.17	0.46	0.71	0.64	19.69
10	233	21	222.5	23	0.10	0.08	1.29	0.42	0.68	0.62	17.78
11	189	12	183.0	17	0.09	0.09	1.07	0.38	0.64	0.59	15.89
12	160	12	154.0	13	0.08	0.09	0.90	0.34	0.60	0.57	14.47
13	135	18	126.0	7	0.06	0.10	0.55	0.31	0.57	0.55	12.75
14	110	13	103.5	6	0.06	0.11	0.53	0.30	0.53	0.55	11.28
15	91	15	83.5	3	0.04	0.12	0.31	0.28	0.50	0.56	9.78
16	73	22	62.0	2	0.03	0.13	0.26	0.27	0.47	0.58	7.82
17	49	19	39.5	3	0.08	0.14	0.56	0.26	0.43	0.60	5.34
18	27	20	17.0	2	0.12	0.15	0.81	0.24	0.40	0.60	2.48

(1) Number of patients at the beginning of an interval
(2) Number of patients "lost" during an interval
(3) Number of patients exposed to a fatal risk during an interval
(4) Number of patients who died during an interval
(5) Relative risk of death during an interval: (4):(3)
(6) Relative risk of death during an interval (control population)
(7) Relative survival curve (5):(6)
(8) Probability of survival until the beginning of an interval
(9) Probability of survival until the beginning of an interval (control population)
(10) Relative survival curve: (8):(9)
(11) Number of expected deaths during an interval: (3):(6)

Two-tailed (one-tailed) test examining differences in mortality rates between the study group and the control population:
By equal weighting of time intervals: $p=0.0000$
By equal weighting of patients: $p=0.000$

Age- and sex-specific death rates for Austria in 1979 were used for calculations (Austrian Federal Bureau of Statistics 1980)

tests are available such as those of MANTEL [24], BRESLOW [3], and GEHAN [10]. Mantel's test is more sensitive for evaluation of late results, whereas the other tests have a higher probability of discovering differences in early follow-up results.

It is advisable to stratify heterogeneous patient data when using these tests in order to obtain unbiased and precise results.

To analyze the dependence of censored variables on ordinal variables, the tests of BROWN et al. [4], O'BRIAN [22], and SCHEMPER [40] are available. The influence of several variables on survival and patency can be described as a mathematical function according to COX [5]. Applications of this model, however, require careful judgement of the constancy of relative risks over time for the variables included.

In such analyses the duration of function, including immediate reocclusion, is registered and evaluated. This resembles the situation with which the patient is confronted. However, if the influence of therapeutic measures alone on the duration of function is studied, then it may be worthwhile to analyze long-term results, omitting immediate reocclusions. Relative survival curves [9] are available (Table 9.2) for comparing mortality between patient study groups and normal populations with corresponding age and sex distributions.

Although the concepts of these methods are easy to understand and the vascular surgeon is able to interpret the results easily and quickly, some should be used only by a biostatistician [23], who can mobilize a wide range of experience for the correct interpretation of the results and who is familiar with the fine points of statistical induction [19]. Furthermore, the biostatistician can provide data processing by computerized systems and employ technical know-how and specialized programs to solve particular problems which are not discussed here.

III. Clinical Studies

Special statistical methods are available for clinical studies [28, 29, 45]. The most important functions of a statistician in clinical studies are:

1. The calculation of necessary sample sizes in order to assess a defined difference in therapeutic effectiveness.
2. Determination of the randomization procedures: The method chosen for random assignment of patients to the various therapy groups should compensate for unknown and disturbing effects and balance the group sizes as well as the prognostic factors over the therapy groups. The method of POCOCK and SIMON [27] has proven to be very useful, especially in its implementation by SCHEMPER [37] in an on-line computer program.
3. Organization of the data acquisition process and of intermediate data analysis, which may lead to discontinuation of the study, are further duties of the statistician. He performs the main analysis and assists in interpreting and presenting the results.

A study report should outline the conditions under which the investigations were made. It should contain the following points:

1. A description of all criteria used in recruiting patients for the study
2. A description of organization and method of randomization in therapy studies
3. Quantitative analysis of completeness of follow-up observations and a statement of reasons for loss of patients during the study
4. Results of power analyses for the tests used
5. Description of statistical methods employed
6. Quantification of the empirical basis (e.g., in follow-up studies, the number of patients who were observed for at least k time periods)

This chapter should have demonstrated that the field of medical statistics deals only in part with arithmetical problems, but primarily with the logic of empirical science [12, 13, 18]. The following citation of MAINLAND [22] should reemphasize the important role of medical statistics: "Research workers' widespread lack of understanding of the rationale of statistical techniques, and the frequent use of statistical tests as a substitute for thoughtful investigational design, meticulous work, and repetition of experiments, justify the antagonism to statistics exhibited by some experiments. To one who has had personal experience of the way in which statistical thinking, as distinct from statistical arithmetic, can promote good investigation, this perversion of statistics is lamentable."

The basic scientific and clinical questions in vascular surgery have not changed much in the last few years. The main points of interest are still the questions concerning indications for surgery, the application of more or less radical procedures, and the choice of reconstructive technique and vessel substitute. Further studies on operative risk, early and late results, and the possibility of limb preservation through a series of operations are necessary. In order to evaluate all relevant data, registration of vascular operations should be organized on a national and international basis by employing computerized data processing. At our institution, favorable experience has already demonstrated the advantages of a computer-assisted documentation system [20].

REFERENCES:

1. Armitage P (1971) Statistical methods in medical research. Blackwell, Oxford
2. Breslow N (1978) Perspectives on the statistican's role in cooperative clinical research. Cancer 41:326–332
3. Breslow N (1970) A generalized Kruskal-Wallis test for comparing K samples subject to unequal patterns of censorship. Biometrika 57:579–594
4. Brown BW, Hollander M, Korwar RM (1974) Nonparametric tests of independence for censored data, with applications to heart transplant studies. In: Proschan F, Serfling RJ (eds) Reliability and biometry. SIAM, Philadelphia, pp 327–354
5. Cox DR (1972) Regression models and life tables. JR Stat Soc B 34:187–220

6. Cutler SJ, Ederer F (1958) Maximum utilization of the lift table method in analyzing survival. J Chronic Dis 8:699–713
7. Dersimonian R, Charette LJ, McPeck B, Mosteller F (1982) Reporting on methods in clinical trials. N Engl J Med 306:1332–1337
8. Dixon WJ, Brown MB, Englman L, Frane JW, Hill MA, Jennrich RI, Toporek JD (1982) BMDP statistical software. University of California Press, Berkeley
9. Ederer F, Axtell LM, Cutler SJ (1961) The relative survival rate: a statistical methodology. Natl Cancer Inst Monogr 6:101–121
10. Gehan EA (1965) A generalized Wilcoxon test for comparing arbitrarily singly censored samples. Biometrika 52:203–223
11. Grabner H, Leihanec J (1976) Das universelle Dokumentationssystem im Rahmen des Informationssystems WAMIS. EDV Medizin Biol 7:53–56
12. Griesser G (1965) Heilkunde und Statistik – Mensch und Zahl. Methods Inf Med 4:114–120
13. Griesser G (1967) Zur Methodik der wissenschaftlichen Arbeit in der Allgemeinmedizin. Med Welt 47:2801–2807
14. Gunta SK, Veith FS, White-Flores SA et al. (1984) System for widespread application of microcomputers to vascular surgery. J Vasc Surg 1:601–604
15. Jacobson JH, Karipineni RC, Weisberg M, Radna R (1980) Description of a universal data entry and retrieval program for vascular surgeons. Surgery 88:766–774
16. Kaplan EL, Maier P (1958) Nonparametric estimation from incomplete observations. J Amer Statist Ass 53:457–481
17. Karmody AM, Fitzgerald K, Branagh M, Leather RP (1984) Development of a computerized vascular registry for large scale use. J Vasc Surg 1:594–600
18. Koller S (1963) Die Aufgaben der Statistik und Dokumentation in der Medizin. Dtsch Med Wochenschr 40:1917–1924
19. Koller S (1963) Systematik der statistischen Schlußfehler. Methods Inf Med 3:113–117
20. Kretschmer G, Wenzl E, Piza F, Polterauer P, Ehringer H, Miner E, Schemper M (1987) The influence of anticoagulant treatment on probability of function in femoropopliteal vein bypass surgery: analysis of a clinical series (1970–1989) and interim evaluation of a controlled clinical trial. Surgery 102:453–459
21. Lawless JF (1982) Statistical models and methods for lifetime data. Wiley, New York
22. Mainland D (1960) The use and misuse of statistics in medical publications. Clin Pharmacol Ther 1:411–422
23. Mainland D (1965) We wish to hire a medical statistican. Have you any advice to offer? JAMA 193:289–193
24. Mantel N (1966) Evaluation of survival data and two new rank order statistics arising in its consideration. Cancer Chemotherapy Reports 50:163–170
25. O'Brien P (1978) A nonparametric test for association with censored data. Biometrics 34:143–250
26. Plecha FR, Avellone JC, Beren EG, DePalma RG, Hertzer NR (1979) A computerized vascular registry: experience of the Cleveland Vascular Society. Surgery 86:826–835
27. Pocock SJ, Simon R (1975) Sequential treatment assignment with balancing for prognostic factors in the controlled clinical trial. Biometrics 31:103–115
28. Pocock SJ (1983) Clinical trials. Wiley, Chichester New York Brisbane Toronto Singapore
29. Rümke ChL (1970) Über die Gefahr falscher Schlußfolgerungen aus Krankenblattdaten (Berkson's Fallacy). Methods Inf Med 9:249–254
30. Sachs L (1974) Angewandte Statistik, 4th edn. Springer, Berlin Heidelberg New York
31. SAS Institute Inc (1982) SAS user's guide: basics. Cary, North Carolina
32. SAS Institute Inc (1981) SAS/Graph user's guide, Cary, North Carolina
33. SAS Institute Inc (1982) SAS/user's guide: statistics. Cary, North Carolina
34. SAS Institute Inc (1982) SAS/FSP user's guide. Cary, North Carolina
35. Schemper M, Funovics J, Puchner M (1981) Computergestützte Patientennachsorge – Darstellung eines Modells und Bericht über 40 Monate Funktionsdauer. In: Adlassnig KP, Dorda W, Grabner G (eds) Medizinische Informatik. Oldenbourg, Wien München, p 69–75
36. Schemper M (1981) Eine Programmsammlung zur statistischen Analyse zensierter Überlebenszeiten. Statistical Software Newsletter 7:118–121
37. Schemper M (1982) Randomisierung für kontrollierte Therapiestudien. Wien Klin Wochenschr 94:604–609
38. Schemper M, Dorda W (1983) Integrierte Datenverarbeitung für klinische Studien. EDV Med Biol 14:65–77
39. Schemper M, Scheiber V (1984) Statistische Standards für klinische Langzeitstudien. Wien Klin Wochenschr 96:361–370
40. Schemper M (1984) Analysis of associations with censored data by generalized Mantel and Breslow tests and generalized Kendall correlation coefficients. Biom J 3:308–318
41. Schemper M (1984) A survey of permutation tests for censored survival data. Commun Statist A 13:1655–1665
42. Stachowiak H (1973) Allgemeine Modelltheorie. Springer, Vienna New York
43. Stokes JM, Slugg WL, Butcher HR (1963) Standard method of assessing relative effectiveness of therapies for arterial occlusive diseases. Ann Surg 157:343–350
44. Troëng Th (1987) The vascular registry – a responsibility for all vascular surgeons? Vascular registry in Southern Sweden (VRISS). Eur J Vasc Surg 1:219–226
45. Victor N, Dudeck J, Broszio EP (eds) (1981) Therapiestudien. Springer, Berlin Heidelberg New York
46. Wagner O (1973) Das Dokumentationssystem der Österr. Ges. für Gefäßchirurgie – Aufbau, Struktur und praktische Anwendung. In: Denck H, Koch G, Piza F, Wagner O (eds) Intestinale Durchblutungsstörungen. Egermann, Wien, pp 211–226
47. Wagner O (1978) Chirurgische Behandlung der arteriellen Durchblutungsstörungen der unteren Extremität – Therapeutische Erfolgsbeurteilung. Med Klin 73:1183–1191
48. Wagner O, Schemper M (1983) Gefäßchirurgie – der chronische Gefäßverschluß der unteren Extremität:

Schwerpunkte chirurgischer Forschung. Chirurg 54:211–220
49. Wagner O, Schemper M (1983) Chronische Durchblutungsstörung der unteren Extremität. Einfluß des Alters auf Sofort- und Spätergebnisse nach Gefäßrekonstruktion. In: Bünte H, Rühland D (eds) Arterielle Durchblutungsstörungen im hohen Lebensalter. Schattauer, Stuttgart New York, pp 193–202 (Ergebnisse der Angiologie, vol 27)
50. Wagner O, Kretschmer G, Piza F, Polterauer P, Schemper M (1984) Hat das Patientenalter einen Einfluß auf die Spätergebnisse von Gefäßrekonstruktionen bei chronischer Durchblutungsstörung der unteren Extremität? In: Piza F, Mavosi L (eds) Angiologie und Geriatrie. Robidruck, Wien, pp 221–229
51. Weber E (1980) Grundriß der biologischen Statistik, 8th edn. Fischer, Stuttgart

10 Postoperative Complications

10.1 Immediate, Early, and Late Complications Following Vascular Reconstruction and Their Treatment (Hemorrhage, Occlusion)

K.L. LAUTERJUNG

CONTENTS

A. Hemorrhage

The time at which hemorrhage occurs points to the possible cause of bleeding. Bleeding in vascular surgery is classified into intraoperative, early postoperative, and late postoperative hemorrhage. For example, anastomotic false aneurysms and infected sutures are almost always causes of late postoperative bleeding (see pp. 167, 173). Prosthetic defects may also be a cause. Compared with extensive operative procedures in general surgery, bleeding in vascular surgery must be expected to occur two to three times more often. Usually most of these complications appear during the intraoperative or early postoperative period [11]. The causes can be classified into two groups:

1. Technical errors
2. Predisposing factors

I. Technical Errors

Technical errors leading to intraoperative or early postoperative hemorrhage must be separated into incorrect methods of tissue dissection and incorrect suturing techniques. However, in some instances, technical errors may lead only to intraoperative or early postoperative bleeding if predisposing factors such as clotting disorders or hypertension are present at the same time.

1. Bleeding During Surgical Dissection

This may occur if the dissection is too traumatic. The main causes are injuries to arterial tributaries and concomitant veins. Injuries of the larger arteries exposed occur less often. The choice of instruments used for dissection under and around the vessel is important. Instead of an Overholt clamp, instruments with less sharply pointed tips should be employed to dissect around the vessel. Umbilical tapes around certain vessels during various procedures, such as dissection of an abdominal aortic aneurysm, may be omitted. The separation of the artery from its concomitant vein may lead to bleeding if both vessels are densely adherent. Even if the surgeon is most careful in dissecting this area, tearing, especially of the venous wall, may occur [23]. The repair of such venous defects by suture is usually difficult and may lead to further tears of either vessel. In such situations, it is advisable to dissect the vein from the artery by first placing tapes around the artery proximal and distal to the site of the adhesion. The dissection of both vessels in scar tissue during a second operation is especially difficult. In such a case, one should abandon the technique of blunt dissection and "carve" the vessels or prostheses out of the scarred tissue with a scalpel.
Hemorrhage may also be caused during preparation of a tissue tunnel in the inguinal region of popliteal fossa for an arterial bypass. Sponge-holding forceps or steel rods should be used only

after a tunnel has been prepared by blunt digital dissection. The only problem with this technique may arise if bidigital dissection is not carried out within the correct layer of tissue.

Arterial wall lesions following the use of a ring stripper for disobliteration, with consecutive intraoperative or early postoperative bleeding episodes, are not always avoidable and are often not discovered immediately. The danger of perforation is high, especially in very extensively calcified vessels. In such cases it is better to choose a different procedure (see p. 381).

Also, lesions caused by the application of a Fogarty catheter are often not discovered immediately. Hemorrhage occurring within the arteries of the lower leg following perforation or wall rupture can often be detected only by intraoperative control angiography. As soon as such lesions are detected, immediate intervention must follow since obliteration of the vessel may occur, owing to an intimal tear or plaque dislocation. Although these complications are not totally avoidable, even if the greatest care is taken, one should not use a metal guide for primary introduction of the balloon catheter. The balloon should be inflated only with the appropriate syringe. Disposable plastic syringes do not glide easily, and one cannot regulate inflation pressure of the balloon carefully enough. For this reason, glass and metal syringes should be used [3, 7].

2. Hemorrhage Due to Incorrect Suture Technique, Bleeding from Suture Holes

Strictly speaking bleeding from suture holes is not really a complication. Maintaining secure compression with gauze for 5–10 min will stop it. One should not suture these leaks prematurely. An additional suture usually worsens the situation. If hemostasis is not achieved by long tamponade or by supplementary suture, the cause is often a clotting disorder. Only adequate substitution of clotting factors or neutralization of heparin can help in such cases. Even in normal cases coagulation problems may occur if platelet function has been impaired by preoperative administration of antiplatelet drugs. Such complications can only be prevented if medication is discontinued early enough before the operation. The chief symptom of such a clotting disturbance is the intraoperative occurrence of capillary bleeding, necessitating the removal of a hematoma in a second procedure. In view of the wide application of antiplatelet drugs, patients should always be asked preoperatively if they take such medication. Because of the prolonged action of these drugs, the period between discontinuation of treatment and surgery must be long enough (3–7 days).

3. Bleeding at the Anastomosis

Bleeding at the anastomosis may occur intraoperatively (e.g., after restoration of blood flow to the arterial vessels), as well as during the early postoperative period. It is almost always due to technical errors made while completing the suture at the anastomosis. The commonest causes, usually recognizable during surgery, are excessively large intervals between stitches or incongruent diameters of prosthesis and artery, leading to the formation of a false aneurysm. Supplementary sutures are necessary in cases where bleeding does not stop after 5–10 min compression.

The same technical errors are the cause of hemorrhaging during the early postoperative period. Arterial hypotension during surgery may disguise technical errors, and as soon as normo- or hypertension returns, bleeding may commence. One example would be the disruption of a thin, fragile vessel wall at the site of the anastomosis as tension increases on the suture during a rise in blood pressure.

A very special and rare complication is the rupture of the suture line at the anastomosis in long bypass grafts spanning the knee joint. In such cases, an intraoperative check of the graft's mobility should be performed by flexing and extending the knee. Otherwise, if the graft is too short or fixed at a certain point, moving the knee from a flexed to an extended position might cause severe injury [13].

II. Predisposing Factors

Predisposing factors of uncontrollable intraoperative and early postoperative hemorrhage are the occurrence of postoperative hypertension in combination with technical errors and disorders of the coagulation system. Clotting disorders can be congenital or acquired. Congenital clotting defects are unlikely in adult patients who have not had a history of these disorders during previous operations. Examination of the coagulation system is absolutely necessary prior to vascular surgery. Usually routine laboratory examinations of prothrombin time, partial thromboplastin time, thrombin time, and a platelet count will suffice.

Intraoperative and early postoperative hemorrhage due to a clotting disorder may be attributed to three causes:

1. Excessively high dose of anticoagulants during and after surgery
2. Dilution of clotting factors owing to transfusion of large amounts of old blood
3. Disseminated intravascular coagulation resulting from shock, infection, and septicemia

Following diagnosis of such disorders – if necessary, by separate examination of each single clotting factor – immediate substitution or neutralization must be performed in order to interrupt the bleeding and prevent the coagulation defect from developing any further [21].

III. Risks of Hemorrhage in Specific Vascular Operation

1. Surgery of the Carotid Artery

Hemorrhage, usually occurring during the early postoperative period, is detected by a swelling of the neck or by increased drainage of blood from the operating area through a drain left near the site of the anastomosis. There are two reasons why early intervention, following immediate reintubation, removal of the hematoma, and search for the cause of bleeding, is absolutely necessary:

1. If the surgeon waits too long, the hematoma may increase to such an extent that the trachea is displaced, making intubation most difficult, if not impossible.
2. If the hematoma is not removed, an infection is more likely to develop, and with it, the possibility of suture arrosion and uncontrollable hemorrhage.

The main cause of hemorrhage is usually a leak at the site of arterial suture that was not detected during surgery under normotensive or hypotensive conditions. Hypertension, which develops in 10% of treated patients as they recover from anesthesia, leads to hemorrhage. Disruption of the suture is also more likely during these blood pressure changes [20]. A ligature may slip off the common facial vein which is usually divided during surgery. Coughing provokes the Valsalva maneuver, causing venous pressure to rise above the systemic arterial blood pressure level. The leak must be oversewn, or the venous stump ligated again.

To prevent wound infection, reintervention should result under perioperative antibiotic cover. Hematoma due to diffuse bleeding because of intraoperative heparinization is rare; one always tries to reach a subtle hemostasis by neutralizing the heparin. However, antiplatelet drugs that have been discontinued too late may lead to diffuse hemorrhage in connection with heparinization, making control difficult during reintervention. In such cases sufficient drainage of the wound and a pressure bandage are often the only measures that can help. When the drainage tubes (Redon) are put in place during the primary or subsequent operations, they should not make direct contact with vein, artery, or anastomosis since the danger of mechanical injury is great. For the same reason, suction at the drains is as a rule out of the question.

2. Surgery of the Subclavian and Vertebral Arteries

Surgery of supra-aortic branches is performed primarily using a supraclavicular approach. Only in those cases where three supra-aortic branches are narrowed or occluded is a median sternotomy preferable for exposure of the aortic arch. Typical bleeding complications usually have their origin in technical difficulties or in unsatisfactory exposure of the surgical anatomy by the supraclavicular approach. Bleeding during supraclavicular dissection of the arteries must be dealt with very carefully as the proximal unexposed portion of the artery is difficult to reach with surgical instruments. If there are problems controlling arterial hemorrhage, the surgeon should not hesitate to obtain better exposure of the surgical area through a median sternotomy. Only if the bleeding is uncontrollable – and this is extremely rare – should division of the clavicle and suture of the proximal subclavian vein be considered. Reunion of the clavicle is achieved by internal fixation (s. p. 529 [17]).

3. Thoracic Aorta

Bleeding following surgery of the thoracic aorta is much easier to diagnose than hemorrhage following abdominal aortic surgery. Postoperative broadening of the mediastinum, constant blood loss over the thoracic drains, radiologic signs of a persisting hemothorax, together with a fall in hemoglobin and hematocrit, make the diagnosis easier. Although it may be difficult to control bleeding of intercostal arteries and many other smaller mediastinal vessels intraoperatively, there remains a high risk of postoperative hemorrhage from vessels which did not bleed during the operation. Vertebrae which are eroded by the pulsation of an aneurysm can bleed intensively and complicate intraoperative control of bleeding. In such situations, the surgeon has the following options for hemostasis: tamponade, suture, bone wax, infrared coagulation. However, a prerequisite is always an intact coagulation system, which must be checked intraoperatively by constant laboratory determinations of clotting values. The blood bank must be able to deliver the necessary blood units, clotting components, and, if necessary, warm blood. The probability that clotting disorders and not technical errors may lead to high blood losses from sutures and surrounding tissues is high. This risk is even higher if, in cases of rupture of the thoracic aorta, additional injuries, such as fractures or liver and spleen rupture, have led to massive bleeding in other parts of the body.

4. Abdominal Aorta

Aortic hemorrhage may occur during the preparation of an infrarenal abdominal aneurysm of the aorta. If immediate control of bleeding cannot be achieved by clamping the aorta at the typical infrarenal site because of an impaired view of the operating area, the aorta should be quickly clamped directly below the diaphragm or above the renal arteries. Infrarenal occlusion is then possible following further preparation of the area.

Furthermore, pressing the aorta against the spine proximal to the rupture site, either by hand or with a large sponge, may prevent severe blood loss. The introduction of a balloon catheter into the aorta may also help to block the proximal inflow tract (see p. 307).

Clamping of the aorta through a separate thoracotomy is also proposed. However, we do not recommend such an approach for the management of massive bleeding because it is too time-consuming.

Dissection around the aneurysm itself should be performed only after clamping of the aorta proximal and distal to the aneurysm. Usually, it is not necessary to put rubber tubing around the proximal part of the aorta. This maneuver has a high risk of intraoperative hemorrhage due to tearing of larger lumbar arteries or veins. Dissection on both sides of the aorta is sufficient for placement of the clamp. Total occlusion of the aorta can be achieved by pressing the clamp against the spine. For the same reasons, a sling should not be passed around the iliac arteries. Anterior and lateral dissection of both arteries is adequate for proper clamping. This avoids venous hemorrhage from the iliac veins, which may be caused by dissection between vein and artery. The risk is especially high in the area of the right common iliac artery, where the iliac vein is almost always tightly adherent to its back wall. If the vein does tear intraoperatively, it should be reconstructed by a continuous suture using 6–0 Prolene. In order to obtain a clear view of the operating site, free of blood, temporary slight pressure on the vein proximal and distal to the defect can be achieved using a larger sponge. The same can be done in tears of the inferior vena cava which is usually adherent to the aorta near the distal portion of the aneurysmal sac [18]. For replacement of the abdominal aorta, only highly porous graft material should be used. In ruptured abdominal aortic aneurysms or following operations of the abdominal aorta with great blood loss, woven prostheses with very fine pores are preferred. Preclotting cannot be performed under such circumstances because a clotting disorder is present. Postoperative hemorrhage from the prosthesis owing to increased fibrinolysis is less likely.

Early postoperative bleeding following operations on the abdominal aorta differs from other bleeding complications in that prompt reintervention is delayed owing to the difficulty of early diagnosis. Inspection of the circumference of the abdomen is not very helpful in the diagnosis of persisting hemorrhage. The patient's abdomen is often greatly distended postoperatively and the retroperitoneal space has a large filling capacity. Great amounts of blood may be taken up by the retroperitoneal space, resulting in tamponade of the bleeding site without a surgical intervention. For these reasons, many surgeons do not drain the abdomen. However, in some cases, temporary drainage of the abdomen for 2–3 days is recommended. The possible need for surgical reintervention can be assessed early enough from the amount of blood emitted by the drains. The time at which surgical intervention may become necessary depends upon the course of blood values (hemoglobin, hematocrit) and the amount of transfused blood. It is important that the surgeon who performed the first operation should evaluate the patient's postoperative condition.

5. Aortoiliac Vessels, Femoropopliteal Vessels

Postoperative hemorrhage in iliac and femoropopliteal vessel segments is easier to detect, its symptoms being swelling, change of skin color, or increased and persistent bleeding through a drain. Usually technical errors occurring during suture or completion of the anastomosis are the cause. Sometimes ligatures may slip off small branches of a vein graft following restoration of blood flow. Reintervention is necessary, not for hemostasis, but to remove the hematoma, which has a high risk of becoming infected and may lead to early occlusion of the graft.

Hemorrhage within lower leg arteries, which is detected intraoperatively by angiography and caused by perforation following embolectomy with a balloon catheter, should always be explored immediately. Otherwise, one must expect impairment of peripheral circulation by dissection.

B. Immediate, Early, and Late Occlusions

The time interval between vascular surgery and a postoperative occlusion is of great importance in finding the cause. Reocclusions can be classified as immediate, early, and late occlusions. Each of these complications must be treated differently.

I. Immediate Occlusion

An immediate occlusion is defined as an obliteration occurring intraoperatively or postoperatively within the first 24 h. It is usually the result of an error in surgical technique or in patient selection. There are three technical errors that may lead to an immediate occlusion:

1. Thrombosis or embolization of the peripheral outflow tract during the operation
2. Obstruction of the peripheral outflow tract due to intimal dissection or dislocation of a plaque
3. Narrowing of the inflow or outflow tract

Conditions leading to a false indication for surgery:

1. Inadequate outflow tract
2. Inadequate influx
3. Construction of a bypass circulation without an adequate pressure gradient

II. Early Occlusion

An early occlusion is defined as a postoperative obliteration occurring later than an immediate occlusion and within 1 year of the operation [23].

This type of occlusion may be caused by technical errors or by a false indication for surgery. In such cases, the errors were not very serious and, owing to anticoagulant therapy, did not produce an immediate occlusion. The probability that such an occlusion is caused by the errors and not by the progression of the underlying arterial disease decreases with time following the first operation.

III. Late Occlusion

Occlusions occurring 1 year or more after the operation are defined as late occlusions. Progression of the patient's underlying arterial disease and tissue changes within the collateral circulation are the most important causes.

1. Diagnosis

a) Immediate Occlusion

An immediate occlusion must be suspected if, after restoration of blood flow, no pulse can be palpated in the periphery or the pulse is weaker than the one found on the contralateral side. An intraoperative angiogram quickly confirms the diagnosis. The cause of an immediate occlusion can be found and corrected during the same operation. It is not advisable to perform postoperative angiography if an immediate occlusion is suspected. Time lost in such a procedure prolongs the duration of ischemia, promotes thrombosis, and increases risk by making additional anesthesia necessary. If intraoperative angiography is not possible, e.g., following reconstruction of supra-aortic branches, diagnosis of an immediate occlusion is confirmed by perturbation and flow measurement [19].

b) Early and Late Occlusions

Diagnostic measures employed to detect early and late occlusions are the same as those used for primary assessment of occlusive arterial disease. Angiography is absolutely necessary for exact diagnosis and localization. Only then is adequate surgical therapy possible. The entire length of the arterial segment should be visualized proximal and distal to the site of primary surgical intervention.

2. Occlusion Following Special Surgical Procedures

a) Supra-aortic Branches, Cerebral Arteries

The most common ischemic complications following procedures on the carotid artery are due to technical difficulties or errors resulting in thrombosis or embolism.

The dislodging of thrombotic or plaque material may be avoided by careful dissection around the carotid artery. Therefore, it is recommended that one dissects the internal and external carotid artery only after placing an umbilical tape around the common carotid artery and cross-clamping it. Only soft vascular clamps should be used for this purpose. Injury to the vascular wall, especially that of the internal carotid artery, promotes the development of a late stenosis. If an intraluminal shunt is introduced, embolization and dissection must be avoided. After removal of the stenosing plaque, no flap should remain at the distal edge of the intima.

If such a step is discovered, it must be fixed by a suture (see p. 469) [12]. After endarterectomy and closure of the arteriotomy, no hint of the now thin elastic wall of the carotid artery should be observed and the elongated segment must be resected or shortened by plication. Direct suture of the arteriotomy always carries the risk of creating a hemodynamically unfavorable reconstruction. Therefore, the arteriotomy is usually closed by vein patch angioplasty. A neurologic deficit developing during the early postoperative period can, but does not have to be, the first sign of an immediate occlusion.

Slight temporary aggravation of a preoperative neurologic deficit following surgery usually improves spontaneously and is therefore not an indication for reoperation. However, if a new large neurologic deficit develops postoperatively one must suspect an immediate occlusion. The most common cause of cerebral ischemia is acute thrombosis at the site of endarterectomy, even though in most cases no cause can be found by arteriography or during reoperation. Patients who are unremarkable neurologically following the operation and then develop a progressive neurologic deficit should be reexplored immediately without previous angiography. Interrupted cerebral blood flow should be restored as fast as possible before cerebral colliquation and permanent brain damage develop.

A hemorrhagic infarct can be avoided by timely reintervention. If reoperation is postponed longer than 2 h after the development of neurologic symptoms, the risk is as high as in surgery of stage III cerebral vascular insufficiency. Reexploration of the operating area, opening of the angioplasty, and removal of the thrombotic material are indicated. If necessary, a Fogarty catheter may be used (see p. 474).

Thrombosis is almost always due to the technical errors mentioned earlier [23].

Late Occlusions and Stenoses (see p. 475). These are diagnosed by the same criteria as primary cerebral vascular disease. The surgical procedures do not differ from those performed during the primary operation.

b) Arteries of the Aortic Arch

Immediate and Early Occlusions. When major branches of the aortic arch are disobliterated, all parts of the thrombus must be completely removed. This prevents cerebral embolism following restoration of blood flow to these vessels. Postoperative cerebral and brachial ischemia almost always signify embolization.

Late Occlusions and Stenoses. Ischemia developing later may indicate recurrent stenoses caused by progression of the patient's underlying disease or by scar tissue formation. Before repeating the operation, the stenosis should be confirmed by angiography. If reintervention is necessary, prosthetic bypass between the supra-aortic branches is preferable. Thromboendarterectomy and angioplasty are often technically too difficult to perform a second time (see p. 508).

c) Thoracic Aorta

Immediate and Early Occlusion. Following operations on thoracic aortic aneurysms of arteriosclerotic or syphilitic origin, immediate postoperative occlusions are very rarely seen. The causes are usually intra-aneurysmal thrombi or dislocated atheromatous debris of an ulcerated plaque which have become dislodged and have entered peripheral arteries. Embolism of mesenteric arteries may lead to impaired perfusion of intra-abdominal organs, and ultimately to intestinal gangrene. This complication is rarely noticed postoperatively because most patients have severe signs of decreased perfusion of intestinal organs after surgery. By contrast, thrombosis and embolism of the lower extremity are diagnosed sooner and treated by simple thrombectomy or early postoperative embolectomy. In these cases, conventional angiography (if necessary, by using the transaxillary approach to prevent injury of the anastomosis) should be performed to confirm the diagnosis.

Late Complications. Following the removal of a thoracic aneurysm and its replacement by a prosthesis, late complications such as stenosis and occlusions are not to be expected. Remnant stenoses are only seen following operations on a coarctation of the aorta. They are almost always a result of inadequate resection of the stenotic aortic segment owing to insufficient mobilization of the proximal and distal ends of the aorta used for anastomosis. If reoperation is necessary because of stenosis, repeated resection may be technically difficult owing to scar tissue formation in the vicinity of the anastomosis or extreme dilatation of the intercostal arteries. In such cases, a prosthetic bypass between the left subclavian artery and the descending aorta is the procedure of choice [4].

Intestinal symptoms such as abdominal pain, as in abdominal claudication, may appear during persistent postoperative arterial hypertension following successful operation of aortic coarctation. Medical treatment of high blood pressure will alleviate intestinal symptoms. If antihypertensive therapy is not successful, postoperative arteritis of the intestinal vessels may develop. This can lead to intestinal infarction. An emergency procedure may be indicated [10, 15, 16].

d) Renal Arteries (see p. 624)

Immediate and Early Occlusions. Immediate and early occlusions following procedures on the renal arteries are almost always a result of technical errors during the operation. Following transaortic thromboendarterectomy of the origin of the renal artery and after distal thromboendarterectomy combined with bypass grafting between the aorta and this artery, a loose intimal flap may lead to immediate occlusion. In a transaortic approach, the probability of not discovering this dissection intraoperatively is much higher. Intraoperative angiography may exclude this complication. Kinks in aortorenal bypass grafts appear after restoration of blood flow. Once detected, they should be removed by shortening the bypass or by reimplantation. Twisted and short grafts that are kinked by light traction on the distal end of the renal artery should be treated in the same manner.

Late Occlusions. The main causes of late complications are thrombosis of the graft and stenosis at the suture line. They occur if the angle at the peripheral and central anastomosis is too large. This creates turbulence at the anastomoses, leading to thrombosis. Stenoses at the suture line are caused by discrepancies in the caliber of the vessels. These complications can be relieved only by renewed anastomosis or patch angioplasty [8].

e) Abdominal Aorta and Aortoiliac Arteries

Immediate and Early Occlusions. Immediate and early occlusions following procedures on the abdominal aorta and iliac arteries are almost always due to poor patient selection or to technical errors. They are more easily avoided in elective procedures involving preoperative angiography of pre- and poststenotic vessels than in emergency procedures, e.g., surgical treatment of a penetrating or perforating abdominal aneurysm. Measures to prevent an immediate or early occlusion comply with the generally accepted rules of vascular surgery. While keeping the aorta clamped, care must be taken not to dislodge thrombi into inadequately perfused peripheral arteries during distal flushing with heparin (see elsewhere). Back bleeding from distal arteries shortly before completing the aortoiliac anastomosis does not prove the absence of distal thrombosis or embolisms. Treatment of choice is thrombectomy through the common femoral artery using a Fogarty catheter. Dissections during open endarterectomy or at the suture line can be avoided by careful surgical technique. In emergency operations without previous arteriography of the peripheral outflow tract, immediate and early occlusions may occur if the arterial run-off is inadequate. The same situation may be encountered in elective procedures, where correct identification of vessel obstruction is not possible owing to insufficient angiographic visualization or underestimation of lesions. The only alternative is to remove the obstructions or extend the bypass grafts beyond the distal obstruction site. The cause of such a complication is usually not diagnosed until after surgery. If possible, confirmation by intraoperative angiography should be obtained and correction undertaken immediately before adherent thrombi unnecessarily complicate reoperation. Both inguinal regions, including the "healthy" side, should always be prepared for surgery since thrombotic material on the diseased side may dislodge and travel to the other side. Usually, technical errors during completion of the distal anastomosis are the cause of narrowing at the suture line or kinks in overlong prostheses, leading to a reduction of blood flow. Both may result in an immediate occlusion.

Late Occlusions. Late occlusions following aortoiliac reconstructions rarely cause acute symptoms of occlusive arterial disease. Immediate reintervention is usually not necessary. There is enough time for adequate diagnostic procedures. Only if the cause of reocclusion is found by arteriography is adequate and successful reintervention possible. Just as in reconstructions of other vascular regions the causes of recurrent thrombosis within the aortoiliac segment are numerous and vary greatly. They differ only qualitatively from factors leading to early occlusion. Surgical reintervention depends on the following circumstances:

1. The nature of the original operative procedure (endarterectomy, bypass grafting)
2. The potential inflow and outflow tracts for a new bypass graft
3. Difficulties in reexposing the occluded vessel segment
4. Risk of reintervention

Following primary thromboendarterectomy of the iliac arteries (open, semiclosed, or closed), a second thromboendarterectomy of the same segment is not indicated. Generally, surgical repair should be a bypass graft anastomosis bridging the previously reconstructed area [5, 6]. The same method of treatment should also be employed following occlusions of primary bypass grafts, independent of their synthetic material. In most cases thrombosis starts at the distal anastomosis, continuing upward through the entire limb of the prosthesis. Correction of the anastomosis with subsequent thrombectomy of the prosthesis alone rarely suffices and does not lead to long-term patency. Therefore, bypassing the distal anastomosis with an autogenous vein (if necessary, taken from the contralateral leg) is the method of choice. If grafting is necessary to span several joints, different graft materials should be combined, e.g., Dacron or PTFE prostheses to bypass the thigh, or vein grafts to bridge the knee joint. Additional stenoses within the outflow tract should also be corrected during the same session.

Repair is performed as follows. First the distal side of the prosthesis is shortened, then thrombectomy is performed. The prosthesis is then lengthened with appropriate material and reconnected to the host artery more distally. In some cases, rerouting the arterial graft must be considered (see p. 539). In high risk patients and in cases of unilateral occlusion of the iliac artery, rerouting of the arterial graft is possible by femorofemoral or axillofemoral bypass grafting [1, 22].

f) Femoropopliteal and Crural Segment

Occlusions of this arterial segment have the same causes as previously described for other vascular regions. Technical errors, wrong assessment of the run-off capacity, and progression of the patient's underlying occlusive disease are common causes. The femoropopliteal and crural arteries are relatively small for the connection of a bypass graft. Thus, the surgeon is more likely to overestimate the run-off capacity. Control of surgical reconstruction can be gained by intraoperative angiography. If the host artery exhibits stenoses distal to the anastomosis, the bypass graft must be extended beyond them. Autogenous vein grafts (from the contralateral leg) should be preferred, especially if joint-crossing reconstructions are performed. Soft PTFE prostheses with annular reinforcement are only a second choice.

If the autogenous material is not long enough to construct a bypass extending beyond the knee, a composite graft consisting of a synthetic prosthesis and an autogenous vein may be used. In such cases, the knee joint itself should be bridged by a venous graft.

Another alternative is a sequential bypass. A synthetic prosthesis is used to construct a bypass extending from the groin to a (disobliterated) segment of the superficial femoral artery proximal to the knee. A second bypass is constructed using an autogenous vein graft that extends from the superficial femoral artery past the knee to the popliteal artery [6].

For the prevention of early and late occlusion it is essential that the vein be handled with care and that there be no stenosing ligatures of its branches or any twisting of its long axis during implantation. As in reocclusions within the aortoiliac segment, treatment of recurrent obstruction following bypass grafting of the femoropopliteal or crural segment should consist of extending the bypass and connecting it further distally to a suitable lower leg artery. If angiography prior to reoperation shows insufficient run-off in the distal portions of the grafted artery, a recurrent occlusion may be prevented by constructing a distal arterial venous fistula in order to increase blood flow to the graft [14].

If reocclusion following reconstruction of the femoropopliteal and crural arteries cannot be relieved, profunda angioplasty can improve the circulation in the extremity [2].

REFERENCES

1. Blaisdell FW (1970) Aorto-iliac arterial substitution utilizing subcutaneous grafts. Ann Surg 172:775
2. Bernhard VM (1977) Profundaplasty. In: Rutherford RB (ed) Vascular surgery. Saunders, Philadelphia London Toronto
3. Dainko EA (1972) Complications of the use of the Fogarty Cath. Arch Surg 102:79
4. Diethrich EB (1973) Complications of procedures of the aortic arch and the thoracic aorta. In: Beebe UG (ed) Complications in vascular surgery, vol 131. Lippincott, Philadelphia Toronto, p 150
5. van Dongen RJAM (1983) Aortoiliakale Rekonstruktionen. In: Carstensen G (eds) Intra- und postoperative Komplikationen. Springer, Berlin Heidelberg New York
6. van Dongen RJAM (1980) Reinterventionen wegen Rezidivverschlüssen nach rekonstruktiven Eingriffen am Aorta-iliaca- und Femoralis Poplitea Abschnitt (operative Taktik und Technik). Langenbecks Arch Chir 352:183–188
7. Fogarty ThJ (1977) The technique of thrombectomy and other uses of the Fogarty catheter. In: Rutherford RB (ed) Vascular surgery. Saunders, Philadelphia London Toronto
8. Foster JH, Dean RH (1973) Complications of visceral arterial procedures. Complications associated with the operative treatment of renovascular hypertension. In: Beebe HG (ed) Complications in vascular surgery. Lippincott, Philadelphia Toronto, p 171
9. Imparato AM, Lin JPT (1967) Vertebral arterial reconstruction: internal plication and vein patch angioplasty. Ann Surg 166:213
10. Lepley D Jr, Flemma RJ, Mullen DC (1981) Complications of surgery of the heart and adjacent great vessels. In: Complications in surgery and their management, 4th edn. Saunders, Philadelphia London Toronto Sydney, pp 367–421
11. Linder FA, Encke A (1966) Die postoperative Nachblutung in der allgemeinen Chirurgie. Langenbecks Arch Klin Chir 316:50
12. Lusby JR, Wylie EJ (1983) Complications of carotid endarterectomy. Symp. on complications of common procedures. Surg Clin North Am – 63/6:1293
13. Müller-Wiefel H (1983) Femoropopliteale Rekonstruktion. In: Carstensen G (ed) Intra- und postoperative Komplikationen. Springer, Berlin Heidelberg New York, p 96
14. Orend KH, Kortmann H, Abendroth D, Becker HM (1985) Die adjunktive AV-Fistel beim femorokruralen Bypass. Fortschr Med 30/46:750
15. Reid HC, Dallechy R (1958) Infarction of ileus following resection of coarctation of aorta. Br J Surg 45:625
16. Ring DM, Lewis FJ (1956) Abdominal pain following surgical correction of coarctation of the aorta. A syndrome. J Thorac Surg 31:718
17. Rob ChG, Beebe HG (1973) Complications of extracranial cerebrovascular procedures. In: High G, Beebe MD (eds) Complications in vascular surgery. Lippincott, Philadelphia Toronto, p 151
18. Rutherford RB (1977) Infrarenal aortic aneurysms. In: Rutherford RB (ed) Vascular surgery. Saunders, Philadelphia London Toronto, p 639
19. Sandmann W, Peronneau P, Kremer K (1983) Caro tischirurgie und Pertubationsmessung. In: Carstensen G (ed) Intra- und postoperative Komplikationen. Springer, Berlin Heidelberg New York
20. Sandmann W (1983) Supraaortische Rekonstruktionen. In: Carstensen G (ed) Intra- und postoperative Komplikationen. Springer, Berlin Heidelberg New York, p 80
21. Silver D (1977) Anticoagulant therapy. In: Rutherford (ed) Vascular surgery. Saunders, Philadelphia London Toronto, p 301
22. Trimble IR (1972) Criteria for femoro-femoral bypass. In: Rutherford RB (ed) Vascular surgery. Saunders, Philadelphia London Toronto (Ann Surg 175:985)
23. Vollmar J (1975) Rekonstruktive Chirurgie der Arterien. Thieme, Stuttgart

10.2 Infections in Vascular Surgery

F. PIZA

CONTENTS

A. General Remarks

Postoperative infections are a typical complication in surgery. In vascular surgery they are of special importance because of the serious sequelae which are possible. They may endanger the extremity involved and even the life of the patient. Their outcome cannot always be predicted, even in the hands of an experienced vascular surgeon.

In contrast to general surgery, superficial infections in vascular surgery more often spread into deeper layers of tissue. A protective tissue layer between the reconstructed vessel and the subcutaneous region or intestine is important to keep superficial infections localized (e.g., skin infections which are most commonly observed in the groin). The interposition of retroperitoneal tissue or omentum, e.g., between an implanted aortic prosthesis and the duodenum or small intestine, is already an important step towards the prevention of an aortoenteric fistula. Alternating incisions are preferred, shielding the surgical area [6].

The groin is the most common site of infection, with superficial and deep infections occurring in a ratio of about 2 or 3:1. This demonstrates the necessity of performing meticulous, layer by layer dissection. The vascular bed is only a short distance away from the skin. A transverse skin incision inhibits the spread of an infection from the outside.

Superficial infections not related to the vascular reconstruction are treated by the usual principles of surgical therapy. Deep infections are much more difficult to treat and must be discussed separately. The frequency of infection in synthetic implants of the aorta and its branches without prophylactic administration of antibiotics ranges from 1.34% to 6%.

B. Prophylaxis

The greater the risk of infection in a vascular surgical procedure, the greater the importance of preventive measures is. Anemia, hypovolemia, hypoxia, diabetes mellitus, obesity, poor nutritional status, cortisone therapy, intercurrent infections, etc. are risk factors for infection [4]. For example, 19% of all synthetic shunts constructed for dialysis of patients suffering from chronic uremia became infected. Local measures consist of thorough skin disinfection and strict observance of asepsis by the operating team and within the operative area. Extensive preoperative invasive diagnostic procedures within the operative area, especially the groin, should be avoided. The prevention of postoperative hematoma, lymphatic fistula, and skin necroses (see the chapter on bone and joint surgery, heart surgery, etc.) is equally important.

It is difficult to establish whether localized latent infections in peripheral necroses of stage IV occlusive arterial disease play a statistically relevant role in the development of severe infections within the inguinal region. Local inflammation and ascending lymphangitis or lymphadenitis found in the advanced stages of vascular disease are potential sources of proximal infection. These should be treated at least preoperatively and basic prophylactic measures undertaken.

One type of prophylaxis is the construction of a distal synthetic graft anastomosis above rather than below the inguinal ligament to prevent infection at the groin. This region is most prone to infection. The first basic method of prophylaxis is systemic administration of antibiotics. During the last few years, the first randomized studies in vascular surgery have shown the actual, positive effect of antibiotic prophylaxis [12, 13]. It has been demonstrated that perioperative administration shortly before and during the operation, with treatment continuing for 2–3 days postoperatively, guaranteed full effectiveness, which is not increased significantly by supplementary local application of antibiotics [12]. The dominance of staphylococcus and the presence of gram-negative bacteria (especially in the inguinal region) would seem to call for the administration of broad spectrum antibiotics [2].

Although local antibiotic prophylaxis alone also exhibited a positive effect [12], systemic administration of antibiotics is preferable, especially in the case of synthetic implants, where bacterial contamination occurs during tunneling. In most cases contamination occurs at the time of grafting [4]. Late infections are spread mainly via the bloodstream. The effectiveness of systemic, intravenous antibiotic administration in the prevention of local infection has been studied by comparing serum antibiotic levels with local levels found in wound secretions [11]. Results show that the maximum antibacterial effect can be expected during the first few hours after application [15]; however, it is directly dependent upon the local blood circulation, the type of tissue, and the type of antibiotic given. Local ischemia has considerable influence on local levels of antibiotic in wound secretions. Whether or not the different adherence of bacteria to different prosthetic materials is clinically relevant remains unanswered. There are, however, reports on the accumulation of antibiotics in the aortic wall [11].

Another step toward prophylaxis of local infections is the commercial availability of vascular prostheses with local antibiotic bonding. Experimental studies have demonstrated that such grafts have considerable resistance to infection.

C. Diagnosis

Superficial infection at the incision site is accompanied by redness and swelling. To determine whether or not the infection has spread to the aorta or the pelvic arteries, diagnostic measures must be employed. Infection may occur at any time during the postoperative period. In an analysis of 128 cases infection appeared 7 months after surgery, on average. The longest time interval observed was 7 years 3 months.

The discovery of a fistula in the inguinal region is certainly a clear indication of chronic infection, especially where synthetic materials have been used. Fistulography usually permits the demonstration of a deep infection around the prosthesis.

Besides clinical signs such as pain, fever, high white blood cell count, increased ESR etc., the demonstration of air or fluid accumulation around the prosthesis by sonography or computed tomography, an enlarged renal pelvis in the intravenous pyelogram, an undiscernible psoas shadow, or a localized distension at the anastomosis signaling imminent rupture in the angiogram may lead one to assume that local infection is present. Especially helpful in diagnosis is a scan using 111 In-labeled granulocytes, which in the hands of an experienced radiologist is a very accurate method of localizing a deep infection. Although diagnostic puncture of the region may be negative in some cases, surgical exposure of the suspected area is the ultimate, totally reliable method for safely excluding infection.

D. Complications of Infection

Early complications of local infection are local abscess formation, hemorrhage, thrombosis, and septicemia. A late complication is false aneurysm developing from septic suture insufficiency [8].

An abscess with or without connection to the reconstruction site can be treated by the basic principles of septic surgery so long as hemorrhage does not occur.

Acute suture insufficiency with increasing swelling and hemorrhage (as in the case of false aneurysms) is the most severe acute complication and should be treated as early as possible. Angiography performed early enough may yield valuable information. If thrombosis occurs in infected prostheses, the danger of bacteremia is great since the contaminated thrombi are an excellent nutritive medium. In such cases, radical excision of the graft is necessary.

Septicemia, the final stage after systemic spread of local infection, seriously endangers the patient's life. The aim is to prevent and successfully treat this state by local revision. This puts high demands on the training and experience of the vascular surgeon.

It should be pointed out that endogenous infections of synthetic prostheses are always possible and can never be excluded as long as pseudointima has formed within the prosthesis. Thus, the patient with an arterial prosthesis must always watch out for infection, even long after surgery, and should consult the vascular surgeon immediately if it occurs. However, a complete uniform growth of pseudointima protects the prosthesis against hematogenic infections to some degree.

Perforations of hollow organs are rare. Of all complications, secondary aortoduodenal or aortointestinal fistula, with hemorrhage inside the gastrointestinal tract, are the most dreaded in local infection. They have a high mortality rate (71%), and repair of the fistula and replacement of the aorta do not necessarily lead to healing of the lesion in all cases. There are several predisposing factors for the development of a secondary fistula: reoperations, inadequate closure of the retroperitoneal tissue over the synthetic prosthesis, false aneurysms, renal infarcts with septicemia, and others. Yet, one of the most important causes is probably local infection. Some 75% of fistulas are located within reach of upper gastrointestinal endoscopy, which is therefore the most important diagnostic method to confirm bleeding. Aortography, usually performed in patients with negative endoscopic results, may additionally discover a false aneurysm. Each aortic anastomosis must be covered with enough connective tissue, if possible in two layers, to separate the aorta from the duodenum and proximal jejunum.

E. General Therapy

General measures, such as the administration of antibiotics following antibiotic sensitivity testing (to determine resistent bacteria and other pathogens), are always undertaken in apparent surgical infection. Systemic antibiotic therapy can rarely be administered alone without additional local treatment of the infected area. Local therapy has priority over systemic therapy, which is only capable of preventing the spread of local infection or additionally combating bacteremia and sepsis.

F. Local Surgical Treatment

The success of local surgical treatment depends on the localization of the infection, secondary complications due to recurrent hemorrhage, the type of primary reconstruction, the number of anastomoses, the patient's general condition, and the experience of the vascular surgeon.

The surgeon must consider several factors when deciding upon surgical repair: the site of the infection (anastomosis or entire prosthesis), virulence, possible bacterial invasion of the pseudointima. For example, hemorrhage caused by infection and leading to severe deterioration of the patient's general condition makes immediate intervention necessary. The patient's general condition also influences the surgeon's decision in trying to save an extremity. Sometimes, the surgeon must choose between the patient's life and saving the extremity. Instead of following general principles, the experienced vascular surgeon will individualize the indication for surgery and adjust treatment accordingly.

Infections of arterial prostheses occur in 1%–2% on average. Here the problem is to cure the infections (removal of foreign matter, drainage, and irrigation) while at the same time avoiding amputation when acute ischemia develops as a result of the local surgical intervention (local ligation).

A new reconstruction within the contaminated area has a double purpose: (1) Cure of the infection by draining the abscess, removing synthetic material acting as a sustaining medium for bacterial infection, local drainage, and irrigation, and (2) at the same time, reconstruction of the arterial vessel using autogenous materials, chiefly veins. The use of absorbable atraumatic suture material may simplify this procedure. In common with other groups, we have employed this combined method successfully in local infections of the pelvic and femoral region. Treatment of a local abscess by drainage and irrigation alone is only possible if the patient's general condition is good and no hemorrhage is present. This treatment may also produce good results in infected regions near an aortic anastomosis. We have observed one cure

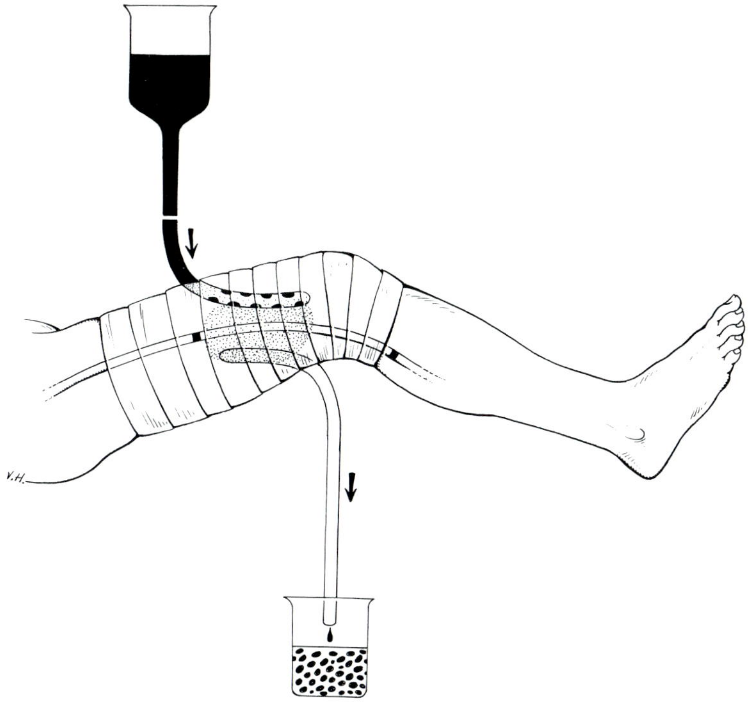

Fig. 10.2.1. Local drainage and irrigation by means of a gravity-fed infusion set

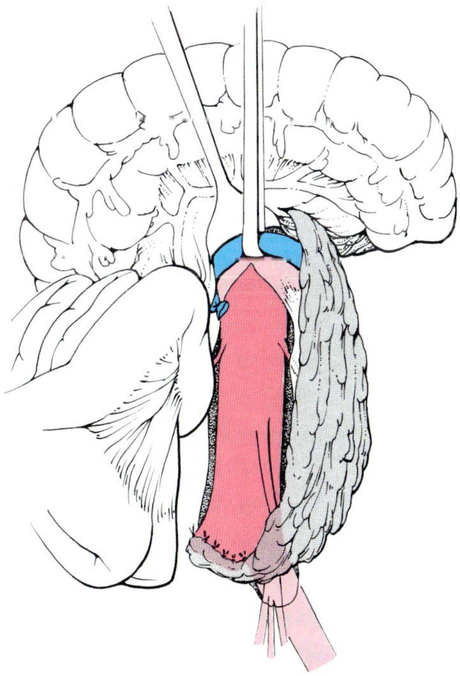

Fig. 10.2.2. Coverage of an infected aortic segment and an infected inguinal arterial reconstruction with greater omentum flap

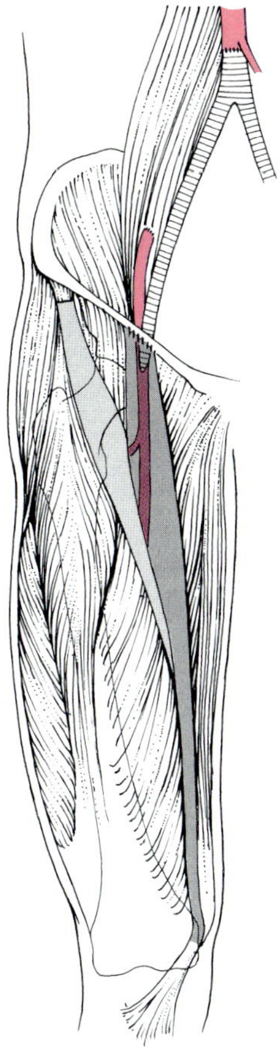

Fig. 10.2.3. Coverage of an infected prosthesis in the groin with the sartorius muscle dissected proximally and displaced medially (LEGUIT and VAN BERGE HENEGOUWEN [10])

of an *E. coli* abscess situated near the proximal portion of a bifurcation prosthesis after many years of follow-up treatment. While irrigation and drainage are performed, continuous flow of irrigating fluid through the infected wound should be checked by maintaining a careful fluid balance (Fig. 10.2.1). Irrigation should be continued for 2–3 days. The drain should be left in place for 3–5 days. The possibility of implanting PMMA chains should be mentioned in this connection.

An important procedure is the covering of an infected vascular segment with greater omentum [3]. This is done by means of a pedicled flap from the transverse colon, vascularized by either the left or right gastroepiploic artery [1]; the flap is lengthened and drawn through a hole in the transverse mesocolon, either down into the retroperitoneal or the femoral region (Figs. 10.2.2, 10.2.3). Coverage with viable tissue and local as well as systemic treatment with antibiotics may cure infection and at the same time preserve blood circulation. In the same manner, transposition of the sartorius muscle [10] and other tissues of the thigh, including flaps from the lower abdomen, are used to cover infections of the groin during the postoperative follow-up period. Local proliferation of connective tissue may lead to shrinkage of the arterial reconstruction following cure of the infection. Then, a secondary procedure may be performed to reconstruct the artery. Surgical management of vascular infections often combines several different procedures.

G. Bypass Procedures

Arterial circulation is interrupted by local ligation in the infected area, and the wound is left open to heal by second intention. This treatment is combined with extra-anatomic bypass procedures in noncontaminated areas for immediate restoration of adequate blood flow to the noninfected area. Bypass should be performed first (see p. 539).

Immediate arterial reconstruction is necessary only if ischemia becomes too severe following ligation of an artery. For example, surgical ligation of the femoral artery within the adductor canal does not necessarily result in total ischemia calling for immediate revascularization. There is time for the infection to heal and for the patient's general condition to improve before revascularization is performed. Sometimes, ameroid or laminaria rings may be installed, causing progressive narrowing of the infected prosthesis. They swell slowly, stimulating the development of collaterals. The occluded prosthesis is then removed in a second operation without extra-anatomic bypass. Suture ligation of arteries within the aortic and inguinal regions causes severe ischemia of the lower extremity. Delayed revascularization following ligation is, therefore, of very high risk and may lead to amputation. The commonest bypass procedure in cases of infected aortic prostheses (48% mortality) is the axillofemoral bypass graft. Infections of the inguinal region are treated by grafting through the obturator foramen. In rare cases, a bifurcation prosthesis is connected proximally to the aorta just below the diaphragm or to the descending aorta. Both sides of the prosthesis are then pulled through a tunnel in the rectus sheath and anastomosed to uninfected arteries distally (Fig. 10.2.4).

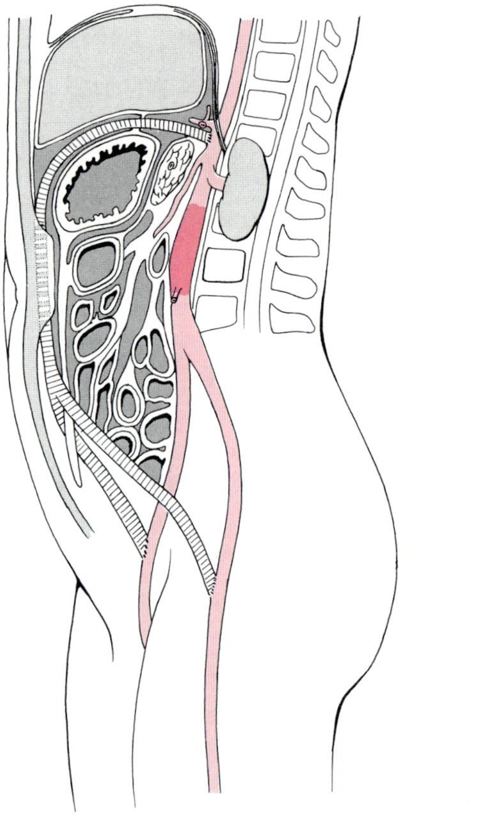

Fig. 10.2.4. Bypass of an infection of the infrarenal aorta; proximal attachment below the diaphragm. Synthetic prosthesis lying in a tunnel of the anterior abdominal wall

Surgical management of perigraft infection, especially if combined with hemorrhage, is summarized as follows:

1. Extra-anatomic bypass, performed according to the basic principles of aseptic vascular surgery
2. Radical revision of the infection site with removal of all foreign material and adequate drainage of the area

Systemic administration of antibiotics will have two effects in such a situation: on the one hand, it is a prophylaxis for the newly reconstructed area, and, on the other hand, it combats infection and sepsis already present.

Although an immediate bypass operation in patients with septic or hemorrhagic shock is an additional risk, it should be performed in view of the catastrophic sequelae following intoxication through ischemic necroses. After aortic ligation, complete ischemia of both legs up to the hips has a mortality rate of about 72%. Immediate revascularization is still the lower risk although it has an average mortality rate of 40% owing to the poor general condition of these patients. Even if revision and reconstruction can be performed during one operation, the outcome of this dreaded complication is often fatal. The mortality rates cited in the literature differ greatly, since they are dependent on several variables: spread of the infection, localization of the synthetic material, number of anastomoses involved, graft thrombosis, etc. In these cases arteriosclerosis, hemorrhage, and sepsis result in severe damage to vital organs. Even though revision of an infection within the inguinal region is easier to perform, the basic problems of management are no different. Quick life-saving decisions are also of the utmost importance.

In contrast, distal infections do not lead to hemorrhagic or septic shock as often (9.9% mortality). However, technical alternatives to a distal anastomosis in an uncontaminated area are very limited. In the case of infection with subsequent hemorrhage, amputation is often necessary. This is the only relatively secure life-saving procedure.

Treatment of choice in secondary aortoenteric fistula is an extra-anatomic bypass and excision of the prosthesis. In a primary fistula of this kind, following spontaneous perforation of an aneurysm into the intestinal lumen, closure of the intestine with resection of the aneurysm and implantation of a bifurcation prosthesis are recommended. Reports on this procedure have demonstrated good results.

The immediate threat from an infected vascular reconstruction is to the patient's limb, but also, secondarily, to his life. And here the boundary line between primary and secondary threat is sometimes very narrow. If the surgeon passes over it, the patient's life will be forfeited. To make the right decision at the right time is one of the greatest responsibilities a vascular surgeon has, demanding the broadest experience and highest degree of technical skill. Because these complications do not occur too often, the surgeon should consult an experienced colleague without delay in order not to make a wrong decision. Schematic aids to decision making, as found in surgical textbooks, are useful for general procedural advice, but they do not necessarily apply in every case. This is why well-organized prophylaxis and individualized treatment of infections are so important.

H. Future Perspectives

Advances in prophylaxis can be expected in the following area:

1. Improvement of surgical management and organization (operating room, postoperative ward, and intensive care unit)
2. Adequate training in general surgery and its subspecialities
3. Antibiotic prophylaxis incorporated in synthetic materials
4. Further refinement of synthetic materials to improve pseudointima formation with prevention of dissections, and within the material a reinforced barrier against bacterial invasion
5. Synthetic materials with local antibiotic binding

Advances in therapy are based on:

1. Further improvement of diagnostic techniques (ultrasonography, scintigraphy, angiography, and others)
2. Adequate training in vascular surgery with special emphasis on the treatment of complications
3. Specific antibiotics with fewer side effects

The poor prognosis of deep infections in vascular surgery, often leading to amputation or even death, totally justify all measures mentioned above and all efforts to improve organization and equipment, despite the costs involved.

REFERENCES

1. Alday ES, Goldsmith HS (1972) Surgical technique for omental lengthening based on arterial anatomy. Surg Gynecol Obstet 135:103
2. Cherry K, Hollier L (1983) Prophylactic antibiotics in vascular Surgery. Pittmann, London, p 10
3. van Dongen RJAM (1983) Vascular protection in reconstructive arterial surgery. In: Liebermann-Meffert D, White H (eds) The greater omentum. Springer, Berlin Heidelberg New York, p 266
4. Goldstone J, Effeney D (1980) Prevention of arterial graft infections. Grune & Stratton, Orlando, p 491
5. Greco R, Harwey R (1980) The role of antibiotic bonding in the prevention of vascular prosthetic infections. Ann Surg 195:167
6. Kessler W (1982) Infektprophylaxe bei arterieller Gefäßrekonstruktion durch queren Leistenschnitt. Angio 5:15

7. Kolb R, Piza F, Thettner O, Tizian C (1975) Gefäßrekonstruktion im infizierten Gebiet unter gezielter Chemotherapie. Acta Chir Austriaca 7:12
8. Koning J, van Dongen RJAM (1981) Treatment of infection after arterial reconstructive procedures. J Cardiovasc Surg 22:291
9. Kretschmer G, Polterauer P, Piza F, Jantsch H (1983) Vorläufige Erfahrungen mit der biologischen Omentumumhüllung als Therapieverfahren infizierter Läsionen in der Gefäßchirurgie. Langenbecks Arch Chir 359:123
10. Leguit P, Van Berge Henegouwen D (1983) The sartorius muscle transposition in the treatment of deep wound infection after vascular surgery in the groin. VASA 12:151
11. Mutch D, Richards G, Brown R, Mulder D (1982) Bioactive antibiotic levels in the human aorta. Surgery 92:1068
12. Pitt H, Postier R, MacGowan W, Frank L, Surmak A, Sitzman J, Bonchier-Hayes D (1980) Prophylactic antibiotics in vascular surgery. Ann Surg 192:355
13. Salzmann G (1983) Infektionsprophylaxe in der Gefäßchirurgie durch perioperative Antibiotikagabe. Ergebnisse einer prospektiven randomisierten Studie. Angio 5:225
14. Surgerman B (1982) In vitro adherence of bacteria to prosthetic vascular grafts. Infection 10:1
15. Walterbusch G, Saathoff M, Hawarich A, Mlasowsky B (1983) Die Abdichtung poröser Gefäßprothesen – eine Gelegenheit zur lokalen Antibiotikaapplikation? Angio 5:239

10.3 Anastomotic Aneurysms

H.M. Becker and H. Kortmann

CONTENTS

A. Causes

In the early days of vascular surgery anastomotic aneurysms were a relatively common late complication (3%–24%) following prosthetic vascular replacement. Most of the anastomotic ruptures were caused by early wear of suture materials (silk!), prosthetic fibers, or texture [1, 2, 3, 6, 7]. After qualitative improvement of these products (Dacron and PTFE prostheses, polyester and polypropylene sutures) the occurrence of late anastomotic aneurysms became rare [2, 17]. Besides mechanical wear, biologic characteristics and technical errors may promote the development of anastomotic aneurysms. The different elasticities of the grafted artery and the prosthesis connected to it cause a mismatch in compliance and exert a very intense mechanical strain upon the anastomosis [9]. Disobliteration and endarterectomy of the arteriosclerotic artery at the suture site should be done very sparingly, if at all. If calcified plaque formation is too extensive and circumferential disobliteration is absolutely necessary, rather larger bites of the arterial wall should be taken during suture of the anastomosis. In large vessels telescopic anastomosis has been very reliable: During the suturing process the prosthesis is pulled slightly into the lumen of the vessel, thereby reinforcing the vessel margin. Favorable hemodynamic conditions at the anastomosis are also important for preventing ruptures of the suture line. A high blood flow with minimal turbulence can be achieved by constructing end-to-side anastomoses at a sharp angle with long and elliptical apertures [11, 12, 18] (see p. 43). Hypertension and clotting disorders, especially during the early postoperative period, promote the development of anastomotic aneurysms [1, 14]. The mycotic aneurysm, usually caused by inadequate aseptic conditions intraoperatively, is a severe complication that almost always leads to removal of the prosthesis. This interrupts blood flow through the reconstruction, making extra-anatomic bypass necessary (see p. 539).

Between 70% and 80% of all anastomotic aneurysms are localized in the inguinal region [10, 11, 13]. There are three reasons for this high rate of incidence. In most cases the prostheses are sutured end-to-side to the femoral artery. This exposes the incorporated rigid prosthetic tube to shearing and bending forces at the hip joint. Furthermore, the groin is highly susceptible to infection because of its neighboring regions and numerous lymphatic vessels [11, 12, 16, 18]. In contrast, anastomotic aneurysms are much less common in pelvic and popliteal regions and also in the aorta and supra-aortic arteries [5, 8]. As a consequence of this statistically confirmed observation, we always prefer iliac connection of prostheses implanted for aneurysmatic disease of the aortic bifurcation.

Today, we use knitted double velour Dacron prostheses for the aortoiliac segment. We prefer the woven Dacron prosthesis in those cases where certain risk factors (advanced age, poor general condition, rare blood group, clotting disorders, emergency procedure) demand impermeability of the prosthesis. Since no true healing takes place at the juncture of the host artery and the prosthesis, the use of nonabsorbable, long-lasting suture material is necessary. Synthetic polyester and polyprophylene sutures are very reliable for this purpose. Beneath the inguinal ligament an autogenous vein graft is the best material for vascular replacement. Pseudoaneurysms of these grafts are a great rarity because true and complete healing between the autogenous graft and the host artery takes place [18]. In cases where a vein is not available, stretched PTFE is used today worldwide. So far, there has been no indication that PTFE has a higher incidence of anastomotic aneurysms than Dacron [2].

A false aneurysm can develop at any suture line. Following endarterectomy and autogenous vein grafting, it is only rarely observed [8]. Likewise, anastomotic aneurysms following reconstructions of the supra-aortic arteries are rare [8]. An aortic aneurysm of the ascending aorta rarely develops owing to the absence of periaortal tissue that could effect tamponade. A postoperative pulsating hematoma in this case leads to cardiac tamponade if it is not discovered early enough. Anastomotic aneurysms of the descending thoracic aorta are often diagnosed only when symptoms of dislocation of neighboring nerves (phrenic nerve, recurrent laryngeal nerve) or hemoptysis, caused by penetration of the bronchial system, occur. Aortoenteric fistulas are very severe complications of the usually asymptomatic suture line aneurysms of the abdominal aorta. The symptoms range from intermittently occurring occult blood loss to severe intestinal hemorrhage leading to hypovolemic shock [2, 4]. Typically, endoscopy does not detect the bleeding site. Anastomotic aneurysms of the pelvic arteries can lead to compression of the neighboring veins with stasis and thrombosis of the affected leg. An expanding pulsating tumor of a false aneurysm following arterial suture at the femoral arteries must not be confused with an inguinal abscess.

B. Diagnosis

Anastomotic aneurysms of limb arteries may often be diagnosed by simple palpation of pulsating tumors in the region of the anastomosis. Anastomotic aneurysms of the aorta, renal, visceral, and pelvic arteries may be visualized by modern noninvasive imaging methods such as ultrasonography and computed tomography. Prior to operative reconstruction, especially of small arteries, angiography is preferred. Diagnosis of small aortoenteric fistulas may pose problems. In these cases, a diverticular marginal contour of the aorta in the angiogram is pathognomonic.

C. Indications for Surgery

The occurrence and rapid advance of an acute anastomotic dehiscence with formation of a pulsating hematoma is extremely painful and must be treated immediately by emergency operation. Delay leads to trophic disturbances of neighboring tissue so that wound necroses and infections must be expected after vascular reconstruction. Prompt intervention is necessary in case of hemorrhage from a leaking suture in a neck artery. Here, there exists an acute danger of asphyxia. The patient must be intubated immediately, and surgery performed. There is very little time left for diagnostic procedures in case of an acutely bleeding aortoenteric fistula or leaking suture of the ascending aorta. If the appropriate acute symptoms are present, laparotomy or thoracotomy are justified. Anastomotic aneurysms developing chronically are surrounded by a wall of fibrotic tissue, fibrin, and adherent stratified mural thrombi. Because they can rupture and embolize, elective resection is indicated as soon as the diagnosis is confirmed.

D. Positioning

The resection of anastomotic aneurysms is usually performed by the same approach as in primary surgery. This is why procedures on the infrarenal aorta, pelvic, and inguinal arteries are done using supine positioning. The suprarenal aorta (segment IV) or the thoracic aorta are exposed with the patient in a semilateral position and slightly rotated according to CRAWFORD: the pelvis and abdomen are left in a supine position, while the thorax is rotated about 45° to the right. For reexposure of supra-aortic arteries, the patient is placed in the usual position. This is also the case in surgical revision of the extremities.

E. Exposure

After excision of the scar, dissection is begun around the inflow and outflow tracts. Umbilical tape is passed around these proximal and distal segments. This is easier 2–4 cm above and below the aneurysmal sac. Following proximal and distal control of bleeding, the false aneurysm is exposed. Where especially massive scar tissue is present from previous operations, the aneurysm is opened directly and a Fogarty balloon catheter used to block inflow and outflow. This technique of intraluminal balloon blockade is especially useful at smaller arterial bifurcations, e.g., at the femoral bifurcation when exposure of the profunda femoris artery is difficult because of severe scar formation (see Fig. 10.3.3c, d). However, in the aorta and great arteries, the surgeon will always try to interrupt blood flow before the aneurysmal sac is divided; otherwise, blood loss will be too great. With the aneurysmal sac open, the anastomosis can be exposed step by step, using the scalpel. One should keep close to the artery in the dissected area in order to avoid injuring veins and nerves.

F. Reconstructions

I. Thoracic Aorta

Following anterolateral thoracotomy, the thoracic aorta is first exposed proximal to the aneurysm. If the anastomotic aneurysm lies just below the aortic arch, the origin of the subclavian artery complicates dissection and in some cases must be sacrificed. The vagus and recurrent laryngeal nerve cross the aortic arch at that point and must be spared by all means (see p. 525). Exposure of the aorta distally is easily achieved by dividing the pleura. Only after proximal and distal bleeding has been brought under control is dissection begun around the pseudoaneurysm. If the anesthetic is properly administered, with subtle reduction of the afterload while taking most careful precautions not to reduce the preload, shunt or bypass techniques can be avoided in the clamping phase. However, under difficult anatomic conditions, one should not hesitate to employ these techniques. Previous hemoptysis is always indicative of aneurysmal penetration of the lung.

Usually, the sixth segment of the left lower lobe is affected. Following blunt as well as sharp separation of both structures and reconstruction of the aorta, resection of the pulmonary segment is necessary. Blood clots are removed from the opened aneurysm and the leaking suture exposed. Aorta and prosthesis around the anastomosis are resected and the continuity of the aorta restored. This basic principle of reconstruction can be applied to all central and peripheral aneurysms. The anastomosis can be repaired by restitching alone only if suture dehiscence is slight and circumscribed and the arterial wall is in intact. In any event, local repair by suture should remain an exception in the operative treatment of anastomotic aneurysms.

II. Abdominal Aorta

Anastomotic aneurysms of the abdominal aorta (Fig. 10.3.1a) are exposed by a transabdominal approach through a median laparotomy extending from the xiphoid to the symphysis pubis, cutting around the umbilicus on the left side. The small intestine is retracted to the right. Typically, a false aneurysm of the proximal aorta may have penetrated the ascending part of the duodenum, just before the duodenojejunal flexure, forming an aortoenteric fistula (Fig. 10.3.2a, c). When the diagnosis has been confirmed, no further exposure is performed. Instead, dissection above the kidneys, preferably cranial to the celiac artery, is continued for better visualization and clamping (Fig. 10.3.2b). The lesser omentum is divided, and the tissue around the aorta is dissected between the sides of the diaphragm. If the origin of the celiac artery is rather high, one should divide the tendinous tissue surrounding the aortic hiatus.

Following systemic anticoagulation with heparin the aorta can be clamped just below the diaphragm. Distal bleeding below the fistula is controlled, the aneurysm is divided, and the fistula is exposed from within the aorta (Fig. 10.3.2c). The visualized duodenal wall defect is closed with a two-row suture (Fig. 10.3.2d). If an aortoenteric fistula is not present, the aortic clamp can be applied below the kidneys following exposure of the left renal vein and dissection of tissue surrounding the aorta in this region (Fig. 10.3.1b). Prior to reconstruction of the aorta, the operating area should be flushed with an antiseptic solution (e.g., 4 g chloramine diluted in 1000 ml lukewarm 0.9% NaCl). The prosthesis and, if necessary, the aorta are resected at the anastomosis (Fig. 10.3.1c, d,

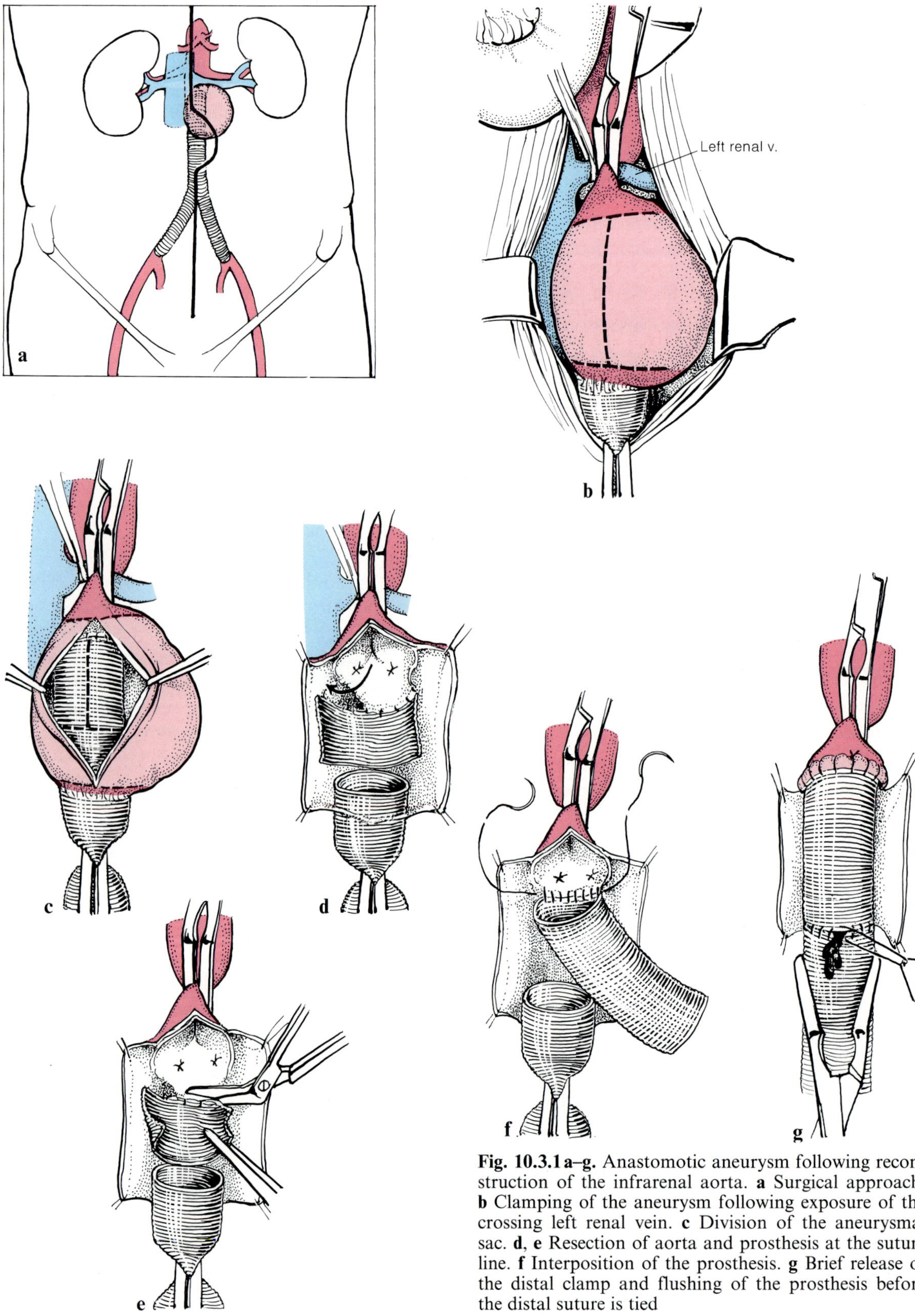

Fig. 10.3.1 a–g. Anastomotic aneurysm following reconstruction of the infrarenal aorta. **a** Surgical approach. **b** Clamping of the aneurysm following exposure of the crossing left renal vein. **c** Division of the aneurysmal sac. **d, e** Resection of aorta and prosthesis at the suture line. **f** Interposition of the prosthesis. **g** Brief release of the distal clamp and flushing of the prosthesis before the distal suture is tied

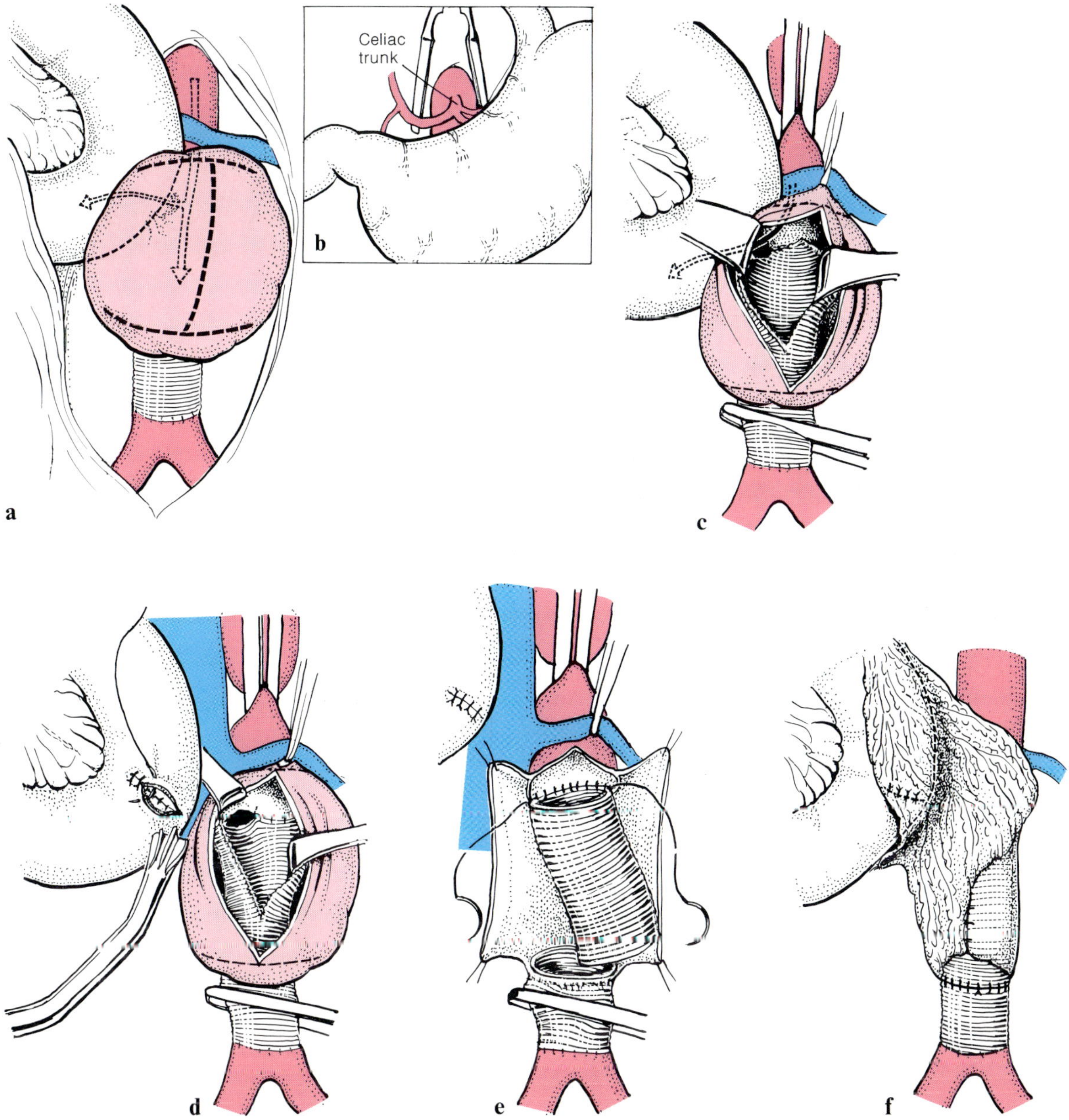

Fig. 10.3.2. a Anastomotic aneurysm with aortoduodenal fistula following reconstruction of the abdominal aorta. **b** Clamping of the aorta above the celiac artery between both crurae of the diaphragm. **c** Division of the aneurysmal sac and prosthesis. **d** Transverse two-row suture of the duodenal wall defect following previous excision. **e** Reconstruction by prosthetic interposition. **f** Pedicled omentum between the proximal anastomosis and the duodenum

e) and the continuity restored by a Dacron graft (Figs. 10.3.1f, g, 10.3.2e). One should perform a continuous suture, taking at least 5–8 mm bites of the aortic margin. This technique securely anchors the suture in the aortic tissue and prevents leakage at the anastomosis. Graft and duodenum must be separated by interposition of soft tissue, for which pedicled greater omentum is best suited (Fig. 10.3.2f). If anastomosis at the proximal infrarenal aortic edge is not successful because of brittle, scarred tissue, the renal arteries are excised together with a Carrel patch and an end-to-side

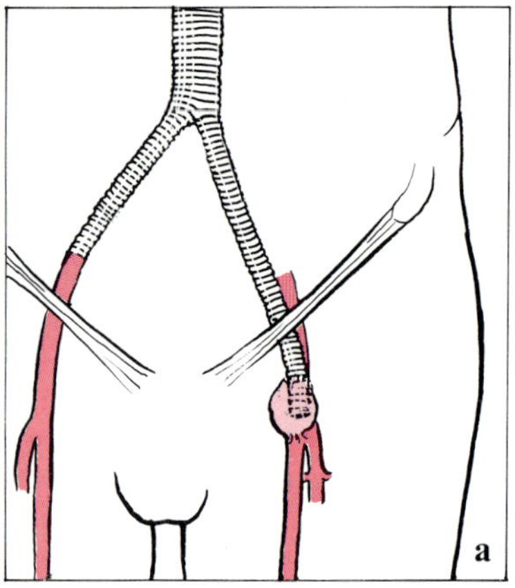

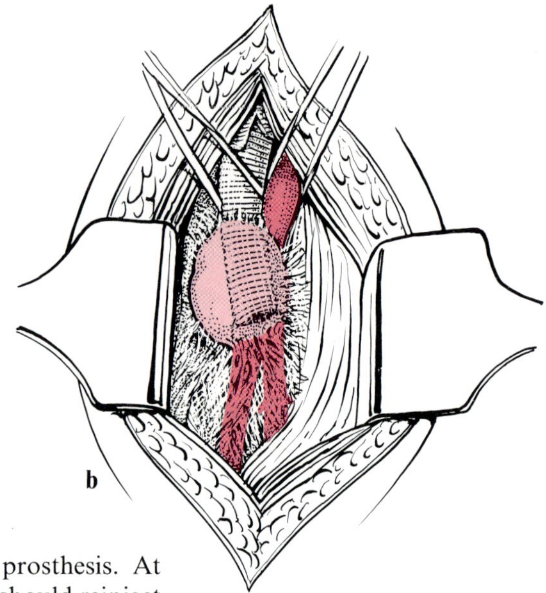

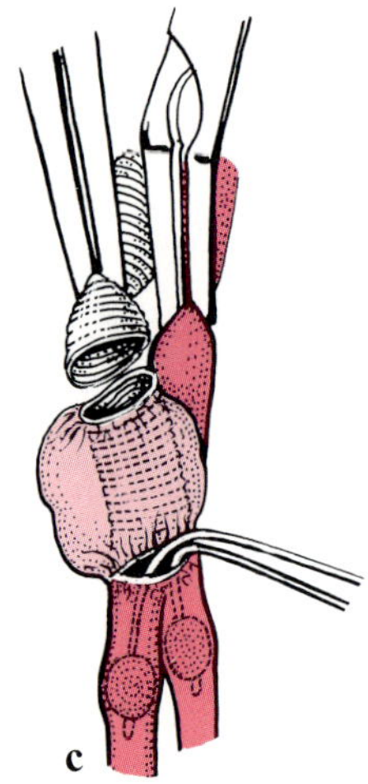

anastomosis reimplanted into the prosthesis. At the beginning of renal ischemia one should reinject cold heparinized normal saline solution (4° C, 1000 units heparin per 20 ml 0.9% NaCl) into both renal arteries.

In the case of an infected anastomotic aneurysm the proximal aortic stump is closed by a 2–0 continuous Dacron suture which is reinforced by an omentum flap (Fig. 10.3.2f). The entire synthetic prosthesis must be removed and the pelvic arteries closed with a 2–0 Dacron suture. An axillofemoral bypass, consisting of 8-mm woven Dacron prostheses constructed prior to laparotomy, reestablishes blood flow to both sides.

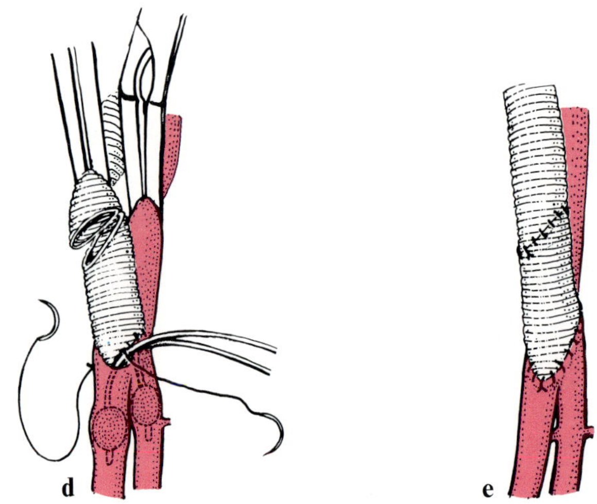

Fig. 10.3.3. a Anastomotic aneurysm of the left femoral artery. **b** Exposure of the aneurysmal sac and proximal passage of umbilical tape around the prosthesis and artery. **c** Bleeding control: proximally by vascular clamps, distally, in case of inadequate dissection, by two inserted Fogarty catheters. **d**, **e** Reconstruction of the graft

III. Femoral Artery

The very common infrainguinal anastomotic aneurysms (Fig. 10.3.3a) are exposed through a femoral incision which is extended cranially. It is advisable first to expose the prosthesis above the pulsating tumor. In an end-to-side anastomosis, the proximal common femoral artery and the external iliac artery must be exposed for complete hemorrhage control, if necessary, by division of the inguinal canal above the inguinal ligament (Fig. 10.3.3b). Then the superficial femoral artery and the profunda femoris artery are exposed distally. Where severe scar tissue formation is present, distal dissection may not be performed, and the technique of intraluminal balloon blockade should be applied instead (Fig. 10.3.3c, d). Following systemic anticoagulation with 10000 units heparin and proximal and distal control of bleeding, the aneurysmal sac is divided and the anastomosis exposed and dissected at the suture line. After trimming of the arterial wall and resection of the torn prosthetic margin, continuity is restored by a synthetic graft. First, the anastomosis between the host artery and the graft is completed, and then the end-to-end anastomosis between both prostheses (Fig. 10.3.3d, e). Just before completion of the distal anastomosis, the balloon catheters are removed and the last sutures tied. To protect neighboring structures, the aneurysmal sac is resected only as far as necessary for good visualization. Wound irrigation, the installation of a Redon drain for 24 h, and layer-by-layer wound closure, with complete subcutaneous coverage of the prosthesis, finish the operation.

G. Postoperative Complications

Postoperative complications following removal of anastomotic aneurysms do not differ from those occurring after reconstructive vascular surgery. However, considering that these procedures represent surgical reinterventions, the risk of local postoperative hemorrhage is increased (usually, oozing from scar tissue, which makes temporary careful drainage necessary). Perioperative prophylactic antibiotics reduce the higher risk associated with secondary wound healing [15].

REFERENCES

1. Baird RJ, Doran ML (1964) The false aneurysm. Can Med Assoc J 91:281
2. Becker HM, Stelter WJ, Kortmann H, Heberer G (1983) Anastomotic arterial aneuryms. Thorac Cardiovasc Surg 31:2
3. Clator H, Birch L, Cardwell ES, Zimmer SL (1956) Suture line rupture of nylon aortic bifurcation graft into small bowel. Arch Surg 73:947
4. Cooley DA, Wukasch DC (1979) Aorto-duodenal fistula. In: Cooley DA, Wukasch DC (eds) Techniques in vascular surgery. Saunders, Philadelphia London Toronto, pp 241–243
5. Courbier R, Larranaga J (1982) Natural history and management of anastomotic aneurysms. In: Bergan JJ, Yao JS (eds) Aneurysms: diagnosis and management. Grune & Stratton, New York, pp 567–580
6. Cutler ED, Dunphy JE (1941) The use of silk in infected wounds. N Engl J Med 244:101
7. Emmrich K, Herbst M, Trenckmann H, Schulz HG, Wohlgemuth B (1982) Severe late complications after operative correction of aortic coarctation by interposition of prosthesis. J Cardiovasc Surg 23:205
8. Giessler R, Gehl H, Heberer G (1968) Das Nahtaneurysma nach alloplastischem Gefäßersatz. Langenbecks Arch Chir 322:992
9. Hollier LH, Batson RC, Cohn J (1980) Femoral anastomotic aneurysms. Ann Surg 191:715
10. Knox NG (1976) Peripheral vascular anastomotic aneurysms: A fifteen-year experience. Ann Surg 183:120–123
11. Knudson JA, Downs AR (1978) Reoperation following failure of aorto-femoral reconstruction. Can J Surg 21:316
12. Nunn DB, Rao N, Renard A (1975) Anastomotic aneurysm. Am Surg 41:281
13. Richardson JV, McDowell HA (1975) Anastomotic aneurysms following arterial grafting: a 10-year experience. Ann Surg 184:179–182
14. Salzmann EW (1965) The limit of heparin therapy after arterial reconstruction. Surgery 57:131
15. Salzmann G (1982) Perioperative antibiotic prophylaxis in vascular surgery. Thorac Cardiovasc Surg 30:36
16. Smith RF, Szilagyi DE (1961) Healing complications with plastic arterial implants. Arch Surg 82:14
17. Starr DS, Weatherford SC, Lawrinc GM, Morris GC (1979) Suture material as a factor in occurence of anastomotic false aneurysms; analysis of 26 cases. Arch Surg 114:412
18. Szilagyi DE, Smith RF, Elliot JP, Hageman JH, Dall'Amo CA (1975) Anastomotic aneurysms after vascular reconstruction: problems of incidence, etiology and treatment. Surgery 78:800–816

10.4 Disorders of Male Sexual Function Following Operative Procedures in the Aortoiliac Region

O. THETTER, A. VON HOCHSTETTER, and R.J.A.M. VAN DONGEN

CONTENTS

A. Introduction

With the continuing development of modern vascular surgery, an increasing number of vascular reconstructions at the site of the abdominal aorta are being performed, even in younger patients. Postoperative sexual dysfunction not present preoperatively is noticed in a significant percentage of patients. The literature reports up to 88%. However, sexual dysfunction following operations in the region of the aorta and iliac arteries is almost always accepted as an unavoidable consequence of limb-saving operative technique and is justified as such to the patient. In the majority of cases, such postoperative impairment of male sexual function is either of *vascular* or of *neurogenic* origin.

B. Vascular Causes of Sexual Dysfunction

Since LERICHE described the syndrome of a thrombosis of the aortic bifurcation named after him, it has been known that a sufficient blood flow within the area supplied by the internal iliac artery is necessary to achieve erection of the penis. The decrease of erectility in patients with occlusive disease of the aorta and of the iliac arteries may already be present 13–18 months before the onset of symptoms of impaired circulation in the lower extremity.

Impairment of sexual function of vascular origin found after operative procedures in the region of the aortic bifurcation must therefore be interpreted by alterations in the hemodynamics of the pelvic blood flow caused intraoperatively or perioperatively. In most cases, this will lead to an insufficient blood supply within the internal iliac artery or its branches (internal pudendal artery, dorsal artery of the penis). A sufficient blood supply of this region, however, is of decisive significance for sustained erection of the penis.

C. Neurogenic Causes of Sexual Dysfunction

Regarding neurogenic sexual dysfunction the detailed report by WHITELAW and SMITHWICK 1951 [20] on the impairment of sexual function following therapeutic removal of various parts of the sympathetic trunk is of great interest. The authors report that high lumbar sympathectomy, with bilateral excision of sympathetic trunk ganglia Th12, L1, and L2, leads to impairment of erection. In contrast, following denervation of the sympathetic trunk ganglia L2 and L3 as well as the hypogastric plexus, one must expect impairment of ejaculation in the sense of "retrograde ejaculation," although erection may be intact. Loss of erection or of correct ejaculation may also be caused by transection of the sympathetic preaortic plexus, depending on the level of the lesion.

Since its appearance this paper has been frequently cited, mainly in the vascular surgical literature, and has thus been responsible for the widespread opinion that there is a lumbar sympathetic pathway for erection. The authors' explanations of the impairment of erection after sympathectomy, however, do not correspond with current physiologic knowledge indicating that erection is regulated by the sacral parasympathetic nervous system [3]. It is generally agreed that the essential source of penile erection is located in the lower part of the sacral spinal cord and only affects the organ and its vessels via the "nervi erigentes" (S2, S3, S4) [3]. However, these neural structures, located within the true pelvis, are usually not injured by the operative procedures mentioned. Subsequent publications also showed that after similar operative procedures it was mainly ejaculation, not erection, that suffered postoperative impairment [1, 6, 8, 13, 16].

In 1965 Harris and Jepson [4] reported on a group of patients with Leriche syndrome, 33% of whom, though sexually potent preoperatively, experienced immediate postoperative "impotence." This fact seemed astonishing since, in all cases of vascular reconstruction, blood flow within the pelvic area had significantly increased. These authors were the first to suggest that operations at the bifurcation may injure the sympathetic nervous network located there.

According to Weinstein and Machleder [19] the type and frequency of postoperative neurogenic sexual dysfunction are directly related to the extent of dissection in the aortoiliac area. They conclude that lesions of the sympathetic hypogastric plexus may be responsible for the impairment. This suggestion is supported by the observation that postoperative impairment of ejaculatory capability are reduced to a minimum when special care is taken of the hypogastric plexus at the site of the terminal aorta during the operative procedure. Vroonhoven [17] found in 1977 that out of 38 patients up to 46% showed postoperative impairment of ejaculation when no special care was taken of the integrity of the hypogastric plexus in this region. This complication rate was significantly reduced in a second group of 37 patients in whom a careful operative technique was employed that aimed at avoiding injury of the plexus. In cases of resection of aneurysms, the complication rate decreased from 48% to 20%, and in patients with claudication, from 18% to 11%.

In 1978, Pircher et al. [11] reported on the largest series so far. Of 318 patients, 148 were preoperatively sexually potent. There were two comparable groups with implantation of an aortobifemoral prosthesis. In the group without complete dissection of the aorta to preserve the sympathetic plexus, postoperative sexual impairment was reduced from 90% to 25%.

In the clinical reports on postoperative sexual disorders the use of the global terms "sexual potency" and "sexual function" without further explanation results in much confusion. Specific reference is rarely made to orgasm, erection, or ejaculation.

D. Physiology of Male Sexual Function

Genital functions in humans include various types of reflexes with complex chronological sequences involving not only sympathetic and parasympathetic, but also somatic reflexes. The knowledge and ideas about male genital reflexes are still very incomplete and have been gained from investigations of healthy people as well as patients whose spinal cord had been injured at the thoracolumbosacral centers of these reflexes. Additional knowledge has been obtained from experiments in several animals [14, 18].

The sequence of male sexual reaction consists of three main phases:

1. Erection
2. Emission
3. Ejaculation

Erection. The erection of the penis is mainly caused by a dilatation of the arteries within the corpora cavernosa penis and the corpus spongiosum penis via cholinergic parasympathetic neurons of the pelvic nerves. The increasing filling inhibits more and more the venous outflow of the corpus cavernosum at the site where the veins penetrate the tunica albuginea and so supports the swelling of the penis.

The mechanism of erection consists of the following six steps [18]:

1. Relaxation of Ebner's cushion. This causes a lowering of resistance in the arteries of the corpus cavernosum.

2. Dilatation of arterial vessels. This results in increased pressure and flow within the corpora cavernosa.
3. Occlusion of the arteriovenous shunts, inhibiting rapid outflow from the arterial system.
4. Relaxation of the smooth muscle of the corpora cavernosa.
5. Occlusion of the venous valves, which allows filling of the corpus cavernosum.
6. Stretching of the vessels, facilitating the increase of pressure and flow.

Visual, olfactory, auditory, and somatoesthetic influences excite the spinal center of erection via the cerebral cortex, the limbic system, and the hypothalamus. The center is located in the sacral spinal cord at the level S2–S4. Sensory peripheral afference is elicited by touching the skin of the genitals as well as the closely packed mechanoreceptors of the glans penis. The afferents run in the pudendal nerve into the parasympathetic spinal center of erection within the segments S2, S3, S4 of the sacral spinal cord. Erection itself is caused exclusively by the parasympathetic nervi erigentes, originating from the pelvic nerves. HABIB [3] succeeded in causing an erection in paraplegic patients by electric stimulation of the roots S2, S3, or S4.

According to the established view of physiology, permanent neurogenic impairment of erection following operations is mainly expected after injury to the parasympathetic nervi erigentes originating at the sacral spinal cord. It has not yet been established whether there is a lumbar sympathetic pathway within the hypogastric plexus that brings about true erection. Operations at the aortoiliac arteries do not touch these parasympathetic nervi erigentes. They run deep in the true pelvis in front of the sacrum and lateral to the rectal ampulla. Therefore, there must be other reasons for the occurrence of postoperative impairment of erection. Most probably, the underlying causes are of hemodynamic origin, resulting in a reduced blood supply to the corpus cavernosum.

Emission and Ejaculation. The term "ejaculation," previously used in a broader sense, should nowadays be divided into visceromotoric emission and somatomotoric ejaculation itself. Seminal emission means the ejection of seminal fluid out of the epididymis, the vas deferens, seminal vesicles, and prostate into the posterior urethra. This occurs by retraction of the smooth muscle of these structures. Simultaneously, the neck of the bladder is closed by the internal vesicle sphincter, inhibiting "retrograde ejaculation" into the bladder. The innervation comes from sympathetic neurons of the thoracolumbar junction. This mechanism is regulated by fibers of the sympathetic center of emission (Th12 to L2) running from the sympathetic trunk to the sexual organs in the pelvis via the hypogastric plexus and the pelvic plexus.

J.L. BUDGE [1] was able to show as early as 1858 that electrical stimulation of the hypogastric plexus causes contraction not only of the inner sphincter of the bladder, but also of the seminal vesicles and the vas deferens. In these experiments, BUDGE could not demonstrate an erection. Postoperatively absent ejaculation or emission, with consequent impotentia generandi, may therefore be explained by the lack of sympathetic innervation at the time of orgasm [19].

The "ejaculatio seminis" itself, however, is initiated by parasympathetic afferents of the internal urethra and the prostate (via pelvic nerves to the sacral spinal cord) as well as by sympathetic afferents of the epididymis and seminal vesicles (via the hypogastric and pelvic plexuses to the thoracolumbar junction of the spinal cord). The ejaculation of sperm from the anterior urethra is finally caused by clonic contractions of the bulbocavernosus muscles, the ischiocavernosus muscles, and the external sphincter urethrae. These muscles are innervated by the genital somatomotoric portion of the pudendal nerve, originating from the parasympathetic center of ejaculation within the sacral spinal cord (S2–S4).

E. Neuro-Anatomy of Male Sexual Function

Anatomy of the Hypogastric Plexus (Fig. 10.4.1). Because ejaculation, and consequently male fertility, is clearly dependent on the lumbar sympathetic trunk and the hypogastric and pelvic plexus, preservation of these structures during operations in the aortoiliac region is necessary [16], but so far, the literature has not provided sufficiently reliable guidelines for avoiding iatrogenic damage to sexual function [7].

The more or less X-shaped sympathetic hypogastric plexus is formed at the level of the aortic bifurcation mainly from two trunks originating from large visceral branches of the cranial lumbar

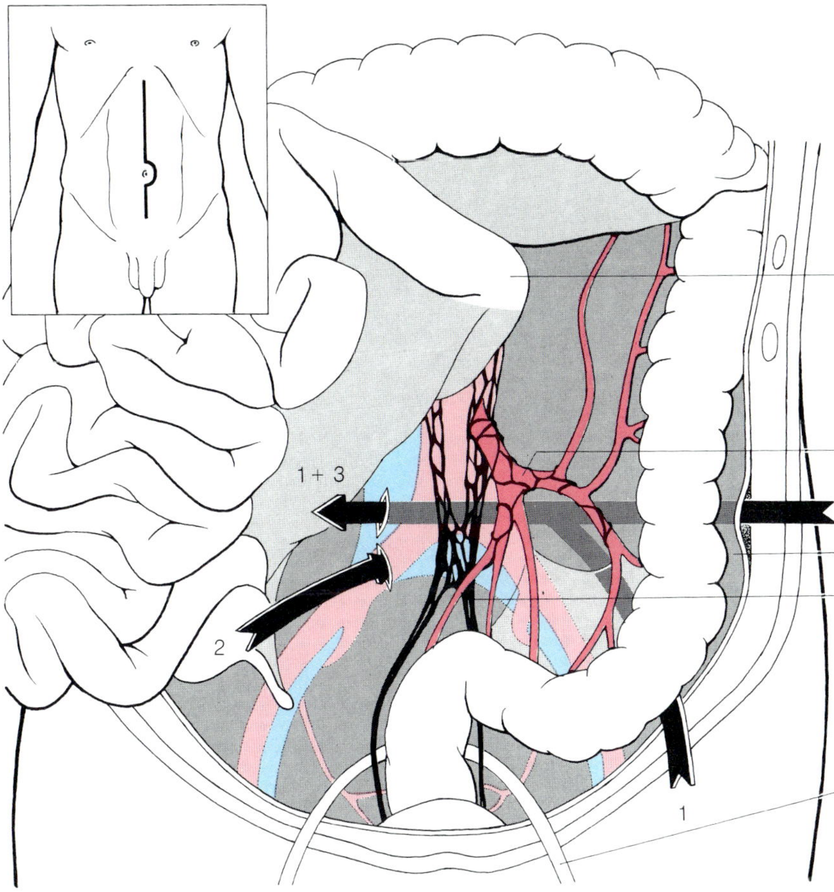

Fig. 10.4.1. Schematic drawing of the infracolic region with the bifurcation of the aorta: *Arrow 1.* transperitoneal-retromesenteric approach: entry into the extraperitoneal space from the intersigmoid recessus, turning to the right between the inferior mesenteric artery and the hypogastric plexus on the one hand and the aorta and inferior vena cava on the other hand, in order to reach the peritoneal cavity through the parietal peritoneum in front of the inferior vena cava. The sigmoid colon is pulled ventrally and cranially to the right; the inferior mesenteric artery and also the hypogastric plexus are lifted off the bifurcation. *Arrow 2.* Direct transperitoneal approach: perforation of the peritoneum next to the right border of the hypogastric plexus, proceeding to the left in order to pass beneath the plexus and the inferior mesenteric artery. *Arrow 3.* retroperitoneal-retromesenteric approach to the hypogastric plexus. The rubber band lies behind the rectum and both pelvic plexuses, as well as in front of the nervi erigentes and the inferior rectal artery

sympathetic trunk (L1, L2). They emerge on both sides of the aorta and becomes united, forming an acute angle in front of the aorta. Additionally, the hypogastric plexus is joined by small strands of the solar and aortorenal plexuses descending in front of the aorta and by the distal lumbar sympathetic trunk. The approximately 1 cm broad, band-shaped nervus plexus (nervus presacralis) crosses the bifurcation in the middle, or often somewhat to the left across the left common iliac artery, and runs in front of the common iliac vein and of the promontorium down into the small pelvis. Here, the plexus separates into two branches (right and left hypogastric plexus) penetrating into the pararectal fatty tissue and then passing anteriorly downward to the pelvic floor, as if riding on the rectum. Here, they form the lumbar sympathetic root of the ganglionic pelvic plexus on both sides. The parasympathetic roots, however, originating in the pelvis from the second to fourth sacral root of the ischiatic plexus, form the nervi erigentes.

Distal to the origin of the inferior mesenteric artery, both lumbar major roots of the hypogastric plexus join together on the anterior wall of the aorta to form an X-shaped plexus. At this site, the plexus, with both its major roots and its two branches, forms a very palpable membrane of sub-

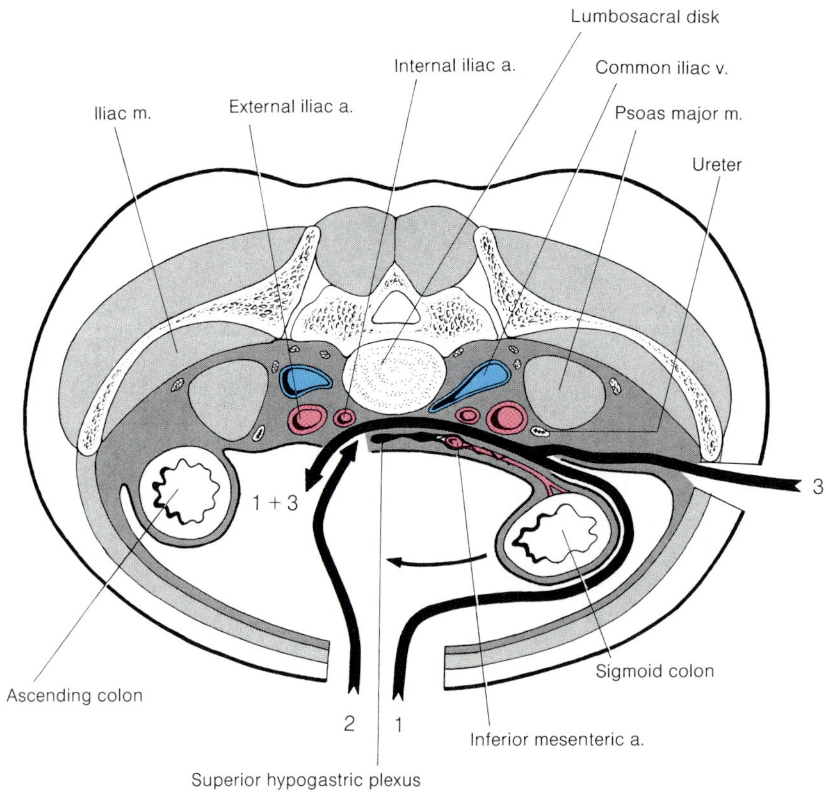

Fig. 10.4.2. Schematic cross section of the abdomen at the level of the sacral junction: the iliac vessels (common iliac vein, external iliac artery, internal iliac artery) are located on both sides in the angle between the psoas major muscle and the lumbosacral disc; behind them are the nerve trunks of the lumbosacral plexus, and anteriorily, lying on the psoas major muscle, the ureter. The hypogastric plexus, situated in front of the vertebral column between the iliac vessels, is attached to the inferior mesenteric artery by vegetative nerve fibers and connective tissue

peritoneal connective tissue attached firmly to the peritoneum. This membrane is easily lifted off its base (aorta, left common iliac vessels, and promontorium). However, fine rami splanchnici lumbalis from the caudal portion of the lumbar sympathetic trunk, of thus far unknown function, may be torn. The plexus lies to the right of the superior rectal artery which descends vertically into the pelvis next to it and is also attached to it by connective tissue. Together with the neural band of the hypogastric plexus, the superior rectal artery, the sigmoid artery, and the whole branched area of the inferior mesenteric artery can be lifted off the base in the layer of secondary adhesions of the mesenterium to the posterior abdominal wall.

F. Diagnosis

During preexamination and planning for reconstructive vascular surgery in the pelvic region, it is important to take an exact history of sexual function. This should include the frequency of sexual intercourse and the ability to achieve an erection and sustain it. Furthermore, the degree of erection and the stability of the erect penis should also be documented as well as any impairment or lack of ejaculation. If impairment of potency is already present before the planned operation, an attempt must be made to determine the psychological, organic, or possibly iatrogenic causes.

Psychological impotence can be distinguished relatively easily by the documentation of spontaneous nocturnal erections using the so-called "stamp ring test." Perforated strips of stamps placed around the penis are torn by unconscious nocturnal erections during the REM phase of sleep, thus providing erectility of the penis. These phases of erection may also be documented by measurements of nocturnal penile tumescence (NPT). If nocturnal erections are verified by these methods, then the impairment of erection reported by the patient is of psychological, not of organic origin [18].

For objective evaluation of erection disorders of vascular origin, several methods of investigations are available by which it is possible to determine blood flow to the corpus cavernosum [2, 5, 12].

1. Impedance plethysmography
2. Control of pulse volume (mean penile arterial pressure)
3. Transcutaneous Doppler ultrasound (systolic penile blood pressure)
4. Aortography
5. Superselective angiography of internal iliac artery and internal pudendal artery
6. Phalloarteriography

Among the noninvasive methods, transcutaneous Doppler ultrasound (estimation of the arterial penile blood pressure) is probably the simplest and most reliable [12]. By means of a Doppler probe and a small blood pressure cuff, this technique allows measurement of pressure in both dorsal penile arteries. The relation of the penile arterial pressure to the blood pressure in the brachial artery is estimated by the penis – brachial index (PBI = BP penis/BP brachial). A fall of PBI below 0.6 indicates impotentia coeundi of vascular origin.

Postoperative measurement is of special importance, as it shows the effect of our reconstructive procedures on the blood supply of the internal iliac region.

The most important preoperative measure is angiographic demonstration of pelvic circulation. Conventional aortography is usually sufficient for high contrast pictures of the iliac vessels. Sometimes, however, it is necessary to inject selectively into the internal iliac artery to better demonstrate the internal pudendal artery. A new method for demonstration of the arteries supplying the corpora cavernosa of the penis is phalloarteriography as described by Michal [10]. This is used to clarify the morphological status of the penile vessels and is therefore an important prerequisite for assessment of a possible microsurgical revascularization of the corpus cavernosum [9].

It should be noted that under certain circumstances a single open internal iliac artery is sufficient for a normal erection. On the other hand, this single artery may show retrograde flow if the common iliac artery of the same side is occluded. Then a steal mechanism exists, in other words an external iliac steal syndrome. This may cause a preexisting erection to fail during intercourse under the increased muscular action of the lower extremity. Such an impotentia coeundi can usually be eliminated once the blood supply to the internal iliac artery has been restored surgically, preserving, of course, the autonomous innervation of the genitalia.

The objective assessment of exclusively neurogenic impairment of sexual function is the task of the neurologist or the urologist. If there is a defect, then, in addition to a neurologic examination there should be a complete urodynamic examination to localize the lesion and determine its degree of severity. The following neurogenic signs should be checked: the tendon-surface reflex, Babinski's sign, cremasteric reflex, perineal reflex, the sensitivity of the outer genitalia, as well as the motility of the anus. A positive bulbocavernous reflex confirms the integrity of the reflex arch between the glans penis, the sensory pudendal nerve, the sacral segments S2 and S4 of the spinal cord, and the motoric pudendal nerve. A thorough investigation of prostatic fluid and urine following masturbation will indicate the degree of impaired emission. In cases of retrograde ejaculation, spermatozoa and fructose will be found in the urine.

G. Operative Technique for Avoiding Postoperative Sexual Disorders

Operative technique used for procedures in the aortoiliac area should be based on the following knowledge:

1. For *erection*, sufficient pressure and flow must be assured within the area supplied by the internal iliac artery. The decisive neural component of erection, the sacral parasympatheticus, is not in the operative field.
2. For *ejaculation*, the sympathetic innervation from the uppermost roots of the hypogastric plexus is essential and must therefore be preserved.

Avoidance of Sexual Disorders of Vascular Origin

For a stable erection, the blood flow supplying the area of the internal iliac artery should be constant, and reconstructive surgical procedures in the aortoiliac region must be planned with this in

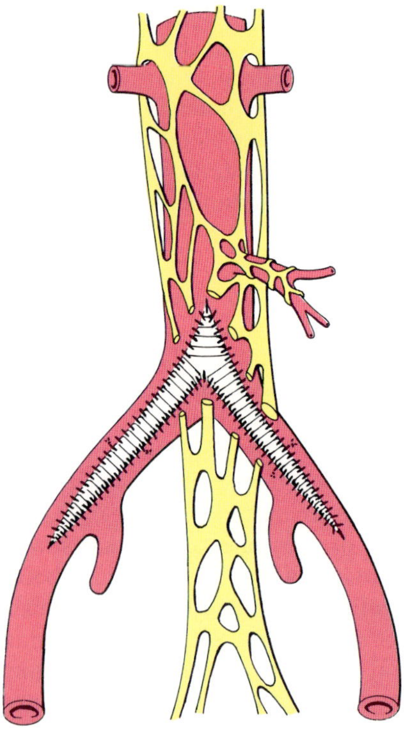

Fig. 10.4.3. Y-patch angioplasty at the bifurcation, endangering the hypogastric plexus

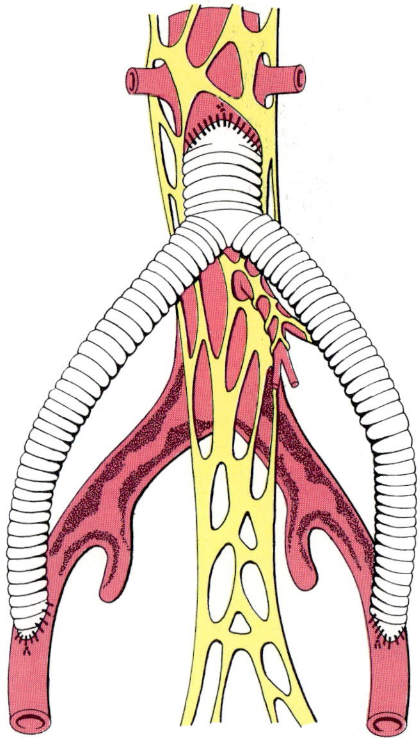

Fig. 10.4.4. Aortobifemoral Dacron bypass (end-to-side). Relation to the hypogastric plexus

mind. In particular, one must insure that bypass procedures are chosen and performed in a way that provides sufficient pressure and flow in the internal iliac artery.

Figures 10.4.3 and 10.4.4 show the dilemma which may be encountered using the *conventional* technique. Both reconstructive procedures for overcoming occlusive disease of the aortoiliac region – open endarterectomy (Fig. 10.4.3) and bypass (Fig. 10.4.4) – most likely cause postoperative sexual dysfunction. Endarterectomy and patch angioplasty facilitate blood flow within the iliac vessels and consequently erectility, but in most cases the hypogastric plexus will be divided by these procedures, resulting in a loss of ejaculation [15].

By contrast, the implantation of prosthesis may avoid injury to the vegetative fibers, but the stenosed internal iliac artery will be completely thrombosed because of stagnation of the blood flow in the pelvic vascular bed after bypassing the bloodstream. This will result in an impairment of erectility clearly vascular in origin.

The shape of the anastomosis, end-to-side or end-to-end, is a very important factor in the blood supply to the pelvis and therefore also in the erectility of the penis. In general it can be said that the end-to-side anastomosis is preferable from this point of view.

Following a proximal end-to-end anastomosis of an aortofemoral Y-bypass, anterograde blood flow into the pelvis will no longer exist after transection of the distal aorta. The result will be complete thrombotic occlusion of the sclerosed pelvic vessels (Fig. 10.4.5). The proximal end-to-side anastomosis of an aortoiliac or an aortofemoral bypass may be possibly sustain blood supply to the internal iliac artery, especially if, in addition, a thromboendarterectomy of the common iliac artery as far as the origin of the internal iliac is performed. The same holds for the distal end-to-side anastomosis, which also improves the blood supply to the pelvis, provided retrograde perfusion into the internal iliac artery is possible, or made possible by thromboendarterectomy of the external and internal arteries.

The operative technique must insure the utmost care. Brisk dissection of the vessels and extensive manipulation of an abdominal aortic aneurysm increase the risk of embolization not only into the periphery, but also into the area supplied by the

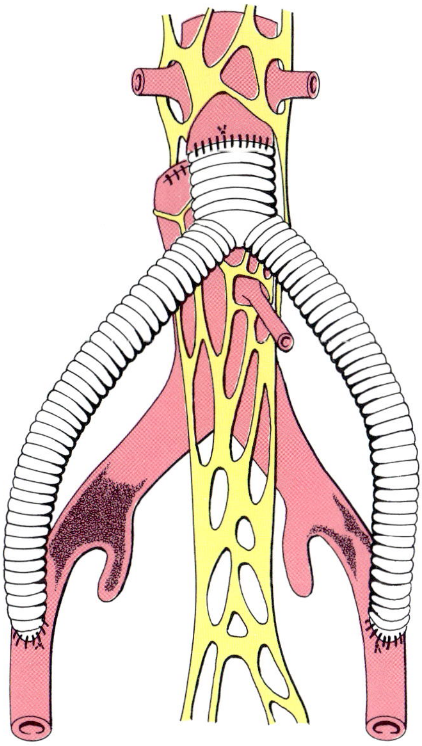

Fig. 10.4.5. Aortobifemoral bypass with proximal end-to-end anastomosis

internal iliac artery. That is why the vessel should be occluded distally by a nontraumatizing clamp as early as possible.

Furthermore, intraoperative formation of thrombi due to stagnation of blood flow within the clamped internal iliac artery must be prevented by the administration of heparin. Finally, before final suturing of the anastomosis or vessel, it is advisable to "flush" all vascular segments with saline solution to remove all clots and atheromatous fragments [2].

H. Retromesenteric Approach to the Aortic Bifurcation Preserving the Hypogastric Plexus

Avoiding Neurologically Caused Sexual Disorders

I. Approach from the Left (Transperitoneal)

When pulling the sigmoid colon with its mesentery ventrally and cranially, there is traction on the junction of the mesenteric and the parietal peritoneum. Here, at the level of the recessus intersigmoideous, the peritoneum is incised medially as far as the left ureter. Then the arteries of the sigmoid colon and rectum, together with the hypogastric plexus, are lifted up in an arch by gradual traction on the sigmoid colon. This arch, consisting of vessels and nerves, extends between the origin of the inferior mesenteric artery and the posterior wall of the rectum and can now be tunneled in a transverse direction from left to right, exposing the area of the bifurcation without injury of the plexus (Fig. 10.4.1 and 10.4.2).

II. Approach from the Right (Transperitoneal)

For exposure of the hypogastric plexus from the right, one only divides the peritoneum medially from the right ureter across the right common and external iliac arteries and feels one's way carefully beneath the peritoneum along the common iliac artery medially and cranially until the right border of the plexus or its right lumbar branch is clearly felt. From there, the plexus, together with the superior rectal artery, may be lifted off the base. Using this technique, free access to the aortic bifurcation is provided from the right side without injury to sympathetic tissue.

III. Retroperitoneal–Retromesenteric Approach

The retroperitoneal approach to the terminal aorta also makes it possible to spare the superior hypogastric plexus by lifting it off the aortic bifurcation and carefully pushing away the peritoneal sac. However, this procedure is more difficult to perform and allows exposure of only a short segment of the aortoiliac junction since the segment is restricted cranially by the lumbar root of the plexus which extends toward the front.

All these procedures are carried out, of course, without any regard for the fine fibers leading caudally to the neural band of the pelvic plexus, which are obviously of no importance for the problems under consideration here.

In the approach to the terminal aorta special attention must be paid to both major lumbar roots of the superior hypogastric plexus, which are clearly visible lateral to the aorta at the level of the inferior mesenteric artery. Cranial to the origin of the inferior mesenteric artery the intermesenter-

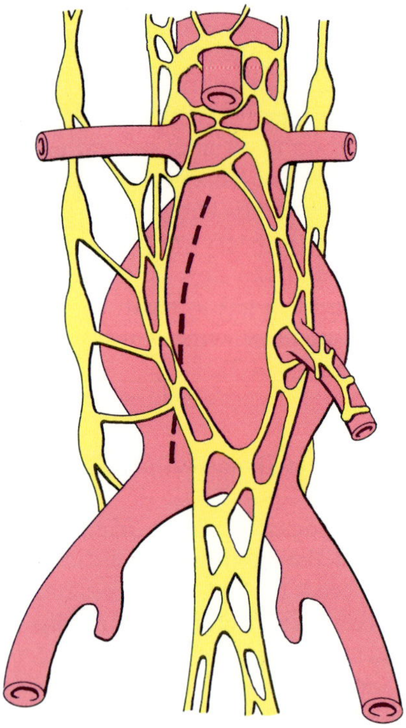

Fig. 10.4.6

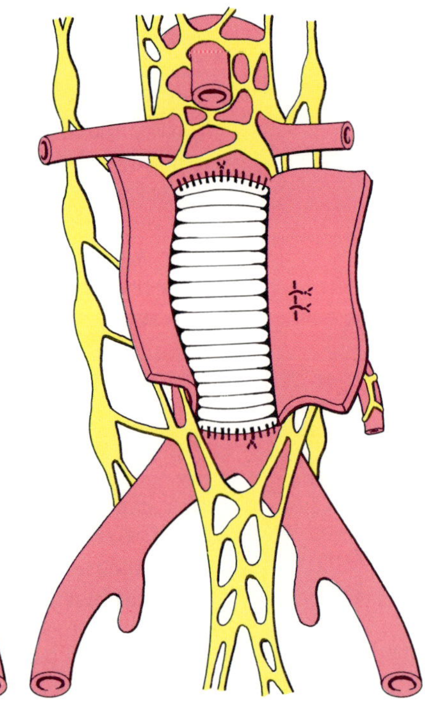

Fig. 10.4.7

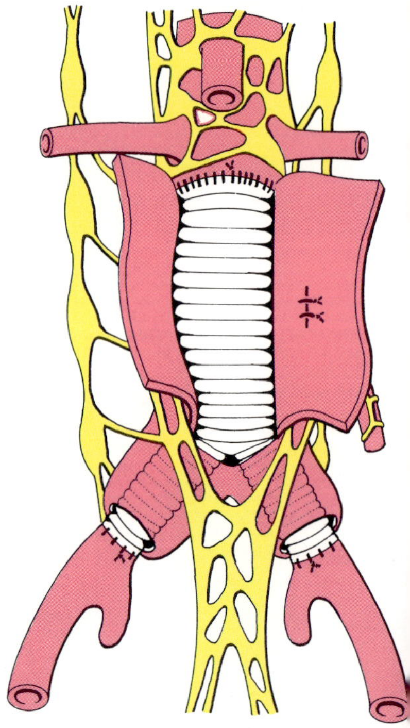

Fig. 10.4.8

Fig. 10.4.6. Aortic aneurysm. Relation to the superior hypogastric plexus. Sparing the plexus by a right paramedian incision

Fig. 10.4.7. Interposition of a prosthesis following resection of the aneurysm saving the hypogastric plexus. The origin of the inferior mesenteric artery is sutured from inside

Fig. 10.4.8. Interposition of a Y-prosthesis following resection of the aneurysm. Both branches of the prosthesis are pulled through the intact iliac arteries and anastomosed end-to-end distally

ic segment of the aorta is more easily accessed with regard to the aortic plexus, as the descending longitudinal fibers of the solar plexus can easily be pushed aside.

When implanting a bifurcation prosthesis or an aortoiliac or aortofemoral bypass, one should always place the proximal anastomosis as far cranially as possible, above the origin of the inferior mesenteric artery. Here, in front of the aorta and between the important roots of the hypogastric plexus, there are only a few insignificant fibers of that plexus. Nevertheless, cranial to the inferior mesenteric artery, one should follow the principle that unnecessary dissection of tissue covering the aorta should be avoided.

Using the above-described approaches to the iliac vessels, it is also possible to anastomose the distal branches of the bypass prosthesis without injury to autonomous tissue.

By the retromesenteric approach, all forms of endarterectomy, with or without patch graft angioplasty, are quite feasible in the region of the pelvic vessels as well as that of the bifurcation and to just below the origin of the inferior mesenteric artery.

Obviously, our effort to save the sympathetic plexus and to maintain the flow within the iliac arteries can only be effective during an elective (planned) surgical intervention. In case of a ruptured aortic aneurysm, quick cross-clamping of the aorta will be necessary for obvious reasons, notwithstanding the considerations discussed above. Consequently, impairment of sexual potency following resection of aneurysms is encountered in a very high percentage of cases.

In cases of elective rather than emergency operations on *aortic aneurysms*, such sequelae can be avoided by various measures. In order to avoid vessel embolization from an aneurysmal sac, it is advisable to cross-clamp both common iliac arteries before manipulating the aneurysm and placing the proximal clamp. Then after incision of the peritoneum, the preaortic plexus and its distal continuation, together with the inferior mesenteric artery and its branches, are drawn up in an arch, providing good exposure of the aortic bifurcation. Dorsal to the plexus, one can now expose the sac of the aneurysm without danger, dissecting upward to just below the origin of the inferior mesenteric artery, where both lumbar roots of the hypogastric plexus pass in front of the aorta. Only cranial to these roots further exposure of the aneurysm in the midline is possible. After carefully pushing the preaortic fibers of the plexus aside, the incision of the aorta is carried out, but only on the *right anterior side* (Fig. 10.4.6), as it is essential that the extraordinarily dense neural network at the origin of the inferior mesenteric artery be spared. Following incision of the aneurysm, the ostium of the inferior mesenteric artery is sutured from inside.

In no case, however, should one attempt to resect the aneurysmal sac. This remains in situ and is sewn together over the implanted prosthesis (Fig. 10.4.7). If the aneurysm includes the iliac arteries, the branches of the prosthesis can be pulled through the uncut iliacal aneurysmal sacs and anastomosed distal to the terminations of the sacs (Fig. 10.4.8).

I. Summary

The recognition of disorders of male potentia coeundi and generandi is gaining increasing significance. Among the long list of organic causes of sexual impairment, several are of special interest for vascular surgery. Primary impairment of sexual potency is found mostly in generalized arteriosclerosis and is operatively correctable only to a very limited degree. In contrast, isolated occlusive processes in the region of the iliac vessels, and especially in the area supplied by the internal iliac artery, can now be corrected surgically. Besides measures for the restoration of sufficient flow within the internal iliac artery, microsurgical techniques for revascularization of the corpus cavernosum have also been reported in the last few years [19, 20].

Impairment of sexual potency occurring after operations in the aortoiliac region has been known for a long time, but without consequences. This fact may be due to the special problem of taking the patient's intimate history. Using modern noninvasive methods of measurement, however, it is possible to document erectility clearly. This in turn makes it possible to determine whether the disorder is psychogenic and to evaluate the surgical result through pre- and postoperative measurement of blood flow.

When performing vascular surgery in the pelvic region, besides the primary goal of improving blood flow to the extremities, one should also aim at preserving normal hemodynamics in the vascular region supplied by the internal iliac artery. It is possible to correct or to avoid impairment of sexual function of hemodynamic origin in a high percentage of cases by an exact assessment of the angiographic findings and by appropriate planning of operative strategy.

In contrast to hemodynamic-vascular causes, postoperative sexual dysfunction resulting from neurologic damage is irreversible. It is particularly important to bear this in mind during retroperitoneal lymphadenectomy, anterior spondylodesis, and interventions in the aortoiliac region, where injury to the sympathetic tissue is to be expected. Using the retromesenteric approach to the aortic bifurcation, the preaortic sympathetic nervous tissue can be carefully lifted and pushed aside. This enables us to minimize the occurrence of ejaculative disorders.

REFERENCES

1. Budge JL (1858) Über das Centrum genitospinale des Nervus sympathicus. Virchows Arch 15:115–126
2. DePalma RG (1980) Impotence as a complication of aortic reconstruction. In: Bernhard VM, Towne JB (eds) Complications in vascular surgery. Grune & Stratton, New York
3. Habib HN (1967) Experience and recent contributions in sacral nerve stimulation for voiding in both human and animal. Br J Urol 39:73–82
4. Harris JD, Jepson RP (1965) Aorto-iliac stenosis: a comparison of two procedures. Aust NZ J Surg 34:211–214
5. Kempczinski RF (1979) Role of vascular diagnostic labor in the evaluation of male impotence. Am J Surg 138:278–282
6. Leiter E, Brendler H (1967) Loss of ejaculation following bilateral retroperitoneal lymphadenectomy. J Urol 98:373–378
7. Maresca C, Ghafar W (1980) The presacral nerve (plexus hypogastricus superior). Anat Clin 2:5–12
8. May AG, DeWeese JA, Rob CG (1969) Changes in sexual function following operation on the abdominal aorta. Surg 65:41–47
9. Michal V, Kramar R, Pospichal J, Hejhal L (1977) Arterial epigastrico-cavernous anastomosis for the treatment of sexual impotence. World J Surg 1:515–520

10. Michal V, Pospichal J (1978) Phalloarteriography in the diagnosis of erectile impotence. World J Surg 2:239–248
11. Pircher W, Stegemann B, Rühland D, Schomacher PH (1978) Potenz nach aorto-femoralem Bypass. Sexualmedizin 7:309–310
12. Queral LA, Flinn WR, Bergan JJ, Yao JST (1979) Sexual function and aortic surgery. In: Bergan JJ, Yao JST (eds) Surgery of the aorta and its body branches. Grune & Stratton, New York
13. Sabri S, Cotton LT (1971) Sexual function following aortoiliac reconstruction. Lancet 2:1218–1219
14. Scharfetter F (1982) Neurology of male fertility disorders. In: Bandhauer K, Frick J (eds) Disturbances in male fertility. Springer, Berlin Heidelberg New York (Handbuch der Urologie. Encyclopedia of urology, vol XVI)
15. Spiro M, Cotton LT (1970) Aorto-iliac thromboendarteriectomy. Br J Surg 57:161–168
16. Thetter O, v Hochstetter A, van Dongen RJAM (1982) Neurogene Störungen der männlichen Sexualfunktion nach Eingriffen im aorto-iliacalen Bereich und deren Vermeidung durch den retromesenterialen Zugang. Angio 4/4:171–177
17. van Vroonhoven ThJMV (1977) Sexual dysfunction after aortoiliac surgery. Vasa 6:226–229
18. Wagner G, Green R (1981) Impotence. Physiological, psychological, surgical diagnosis and treatment. Plenum Press, New York
19. Weinstein MH, Machleder HI (1975) Sexual function after aorto-iliac surgery. Ann Surg 181:878–790
20. Whitelaw GP, Smithwick RH (1951) Some secondary effects of sympathectomy. N Engl J Med 245:121–130

11 Anesthesia in Vascular Surgery

H. KUPPE and E. MARTIN

CONTENTS

A. Introduction

Arteriosclerosis of the coronary, cerebral, or peripheral vessels is one of the most frequent causes of increased perioperative morbidity and mortality in Western Europe and North America. The exact cause of arterial occlusive disease still remains unclear. However, there is no doubt that certain risk factors are of decisive significance for the development and progression of the underlying disease (see Table 11.1).

Table 11.1. Classical risk factors

Age	Diabetes mellitus
Sex	Obesity
Hypertension	Hyperuricemia
Hyperlipoproteinemia	Inactivity and
Excessive cigarette smoking	genetic factors

In patients undergoing vascular procedures, often the biologic age does not correspond with the actual age. The multiple concomitant diseases of these patients with impaired organ function are considered to be the result of the effective risk factors.

Exact preoperative knowledge of circulatory conditions during the preoperative anesthesiologic evaluation and therapy of correctable abnormalities significantly determine the operative success.

B. Preoperative Evaluation and Assessment of Risk

I. Coronary Artery Disease

Coronary artery disease represents a clinical syndrome consisting of angina, coronary insufficiency, and myocardial infarction. Among the significant sequelae and complications are congestive heart failure, dysfunction of the papillary muscle, ventricular aneurysm, arrhythmia, and sudden cardiac death.

The perioperative mortality in patients with coronary artery disease is increased two- to threefold. Patients with coronary artery disease are especially sensitive to perioperative myocardial ischemia. Events during the anesthesia may induce myocardial ischemia by an imbalance between oxygen supply and oxygen consumption of the myocardium.

For patients undergoing vascular surgery the evaluation of cardiovascular disorders is crucial as it may allow conclusions to be drawn regarding impairment of myocardial function and thereby provide a basis on which to decide whether cardiac functional capacity can be improved by preoperative drug therapy. The indication for invasive monitoring is a result of the preoperative collection of findings and the diagnosis of preexisting diseases. Furthermore, asymptomatic patients may already show a significantly reduced cardiac reserve.

Coronary artery disease must be assumed, even when no clinical symptoms are present and only predisposing factors are found. Smokers have a twofold risk of cardiac complications. The combination of smoking and hypertension results in a fourfold increased risk, and combination of smoking, hypertension, and hyperlipoproteinemia produces an eightfold increase [8]. The diagnosis of coronary artery disease is based on the history of angina or electrocardiographic verification of the myocardial ischemia. Angina is often described as a painful retrosternal sensation or pressure. Attention should be paid to the frequency and the duration of the attacks. Patients with unstable angina and impaired exercise tolerance may have the same operative risk as patients with acute infarction. Possible concomitant coronary artery disease may be missed owing to the clinically dominating symptoms of peripheral vascular disease, including intermittent claudication and the pain related to ischemia.

The risk of cardiac infarction is in close correlation with the pathologic changes of the ECG, according to the Framingham study. The signs of left ventricular hypertrophy are present prior to cardiovascular death in 45% of cases and mean more than a tenfold risk of sudden cardiac death. Premature ventricular contractions are often the cause of a sudden cardiac death when left ventricular dysfunction is present. It should be treated before surgical intervention whenever possible.

The final diagnosis of latent coronary insufficiency is made by the treadmill ECG. Despite severe changes of the coronary arteries, the resting ECG is normal in 50% of cases. The ischemic changes are mostly found in leads V4–V6. Here, a depression of the ST segment by 0.1 mV is considered as a direct indication of myocardial ischemia. But even here the proportion of false-negative findings is still 20–30% [28]. A persistent angina following myocardial infarction increases the postoperative morbidity and mortality two- to fourfold. Changes of the left ventricular wall, e.g., agenesia and dyskinesia, are often found in patients with coronary artery disease by means of ventriculography or noninvasive techniques such as ultrasound.

Patients with coronary artery disease show another peculiarity. They have a diminished regulation of blood volume and often show a deficit of plasma volume, despite normal red cell volume. Consequently, these patients present with a relatively high hemoglobin level while the circulating plasma volume is reduced. The high concentration of hemoglobin is merely a result of a so-called "hypovolemic" hemoconcentration. Therefore, during perioperative fluid therapy a rapid drop in hemoglobin and hematocrit levels is frequently observed, making careful control of these two parameters mandatory.

Improvements in anesthesia reduced the incidence of reinfarction from almost 100% in 1962, to 6% in 1978 [8, 29]. However, when an operation is performed within the first 3 months after an infarction, the incidence of reinfarction is 36%; if the operation comes 4–6 months afterward, the incidence is 26%. In a study by RAO, these rates of infarction were decreased by invasive cardiac monitoring from 36% down to 5.7% and from 26% to 2.3%, respectively [23]. The long-term prognosis for patients with concomitant disease such as arterial hypertension, arrhythmias, or temporary renal failure is poor.

II. Arterial Hypertension

In a high percentage of patients (up to 60% of surgical patients) a severe arterial hypertension is found with values greater than 180/100 mmHg, a diastolic pressure over 100 mmHg being the decisive pathologic parameter. Slight hypertension, with diastolic values between 90 and 100 mmHg without signs of cardiac, renal, or cerebrovascular involvement, does not seem to increase the frequency of postoperative complications following surgical intervention. The frequency of cardiovascular complications is proportional to the degree of hypertension [5, 23]. The diagnosis of hypertension is missed in 50% of patients; 50% of the diagnosed patients are not treated, and 50% of the treated patients are given inadequate treatment. Arterial hypertension in patients with vascular disorders is only one factor in the increased mortality in this group of patients. Myocardial infarction determines the degree of this complication in hypertensive patients. An analysis of the factors leading to mortality reveals a high incidence of myocardial infarction, about 60%. Some 30%–40% of patients die of cerebrovascular complications and 10% from other causes [5].

The cardiac complications of arterial hypertension are coronary artery disease and left ventricular hypertrophy. The cerebral complications of arterial hypertension include transient ischemic attacks and frank strokes. An impairment of renal function may also be caused by hypertension. For the diagnosis of these manifestations, urea and creatinine concentrations must be measured. However, significantly elevated values will be found only if the impairment of the function is about 70%. Serum electrolyte, urea, and creatinine should therefore be measured, together with the creatinine clearance. Furthermore, careful analyses of the urine are necessary, and attention must be paid to an elevation of serum proteins in the urine.

Some 90% of hypertensive patients are suffering from primary, or essential, hypertension. One should always attempt to evaluate the cause of the hypertension. Renal or possible endocrine causes should be eliminated. The treatment of arterial hypertension possibly increases life expectancy and reduces the rate of cardiac, cerebrovascular, and renal complications. Exact knowledge of the pharmacology of antihypertensive drugs is necessary, as some drugs, e.g., the thiazides, may cause hyperuricemia and hyperglycemia. Withdrawal of antihypertensive drugs may cause a severe hypertensive crisis. Therefore, it is necessary to continue administering them until the day of the operation [21].

Also, the sudden withdrawal of beta-blockers as antihypertensive drugs may aggravate angina. Investigations of beta-blockers and their withdrawal 24–48 h before the operation showed circulatory instability and increased risk of arrhythmias and hypertensive crisis [26]. Continuation of therapy with beta-blockers is therefore indicated in patients with vascular disease [14, 15]. These substances exert a protective effect on the myocardium by decreasing the heart rate as well as the arterial pressure. In animal experiments, they reduced the degree of ischemic damage following coronary artery occlusion [17], and they should also reduce the negative inotropic effect of anesthetics on the myocardium in humans [8].

III. Congestive Heart Failure

The diagnosis and treatment of congestive heart failure is necessary before an elective surgical intervention, as failure of the right or left ventricle during surgery represents a severe complication. According to some authors [8] preoperative administration of digitalis may reduce the negative inotropic effect of anesthetics on the myocardium. However, it should be noted that for some authors perioperative application of digitalis is justified only in the presence of congestive heart failure and atrial fibrillation or atrial flutter [28]. Preoperative digitalization may reduce the tendency to arrhythmias, especially fast supraventricular arrhythmias [20]. Other authors have found an unchanged – or even an increased – incidence of arrhythmias [5]. The risk of digitalis-induced arrhythmias is increased in the presence of electrolyte disorders or metabolic alkalosis. Therefore, digitalis should be used only in cases of clinically manifest congestive heart failure, until the evening prior to the operation. Routine administration of digitalis before operations, especially before major abdominal or intrathoracic procedures must be viewed critically. Digitalis is not used for compensation of the negative inotropic effects of anesthetics.

IV. Cerebrovascular Diseases

Evaluation should be performed carefully to detect possible events with transient neurologic functional defects. Transient ischemic attacks are often of short duration. In case of stenoses of carotid artery segments, short hemipareses are noted, often together with a hemianopia. In cases of stenoses of segments of the vertebral artery, the most frequent clinical symptoms are attacks of vertigo and a repeated tendency to fall.

During a longer sustained hypertensive phase, a cerebrovascular accident may occur intraoperatively [13]. Besides postoperatively occurring myocardial infarction the postoperative stroke has a high mortality of 50% [22]. The mortality in patients with preexisting cerebrovascular diseases undergoing surgical procedures of the coronaries is relatively high. The incidence of cardiac and cerebrovascular complications can be minimized by performing the procedure on the coronaries and the endarterectomy of the carotid artery simultaneously [22]. This should be taken into consideration in patients with preexisting cerebrovascular diseases and with correctable coronary artery stenoses.

V. Assessment of Risk

Careful preoperative evaluation enables one not only to confirm the diagnosis, but also to determine the severity and degree of preexisting cardiovascular disease with respect to the increased perioperative morbidity and mortality. Table 11.2 shows a point system for determination of postoperative cardiac complications according to GOLDMAN [11]. It allows preoperative computation of risk for noncardiovascular operative procedures. These play a significant role in the safe management of patients with coronary artery disease and arterial hypertension. The possible hazards of a blockade of β-receptors, however, should not be ignored. In patients with congestive heart failure, arterioventricular conduction defects, asthma, or anemia, beta-blocker therapy is indicated.

Occasional bradycardia following withdrawal of neuromuscular blockade by neostigmine has been noticed in patients on long-term medication [8].

Table 11.2. Preoperative computation of cardiac risk according to GOLDMAN [11]

Criteria	Point scale
1. History	
1. Age more than 70 years	5
2. Myocardial infarction within the last half year	10
2. Physical examination	
1. Gallop rhythm	11
2. Aortic stenosis	3
3. ECG	
1. Rhythm other than sinus	7
2. More than five premature ventricular contractions (time?)	7
4. General laboratory evaluation	
$pO_2 < 60$ mm Hg, $pCO_2 > 50$ mm Hg, Potassium 3.0, $HCO_3 < 20$ mequiv./l, BUN > 50 or creatinine > 3.0 ml/dl, abnormal SGOT, chronic liver disease	3
5. Operation	
1. Intraperitoneal, intrathoracic procedure	3
2. Emergency procedure	4

Table 11.3. Multifactorial risk index affecting perioperative cardiac complications

Class	Points	Minor or no complications (%)	Life-threatening complications (%)	Cardiac causes of death (%)
I	0–5	532 (99)	4 (0.7)	1 (0.2)
II	6–12	295 (93)	16 (5)	5 (2)
III	13–25	112 (86)	15 (11)	3 (2)
IV	25	4 (22)	4 (22)	10 (56)

The high incidence of life-threatening complications during anesthesia in patients with cardiovascular diseases is shown in Table 11.3. It often seems that anesthesia itself and the immediate postoperative phase are without problems. The major cardiac complications usually do not occur in the early postoperative phase. Besides a thorough evaluation prior to surgery, with appropriate preparation and careful intraoperative monitoring, patients must also be closely monitored in the postoperative phase in order to reduce the number and severity of cardiac complications.

C. Effect of Anesthetics on Circulation

There are numerous studies of the influences of anesthetics on the heart and circulation [3]. When analyzing these data, the following points should be taken into consideration. There is interaction between the drugs and the anesthetics used. Additive and potentiating effects, but also counteracting effects are possible. However, it must be pointed out that the individual patient may have a peculiar sensitivity to the various anesthetics and their cardiovascular effects. Therefore, careful supervision of the fluid status, the age, and the degree of underlying concomitant diseases is of utmost importance for selection of the correct anesthetic in the properly reduced dosage.

In principle, dose-dependent volatile anesthetics as well as drugs used for intravenous induction of anesthesia reduce the contractility of the heart. Some directly affect the vessels regulating resistance and capacity or change the response of those vessels to adrenergic stimuli. Comparing volatile anesthetics with intravenous ones, it seems evident that the former may be better controlled; on the other hand, intravenous anesthetics offer more protection against operative stress.

Barbiturates used for induction of anesthesia cause a marked reduction of contractility and filling pressures and, overall, diminished oxygen consumption by the heart. The application of fentanyl alone to induce anesthesia is not justified. The combination of fentanyl with, e.g., diazepam for induction, has attracted wide interest. Sufficient analgesia, combined with a slight reduction of arterial pressure, heart minute volume, and filling pressures is considered favorable.

Among the numerous anesthetics for induction, etomidate has the least influence on the cardiovascular system. In vascular surgery, it is predominantly volatile anesthetics that are used for continuing anesthesia. Through the combination of small amounts of analgesics (e.g., fentanyl) and volatile anesthetics like enflurane, halothane, and isoflurane, adequate protection against sympathicoadrenergic reactions and an appropriate depth of anesthesia can be sustained [7]. Reduced myocardial oxygen consumption at an appropriate dosage and an increase in the coronary reserve speak in favor of volatile anesthetics. On the other hand, in critical situations (massive blood loss) the additive effect of diminished contractility owing to hypovolemia as well as to the anesthetics must be taken into consideration. The volatile anesthetics rapidly cause a significant, but reversible myocardial depression in critical situations. Animal experiments have shown that the degree of severe ischemic damage may be reduced by the use of inhalation anesthetics. All volatile anesthetics cause a dose-dependent reduction of cardiac output. The increased dilatation of arterioles and the reduced tendency to arrhythmia with enflurane and isoflurane are considered to be an advantage. By comparison, intraoperatively administered analgesics such as fentanyl and morphine have a minimal effect on left ventricular function. The ability of the various analgesics to depress contractility is listed in Table 11.4.

However, inhalation anesthetics are considerably easier to handle from the point of view of their control. Morphine is used at a dose of 0.5–3 mg per kilogram body weight when left ventricular function is impaired. Fentanyl, at a dose of 0.0015–0.007 mg per kilogram body weight, shows a minimal influence on circulation with adequate protection against adrenergic stimuli. Postoperative analgesia is provided by intravenous anesthetics during the immediate postoperative phase. In contrast, inhalation anesthetics wear off rapidly, so that one has to change to intravenous analgesic therapy with possible negative side effects. But this leads to problems if it becomes necessary to use naxolone to antagonize the intravenous analgesics, as naxolone can cause pulmonary edema in the presence of heart failure.

Table 11.4. Determinants of myocardial oxygen supply and of myocardial oxygen consumption

Myocardial oxygen supply	Myocardial oxygen consumption
Coronary perfusion pressure	Myocardial contractility
Coronary vascular resistance	Left ventricular wall tension
Oxygen content: Hb	Heart rate
paO_2	Afterload
SaO_2	

D. Anesthesia in Patients with Coronary Artery Disease

In order to minimize risk, anesthetic technique must aim at minimal impairment of ventricular function and the prevention of myocardial ischemia. In the presence of coronary artery disease, a more extensive collection of data is necessary. Besides the patient's clinical tolerance of stress, exact data should be obtained concerning recent heart attacks as a clear correlation between recent heart attack and perioperative mortality has been found [11, 23]. Moreover, the current medication and the effectiveness of the therapy should be checked. Based upon the preoperative findings, a clinical classification of patients is possible. Patients with coronary artery disease are then classified primarily into two categories.

1. Patients with signs and symptoms of coronary artery disease and good left ventricular function at rest
2. Patients with signs and symptoms of coronary artery disease and diminished left ventricular function under exercise

This classification is clinically valid. The significant difference between the two groups of patients is their different tolerance to stress. Both groups show adequate left ventricular function at rest. Some of these patients will suffer from angina,

Table 11.5. Possible indications and contraindications for regional anesthesia

1. Indication for regional anesthesia
1. Urgent operative procedures in patients who are not n.p.o.
2. Metabolic disorders, liver and renal diseases
3. Diabetes mellitus
4. Significant impairment of pulmonary function

2. Relative indication
1. Heart failure and cardiovascular diseases
2. Cerebrovascular diseases

3. Absolute contraindication
1. Noncooperative patients
2. Anesthesiologist's lack of experience in the use of regional anesthesia and in coping with unforeseen incidents
3. Hypovolemia
4. Clotting disorders
5. Infection at the site of puncture
6. Allergy to local anesthetics

4. Relative contraindications
1. Severe general infection
2. Neurologic diseases
3. Certain concomitant diseases (severe hypertension and use of spinal or peridural anesthesia)
4. Heart failure, cardiovascular disease, and preexisting cerebrovascular disease

Table 11.6. Relative ability of various analgesics to depress contractility according to STRAUER [28]

	Equianalgesic doses		Blood concentrations resulting in a 50% – depression of contractility (μg/ml)	Relative ability to depress contractility
	(mg)	Ability		
Morphine	10	1	2000	1
Fentanyl	0.1–0.2	50–100	50–100	2–4
Piritramide	5–10	1–2	1000	1–2
Pentazocine	30	0.3	50	100–200
Meperidine	70	0.1–0.2	100	100–200
Tilidine	100	0.1–0.4	400	10–50

a long-lasting hypertension, but without signs of chronic impairment of left ventricular function. Only under exercise can diminished cardiac output be noticed [4].

Keeping a balance between myocardial oxygen supply and oxygen consumption in order to prevent myocardial ischemia is the essential aim of safe and careful anesthesiologic technique.

In Table 11.5, the essential determinants of myocardial oxygen supply and oxygen consumption are shown. This balance can be kept by avoiding hypotension, hypertension, and hypoxia and by drug control of the determinants of myocardial oxygen consumption (heart rate, preload, afterload, contractility). Heart rate and diastolic filling seem to play a major role. Numerous investigators have shown that myocardial oxygen consumption per heart beat remains constant within the physiologic range during unaltered preload and afterload.

The deleterious effect of tachycardia derives from the reduced filling time during diastole and the diminished diastolic coronary perfusion time. An increased preload not only increases myocardial oxygen consumption, but also worsenes perfusion of the endocardial and subendocardial layers. Myocardial ischemia can be avoided by the precise use of drugs to influence the determinants of increased myocardial oxygen consumption.

As mentioned earlier, medical therapy already underway preoperatively should be continued until the time of the operation as many of the drugs are also used intraoperatively. To avoid myocardial ischemia, a sufficiently deep phase of anesthesia with stable hemodynamics should be attempted. Today, there are no data proving that certain anesthetics or anesthesiological techniques are preferred in patients with cardiovascular diseases. Therefore, it is not possible to recommend any particular anesthesiological procedure as being suitable for all patients undergoing vascular surgery. When choosing the type of anesthesia for an elective operative procedure some important criteria have to be considered:

1. Type and localization of the procedure
2. Current general condition of the patient
3. Urgency of the operation
4. Necessity of postoperative analgesic therapy

For a number of operations in vascular surgery regional anesthesiological techniques in the lower extremity and the lower abdomen seem to have advantages (only slight impairment of the vital functions such as respiration, consciousness, and circulation: effective intraoperative blockade of pain, early mobilization of the patient, improvement of regional blood flow). The list of indications and contraindications of regional anesthesia is given in Table 11.6.

Bearing in mind that patients undergoing vascular surgery present with significant concomitant diseases and advanced age, the indication for regional anesthesia seems to be limited. Especially with spinal anesthesia, patients with chronic isotonic dehydration will be subject to a dangerous drop in blood pressure and cardiac output, owing to the diminished peripheral resistance that results from the regional blockade. The occurrence of angina attacks and ventricular fibrillation as a result of myocardial ischemia has been described. In this group of patients, therefore, one must proceed cautiously and critically when deciding whether regional anesthesia is indicated. So far, there is no clinical study confirming that mortality has been reduced by regional procedures such as spinal anesthesia and peridural anesthesia as compared with general anesthesia.

E. Monitoring

In general, when supervising these patient groups, the cardiovascular system is of primary importance because of the presence of concomitant disease. The only currently available clinical noninvasive method for the detection of ischemia is the use of the II of V_5 recording of the ECG. Timely detection and direct therapy are at the center of the anesthesiologist's efforts. However, it should be pointed out that ST changes in the ECG represent relatively late signs of myocardial ischemia.

The effects of ischemia on the left ventricular function are shown in Fig. 11.1.

Based on these facts, the filling pressures of the heart are of special importance. Preoperatively determined values prior to elective surgery may be used as guidelines for intraoperative monitoring. Therefore, during major vascular surgery, it is advisable to measure not only right ventricular filling pressure (CVP), but also left ventricular filling pressure by means of a Swan-Ganz catheter since significant myocardial stress has to be expected in the operative procedure (clamping, declamping). Another possibility for detection and assessment of the actual hemodynamic situation is to draw so-called curves of ventricular function. If one relates the left ventricular ejection capacity, measured as heart index, to the left ventricular filling pressure, then an instantaneous Frank – Starling curve is obtained. The determination of these curves for the measurement of myocardial tolerance to volume and for the control of therapy with vasodilators is of great importance for the

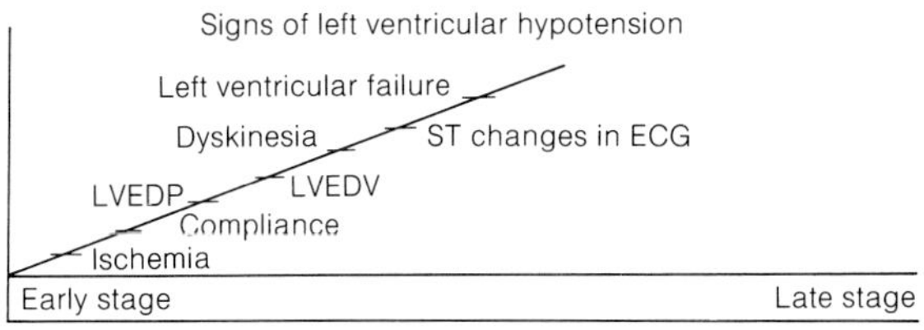

Fig. 11.1. Time course of signs of left ventricular hypotension

intraoperative monitoring of fluid therapy. The diagnosis of a beginning left-sided heart failure can be obtained by the continuous recording of the pulmonary capillary wedge pressure, and therapy can be initiated early. Therapy in high-risk patients is optimized by extended monitoring. Several drugs are available. Mainly vasodilators and calcium antagonists are used. Sodium nitroprusside and nitroglycerin are the most frequently used drugs for the treatment of hypertensive crisis with increased left ventricular filling pressures.

F. Anesthesia for Operative Procedures in the Aorta

I. Physiologic Changes

Myocardial infarction, renal failure, and stroke are the major causes of postoperative morbidity and mortality in patients undergoing operations on the aorta. Stable circulation, controlled fluid therapy, adequate depth of anesthesia, and the control of renal function are the essential parameters of intraoperative monitoring. The sudden increase of the peripheral resistance after clamping of the aorta causes a significant increase of the mean arterial pressure and an acute increase of the left ventricular afterload with the risk of acute left-sided heart failure in patients with latent insufficiency. The increased left ventricular afterload leads to increased myocardial oxygen consumption. As a consequence of the functional deterioration of the left ventricle, there will be a drop in the heart index. The pressures in the right ventricle remain almost unchanged [25]. An increase in oxygen consumption due to the increased left ventricular wall tension is added to the previously mentioned increase in the afterload. Following clamping of the aorta, arrhythmias and ST segment changes may occur as a result of myocardial ischemia [24].

Table 11.7. Coping with ischemia during cross-clamping of the aorta

Clinical causes and sequelae of ischemia	Treatment
Increased arterial blood pressure	1. Change of depth of anesthesia 2. Vasodilators 3. Beta-blockers
Increased heart rate	1. Change of depth of anesthesia 2. Fluid therapy 3. Beta-blockers
Increased CVP or PCWP	1. Vasodilators 2. Volume restriction 3. Diuretics 4. Positive inotropic substances
Hypotension	1. Change of depth of anesthesia 2. Volume therapy 3. Positive inotropic substances 4. Volume restriction 5. Vasopressors
Arrhythmia	1. Change of depth of anesthesia 2. Control of electrolytes 3. Antiarrhythmic drugs 4. Beta-blockers 5. Calcium antagonists

Various kinds of therapy for dealing with ischemia are listed in Table 11.7. Vasodilators occupy a prominent position in the treatment of acute left-sided heart failure. As a result of the decrease in peripheral resistance, there will be a reduction of the afterload (decrease in mean aortic pressure), a drop in left ventricular and diastolic pressure, and an increase in stroke volume.

Vasodilators that have proven effective for such therapy include: sodium nitroprusside, nitroglycerin, hydralazine, aminophylline, and urapidil. Nitroglycerin is preferred because of its great therapeutic range. Infusion of nitroglycerin normalizes pulmonary capillary wedge pressure, which should be adjusted to the preoperatively determined value. Overall, the balance between oxygen supply and oxygen consumption is considerably influenced by the reduction of the preload and afterload.

Furthermore, occlusion of the aorta causes a decrease of renal blood flow and a shunting of intrarenal blood flow from the cortex to the outer medulla. It is unclear whether a beginning tubular necrosis can be controlled by the application of mannitol. The prophylactic application of hyperosmolar solutions and diuretics before clamping is handled differently in different institutions.

Reopening of the peripheral arterial vascular bed often leads to significant hypotension – described as declamping shock – which is the result of either a relative hypovolemia or an impaired arteriovenous compliance of the vascular system as a result of local acidosis [19, 24]. Also there is a release of vasoactive substances such as bradykinin, serotinin, and prostaglandins, which are seen as factors of declamping shock. The most frequent change is a pronounced metabolic acidosis and a sometimes inadequate circulating blood volume.

Increased hydrogen ion concentrations in the peripheral vascular bed prevent a vasoconstrictor response and cause dilatation of the peripheral vascular bed with resulting hypotension. It is unclear to what extent factors are released from the peripheral vascular bed that have an immediate depressant effect on the myocardium. Persistent hypotension may lead to hypoxic myocardial failure and to a permanently inadequate coronary perfusion.

Acute hypotension can be prevented to some extent by gradual declamping of the aorta. Close cooperation between the surgeon and the anesthetist is necessary. The degree of the declamping syndrome is diminished by careful monitoring, early correction of disturbances of the acid-base balance, maintenance of an adequate circulating volume, and possibly also by the use of vasopressor substances. An increase in load can be avoided by ascertaining the left ventricular filling pressures. Hemodilution leads to reduced blood viscosity and improved microcirculation in arteriosclerosis. Another aim is the maintenance of renal function by an adequate blood volume. Any temporary change in the renal blood flow may cause parenchymal damage with possible necrosis of the cortex. Two aspects are important in the maintenance of renal function: the maintenance of an adequately circulating blood volume, and the possibility of suppressing sympathetic adrenergic activity and the resultant release of hormones. Increased sympathetic adrenergic activity releases the antidiuretic hormone ADH. It is controversial to what extent a thoracic epidural blockade can stabilize the renal function.

II. Anesthesiologic Procedures

Operations on the aorta may be performed electively or in response to a life-threatening emergency. The following approach is recommended for elective cases:

1. ECG monitoring
2. Large intravenous catheters for fluid therapy
3. Continuous recording of arterial blood pressure via the radial artery
4. Central venous catheter
5. Possibly Swan-Ganz catheter
6. Foley catheter for recording urinary output
7. Nasogastric tube

Furthermore, a sufficient number of blood units should be in reserve in case a massive transfusion becomes necessary.

1. Procedures in Case of a Ruptured Aneurysm

Patients with a penetrating or ruptured aneurysm are extremely hypovolemic, have often had a long trip to the hospital, and present with the clinical signs of hemorrhagic shock with early symptoms of acute respiratory insufficiency.

Basic laboratory testing must be done as quickly as possible. All venous and arterial catheters should be inserted prior to local anesthesia. If possible, a sufficient number of blood units, red blood cell concentrates, and fresh frozen plasma should be prepared. Blood volume should be restored before anesthesia if at all possible.

If this is impossible, the immediate surgical intervention is the only means of controlling massive bleeding. In case of penetrating aneurysms, induction of anesthesia should be performed on the table after cleaning the patient's skin with antiseptics. A sudden change in intra-abdominal pressure following relaxation, or as a result of pain relief, may result in a hazardous drop in blood pressure in the case of penetrating aneurysms. Retroperitoneal hematomas may induce ileus with the high risk of aspiration. The anesthesiologist should therefore employ the technique of ileus induction. Hypovolemia and diminished tissue perfusion lead to metabolic acidosis which must be corrected. When correcting acidosis one must be alert to the possibility of hypokalemia. By use of a cell saver (autotransfusion), massive transfusion of homologous blood, with its complications, can be reduced.

2. Procedure in Case of Dissecting Aneurysms of the Thoracic Aorta

In the majority of such cases primary treatment is conservative, using controlled hypotension. If surgical intervention is indicated, the duration of clamping is a decisive factor. If clamping time exceeds 20 min, irreversible damage to the spinal cord (anterior spinal artery syndrome) or to the kidneys must be expected. In dealing with the excessive increase in pressure produced by clamping the thoracic aorta, carefully controlled induced "hypotension" under sodium nitroprusside minimizes the risk of myocardial ischemia or damage to the cerebrum. Sodium nitroprusside [30] is the drug of choice because of the immediate onset of its effect and the good control; with nitroglycerine, our experience shows that an adequate pressure reduction during clamping of the thoracic aorta is much more difficult to achieve. Postoperative pain relief and adequate antihypertensive therapy may be achieved eventually by thoracic epidural anesthesia.

G. Anesthesia for Acute Arterial Occlusions

The cause of an acute occlusion is the detachment of a mural thrombus. Problems with anesthesia are the result of preexisting cardiovascular disease. The reactive increase in pressure following acute occlusion of the aortic bifurcation may cause increased myocardial oxygen consumption and left ventricular failure. After declamping, the usually uncorrected metabolic acidosis resulting from the occlusion may lead to irreversible hypotension. Correction of metabolis acidosis takes absolute priority in treatment. In all cases, electrolyte balance must be monitored very carefully and necessary electrolytes must be substituted as a Tourniquet syndrome may result if ischemia persists too long. The greatest danger is postischemic hyperkalemia which may result in irreversible cardiac arrest.

Close control of potassium, possibly glucose-insulin infusion and a gradual release of arterial blood flow should be performed as precautionary measures. Blood loss is usually not very marked; therefore, any attempt to correct hypotension by means of fluid therapy may cause iatrogenic left heart failure. Registration of central venous pressure seems to be necessary in patients with impeding left heart failure since under these circumstances patients have pronounced dehydration. In vascular patients with apparent or suspected coronary artery disease, hematocrit should not be lower than about 35 g% and hemoglobin about 12 g%.

In cases of occlusion of the mesenteric arteries, symptoms of bowel infarction or ileus are clinically predominant.

This requires an anesthesiological procedure aimed primarily at preventing aspiration. However, preparatory measures should be described in the preceding sections.

H. Anesthesia in Cases of Venous Occlusion

Iliofemoral thrombectomy is the emergency procedure for acute occlusion of the pelvic venous system. Surgical trauma during the operation is judged as minor; however, blood loss may be considerable. The danger of a pulmonary embolism as a result of dislodging a thrombus during surgical dissection can be minimized by placing the patient in the upright position and by artificial respiration with high positive end-expiratory pressure. The effects of high end-expiratory pressure on hemodynamics have to be considered (hypotension, reduced blood flow to liver and kidneys). The recording of central venous pressure and the monitoring of respiratory pressure are therefore absolutely necessary for early detection of pulmonary embolism. Monitoring of the pulmonary arterial pressure represents an optimal procedure, but is not absolutely necessary.

I. Anesthesia for Operative Procedures on the Carotid Artery

I. Pathophysiologic Changes

Stenoses of the carotid artery are usually found in the higher age groups, with males contributing over 80%. Owing to multiple medical problems, this group of patients shows an increased risk under anesthesia. Arterial hypertension with increased systolic pressure is a significant factor in the development of a CVA [1]. Neurologic deficits will occur in 6%–8% of patients. The cause is the embolization of an atheromatous plaque during surgical dissection. Also, acute changes in arterial pressure are thought to be responsible for the degree of neurologic deficit [1]. If the patients are operated on within 1 month after an episode of cerebral ischemia and are still suffering partially from persisting neurologic deficits, the operative intervention carries a high risk of further worsening of the neurologic deficit. Most patients undergoing operative procedures on the carotid artery are older patients with generalized arterial disease. Owing to the arteriosclerotic changes of the vessel, the capability of the vascular system for autoregulation has ceased. Cerebral perfusion becomes dependent on the systemic pressure. Hypotension therefore limits oxygen supply to the cerebrum. Simultaneously, the risk of thrombosis with obstruction of the intracranial vascular system may be increased by diminished blood velocity. Postoperative hypertension increases the risk of bleeding, which may result in cerebral infarction [9]. Hypertension with values over 200 mmHg is found in 33% of patients [1]. Some authors recommend the preoperative application of beta-blockers or calcium antagonists. The cause of intraoperative hypertension is unknown, but it seems to be the denervation of the carotid sinus [9]. Infiltration of the carotid sinus with 1% lidocaine solution seems to influence not only hypertension and bradycardia, but also the incidence of postoperative hypertensive reactions.

Sufficiently deep anesthesia may exert a protective effect on healthy nervous cells by reducing oxygen consumption. The oxygen supply should therefore be adapted to the metabolic requirements at all times. The application of 100% oxygen is not routinely necessary. Controlled artificial respiration guarantees sufficient oxygenation and the exact adjustment of CO_2 pressure to preoperative values. During clamping of the carotid artery, oxygen supply is dependent on the effectiveness of intracranial collaterals [16]. The stump pressure of the internal carotid artery, which is the pressure, after clamping, distal to the clamp, may indicate a sufficient collateral blood supply, but is not an exact indicator of the collateral flow in the ischemic area. Systemic arterial pressure, CO_2 pressure, and anesthesia influence the relation of carotid occlusion pressure and regional blood flow. The acceptable occlusion pressure is estimated at 60 mmHg. Cerebral venous oxygen saturation seems to be a more precise parameter of the effectiveness of collateral blood supply, according to some authors.

II. Oxygen Supply to the CNS

For the preservation of autoregulation, arterial pressure should no doubt be kept within the physiologic range of each individual patient. A slight increase in pressure of 15%–20% of the basal value seems to be advantageous according to some authors [6]. It is not known to what extent induced hypertension will actually result in an improvement of the ischemic areas. Furthermore, vasopressor agents should be used only with the greatest care in patients with coronary artery disease. A further improvement of perfusion seems to be possible by reducing blood viscosity. To what extent the use of low molecular dextran improves oxygen supply within the damaged vascular area is not settled [9].

Hypercapnia increases cerebral blood flow. If the arterial CO_2 pressure exceeds 45 mmHg, autoregulation becomes impossible. An intracerebral steal phenomenon will occur within the ischemic area. In the damaged region, owing to the anerobic metabolism, there will be an increase of H ion concentration and of vasomotor paralysis with loss of reaction to changes in CO_2. There should be a shunting of blood flow into areas of lowest resistance. The degree of shunting depends on vasodilation in the appropriate vascular bed, on the capacity of the collateral circulation, and possibly on increase of flow within other vessels. It is questionable whether hyperventilation has a favorable effect on cerebral blood flow since cerebral areas damaged by ischemia lose their responsiveness to CO_2, resulting in further shunting by the intracerebral steal phenomenon [2, 9].

Furthermore, as the intracranial volume increases, the capability of outer regulation of the vessels decreases and the occlusion pressures decrease. The result is a reduced perfusion. In each case, it is not known how the vessels in the ischemic area will react to changes in CO_2 and to what extent reduction of CO_2 partial pressure will decrease the global cerebral blood flow.

III. Anesthesiological Management for Operative Procedures on the Carotid Artery

During anesthesia, oxygen consumption is reduced. A further reduction in metabolism can be achieved by the use of barbiturates. It remains to be demonstrated, however, whether barbiturates effectively protect the cerebrum against ischemic damage. Reducing cerebral metabolism provides some protection against local ischemia; therefore, in many centers, a bolus of 4–5 mg/kg thiopental is given before clamping of the carotid artery [18].

It is still not clear which anesthetic is the most favorable for vascular procedures on the carotid artery. Halothane and enflurane cause cerebral vasodilatation; the lower limit for perfusion of the hemispheres under normal ventilation is calculated to be 15–18 ml per 100 g per min. In most centers, small concentrations of halothane and enflurane, together with nitrous oxide oxygen is recommended. Also, on the application of fentanyl and dehydrobenzperidol, no significant increase in cerebral blood flow and in the occlusion pressure of the carotid artery was found. Anesthesiological management during thromboendarterectomy is summarized in Table 11.8.

General anesthesia should provide sufficient protection by effective blockade of sensory and autonomic reflexes. Cardiovascular stability is the most important factor. Early postanesthetic recov-

Table 11.8. Anesthesiological management during thromboendarterectomy of the carotid artery

Careful history

1. Evaluation of risk factors
2. Medical correction or continuation of antihypertensive beta-blocker or digitalis therapy

Maintenance of cerebral perfusion

1. Avoiding hypotension and bradycardia
2. Normocapnia
3. Application of shunt

Monitoring

1. ECG
2. Arterial pressure, continuously
3. EEG, when possible
4. Occlusion pressure of the carotid artery
5. (Cerebral blood flow and sensorially evoked potentials)

Close postoperative monitoring

1. Maintenance of normal blood pressure
2. Free airways (rebleeding)
3. Serial neurologic checks

ery is essential for immediate assessment of possible neurologic changes. Local anesthesia for operative procedures on the carotid artery is favored by some authors [31]. The theoretical advantages are minimal cardiac or respiratory impairment and immediate registration of neurologic change. Overall, however, general anesthesia seems to be more satisfactory because of the significant reduction of stress that is achieved. A potential obstruction of the airway owing to bleeding can be dealt with better under general anesthesia.

The administration of 10000 units of heparin before clamping improves cerebral blood flow. In order to maintain a sufficient oxygen supply during clamping of the carotid artery, many surgeons insert shunts. Today, there is no clear criterion as to which patients require shunts. The measurement of the occlusion pressure of the carotid artery is not a reliable parameter. Measurement of the regional cerebral blood flow and that of the affected hemisphere or a complete EEG recording is necessary before a decision can be made regarding the use of shunt. Data obtained from various surgical centers show the same results both with and without routine use of a shunt.

Also in doubt are attempts to reduce neurologic complications by giving 3 × 8 mg dexamethasone. At present there is no possibility of avoiding the embolization of atheromatous material. Only careful surgical dissection can minimize these hazardous complications.

K. Postoperative Supervision

Postoperative therapy has to be seen as an integral part of the total therapeutic concept. Its extent should be recognized and determined preoperatively, or at the very latest intraoperatively. Numerous preexisting risk factors are always involved; therefore the administration of the anesthetic, the adequate substitution of fluid, and the monitoring and treatment of cardiac function and metabolism – all of these – assume great importance alongside the operative procedure itself. Efforts in the postoperative phase should concentrate on accurate recognition of the effects of acute disorders and on their appropriate treatment.

Many kinds of postoperative complications are possible. The postanesthetic recovery phase after the operation is the first critical postoperative phase for the patient.

Table 11.9. Postoperative complications

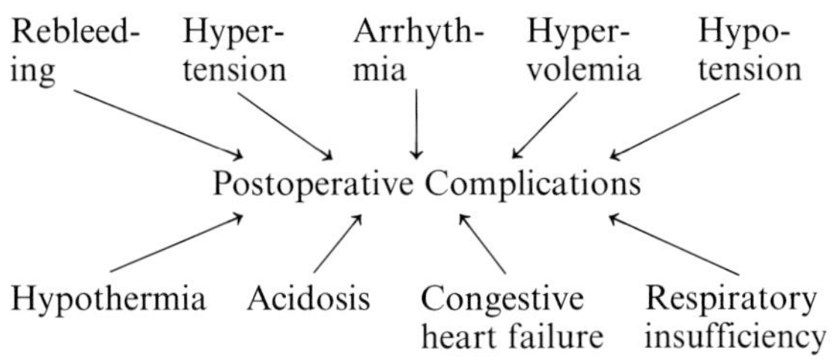

The recovery phase is characterized by an increased adrenergic reaction immediately after extubation. The causes of this are: a decrease in the depth of anesthesia, an increase in pain sensation, insufficient oxygenation with simultaneous hypercapnia, and, in addition, the increased release of catecholamines following induced hypotension by means of vasodilators. Close monitoring during this phase often reveals hypertensive blood pressure values and tachycardia, which usually constitute a critical situation for the patient with coronary artery disease. Such patients therefore demand special care in the recovery phase.

The transitional phase from the operating room to the recovery room is one of the weakest links in the postoperative chain of supervision. The possibilities for complication in the recovery room are numerous. They can be divided into those that occur often and those that are rare.

Rebleeding is rare. When it does occur it can be acutely life threatening, especially in patients who have undergone operations on the carotid artery because of the extreme difficulty of reintervention under these circumstances and the risk of hypoxic cardiac arrest. One must therefore be alert to the occurrence of stridor while monitoring the patient following disobliteration of the carotid artery. More frequent, and of great importance during the postoperative period, are hypertensive crises.

The causes of postoperative arrhythmias, which occur often, are mainly disturbances in electrolytes, anemia, hypoxia, and hypovolemia. The control of potassium, hemoglobin or hematocrit, and blood gases and the measurement of central venous pressure may help to disclose the causes and to indicate appropriate therapy. Also, hypertensive crises are often associated with arrhythmias. In such cases, antihypertensive medication is indicated. Other causes of arrhythmia, such as heart failure, pulmonary embolism, atelectasis, and pneumonia, are rather rare, but require intensive therapy.

Following surgical treatment of aneurysms, hypovolemia often occurs. This can be partially explained by the intraoperative use of vasodilators, but may also be the result of an underestimated blood loss.

For better monitoring and control of fluid therapy, the use of a Swan-Ganz catheter intraoperatively as well as postoperatively has been recommended in these patients.

Preoperatively initiated medical therapy with digitalis, beta-blockers, nitro-preparations, and antihypertensive drugs must be continued in an appropriate manner. Postoperatively, the therapy should be continued only when hypovolemia, anemia, and hypertensive crisis have been corrected and the circulatory function stabilized.

Although there are different opinions regarding the necessity and the effect of postoperative ventilation, patients with a Y-prosthesis are routinely kept on the respirator postoperatively. The duration of ventilation is usually about 18–24 h. The necessity of postoperative ventilation is the result of numerous risk factors. It is known that age, overweight, and heavy smoking in the presence of severe abdominal pain decrease the functional residual capacity, while increasing the occlusive capacity. When the occlusive capacity exceeds the functional residual capacity, atelectasis develops, resulting in ventilatory and perfusion disorders. Furthermore, ventilatory stimulation is significantly diminished by volatile anesthetics and by analgesics during a phase in which hypoxia is not a rare event.

Today, the question must remain open whether postoperative ventilation can prevent pneumonia. However, one thing is certain: in cases of hypothermia following massive transfusion, where a patient with impaired cardiac function is receiving medication to improve circulation, the risk will be greater if such a patient is exposed to the additional danger of respiratory insufficiency.

I. Postoperative Monitoring

It is difficult to make a general statement. According to Greenberg [12], the extent and frequency of monitoring should be adjusted for the various risk groups.

The first step, basic monitoring, helps to define stability of organ functions and deviations. Frequency and extent of measurements will vary according to the operation and the patient's condition (Table 11.10a).

The second step, extended monitoring, is indicated when preexisting risk factors and the type of operation may cause pathologic changes in organ function (Table 11.10b).

In principle, the parameters listed for basic monitoring will be determined more frequently. Additionally, the monitoring will be more invasive, e.g., through a central venous catheter. In general, patients with a Y-prosthesis will be in that category. In all cases where severe hemodynamic disorders are to be expected or have occurred, or where manifest organ failure is present, the third step, i.e., differential monitoring, is indicated (Table 11.10c).

Preoperative evaluation and therapy, the operative procedure itself, and the anesthetic phase – none of these can be regarded as successful unless the patient recovers without serious complications. Monitoring that is appropriate to the procedures

Table 11.10a. Basic monitoring

Intensive care unit	Laboratory findings
Blood pressure, pulse	Serum electrolytes
Respiratory rate	Blood glucose
Body temperature	Hemoglobin and Hematocrit
Fluid intake	Blood gas analysis
Urine volume	Chest X-ray
Blood and fluid loss	

Table 11.10b. Extended monitoring

Intensive care unit	Laboratory data
Ventilatory parameters	Venous O_2 saturation
Central venous pressure (CVP)	Serum and urine osmolarity
Arterial pressure	Electrolytes
Neurologic findings	Leukocytes and platelets
	Coagulation, lactate serum protein
	Colloid osmotic pressure (COD)
	Enzymes

Table 11.10c. Differential monitoring

Intensive care unit	Laboratory data
1. Measurements by Swan-Ganz catheter	Special investigations
2. Determination of intracranial pressure	

and measures that come before it is a necessary prerequisite to effective postoperative therapy.

Following major vascular surgery, routine postoperative ventilation has proven to be beneficial. The aims of recovery room and intensive care therapy are: gradual reduction of the maximal stress of operative intervention, detection and prevention of life-threatening complications, and converting an operative success into a personal success for the patient.

It should be reemphasized that the anesthesiologist can minimize the complication rate in multimorbid patients by a comprehensive preoperative workup of patients undergoing vascular surgery, by appropriate intraoperative monitoring, and by careful postoperative care. Anesthesia in patients with vascular surgery is an ongoing challenge.

REFERENCES

1. Asiddao CB, Donegan JH, Whitezell RC, Kalbfleisch JH (1982) Factors associated with perioperative complications during carotid endarterectomy. Anaesth Analg 61:631
2. Baker WH, Rodman JA, Barnes RW, Hoyt JL (1976) An evaluation of hypocarbia and hypercarbia during carotid endarterectomy. Stroke 715:451
3. Bland JHL, Lowenstein E (1976) Effect of halothane on myocardial ischaemia. Anesthesiology 45:287
4. Braunwald E (1971) Control of myocardial oxygen consumption: physiologic and clinical considerations. Am J Cardiol 27:146
5. Bulpitt CJ, Beilin LJ, Clifton P, Coles EC, Dollery CT, Gear JSS, Harper GS, Johnson BF, Munro-Faure AD (1979) Risk factors for death in treated hypertensive patients. Lancet 2:134
6. Fan FC, Chen RYZ, Chien S, Correll JW (1981) Bypass blood flow during carotid endarterectomy. Anesthesiology 55:305
7. Francis CM, Lowenstein E, Davis WL, Foex P, Ryder WA (1980) Effect of halothane on the performance of myocardium supplied by a narrowed artery. Br J Anaesth 52:236
8. Foex P (1981) Preoperative assessment of the patients with cardiovascular disease. Br J Anaesth 53:731
9. Frost EAM (1981) Anaesthetic management of cerebrovascular disease. Br J Anaesth 53:745
10. Goldman L, Caldera DL (1979) Risks of general anesthesia and elective operation in the hypertensive patient. Anesthesiology 50:185
11. Goldman L, Nussbaum SR, Southwick FS, Korgstar D, Murray B, Burke DS, O'Malley TA, Gorrol AH, Caplan CH, Nolan J, Carabello B, Slater EF (1977) Multifactoral index of cardiac risk in noncardiac surgical procedures. N Engl J Med 297:845
12. Greenberg AG, Peskin GW (1978) Monitoring in the recovery room and surgical intensive care unit. In: Saidman LJ, Tysmith N (eds) Monitoring in anesthesia. Wiley, New York, p 221
13. Grundy BL, Sanderson AC, Webster MV (1981) Hemiparesis following carotid endarterectomy: comparison of monitoring methods. Anesthesiology 55:462
14. Howat DDC (1981) Cardiac disease, anesthesia and operation of the cardiac patient. Br J Anaesth 43:288
15. Kaplan JA, Wells PH (1981) Early diagnosis of myocardial ischemia using the pulmonary arterial catheter. Anesth Analg 60:789
16. McKay RD, Sundt TH, Michenfelder JD, Gronet GA, Messick JH, Sharbrough FW, Piepgras DG (1976) Internal carotid artery stump pressure and cardial blood flow during carotid endarterectomy. Anesthesiology 45:390
17. Manners JB, Walters FJM (1979) Beta adrenoceptor blockade and anaesthesia. Anaesthesia 34:3
18. Michenfelder JD, Theye RA (1973) Cerebral protection by thiopental during hypoxia. Anesthesiology 39:510
19. Modig J, Kolstad K, Wigren A (1978) Systemic reactions to tourniquet ischaemia. Acta Anaesth Scand 22:609
20. Moss JJ, Schwartz PJ (1979) Sudden death and the idiopathic long Q-T syndrome. Am J Med 66:7
21. Prys-Roberts C (1979) Hemodynamic effects of anesthesia and surgery in renal hypertensive patients receiving large doses of beta-receptor antagonists. Anesthesiology 51:122
22. Prys-Roberts C (1981) Cardiovascular monitoring in patients with vascular disease. Br J Anaesth 53:767
23. Rao TLK, Jacobs KH, El-Etr AA (1983) Reinfarction following anesthesia in patients with myocardial infarction. Anesthesiology 59:6
24. Reiz S, Peter T, Rais O (1979) Hemodynamic and cardiometabolic effects of infrarenal aortic common iliac artery declamping in man, an approach to optimal volume loading. Acta Anaesthesiol Scand 23/6:579
25. Schmucker P, Franke N, Vogel H, Martin E, Ackern K van, Laubenthal H, Becker HM (1982) Hämodynamische Veränderungen bei der Operation infrarenaler Bauchaortenaneurysmen. Anaesthesist 31:155
26. Slogoff S, Keats AS, Ott E (1979) Preoperative propanolol therapy and aortocoronary bypass operation. JAMA 240:1487
27. Sorensen HB, Engell HC (1978) Preoperative haemodynamic evaluation of patients submitted for major surgery. Acta Anaesthesiol Scand 22:391
28. Strauer BE (1982) Fortschritte der kardiovaskulären Pathophysiologie. In: Peter K, Jesch F (eds) Inhalationsanaesthesie heute und morgen. Springer, Berlin Heidelberg New York, p 63
29. Tarhan S, Moffitt EA, Taylor WE (1972) Myocardial infarction after general anaesthesia. JAMA 220:1451
30. Taylor TH, Styles H, Lamming AJ (1970) Sodium nitroprusside as hypertensive agent in anaesthesia. Br J Anaesth 42:859
31. Whittemore AD (1980) Carotid endarterectomy: an alternative approach. Arch Surg 180:940

Special Section

12 Vascular Deformities

12.1 Atypical Coarctation of the Aorta

G. Heberer and H. Denecke

CONTENTS

A. Etiology and Anatomy

The clinical term "atypical coarctation" of the aorta as compared with "typical coarctation" refers to those stenoses lying within the aortic segments II–IV. The etiology can be very difficult to establish. However, this is not a significant factor in either the decision to operate or in the choice of the reconstructive procedure.

The most common causes are inflammatory diseases such as Takayasu aortitis, aortoarteritis and granulomatous aortitis [5, 6, 7]. Hypoplastic types are classified as congenital defects [3, 4, 8]. Congenital nature especially has to be considered if long hypoplastic segments are found and macroscopic and microscopic post inflammatory lesions are absent (Table 1).

Table 12.1.1. Classification and topographic description of the aortic segments

Segment	Description	Topography
I	Ascending aorta	To brachiocephalic trunk
II	Aortic arch	To left subclavian artery (incl.)
III	Descending aorta	To phrenic hiatus
IV	Middle aorta	To renal arteries (incl.)
V	Infrarenal aorta	To bifurcation

For the operative procedure, clinical symptoms as well as localization and extent of the stenosis is taken into consideration. Not the etiology, but the pathoanatomic extent and the pathophysiologic degree of the stenosis is important. Figure 12.1.1. shows the most common thoracoabdominal stenoses of the aorta encountered in clinical practice. The topographic classification given by Ueno (1967) contains the aortic arch syndrome (type I), stenoses of the renal arteries but without adjacent aortic involvement and infrarenal aortic stenosis without concomitant hypertension [11]. All of these types of stenoses may occur in aortitis, but do not belong to the proper group of atypical aortic coarctation.

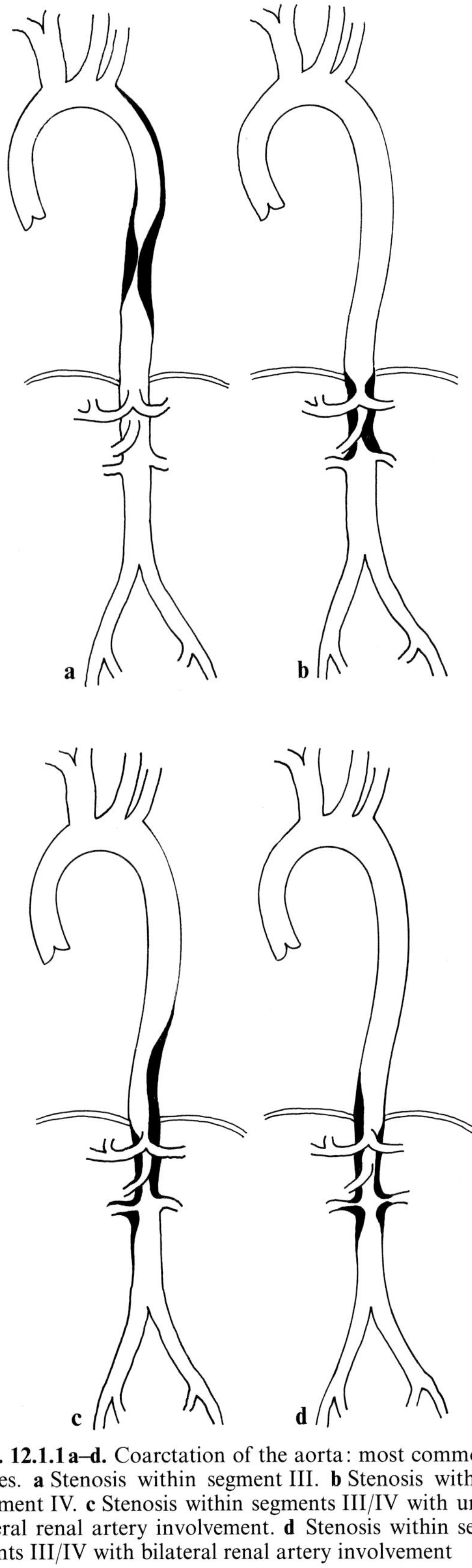

Fig. 12.1.1 a–d. Coarctation of the aorta: most common types. **a** Stenosis within segment III. **b** Stenosis within segment IV. **c** Stenosis within segments III/IV with unilateral renal artery involvement. **d** Stenosis within segments III/IV with bilateral renal artery involvement

B. Indications

The clinical symptoms of an atypical coarctation of the aorta are caused by impaired perfusion of the poststenotic region. Extensive collateral systems, however, may compensate the stenosis and maintain organ function. For example, weakened or absent pulses in the lower limb do not necessarily constitute clinical or functional manifestation of circulatory impairment. Claudication occurs in only 14% of cases [3].

High arterial blood pressure is the cardinal symptom and main indication for surgery. In most cases, hypertension is caused by impaired renal blood supply. The renal arteries are included in the stenotic process in 33%–80% of patients. Often, bilateral stenoses are present [4, 5]. If the stenosis is localized just above the renal arteries, the resultant hypertension corresponds to that caused by bilateral renal artery stenosis ("two kidneys – two stenoses" type, which is pathophysiologically identical to Goldblatt's one-kidney hypertension). Chronically, renin release will be suppressed. This type of renovascular hypertension may be relieved simply by constructing a thoracoabdominal bypass with distal anastomosis to the infrarenal aortic segment. Failing blood pressure normalization may be due to intrarenal arteriosclerosis, which already may have developed in elder patients.

In cases of juxtarenal aortic stenoses with deminished blood flow in a single artery, the resulting hypertension corresponds to that caused by unilateral renal artery stenosis (i.e., two kidneys – one stenosis type pathophysiologically identical to the so-called two-kidneys hypertension). Besides correction of the aortic stricture, the blood flow to the renal artery also must be reestablished.

An additional aortic stenosis below the renal arteries (segment V) is significant only if it threatens to obstruct retrograde blood flow to the renal arteries following establishment of a thoracoabdominal bypass with distal anastomosis caudal to the stenosis in question.

Stenoses of the visceral arteries seldom lead to true symptoms of intestinal angina.

Since without treatment the atypical coarctation of the aorta bears a poor late prognosis [7], revascularization is always indicated. The main causes of death in these mostly young patients are heart failure and strokes as a consequence of persistent arterial hypertension.

C. Positioning and Surgical Approach

The most favorable approach in a thoracoabdominal procedure is that described by CRAWFORD. The upper left portion of the patient's body is elevated and rotated toward the right (Fig. 12.1.2a). The incision extends from the midline of the lower abdomen to the umbilicus and from there to the left costal arch into the seventh interspace. The costal arch is divided. The diaphragm is transected dorsolaterally to the hiatus tendineus. The phrenic nerve and its innervating branches are spared, together with the largest portion of the diaphragm on the medial side. The spleen, the left colon, the left kidney, and the intestine are retracted medially i.e., to the right. This permits full exposure of the entire aorta, starting at the origin of the subclavian artery down to the iliac arteries. This visualization is especially favorable for the completion of the distal anastomosis and for the reconstruction of the abdominal aorta using a dorsolateral approach.

Fig. 12.1.2a, b. Position and approach. **a** As described by CRAWFORD in a right semilateral position. **b** Separate thoracic and abdominal incisions

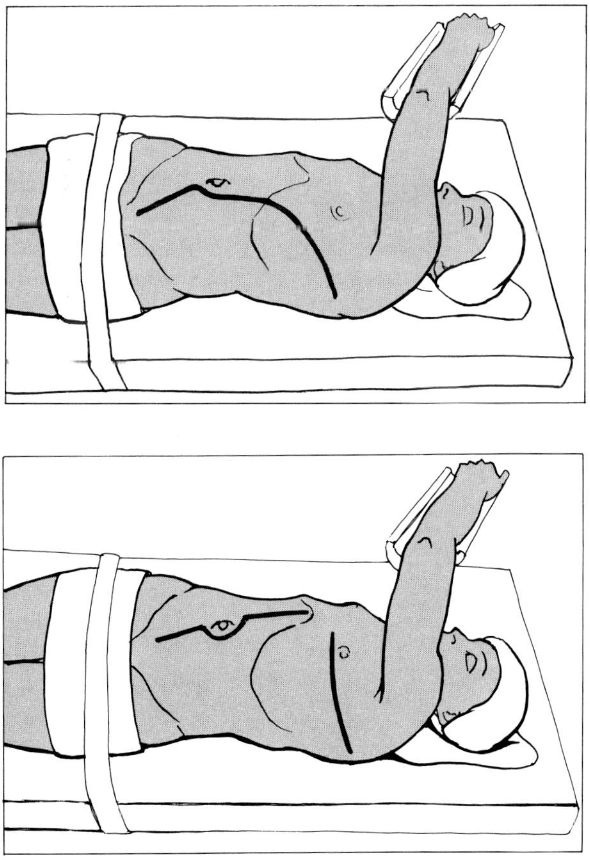

If the thorax and the abdomen are opened separately, an approach is made through the fifth interspace with the upper left portion of the body elevated and rotated toward the right (Fig. 12.1.2b). By retracting the lung medially, the descending aorta is well exposed. The abdomen is opened by a large midline incision. This incision should extend all the way up to the xiphoid process, especially if revascularization of the renal arteries is planned. Just as during exposure for renal artery revascularization, the transverse colon and the greater omentum are retracted upward and the small intestine is wrapped in a moist towel and retracted to the right (see p. 613). The broad retractor of the VOLLMAR type has proven very useful in holding the full length of the mesenteric root away from the aorta.

In stenoses of the descending aorta extending far upward or in a procedure done in a simple supine position the proximal end of the graft is connected to the ascending aorta. Exposure is transsternal by median incision [1]. Similarly, the infrarenal aorta is exposed for distal anastomosis by median laparotomy.

D. Technique of Exposure and Reconstruction

I. Thoracoabdominal Bypass

The anastomosis at the thoracic aorta does not cause any special problems. A woven or monofilament 3-0 suture is used. Woven prosthetic material is preferred. Usually, the aorta is cross-clamped proximally and distally so that a short segment is totally occluded on both sides. The anastomosis is performed on the anterior wall (Fig. 12.13a). Sometimes, lateral partial clamping may be adequate (Fig. 12.1.3b). After leakage at the anastomosis has stopped, the prosthesis is pulled through the diaphragmatic hiatus downward into the abdomen. In separate thoracic and abdominal approaches, a channel is created on the left side of the aorta through the diaphragm and the retroperitoneum posterior to the pancreas (Fig. 12.1.3c).

The distal end-to-side anastomosis to the abdominal aorta is performed in the infrarenal aortic

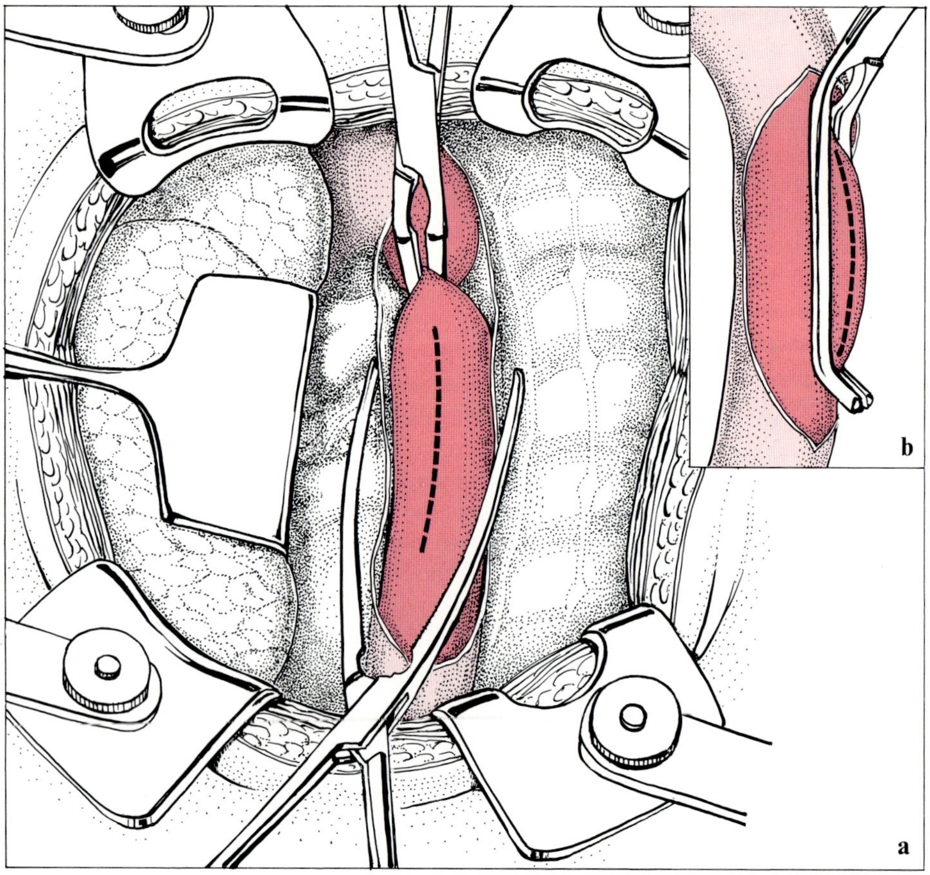

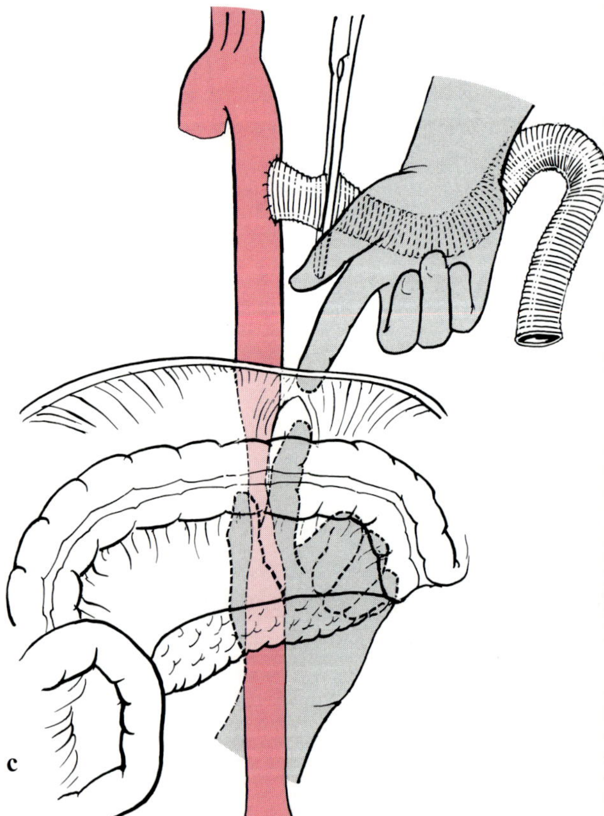

Fig. 12.1.3a–e. Thoracoabdominal revascularization (separate thoracic and abdominal approaches). **a** Total proximal and distal occlusion of the thoracic aorta for proximal anastomosis to its anterior wall. **b** Longitudinal clamping of the thoracic aorta for proximal lateral anastomosis. **c** Dissection of the diaphragm for retroperitoneal placement of the prosthesis. **d** Distal anastomosis to the infrarenal aortic segment. **e** The ascending aorta may also be chosen for the thoracic anastomosis (following a median sternotomy approach)

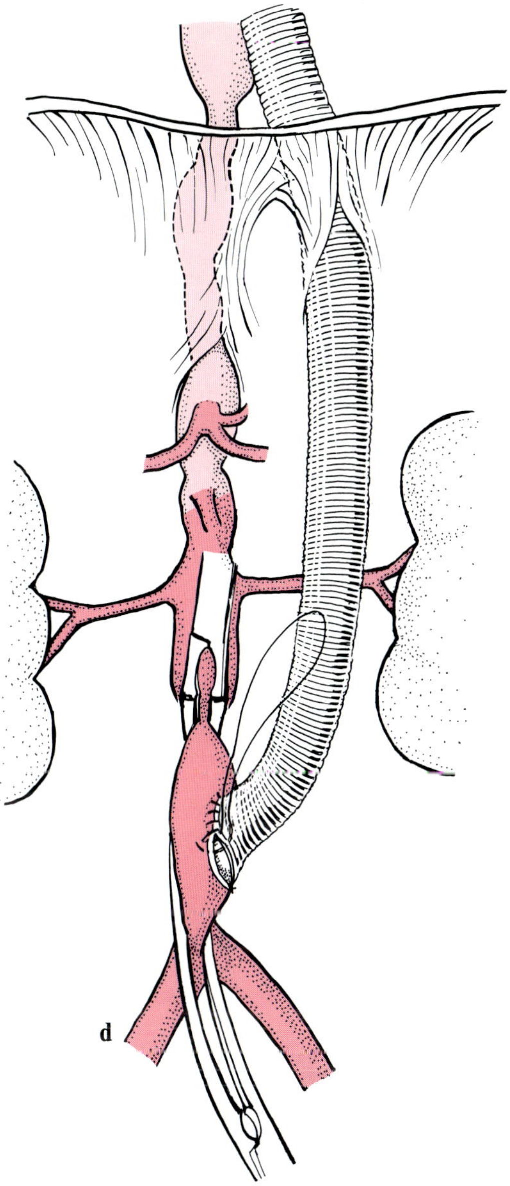

d

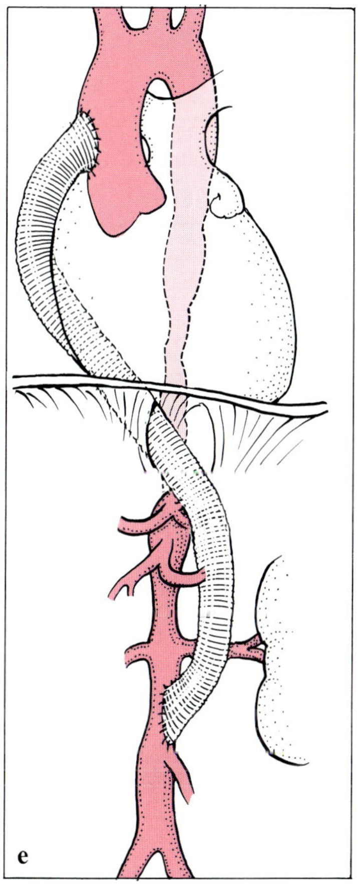

e

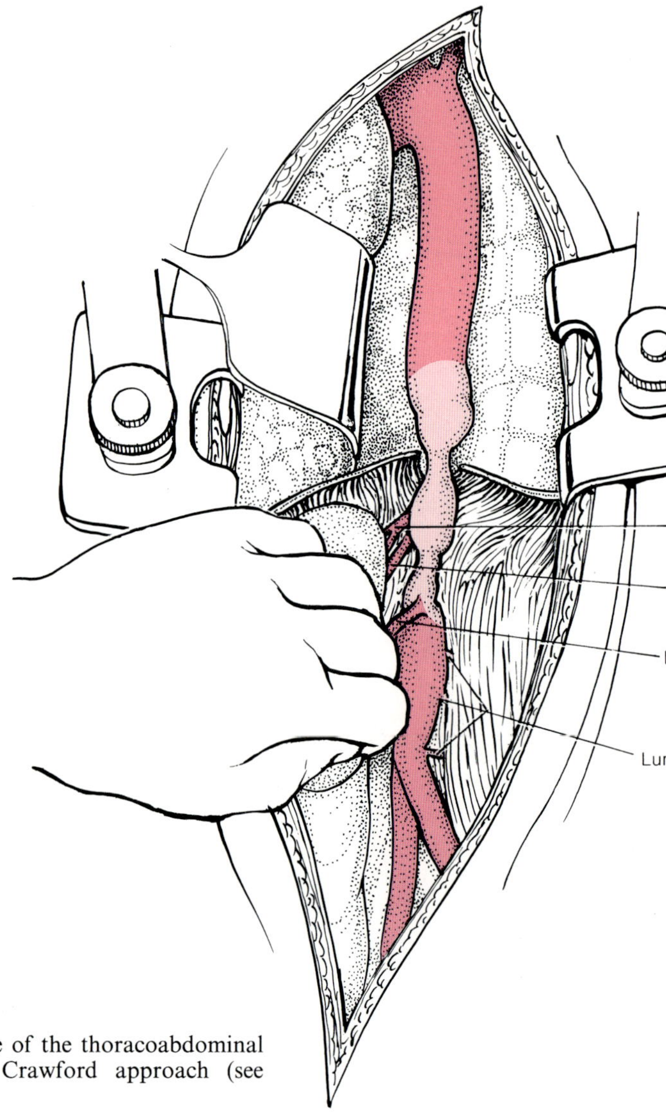

Fig. 12.1.4 The best exposure of the thoracoabdominal aorta is achieved by the Crawford approach (see Fig. 12.1.2a)

segment, i.e., segment V (Fig. 12.1.3d). If the lumen of the aorta is of normal width, a partial section of its wall may be clamped longitudinally. However, in this segment the aorta is often slightly hypoplastic or its walls are thickened. Then, total cross-clamping with a straight, angled, or curved aortic occlusion clamp proximal and distal to the site of anastomosis is preferred. Depending on how far distally the lesions extend, the iliac arteries or femoral arteries may have to be connected to the aorta with a bifurcation prosthesis. We have had to perform such a distal connection in only 2 of 19 patients.

A transdiaphragmatic channel must also be created for an ascending abdominal bypass (Fig. 12.1.3e). This maneuver is not necessary in the Crawford approach, which offers the best exposure of the thoracoabdominal aorta (Fig. 12.1.4; see pp. 314, 356).

II. Renal Artery Anastomosis

The technique for revascularization of the renal arteries is the same as for surgical management of renovascular hypertension (see p. 616 ff.). If normal renal perfusion is guaranteed by the diversion of blood to the infrarenal aorta, a simple thoracoabdominal bypass is sufficient. It is also adequate if no hemodynamically significant stenosis obstructs retrograde aortic blood flow beneath or at the level of the renal arteries (interrenal or jux-

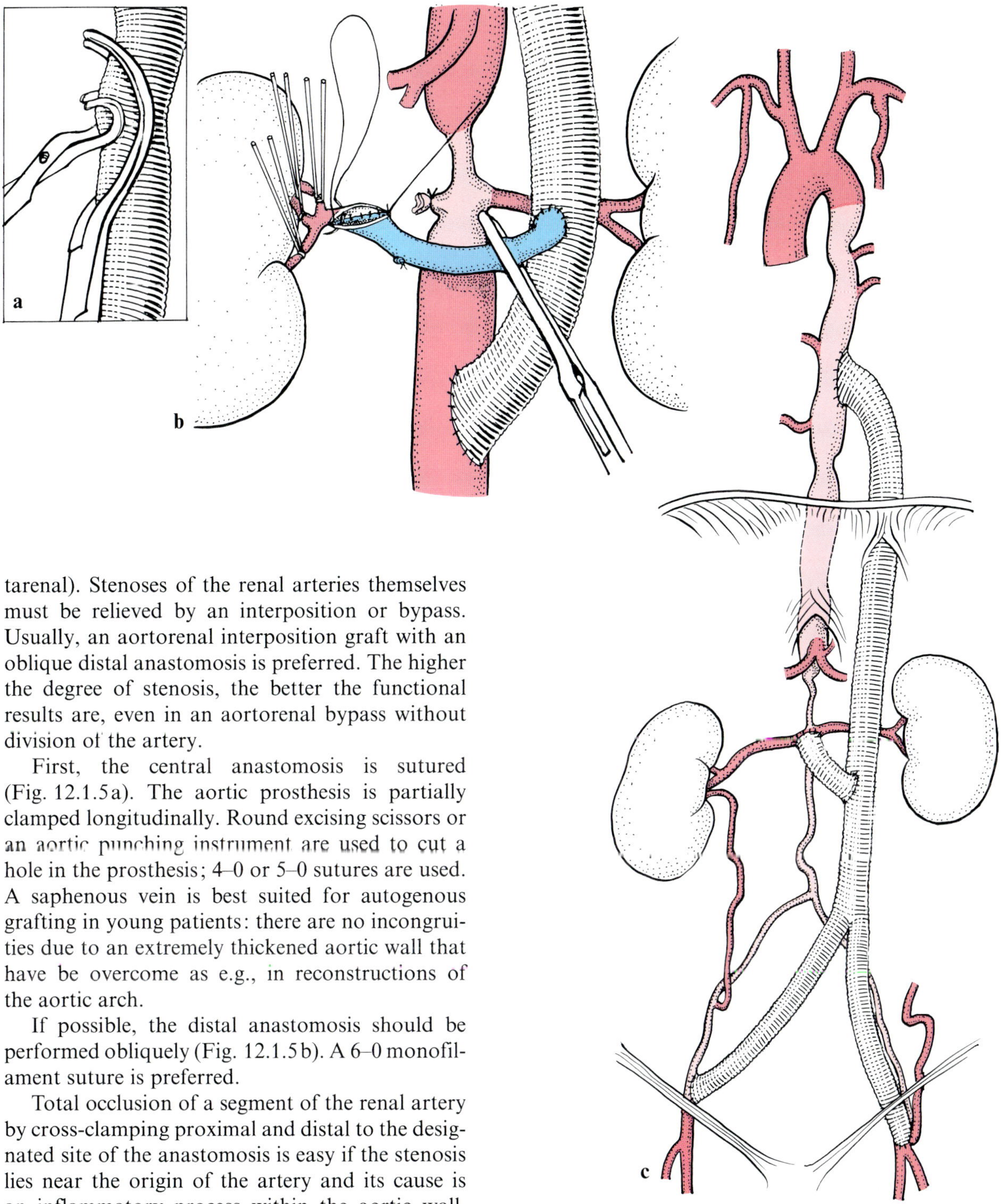

tarenal). Stenoses of the renal arteries themselves must be relieved by an interposition or bypass. Usually, an aortorenal interposition graft with an oblique distal anastomosis is preferred. The higher the degree of stenosis, the better the functional results are, even in an aortorenal bypass without division of the artery.

First, the central anastomosis is sutured (Fig. 12.1.5a). The aortic prosthesis is partially clamped longitudinally. Round excising scissors or an aortic punching instrument are used to cut a hole in the prosthesis; 4–0 or 5–0 sutures are used. A saphenous vein is best suited for autogenous grafting in young patients: there are no incongruities due to an extremely thickened aortic wall that have be overcome as e.g., in reconstructions of the aortic arch.

If possible, the distal anastomosis should be performed obliquely (Fig. 12.1.5b). A 6–0 monofilament suture is preferred.

Total occlusion of a segment of the renal artery by cross-clamping proximal and distal to the designated site of the anastomosis is easy if the stenosis lies near the origin of the artery and its cause is an inflammatory process within the aortic wall. If the stenosis lies within a peripheral portion of the renal artery, well-soaked, pliable catgut threads are placed around the segmental arteries and tightened.

Bilateral renal artery stenoses are revascularized on both sides during the same operation, e.g.,

Fig. 12.1.5a–c. Connection of the renal arteries. **a** Excision of the prosthesis for the central anastomosis. **b** In long renal artery stenoses, a wide peripheral anastomosis is performed. **c** Possible connection of both renal arteries by a common prosthetic interposition graft with a common prosthetic interposition graft (see p. 619).

The special techniques of renal artery revascularization are individually adapted to the many different variations of vascular diseases. In a 23-year-old patient we were able to revascularize both renal arteries by connecting them to an unstenosed juxtarenal aortic segment (Fig. 12.1.5c). The correction of a renal artery stenosis by percutaneous angioplastic dilatation must be considered [10] (see p. 121); however, we always prefer additional revascularization during the same operation.

III. Techniques of Interposition

Replacement and also direct enlargement of the back wall of the stenotic aorta is technically possible only by the Crawford approach. This means that the distal anastomosis is sutured onto the stenosed segment as in patch graft angioplasty (Fig. 12.1.6). The best way of preventing back bleeding from the organ arteries (renal arteries, celiac artery, superior mesenteric artery) is the in-

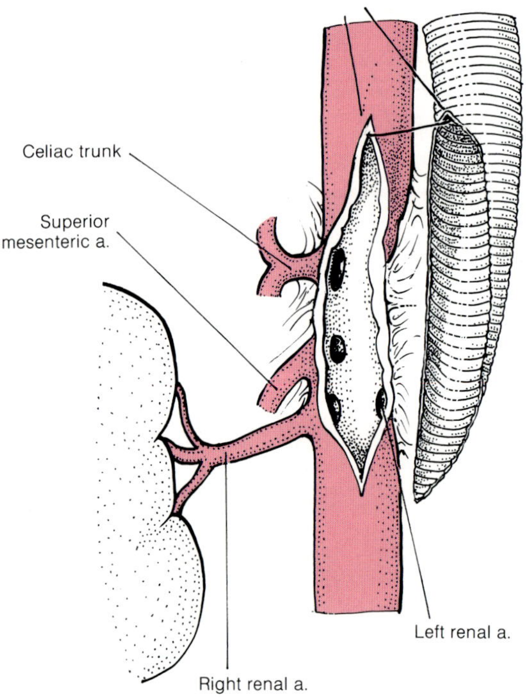

Fig. 12.1.6. Distal anastomosis similar to patch graft angioplasty in segments IV and possibly V

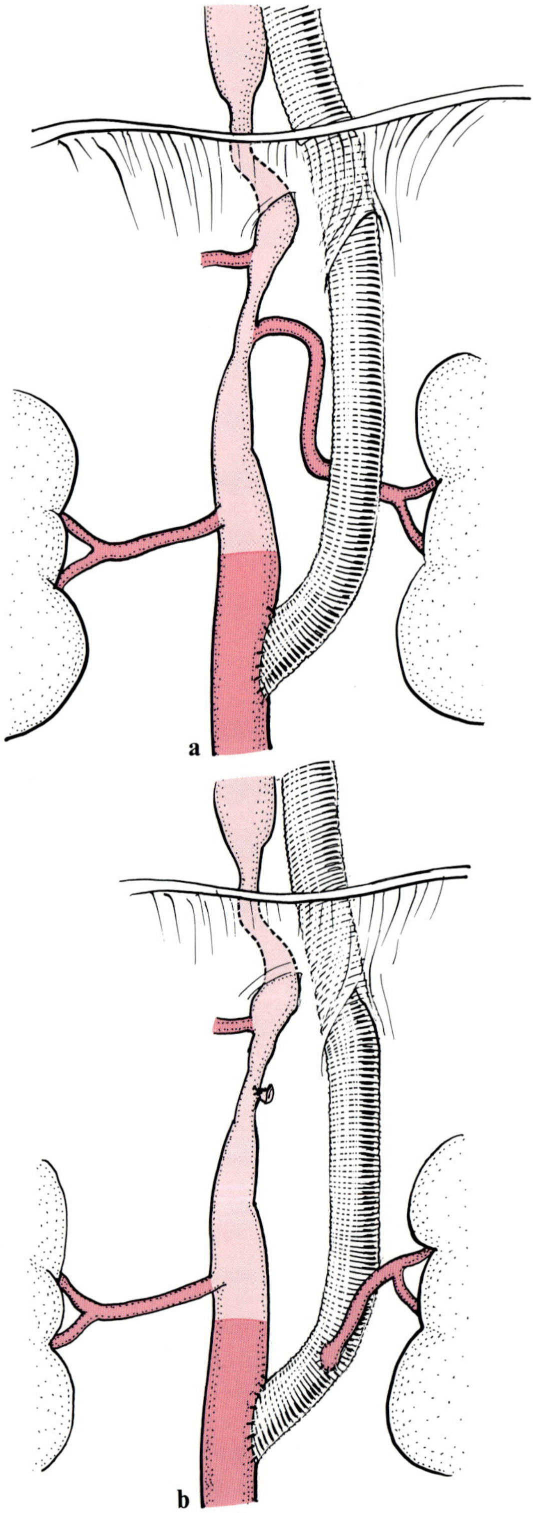

Fig. 12.1.7. **a** Persistent renovascular hypertension following aortoaortic bypass. Diminished blood flow to the left kidney remaining in spite of throcoabdominal pressure equalization. **b** Reimplantation of the left renal artery into the prosthetic bypass graft

sertion of a Fogarty balloon catheter following local heparinization.

If it is not possible to revascularize the stenotic region using this technique, all the arteries of each organ must be connected to the prosthesis separately. In such a case, the aorta may be replaced by an interposition graft instead of a bypass graft. Graft interposition is especially preferred if the lesion shows aneurysmal enlargement [1]. However, all of our 19 patients had only stenotic lesions.

It is rarely necessary to revascularize the celiac artery or the superior mesenteric artery [5]. This is why the technique of direct enlargement, using an oblique distal anastomosis similar to a patch graft, is preferred. If prosthetic replacement of the aorta is necessary, the visceral arteries should be reimplanted into the prosthesis with a large cuff of anterior aortic wall tissue around them (see p. 318).

E. Reintervention

Persistent high blood pressure is caused by residual or newly developed impairment of renal blood supply (Fig. 12.1.7a). However, hypertension caused by parenchymal disease of the kidney may already have been present during the primary operation. Another possibility is that an additional, functionally significant stenosis may not have been revascularized. Angiographic methods as well as the direct or indirect measurement of renin release may answer the question whether a functionally significant stenosis is present, which would be an indication for reoperation. In some cases the reimplantation of a renal artery (Fig. 12.1.7b), an aortorenal interposition, or an iliorenal bypass may lead to normalization of perfusion.

The treatment of anostomotic aneurysms is described in Chap. 10.3.

REFERENCES

1. Crawford ES, Crawford JL (1985) Diseases of the aorta. Williams and Wilkins, Baltimore London
2. Denecke H (1979) Renovaskulärer Hochdruck. Klinische Untersuchungen zur Spätprognose nach operativer Behandlung und tierexperimentelle Studien zu intrazellulären Elektrolytkonzentrationen. Med Habil (München)
3. Heberer G, Schildberg FW, Becker HM, Stelter WJ, Zumtobel V (1975) Die typische suprarenale Aortenstenose als Ursache eines juvenilen Hypertonus. Dtsch Med Wochenschr 100:649
4. Hejhal L, Heinal J, Firt P (1973) Coarctation of the abdominal aorta. J Cardiovasc Surg 14:168
5. Liu Y-Q, Diu J-H (1984) Aorta-Arteritis: a collective angiographic experience 244 cases. Inter Angio 3:487
6. Lupi-Herrera E, Sanchez-Torres G, Marenshamer J, Misireta J, Horwitz S, Vela JE (1977) Takayasu's arteritis. Clinical study of 107 cases. Am Heart J 93:94
7. Marooka S, Ito I, Yamaguchi H, Takeda T, Saito Y (1972) Follow-up observation of aortitis syndrome. Japn Heart J 13:201
8. Saveuse N, Goupil-Colliard M, Bacourt F, Tscherdakoff P (1983) Coarctations de l'aortae abdominale: diagnostic, pathogénie, treitement médical ou chirurgical. Presse Med 12:1475
9. Scott HW, Dean RH, Boerth R, Sawyers JL, Meacham P, Fisher D (1979) Coarctation of the abdominal aorta. Ann Surg 189:746
10. Tan AT, Chia BL, Tan LK, Gwee HM (1983) Successful angioplasty of renal artery stenosis due to aorto-arteritis. Cardiology 70:213
11. Ueno A, Avane Y, Wakabayachi A, Shimuzu K (1967) Successful operated obliterative brachiocephalic arteritis (Takayasu) associated with the elongated coarctation. Jpn Heart J 8:538

12.2 Congenital Malformations of the Iliofemoral Artery

J. GREEBE and R.J.A.M. VAN DONGEN

CONTENTS

A. Embryology

In order to understand congenital malformations of the iliofemoral artery, some preliminary remarks on the embryologic development are in order. The first vessels originate from a preexisting vascular network [4]. These unite to form several vascular trunks of different caliber [5, 11].

From the umbilical artery, which is a branch of the dorsal aorta, a tributary develops, the so-called axial artery, which runs down the dorsal side of the embryo lateral to the sciatic nerve (Fig. 12.2.1). At a later stage, the axial artery can be divided into three segments: a proximal (sciatic artery), a middle (deep popliteal artery), and a distal segment (the embryonic interosseal artery). Later, the external iliac artery arises from the umbilical artery proximal to the origin of the axial artery (Fig. 12.2.2).

The inferior epigastric artery and the proximal portion of the femoral artery arise from the external iliac artery. A large trunk, which develops from the ventrally located femoral network, comprises the middle portion of the femoral artery (Fig. 12.2.2). Its distal portion evolves from the superior communicating branch, running back through the hiatus tendineus (Fig. 12.2.2).

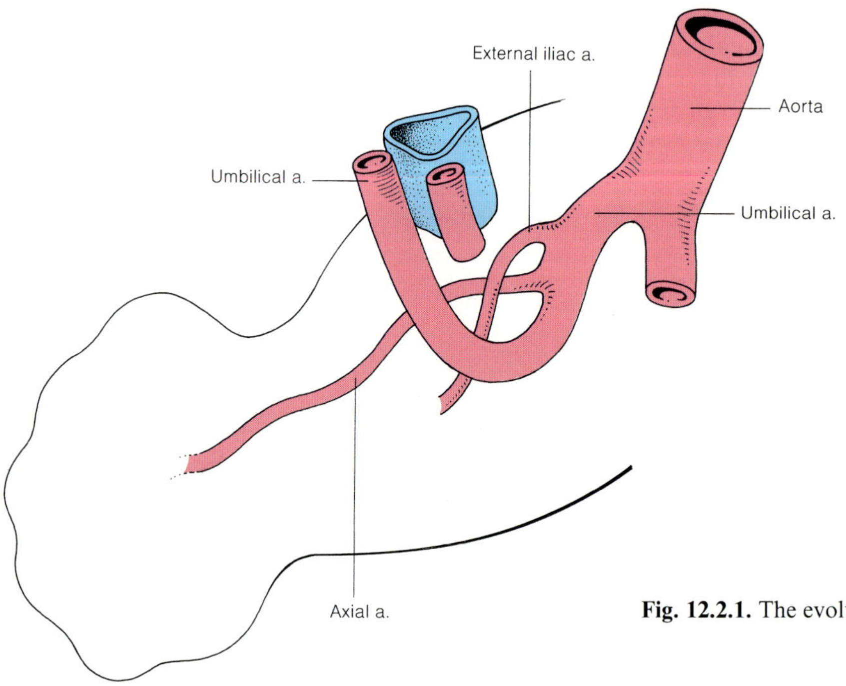

Fig. 12.2.1. The evolution of the iliofemoral artery

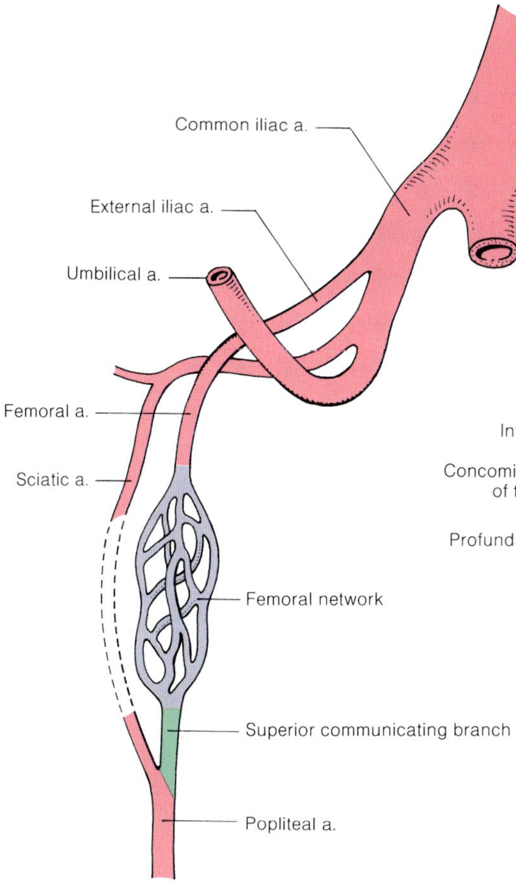

Fig. 12.2.2. The development of the iliofemoral artery

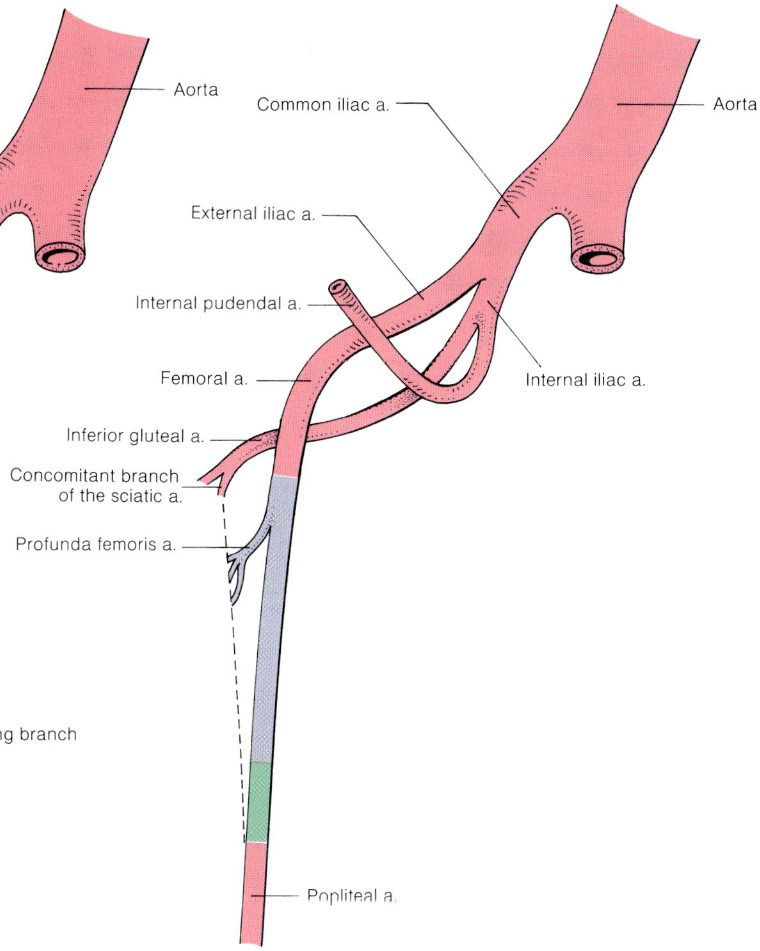

Fig. 12.2.3. The formation of the adult iliofemoral artery

A second large branch of the femoral artery, the profunda femoris artery, arises from the femoral network. Its terminal branches form the network of the sciatic artery. The greater part of this artery disappears during the formation of the femoral vessels (Fig. 12.2.3).

The proximal portion of the sciatic artery remains, forming the inferior gluteal artery, together with the concomitant branch of the sciatic nerve. The deep popliteal artery develops into the proximal portion of the adult popliteal artery later on.

Following birth, as soon as blood circulation through the placenta is interrupted, the caliber of the internal iliac artery decreases. Thereafter the external iliac artery is the direct continuation of the common iliac artery.

B. Special Pathologic Anatomy

Numerous congenital arterial anomalies in the pelvic region and the lower extremities are reported in the literature [10, 12]. Only three anomalies lead to clinical symptoms [1, 3, 5, 6, 7, 8, 9]. These are:

a) Aplasia: The artery is totally absent (Fig. 12.2.4)
b) Atresia: The artery is present, but it has no lumen. Only a solid vascular cord exists (Fig. 12.2.5).
c) Hypoplasia: The artery is present and has a lumen, which is extremely narrow (Fig. 12.2.6).

Combinations of these three types may be found in the same patient (Fig. 12.2.7).

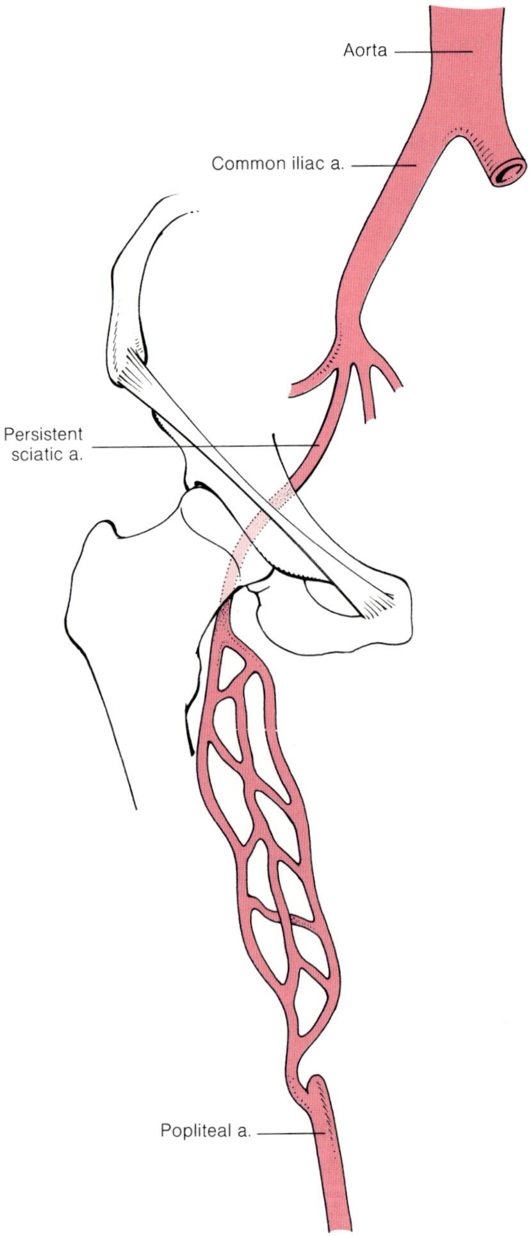

Fig. 12.2.4. Aplasia of the iliofemoral artery

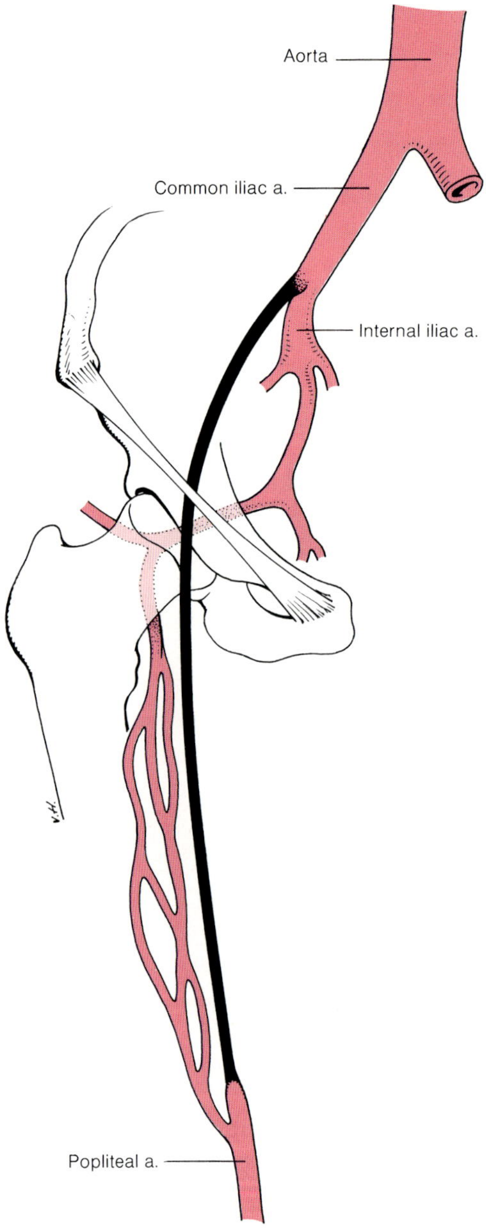

Fig. 12.2.5. Atresia of the iliofemoral artery

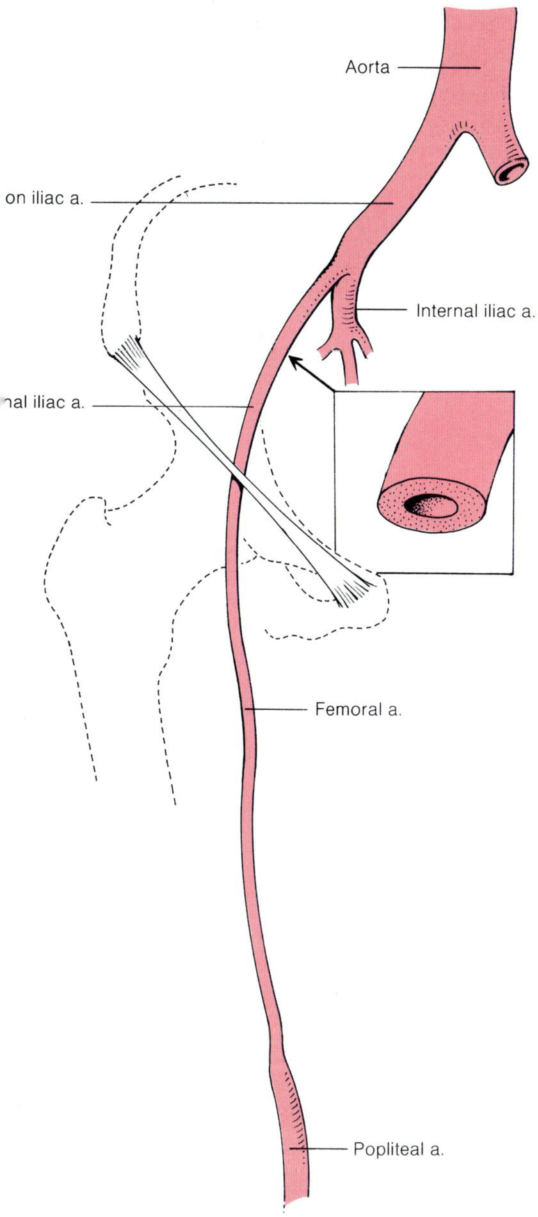

Fig. 12.2.6. Hypoplasia of the iliofemoral artery

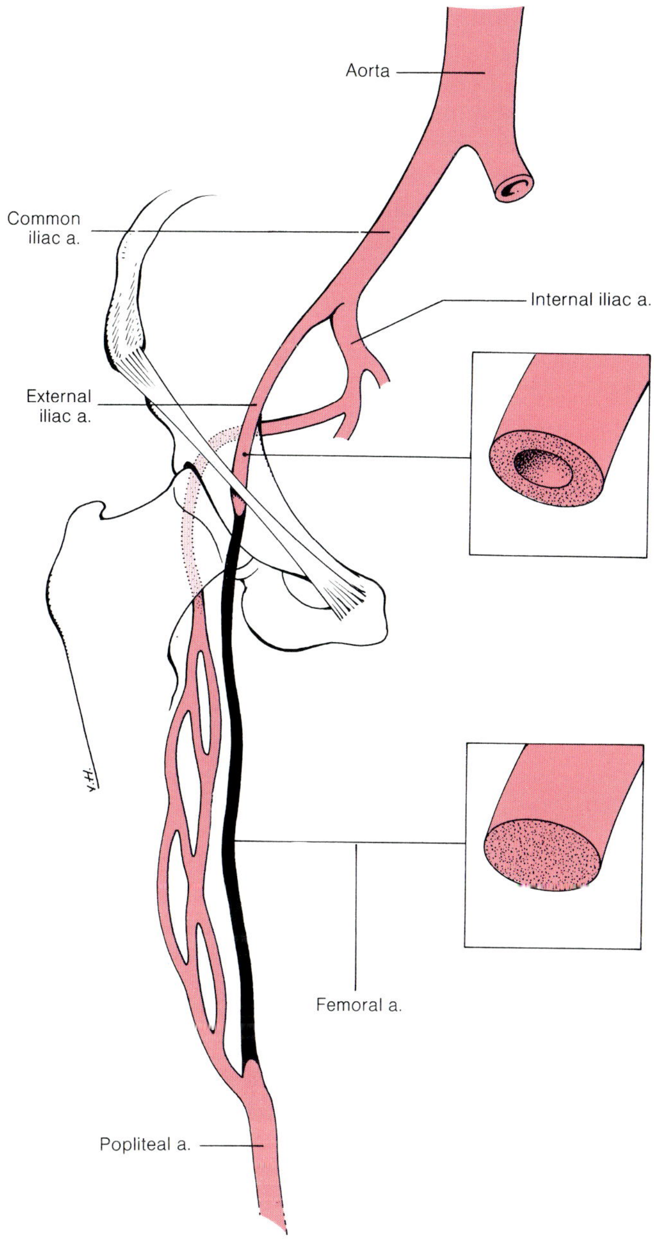

Fig. 12.2.7. Hypoplasia of the external iliac artery and atresia of the femoral artery

C. Indications for Reconstructive Procedures

The indication for operative reconstruction depends on the clinical picture. If an anomaly is discovered by chance and the patient is asymptomatic, operative correction is not indicated.

Clinical stages III and IV are absolute indications for surgery.

Stage II disease may make a reconstruction necessary, depending on the extent of the anomaly and shortening of the leg, walking disability, and the age of the patient. In cases of severe anomaly or shortening, reconstruction may be indicated even in young patients. If only slight intermittent claudication is present, a reconstructive procedure may be postponed until the patient reaches adulthood.

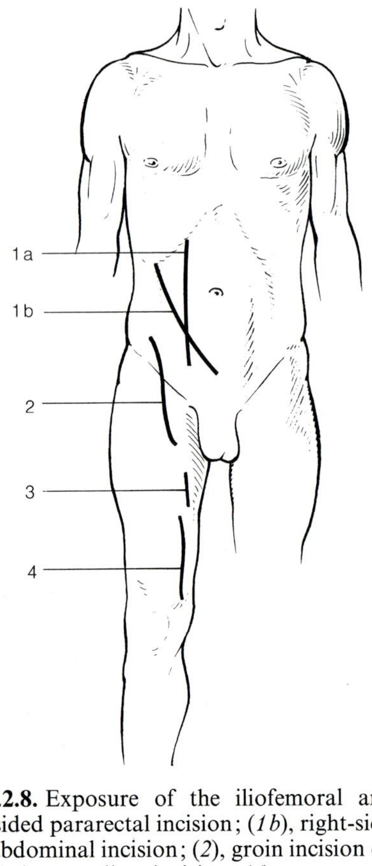

Fig. 12.2.8. Exposure of the iliofemoral artery. (*1a*), Right-sided pararectal incision; (*1b*), right-sided oblique lower abdominal incision; (*2*), groin incision on the right side; (*3*), intermediate incision; (*4*), supragenual incision

Fig. 12.2.9. Topography of the common and internal ▷ iliac arteries with the external artery missing

D. Surgical Approach and Exposure

Surgical approach and exposure of the iliac artery and femoral artery are described in Chap. 17.5.D. (see p. 379, 380, 392; Fig. 12.2.8).

Aplasia or other forms of congenital anomaly may be ascertained only following exposure of the area involved.

In aplasia, no arterial rudiments whatsoever are found (Fig. 12.2.9). In atresia, a thin solid cord with no lumen is present instead of a normal artery (Fig. 12.2.10). In hypoplasia the artery is very small and has a very narrow lumen. Atretic or hypoplastic vessels are never located ectopically.

E. Reconstructive Techniques

Only bypass methods may be considered in vascular malformations of the iliofemoral artery. They do not differ from those applied in multilevel occlusions (see p. 432, Chap. 17.5). Preferably, the undeveloped vascular segments are bridged with a great saphenous vein graft. Such an autogenous vein graft grows together with the rest of the body and is therefore the material most suitable for use in young patients.

Because a long graft is needed for replacement between the aorta or common iliac artery and the

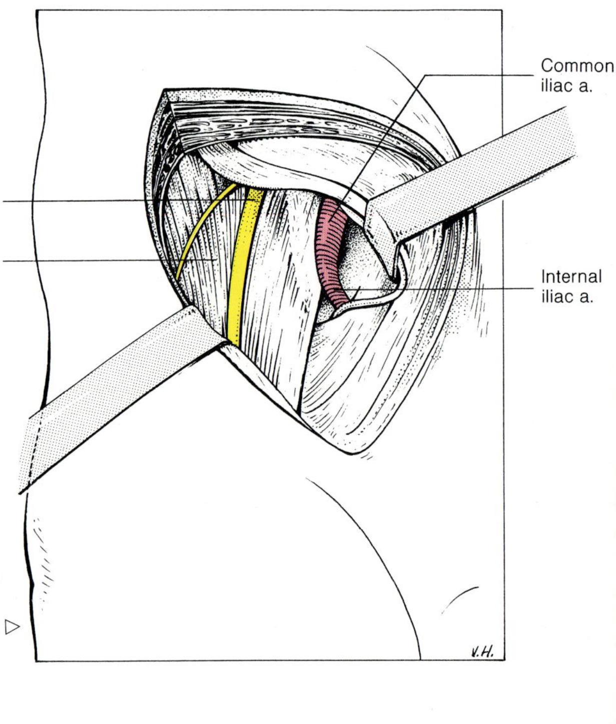

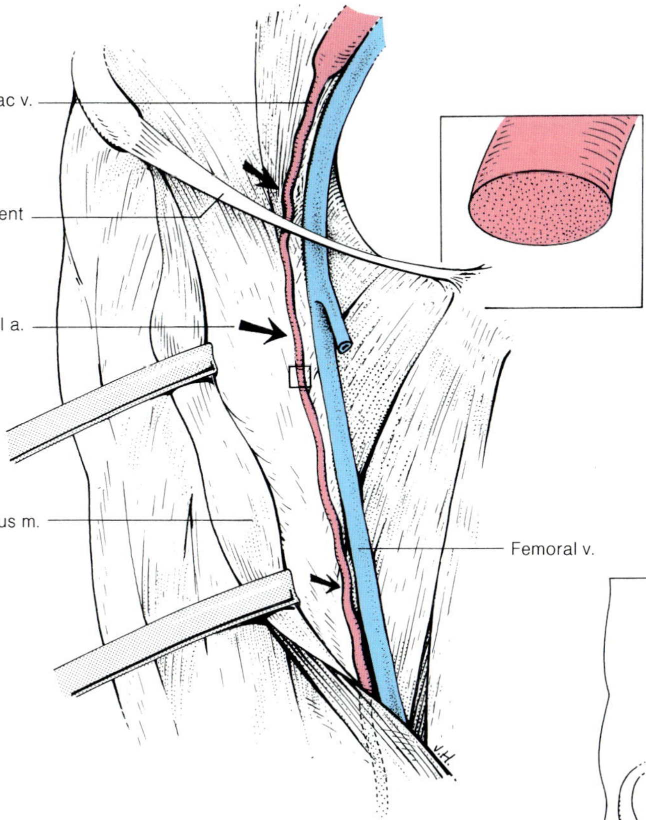

Fig. 12.2.10. Topography of the atretic iliofemoral artery

Fig. 12.2.11. Iliopopliteal bypass composed of two great ▷ saphenous veins with a patch graft

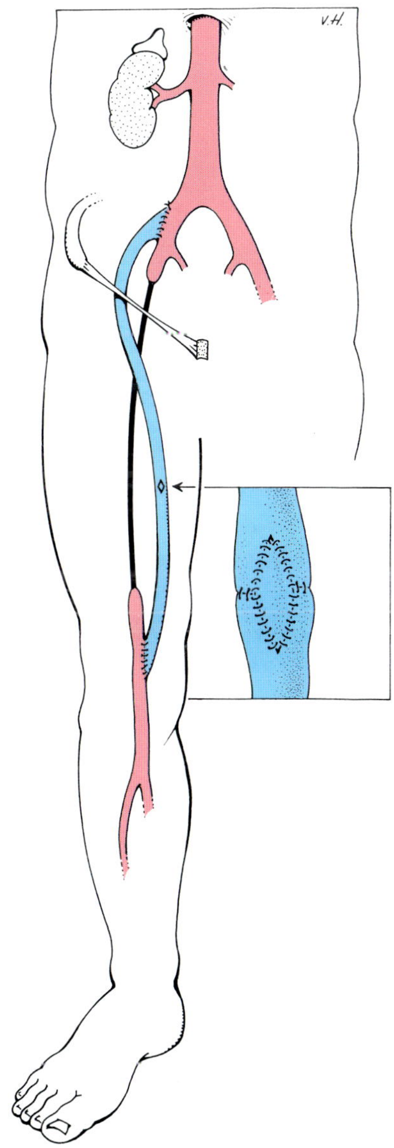

popliteal artery, it is often necessary to combine the great saphenous vein of both legs in a single graft (oblique end-to-end anastomosis or right-angled end-to-end anastomosis with patch graft) (Fig. 12.1.11) [2].

If the great saphenous veins are not suited for total bypass, a composite bypass must be employed to reconstruct the iliac segment with alloplastic or homologous material. The femoral segment sould always be reconstructed with autogenous material, if possible.

If no autogenous material is available, the entire length of the undeveloped artery must be bridged with a synthetic prosthesis.

If arterial reconstruction is not possible, an attempt should be made to compensate incongruities in limb length. In young patients, stapling of the distal femur epiphysis may be performed to inhibit growth of the healthy leg. In adults, orthopedic techniques for reducing limb length may be considered.

REFERENCES

1. Cowie ThH, the Hellar NJ, the Lean N, Smith G (1960) Unilateral congenital absences of the external and femoral arteries. Br J Radiol 33:520
2. van Dongen RJAM (1970) A photographic atlas of reconstructive arterial surgery. Springer, Berlin Heidelberg New York
3. Dumanian AV, Frahm CHJ, Benchik FA, Wooden ThF (1965) Intermittent claudication secondary to congenital absence of iliac arteries. Arch Surg 91:604
4. Evans HM (1909) On the development of the aorta, cardinal and umbilical veins and the other blood vessels of vertebral embryos from capillaries. Anat Rec 3:498
5. Greebe J (1977) Congenital anomalies of the iliofemoral artery. J Cardiovasc Surg 18:317–323
6. Howard JM, Gaudelock WJ, Couwes CM (1957) Congenital atresia of the external iliac artery. Arch Surg 75:296
7. Kunst AB (1971) Hypoplasia van de arteria iliofemoralis. NTv G 115:307
8. Kunst AB, Zimmermann AE (1970) Congenital hypoplasia of the iliofemoral artery. J Cardiovasc Surg 11:393
9. Rob CG, Owen K (1958) Congenital hypoplasia of the iliac arteries. Postgrad Med J 34:391
10. Senior HD (1918/1919) An interpretation of the recorded arterial anomalies of the human leg and foot. J Anat 53:130
11. Senior HD (1919) The development of the arteries of the human lower extremity. Am J Anat 25:55
12. Senior HD (1925) An interpretation of the recorded arterial anomalies of the human pelvis and thigh. Am J Anat 36:1

12.3 Congenital Arterial and Arteriovenous Dysplasia

R.J.A.M. VAN DONGEN

CONTENTS

A. Introduction

Angiodysplasias are a combination of several different congenital malformations. They are polydysplasias with arterial, venous, capillary, and lymphatic components. Pathologic changes involve not only the vascular systems, but all other tissues as well: skin, connective tissues, bones, cartilage, and nerves. The classification of the different clinical pictures is based mainly on the vascular system predominant in each type of angiodysplasia [10, 11, 13, 16, 19].

The treatment of angiodysplastic anomalies is sometimes palliative, symptomatic, or cosmetic (reduction of the difference in length between the limbs, surgery of varices, extirpation of hemangiomas, lymphangiomas, and other vascular and connective tissue proliferations localized on the body's surface). Most therapeutic measures are focused on the arterial components of the anomaly, on arterial hypervascularization, vascular proliferations, and especially on pathologic arteriovenous shunts. The aim of treatment is not only to eliminate active arteriovenous fistulas and vascular proliferations by resecting and inducing obliteration, but also to minimize hypervascularization. These therapeutic measures are not suited to angiodysplastic changes that are limited to the venous system.

B. Indications for Treatment

Angiodysplastic malformations with involvement of the arterial system may be treated by percutaneous or operative measures, whether or not dysplastic arteries, hemangiomatous proliferations, hypervascularization, or arteriovenous shunts are present.

Treatment is especially important in hemodynamically significant arteriovenous shunts, as in the F.P. Weber syndrome. Vascular malformations in this syndrome cause growth disorders (gigantism) and may lead to monstrous malformations and malfunctions of the limbs. Compression with subsequent injury of the neighboring nerves may sometimes cause intolerable pain. Arteriovenous shunts may have considerable effects on total body circulation, with possible cardiac and vascular decompensation. Sometimes, skin ulcers develop from the pressure of underlying phlebectasias. Reduced perfusion of the distal portions of the limbs may lead to gangrene. Angiomatous proliferations may destroy connective tissue and bone to such an extent that a malignancy is mistakenly assumed. Sometimes amputation is the only way of relieving the patient's suffering [9].

The treatment of congenital malformations is indicated in all cases in which arteriovenous shunts have led to these complications. The most important goal is to normalize the patient's hemodynamic state and to reduce the shunt volume by eliminating the arteriovenous shunts.

However, measures to eliminate asymptomatic, hemodynamically significant arteriovenous fistulas and dysplastic vessels are also indicated. No effective conservative treatment and no spontaneous cure exist. On the contrary, the vascular proliferations have an unpredictable tendency to progress, with the risk of later complications such as skin ulcers, gangrene, or nerve injuries. Once such complications have occurred, the prospect for complete cure is poor.

Treatment should begin as soon as possible. The longer one waits, the more extensive the satellite circulation and the destruction of the involved tissue will be. Early treatment minimizes secondary changes such as gigantism.

In mixed angiodysplasias of the extremities venous and lymphatic malformations occur, together with dysplasia of the arteries. In such cases not all arteries of the extremity are altered pathologically. Usually, only a single artery, e.g., one of the three lower leg arteries, shows pathologic changes. Obliteration of this single artery and all of its branches may be indicated, whether or not arteriovenous fistulas are demonstrable.

C. Preoperative Examinations

Quantitative measurement of shunt volume is essential for determining whether or not hemodynamically significant arteriovenous fistulas are present. This can be done by any isotope laboratory. Comparisons of the two limbs with respect to venous oxygen saturation should always be performed, but the results may not always allow an accurate assessment of the magnitude of the shunting. Other examinations, such as Doppler ultrasonography, venous occlusion, plethysmography, thermography, thermodilution, or isotope clearance methods likewise fail to yield a clear-cut assessment. Cardiac examinations, such as measurement of the cardiac minute volume and stroke volume, should not be omitted.

Arteriograms of high quality are an essential precondition for every kind of treatment, particularly when embolization therapy is intended. The importance of carefully performed arteriographic investigation cannot be overemphasized. It is essential to delineate the precise nature and extent of disease and to know precisely the anatomic situation of the clew of vessels. It is essential to know which branches must be excised or obliterated and which vessels have to be preserved to prevent ischemic damage, especially where malformations of the face, the feet and hands, or the toes and fingers are concerned. Visualization of details, optimal sharpness, dense opacification and right projection are required. The main arteries of the forearm and lower leg must be visualized separately.

Arteriograms showing a mass of abnormal, tortuous, and dilated arteries and veins cluttering the affected area, with accumulation of the contrast medium in area of the fistulas, are interesting pictures and may give an impression of the extent of the lesion, but such arteriograms are useless for performing an embolization because it is impossible to see any anatomic detail.

Selective, often superselective filling is necessary, and for the study of the anatomic situation the exposures in the early phase of filling are especially important. Each branch must be visualized in full anatomic detail. It must be possible to make an anatomic analysis of the complex circulatory pattern. The study of the distribution of the feeding vessels and of the vessels of the malformation itself is possible only if in the early seconds after the injection of the dye, a rapid series is made with at least three exposures to the second.

Some other measures contribute to a better insight into the anatomic situation:

- The projection must be such that the topography is clearly visualized (lower arm in supination, lower leg in internal rotation, hand and foot lying flat on the X-ray table, foot also visualized in a lateral projection).
- Stereoscopic pictures or X-rays in different projections allow for a better assessment of the morphological conditions.
- The angiodysplastic area resembles a blood sponge! A relatively large amount of contrast medium must be injected under high pressure.
- In order not to miss the early arterial phase, the X-ray sequence should be started before the contrast medium reaches the dysplastic area.
- Arteriographic X-rays of the inflow tract arter-

ies and the neighboring vascular regions are necessary.

Needless to say, digital subtraction angiograms are unfit for use. It is impossible to see any details, and it is also impossible to decide on the ground of DSA pictures which branches have to be eliminated. Conventional arteriograms are required.

D. Methods of Treatment

In the past, many operative procedures have been suggested. Only one of these may be termed curative. Some others have palliative value. Most of them are senseless.

I. Total Extirpation

The only curative therapy available is total excision of the entire angiodysplastic vascular convolution, with all of its arteriovenous shunts. But such a treatment is only rarely possible, e.g., in the racemose angioma of the scalp. In such cases, ligation of the feeding arteries (frontal artery, supraorbital artery, temporal artery, posterior auricular artery, and occipital artery) on both sides, and extirpation of all ectatic fistulous vessels will bring about a definitive cure. In localized tumorous angiodysplastic lesions of other body regions, total extirpation also leads to cure [11].

II. Interruption of the Afferent Arteries

Ligature of the afferent arteries is a senseless procedure. Unfortunately, it is still performed. Even if arteriography shows that dysplastic and arteriovenous vascular changes are fed by only a single artery, ligation of this artery will be useless. Neighboring arteries take over perfusion of the angiodysplastic region through collaterals in only a short time. In arteriovenous dysplasia within the area of a lower arm or lower leg artery an additional distal ligature is usually recommended, which, of course, has no effect whatsoever on the results. Ligature of a main artery in the shoulder, upper arm, pelvic, or thigh areas is sometimes performed. Such a procedure is absolutely useless and should be regarded as a therapeutic mistake [2, 12, 15].

III. Operations on the Venous System

Surgery on the venous drainage system (removal of varices, sclerotherapy, ligation of veins, and other operations on the efferent side of the angiodysplastic area) do not substantially influence shunt volume and beyond this have only a transient effect. Such procedures are useless. The removal of varicose veins is a cosmetic operation. In such cases one must expect the formation of new phlebectasias within a short time after surgery.

IV. Skeletation of the Main Vessels

In the last 10 years, a method called the "skeletation operation," suggested by Malan [12] and propagated by Vollmar [20], has often been applied in congenital arteriovenous dysplasias of the extremities. All branches of the main artery and vein within the vascular anomaly are ligated and eventually divided. Blood supply to the angiomatous tissue is not reduced because collaterals develop from the neighboring body regions. These take over the perfusion of the tissue and of the fistulous convolution as well, which remains unchanged. Although shunt volume is reduced by extensive skeletation of a long segment of the main vessel immediately following the operation, it only takes a few weeks or months until blood supply to the fistulous vessels is furnished by neighboring or even sometimes remote body parts, thus leading to a second rise in shunt volume [3, 5]. Growth of the malformation progresses because not only new arterial collaterals, but also venous ones are formed. Superficial varicose veins spread out. Sometimes clinical symptoms also increase. Then, further skeletation of the proximal and distal vascular regions is performed. The result, again, is only temporary. In the long run, the results of skeletation alone are unsatisfactory.

An additional disadvantage of this method is that it can only be applied in larger limb arteries. Skeletation of lower arm and lower leg arteries demands great preparatory effort, and the results are disappointing. Arteriovenous fistulas in other body regions are not at all suited to this kind of treatment.

V. Resection of the Main Artery and Replacement by a Prosthesis or Graft

An alternative to skeletation is the resection of a long segment of a main artery and its replacement by a prosthesis (subclavian artery, common and external iliac arteries) or a venous graft (brachial artery, femoropopliteal artery) [9]. In this procedure, not only are the feeding branches arising from the main artery eliminated, but the formation of new vessels (vasa vasorum? small overlooked branches?) which, following skeletation, branch off from the main artery in the vicinity of the malformation is also prevented. However, collaterals from neighboring vascular regions develop quickly, so that this method of treatment is not superior to others.

VI. Percutaneous Catheter Embolization

Percutaneous catheter embolization makes it possible to occlude the vessels of a pathologically altered area, excluding the entire dysplastic vascular lesion from systemic blood circulation [6, 7, 8, 14, 15, 18]. This method, which has found general acceptance in the last few years, has the advantage of avoiding difficult and time-consuming operations and in most cases can be repeated in the event of recurrences. However, transcatheter embolization alone is of limited value. This method has several disadvantages and limitations:

1. It is not always possible to reach the feeding vessels of the angiodysplastic complex because of the presence of coils and kinks in the main trunk.
2. Most feeding vessels are of small, often microscopic size and cannot be selectively catheterized.
3. The embolizing particles cannot be brought deep enough into the nidus of the lesion.
4. The multiplicity of feeding vessels and arteriovenous connections makes it unlikely that all vessels of the pathologic process will be occluded.
5. The percutaneous procedure entails the inadvertent risk of distal reflux of particles, causing unintentional embolic occlusion of peripheral arteries.
6. Because the embolizing particles used in the transcatheter procedure are relatively small, they may pass through the large-sized arteriovenous connections.

Embolization will be successful if all feeding vessels and all vessels of the angiodysplastic bulk are eliminated, but this is not possible using the percutaneous technique alone. Every residual vessel of the malformation, every arteriovenous connection, will increase slowly in size, resulting in clinical recurrence. Using percutaneous embolization, only a partial obliteration is obtained. It is on a level with partial resection.

Transcatheter embolization may be useful in the treatment of arteriovenous malformations in locations such as the spinal cord and cerebral vessels, which are poorly treated by surgery.

The percutaneous technique has been recommended as a preoperative adjunct to decrease the vascularity of the lesion and facilitate subsequent surgical treatment. In many cases, however, transcatheter embolization destroys access routes for operative embolization because feeding vessels become blocked. Preoperative percutaneous embolization should be used chiefly when complete excision of the malformation is intended; only in exceptional cases should it be used prior to operative embolization.

VII. Operative Embolization, Combined Methods

In order to achieve satisfactory and long-lasting therapeutic results, it does not suffice to interrupt afferent and efferent vessels, i.e., to eliminate inflow and outflow. Neither is it sufficient merely to obliterate parts of the dysplastic vascular tumor by catheter embolization. The aim of treatment of arterial and arteriovenous dysplasia must be to eliminate all pathologic vessels, to exclude the entire arteriovenous convolution from the systemic circulation, and to obliterate the pathologic vessels of such an angiomatous conglomeration by inducing thrombosis.

1. Therapeutic Concept

The total therapeutic concept not only includes a combined operative technique, but also a percutaneous method (Fig. 12.3.1).

The surgical components of this concept are:

1. Extirpation of the dysplastic vessels and angiomatous tissue as extensively as is feasible
2. Embolic obliteration of all remaining vessels within the pathologic area through all feeding branches of the main artery
3. Skeletation of long segments of the main vessels

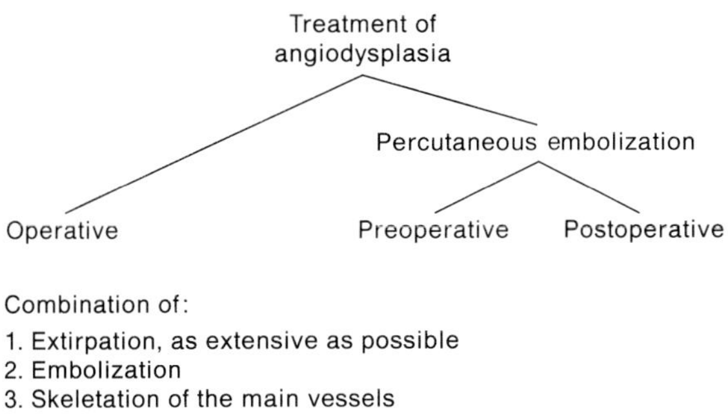

Fig. 12.3.1. Therapeutic algorithm of arterial and arteriovenous dysplasia

Sometimes percutaneous catheter embolization is performed preoperatively. Small solid particles are introduced into the feeding branches in order to obliterate as many of the small vessels of the angiomatous conglomerations as possible. This minimizes blood loss during subsequent surgery and resection of pathologic tissue. Beyond this, it facilitates the introduction of embolizing material during surgery through reduction of backward blood pressure, which allows the embolizing material to reach the smallest vessels in the center of the angiomatous convolution. If postoperative control arteriography demonstrates that angiomatous vessels are still patent, percutaneous embolization is repeated. Late recurrences are also obliterated by percutaneous catheter embolization.

2. Embolic Material

Various materials have been utilized as embolic agents, including autogenous blood clot, plastic and metallic microspheres, polyvinyl alcohol, gelatine sponge, tissue adhesive, and fibrin seal.

Gelatin sponge (Gelfoam) and autogenous blood clot made with epsilon amino caproic acid, have the disadvantage of being resorbable. They produce temporary occlusion for a period of weeks and are therefore unusuable.

Silicone polymer and the tissue adhesive isobutyl-2-cyano acrylate are permanent agents. However, the last agent polymerizes immediately on contact with blood, and it is impossible to ensure its travel into the core of the malformation. Silicone polymer injected into one feeding vessel may be washed out of the malformation by other supplying vessels and not retained in the nidus of the vessel clew.

Liquid materials like fibrin seal (Tissucol) are no longer used because of serious vascular and neurologic complications which may be caused by ischemic damage to peripheral tissues and nerves. Damage to the nerves is due to obliteration of the vasa nervorum, the vessel network around the nerves.

Coils and detachable balloons have also been used for permanent embolic occlusions, but they cannot be used for embolization of angiodysplastic malformations. They obliterate only the feeding vessels; they do not produce obliteration of the vascular elements of the pathological clew itself and the arteriovenous connections.

Embolic agents should fulfill the following requirements:

1. They should be nonresorbable to minimize the likelihood of vessel recanalization.
2. They should be biocompatible.
3. They should be able to enter into and ablate the interstices of the arteriovenous malformation.
4. They should not be liquid.

Polyvinyl alcohol (Ivalon) and silicone microspheres are permanent agents with proven inert properties, satisfying all prerequisites. We currently use only Ivalon foam suspended in a syringe with diluted contrast medium and silicone microspheres with diameter 1–4 mm put into a container.

3. Technique of Embolization

Prior to surgery, the patient receives a Foley catheter. The main artery whose branches supply the angiomatous convolution is exposed over a long distance, carefully sparing all branches. Vessel loops are passed around all these branches. Angiomatous tissue is removed as far as the anatomic situation allows.

The arteriograms are used to judge which tributaries must be considered for embolization. Figure 12.3.2 shows the embolizing system.

The embolizing material is injected through specially constructed cannulas which are transluminally introduced into the different tributaries following longitudinal arteriotomy of the main artery. They are fixed in place by tightening tapes around them (Fig. 12.3.3). One arm of a three-way stopcock system is connected to a transparent plastic container which holds the embolizing material. The other arm is attached to an infusion under pressure. The whole system of container, connecting tubes, stopcocks, and cannulas must

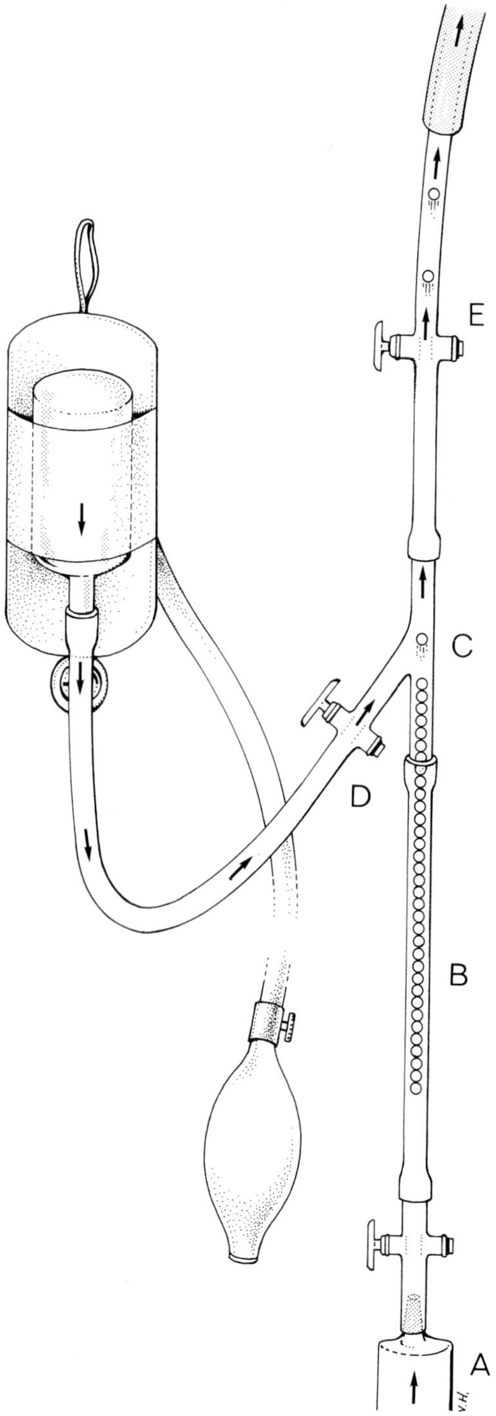

Fig. 12.3.2. Embolizing system. The embolizing material which fills the plastic container (*B*) is slowly injected using a syringe filled with fluid (*A*). As soon as a particle reaches point (*C*) it is carried away by the fluid stream (*D*) under pressure and shot far into the angiomatous convolution through a special cannula (*E*). All parts of the system (container, connecting tubes, stopcocks, and cannulas) form one smoothly interconnecting system

be absolutely free of any narrowings and irregularities, otherwise the particles will stagnate.

For the injection of Teflon or silicone spheres, systems with different internal diameters should be available. They should be chosen according to the diameter of the spheres used for embolization. A syringe is used to inject the embolizing material slowly into the three-way tube system. The particles are carried away by the fluid stream. This ensures that embolizing particles enter the embolizing cannula one by one and from there shoot into the pathologic vessels and feeding arterial branches under the hydraulic pressure of the infusion fluid. They can reach the smallest vessels in the center of the angiomatous tissue without difficulty.

It is important that backward pressure be as low as possible during injection of the embolizing material. Backward flow pressure has already been reduced by preoperative catheter embolization. It can be lowered further by clamping the main artery as far proximally as possible during injection of the material, if necessary by blocking it with an intraluminally introduced balloon catheter (Fig. 12.3.3).

After embolization of all branches supplying the angiomatous convolution, the arteriotomy of the main artery is closed with ultrafine atraumatic suture material. Thereafter, skeletation of the main vein is performed. Then, all nonembolized tributaries of the main artery are ligated at their origins. These branches are obliterated by injecting extremely small polivinyl alcohol particles.

In mixed angiodysplasias which have only microfistulas or no arteriovenous fistulas at all, one may consider obliterating the main artery (one of the lower leg or forearm arteries) with all of its tributaries. The caliber of the artery to be obliterated is sometimes so small that the embolizing system cannot be employed. In such cases, embolization is performed using a polyethylene tube which is advanced as far as possible into the vessel. The embolizing material is then injected under pressure while the tube is slowly withdrawn. This maneuver usually succeeds in obliterating not only the main vessel, but also its finest tributaries.

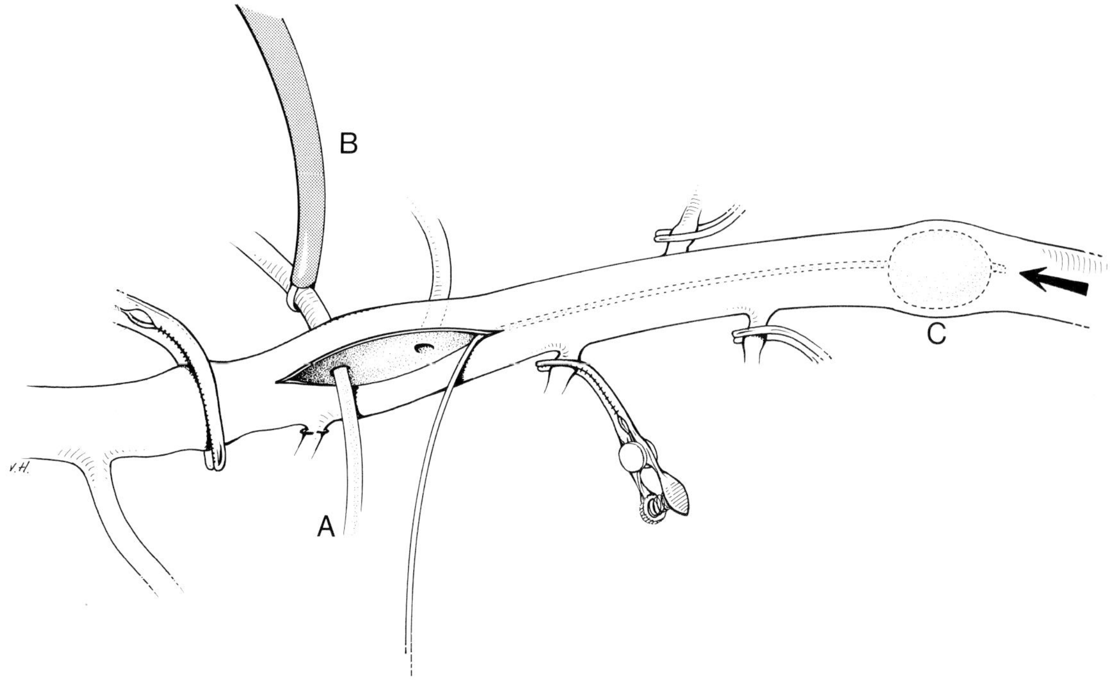

Fig. 12.3.3. Following longitudinal arteriotomy of the main artery the embolization cannula (*A*) is introduced transluminally into the various branches and fixed with the aid of a ligature (*B*) (Vesselclud). The main artery itself is blocked as far proximally as possible with an intraluminally introduced balloon catheter (*C*)

E. Basic Principles in the Treatment of Angiodysplasia at Different Locations

The technique of embolization is chiefly dependent on the location of the angiodysplastic malformation. The anatomic relationships between the arteries supplying the angiodysplastic regions make it necessary to vary the tactics and technique of embolization. At each possible location, attention must be paid to details which are closely related to the topographic situation. Some commonly occuring locations will be discussed in detail.

I. External Carotid Artery

An angiodysplastic process localized in the area perfused by the external carotid artery and its branches are always additionally supplied by the contralateral side. Treatment must therefore always be bilateral. The question of which branches of the external carotid artery supply the angiodysplastic lesion with blood must be answered with reference to the detailed angiograms. After exposure of the carotid bifurcation and branches of the external carotid artery, all tributaries leading to the malformation are selectively embolized using silicone spheres (except when embolizing the lingual artery). The two branches originating nearest to the main nutritive tributaries are also obliterated. Although they do not directly supply the dysplastic area with blood, they could develop collaterals which would nullify the effect of embolization. During injection of the embolizing material, the external carotid artery is clamped at its origin. On the contralateral side, only those branches are embolized which directly lead to the dysplastic region. The arteries adjacent to the main nutritive artery are not obliterated.

II. Shoulder and Upper Arm

Most arteriovenous dysplasias of the shoulder and arm regions are of the F.P. Weber type. They are supplied not only by the axillary and brachial arteries, but also by branches of the subclavian artery and proximal forearm arteries. Often, the intercostal arteries also participate in feeding the pathologic process via the lateral thoracic artery. In order to avoid the necessity of extensive exposure and dissection of the arteries, the internal thoracic artery, the thyrocervical and costocervical trunks, the transverse cervical and suprascapular arteries, and all smaller branches of the subclavian artery are first embolized percutaneously. In the same manner, the superior and inferior collateral arteries, the radial and ulnar recurrent arteries, and, if possible, also the recurrent interosseal artery are obliterated percutaneously by injecting polyvinyl alcohol granules. During the subsequent operation, the axillary artery and the proximal half of the brachial artery are exposed along their entire length. Dysplastic, sometimes aneurysmally enlarged segments of their branches are resected as far as possible. All branches leading to the arteriovenous malformation are embolized with polyvinyl alcohol granules and silicone spheres. Special attention is paid to the lateral thoracic artery.

Finally, skeletation of a long segment of the main vessels is performed, during which the tributaries are obliterated peripherally with fine polyvinyl alcohol particles.

III. Internal Iliac Artery and Profunda Femoris Artery

In patients with arteriovenous dysplasia localized in the area perfused by the internal iliac artery, many other arteries of neighboring or remote regions are almost always contributors: the branches of the external iliac artery on both sides, the contralateral internal iliac artery and its branches, the lower lumbar arteries, the median sacral artery, even the inferior mesenteric artery via the superior rectal artery and the lower branches of the profunda femoris artery. On the other hand if the angiodysplastic lesion is situated in the area perfused by the profunda femoris artery, all branches of the internal iliac artery are involved, especially the inferior gluteal artery. The branches of the external iliac artery also belong to the feeding vessels. The situation becomes extremely complicated if the angiodysplastic lesion is supplied by both the internal iliac artery and the profunda femoris artery. In such cases, multiple operative and percutaneous treatments are necessary to eliminate and obliterate the entire angiodysplastic malformation.

Treatment is performed in two sessions and consists of the following sequences: during the first operation, the contralateral external iliac artery and the proximal portion of the internal iliac artery are exposed. The external iliac artery is skeletized and its branches embolized with polyvinyl alcohol granules. The tributaries of the anterior branches of the internal iliac artery, which also take part in perfusing the angiodyplastic area, are embolized separately using polyvinyl alcohol granules and silicone spheres. During a second surgical procedure, performed 2 weeks later, the same treatment is done on the diseased side, but embolizing all branches of the internal iliac artery. The ipsilateral profunda femoris artery and its branches are treated in the same manner.

Care must be taken in embolizing the inferior gluteal and profunda femoris arteries. Both arteries take part in the blood supply of the sciatic nerve. Total obliteration of all side branches of these arteries may cause ischemic damage of the nerve, resulting in peripheral nerve palsy, particularly if liquid embolic agents are used.

Moreover, the inferior gluteal arteries supply the cavernous bodies via the internal pudendal arteries. Embolization of these arteries on both sides endangers the erectile function of the penis. Obliteration of the inferior gluteal artery should be restricted to the distal part of this vessel, beyond the origin of the branch leading to the sciatic nerve.

IV. Hand, Finger, Foot, and Toe

The more distally angiodysplastic lesions are localized, the more delicate and difficult treatment will be. In order to make the decision as to which arteries and branches can be eliminated by excision, ligation, and embolization and which must be spared, one must have excellent arteriograms at one's disposal.

Treatment of lesions of the hand, foot, fingers, or toes requires visualization of the arches with all their branches. Dysplastic vessels must be excised and other branches must be embolized with polyvinyl alcohol foam or silicone microspheres in such a way that at least one normal digital artery for each finger or toe is saved in order to prevent ischemic damage. All residual vessels are eliminated or treated by skeletation.

Good permanent results can be obtained and ischemic damage avoided by careful dissection and meticulous technique.

F. Postoperative Complications

There are two major types of complication that can be expected following the combined method of treatment.

Ischemic complications may occur following the treatment of angiodysplasias of the hand, finger, foot, and toe regions if certain arteries outside the pathologic area important for the perfusion of fingers and toes are not spared. Blood supply to the periphery must be preserved.

It cannot be stressed often enough that one should not embolize distally located vascular malformations if the available angiograms are not of high quality. "Blind" embolization of peripherally localized angiodysplasias cannot be recommended today.

Even if perfect arteriograms are available and those branches are carefully saved which are vitally important for the preservation of fingers and toes, ischemic complications do occur in a few cases. They are probable only if ischemic lesions in the form of necrosis or gangrene are present prior to treatment. Such distally localized dysplasias, combined with ischemic lesions, should be handled with special care. Limited amputations at the boundary line may be necessary in such cases.

Neurologic complications, such as functional disorders of peripheral nerves, especially of the peroneal nerve and the sciatic nerve, are rare. They are undoubtedly due to ischemia (embolization of the profunda femoris artery or inferior gluteal artery). Functional losses which might occur are seldom far-reaching and are usually reversible.

G. Reinterventions

Routine control angiography is of critial importance following the embolization of an angiodysplastic lesion. Such a control examination should be done a few weeks after treatment. Remnants of the vascular malformation can then be treated by percutaneous catheter embolization.

Recurrences discovered angiographically during the late postoperative course are treated primarily by percutaneous embolization. Usually what is found in such cases are branches running from neighboring regions to the outer limits of the initial malformation. These branches can be easily embolized percutaneously. Following correct treatment by the combined method, such recurrences are relatively rare.

REFERENCES

1. van Dongen RJAM (1983) Therapie der angeborenen arteriovenösen Angiodysplasien unter besonderer Berücksichtigung der operativen Embolisation. Angio 5:169
2. van Dongen RJAM (1985) Angeborene arteriovenöse Dysplasie: Behandlungsindikation, angiographische Dokumentation, kombinierte percutane und operative Behandlung. Chirurg 56:65
3. Ehrenfeld WK (1976) Diskussionsbemerkung. Surgery 79:11
4. Elliot JP Jr, Hageman JH, Szilagyi E, Ramakrishnan V, Bravo JJ, Smith RF (1980) Arterial embolization. Problems of source, multiplicity, recurrence, and delayed treatment. Surgery 88:833
5. Florack G, Sandmann W, Müller H, Lerut J, Kremer K (1980) Arteriovenöse Fisteln – Möglichkeiten und Grenzen der operativen Behandlung. Angio 2:47
6. Frileux C, Blonstein A (1976) Embolisation therapeutique pour anévrisme cirsoide récidive de la main. J Mal Vasc 1:47
7. Grace DM, Pitt DF, Gold RE (1976) Vascular embolization and occlusion by angiographic techniques as an aid or alternative to operation. Surg Gynecol Obstet 143:469
8. Joyce PF, Sundaram M, Afzal Riaz M, Wolverson MK, Barner HB, Hoffmann RJ (1980) Embolisation of extensive peripheral angiodysplasias. Arch Surg 115:665
9. Konrad EA, Stiegler H, Meister P, Becker HM (1980) Das P.F. Weber-Syndrom; Umschriebener Riesenwuchs der unteren Extremität mit kongenitalen arteriovenösen Fisteln. Vasa 9:331
10. Malan E, Puglionisi A (1964) Congenital angiodysplasias of the extremities; generality and classification; venous dysplasias. J Cardiovasc Surg 5:87
11. Malan E, Puglionisi A (1965) Congenital angiodysplasias of the extremities; arterial, arterial and venous, and haemolymphastic dysplasias. J Cardiovasc Surg 6:255
12. Malan E (1965) Surgical problems in the treatment of congenital arteriovenous fistulae. J Cardiovasc Surg [Suppl]:251
13. May R, Nissl R (1970) Beitrag zur Klassifizierung der „gemischten Angiodysplasien". ROFO 113:170
14. Natali J, Merland JJ (1976) Superselective arteriography and therapeutic embolisation for vascular malformations (angiodysplasias). J Cardiovasc Surg 17:465
15. Olcott C, Newton TH, Stoney RJ, Ehrenfeld WK (1976) Intra-arterial embolization in the management of arteriovenous malformations. Surgery 79:3
16. Pratesi F (1972) Classification of angiopathic diseases of the limbs. Folia Angiologica 20:193

17. Rickets RR, Finck E, Yellin AE (1978) Management of major arteriovenous fistulas by arteriographic techniques. Arch Surg 113:1153
18. Stillman RM, Powers JC, Fitzgerald JF (1977) Cosmetic excision of an isolated extracranial arteriovenous malformation using Gelfoam embolization. Br J Surg 64:784
19. Vollmar JF (1974) Zur Geschichte und Terminologie der Syndrome nach F.P. Weber und Klippel-Treaunay. Vasa 3:321
20. Vollmar JF, Stalker CG (1976) The surgical treatment of congenital arteriovenous fistulas in the extremities. J Cardiovasc Surg 17:340

13 Peripheral and Abdominal Arterial Injuries

A. ZEHLE

CONTENTS

A. General Considerations

I. Introduction

Peripheral arterial injuries are of special significance because, in addition to the threat they may pose to the life of the patient, they can also cause irreversible secondary trauma to the extremities or to the brain, thereby precluding the possibility of complete rehabilitation.

Vascular injuries occur in 0.9%–4% of trauma victims [5, 19, 21]. However, the incidence is significantly higher in patients with multiple injuries, about 7%–10% [22, 63].

Approximately one third of arterial injuries are caused by cardiologic or radiologic diagnostic procedures and less frequently by operative procedures [24].

In war, the mean incidence of arterial injuries is 2%–2.4%. In the Vietnam war, the distribution of 1000 vascular injuries was: carotid artery 5%, upper extremity 34%, and lower extremity 57%. Only 4% of the injuries were within the thorax or abdomen [45]. A survey of the distribution of peripheral vascular injuries is given in Table 13.1.

According to HEBERER [19], perforating and nonperforating as well as open and closed arterial injuries have to be distinguished. A sharp penetrat-

Table 13.1. Distribution of vascular injuries in civilian and military series [3, 10, 44, 45, 49, 61]

	Civilian injuries		Military injuries	
	n	%	*n*	%
Internal/common carotid artery	68	4.4	50	5.0
Vertebral artery	6	0.4		
Subclavian artery	67	4.4	8	0.8
Axillary artery	75	4.8	59	5.9
Brachial/cubital artery	219	14.2	283	28.3
Radial/ulnar artery	187	12.1		
Aorta/ innominate artery	62	4.0	3	0.3
Hepatic artery/celiac trunk	9	0.6		
Splenic artery	3	0.2		
Superior, inferior mesenteric artery	19	1.2		
Renal artery	30	1.9		
Abdominal aorta	52	3.4	3	0.3
Common/external iliac artery	171	11.1	26	2.6
Internal iliac artery	9	0.6		
Common femoral artery	135	8.8	46	4.6
Profunda femoris artery	24	1.6		
Superficial femoral artery	221	14.4	305	30.5
Popliteal artery	95	6.2	217	21.7
Anterior, posterior tibial artery and peroneal artery	85	5.5		
	1537		1000	

RICH [45] only reports injuries of major arteries so that there are no data on vascular injuries of the distal upper and lower extremity ing trauma is caused by gunshot and stab wounds, cuts, penetrating foreign bodies, and fractured bones and may result in a small laceration or clean division, or even large lacerations with greater defects.

Nonperforating arterial injuries are mainly caused by contusion, e.g., by dislocation of bones following fracture or luxation and may result in injury of the inner surface of the artery with bleeding into the vessel wall, intimal disruption with secondary thrombotic occlusion, or traumatic dissection. Compression by a subfacial hematoma or edema by dislocated bone fragments or casts may cause arterial insufficiency and secondary thrombosis.

Indirect injuries are lacerations and disruption caused by distension (e.g., rupture of the aorta by rapid deceleration). Traumatic arterial spasm is rare [16, 21, 63].

Clinically significant *late complications following vascular injuries* are arterial thrombosis, false aneurysm, arterial aneurysms, and arteriovenous fistulas (Table 13.2).

Table 13.2. Classification of arterial injuries [c.f. 21, 33, 69]

I. Direct injuries

1. *Penetrating trauma*
   a) Cuts, stab and gutshot wounds
   b) Iatrogenic (angiography, cardiac catheter, operations, intra-arterial injection)
2. *Blunt trauma*
   a) Contusion (thrombosis)
   b) Compression (hematoma, fractures)
   c) Constrictions (constricting dressings)

II. Indirect injuries

1. Lacerations by distension
2. Deceleration (thoracic aorta)
3. Arteriospasm

III. Late complications

1. Acute thrombosis
2. Infections
3. Peripheral edema, tourniquet syndrome
4. False aneurysm
5. Arterial aneurysm
6. Arteriovenous fistula

II. Diagnosis

Patients with deep penetrating and also with severe blunt injury of extremities should have a careful physical examination to exclude arterial injuries during the initial management.

In case of an *open penetrating* arterial injury the diagnosis is usually easily made when the mechanism of trauma and the direction of the wound are taken into consideration. A large hematoma or massive bleeding may be absent when both ends of the injured artery are rolled in and an early thrombosis has occurred.

Blunt arterial injuries are more difficult to diagnose. Peripheral ischemia distal to the injury is the sure sign in diagnosis. Absence of peripheral pulses with lack of sensitivity and of spontaneous movements probably point to an injury of peripheral vessels. The color and temperature of the skin and the filling of veins may provide additional significant information.

Arteriospasm and a reduction of arterial perfusion in the case of traumatic shock must be excluded through differential diagnosis.

A significant diagnostic measure is *Doppler ultrasonography*. In the region of the extracranial vessels, the flow direction of the supraorbital artery may be of great help, while the measurement of the blood pressure of the distal extremity compared with that of the healthy brachial artery significantly adds to the diagnosis of vascular injuries of the extremities. In case of peripheral vascular injuries of the extremities, the blood pressure is usually measured over the radial/ulnar artery or the anterior/posterior tibial artery. Vascular injury is likely to be present when the blood pressure in the injured extremity is not measurable by Doppler ultrasonography or when the values thus obtained are 50% lower than the systemic blood pressure. Doppler ultrasonic examination is absolutely necessary for the evaluation of a severely injured patient if vascular injury is suspected clinically.

Where there is a clear clinical indication for operative exposure of the injured vessel because of massive bleeding or hematoma, preoperative *arteriography* is usually unnecessary and may only cause an unnecessary prolongation of ischemia. Therefore, one should consider intraoperative angiography (documentation and assessment of the needed repair, exclusion of other simultaneous lesions). If the diagnosis of vascular injury, based on the clinical criteria mentioned, cannot be made with sufficient certainty, and if there is persistent ischemia despite adequate treatment for shock, then an arteriographic evaluation should be performed within 2–3 h.

Angiography is of special importance in cases of suspected peripheral ischemia, blunt abdominal trauma, and concomitant fractures of the extremities in typical locations (supracondylar fracture of the humerus, supracondylar fracture of the femur, fracture of the tibial head, and fracture of the lower leg) [36, 39, 56].

III. Initial Management

Massive bleeding requires immediate provisional hemostasis at the site of the accident.

Control of bleeding from injured *carotid arteries* or the subclavian artery is only partially successful by digital compression. The prognosis is very much dependent on the speed of transportation to a hospital equipped to manage such injuries. Temporary control of bleeding of *vascular injuries of the extremities* is performed by various methods.

Because of the threat of damage to muscles, veins, and nerves, a tourniquet should be applied to an extremity only if there is no other possibility of controlling the bleeding. Also, clamping of the pulsating artery should be avoided because of the increased risk of infection and of trauma to the vessel ends. No operation should be performed at the site of the accident!

The method of choice is digital compression applied proximally or at the injury, or pneumatic compression applied to sterile wound dressings, e.g., by means of a blood pressure cuff [27] at pressures above the systolic value. Early intubation and fluid replacement are essential for stabilization of the patient's condition; otherwise, definitive management will not be possible.

IV. Operative Technique and Adjuvant Therapy

Conservative management of peripheral vascular injuries is only allowed when there is no significant bleeding or when restoration of function will not be improved by the vascular repair (e.g., axillary artery injury in case of disruption of the nerve plexus without peripheral ischemia of the arm).

Ligature of extracranial arteries may cause ischemia of the central nervous system in a high percentage of cases, and ligature of arteries of the extremities may lead to amputation [11, 24] (Table 13.3).

Table 13.3. Percentage of ischemic damage to the central nervous system and to parenchymatous organs of amputation of extremities following arterial ligature [3, 9, 11, 24]

Ischemia of the central nervous system (%)		*Amputations (%)*	
Innominate artery	5	Subclavian artery	29
Common carotid artery	14–24	Axillary artery	43
Internal carotid artery	40	Brachial artery (cranial)	56
Vertebral artery	5	Brachial artery (caudal)	26
		Radial artery	5
Organ ischemia (%)		Ulnar artery	1.5
Celiac trunk	0	Radial and ulnar artery	39
Common hepatic artery	<10	Common iliac artery	54
Proper hepatic artery	12	Internal iliac artery	0
Left hepatic artery	36	External iliac artery	47
Right hepatic artery	<100	Common femoral artery	81
Superior mesenteric artery	100	Profunda femoris artery	0
Inferior mesenteric artery	1.5	Superficial femoral artery	55
Renal artery	100	Popliteal artery	73
		Anterior tibial artery	8.5
		Posterior tibial artery	13.6
		Peroneal artery	14.3
		Anterior and posterior tibial artery	69
		Posterior tibial and peroneal artery	40

Therefore, repair of peripheral vascular injuries is usually necessary and urgent, independent of their localization, because the time between the onset of ischemia and definitive vascular repair is just as decisive for the prognosis as are the localization and the concomitant injuries.

The management of peripheral vascular injuries follows the principles of reconstructive vascular surgery, depending on the type of injury (see Chap. 4). Only trauma-specific technical principles will be outlined here in more detail.

Clean stab wounds are repaired by direct interrupted over-and-over sutures, placing the needle from the outside in and from the inside out. The suture material is monofilament 5–0 to 7–0 vascular suture (Fig. 13.1.a). When a direct suture is impossible because the cut is irregular, continuity may be restored by a limited resection and an end-to-end anastomosis (Fig. 13.1.b). Longitudinal injuries may be repaired by a direct suture only when

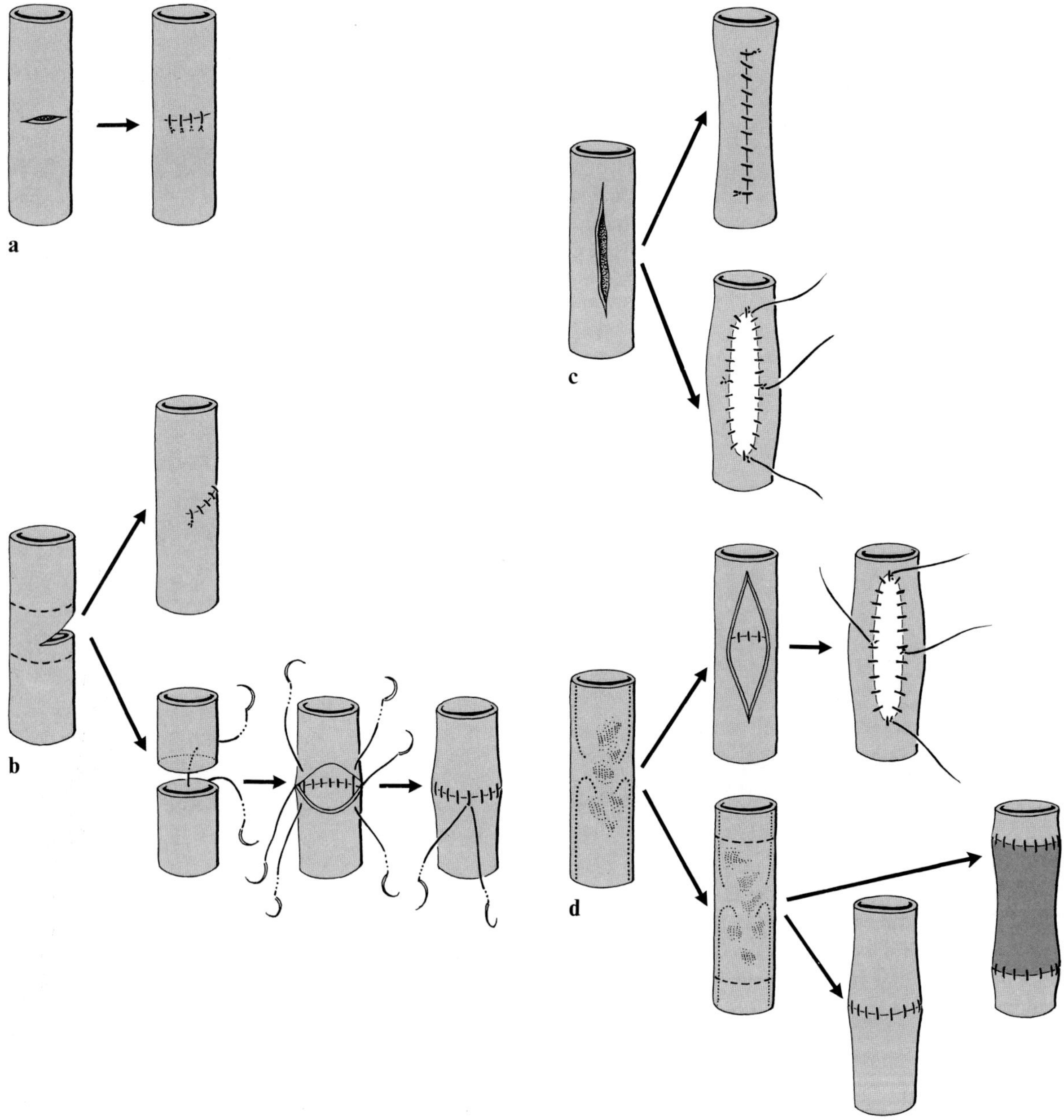

Fig. 13.1 a–d. Operative repair of peripheral arterial injuries. **a** Clean transverse cut. Operative technique: over-and-over interrupted suture. Suture material: 6–0 monofilament polyamide (Prolene) or monofilament polyglycolic acid (PDS). **b** Oblique larger cut. Technique: continuous over-and-over suture, corner sutures, placing the suture from the inside out. Suture material: double monofilament polyamide, size 6–0. Alternatively: resection and end-to-end anastomosis. **c** Longitudinal cut. Technique: direct continuous suture (as in **b**), alternatively: venous patch graft. Suture material: as in **b. d** Blunt vascular injury with involuted intimal tear. Technique: longitudinal incision, intima fixation, venous patch graft. Alternatively: resection and end-to-end anastomosis or resection and interposition of venous graft. Suture material: as in **b**

there is a large diameter and a clean cut. However, it usually makes more sense to utilize a venous patch graft (Fig. 13.1c).

Blunt, nonperforating vascular injuries with involuted intimal tear require exposure of the injured area using a large incision, fixation of the intima, and closure of the incision by a venous patch graft or by resection of the injured segment and its replacement by a graft (Fig. 13.1d).

Longitudinal, clean lacerations of smaller vessels with a diameter less than 5 mm should be repaired principally by venous patch graft angioplasty (Fig. 13.2a). More severe injury of the artery,

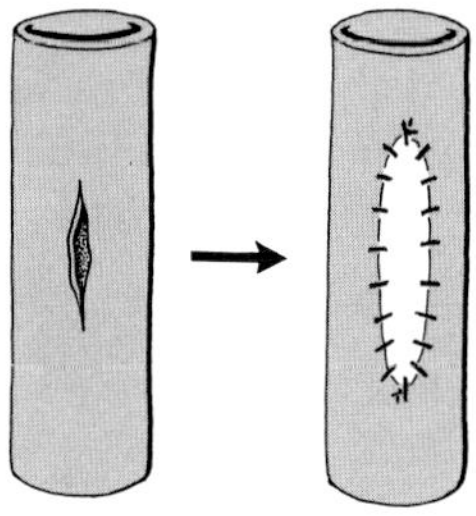

a

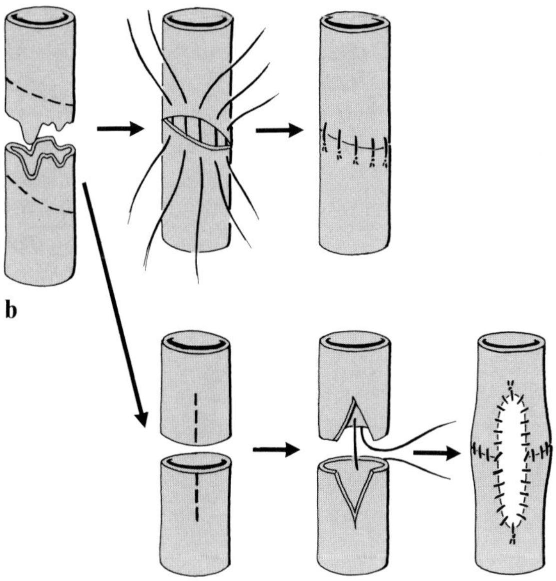

b

Fig. 13.2a, b. Operative repair of small peripheral arteries. **a** Longitudinal stab wound. Technique: venous patch graft, suture material 7–0 double monofilament polyamide (prolene) using a small needle (BV 1). Interrupted suture technique. Suture distance 1 mm. **b** Division: technique: beveled resection and end-to-end anastomosis with interrupted sutures. Alternatively: longitudinal incision of the anterior wall of both vessel ends. Suture of the posterior wall with interrupted sutures end-to-end and extension of the anterior wall by means of a patch graft (VAN DONGEN technique)

or clean division, requires an end-to-end anastomosis with interrupted sutures of monofilament 6–0 and 7–0. Both vessel ends should be beveled before being sutured. Enlargement of the anastomosis is also possible by means of the anastomotic technique described by VAN DONGEN (Fig. 13.2b). Table 13.4 gives an overview of the techniques described in the most important papers.

Besides the technical considerations mentioned, repair of peripheral vascular injuries should adhere to the following principles:

1. Vascular reconstruction as early as possible. If ischemia persists, postoperative edema is a danger; if ischemia lasts longer than 6 h, a tourniquet syndrome may occur.
2. Sufficient exposure and mobilization of the injured vessel to allow for proper evaluation of the extent of injury and to provide approximation of both vascular ends without tension.
3. Use of autogenous saphenous vein from the noninjured extremity whenever a primary end-to-end anastomosis is impossible. Alternatively, Dacron double velour prostheses may be used for larger arteries although the risk of infection is higher. For smaller arteries, thin-walled PTFE prostheses are preferred.
4. Before the anastomosis is performed, a careful distal thrombectomy with a Fogarty catheter should be carried out in all cases, despite backflow, and the vessel ends to be anastomosed should be dilated carefully (alternative: intraoperative angiography as a control of the periphery).
5. The best long-term results are achieved with end-to-end anastomosis and interrupted sutures [71].
6. Regional distal and proximal heparinization is required (for instance 5000 IU heparin in 100 ml 0.9% NaCl solution and injection of 10–20 ml proximally and distally).
7. Larger concomitant veins should also be repaired whenever possible.

Table 13.4. Operative technique in vascular injuries

Operative technique	Civilian injuries [3, 10, 44, 57]		Military injuries [45]	
	n	%	n	%
Lateral suture	190	26	87	9
End-to-end anastomosis	260	35	377	38
Venous graft, in-line or bypass	114	15	459	46
Fabric prostheses	32	4	4	0.4
Thrombectomy, patch graft angioplasty	34	5	–	–
Fixation of the intima	3	0.4	–	–
Ligature	63	9	15	1.5
Others/undetermined	40	5	58	6
	736		1000	

8. All grafts should be covered with healthy tissue; if this is not possible, they should be placed extra-anatomically.
9. The injured extremity should be sufficiently immobilized postoperatively.
10. An early fasciotomy is essential especially when there is simultaneous muscle and bone injury or ischemia of longer duration.

V. Vascular Injuries in Children

Juvenile vascular injuries are increasing in frequency and are very serious because of a child's lesser capacity to compensate larger losses of blood. Mortality is about 13%; however, for purely peripheral arterial injuries it is zero. The commonest localization is the brachial artery and the superficial femoral artery [38].

In *infants*, vascular repair of extremity arteries is seldom successful, owing to the extreme contractility of the arterial wall [42].

On the other hand, good spontaneous formation of collaterals allow ligatures in areas where in adults gangrene would be likely. Nevertheless, longitudinal growth of the extremity is impaired [22, 38, 60]. Therefore, it is advisable to do a secondary reconstruction before the last growth stimulus whenever a primary reconstruction was impossible or unsatisfactory [42].

In *older children* vascular injuries are repaired as in adults. However, the following principles must be observed:

1. Any suspicion of arterial injury should be checked out by angiography since in juveniles such lesions may cause only a sensation of cold and a short period of pain.
2. The reconstruction should then always be performed within the time of ischemic tolerance.
3. Microsurgical suture technique (magnifying glass or microscope, monofilament 10–0 to 7–0 suture material) is required. The anastomosis should be performed with interrupted sutures and be tensionless, which means that it should be placed so that it may expand in length and width. A venous bypass or interposition can therefore be longer in juveniles than in adults. Running sutures will cause stenosis during growth.
4. Prosthetic material should not be implanted, or only for vital indications.
5. Routine follow-up until cessation of longitudinal growth is required to diagnose shrinking of the anastomosis and to allow corrections before the onset of growth retardation [22, 42].

VI. Concomitant Injuries

The close anatomic relationship of arteries, veins, and nerves, especially in the extremities, usually causes simultaneous injuries of these structures. Table 13.5 summarizes data from various authors on the incidence of concomitant injuries following arterial trauma. Clean division of a vessel together with an additional blunt trauma and large concomitant injuries are typical for high velocity gunshot wounds.

Table 13.5. Frequent concomitant injuries of peripheral vascular trauma

	Vascular injuries	Concomitant injuries		
		Bone, joints	Vein	Nerve
DRAPANAS [10]	266	19	93	23
HEBERER [21]	118	39	52	19
LINDER [33]	145	20	104	36
SMITH [58]	127	24	51	57
	616	102 (17%)	300 (49%)	135 (22%)
RICH [45]	1000	285 (28%)	377 (38%)	424 (42%)

1. Venous Injuries

In war, venous injuries are reported as concomitant to arterial trauma in 34%–38% of cases [45]. In civilian series an incidence of 14%–66% is reported, depending on the predominant type of trauma [3]. Ligation of concomitant veins is only allowed distal to the knee and the cubital area. Proximal to these regions, reconstruction must be performed. The priority of repair is evaluated differently. The advantage of a primary repair of the artery is reduction of ischemic time. A disadvantage may be greater peripheral venous congestion and venous bleeding after arterial declamping. Whenever time allows, venous repair should therefore be done first. Details of venous reconstructions are described in Chap. 27.1.

2. Nerve Injuries

Neural injuries in combat are found to be concomitant to arterial trauma in 27%–42% of cases [45]. This exceeds the incidence of civilian nerve injuries, which is about 22%. These concomitant injuries should be treated definitively together with vascular injuries, in one operation. The functional capability of the injured extremity depends more on successful restoration of the nervous function than on vascular reconstruction.

Nerve suturing done with the aid of the microscope at the first operative session, along with the procedure on the injured arteries, produces better results than those obtained in a secondary reconstruction. Primary reconstruction, however, can be undertaken only if the patient's condition allows prolongation of the operative time.

3. Soft Tissue, Bone, and Joint Injuries

For the prognosis in the case of an injured extremity, larger *soft tissue defects* are also of significance (decollement, muscle contusion, ruptured ligaments). They occur predominantly following blunt trauma, with an incidence of about 26%–29% [3]. In particular, these injuries bring with them a higher risk of infection following arterial reconstruction.

Rarely, *dislocations* cause blunt hyperextension trauma to adjacent arteries (Fig. 13.3). Examples of this are dislocation of the shoulder (luxatio erecta) [29] and luxation of the elbow and the knee [33]. When such a dislocation is accompanied by peripheral ischemia, careful respositioning should first be performed. If there is no improvement of peripheral circulation, angiography and exposure of the appropriate vessel is required. If the joint injury requires major reconstruction, then arterial repair has priority. The joint may first be immobilized temporarily and then reconstructed in a second session with less time pressure on the surgeon.

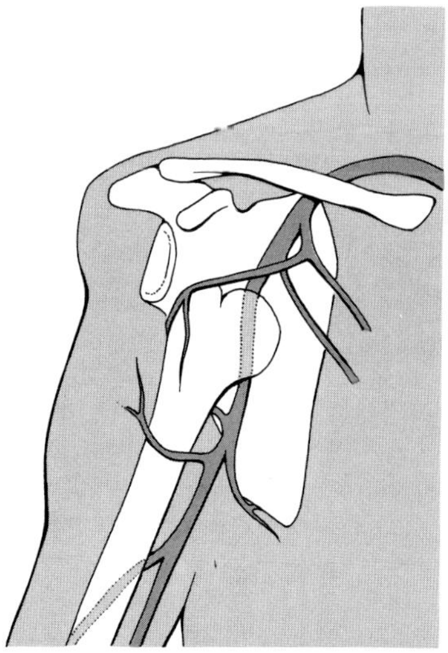

Fig. 13.3. Blunt hyperextension trauma of the axillary artery as a result of anterior dislocation of the shoulder

Fractures are found in 27%–28% of cases (Table 13.5) as concomitant injuries following peripheral vascular trauma and are frequently the cause of them. Fractures pierce the artery or cause hyperextension with tearing of the intima and involution of the intimal flap, or may even cause division. Juxta-articular fractures of long bones, e.g., supracondylar fractures of the humerus or the femur, are very likely to produce such arterial injuries [12, 70].

Regarding the conduct of the operation, it is sometimes advisable to repair the vessel initially to keep peripheral ischemia as brief as possible. On the other hand, it may be advisable to perform the reconstruction of the bones first and to accept a longer ischemic time because of the risk of injuring the reconstructed vessel while subsequently repairing the bones [48, 58, 70]. This approach has become widely accepted. Only in cases of a longer ischemic period should this principle be disregarded and the artery reconstructed first [16]. Alternatively, arterial blood flow may be provided by a temporary intraluminal shunt [14].

In war, the preferred method of immobilization is external fixation because of its lower risk of infection [46]. In the civilian sector this technique of osteosynthesis is sometimes preferred, especially where ischemia is protracted [17]. Generally, reconstruction of the bones is performed according to the principles of the ASIF (Association of the Study of Internal Fixation) [1, 65] using internal osteosynthetic material.

These injuries to soft tissue, joints, and bones, especially following severe blunt closed trauma, attract such attention that sometimes the arterial injury is missed or diagnosed too late. This is the main reason for an amputation rate of 28%–50% following these multiple injuries [13, 70]. The unfavorable prognosis may be significantly improved and the rate of amputation dramatically reduced if arterial injury is always considered in cases of multiple injuries [22].

B. Special Section

I. Brachiocephalic and Carotid Vascular Injuries

1. Common Carotid Artery, External, and Internal Carotid Artery

Injuries of the carotid artery and its branches are rare. The predominant form is penetrating trauma. The site of injury is the common carotid artery in 50% of cases [2] and the external and internal carotid artery, each in 25% [67]. Upon admission to hospital, about 20% of patients present with severe, 10% with slight, and 70% with no neurologic deficit [2, 67]. Patients with hypotension and acute bleeding from a suspected carotid artery injury should be operated on immediately. The life-saving control of bleeding has absolute priority over diagnostic measures. Delaying the operative revision runs the risk not only of exsanguination but also, if there is bleeding into the thorax, of lethal compression of the airways.

The evaluation of patients following sharp or severe blunt lateral trauma of the neck should also include consideration of a potential carotid artery injury, especially in the presence of a large hematoma. Horner's syndrome, or contralateral neurologic deficits [31, 35]. If circulation is stable and there is no evidence of compression of the airways, diagnostic measures are completed by a cerebral ultrasonic Doppler examination.

In the case of a wound above the angle of the mandible and below the clavicle, arteriography should be performed [34]. Whenever possible, digital subtraction arteriography should be carried out [47]. Computed tomography should reveal whether there are necroses in the brain in cases of severe neurologic deficit.

The following *guidelines* for the management of carotid artery injuries are generally accepted:

1. If there is no neurologic deficit, reconstruction should be performed. Ligation is allowed only exceptionally, when a high internal carotid artery injury is technically not reconstructible. Repair gives good results in over 91% of cases as compared with only 66% without reconstruction [67].
2. Reconstruction should also be performed in cases of neurologic deficit (hemiplagia, aphasia, brief loss of consciousness). In 34% of patients, symptoms are improved, in contrast to 14% without reconstruction [67].
3. If the patient is in a state of unconscious shock or in a coma, the prognosis is bad and so some authors recommend ligature. Despite different opinions [5, 29], UNGER [67] stresses that there is no statistically proven basis for not performing a reconstruction under these circumstances.

Ligature is indicated:

a) If anterograde flow is absent in a comatose patient [67]
b) Following extensive cerebral destruction, as indicated by computed tomography
c) If the reconstruction is technically impossible

The carotid artery may be exposed by extending the existing wound longitudinally from the earlobe down to the jugular (Fig. 13.4a). The carotid arteries are exposed by sweeping the sternocleidomastoid muscle and the jugular vein laterally and dividing the venous tributaries that run medially (see p. 468). The external carotid artery may be ligated. The common and internal carotid arteries are reconstructed.

In most cases injuries of the common carotid artery can be repaired by direct suture (Fig. 13.4b). Besides heparinization, no other protective measures are required.

If resection is necessary for treatment of an injury in the area of the carotid bifurcation, an intraluminal shunt should be used (Fig. 13.4c, d; see p. 471).

If the injury is close to the base of the skull so that vessel cannot be clamped above the site of the injury, then the artery may be occluded by a Fogarty catheter inserted through an additional incision at the carotid bifurcation (Fig. 13.4e). Alternatively, it may also be possible in the case of a smaller high injury to insert an intraluminal shunt at the carotid bifurcation and push it upward, completely occluding the lumen of the peripheral internal carotid artery. This way, no further peripheral occlusion or clamping is required; intracerebral blood flow is provided for by the shunt (Fig. 13.4f).

2. Vertebral Artery Injuries

These are very rare injuries with a relative incidence of 1%. According to the literature, damage to the central nervous system will be encountered in 8% of cases [11]. Exploration of the vertebral artery in its proximal portion is performed using the same approach as for the subclavian artery in its distal portion, namely, through a longitudi-

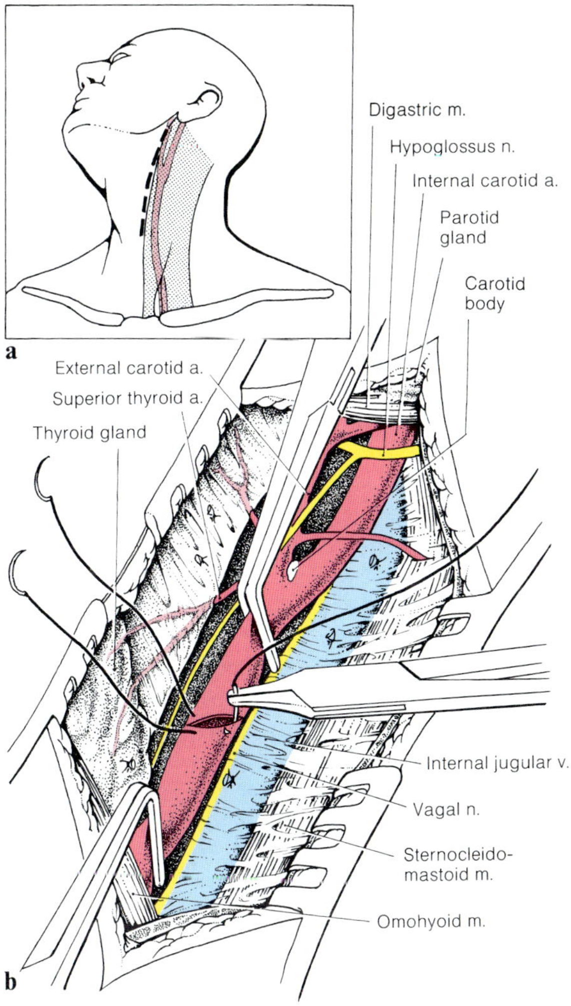

Fig. 13.4a–f. Operative technique for carotid artery injuries. **a** Line of incision for access to the common, external, and internal carotid arteries. **b** Common carotid artery injury. Technique: continuous over-and-over suture. Direction of corner sutures from inside out. No protective measures required. Suture material: 6–0 monofilament double suture material (Prolene, PDS), suture distance about 1 mm. **c** Injury at the carotid bifurcation with irregular margin and loss of tissue. Technique: resection of the injured vessel wall as first step. **d** Insertion of an intraluminal shunt and end-to-end anastomosis. In the second step, a corner suture is placed on the posterior surface, followed by continuous over-and-over sutures around on both sides, meeting on the anterior surface. Suture material is the same as in **b. e** Internal carotid artery injury close to the base of the skull. An additional incision in the area of the carotid bifurcation is made, a Fogarty catheter is pushed forward, and the internal carotid artery is occluded, followed by suture of the injury (technique as in **b**). **f** Internal carotid artery injury above the bifurcation. Through an additional incision made at the area of the bifurcation an intraluminal shunt can be inserted. If the shunt is thick enough, back flow from the internal carotid artery is avoided. The injury can then be repaired without clamping of the internal carotid artery

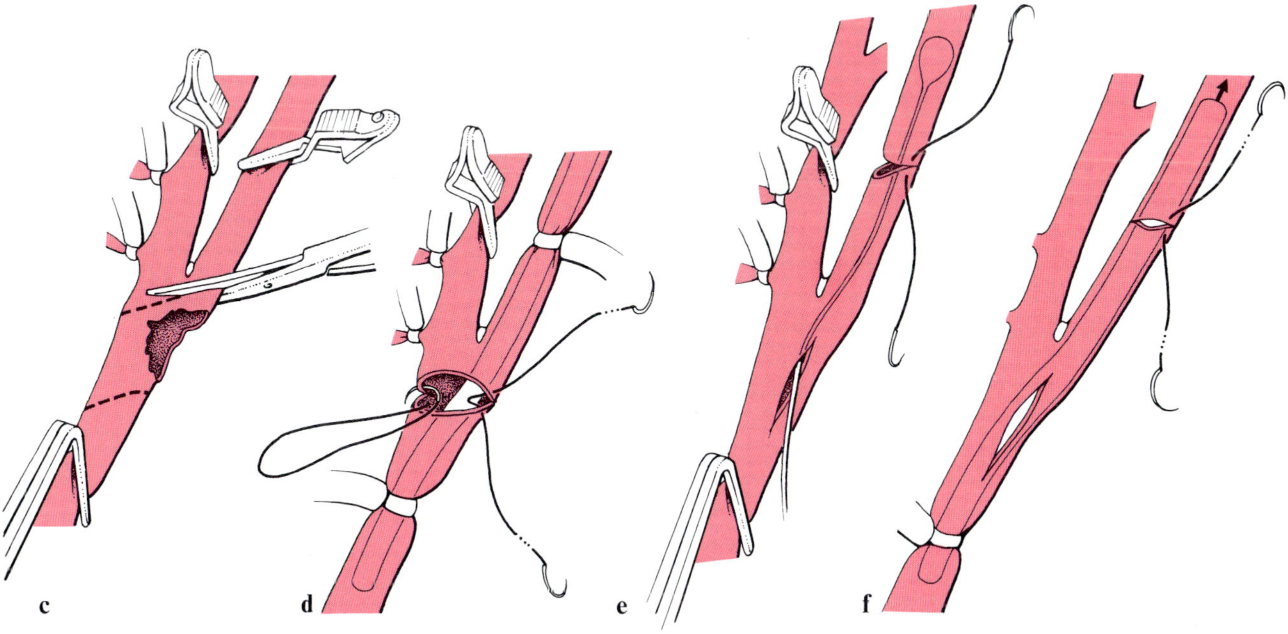

nal incision along the sternocleidomastoid muscle. Reconstruction is the exception; ligation is the therapy of choice.

II. Vascular Injuries of the Upper Extremity

1. Subclavian Artery

Because the subclavian artery is well protected, it is rarely injured (Table 13.1).

Injuries may occur from shooting or stabbing (penetrating trauma). A fractured clavicle or a distal fragment of a fractured first rib may penetrate the vessel. Injury may also occur by massive hyperextension of the arm (blunt trauma). The latter is usually accompanied by disruption of the plexus so that the indication for reconstruction of the artery may not be absolute when severe ischemia is absent [8].

Massive hematoma at the site of the clavicle and absent pulse of the axillary artery, confirmed by measurable difference of arterial blood pressure or Doppler pressure, make the diagnosis easy. However, subclavian artery injuries may be missed because peripheral ischemia of the arm is usually ameliorated by the highly effective collateral system in the region of the shoulder. Angiographic demonstration of the aortic arch, including its branches, by means of a Seldinger catheter or transvenous digital subtraction angiography (DSA) confirms the diagnosis.

Repair of injuries to the first third of the subclavian artery requires proximal exposure in order to be able to cross-clamp the vessel at its takeoff from the innominate artery or on the left near the aorta. Exposure of the first portion of the right subclavian artery is achieved by a supraclavicular transverse incision dividing the clavicular and sternal insertion of the sternocleidomastoid muscle and by an upper sternotomy. On the left side, exposure is made by a thoracotomy at the second interspace (see Chap. 15.5).

When the distal arterial segment is injured, the vessel may be exposed by an angulated supraclavicular incision passing through the scalenus muscles. Special care must be taken of the branches of the cervical plexus. The arm is adducted in order to get the clavicle into the most caudal position.

The *peripheral segment of the vessel* exposed by a transverse incision just under the clavicle, dividing the pectoralis muscle. The arm has to be adducted in order to draw up the clavicle. This incision may be extended to the axilla, dividing the major and minor pectoralis muscle. However, it seems more reasonable to expose the axillary artery by an additional curved incision in the axilla and to tunnel the pectoralis muscle. When the injury is circumscribed, direct suture is the method of choice. When this does not seem to be safe enough, resection with end-to-end anastomosis is the method of choice [8, 37].

In rare cases, a bypass is required, primarily using autogenous saphenous vein. The mortality rate with these rare arterial injuries is reported to be between 0% [70] and 25% [10]. When ligating the artery, an amputation rate of 29% is encountered (Table 13.3). Following reconstruction, the amputation rate is about 6% [10].

2. Axillary Artery

Besides gunshot and stab wounds, the *causes* of injuries to the axillary artery are the anterior dislocation of the shoulder and luxatio erecta, with an incidence of 810:1 [17]. In most cases, there was a prior intimal lesion with subsequent thrombosis. The relative incidence of axillary artery injuries is 5%–6% of all peripheral vascular injuries in peace and war (Table 13.1).

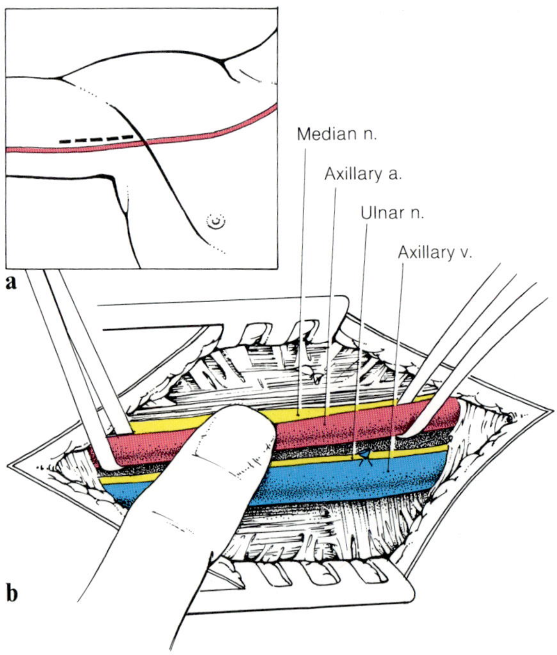

Fig. 13.5. a Line of incision for exposure of the axillary artery. **b** Anatomy following dissection of skin and subcutaneous tissue. Tapes are placed around the axillary artery

Diagnosis is usually made without difficulty because of the artery's superficial location and the mechanism of injury.

Exposure of the vessel is achieved by means of a curved incision in the axilla, extending into the sulcus bicipitalis medialis. The arm is abducted (Fig. 13.5a, b). In this area, collateral flow is not sufficient and therefore reconstruction is absolutely mandatory. Following ligature, the amputation rate is about 43% (Table 13.3).

Direct reconstruction is possible in two thirds of patients. In one third of patients, an interposition of saphenous vein is required [37]. The amputation rate following reconstruction is 0%–8%, with very low mortality [10, 37].

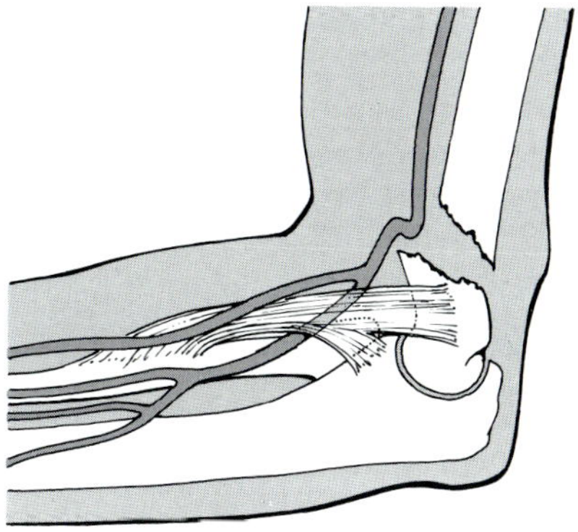

Fig. 13.6. Injury of the distal brachial artery in the presence of a supracondylar fracture of the humerus

3. Brachial Artery

Brachial artery injuries are caused by gunshot and stab wounds (knife, glass) and by blunt trauma following fractures of the humerus. The relative *incidence* is 80% in civilian life and 29% in war (Table 13.1). Following ligation of the vessel, an amputation rate of up to 26% is reported, depending on the concomitant injuries [19]. Therefore, reconstruction is mandatory. Only in cases of incomplete ischemia may reconstruction be delayed because of the relatively good collateral flow [3].

Exposure is made through a longitudinal incision in the sulcus bicipitalis medialis, where the vessel is palpated throughout its whole length. Care should be taken of the median nerve, running in the middle of the upper arm directly in front of the artery (Fig. 13.7a, b). Following reconstruction according to the principles mentioned above, there is an amputation rate of 3%–6% [10].

The distal brachial artery (cubital artery) may be sharply injured by a supracondylar fracture of the humerus. Besides this possibility, the peripheral fragment of the fractured humerus may injure the vessel (Fig. 13.6). For the fractures mentioned the incidence is only 560:1 [17]. Among children, however, this injury assumes greater importance; with a relative incidence of up to 22%, it must be regarded as a typical peripheral arterial injury for that group. If it is not repaired, the risk of amputation is 25% [19], and especially in children there is the additional risk of Volkmann's contracture.

Exposure of the distal brachial artery is achieved through an S-shaped incision in the elbow (Fig. 13.7c). The antecubital fascia is divided. The artery is just underneath. If the pronator teres

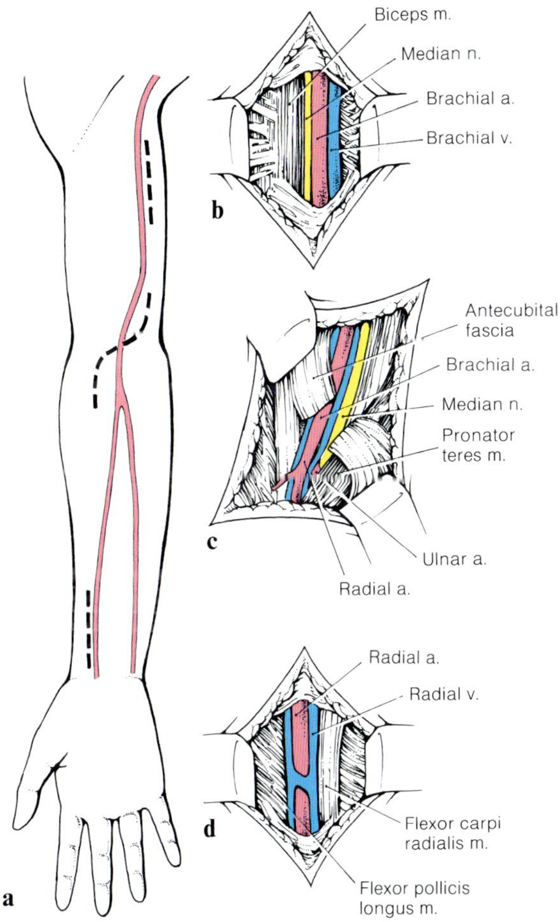

Fig. 13.7. a Lines of incision for exposure of predisposed arteries of the arm. **b** Exposure of the brachial artery in the sulcus bicipitalis medialis. **c** Antecubital region. The antecubital fascia is divided. The pronator teres muscle covers the ulnar artery distal to its origin. **d** Exposure of the distal radial artery

muscle inserts a few centimeters above the medial epicondylus, it covers the artery and must therefore be mobilized appropriately.

Operative therapy consists of a longitudinal incision, intima fixation, and enlargement by a small venous patch. Alternatively, resection and end-to-end anastomosis may be carried out. In children, microsurgical suture techniques should be applied (magnifying glass, appropriate instruments, and 7–0 suture material).

4. Forearm Arteries

Injuries of the forearm arteries are among the most frequent peripheral arterial injuries, with an incidence of 27% (Table 13.1). Beside cuts and stab wounds, often from attempted suicide, severe sharp and blunt trauma with fractures of the bones of the forearm are the causes. The localization of these injuries is mainly at the wrist (Fig. 13.7a, b).

Following division of one of the two forearm arteries, a ligature may be placed; this is the most frequently used method of management. Disturbed peripheral circulation results in only 1%–5% (11). Where reconstruction does not involve great difficulty, e.g., in cases of clean division of the peripheral radial artery, reconstruction is preferred over ligation. Maintaining the function of this vessel may be of significance later.

When both the radial and ulnar artery are injured, reconstruction of at least one of the forearm arteries is absolutely necessary. Following ligation or failure of reconstruction the amputation rate is 39% [9]. The repair should be performed by direct suture, resection, and end-to-end anastomosis, or vein interposition. Because of the small caliber, the peripheral greater saphenous vein should be taken. Microsurgical suture technique is required.

III. Abdominal Arterial Injuries

About 30% of all patients with multiple injuries today show blunt or penetrating abdominal injuries. However, HEBERER et al. [22] found among 407 patients with multiple injuries, of whom 118 had undergone laparotomy, only 3 injuries of the abdominal aorta and its major branches. TREDE [63] saw only 5 abdominal vascular injuries in 424 patients with multiple injuries, all of these involving the renal artery.

Despite the fact that these injuries are rare, in most cases sharp or blunt trauma of the abdomen is fatal, extensive vascular injury is the cause. The mortality is about 30%–60%, depending on the site and type of injury. The mortality increases therefore when multiple intra-abdominal injuries have occurred instead of a single vascular injury [26]. The symptoms are those of concomitant shock. About 50% of these patients reach the hospital with no measurable blood pressure [26, 32, 40].

One should observe the following rules for the prophylaxis and therapy of shock:

1. Massive transfusions should be supplemented in at least the proportion of 4:1 by administration of fresh frozen plasma.
2. Autotransfusion (for instance Hemonetics Cell Saver) should be supplemented by fresh frozen plasma, fresh blood, or platelet concentrates.
3. Hypothermia below 32° C must be avoided by adding warmed blood and by means of a heating cushion on the operative table. Infusions should be warmed to 40° C and these solutions should also be used for abdominal lavage.
4. A pH below 7.20 must be avoided by infusion of Ringer's lactate and, if necessary, bicarbonate.
5. As an immediate operative measure one may start with a left-sided anterolateral thoracotomy and reduce the flow in the thoracic aorta to minimize blood loss during the subsequent laparotomy [26, 32].

The group led by MOORE [26, 40] recommends this procedure for patients suffering from myocardiac arrest after the primary treatment or whose blood pressure does not rise above 80 mm Hg despite appropriate therapy.

1. Abdominal Aorta

Penetrating gunshot or stab wounds of the abdominal aorta usually cause sudden death by massive bleeding. For this reason DE BAKEY [9] reported that only 12 injuries of the abdominal aorta reached the vascular surgical unit out of more than 1000 military arterial injuries. The prognosis is especially unfavorable in cases of aortic injuries with access to the free abdominal cavity. In case of dorsal injury, however, the retroperitoneum may provide temporary tamponade. Blunt injuries of the aorta caused by force acting on a small area (contact with steering wheels, seat belts –

„seat belt aorta“ – [4], gun butts) are ten times less common than sharp lesions [7]. They result in acute occlusion by dissection and thrombosis. Iatrogenic injuries are noticed during operations on intervertebral disks or during angiography.

Only if the patient is hemodynamically stable will there be time for thorough *diagnosis*. Today, modern ultrasound devices can localize a large hematoma in the shortest time and allow estimation of the level of injury. Computed tomography and angiography, and whenever possible digital subtraction angiography, may be used as time permits.

The best *operative* approach is provided by a median laparotomy. This type of incision can eventually be extended cranially by means of a median sternotomy. After insertion of the Rochard retractor and a large transverse retractor, the whole abdominal aorta can be approached easily. The *diaphragmal* aorta is exposed subhepatically following division of the lesser omentum approaching from the right. The more caudal suprarenal *„visceral“* aorta is best approached by mobilization of the left colon, moving it to the right (Fig. 23.3). Injuries of the upper abdominal aorta, of the celiac trunk, and of the left renal artery are repaired using this approach.

The right renal artery, especially in cases of suspected concomitant injury of the vena cava or of the renal vein, is dissected from the right by moving the right colon to the left.

The typical approach to the infrarenal aorta in patients suffering from arterial occlusive disease is mobilization of the small bowel to the right and incision of the retroperitoneum just left of the duodenum.

The aorta is exposed while compressing the site of injury by hand. Careful dissection of periaortic tissues may be omitted when proximal control of the aorta by a straight vascular clamp can be achieved. For distal cross-clamping of the aorta, a curved or right-angled vascular clamp is best applied, simultaneously occluding lumbar tributaries originating from the posterior vessel wall. With this technique, the aorta will not be compressed so much as when a Satinsky clamp is applied. Repair of the aortic injury is thereby greatly facilitated.

The most commonly used reconstructive procedure is direct suture, perhaps with a venous patch graft angioplasty. The reason may well be that patients with more severe injuries requiring a more complicated repair do not reach hospital.

In perforating injuries of the aorta, one must not forget to reconstruct the posterior wall as well. It may be necessary to suture the posterior wall from the inside after a longitudinal incision of the anterior wall.

The results of treatment of abdominal aortic injuries show a mortality of 50%–60% [3, 26, 32]. The mortality is especially high (75%–90%) in patients with injuries of the „visceral“ aorta. Infrarenal aortic injuries have a somewhat more favorable mortality following reconstruction (53%) [26, 32].

2. Celiac Trunk and Hepatic Artery

Injuries of the celiac trunk and the hepatic artery comprise about 10% of all abdominal arterial injuries. Generally, the incidence is 0.6% of all arterial injuries. The operative approach is the same as for the abdominal aorta. The vessels are exposed below the liver following division of the lesser omentum und dissection of the hepatoduodenal ligament. The celiac trunk may be ligated without risk just distal to its origin [11]. Following ligation of the common hepatic artery, ischemic complications are encountered in less than 10%. Lim [32] reported in a collective series of 345 patients a total mortality of 3.7% caused by secondary liver failure. Ligation of the proper hepatic artery will result in ischemic hepatic failure in 12%, ligation of the left hepatic artery in 36% [11]. Therefore, whenever possible peripheral hepatic artery injuries should be reconstructed. Ligation of the proper hepatic artery or the right hepatic artery should be combined with a cholecystectomy (the postoperative development of an empyema of the gallbladder is favored by secondary sequelae of shock). The principles of this reconstruction include lateral suture, venous patch graft angioplasty, or venous interposition. The period of ischemia tolerated by the liver is reported to be 30 min [48]. However, this is only true for total occlusion of the blood flow to the liver. Therefore, when performing reconstruction, which usually takes longer than this, special attention must be paid to maintaining blood flow in the portal vein.

3. Superior and Inferior Mesenteric Artery

Both intestinal arteries also make up approximately 10% of abdominal vascular injuries. These injuries are mostly accompanied by severe injuries of the pancreas, intestine, and mesenterium. Division of the main branch of the superior mesenteric artery will cause extensive bowel ischemia owing to the absence of collaterals, except in the presence of chronic arterial occlusive disease. Therefore, reconstruction is absolutely necessary. For the small bowel the time of warm ischemia is also short, about 1 h [48]. A successful reconstruction, however, is still possible after 2–3 h.

Reconstruction is performed by lateral suture, venous patch graft angioplasty, or aortomesenteric venous bypass. Following reconstruction, intestinal blood flow may be tested by means of intraoperative ultrasound or by injection of a fluorescent dye under ultraviolet light [7]. Even with this technique, a second-look operation is obligatory within 24 h, because during the postoperative phase segmental small bowel ischemia and necrosis are not recognizable with sufficient certainty prior to the onset of fatal complications. The mortality rate for injuries of the superior mesenteric is high, 33%–57% [7, 32], owing to the usually severe concomitant injuries. The inferior mesenteric artery may be ligated just distal to its origin. There will be no complications if the other mesenteric arteries are patent.

4. Renal Artery

Injuries of the renal artery mainly occur following severe blunt abdominal trauma. Besides direct trauma, a contrecoup effect may stretch the renal artery and result in an occlusion due to intimal damage with thrombosis.

Renal artery injuries are rare, 1.9% of 1583 vascular injuries (Table 13.1). However, they represent about 14% of abdominal vascular injuries. Diagnostic signs may include pain in the side, hematuria, or a negative early urogram. The diagnosis is confirmed by aortography. The most useful technique is digital subtraction angiography. However, the small ischemic tolerance of the kidney, less than 1 h, makes treatment very urgent and does not allow time-consuming diagnostic procedures. Therefore, if there is adequate suspicion, laparotomy should be performed.

The operative details are described in the appropriate chapter (see p. 609 ff.). The decision as to whether a reconstruction is logical and technically feasible or whether a primary nephrectomy should be carried out depends on any additional parenchymal or renal vein injuries.

An attempt at reconstruction may be made extending beyond the ischemic tolerance time since the renal blood supply can be maintained by vessels of the capsula and since in favorable cases, renal arteries can be reconstructed successfully, even after several days [53, 66]. However, this attempt should be undertaken only if the contralateral kidney is healthy and if circulation is stable. The high mortality (see below) obliges one to consider whether the additional prolongation of operating time as compared with nephrectomy can be justified.

Favorable conditions for a reconstruction are proven flow in the renal arteries, diagnosed preoperatively by angiogram or intraoperatively, and simple lesions caused by penetrating trauma. Intraoperatively, the ischemic time may be prolonged and the blood flow to the kidneys demonstrated by perfusing the kidney through an intraluminal catheter, using a cooled solution (25 ml low molecular weight dextran + 25 ml Ringer's solution + 1000 IU heparin at 4° C). If the kidney completely loses its color, larger infarctions or rupture of polar arteries can be excluded. Otherwise, incomplete revascularization and subsequent nephrogenic hypertension can be expected, which in 85% of these cases entails secondary nephrectomy [66].

As *reconstructive procedures*, lateral suture, venous patch graft angioplasty, venous interposition, and perhaps aortorenal bypass may be performed (see p. 616ff.).

The results show a mortality of 37% [66]. Only 10% of kidneys following arterial injuries and about 40% of kidneys after revascularization may be saved.

5. Iliac Arteries

Lying deep within the small pelvis, the iliac arteries are anatomically well protected; nevertheless, injuries to these arteries are relatively frequent (Table 13.1; 30% of all abdominal arterial injuries [26]).

Blunt trauma is the result of direct force in or above the groin and of pelvic fractures. Among sharp traumas iatrogenic injuries are of greater importance, especially in the distal portion of the artery. Injuries during angiography or during operative procedures such as appendectomies, gynecologic and orthopedic operations (endoprostheses) have been reported.

Ligation of the common iliac artery leads to amputation in 53.8% and ligation of the external iliac artery requires it in 46.7% [11]. Also, extremely severe necroses of the gluteal region have been described. Reconstruction is therefore obligatory.

Exposure of the vessel begins either transperitoneally, from a medium or paramedian incision, or extraperitoneally, through an oblique incision in the side extending down to the groin and providing very good exposure.

The *principles of reconstruction* are direct suture, venous patch angioplasty, and saphenous vein interposition. Even though the approach is relatively easy and the diameter of the vessel is favorable for rapid reconstruction, the mortality is still high, 30%–40% [3, 24, 26]. The underlying reason is frequent concomitant vein injury, which, especially in the true pelvis, can cause bleeding that is difficult to control.

IV. Vascular Injuries of the Lower Extremity

1. Common Femoral Artery

Because of its length of only 5 cm and its relatively protected position, injuries of the common femoral artery have a relative incidence of only 5% (Table 13.1). In civilian series, stab wounds, gunshot wounds, and iatrogenic injuries are mainly responsible. Catheterization of vessels or of the heart cause vascular injury in 0.12% of cases [25]. However, common femoral artery injuries account for about 50% of all iatrogenic vascular injuries [25].

Blunt trauma is caused by impalement and by bicycle handlebar and sled injuries.

The diagnosis of an injury to these superficial vessels is easy in that sharp trauma causes bleeding and formation of hematomas while blunt trauma causes peripheral ischemia. Additional diagnostic procedures beyond routine examination with a Doppler ultrasound probe are seldom necessary.

The technique of *exploration* is known from the treatment of arterial occlusive disease (see p. 392). In cases of severe bleeding, it is advisable to expose first the external iliac artery by an extraperitoneal approach above the inguinal ligament in order to control the bleeding.

The preferred method of *reconstruction* is direct suture, excision of the lacerated vessel wall and suture with a venous patch graft. Less often, an end-to-end anastomosis or interposition is performed. The greater saphenous vein may be used. If its diameter is significantly smaller than that of the common femoral artery, the vein can be tailored so that two venous segments of the same length are slit longitudinally and sutured together along the longitudinal edges. The circumference of the graft is thus doubled [70]. When the common femoral artery is ligated, the extremity is lost in over 80% (Table 13.3). Revascularization is usually successful. Some deaths result from exsanguination, shock due to fluid loss, or from severe concomitant diseases [3].

2. Profunda Femoris Artery

The profunda femoris artery is thought to be virtually invulnerable [45]. However, when the vessel is injured it should be reconstructed [24]. Ligation may result in extensive destruction of the femoral musculature with renal failure and death, despite palpable pulses at the foot [24].

3. Superficial Femoral Artery

Injuries of the superficial femoral artery are of special quantitative significance, with an incidence of 20% in peace and 30% in war. The major causes are: gunshot and stab wounds (including accidental wounds self-inflicted by butchers), work-related crushing injuries, and especially blunt injuries sustained in motorcycle accidents, frequently associated with fractures.

The clinical *symptoms* depend upon the etiology. The pulsating hemorrhage in cases of trauma has to be controlled immediately without further diagnostic procedures. Every closed femur fracture requires an angiologic examination to exclude blunt vessel injuries. A cool, pale, and pulseless limb may be misdiagnosed because of shock or because of being masked by collaterals. If there is doubt, angiography is absolutely indicated [48]. The exposure of the vessel begins along the ventral edge of the sartorius muscle with a longitudinal incision. The proximal and distal healthy vessel segments must be exposed, if necessary by division of Hunter's canal (Fig. 13.8a, b).

Reconstructive procedures are employed according to the extent of the vascular injury and may consist of direct suture, end-to-end anastomosis, or the interposition of saphenous vein harvested from the healthy extremity. Concomitant venous injuries must be diagnosed and reconstructed, either before or after the arterial repair, depending on the situation (Fig. 13.8c).

Ligation is no alternative to reconstruction of this vessel segment. The amputation rate is 55%

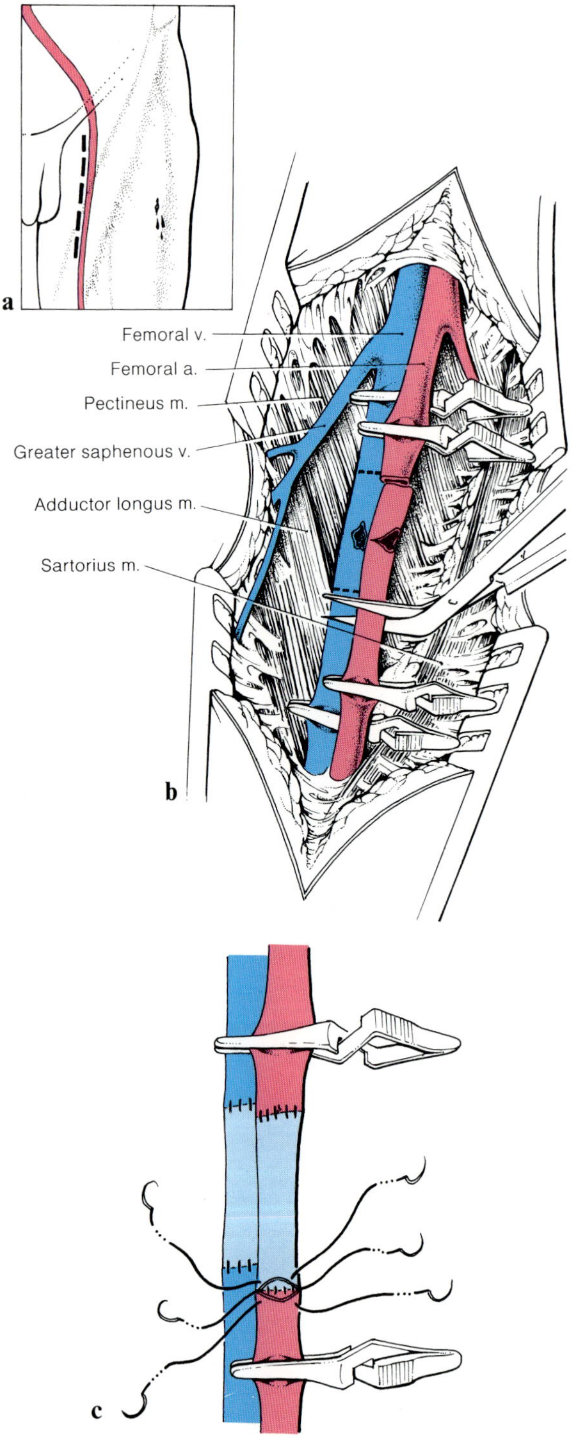

Fig. 13.8. **a** Incision for the exposure of the proximal superficial femoral artery. A line from the middle of the inguinal ligament to the condylus tibialis femoris can serve as a guide, as can the sartorius muscle. **b** The sartorius muscle is retracted laterally and the deep fascia divided. The subsartorius canal is still intact and may be divided if necessary. **c** The repair of the injured femoral artery and vein by venous interposition graft

(Fig. 13.2 [11, 13]). The results of reconstruction are good. BURRI [3] reports that of 26 traumatized patients presenting superficial femoral artery injuries there were 3 deaths due to shock, staphylococcus sepsis, and fat embolization, as well as pulmonary complications. During the long-term follow-up, 21 of the 23 patients who survived were considered to be cured. There was one amputation and one partial recovery.

4. Popliteal Artery

Popliteal artery injuries are of significance because of their relative incidence of 20% in war and 10%–20% in civilian series [59].

They are caused by blunt trauma, such as posterior luxation of the knee, epiphysiolysis of the distal end of the femur, supracondylar fracture of the femur, and tibial head fracture. The incidence of concomitant vascular injuries following such trauma is reported to be 23% [3] (Fig. 13.9, 13.10).

Penetrating trauma, such as gunshot wounds, are rare in central Europe; however, in the series reported on by SNYDER [59] they constitute 75% of the 110 collected cases of knee trauma.

Ligation of the popliteal artery may result in amputation in 73%–75% because the collateral vessels may be affected as well [9, 12].

The early diagnosis of a popliteal artery injury is therefore very important because ischemic time plays an important role in the prognosis [22].

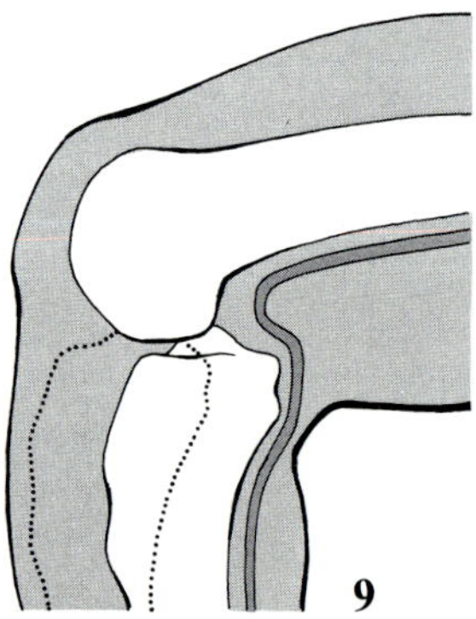

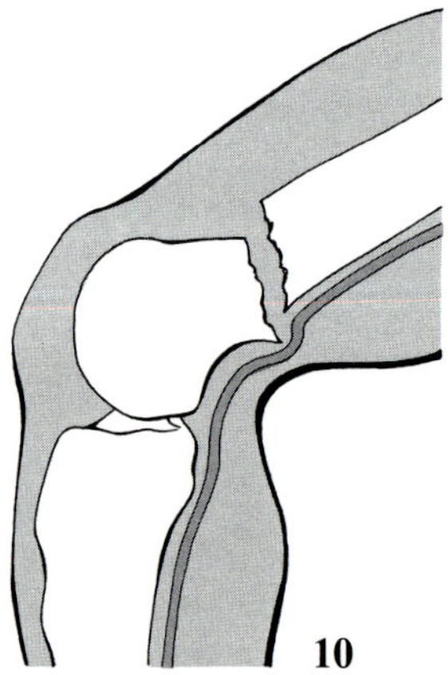

Fig. 13.9. Blunt trauma of the popliteal artery by posterior luxation of the knee

Fig. 13.10. Blunt trauma of the popliteal artery by supracondylar fracture of the femur

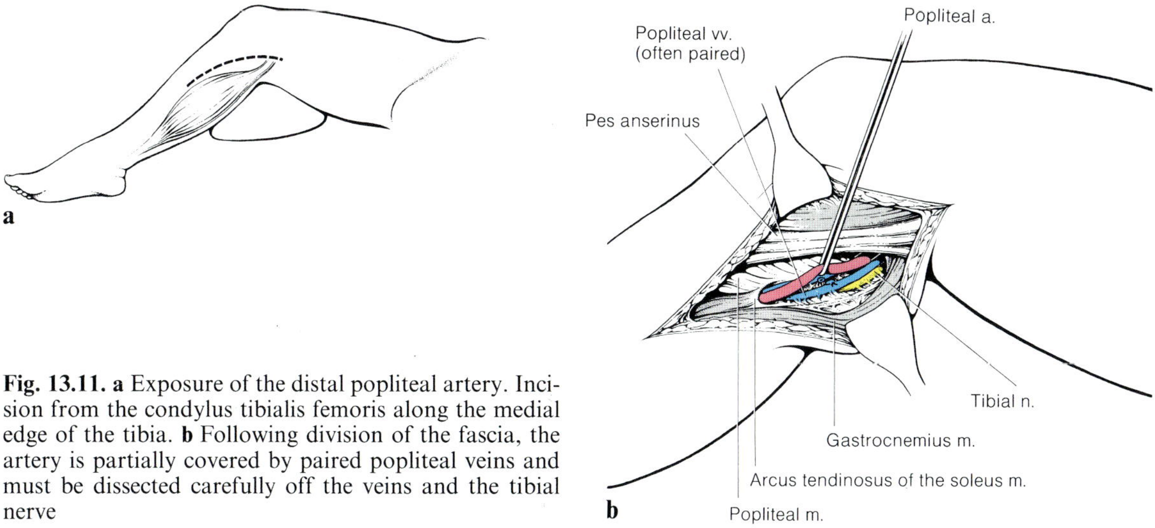

Fig. 13.11. a Exposure of the distal popliteal artery. Incision from the condylus tibialis femoris along the medial edge of the tibia. **b** Following division of the fascia, the artery is partially covered by paired popliteal veins and must be dissected carefully off the veins and the tibial nerve

Open trauma in the region of the knee should be managed by immediate surgery. Vascular injury must be excluded or confirmed; reconstruction should take place. Closed trauma requires immediate angiography whenever there is clinical suspicion of vascular injury so that the artery can be reconstructed within 6 h.

In the operative approach to the first popliteal segment, a medial longitudinal incision is chosen similar to that used for the exposure of the superficial femoral artery (Fig. 13.11, see p. 394). The distal popliteal segment is exposed by means of a longitudinal incision along the medial tibial crests. The gastrocnemius muscle is retracted and the tendon of the semitendinosus muscle and of the gracilis muscle is divided. The incision can be extended proximally and distally in order to expose the second popliteal segment of the trifurcation (Fig. 13.11 a, b). This approach is regarded as the standard reconstructive procedure in surgery of arteries. It is preferred to the dorsal approach through an S-shaped skin incision of the fossa poplitea that is chosen for the operative repair of minor popliteal aneurysms (see p. 281 ff.).

The reconstructive principles include the procedures already mentioned; however, saphenous vein interposition or saphenous vein bypass are preferred. The saphenous vein graft should be harvested from the healthy limb so as not to endanger venous flow in the injured limb. Furthermore, a concomitant lesion of the ipsilateral greater saphenous vein will then be irrelevant to the arterial reconstruction. Despite reconstruction, the rate of amputation following popliteal artery injuries was still 29% in the Vietnam war [9]. Civilian series show similar, or somewhat better results [12, 15].

Of great importance are the diagnosis of concomitant venous injuries and their reconstruction (see Chap. 27.1). Furthermore, a fasciotomy should always be carried out (see Chap. 24.3). Both measures may improve the results of subsequent reconstruction of vascular injuries of this segment [12, 24, 37, 59].

5. Lower Leg Arteries

Isolated injuries of a lower leg artery may be managed without reconstruction, by ligature. An amputation rate of 8.5% is reported following injuries of the anterior tibial artery, and of 14% following injury of the posterior tibial artery [11]. However, the major reason for these results may be the peculiarities of data collection and the evaluation of the results of war injuries rather than the vascular injury itself. When all three lower leg arteries are injured, reconstruction has to be performed; otherwise, there is an amputation rate of 70% [9]. This type of injury, however, is rare and usually occurs only in traumatic amputations (see Chap. 14). For its repair, special knowledge of microsurgical reimplantation is necessary, besides knowledge of the approaches. Details will not be discussed here because of the rare incidence of these injuries and the description of reimplantation techniques in Chap. 14.

A long saphenous vein bypass to the posterior tibial artery seems to have the most favorable results [16].

C. Sequelae

I. Recurrent Thrombosis

Early recurrent thrombosis following reconstructions of vascular injuries depends on the severity of concomitant injuries. The larger the tissue trauma, e.g., following gunshot wounds with high velocity bullets, the higher the rate of recurrent thrombosis is [16]. In war, it is 19.3% (193 of 100 patients) with an amputation rate of about 25% (75). In civilian series, this complication is significantly less common, 1.4%–9.2% [44, 53].

When recurrent thrombosis is suspected on clinical grounds, early angiography is required. If the diagnosis is confirmed, one has to decide on the basis of clinical condition whether a reoperation is justified or whether one should amputate immediately so as not to endanger the patient's life [16].

The particular operative approach is dependent on the type of primary reconstruction and must be selected according to the circumstances of the individual case. Approximately half of early recurrent occlusions can be reconstructed again [42].

For the diagnosis, the decision to operate, and for therapy of late occlusions, the same principles apply as in the treatment of chronic arterial occlusive disease. If there are clinical symptoms, a special argument for reconstruction of late occlusions is that concomitant injuries have healed in the meantime and that the arterial system is most likely healthy, so that another reconstruction seems to have a better chance than it would in the case of chronic arterial occlusive disease.

II. Infection

With antibiotic prophylaxis and careful operative technique the rate of infection following arterial reconstructions nowadays is low. It has decreased from about 3% [20] to below 1%.

Following vascular injuries, infection of the graft is favored by trauma-related contamination of the wound and by the extensive destruction of tissue that results not only from the trauma itself, but also from posttraumatic ischemia with subsequent muscle necrosis. Following manifest infection, the chief danger is vessel rupture with massive bleeding. Following war injuries, this life-threatening chain of complications occurs in about 4.6% [45]. In civilian series, the infection rate is approximately 3.5% [44].

For prophylaxis careful wound debridement, excision of nonvital tissue, drainage, and adequate postoperative immobilization during the initial management are required.

Whenever possible, segments of autogenous saphenous vein should be used for grafts. Exceptionally an alloplastic vascular prosthesis, e.g., a PTFE prosthesis, may be used, provided it can be covered with healthy tissue [21, 22].

An extra-anatomic bypass may have to be chosen.

Broad-spectrum antibiotic therapy is advisable for several days. It should also be directed against anaerobic bacteria.

In case of a deep wound infection, the wound should be opened wide and revised surgically. Afterward, rinsing and suction drainage may be performed. If the vessel ruptures due to the infection or if there is a primary rupture, proximal and distal ligature of the artery must be performed. The wound is either closed, applying rinsing and suction drainage, or an antiseptic treatment is carried out. Peripheral circulation is restored by an extra-anatomic bypass, passing through noninfected tissue (see also Chap. 10.2). In cases of peripheral vascular injury with massive infected tissue necrosis and secondary infection of the reconstruction, the indication for early amputation is critically important for the further course of the disease.

An infection with anaerobic bacteria (e.g., gas gangrene) must be diagnosed at the earliest possible time and the appropriate measures must be taken.

III. Torniquet Syndrome, Compartment Syndrome

The discontinution of peripheral blood flow causes significant injuries of the organ systems supplied by this vessel. After only 30 min of ischemia paresthesia and hypesthesia may occur as symptoms of incipient nerve damage. There may be irreversible loss of sensitivity after 12 h of ischemia.

Disturbances of vessel function are noticed after 2 h of ischemia and will cause complete loss of functions after 4–12 h. This is usually irreversible after 1 h of ischemia. The term "tourniquet syndrome" usually summarizes organ manifestations occurring after reperfusion of an extremity following longer ischemia (more than 4–6 h). The common sequelae are the result of the inflow of potassium, acidic metabolic products, and myoglobin into the organism, and of hemoconcentration due to the peripheral edema [24, 62]. Hyperkalemia, acidosis, and lack of fluid may cause severe damage to cardiac and renal functions, with eventual cardiac arrest or renal failure. The best therapeutic measures are sufficient fluid replacement, early administration of bicarbonate, and dopamine.

Postischemic edema causes a local increase of subfascial tissue pressures from 0–5 mmHg to more than 40 mm Hg [52]. This additionally impairs circulation and function of the appropriate musculature (compartment syndrome). Muscle necrosis and late sequelae threaten when no other measures are performed [28]. The commonest site for a compartment syndrome is the anterior tibial compartment [64]. However, it may also develop at the upper extremity in the compartment of the flexor muscles of the forearm and also in other muscle compartments of the lower extremity. Strangulation dressings have to be split. Too much elevation of the leg must be avoided as it would further worsen peripheral circulation. The therapy of choice is fasciotomy with wide opening of the appropriate compartments [43].

Following vascular injuries, especially in the region of the popliteal artery, decompression by fasciotomy should be performed primarily. When there is a significant compartment syndrome the skin should not be closed. It should stay open and be closed secondarily by a plastic surgical procedure (see also Chap. 24.3).

IV. Arterial Aneurysm, False Aneurysm

True arterial aneurysms resulting from vascular injuries have been reported [3], so seldom, however, that they play practically no role. The repair should be performed according to the principles of aneurysmal surgery. Following stab wounds or gunshot wounds, "false aneurysms" or "pulsating hematomas" are found much more frequently.

The wound canal is outwardly closed, and so the hematoma develops within the soft perivascular tissue. Its periphery coagulates, but inside it is still perfused and shows turbulence. This injury is a typical iatrogenic one following cardiac catheterization or catheter angiography at the groin.

Repair begins with exposure of the proximal and distal segment of the injured vessel. After cross-clamping, the false aneurysm is opened, perhaps resected, and the site of perforation of the artery, which is usually small, is then closed by direct suture. Alternatively, excision of the traumatized vascular segment and venous patch graft angioplasty may be performed.

V. Arteriovenous Fistula

In war, traumatic arteriovenous fistulas develop in 90% as a result of shell splinter wounds and splinters from bombs [68]. In civilian life, stab, gunshot, or iatrogenic wounds are responsible.

Significant late sequelae include: reduced perfusion [24, 27]; central angiectases of the afferent arteries and efferent veins, which may often extend to the heart; and cardiac dilatation and insufficiency due to the chronic volume load [27].

Traumatic arteriovenous fistulas occur in regions where artery and vein are close together and susceptible to simultaneous injury. In a collective series of 593 arteriovenous fistulas [19], the femoral artery is involved in 24%, the carotid artery in 8%, the axillary artery in 6%, and the brachial artery in 5%.

One has to distinguish "uncomplicated" fistulas, consisting of slightly altered afferent and efferent vessels, the vessel walls at the site of the fistulas being close together, from short narrow fistulas, with a false aneurysm in between or with aneurysmal degeneration of the vessels.

If a fistula is suspected, the diagnosis is easily made in the early stages. Fistulas of the extremities, when hemodynamically effective, always emit pulse-synchronous "machine noise". When the shunt volume is large and the adaptation of the organism has been long enough, compression may cause a decrease in pulse rate and an increase in blood pressure (Nikoladoni-Branham sign).

As a complement to physical examination and auscultation, Doppler ultrasound investigation is important. The diagnosis is confirmed by arteriography. It seems that digital subtraction angiography with intravenous injection can also be used [30]. This procedure allows identification of the fistula; if necessary, selective angiography can be performed as a second step for further preoperative evaluation.

The indication for operative removal of a posttraumatic arteriovenous fistula is given generally because of the threat of local and systemic sequelae [18, 19, 23, 41, 68, 70]. When operating, one

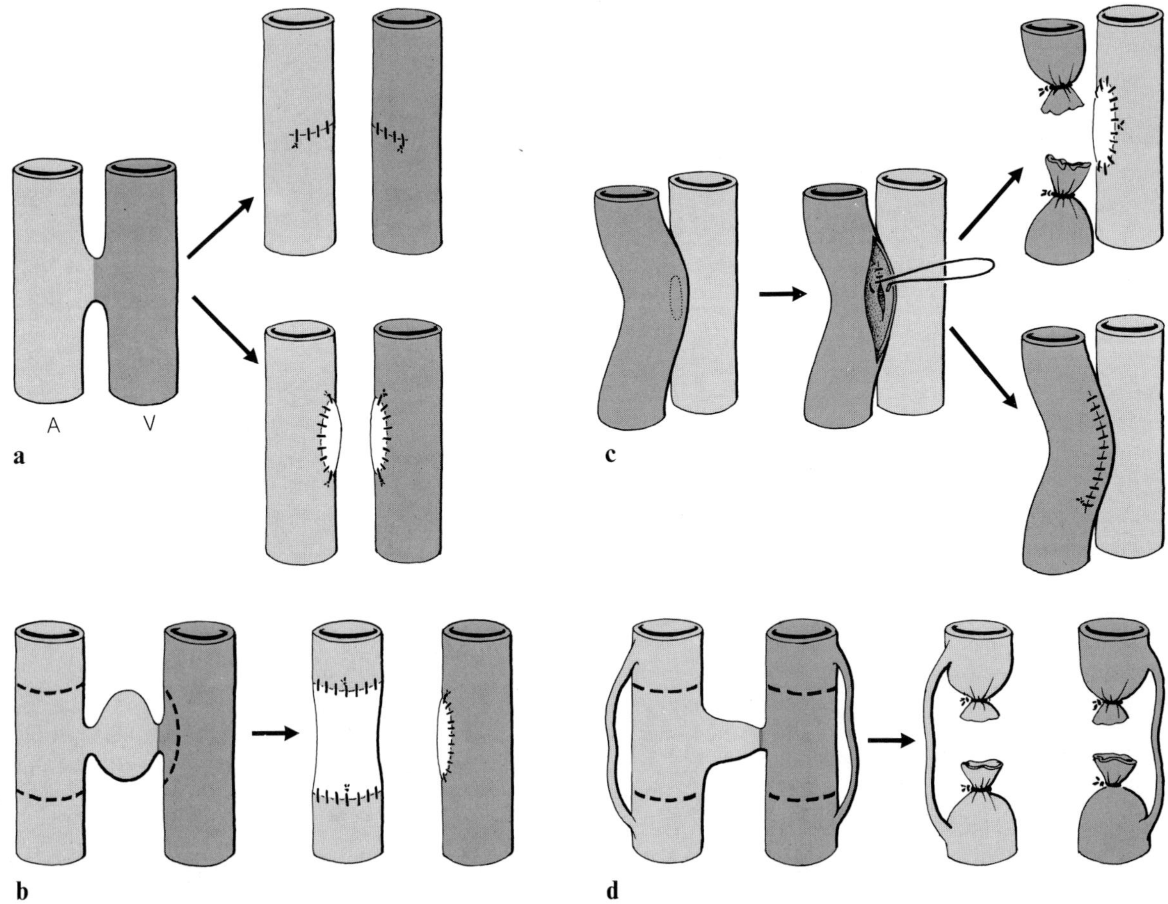

Fig. 13.12 a–d. Operative repair of arteriovenous fistulas [as described in 25, 49]. **a** Short arteriovenous fistula. Division and direct suture of artery and vein. Alternatively: reconstruction of each vessel by means of a venous patch graft. **c** Arteriovenous fistula with an interposed false aneurysm. Resection of artery and saphenous vein interposition. Closure of vein by patch graft. **b** Transvenous suture of arteriovenous fistula. *Above right:* in small peripheral vessels, the vein be ligated. *Lower right:* in larger vessels, direct suture of the vein following transvenous suture of the artery. **d** Bramann's method of quadruple ligation and excision. Only suitable for peripheral fistulas

should dissect very carefully because, owing to the thinness of the venous walls and the fragility of the artery in conjunction with trauma-induced indurations, the anatomy may be difficult to identify and massive bleeding may occur. First, all afferent and efferent vessels should be dissected and tape placed around them in order to provide sufficient control of bleeding if necessary [41].

The simplest operative procedure is division of the fistula and lateral suture of artery and vein. If the closure is not possible without stenosing the vessel, it is done by means of a venous patch graft angioplasty (Fig. 13.12a).

An isolated false aneurysm between the vessels should be resected. Afterwards, one decides whether a lateral suture is possible or whether the artery must be resected and a graft interposed (Fig. 13.12c). When there are elongations or aneurysms of the vessels, their degree will decide further procedure. If the artery alone shows an aneurysm, then, following resection of the fistula and of the aneurysm, continuity can be restored either by direct end-to-end suture or by means of a graft (vein, fabric prosthesis). Venous aneurysms can be resected and replaced by interposition grafts: a Dacron or PTFE prosthesis if the venous diameter is large, or a saphenous vein graft if the diameter is small.

Transvenous suture of the arterial opening using the Matas-Bickham technique is indicated for small vessels (forearm, lower leg) where lateral longitudinal suture of the artery is forbidden. Transvenous suture is also indicated in larger arteries when it is impossible to dissect the artery sufficiently because of its firm attachment to its surroundings (Fig. 13.12c) [19]. Bramman's method of quadruple ligation and excision should be performed only with smaller vessels. It can also be used where peripheral circulation is sustained by sufficient collateral flow and where the effort of reconstructing artery and vein does not seem to be justified. This procedure is not feasible proximal to the knee and the elbow (Fig. 13.12d) [19, 41].

In the presence of compensated relative and severe cardiac failure (grading according to ASCHENBRENNER), the attitude of surgeons regarding the feasibility of a later operation for arteriovenous fistulas was formerly one of hesitation. Such hesitation, however, is no longer justified. Here also, the aim should be the repair of all reconstructible vessels, including the vein [18].

REFERENCES

1. Allgöwer M, Border JR (1983) Management of open fractures in the multiple trauma patient. World J Surg 7:88–95
2. Bergentz SE, Bergquist D, Ericsson BF (1983) Vascular trauma. Acta Chir Scand 149:1–10
3. Burri P (1973) Traumatologie der Blutgefäße. Huber, Bern Stuttgart Wien
4. Clyne CAC, Ashbrooke EA (1985) Seat-belt aorta: isolated abdominal aortic injury following blunt trauma. Br J Surg 72:239
5. Cohen A, Brief D, Mathewson C (1970) Carotid artery injuries. Am J Surg 120:120–214
6. Cooley DA, Wukasch DC (1979) Techniques in vascular surgery. Saunders, Philadelphia
7. Courcy PA, Brotman S, Oster-Granite ML, Soderstrom CA, Siegel JH, Cowley RA (1984) Superior mesenteric artery and vein injuries from blunt abdominal trauma. J Trauma 24:843–845
8. Criado FJ, Wilson TH (1981) Axillary artery injuries: importance of early recognition. Injury 12:491–494
9. De Bakey ME, Simeone FA (1946) Battle injuries of the arteries during the second world war, an analysis of 2471 cases. Ann Surg 123:534–579
10. Drapanas T, Hewitt RL, Weichert RF, Smith AD (1970) Civilian vascular injuries: a critical appraisal of three decades of management. Ann Surg 172/3:351–360
11. Ehrichs E (1983) Die Unterbindung großer Gefäße. In: Eisemann B (ed) Prognose chirurgischer Erkrankungen. Enke, Stuttgart
12. Fabian TC, Turkleson ML, Connelly TL, Stone HH (1982) Injury to the popliteal artery. Ann J Surg 143:225–228
13. Fischer H (1977) Gefäßverletzungen. Akt Traumatol 7:221–226
14. Flint LM (1976) Injuries to major vessels: an overview of current concepts. Heart Lung 5/2:301–304
15. Franke F (1981) Erfahrungen bei arteriellen Gefäßverletzungen. Angio 3:313–316
16. Gaspar MR (1981) Arterial trauma. IN: peripheral arterial disease, 3rd edn, pp 124–157
17. Gaudernack T (1977) Periphere Gefäßverletzungen. Unfallheilkunde 80:515–521
18. Heberer G (1961) Probleme der Spätoperation traumatischer arterio-venöser Fisteln. Langenbecks Arch Chir 298:354–363
19. Heberer G, Rau G, Löhr HH (1966) Aorta und große Arterien. Springer, Berlin Heidelberg New York
20. Heberer G, Zehle A, Chorus A (1971) Wundheilungsstörungen in der rekonstruktiven Arterienchirurgie. Chirurg 42:337–346
21. Heberer G (1972) Verletzungen der Gliedmaßenschlagadern. Langenbecks Arch Chir 332:307–315
22. Heberer G, Becker HM, Dittmer H, Stelter WJ (1983) Vascular injuries in polytrauma. World J Surg 7:68–79
23. Heerklotz I, Basche S, Großmann K, Lauten A (1982) Klinisches und angiographisches Erscheinungsbild der traumatischen peripheren arteriovenösen Fisteln. Z Gesamte Inn Med 37,2:777–780
24. Heinrich P, Oschatz R, Willenberg E (1982) Arterienverletzungen. Urban u. Schwarzenberg, München Wien Baltimore
25. Janisch K, Bürger K, Hübner R (1974) Iatrogene Gefäßverletzungen. Dtsch Ges Wesen 29:1366–1368
26. Kashuk JL, Moore EE, Millikan JS, Moore JB (1982) Major abdominal vascular trauma – a unified approach. J Trauma 22/8:672–677
27. Kremer K (1959) Chirurgie der Arterien. Thieme, Stuttgart
28. Lanz U (1982) Folgezustände des Kompartmentsyndroms an den unteren Extremitäten. Langenbecks Arch Chir 358:237–242
29. Ledgerwood AM, Mullins RJ, Lucas CE (1980) Primary repair vs ligation for carotid artery injuries. Arch Surg 115:488–493
30. Leininger RG, Hillmann BJ, Pond GD (1982) Digital intravenous angiographic diagnosis of post-traumatic arteriovenous fistula. Urol Radiol 4:251–253
31. Lieckweg WG, Greenfield LJ (1978) Management of penetrating carotid arterial injury. Ann Surg:587–592
32. Lim RC, Trunkey DD, Blaisdell FW (1974) Acute abdominal aortic injury. Arch Surg 109:706–711
33. Linder F, Vollmar J (1965) Der augenblickliche Stand der Behandlung von Schlagaderverletzungen und ihrer Folgezustände. Chirurg 2:55–63
34. Lundy LJ, Mandal AK, Sister MAL, Alexander JL (1978) Experience in selective operations in the management of penetrating wounds of the neck. Surg Gynecol Obstet 147:845–848
35. Mavroudis C, Roon AJ, Baker CC, Thomas AN (1980) Management of acute cervicothoracic vascular injuries. J Thorac Cardiovas Surg 80:342
36. McDonals EG, Goodmann PHL, Winestock DP

(1975) The clinical indications for arteriography in trauma to the extremity. Arch Surg 116:45–47
37. McNamara JJ, Rief DK, Beasley W, Wright JK (1969) Vascular injury in Vietnam combat casualties. Ann Surg 178:143–147
38. Meagher DP, Defore WW, Mattox KL, Harberg FJ (1979) Vascular trauma in infants and children. J Trauma 19:532–536
39. Menzoian JO, Doyle JE, Lo Gerfo FW, Cantelmo N, Weitzmann AF, Sequiera JC (1983) Evaluation and management of vascular injuries of the extremities. Arch Surg 118:93–95
40. Millikan JS, Moore EE (1985) Critical factors in determining mortality from abdominal aortic trauma. Surg Gynecol Obstet 160:313–316
41. Müller-Wiefel H (1979) Arteriovenöse Fistel. In: Breitner B (ed) Operationslehre, Eingriffe an den Arterien, vol IV/I. Urban & Schwarzenberg, München Wien Baltimore, pp 149–151
42. Navarre JR, Cardillo PJ, Gorman JF, Clark PM, Martinez BD (1982) Vascular trauma in children and adolescent. Am J Surg 143:229–231
43. Oestern HJ, Echtermeyer V (1982) Behandlung des Kompartmentsyndroms und Ergebnisse. Langenbecks Arch Chir 358:227–232
44. Perry MO, Thal ER, Shires GT (1971) Management of arterial injuries. Ann Surg 173:403–408
45. Rich NM, Baugh JH, Hughes CW (1979) Acute arterial injuries in Vietnam: 1000 cases. J Trauma 10:359–369
46. Rich NM, Metz CHW, Hutton JE, Baugh JH, Hughes W (1971) Internal versus external fixation of fractures with concomitant vascular injuries in Vietnam. J Trauma 11:463–473
47. Russel JB, Watson TM, Modi JR, Lambeth A, Summer DS (1983) Digital subtraction angiography for evaluation of extracranial carotid occlusive disease: comparison with conventional arteriography. Surgery 94:604–611
48. Sandmann W (1984) Gefäßverletzungen. In: Kremer K, Müller E (eds) Die chirurgische Poliklinik. Thieme, Stuttgart New York
49. Sharma PVP, Babu SC, Shah PM, Clauss RH (1985) Changing patterns in civilian arterial injuries. J Cardiovasc Surg 26:7–11
50. Schlosser V, Spillner G, Urbaniy B (1981) Schußverletzungen des cardiovasculären Systems. Angio 3:299–304
51. Schlosser V, Kuner EH, Spillner G (1978) Ursache von Gefäßverletzungen bei alloplastischem Hüftgelenkersatz. Chirurg 49:180–183
52. Schmidt-Neuerburg KP (1982) Diagnose und Differentialdiagnose des Kompartmentsyndroms. Langenbecks Arch Chir 358:221–226
53. Schneiders H, Medrano J, Böttcher J (1976) Zur Diagnostik und Behandlung von Gefäßverletzungen. Unfallheilkunde 79:241–249
54. Schweiberer L, Dambe LT, Klopp F (1978) Die Mehrfachverletzung: Schweregrad und therapeutische Richtlinien. Chirurg 49:608–614
55. Shaftan GW (1983) The initial evaluation of the multiple trauma patient. Survery 7:19–25
56. Sirinek KR, Levine BA, Gaskill HV, Root HD (1981) Rasssessment of the role of routine operative exploration in vascular trauma. J Trauma 21:339–344
57. Sirinek KR, Gaskil HV, Dittmann I, Levine BA (1983) Exclusion angiography for patients with possible vascular injuries of the extremities. – A better use of trauma center resources. Surgery 94,4:598–603
58. Smith RF, Elliott JP, Hagemann JH, Szilagyi DE, Xavier AO (1974) Acute penetrating arterial injuries of the neck and limbs. Arch Surg 109:198–205
59. Snyder WH (1982) Vascular injuries near the knee: an updated series an overview of the problem. Surgery 91:502–506
60. Steiner E, Flora G (1977) Wachstumsstörungen nach Gefäßverletzungen bei Jugendlichen. Med Wochenschrift, Wien, 127:745
61. Stelter WJ, Kortmann H (1981) Gefäßverletzungen und arteriovenöse Fisteln. In: Heberer G, Schweiberer L (eds) Indikation zur Operation, 2nd edn. Springer, Berlin Heidelberg New York, pp 317–322
62. Stock W, Geppert E, Zehle A (1975) Das Tourniquet-Syndrom als bedrohliche Komplikation nach Embolektomie bei Sattelembolie. Thoraxchir 23:324–329
63. Trede H, Thiele HH, Hagmüller E, Reiber M (1985) Begleitverletzungen an Gefäßen bei Polytrauma. In: Ungeheur E (ed) Das Polytrauma. Urban & Schwarzenberg, München Wien Baltimore
64. Tscherne H (1982) Das Kompartmentsyndrom. Langenbecks Arch Chir 358:243–244
65. Tscherne H, Oestern HJ, Sturm J (1983) Ostheosynthesis of major fractures in polytrauma. World J Surg 7:80–87
66. Turner WW, Snyder WH, Fry WJ (1983) Mortality and renal salvage after renovascular trauma. Am J Surg 146/6:848–851
67. Unger SW, Tucker WS, Mrdeza MA, Wllons HA, Chandler JG (1980) Carotid arterial trauma. Surgery 87/5:477–487
68. Vollmar J (1964) Traumatische arterio-venöse Fisteln (Erfahrungsbericht über 190 Fälle). Zentralbl Chir 89:1930–1939
69. Vollmar J (1976) Gefäßverletzungen. Chir Gegenwart IV:2–25
70. Vollmar J (1982) Rekonstruktive Chirurgie der Arterien, 2nd edn. Thieme, Stuttgart New York
71. Wicky B, Largiader J, Pouliadis G, Zollikofer C (1984) Klinische und angiographische Verlaufskontrolle und Gefäßverletzungen großer Extremitätenarterien. Chirurg 55:244–248

14 Replantation of Peripheral Body Parts (Microreplantation)

E. BIEMER

CONTENTS

A. Definitions and Nomenclature

I. Amputation

An *amputation* is the total separation of all, or almost all, anatomic structures from the body; only very few connections to the body may remain. No sign of blood circulation is present.

II. Replantation

A replantation is the operative reconstruction of all structural connections. The most important, of course, is the vascular connection because only this guarantees the vitality of the peripheral part as well as healing after surgery. Today, the surgeon always tries to reconstruct all functional structures with the greatest possible degree of anatomic correctness. The time interval between amputation and replantation – the period of total interruption of blood circulation – is incorrectly called the *ischemic time*. The term *anoxemia* is more accurate. By cooling the amputated part down to 4° C this period may be prolonged without irreversible damage that would jeopardize the success of replantation (in fingers almost 24 h). In principle, however, the shorter the time of anoxemia, the higher the rate of healing is.

III. Total and Subtotal Amputation

A peripheral body part may be totally separated from the body. This is called "total amputation". If tissue connections to the body, such as tendon fibers remain, such an injury is then called a "subtotal amputation."

According to the connecting structure, we differentiate the following types of subtotal amputation:

Type I	bones
Type II	extensor tendons
Type III	flexor tendons
Type IV	nerves
Type V	skin connections

IV. Macro- and Microreplantations

Because there are important technical and clinical differences between the replantation of an arm and a thumb, we distinguish between the following two groups:

1. Macroreplantations: proximal to the wrist or ankle joints.

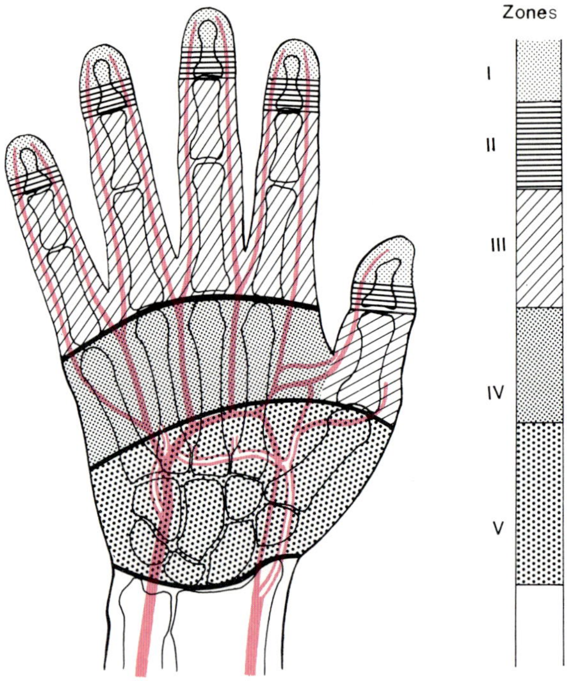

Fig. 14.1. Zones of amputation in the hand

2. Microreplantations: distal to the wrist or ankle joints. Other amputations, such as scalping injuries and ear and nose amputations, also belong to this group if replantation requires microsurgical techniques.

V. Classification of Hand Amputations

According to the level of amputation, we distinguish five hand zones (Fig. 14.1). This classification is important for the surgical indication and operative technique. Therefore, it will be referred to in the corresponding sections.

B. Indications for Replantation

Today, replantation is indicated as a matter of course in every amputation. Factors limiting immediate surgical treatment include poor general condition or severe concomitant injuries. Life-threatening conditions always have priority over replantation! Furthermore, it is impossible to replant body parts which have been totally destroyed.

In addition to these criteria, certain functional aspects of the hand must be considered. These have developed from the evaluation of long-term results:

Absolute indications:
- Thumbs
- Several long fingers
- Midhand
- Hand
- Amputations in children (there is one restriction, determined by the long-term results; see below)

Relative indications:
- End phalanx
- A single finger

No indications:
- Single fingers in patients who work outdoors (intolerance to cold)
- Replantation of a single finger with a destroyed large joint (proximal joint, middle joint)

This classification is not a rigid scheme. It is intended to serve as an orientation. As a matter of principle, in the last two groups the final decision should be made only after consultation with an experienced hand surgeon. Aesthetic and psychological aspects must always be considered.

The long-established rule that *amputations in children* are always *absolute indications* for surgery must be revised today. It has been shown that replanted body parts always show considerable *growth retardation*. Moreover, deformations commonly develop later on, owing to *partial injury to the epiphysis*. Children also have a large adaptive capability and can, for example, completely compensate for a missing finger. Replants that show strong growth retardation or that have healed in the wrong position often make complicated secondary surgery or reamputation necessary.

C. Technique of Replantation in the Hand

In principle, replantation always involves reconstruction of all functional structures. This means that total surgical repair is done in one session. If the destruction of tendons and nerves does not allow reconnection, nerve transplantations or nerve and tendon transfers should be performed, if necessary.

In some cases, silicone rods may be implanted to pave the way for tendon transplantation at a later time. Total primary surgical repair shortens the time of treatment in the long run and reduces the number of secondary operations, which are usually very difficult.

I. General Preparation of the Injured Patient for Replantation

After the patient has been informed of the necessity of surgical reconstruction, a complete general medical examination should follow. This means:

a) Laboratory examinations: electrolytes, hemoglobin and hematocrit, blood typing, and parameters of coagulation. These values are necessary because amputation often leads to severe hemorrhage; and general anesthesia, together with infusion therapy, may lead to electrolyte shifts. Furthermore, they are needed as control values, especially if heparinization is necessary during and after surgery.
b) Past history: chronic diseases, medication, clotting disorders, diabetes mellitus, etc.
c) X-rays of the injured limb and of the amputated body part.
d) ECG and chest X-ray.
e) Tetanus immunization.

II. Surgical Procedure

The patient must be positioned carefully and comfortably on the operating table since surgery of the upper extremity under *plexus anesthesia* (axillary plexus) takes about 9–10 h. In our experience, the patient can lie very comfortably on his/her normal ward bed during the operation.

As the patient is being prepared for surgery, the surgeon can begin the dissection of the totally amputated body part. All of the structures which have to be reconnected are carefully exposed and marked, the arteries with clips, the nerves with 6–0 nylon sutures, the flexor tendons and extensor tendons with 4–0 nylon sutures.

We recommend small longitudinal incisions of the skin over the neurovascular bundles for better orientation. The triangular skin flaps are retracted and held in place by suturing them directly to the skin surface. Following internal fixation, a rhomboid skin defect is formed which provides good exposure of vascular anastomoses and nerve sutures.

Moreover, these longitudinal incisions interrupt the circular scars on the finger (Fig. 14.2).

1. Wound Excision and Markings

The *identification and marking* of structures within the amputated stump under magnification is extremely important. Following internal fixation, it is usually not possible to find vessels or nerve stumps. *Wound excision* is performed only after structures are marked. All injured tissue should be removed.

The foremost rule in replantation surgery is:

When connecting tissues to one another, connect only "viable with viable."

The severest complication following replantation is circular connective tissue necrosis in the area of the anastomosis. Trimming of the vascular ends and nerve stumps is done under the microscope. The stronger magnification of this instru-

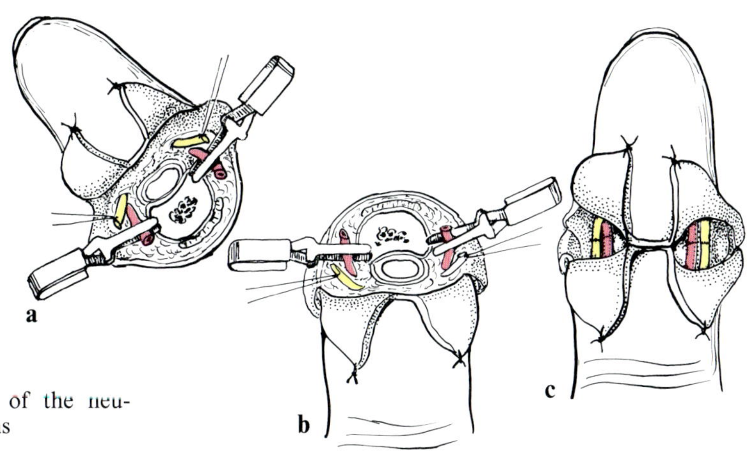
a b c

Fig. 14.2a–c. Visualization and marking of the neurovascular bundles by longitudinal incisions ment allows for a better assessment of the fine structures.

Bones must be shortened and their surfaces smoothed before one is able to reconnect all structures. Excessive shortening must be avoided, however, especially in the thumb. Vascular defects should not be compensated by further shortening of the bone, rather, they are an indication for microsurgical vein interposition. For replantations in the hand, the following order of reconstruction has been established:

1. Internal fixation
2. Suture of the flexor tendons
3. Suture of the tendon sheaths
4. Anastomosis of both volar finger arteries
5. Suture of both volar finger nerves
6. Suture of the extensor tendons
7. Anastomosis of 1–2 dorsal veins per finger
8. Loose skin adaptation

2. Internal Fixation (Fig. 14.3a–e)

Central intramedullary Kirschner wire (Fig. 14.3a)

Advantages: Quick, simple, always applicable. Rotation makes vascular anastomosis easier. The wire can be easily removed.
Disadvantages: No exercise stability of the internal fixation, no rotational stability. In most cases, neighboring joints must also be fixed.

Two short, crossed drill wires (Fig. 14.3b):

Advantages: Greater stability, including rotational stability. Relatively simple technique. Easily removed.
Disadvantages: Not applicable in severe infractions of the bones and near joints. It is often necessary to include neighboring joints. No exercise stability.

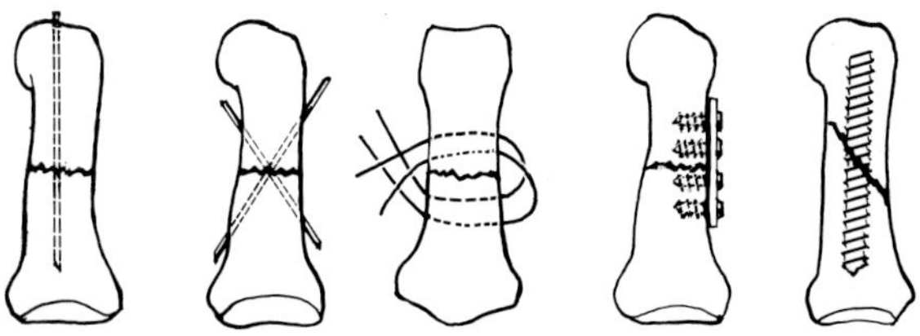

a **b** **c** **d** **e**

Fig. 14.3a–e. Internal fixation in replantations of the hand. **a** Simple intramedullary Kirschner wire, **b** crossed Kirschner wires, **c** two transosseus wire sutures, **d** miniplate and screws, **e** intramedullary screw fixation

Transosseous wire sutures with temporary intramedullary central Kirschner wire fixation (Fig. 14.3d):

Advantages: Good compression and exercise stability.
Disadvantages: Complicated technique, can only be used in fractures which are not next to joints. Not applicable where there are extensive infractions or multiple bone fragments. Removal of the osteosynthetic material is difficult or impossible.

Plates and screws (AO small fragment instrumentarium) (Fig. 14.3d):

Advantages: Absolute exercise stability.
Disadvantages: Only applicable in the metacarpal region. Cannot be used with infractions or multiple bone fragments, also not near joints. A long segment of the bone must be exposed. Complicated and time-consuming method: The material must be removed in a second operation.

Intramedullary screw fixation (Fig. 14.3e):

Advantages: Absolute exercise stability with good compression.
Disadvantages: Applicable only in the middle third of the phalanx. Not possible with infractions or multiple bone fragments. A large metal body must remain permanently in the bone (danger of metallosis).

Selection of the most suitable osteosynthetic material is made according to the particular requirements in each individual case.

3. Suture of the Flexor Tendons

Although finger amputations occur within the area described by BUNELL as "no man's land", primary reconstruction of all parts of the flexor apparatus is the aim. The deep and superficial flexor tendons are sutured with a Kessler suture, followed by additional fine adaptation (Fig. 14.5). A 4–0 woven synthetic suture and two straight needles are used. A 6–0 to 7–0 monofilament nylon suture is used for continuous fine adaptation. One should also attempt to adapt the tendon sheath and periosteum lying beneath the tendons. Both tendon stumps are held in place by the BIEMER tendon adapter (Fig. 14.4).

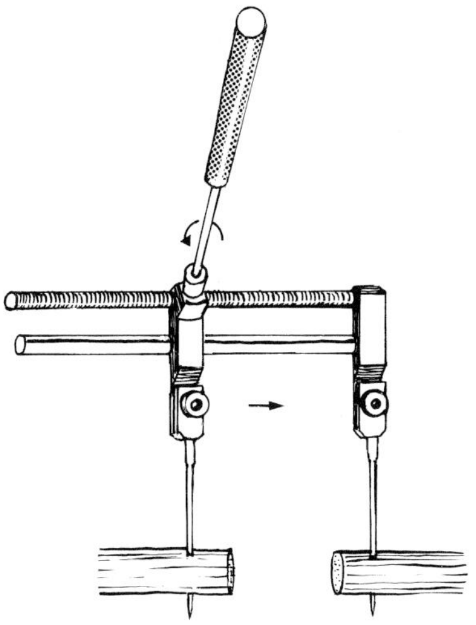

Fig. 14.4. Tendon adapter according to BIEMER (Aesculap Company)

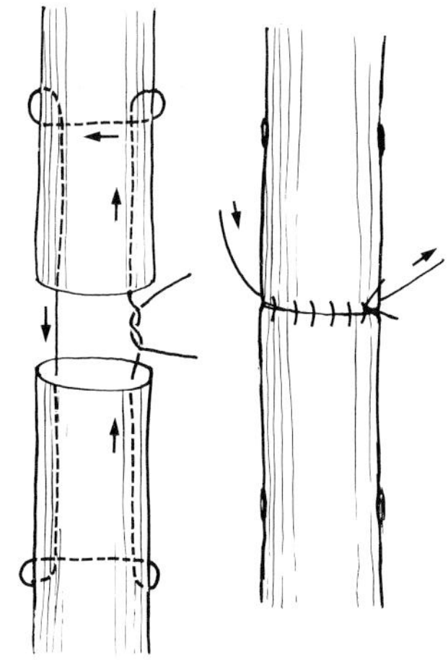

Fig. 14.5. Kessler suture with fine adaptation of the flexor tendon

4. Arterial Anastomosis

As a matter of principle, both volar finger arteries should always be anastomosed to maximize perfusion. In thumbs and index fingers, the radial arteries are often very weak or sometimes not even present. In such cases, only the ulnar vessels can be anastomosed.

The stumps must lie opposite one another, loosely and without tension. Double clamps or vascular adaptors are not used in our clinic. The anastomosis is then performed as described in the chapter on suture techniques.

5. Nerve Suture

The sensory finger nerves may be separated into 1–3 fascicles. This allows a true interfascicular or a perineural suture to be performed.

Only 2–3 epiperineural sutures are usually placed; further divisions are not made (Fig. 14.7). Just as with tendons, the nerve stumps may be held by a BIEMER nerve adapter (Fig. 14.6).

It is difficult to connect the motor fibers of the median nerve and the ulnar nerve in amputations of the entire hand. In these large nerves a perineural suture of each fascicular bundle should be performed (Fig. 14.7).

6. Suture of the Extensor Tendons

After connecting all structures on the palmar side the hand is turned over and the extensor tendons are reconstructed. If possible, all parts should be adapted with 4–0 to 5–0 monofilament nylon sutures.

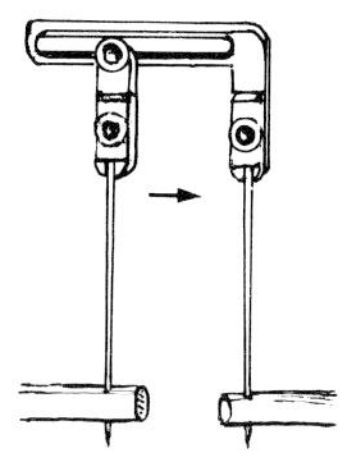

Fig. 14.6. Nerve adapter according to BIEMER (Aesculap Company)

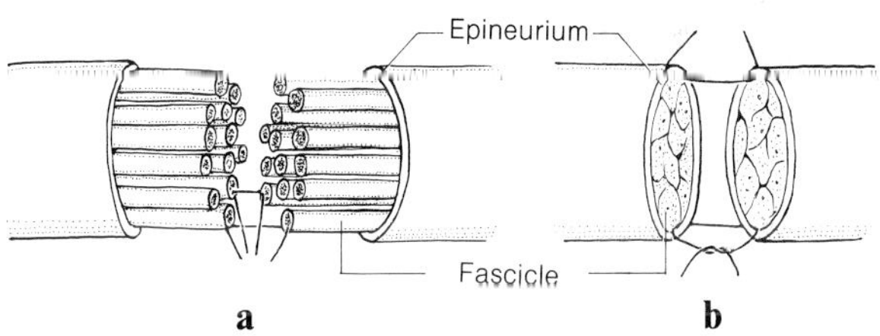

Fig. 14.7. a Interfascicular suture in polyfascicular nerves. **b** Epineural suture of an oligofascicular nerve

7. Venous Anastomoses

The one or two larger veins exhibiting the strongest back flow should be identified in each finger. They are then marked with clips and stabilized. If no corresponding venous stumps can be found, oblique connections can be constructed by implanting small vein graft interpositions. Because there is very little tissue between these veins and the skin, tendons, and bones, no tension should remain on the venous anastomoses.

Careful ligation or coagulation of all other bleeding veins prevents recurrent hemorrhage and raises flow velocity up to arterial values in the one or two venous connections thus constructed. We think this is a good prophylaxis of venous thrombosis. Therefore, we do not create more than two well-functioning venous anastomoses.

8. Skin Suture

Adaptation of the skin is achieved with only a few loose stitches. The anastomotic sites should be covered by skin. However, it has been shown that in some cases, it is better to keep venous interpositions uncovered, rather than achieve skin closure under tension. Free skin transplants or local flaps may be used.

For the prevention of circular scars, small skin incisions or Z-plasty are useful techniques.

9. Wound Dressing

The wound dressing should not constrict or strangulate any part of the wound area. We use lubricated strips of gauze and wrap them smoothly in cotton. A loose gauze bandage holds the dressing material in place. This creates a loose and absorbent wound dressing. All finger tips must remain uncovered so that their appearance can be judged at all times. We do not use splints or plaster casts any more because we have seen repeated injuries due to compression (Fig. 14.8).

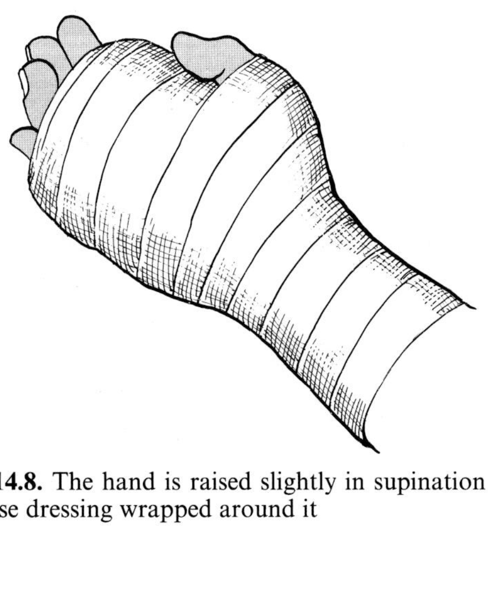

Fig. 14.8. The hand is raised slightly in supination with a loose dressing wrapped around it

The dressing should be changed only when absolutely necessary. If a dressing becomes completely soaked with fresh or dry blood, it must always be removed, otherwise, it may cause constriction of the wound area.

10. Medication

The reader is referred to Chap. 6.6 on microvascular surgery.

11. Postoperative Care

Because most vascular thromboses occur within the first 24 h, the patient must be *routinely monitored* following each replantation, in order to detect circulatory disorders quickly and, if necessary, to reintervene. Several instruments are used for this purpose: temperature recording instruments, plethysmography, Doppler ultrasound, percutaneous PO_2 measurements, thermography, etc. In our experience, and in the experience of other centers worldwide, clinical observation is the most secure and reliable method. Therefore, the replanted body part should be inspected every 2 h. Nail pressure, temperature measurements, and, if necessary, puncture of the skin with a small lancet afford control of perfusion. If there are any signs of reduced blood circulation or venous stasis, the wound dressing and the skin sutures must be checked first in order to detect possible compression from the outside. If the condition does not improve within a very short period of time, a *reoperation* is indicated.

If the venous drainage system does not function properly and stasis cannot be relieved, there is still a chance of improvement by making several incisions under heparinization for the purpose of letting the congested blood flow out of the reconstructed body part. Leeches may also be placed on the congested area. Of course, during such a procedure, constant hemoglobin and hematocrit checks must be made, since in some instances blood loss may be considerable.

D. Specific Considerations in Different Mechanisms of Amputation

I. Cutting Amputation

A cutting amputation is an injury caused by a narrow-edged and relatively sharp object and producing minimal traumatization at the line of amputation. Circular saw amputations are the commonest injuries of this type.

A relatively smooth cutting amputation offers the most favorable conditions for replantation. As a result of the fact that the bone is only very slightly shortened, it is usually possible to effect vascular anastomoses, and nerve and tendon sutures as well, that are free of tension. In oblique amputations, which are common injuries of the left thumb among right-handed persons with a circular saw, the tangentially injured volar vessels must often be bridged by venous interposition grafts so that the thumb does not become too short.

II. Crushing Amputation

In a crushing amputation, the entire crushed tissue zone must be resected. In these areas the vessel walls are damaged so badly that vessel occlusion is caused by intimal lesions. Furthermore, necrosis of the connective tissue or skin surrounding the area of anastomosis almost always leads to thrombosis. In subtotal crushing injuries, this mandatory resection is often not performed in an effort to preserve structures. Existing skin bridges in particular make replantation easier because of their vein connections.

However, in many cases, we have found that these preexistent vein connections have been damaged so badly that they play no important functional role in limb preservation. Instead, we have found them to be obstructed by thrombosis during the postoperative course. Therefore, in subtotal crushing injuries, it is often better to convert a subtotal amputation into a total smooth cutting amputation by resecting the entire crushed zone first and then performing replantation.

III. Evulsion Amputation

This type of injury is the most unfavorable condition for replantation. The main problem in such amputations is that the various structures are not separated at the same level; instead, some are torn more proximally and some more distally.

We have observed that, in these amputations, the flexor tendons usually tear at sites which lie high up near the origins of the forearm muscles, and that the extensor tendons are divided at the level of bone fractures. The neurovascular bundle is usually injured at different levels. The nerves are almost always longer than the vessels. The dorsal veins tear at the edge of the skin remants, which differ considerably in length. Evulsion injuries most commonly occur at the thumb.

In most cases arterial reconstruction is possible by means of vein interposition grafts. Sometimes, revascularization is only possibly by reconnection of the superficial branch of the radial artery in the tabatière. The flexor tendon of the thumb, which usually tears far up near the origin of the forearm muscles, may be replaced by a subcutaneously displaced superficial flexor tendon of a long finger. In cases where the thenar muscles are still well preserved and primary arthrodesis of the proximal thumb joint is performed, the thumb may still show good function without replacement of the flexor tendons.

The problem of resensibilization must be individualized. Transfer of the ulnar finger nerves or connection to a dorsal branch of the radial nerve is possible. These maneuvers may achieve excellent protective sensibility in the thumb.

IV. Skeletizing Amputation

Skeletizing injuries are characterized by the preservation of the skeletal and tendinous apparatus.

Only the surrounding soft tissue coat is pulled off. Such a mechanism can be seen in accidents involving rollers, e.g., in pressing machines, where the extreme tip of the finger gets stuck in the machine, and the coat of soft tissue around the finger is torn off like a glove.

Another mechanism is encountered when a finger ring gets stuck. The ring scrapes the soft connective tissue off the finger.

In both cases *severe injury of the amputated integument* results, either as a consequence of the crushing between the rollers or the scraping and pushing of the ring. Peripheral bone parts of varying length may be ripped off, together with the skin covering.

The reconstruction of such circular stripping of the skeletal apparatus is possible only by means of pedicled flaps or cuffs in step-by-step operations. In some cases, the neurovascular bundle is amputated over the tendons along with the soft tissue integument, making true replantation possible. If such a reconstruction is successful, very good aesthetic and functional results can be expected as the joints and tendons remain uninjured.

V. Severe Combined Forms of Amputation

These types of amputation are a combination of crushing, tearing, or other mechanisms of injury.

They are among the most difficult problems in replantation surgery. Vessels are not only separated at the amputation line, but also distally within the amputated body part. Additional massive crushing of the amputated parts or of the proximal portions of the stump almost always lead to massive edema and, as a consequence, to extensive scar formation which limit functional results in the long run. At least the *main zone of injury must be resected* in these patients. If necessary, vein interpositions within the arterial as well as the venous system must be constructed on a large scale. In many cases, simultaneous *nerve transplantation* is also necessary.

Longer, destroyed portions of tendons must undergo secondary reconstruction, which may be prepared for implanting silicone rods at the time of replantation.

E. Heterotopic Replantations (Primary Finger Exchange)

In *multiple amputations* in which the parts are almost completely destroyed or not present at all, the general principles of hand reconstruction must be observed.

Since the hand is a grasping organ, one must always attempt to restore its grasping function. For example, if all the fingers and the thumb are amputated, and the thumb cannot be replanted, the amputated index finger should be used for reconstruction of the thumb. A dispensable amputated index finger or another finger which is so severely destroyed at its proximal joint that replantation is not indicated are most suited for this purpose.

The thumb is reconstructed first, then the ulnar finger (ring, or little finger), and finally the other fingers, if possible.

F. Postoperative Physiotherapy

Of the utmost importance for later function of the hand is postoperative physiotherapy. In our hospital, this is performed according to the following scheme, provided no problems are encountered during recovery:

Passive treatment: starting on day 3–4
Active treatment: starting in week 3
Provisional exercise: after removal of implanted Kirschner wires

G. Microreplantations of Other Parts

I. Scalping Injuries

These injuries are always an *absolute indication* for replantation. Usually, the scalp is ripped off at the periosteum. First, it is shaved and cleansed. The veins are easily identified on the bottom surface of the scalp. The arteries are harder to find since they run subcutaneously.

The temporal and occipital arteries are best suited for anastomosis. To ensure blood circulation after a total scalping injury, anastomosis of only one artery is sufficient. The "watershed" at the top of the head, which has often been postulated by several investigators, does not exist.

II. Injuries of the Face

Sometimes, in children parts of the lip or entire portions of the middle face have been bitten off by dogs. In these injuries, the vessels must be searched for according to their topographical positions. The results achieved so far in these operations justify the absolute indication for replantation in such cases.

III. Amputation of the Penis

This is a very rare form of amputation which is usually the result of self-mutilation by a psychiatric patient. The vessels are larger and easily identified. In order to achieve good circulation to the glans penis, not only the dorsal vessels should be reconnected, but also the central ones. Of course, nerve suture is absolutely necessary.

IV. Peripheral Amputations of the Foot

Amputations distal to the ankle joint are also very rare. Replantation is only indicated in smooth cutting amputations.

In amputations of the toes, the large toe alone is sometimes replanted for aesthetic reasons. This remains, however, a relative indication.

In metatarsal and foot amputations, shortening of the foot should not be too extensive. Furthermore, there must be a possibility of resensibilizing the amputated part. The vessels are large and easy to anastomose. All other structures are repaired as anatomically as possible.

REFERENCES

1. Biemer E (1977) Replantation von Fingern und Extremitätenteilen. Technik und Ergebnisse. Chirurg 48:353
2. Biemer E, Duspiva W (1977) Komplikationen bei der Replantation abgetrennter Gliedmaßen. Handchirurgie 9:67
3. Biemer E, Duspiva W, Herndl E, Stock W, Ramatschi P (1977) Early experiences in organising and running a replantation service. Br J Plast Surg 31:9
4. Biemer E, Duspiva W (1978) Erfahrungen nach über 272 Replantationen peripherer Extremitätenteile mit mikrovaskulären Anastomosen. Z Orthop 116:587
5. Biemer E (1979) Indikation zur Replantation peripherer Körperteile (Mikroreplantation). Unfallheilkunde 82:224–231
6. Biemer E, Duspiva W (1980) Rekonstruktive Mikrogefäßchirurgie. Springer, Berlin Heidelberg New York
7. Biemer B, Stock W, Duspiva W (1983) Replantationen an der unteren Extremität. Chirurg 54:361–365
8. Buncke HJ, Buncke CM, Schulz WP (1966) Immediate Nicoladoni procedure in the rhesus monkey, or hallux-to-hand transplantation, utilizing microminiature vascular anastomoses. Br J Plast Surg 19:332
9. Duspiva W, Biemer E, Herndl E, Stock W, Alberti I (1979) Knochenheilung in der Replantationschirurgie der Hand. Fortschr Med 97:953
10. O'Brian BMcC, McLeod AM, Miller GDM, Newing RK, Hayhurst JW, Morrison WA (1973) Clinical replanation of digits. Plast Reconstr Surg 52:490
11. Meyer VE (1983) Replantationschirurgie der oberen Extremität. Huber, Bern Stuttgart Wien
12. Schmidt-Tintemann U, Biemer E, Duspiva W (1976) Replantationen abgetrennter Finger, Daumen und Hände durch Mikrogefäßchirurgie. Dtsch Ärzteblatt 20:1367
13. Tamai S (1974) Present status and prospect of limb and finger replantation. Surg Diag Traet 6:547

15 Arterial Aneurysms

15.1 Arterial Aneurysms of the Extracranial Supra-aortic Branches and the Upper Extremities

D. RAITHEL

CONTENTS

A. Anatomy and Etiology

Anatomy. See Chaps. 2.1, 2.2, 7.1, 8, and 10

I. Aneurysms of the Supra-aortic Branches

Aneurysms of the extracranial carotid artery are very rare and are limited mainly to the common carotid artery and the internal carotid artery [1, 4–7, 9, 10]. In regard to etiology, traumatic aneurysms are predominant, followed by arteriosclerotic ones. Luetic aneurysms are a rarity nowadays.

Furthermore, aneurysms have been noticed following cystic medial necrosis, fibromuscular dysplasia, and other congenital malformations.

II. Aneurysms of the Upper Extremities

Aneurysms of the subclavian artery, which are relatively frequent and mainly caused by a cervical rib, represent a poststenotic dilatation [2, 3]. They are seldom of arteriosclerotic origin. Also, tuberculosis located at the apex of the lung with perisubclavian inflammation may cause an aneurysm. In Marfan's syndrome, the subclavian artery is one of the preferred localizations.

Aneurysms of the brachial artery are mostly of traumatic origin or caused by transbrachial catheter angiography. Injuries also play a role in the development of aneurysms of forearm arteries

Rarely, aneurysms of large supra-aortic branches in combination with other peripheral aneurysms are observed.

B. Indication for Operation

The indication for operation is based on all of the findings, the age, and the general condition of the patient.

In contrast to central or peripheral aneurysms of the lower extremity, thromboembolic complications have to be mentioned first; the risk of aneurysm rupture is low. According to a survey of the literature by HOBSON et al. [3] 86% of the aneurysms of the axillosubclavian arteries cause peripheral embolizations. Some 19% of patients showed concomitant neurologic symptoms, pressure injury of the brachial plexus being commonest.

Therapy is indicated in patients with aneurysms that cause embolization, especially aneurysms of arteries supplying the brain. In the case of a ruptured or nonruptured aneurysm, we also consider it an indication for operation when there is compression of adjacent nerve structures with neurologic deficit. In case of a thrombosed aneurysm, operation is indicated only when the blood flow in the organs supplied by that artery is diminished, e.g., in the presence of cerebrovascular insufficiency. If thrombosis remains asymptomatic, operative therapy is not indicated.

Where the aneurysm is associated with a stenosis of the carotid artery above or below the aneurysm, the indication for operation of both lesions is urgent.

Younger patients may be *treated prophylactically* (in order to prevent the complications mentioned) when the aneurysm can be removed relatively easily and with minimal risk.

When judging whether surgery is indicated, we consider arteriographic findings to be important: ulcerative changes of the vessel wall and thrombotic deposits are factors favoring surgery (this is especially true for aneurysms of the carotid artery); if the vessel wall is smooth, one may wait [8].

Aneurysms located directly at the base of the skull in the distal portion of the extracranial internal carotid artery are difficult to dissect, and the reconstruction following resection of such an aneurysm is a problem. In such cases two procedures may be considered:

1. Ligation of the proximal internal carotid artery with simultaneous extra-intracranial anastomosis
2. "Gradual" carotid occlusion with an ameroid ring

C. Positioning

For operative procedures of the carotid arteries the patient is always placed in a supine position with the head slightly turned to the side opposite that of the operation.

The same is true for procedures on the axillary and subclavian arteries. The arm of the patient, however, should also be fixed in an abducted position, thereby allowing a graft to be anastomosed peripherally, if necessary.

For a transaxillary operation on a subclavian aneurysm, the patient is placed in the lateral position.

For correction of aneurysms of the upper extremity the arm is also abducted, rotated externally, and secured on an arm board.

In our opinion, the possibility of repair by means of a saphenous vein interposition ought to be considered. For that purpose, both inguinal regions as far as the middle of the femur should be draped for harvesting the greater saphenous vein.

D. Operative Exposure

The choice of operative procedure and consequently also of operative exposure is dependent upon the localization and the size of the aneurysm. As a matter of principle, it is important that exposure be as generous as possible for repairs with low risk [8, 11].

Innominate aneurysms are corrected by median sternotomy. The mediastinum may be widely exposed by the use of a rib retractor at the region of the manubrium sterni. This provides for secure cross-clamping at the origin of the innominate artery (Satinsky clamp; Fig. 15.1.1 b). For aneurysms of the common carotid artery located close to the origin, a partial median sternotomy may be sufficient (Fig. 15.1.1 a).

The carotid bifurcation is exposed by an incision at the anterior border of the sternocleidomastoid muscle with possible extension of the incision posteriorly (Fig. 15.1.3 a).

Subclavian aneurysms on the right side are exposed by supraclavicular incision, perhaps in combination with a partial median sternotomy (Fig. 15.1.6 a).

Subclavian aneurysms on the left side, located centrally, require exposure through the third interspace, with tapes placed around the aorta, the subclavian artery, and the vertebral artery, and a Satinsky clamp placed tangentially on the aorta, excluding the subclavian artery (Fig. 15.1.5 a, b). Smaller extrathoracic subclavian aneurysms may be resected using a supraclavicular approach alone. Surgeons who are familiar with the transaxillary resection of the first rib may prefer the transaxillary approach to subclavian aneurysm.

Aneurysms of the vertebral artery are exposed by a supraclavicular approach, following division of the anterior scalenus muscle, with preservation of the phrenic nerve (Fig. 15.1.6 a).

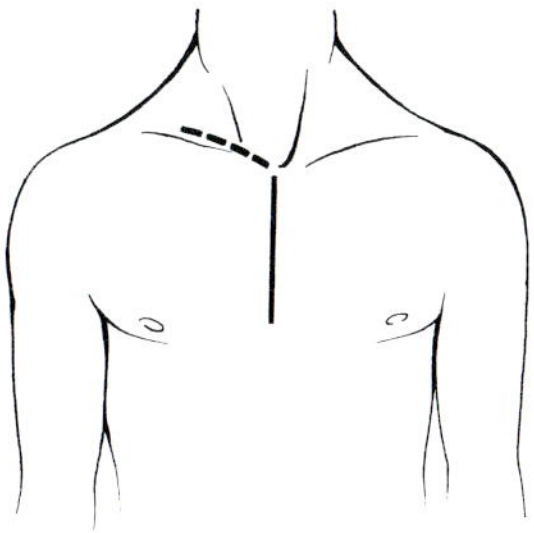
a

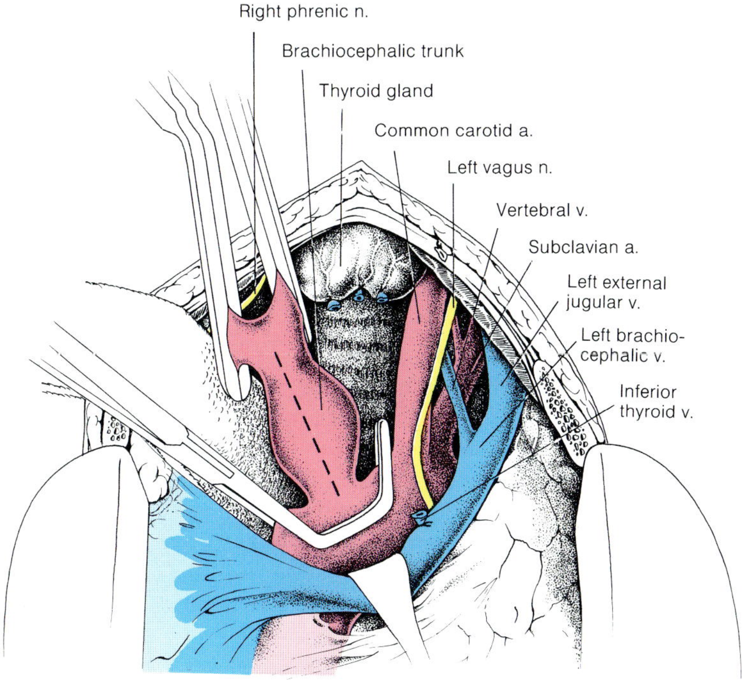

b

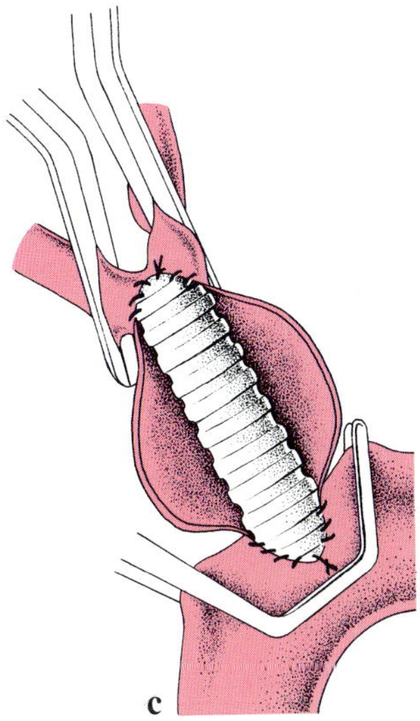
c

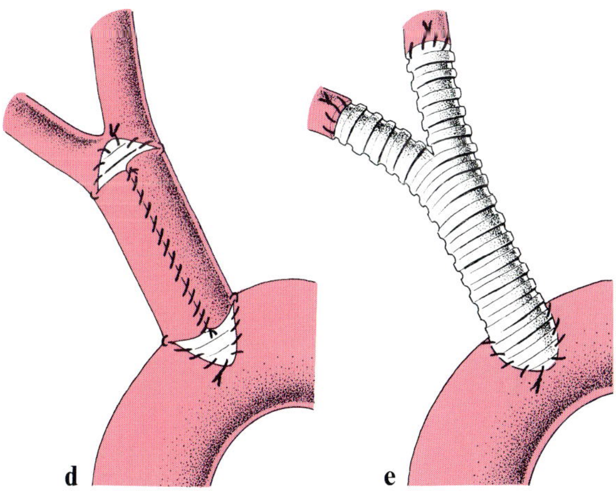
d e

Fig. 15.1.1. a Median sternotomy with possible supraclavicular extension to expose the innominate artery. **b** Exposure of the innominate artery and exclusion using a Satinsky clamp on the aortic arch. **c** Interposition of a straight prosthesis (8 mm). **d** The prosthesis is inclosed in the aneurysmal sac. **e** Interposition of a bifurcation prosthesis (14 × 8 mm)

Aneurysms of the axillary artery and of the subclavian-axillary junction are best exposed by an infraclavicular incision. A transaxillary approach with resection of the first rib is also recommended (see p. 559).

Proximal aneurysms of the *brachial artery* are exposed by an incision in the medial upper arm, following the course of the sulcus bicipitalis medialis.

For exposure of distal brachial aneurysms, an S-shaped incision in the elbow is recommended, dividing the fascia of the tendon of the biceps muscle.

E. Operative Techniques

I. Innominate Aneurysms

The operation is performed under systemic heparinization.

Following median sternotomy, the ascending aorta, the innominate artery, and the subclavian and common carotid arteries are exposed (Fig. 15.1.1 b).

While dissecting, one should pay particular attention to the innominate vein, which may be adherent to the aneurysm.

The origin of the innominate artery is clamped off by placing a Satinsky clamp tangentially on the ascending aorta. Following cross-clamping of the common carotid artery and the right subclavian artery, the aneurysm is opened and thrombi are removed (Fig. 15.1.1b).

The aneurysm may extend into the subclavian or the common carotid artery. In these cases a bifurcation prosthesis (14 × 8 mm) or a straight fabric prosthesis (8 mm) must be interposed in either an aortocarotid or aortosubclavian position, as the case may be (Fig. 15.1.1c–e).

If a straight prosthesis is interposed, either the subclavian artery or the common carotid artery must be anastomosed end-to-side.

The central anastomosis with the ascending aorta is beveled end-to-side; the distal anastomosis should be beveled end-to-end.

Following the suture of both anastomoses, the prosthesis is covered by closure of the remaining wall of the aneurysm (Fig. 15.1.1d).

II. Aneurysms of the Common Carotid Artery

Aneurysms close to the origin of the common carotid artery may be corrected on the right side by a partial medial sternotomy. On the left side, thoracotomy in the third interspace is required if the lesion is localized proximally (Fig. 15.1.2a).

The aim of dissection is to achieve the most generous exposure possible. This means that a tape must be placed around a healthy segment of the vessel in order to avoid intraoperative cerebral embolization (Fig. 15.1.2b).

One seldom succeeds in approximating both ends of the common carotid artery without tension following resection. The safest procedure is interposition of an 8-mm prosthesis (Fig. 15.1.2c).

An autogenous segment of the saphenous vein should not be used in this position because of its smaller caliber.

III. Aneurysms of the Carotid Bifurcation and the Internal Carotid Artery

When exposing the carotid bifurcation, the incision may sometimes have to be extended cranially and posteriorly to achieve sufficient exposure (Fig. 15.1.3a).

First, a tape is placed around the common carotid artery, then around the external carotid artery and its proximal tributaries, and finally around the internal carotid artery (Fig. 15.1.3b). In order to avoid intraoperative microembolization during

Fig. 15.1.2. a Exposure of the right carotid bifurcation. **b** Exposure of a common carotid artery aneurysm. **c** Reconstruction by interposition of an 8-mm prosthesis

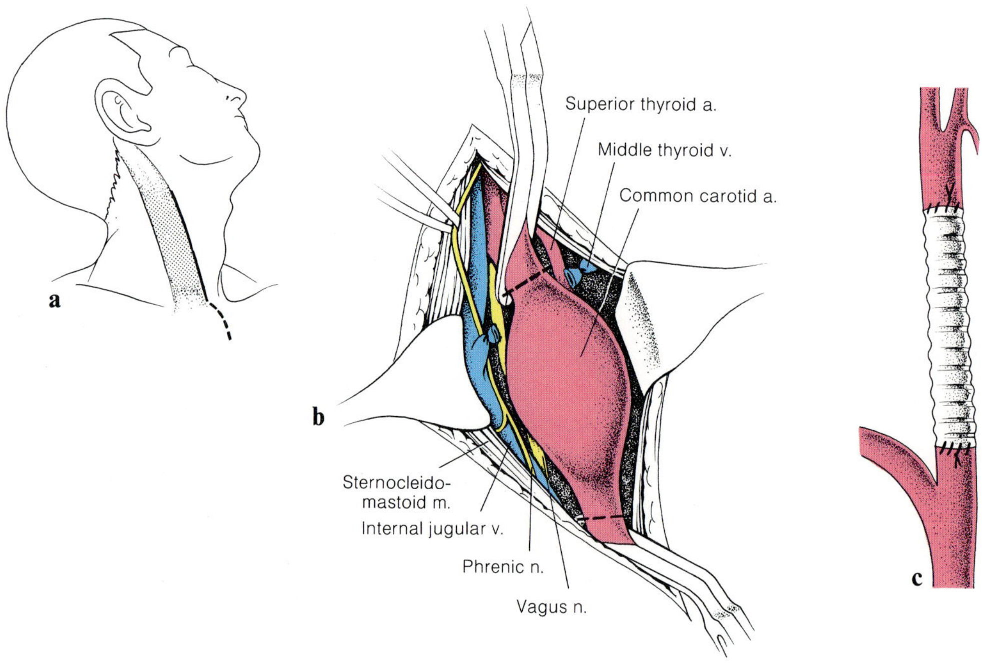

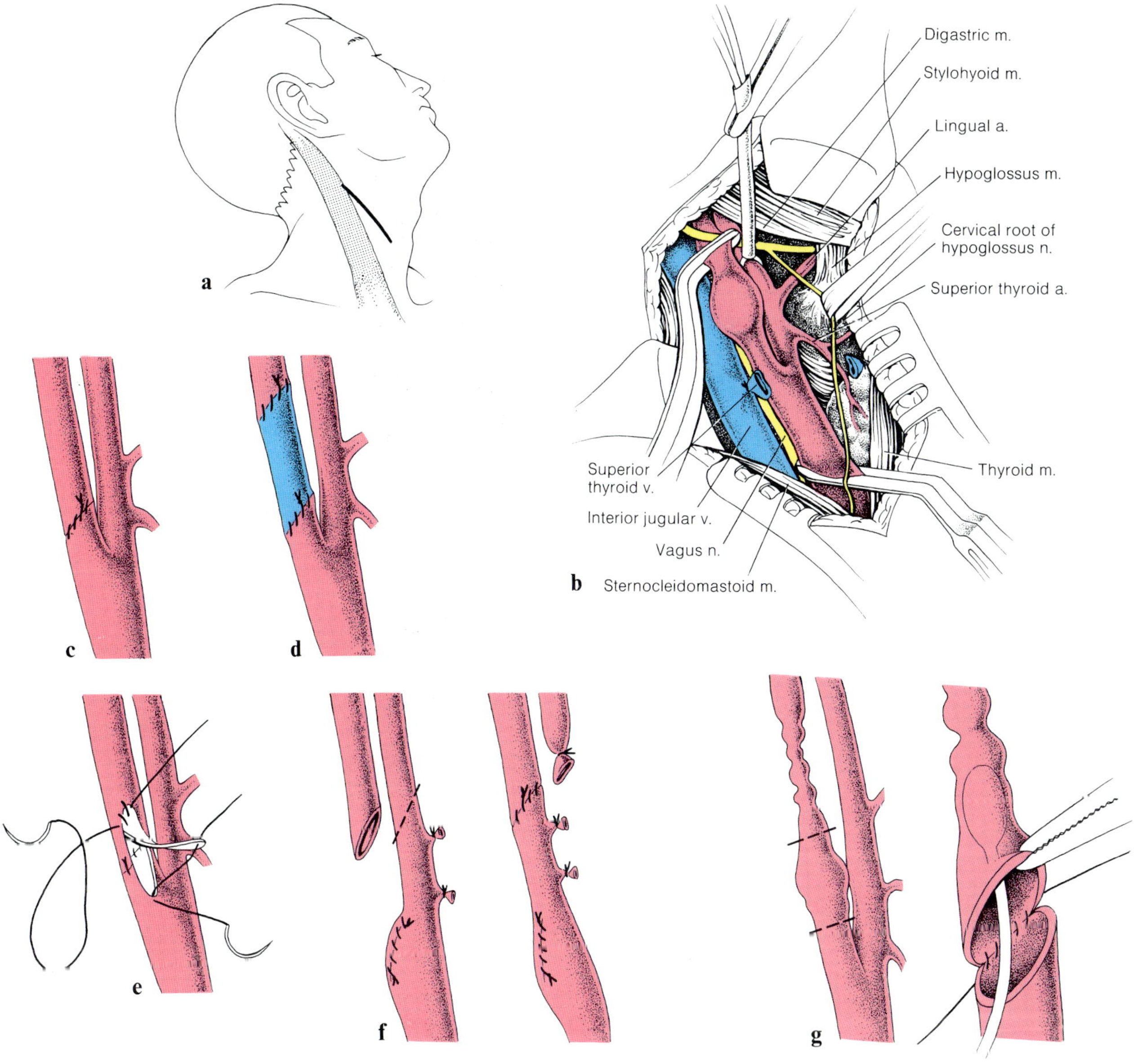

Fig. 15.1.3. a Exposure of the carotid bifurcation. **b** Exposure of the internal carotid artery aneurysm. **c** Partial resection of the carotid artery with end-to-end anastomosis. **d** Interposition of a saphenous vein segment. **e** Partial resection of the carotid artery with partial suture of the posterior wall and closure of the anterior wall by means of a patch graft. **f** Resection of the carotid artery aneurysm followed by division of the external carotid artery and suture of the proximal stump with subsequent reinsertion of the internal carotid artery into the proximal segment of the external carotid artery. **g** Partial resection followed by dilatation of the internal carotid artery and end-to-end reanostomosis

mobilization of the aneurysm, dissection should be done with extreme care.

Depending on the size of the aneurysm, complete removal with end-to-end anastomosis or graft interposition are performed (Fig. 15.1.3c, d).

Fabric prostheses should not be implanted in this position. If it is not possible to restore continuity following resection of the aneurysm by an end-to-end anastomosis, interposition of a saphenous vein is recommended (Fig. 15.1.3d).

The complete excision of large aneurysms cannot be recommended because their walls are often adherent to surrounding nerves.

When correcting aneurysms of the carotid artery, one should also keep in mind that the afferent or efferent segment is often stenosed by an arteriosclerotic plaque. Such stenoses must be considered when correcting the aneurysm. Resection and end-to-end anastomosis of carotid bifurcation aneurysms may cause anastomotic stenosis. In order to achieve a tensionless anastomosis it has been found useful to divide the internal and external carotid arteries. The cranial ends of both arteries are partially sutured at the posterior wall and an incision is made at the anterior wall. This funnel-shaped inflow will then be anastomosed end-to-end with the common carotid artery. The anterior wall is closed using a patch graft (Fig. 15.1.4a–d).

Alternatively, graft interposition following transection and ligation of the external carotid artery is possible (Fig. 15.1.4e).

Difficulties may arise in controlling the cranial segment of the internal carotid artery. We have found it useful to occlude the vessel temporarily with a Fogarty balloon catheter.

In the region of the carotid bifurcation and the internal carotid artery, other reconstructive methods may be also considered.

Fig. 15.1.4. a Resection of an aneurysm at the carotid bifurcation. **b–d** Reestablishment of vessel continuity by tailoring a common orifice using internal and external carotid arteries and reanastomosis at the anterior wall using a patch graft. **e** Reconstruction of a carotid bifurcation aneurysm by interposition of a prosthesis between the common and internal carotid arteries and division of the external carotid artery

1. Resection in Continuity

Following proximal and distal clamping, the aneurysm is resected. In the case of small saccular aneurysms, the internal carotid artery is beveled and anastomosed end-to-end with 6–0 interrupted sutures (Fig. 15.1.3b, c). It is important to free the internal carotid artery of the perivascular tissue in order to provide a tensionless anastomosis. Excessive tension on the anastomosis will always lead to restenosis.

If there is too much tension, resection and continuity may be achieved by division of the internal carotid artery at the carotid bifurcation and closure of the proximal stump. The distal stump is then reanastomosed end-to-end with the proximal segment of the divided external carotid artery (Fig. 15.1.3f).

2. Saphenous Vein Interposition

If resection in continuity fails, an autogenous saphenous vein graft should be interposed (Fig. 15.1.3d). Following excision of the aneurysm – leaving the posterior wall intact in the case of larger lesions – an autogenous saphenous vein graft is interposed end-to-end. When suturing the anastomosis, one should be careful to compensate the difference in vessel diameter, at least that of the common carotid artery. This may be done either by a beveled end-to-end anastomosis, or, better, by enlarging the anterior wall using a small vein patch.

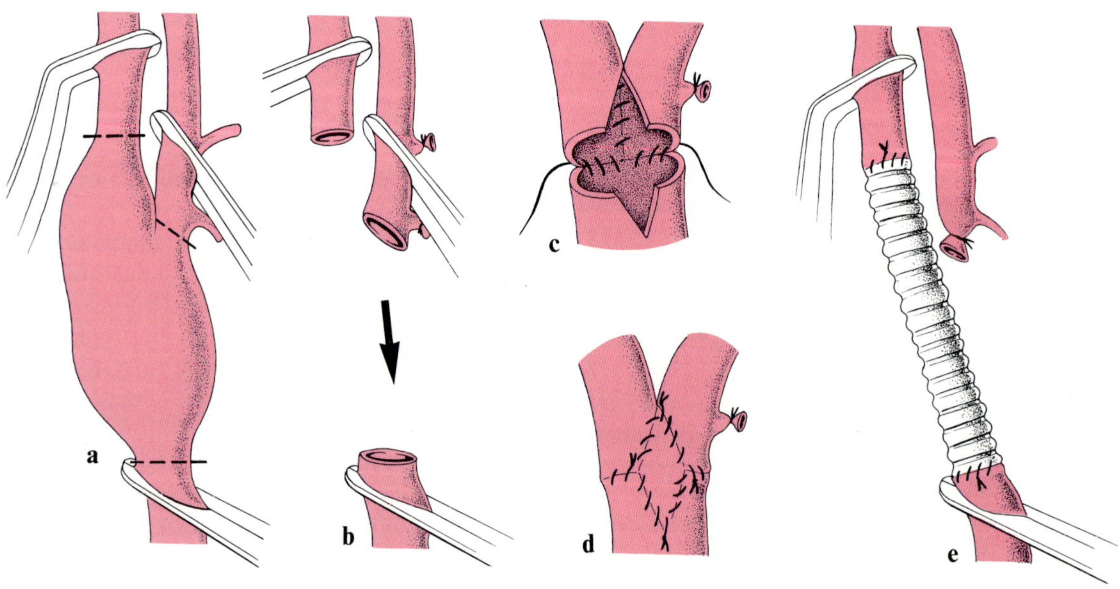

For this purpose, the anterior wall of the common carotid and the internal carotid arteries is incised. The posterior wall is sutured half way around with a continuous suture. Then the autogenous vein patch is implanted to enlarge the anastomosis (Fig. 15.1.3e).

Experience shows that it is better to perform the cranial anastomosis first. This is easily done using a freely mobile graft.

In the case of a fibromuscular dysplasia, besides resection of the saccular aneurysm, dilatation of the adjacent cranial segment of the internal carotid artery may be necessary (Fig. 15.1.3g). In this case, the stenosed segment of the internal carotid artery is dilated carefully with so-called coronary dilators (Garrett dilators) before completion of the cranial anastomosis.

IV. Aneurysms of the Subclavian and Axillary Arteries

Correction of central aneurysms of the subclavian artery on the left side is done by means of a thoracotomy in the third interspace. On the right side, the approach is by way of a total or partial median thoracotomy with extension of the incision supraclavicularly and to the right.

Interposition of a prosthesis (8 mm) end-to-end has proven effective. Complete excision of large aneurysms is not recommended. We prefer to leave the posterior wall of the aneurysm and to use the remaining portion of the sac or wrap the prosthesis (Fig. 15.1.5a, b).

For the correction of peripheral subclavian or axillosubclavian aneurysms, a transaxillary approach is preferred. The technique is described on p. 565.

Alternatively, these aneurysms may be treated using a supraclavicular approach, and under certain circumstances by division of the clavicle (Fig. 15.1.6a–c). Often, osteotomy alone, instead of clavicular resection, is sufficient to provide good exposure.

Following division of the platysma and the clavicular portion of the sternocleidomastoid muscle, dissection is performed medially in the direction of the jugular vein. The phrenic nerve is retracted medially. Division of the anterior scalenus muscle provides good exposure of the subclavian artery with the aneurysm. The lateral limitation consists of the brachial plexus (retraction). Medially, there

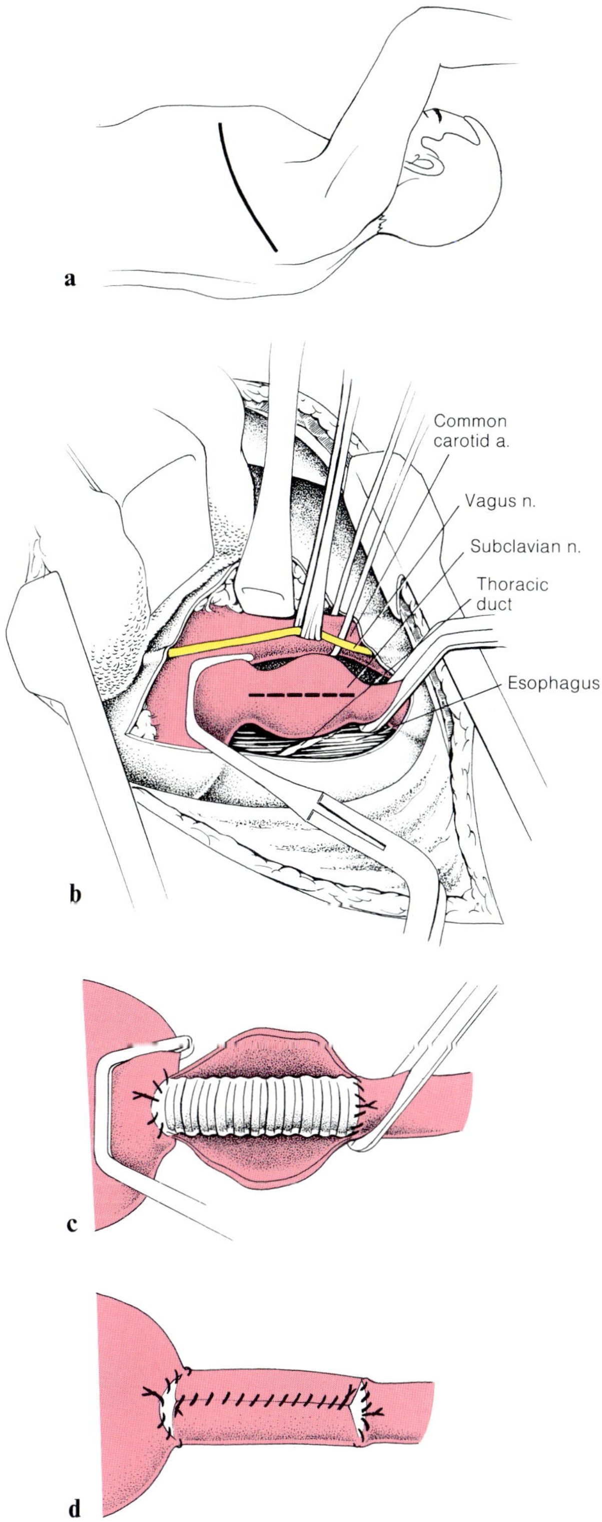

Fig. 15.1.5. **a** Exposure of the subclavian artery in the third interspace. **b** Exposure of the left subclavian artery by placing a Satinsky clamp tangentially on the aortic arch. **c** Interposition of a prosthesis. **d** Covering the prosthesis

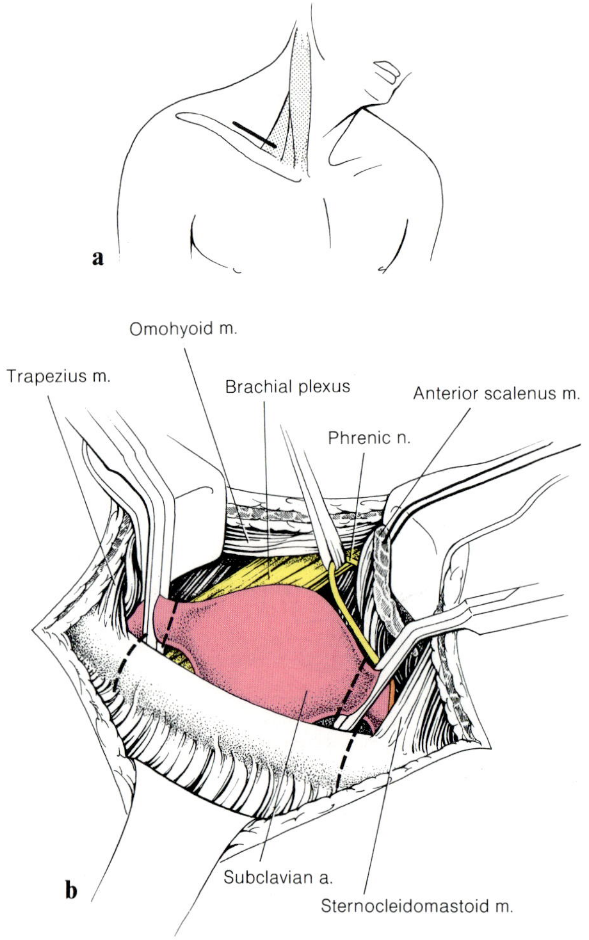

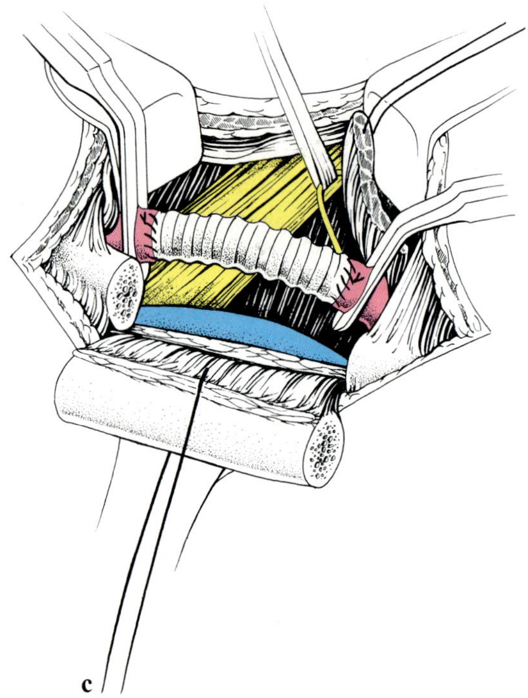

Fig. 15.1.6. **a** Supraclavicular approach to expose a peripheral aneurysm of the subclavian artery. **b** Exposure of an aneurysm of the subclavian artery. **c** Interposition of a prosthesis

Fig. 15.1.7. **a** Supraclavicular and axillary approach to expose an aneurysm of the subclavian artery. **b** Interposition of a prosthesis in a subclavian-axillary position

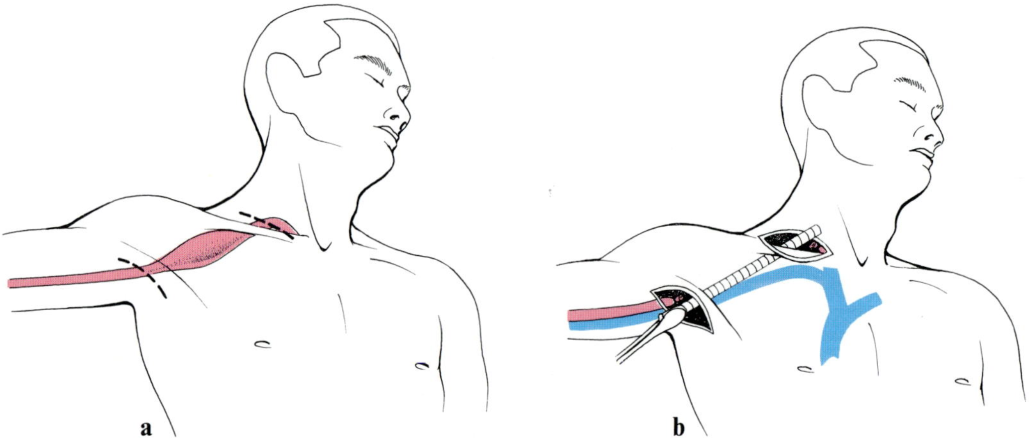

is the risk of injury to the recurrent nerve and, on the left side, to the thoracic duct.

For the treatment of aneurysms of the axillary artery of the subclavian axillary junction, it is not absolutely necessary to resect the clavicle. With an infraclavicular incision, the aneurysm can be resected and a prosthesis or a vein graft interposed (Fig. 15.1.7a, b).

When peripheral embolization has occurred from a subclavian or an axillary artery aneurysm, an embolectomy may be performed in the same session, possibly in combination with a sympathectomy.

V. Vertebral Artery Aneurysms

Extracranial aneurysms of the vertebral artery are rare and mostly of traumatic origin. Exposure begins with a supraclavicular incision, similar to that for the exposure of the subclavian artery. Where reconstruction is not required, simple ligation of the vertebral artery, just distal to its origin and again just cranial to the aneurysm, is sufficient (Fig. 15.1.8a, b).

Fig. 15.1.8. a Supraclavicular approach for exposure of the vertebral artery. **b** Ligation of the vertebral artery in a case of aneurysm

If reconstruction of the vertebral artery is required (stenosis or occlusion of the contralateral vertebral artery), transection of the vertebral artery distal to the aneurysm and reinsertion of the distal stump into the common carotid artery is recommended.

In such cases, the vertebral artery is best exposed through a longitudinal incision at the anterior border of the sternocleidomastoid muscle. Between the jugular vein on the one side and the common carotid artery and the vagal nerve on the other, the vertebral vein is exposed in depth and divided between ligatures. The vertebral artery lies behind the divided vein. The artery can be dissected without difficulty in the direction of the subclavian artery as far as the aneurysm. There, the vertebral artery is divided. The proximal stump is ligated and the peripheral stump anastomosed to the common carotid artery end-to-side.

VI. Brachial Artery Aneurysms

Smaller aneurysms of the brachial artery may be resected and the vessel ends anastomosed end-to-end (Fig. 15.1.9a, b). With larger aneurysms, vein interposition is preferred, in order to achieve a tensionless anastomosis. In these cases, a vein graft may be harvested from the arm (Fig. 15.1.9c).

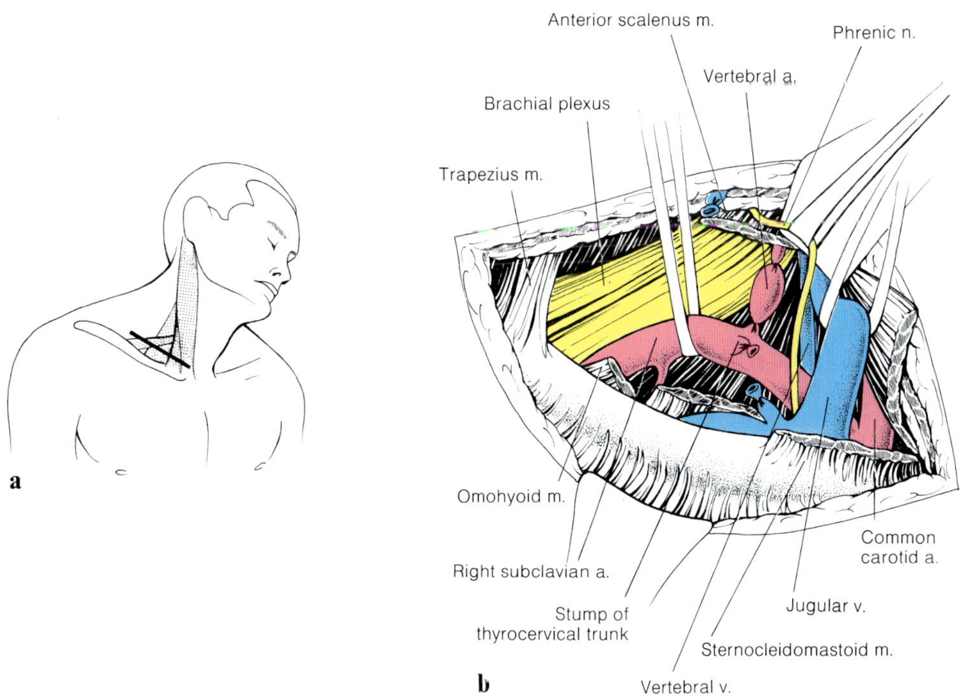

a

b

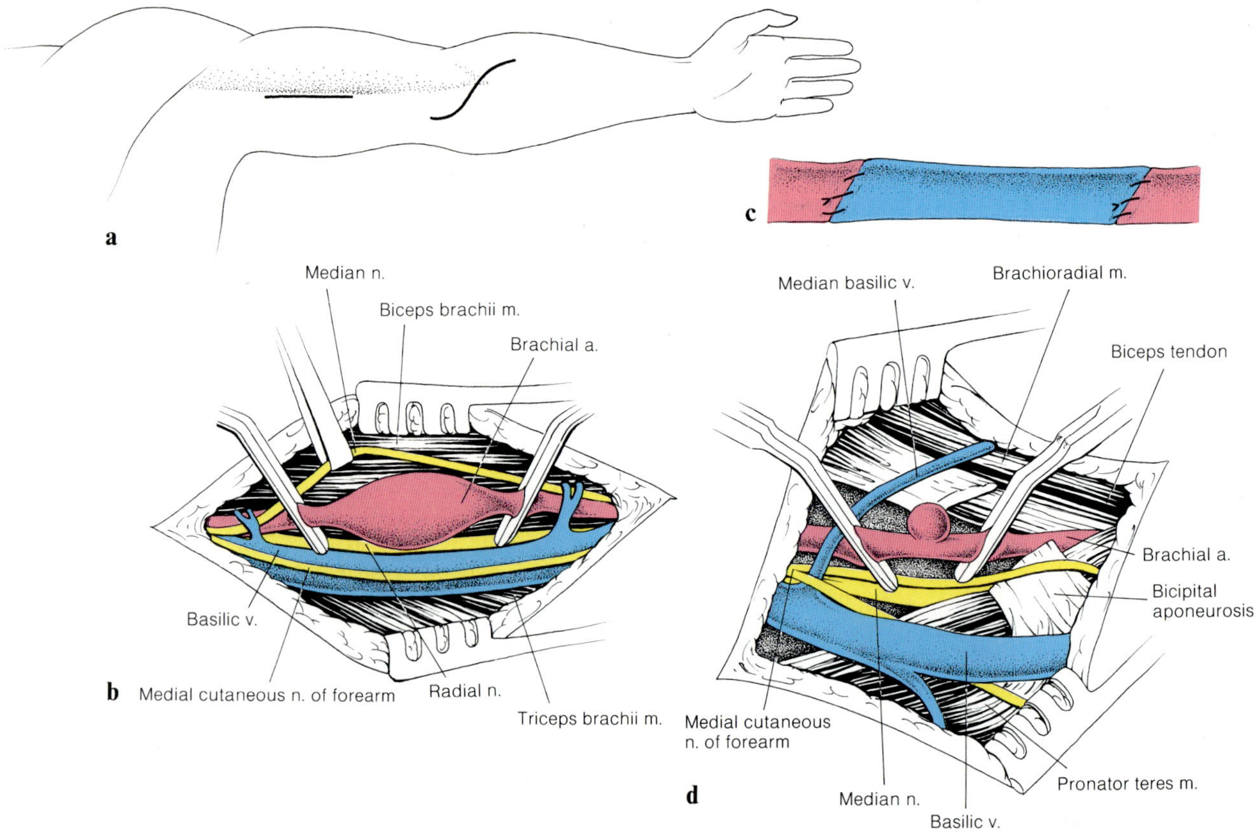

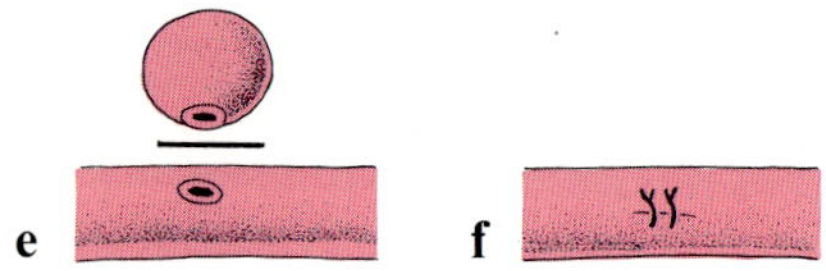

Fig. 15.1.9. a, b Exposure of the brachial artery. **c** Vein interposition following resection of an aneurysm of the brachial artery. **d–f** Resection of an aneurysm of the brachial artery and reconstruction of the brachial artery by vascular suture

In case of a false aneurysm, one may succeed in closing the artery with interrupted sutures after removal of the thrombi. However, parts of the arterial wall have to be resected here as well (Fig. 15.1.9d–f).

VII. Aneurysms of the Radial and Ulnar Arteries

These aneurysms can be resected following ligation. A resection and primary reanastomosis is necessary only when both arteries are occluded.

F. Intraoperative Protective Measures – Possible Complications – Follow-up

For maintenance of cerebral blood flow during correction of extracranial aneurysms of the carotid artery, the same guidelines hold as for the entire spectrum of carotid artery surgery [8]. In our opinion securing constant circulatory parameters during cross-clamping is of the greatest practical significance. Today, we no longer use an intraluminal shunt in carotid artery surgery.

When a shunt is used, the following technique can be recommended:

Following cross-clamping of the carotid artery, incision, and removal of thrombotic material from the aneurysm, a graft is placed over the shunt. The shunt itself is then inserted upward into the carotid artery, flushed with the bloodstream in the cranial carotid artery, and finally fixed by a tourniquet.

With the shunt in place, cranial and caudal anastomoses are performed. Before completion of the proximal anastomosis, the shunt is removed.

Of the possible complications, the most important are:

1. Ischemic cerebral injury
2. Cerebral or peripheral embolization
3. Recurrent thrombosis
4. Local injury of nerves and adjacent vessels

Although the majority of patients tolerate cross-clamping of the carotid artery without special protective measures, ischemic cerebral injuries have been observed in a small percentage, despite the use of an intraluminal shunt. A reoperation is not required if patency can be demonstrated following reconstruction. The treatment is purely conservative, i.e., in accordance with the principles for treatment of cerebral vascular insufficiency. Improper manipulation during the operation may cause embolization into the cerebral circulation or the extremities.

In such cases, an embolectomy using a Fogarty balloon catheter is possible only in the region of the arm.

To avoid such embolizations, manipulation of the aneurysms must be kept to an absolute minimum. Inflow and outflow segments must be generously exposed. If early reocclusion by thrombosis occurs, one should immediately reoperate to prevent further ischemia. Usually, the cause is a technical failure at the site of the anastomosis.

Local nerve injuries are caused mostly be retraction. Injuries to concomitant vessels may be avoided by proper dissection.

Follow-up: In very few cases, postoperative anticoagulation is recommended.

G. Reoperations

Reoperation is indicated if, following treatment of an aneurysm of the upper extremity, peripheral circulation worsens. Reoperation is also indicated following correction of an extracranial aneurysm of the supra-aortic branches if transient ischemic attacks are observed.

In any case, angiography must be performed in order to reveal the site of reconstruction. Reintervention is indicated when the graft is occluded or when there is extreme narrowing of the anastomosis that could result in complete occlusion.

The operative procedure is similar to primary vascular reconstruction. The exposure of the original operative field may well cause problems in the region of the carotid artery and with aneurysms close to the aortic arch. The risk of injury to concomitant structures is high.

Replacement of the graft is recommended. From the point of view of long-term results, patch graft angioplasty is not advisable in such cases.

REFERENCES

1. Beall AC, Crawford ES, Cooley DA, DeBakey M (1962) Extracranial aneurysms of the carotid artery. Report of seven cases. Postgrad Med 32:93
2. Hobson RW, Sarkaria J, O'Donnell J, Neville W (1979) Atherosclerotic aneurysms of the subclavian artery. Surgery 85:358
3. Hobson RW, Israel MR, Lynch ThG (1982) Axillo-subclavian arterial aneurysms. In: Bergan JJ, Yao JST (eds) Aneurysms – diagnosis and treatment. Grune & Stratton, New York
4. Johnson JN, Helsby CR, Stell PM (1980) Aneurysm of the external carotid artery. J Cardiovasc Surg 21:105
5. Kaupp HA, Haid SP, Juravy MN, Bergan JJ, Trippel OH (1972) Aneurysms of the extracranial carotid artery. Surgery 72:946
6. McCollum CH, Wheller WG, Noon GP, DeBakey ME (1979) Aneurysms of the extracranial carotid artery. Twenty-one years experience. Am J Surg 137:196
7. Perdue GF, Pellegrine RV, Arena S (1981) Aneurysms of the high internal carotid artery: A new approach. Surgery 89:268
8. Raithel D (1977) Cerebrale Insuffizienz durch extracranielle Gefäßverschlüsse. perimed-Verlag, Erlangen
9. Rhodes EL, Stanley JC, Hoffmann GL, Cronenwett JL, Fry WJ (1976) Aneurysm of extracranial carotid arteries. Arch Surg 111:339
10. Trippel OH, Haid SP, Kornmesser TW, Bergan JJ (1982) Extracranial carotid aneurysms. In: Bergan JJ, Yao JST (eds) Aneurysms diagnosis and treatment. Grune & Stratton, New York
11. Vollmar J (1982) Rekonstruktive Chirurgie der Arterien. Thieme, Stuttgart New York

15.2 Aneurysms of the Lower Extremity

H. DENECKE and E. PRATSCHKE

CONTENTS

A. Anatomy

True aneurysms of the lower extremity occur as individual lesions or as part of a general aneurysmal vascular disease in combination with lesions at other sites. They are almost exclusively of arteriosclerotic origin.

Iliac artery aneurysms are predominantly associated with aortic aneurysms. Femoral artery aneurysms and popliteal aneurysms are often bilateral. In up to 80% these lesions occur bilaterally or are found together with aneurysms of other vascular segments, especially of the aorta [3, 6, 7, 10]. Surgical anatomy of aneurysmatic arteries does not differ from that of arteries which are stenosed. However, by exerting compressive force expanding aneurysms may cause adhesions and indurations of the surroundings, so that extensive dissection can pose a danger to adjacent structures, (e.g., veins, nerves, ureter).

Therefore, it is a peculiarity of surgery of aneurysms that complete dissection should be abandoned. In many cases, partial resection is sufficient and reconstruction may be performed by "inlay" techniques or bypass procedures.

B. Indications

Surgical intervention for the elimination or an aneurysm in the region of the pelvis or the lower extremity is indicated because of the danger of thromboembolization with subsequent ischemia. In our own patient groups preoperative thromboembolization had occurred in 57 (31%) of 184 patients with aneurysms of the iliaco-femoral vascular system. In 16% amputation was necessary. Limb preservation was possible in only half the patients suffering from embolization. As compared with large aortic aneurysms, the risk of rupture of aneurysms of the lower extremity is smaller [9]. Therefore, small fusiform aneurysms may be observed for a time if the patient presents with significant general risk factors. Ultrasonography provides an outstanding tool for exact assessment and control of growth and possible formation of thrombi.

Bilateral aneurysms are managed metachronously, priority being given to the symptomatic side. If aneurysms are present in different vascular systems, the indication for surgery will depend on the urgency. Aneurysms with a high risk of rupture, such as aortic aneurysms, must be operated on first because of the greater danger to the patient's life. The reality of this risk is brought home by the fact that the operative mortality from popliteal aneurysms depends significantly on postoperative ruptures of aortic aneurysms [8].

For all aneurysms, preoperative angiography is indispensable for planning the operation and for evaluating the extent of revascularization. Visualizing the distal vascular system and estimating outflow are important for successful revascularization [5].

C. Incisions and Operative Approach

I. Common Iliac Artery Aneurysm, Internal Iliac Artery Aneurysm

The transperitoneal approach through a large midline incision is preferred for combined aneurysms of the aorta and the iliac arteries. It is not different from the approach used for other reconstructions in this vascular region (see p. 378). The same holds true for the extraperitoneal approach to unilateral iliac artery aneurysms (see p. 380). The incision is made pararectally and extends to a point just below the lowest point of the costal arch. The fascia of the external oblique muscle, the internal oblique muscle, and the transverse abdominal muscle are divided and the rectus abdominus muscle, together with the peritoneal sac, is retracted medially. During blunt dissection of the peritoneal sac out of the iliac fossa care should be taken not to dissect too far laterally and dorsally along the psoas muscle. Otherwise, the cavity is enlarged unnecessarily. The retractor should be provided with two jaws of different length, the longer one being placed medially (Fig. 15.2.1a, b).

The ureter crosses above the iliac bifurcation. Particular attention must be paid to the iliac vein, as it is often firmly adherent to the aneurysm and therefore easily injured. With the extraperitoneal approach, the distal aorta, the total iliac vascular system, and the internal iliac artery can be well exposed. If the whole length of the iliac artery has to be replaced, a separate incision is made in the groin to expose the upper common femoral artery for distal anastomosis (see next section).

II. Common Femoral Artery Aneurysm

The incision is made longitudinally across the groin (from approximately 6 cm above to about 6 cm distally) and somewhat lateral to the pulse (Fig. 15.2.3a). Usually, the pulsatile vessel is easily palpable and may be used as a guideline. When the abdominal wall is very fat, incision of the skin and the subcutaneous tissue sometimes has be extended further upward.

The lymph nodes are pulled medially. When sharp dissection is performed, one should carefully ligate to avoid postoperative fistulas. The profunda femoris artery is exposed over a distance of 1–2 cm. A small vein close to the origin to the profunda femoris artery must always be divided and ligated. When the aneurysms are located higher, a separate extraperitoneal approach to the external iliac artery is necessary by a suprainguinal incision.

III. Superficial Femoral Artery Aneurysm

Aneurysms of the superficial femoral artery are exposed by direct incision above the course of the artery or aneurysm. Usually, these aneurysms are long. Exposure is then made through two separate incisions above the femoral bifurcation (longitudinal incision in the groin) and above the distal segment of the femoral artery medially and proximal to the knee (Fig. 15.2.4a).

IV. Popliteal Aneurysm (Fig. 15.2.5a, b)

The medial approach is most frequently used. The patient is in a supine position. The knee is flexed at 30° by placing drapes underneath it. The knee itself should be free, at least on the medial side. This way, there is no compression on the operative field from below.

This approach is especially advantageous with large aneurysms. The incisions are made above and below the knee. The greater saphenous vein is carefully preserved, smaller tributaries being ligated. Following division of the sartorius muscle at its insertion, the deep fascia is incised dorsal to the bone. In the fatty tissue of the popliteal fossa, the bundle of vessels and nerves is found. The vein (often doubled) usually lies adjacent to the artery or the aneurysm and must therefore be dissected carefully. This approach provides exposure of the proximal third of the popliteal artery, or the upper branch of the aneurysm.

For good exposure, we prefer the Gilby retractor. For the separate approach to the distal popliteal segment, the medial portion of the gastrocnemius muscle is pulled downward. Following retraction of the soleus muscle, the neurovascular bundle is exposed. Also in this position, the Gilby retractor is of advantage. In the distal third of the popliteal artery there are no major tributaries. The exposure is therefore simple. Early cross-clamping or early ligature is advisable in order to avoid intraoperative embolization. If the origin of the anterior tibial artery must be exposed further distally, the medial portion of the gastrocnemius muscle, as well as the tibial insertion of the soleus muscle, have to be partially divided. However, this procedure, with two separate incisions for the upper and lower third of the popliteal artery, avoids a continuous medial exposure with division of the gracilis, semitendinosus, and semimembranosus muscle as well as the medial portion of the gastrocnemius muscle. Smaller popliteal aneurysms may be managed using a dorsal approach by a single incision. The patient lies prone with the ankle supported by a roll. The incision is best made starting laterally and above and running transversely through the popliteal fossa, and finally downward on the medial side (according to the course of the vessel!) (Figs. 15.2.6a). A simple longitudinal incision may be used. Following division of the posterior popliteal fascia, the fossa poplitea with the fatty tissue and the neurovascular bundle is exposed between both portions of the muscle (Fig. 15.2.6b). The nerve branches, passing distally and sometimes crossing, have to be dissected carefully to avoid injury. The dissection of the popliteal vein or the short saphenous vein may be difficult.

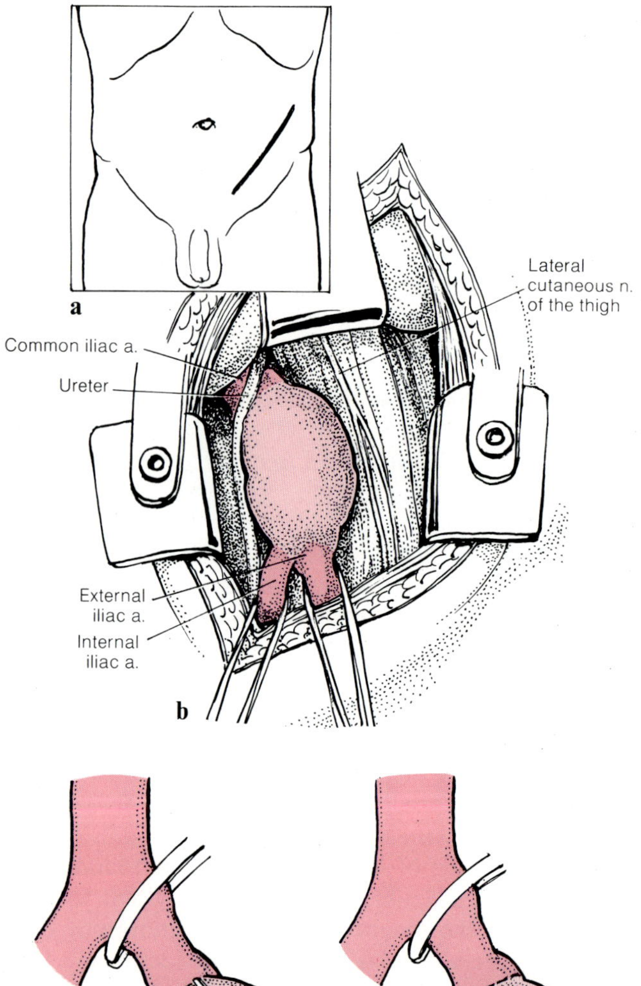

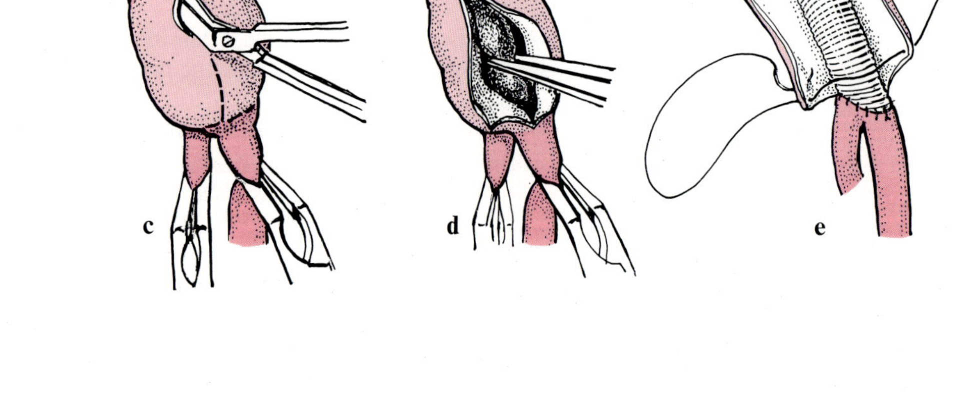

Fig. 15.2.1 a–e. Common iliac artery aneurysm. **a** Incision for the extraperitoneal approach. **b** Exposure of the common iliac artery. The peritoneal sac is shifted medially and cranially. The deeper jaw of the retractor is on the medial side. **c** Following local heparinization, the clamps are first placed distally and then proximally; the aneurysm is incised longitudinally. **d** Removal of thrombotic material. Transverse incisions of the anterior wall made proximally and distally, so as to form two closable flaps. The posterior wall remains in situ (preservation of the vein, better fixation of the sutures, more rapid dissection). **e** Following the anastomosis (posterior wall using inlay technique), the remaining wall of the aneurysm is trimmed. The prosthesis is covered using a running suture

D. Technique of Reconstruction

I. Iliac Artery Aneurysm

The aneurysm usually has a well-defined neck at the origin of the iliac artery, providing a good possibility for anastomosis at the bifurcation, much as in the case of an infrarenal aortic aneurysm just below the renal arteries (Fig. 15.2.1c). The distal aorta, however, must be exposed to such an extent that it can be clamped rather far upward, as arteriosclerotic plaques often make it impossible to clamp the iliac artery close to the lesion. The posterior wall of the aneurysm is not dissected completely, but remains in situ; by restricting dissection in this manner, one is less apt to injure the vein. Early distal cross-clamping is important for avoiding embolizations [5]. The sac of the aneurysm is incised longitudinally on the anterior wall and then transversely at the proximal and distal ends, resulting in two flaps resembling the wings of a door. Usually, the vessel does not have to be divided completely, either for the upper or the lower anastomosis. If the vessel walls are thin, it is important to preserve the posterior wall, thereby providing more "material" for a reliable suture. The free portions of the wall are shortened or partially resected, depending on the size of the aneurysm. However, sufficient material should be left to cover the prosthesis with these "wings" (Fig. 15.2.1c–e).

The iliac vein, lying adjacent to the aneurysm, must not be injured, either in making the transverse incisions or during suturing. The most favorable procedure for revascularization is graft interposition. The suture is made with 3–0 or 4–0 nonabsorbable suture material starting from the posterior wall and continuing around on both sides to the anterior wall. The smaller the vessel or the diameter of the anastomosis, the greater the hemodynamic advantages of a beveled anastomosis will be (see p. 59ff.). The prosthesis is placed into the lumen of the aneurysm and pulled underneath the ureter. The distal anastomosis is also beveled. Whenever possible this anastomosis should be placed into the iliac bifurcation so that perfusion of the internal iliac artery is maintained (Fig. 15.2.1e).

II. Internal Iliac Artery Aneurysm

Ligature for exclusion of aneurysms of the internal iliac artery can be performed on one side. Ligation of both internal iliac arteries results in a high risk of extensive necrosis of pelvic and gluteal tissue. This is always lethal. Therefore, at least on one side, revascularization is necessary, e.g., using a prosthesis (Fig. 15.2.2a–c).

III. External Iliac Artery Aneurysm

Isolated aneurysms of the external iliac artery are rare. Usually, these are long aneurysms, extending into the common iliac artery or even into aneurysms of the abdominal aorta. In those cases the long bifurcation prostheses are anastomosed to the common femoral arteries just below the inguinal ligament. This segment is exposed by a separate incision in the groin. Care should be taken to save at least one internal iliac artery.

IV. Common Femoral Artery Aneurysm

In this region, aneurysms are best replaced by fabric prostheses (for instance double-velour, 6 or 8 mm in diameter). One should attempt to achieve an anastomosis to the profunda femoris artery (Fig. 15.2.3b, c), beveling the anastomosis as much as possible. The anastomosis is best performed using the inlay technique (Fig. 15.2.3d–f). If, as is often the case, the superficial femoral artery is thrombosed, the thrombotic material should be evacuated. Once this has been done, anastomosis with both femoral arteries can be performed. Nonabsorbable 5–0 or 6–0 suture material is best suited for this purpose.

If proximal anastomosis with the external iliac artery is necessary, the inguinal ligament may be incised. Higher anastomoses require exposure of the external iliac artery above the inguinal ligament through a separate incision.

V. Superficial Femoral Artery Aneurysm

Small aneurysms of the superficial femoral artery are resected and, insofar as possible, replaced by a saphenous vein graft. Larger aneurysms, and in particular longer ones, are replaced by a graft run-

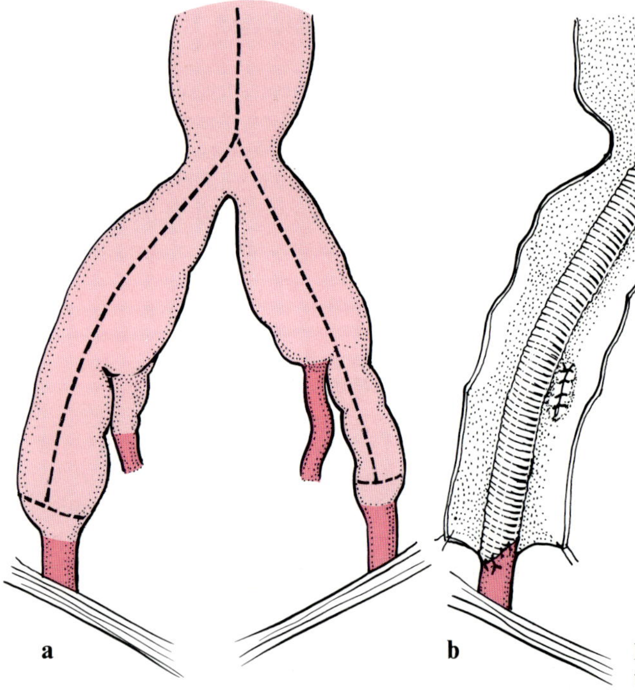

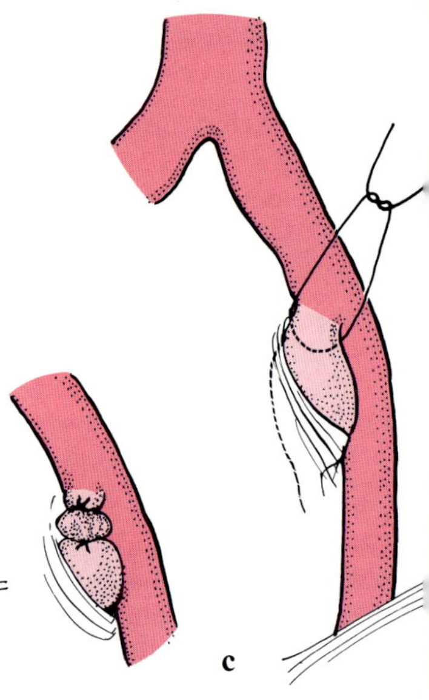

Fig. 15.2.2 a–c. Iliac artery aneurysms. **a** Incision to open the vessel in the case of extensive aneurysmal dilation of the aortoiliac region. **b** Bi-iliac prostheses using the inlay technique. To maintain the blood flow to the pelvic organs, at least one internal iliac artery must be anastomosed or preserved. **c** Unilateral aneurysms of the internal iliac artery may be ligated

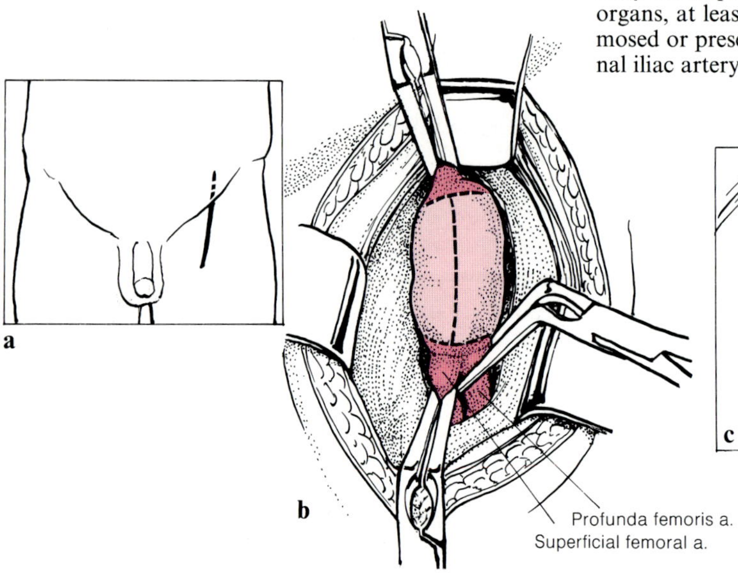

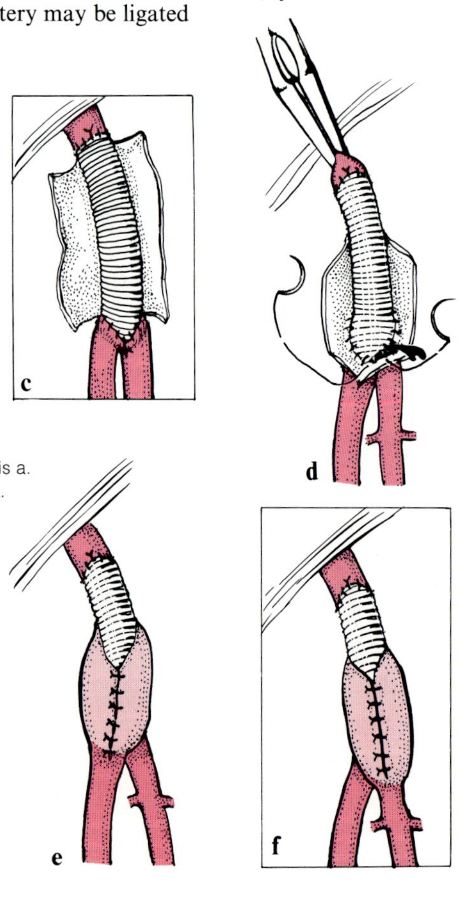

Fig. 15.2.3 a–f. Common femoral artery aneurysm. **a** Incision across the unilateral groin, somewhat lateral to the pulse. **b** Cross-clamping, first of the distal vessels, then of the proximal vessels, and "wing"-incision of the aneurysm. **c** Interposition of prosthesis, partially applying the inlay technique. The distal anastomosis should include the lumina of both femoral arteries. **d** The distal anastomosis of the prosthesis using a complete inlay technique (less dissecting effort, more material for the suture, less risk of injury to the vein). **e, f** Using the inlay technique, the incision is made into the vessel with the lesser outflow (exception: planned profundaplasty to widen the stenosed origin of that artery)

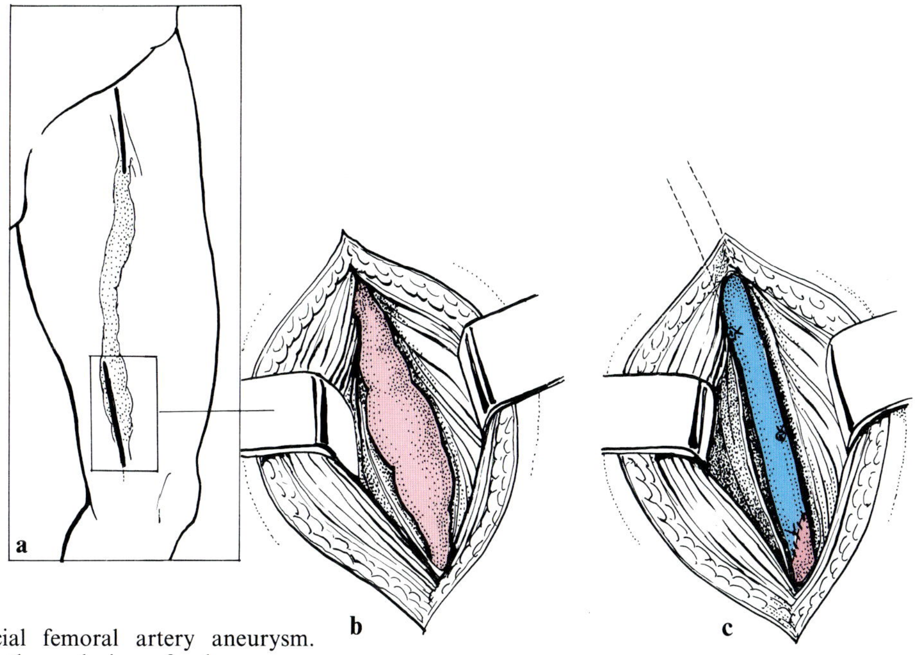

Fig. 15.2.4a–c. Superficial femoral artery aneurysm. **a** Separate incisions for the exclusion of a long aneurysm. **b** Medial approach to the distal superficial femoral artery or the upper third of the popliteal artery. **c** Beveled distal end-to-end anastomosis with a saphenous vein graft

ning from the femoral bifurcation to the proximal popliteal artery.

Here too, early distal cross-clamping of the vessel is necessary because of the risk of embolization (Fig. 15.2.4a–c).

VI. Popliteal Aneurysm

Only very small popliteal aneurysms are resected completely, and only when the dissection is easy to perform. However, adjacent structures (popliteal vein, nerve) are often adherent, posing the risk that dissection will result in lesions that would in turn increase the risk of thrombosis and pulmonary embolism. Therefore, the dissection and ligation of surrounding venous structures is limited to the provision of access for clamping, ligature, or incision of the aneurysmal sac. In both approaches (dorsally or medially) the distal segment is cross-clamped first (Figs. 15.2.5b and 15.2.6b). Both anastomoses are beveled and sutured end-to-end (Figs. 15.2.5c–e and 15.2.6e). The material of choice is saphenous vein. For grafts crossing joints, double-velour or ring-enforced Goretex (8 mm/6 mm) may also be used. Larger aneurysms are bypassed or partially resected, inserting the prosthesis into the opened lumen (Fig. 15.2.6c–d). Tributaries are suture-ligated from the inside. In this way, one also avoids the ligation of the collaterals, which would be necessary when dissecting the aneurysm from the outside. This may also be important for limb preservation in the presence of a thrombosed aneurysm.

For large aneurysms, however, it is more convenient to use the medial approach above or below the knee. The anastomosis is beveled and performed in the upper or lower third of the popliteal artery using 5–0 or 6–0 Prolene.

Either the aneurysm is bypassed or a graft is interposed through the sac of the aneurysm. Before completion of the distal suture, a Fogarty catheter is passed through the outflow tract to remove possible emboli. Operative results may also be documented by intraoperative angiography, which will also disclose peripheral emboli. The wound can be closed without drainage if bleeding has been arrested completely. Divided muscles are again approximated by sutures. However, this is only necessary following the continuous exposure of the popliteal fossa from the medial side.

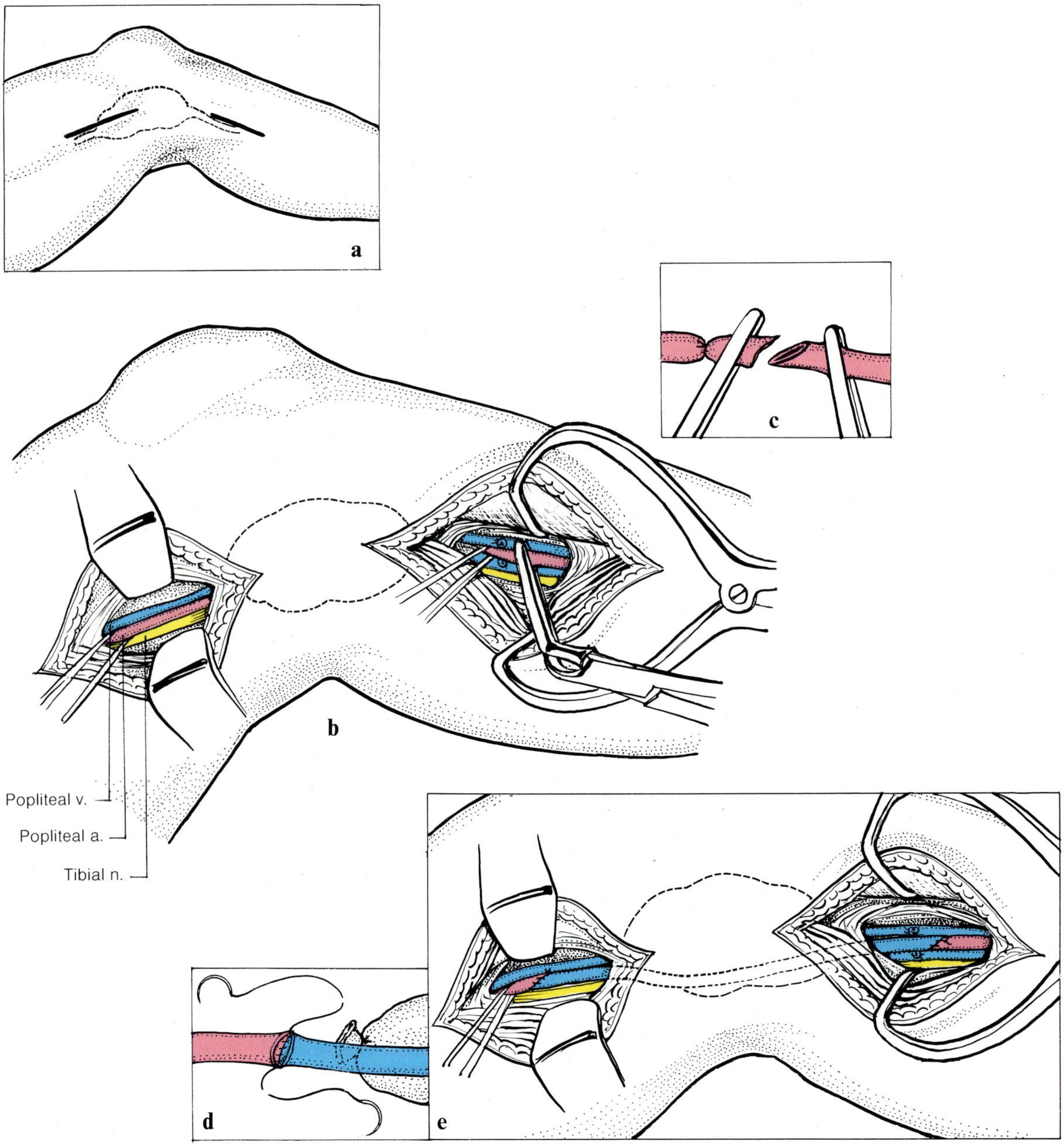

Fig. 15.2.5 a–e. Popliteal aneurysm: medial approach. **a** Two separate incisions, the knee being slightly flexed. **b** Exposure of the popliteal artery in the upper and in the lower third with concomitant veins and nerves. Early distal cross-clamping! **c** End-to-end anastomosis of the afferent artery to the saphenous vein graft. The aneurysm is excluded. **d** Distal anastomosis is considerably beveled. **e** Bypassing the excluded aneurysm with a vein graft

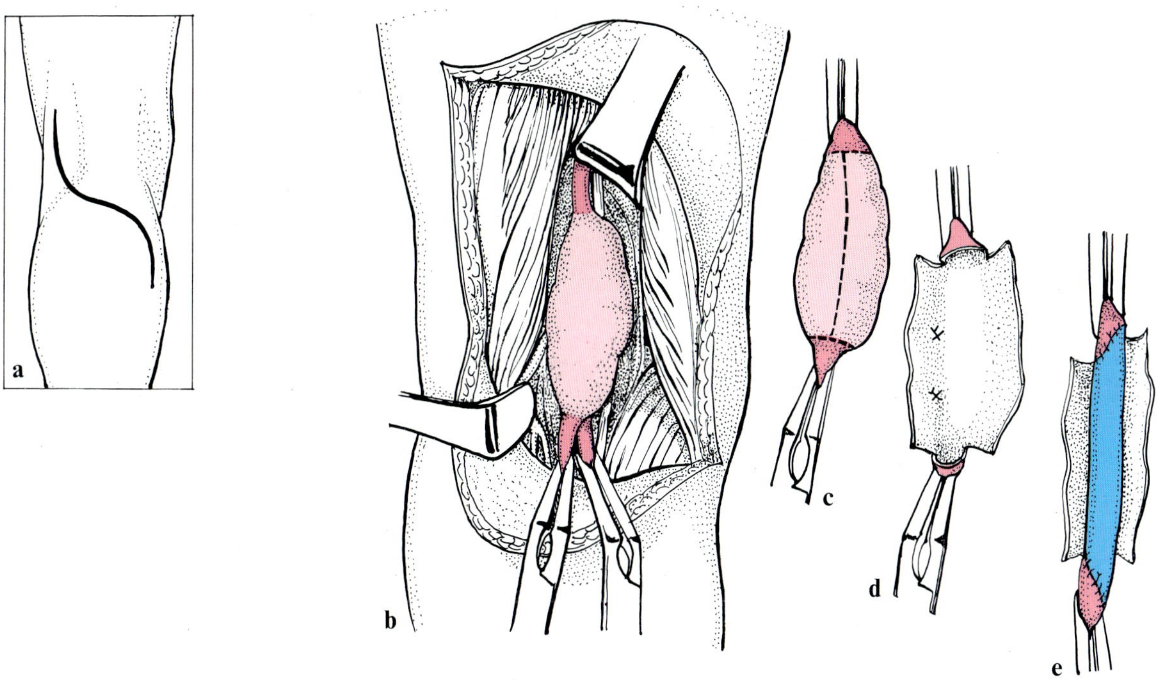

Fig. 15.2.6 a–e. Popliteal aneurysm: dorsal approach. **a** Skin incision from lateral and above, downward medially. **b** After careful exposure distally, the efferent vessels are cross-clamped early. **c** The aneurysm is opened and partially resected. **d** Suture ligation of arterial tributaries from the inside avoids dissection and injury of veins or nerves adjacent to the aneurysm. **e** Extremely beveled anastomosis with a saphenous vein graft

E. Postoperative Complications and Reoperations

The most frequent postoperative complications are caused by embolization of thrombotic material. Therefore, before completing the distal anastomosis, the outflow should always be controlled by a Fogarty catheter (when in doubt intraoperative angiography must be added). In order to avoid thrombosis within the clamped-off segment, intraoperative systemic heparin (5000–10000 IU i.v.), or better, additional local heparinization into the afferent segment is required (5000 IU heparin in 100 ml 0.9% sodium chloride solution; 20 ml injected into the clamped-off vessel). The outflow is important. Large aneurysms have a known tendency to coagulate. Treatment of late complications, e.g., anastomotic aneurysms, does not differ from that following procedures for stenotic lesions.

REFERENCES

1. Cooley DA, Wukasch DC (1979) Techniques in vascular surgery. Saunders, Philadelphia London Toronto
2. Eisenmann JJ (1967) The isolated iliac artery aneurysm. Vasc Surg 1:202
3. Graham LM, Zelenock GB, Whitehouse WM, Erlandson EE, Dent TL, Lindenauer SM, Stenley JC (1980) Clinical significance of arteriosclerotic femoral artery aneurysms. Arch Surg 115:502
4. Heberer G, Reidemeister JChr (1974) Aneurysmen und Elongationen der Arterien. In: Heberer G, Rau G, Schoop W (eds) Angiologie, 2nd edn. Thieme, Stuttgart, p 555
5. Heberer G, Rau G (1966) Aorta und große Arterien. Springer, Berlin Heidelberg New York
6. Kremen J, Manzoian JO, Carson JD, Bush HL, Lo Gerfo FW (1981) Atherosclerotic aneurysms of the superficial femoral artery: a literature review and report of six additional cases. Am Surg 47:338
7. Lowry SF, Kraft RO (1979) Isolated aneurysms of the iliac artery. Arch Surg 113:1289
8. Madden JL (1964) Atlas of techniques in surgery, 2nd edn. Appleton Century Crofts, New York
9. Vollmar J (1975) Rekonstruktive Chirurgie der Arterien, 2nd edn. Thieme, Stuttgart
10. Whitehouse WM, Akefield TW, Graham LM, Kazmers A, Zelenock GB, Cronenwett JL, Dent TL, Lindenauer SM, Stanley JC (1983) Limb-threatening potential of arteriosclerotic popliteal artery aneurysms. Surgery 93:694
11. Wychulis AR, Spittell JA, Wallace RB (1970) Popliteal aneurysms. Surgery 68:942

15.3 Visceral Arterial Aneurysms

D.P. VAN BERGE HENEGOUWEN
and R.J.A.M. VAN DONGEN

CONTENTS

A. Introduction

Most aneurysms of the visceral arteries are found accidentally in an asymptomatic stage of development. Routine angiography for the diagnosis of vascular, gastroduodenal, and oncologic disease may reveal them. They pose a serious threat, owing to the possibility of rupture or of peripheral thromboembolization. Opinions differ regarding the necessity for conservative versus operative treatment [2, 11, 15, 17]. Since the etiology, symptoms, and management of aneurysms depend on their localization, a discussion of their occurrence in individual arteries is not only reasonable, but indispensable.

The incidence of visceral arterial aneurysms is 0.1% in autopsy series. The distribution for the various arteries is shown in Table 15.3.1.

Table 15.3.1. Distribution of visceral arterial aneurysms

	(%)
Splenic artery	51
Hepatic artery	17
Renal artery	12
Superior mesenteric artery	7
Jejunal, ileal, and colic arteries	5
Gastric and gastroepiploic arteries	3.9
Gastroduodenal and pancreaticoduodenal arteries	0.4
Celiac trunk	3.5
Inferior mesenteric artery	0.01

B. Splenic Artery Aneurysms

I. Prevalence, Pathology, Indications

Among visceral arterial aneurysms, those of splenic artery are the most frequent (58%). As early as 1770, BEAUSSIER [1] described a splenic artery aneurysm. Since then, a total of about 1500 have been described. In autopsy series, the ratio is approximately 0.07%, increasing significantly with age. In the earlier literature, there are numerous reports of ruptured splenic artery aneurysms in pregnant women. It is almost exclusively found in multiparae with six or more pregnancies. In more recent publications, however, aneurysms are described more often in older patients. It is supposed that these changes in patient groups may be the result of a reduction in the number of pregnancies per woman.

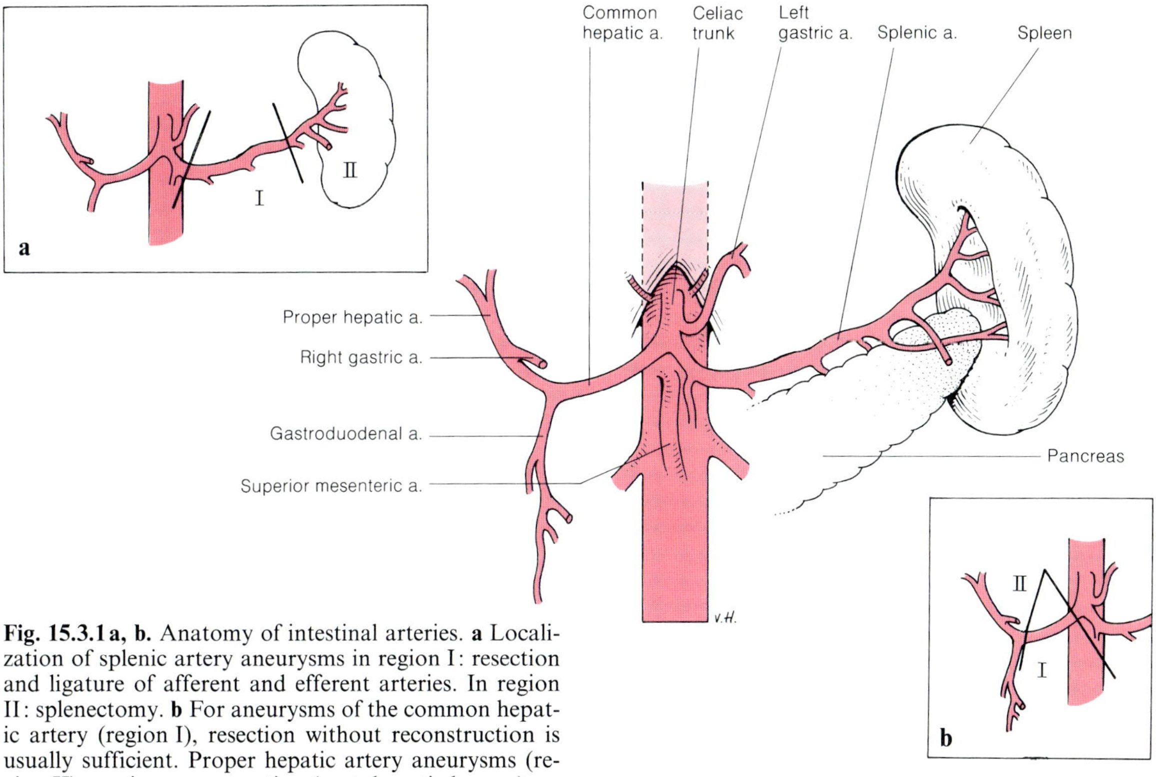

Fig. 15.3.1 a, b. Anatomy of intestinal arteries. **a** Localization of splenic artery aneurysms in region I: resection and ligature of afferent and efferent arteries. In region II: splenectomy. **b** For aneurysms of the common hepatic artery (region I), resection without reconstruction is usually sufficient. Proper hepatic artery aneurysms (region II) require reconstruction (aortohepatic bypass)

Degeneration of the media is thought to be of etiologic significance. In the case of saccular aneurysms it is thought that hormonal changes during pregnancy cause irreversible injury to the vessel wall, which becomes progressively worse during subsequent pregnancies.

Boijsen et al. [3] are of the opinion that the possibility of functional arteriovenous anastomoses in the spleen may play a role in this mechanism. A connection between fibromuscular dysplasia and degeneration of the media is discussed by Stanley et al. [13, 14]. In the higher age group the second major cause, arteriosclerosis, gains significance. Congenital or mycotic aneurysms of the splenic artery, however, are rare [5, 9, 14].

The incidence of rupture of splenic artery aneurysms is low, about 3% [6]. The phase preceding rupture is frequently characterized by an expansive growth of the aneurysm with increase of abdominal symptoms and perhaps also peritoneal signs. The pancreas may also be involved. The mortality of ruptured splenic artery aneurysms is high. In earlier references, 100% is reported, in recent series about 25% [14].

II. Management

1. Positioning

The patient is in a supine position with the left side elevated. In principle, there are two types of treatment, depending upon the localization: (1) splenectomy, (2) resection of the aneurysm and ligature of afferent and efferent arteries (Fig. 15.3.1 a). Only resection is described here.

2. Operative Approach

Extended subcostal incision on the left side. The extension of the skin incision should correspond with the localization of the aneurysm, either more medially or more laterally (Fig. 15.3.2 and see p. 592).

3. Intra-abdominal Approach

The lesser sac of the omentum is opened along its greater curvature. The tributaries of the gastroepiploic artery are divided between ligatures.

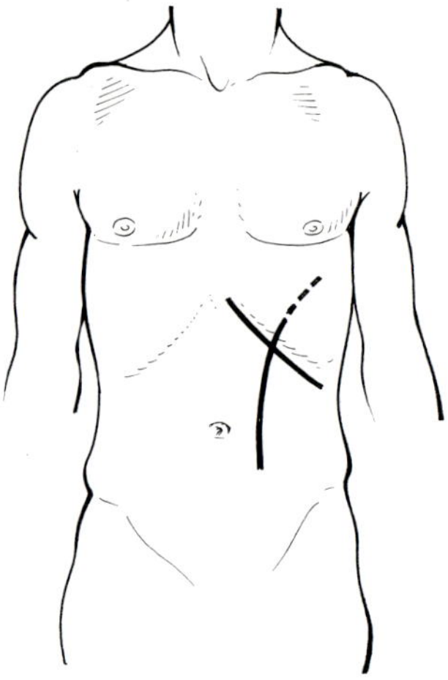

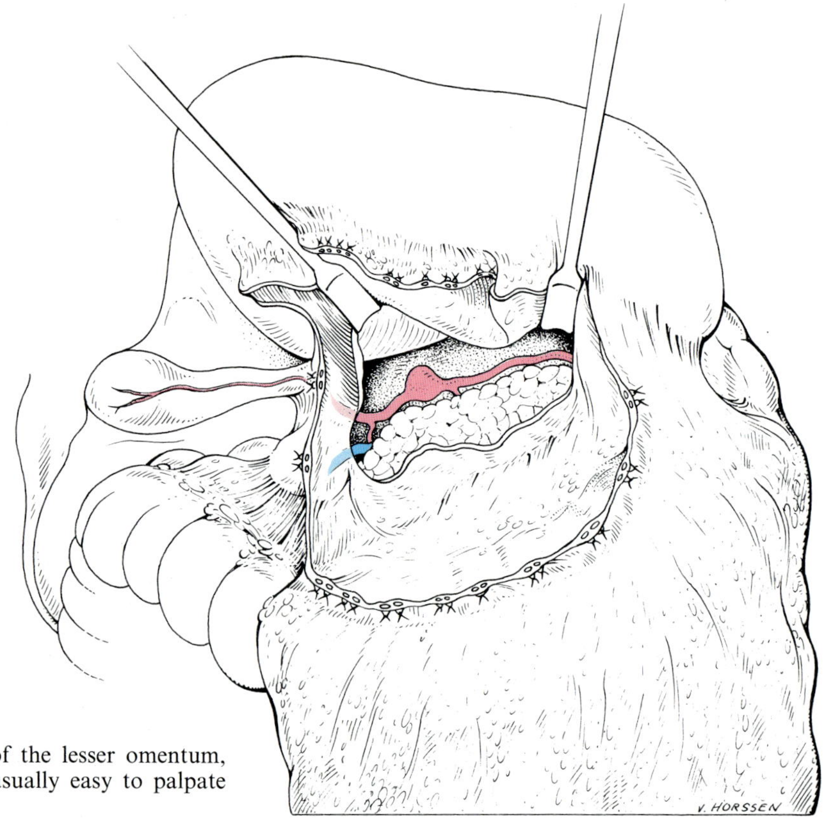

Fig. 15.3.2. Following opening of the lesser omentum, the splenic artery aneurysm is usually easy to palpate and to dissect

The dissection is continued along the greater curvature, because more caudal the vascularization of the colon may be endangered. The lateral short gastric arteries should be preserved. In the lesser sac of the omentum, the splenic artery may be palpated behind the upper border of the pancreas. The aneurysm is often easy to localize. The splenic artery is exposed and ligated proximal and distal to the aneurysm. One should pay special attention to small branches of the splenic artery that supply the pancreas and also have to be ligated. If resection of the aneurysm is difficult because of its localization in the pancreatic tissue, it should not be forced, owing to the risk of a pancreatic fistula or of postoperative pancreatitis. Aneurysms located more medially require opening of the lesser omentum (Fig. 15.3.2).

C. Hepatic Artery Aneurysms

I. Prevalence, Pathology, Indications

Hepatic artery aneurysms are the second most common, comprising 20% of all visceral arterial aneurysms. One should be wary of these lesions because of the great danger of rupture. Formerly, aneurysms of this artery were usually diagnosed as mycotic in nature; however, owing to the introduction of antibiotics, mycotic lesions are seen less frequently [5]. Besides arteriosclerosis, degeneration of the media along with trauma figure most prominently in the etiology. Also, in patients suffering from periarteritis nodosa, this artery frequently shows aneurysms [14, 16].

The risk of rupture of a hepatic artery aneurysm is reported to be 44%–80%, with an extremely high mortality. The type of management depends on whether the aneurysm lies in the common hepatic artery or the proper hepatic artery (Fig. 15.3.1 b). In the first case, blood flow to the liver is maintained through collaterals of the gastroduodenal and pancreaticoduodenal arcades.

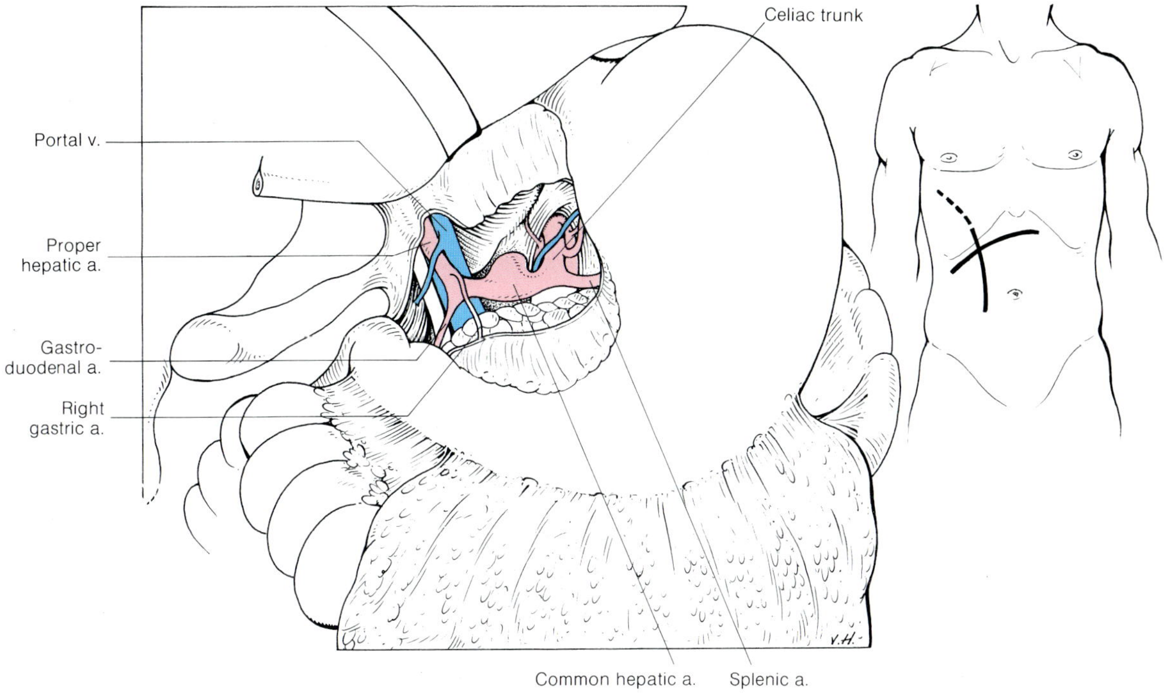

Fig. 15.3.3. After opening of the lesser omentum, the common hepatic artery with the aneurysm is dissected

Resection of the aneurysm without vascular reconstruction is therefore possible. However, if the aneurysm includes the proper hepatic artery, blood flow to the liver must be restored again.

Intrahepatic aneurysms can be exposed only with great difficulty. In some cases, a proximal ligature in combination with embolization of the aneurysm may be indicated. For all of these procedures, however, precise preoperative determination of local blood supply is essential. Using isotopes, one can determine to what extent the hepatic artery and the portal vein are responsible for blood flow and oxygen supply to the liver. Then, depending on this distribution, in difficult cases a procedure such as embolization may be performed for intrahepatic aneurysms.

II. Management

1. Operative Approaches

Exposure of the common hepatic artery as well as the proper hepatic artery is achieved through a right subcostal incision, extending to the left half of the body. A second approach is a right pararectal thoracophrenic laparotomy. By displacing the liver cranially and dorsally, one may dissect far into the hilus of the liver, even into the parenchyma.

2. Aneurysms of the Common Hepatic Artery

The lesser omentum is opened along the lesser curvature of the stomach (Fig. 15.3.3). Often, the aneurysm is already palpable. Proximally, the common hepatic artery branching off from the celiac trunk is exposed and a tape placed around it. Distally, the proper hepatic artery, the gastroduodenal artery, and the right gastric artery are exposed and tapes placed around them as well. The proper hepatic artery lies in the hepatoduodenal ligament, framed by the portal vein and bile duct. Following exposure of the vessels the common hepatic artery is ligated proximally and distally to the aneurysm. The aneurysm is then dissected. The circulation of the collaterals via the pancreaticoduodenal arteries and the gastroduodenal artery is sufficient to supply the liver.

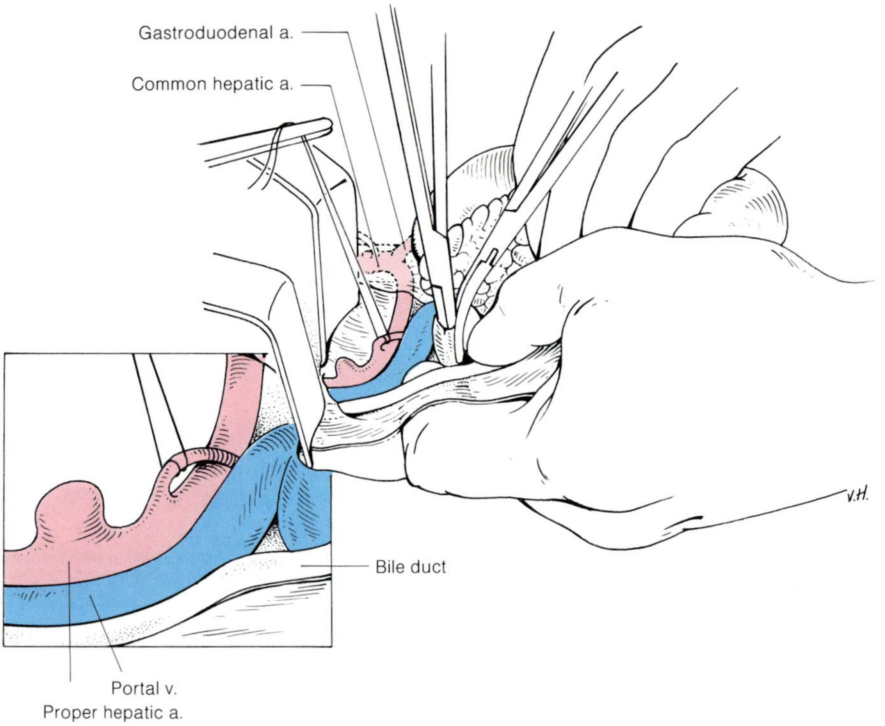

Fig. 15.3.4. The proper hepatic artery is exposed at the hepatoduodenal ligament. Care must be taken with the adjacent structures, the portal vein, and the bile duct

3. Aneurysms of the Proper Hepatic Artery

For exposure a supracolic approach is chosen. First, the hepatoduodenal ligament is dissected within the hilus of the liver. The proper hepatic artery lies in its dorsomedial portion. While dissecting the artery, therefore, first the bile duct and then the portal vein must be identified (Fig. 15.3.4). In the proximal region, temporary ligatures or tourniquets are first passed around the common hepatic artery, the gastroduodenal artery, and the right gastric artery. The aneurysm itself must be dissected very carefully without being ruptured, especially in the case of a mycotic aneurysm. Distal to the sac of the aneurysm, the hepatic artery is dissected over a length of at least 2 cm, so that an end-to-end anastomosis with a venous graft is possible.

Next, the proximal infrarenal abdominal aorta is exposed (see p. 594; see Fig. 15.3.4). The greater saphenous vein graft, which should have been harvested beforehand, is anastomosed to the infrarenal aorta end-to-side, the aorta having been previously cross-clamped with two straight clamps. An oval incision about 7 mm in diameter is tailored in the anterior aortal wall. This may also be performed with a punching device. The anastomosis itself is made with a 6–0 continuous suture. When tailoring the end of the vein graft for the anastomosis, one should take care to have the inflow as funnel shaped as possible in order to avoid late aneurysms due to a bad inflow. The aorta is then unclamped and the vein graft cross-clamped.

The tunnel between the infrarenal aorta and the hepatoduodenal ligament is created by blunt dissection. The index finger of the right hand dissects above the left renal vein, below the superior mesenteric artery, and ventral to the head of the pancreas in the direction of the opened hepatoduodenal ligament (see p. 218). Following slight dilation of the tunnel with the index finger of the left hand, the filled vein graft is passed through.

The proper hepatic artery is ligated proximal to the aneurysm. A small bulldog clamp is placed as distally as possible near the branching of the proper hepatic artery. The aneurysm is incised and resected as far as possible. If surrounding structures are endangered, one should not use excessive force. The distal proper hepatic artery is incised

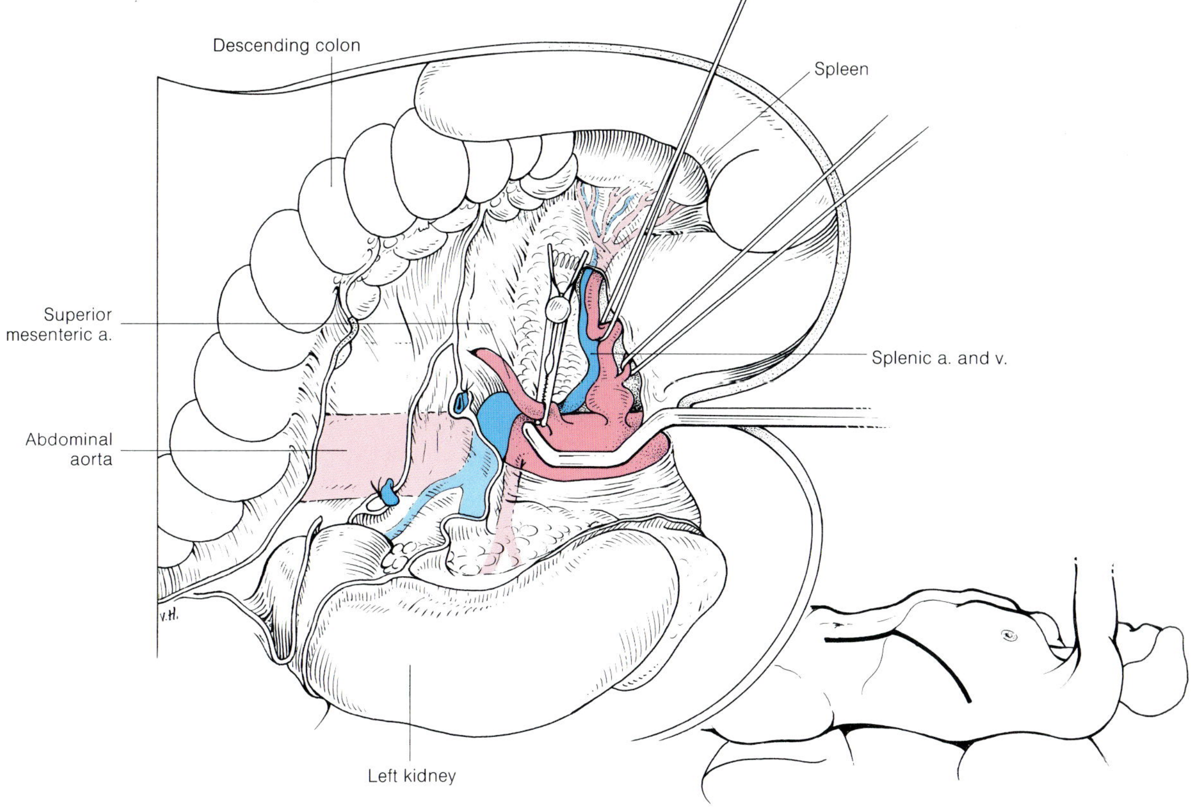

Fig. 15.3.5. Celiac trunk aneurysm. Between the aorta and the celiac trunk aneurysm, there is relatively little space for cross-clamping. Therefore, the aorta should be well dissected primarily above and below

on its ventral side for about 1 cm. The vein graft is measured to the correct length. The anastomosis is then performed using 7–0 suture material, starting at the corner of the side towards the vena cava. After restoration of circulation, blood flow is checked by Doppler ultrasound or electromagnetic flow probe. The operation in this region is finished by placing a drain and covering the bypass with the surrounding retroperitoneal tissue.

D. Celiac Trunk Aneurysms

I. Prevalance, Pathology, Indications

Celiac trunk aneurysms usually develop out of poststenotic dilatations of an arteriosclerotic or congenital stenosis at the origin of the trunk. Other, rarer causes are syphilis, trauma, or inflammatory disease. When considering whether operative revision is indicated, the high incidence of rupture has to be weighed against the operative risk. It must be confirmed by preoperative angiography that the superior mesenteric artery and the pancreaticoduodenal arcade are intact. In these cases, removal of the aneurysm without further reconstruction is sufficient.

II. Management

1. Positioning

Supine position, with the left side elevated (see p. 592).

2. Operative Approach

Left thoracoabdominal incision (see p. 592).

3. Intra-abdominal Approach

Following division of the skin, the subcutaneous tissue, and the fascia of the transverse muscle, the incision is continued through the costal arch and the intercostal muscles, finally incising the diaphragm. The left flexure of the colon, spleen, and pancreas are mobilized and retracted medially, together with the stomach (see Fig. 22.5a, c, p. 594). The left renal vein lies farthest caudal in the operative field. The aorta is easy to palpate. The periaortic tissue is dissected cranial to the left renal vein; then, the aorta and its branches, the superior mesenteric artery, and the celiac trunk are dissected. Exposure of the neck of the aneurysm may be difficult as the celiac trunk may lie directly on the anterior wall of the aorta (Fig. 15.3.5). Therefore, it is important to expose the proximal aorta beforehand so far that it can be cross-clamped in case of emergency. Also, all tributaries of the celiac trunk should be dissected peripherally and tapes placed around them.

In most cases resection and ligation of the remaining arterial stumps are sufficient for management of the aneurysms. The collateral circulation via the pancreaticoduodenal arteries will already have taken over the blood supply of the organs in the upper abdomen in the vast majority of cases. However, if the superior mesenteric artery is occluded or highly stenosed, reconstruction is necessary. Two procedures are possible: either hepatic artery bypass from the aorta to the common hepatic artery (see p. 603) or insertion of the splenic artery into the aorta (see p. 599). A drain is placed in the operative field. The retroperitoneal incision is closed by interrupted sutures. We sew the diaphragm with continuous absorbable suture. A chest tube is placed in the pleural cavity, and the outer wounds are closed in the usual fashion.

E. Renal Artery Aneurysms

I. Prevalence, Pathology, Indications

Renal aneurysms are found in 1 of 9000 autopsies. The causes are arteriosclerosis and fibromuscular dysplasia, and, less commonly, periarteritis nodosa and trauma. In 15% of all cases, aneuryms are found on both sides. An operation is indicated when there is danger of embolization into the kidneys. The risk of rupture, however, is low [15].

II. Management

Positioning and operative approaches are described in the chapter on renal arteries (see p. 609). In cases of small saccular aneurysms, resection and patch graft angioplasty are sufficient. Larger, fusiform aneurysms require resection with subsequent interposition of a greater saphenous vein graft. This is first harvested in the groin and then anastomosed side-to-end to the distal abdominal aorta (see p. 618). Following clamping, the aneurysm is resected and the kidney flushed with heparinized saline solution or cold 10% glucose solution. The distal stump of the renal artery is dilated slightly by means of bulldog clamps and beveled for the end-to-end anstomosis. This is performed using a 7–0 continuous suture. After restoration of flow, the cross-clamped proximal renal artery is sutured first. If the renal artery aneurysm is on the right side, reconstruction follows the same principles. The bypass is placed ventral to the inferior vena cava.

F. Superior Mesenteric Artery Aneurysms

I. Prevalence, Pathology, Indications

Superior mesenteric artery aneurysms are rare. In the literature, just over 100 have been described [5]. In contrast to other visceral arteries, almost 50% are of mycotic origin. Therefore, one should consider the possibility of a superior mesenteric artery aneurysm when a patient with a history of sepsis presents with a pulsatile tumor and a murmur in the upper abdomen. Also, patients in whom mycotic aneurysms have been diagnosed in other regions should have additional angiographic evaluation of the superior mesenteric artery. DE BAKEY and COOLEY [4] described the successful resection of a superior mesenteric artery aneurysm with ligation of both arterial stumps. This procedure can be performed only if there is sufficient collateral circulation between the jejunal arteries proximal to the aneurysm and the ileac branches distal to the aneurysm.

To answer this question, good selective angiography of the superior mesenteric artery is necessary [2]. If the aneurysm is of mycotic origin, it is important to identify the underlying microorganism preoperatively. Here, careful evaluation of the history may help. The primary disease, with its characteristic bacteria, may point in the right direction. In former times, streptococci were predominant. Today, infections with *Staphylococcus aureus* are predominant. Also, other microorganisms, such as gonococci, salmonella, and bacteroides have been cultured from mesenteric aneurysms. MREYEN [8] even reported a myotic aneurysm of the superior mesenteric artery of tuberculous origin.

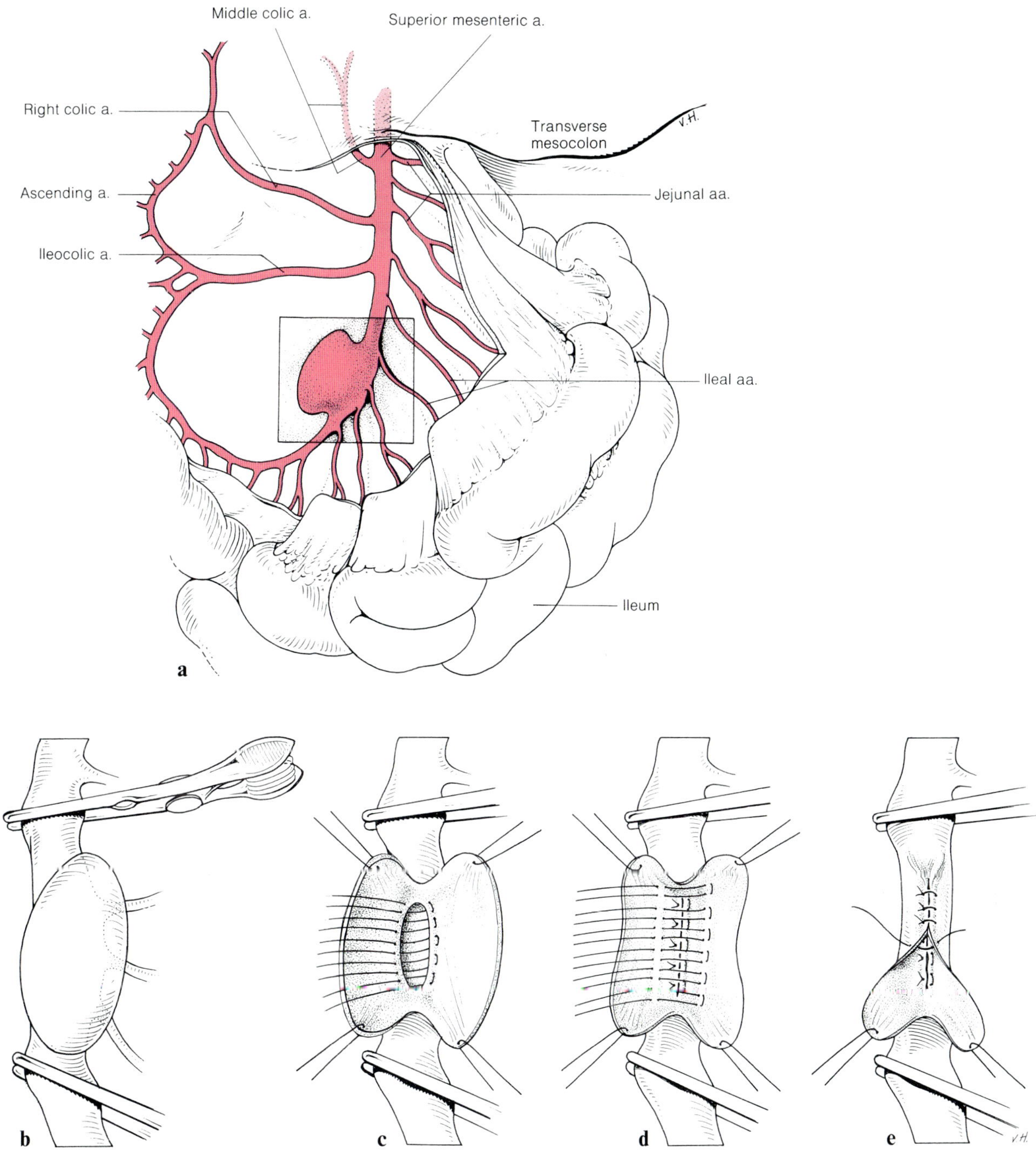

Fig. 15.3.6. a Aneurysmorrhaphy of a mycotic aneurysm of the superior mesenteric artery. **b** Cross-clamping. **c** First layer of mattress sutures. **d** Second layer of mattress sutures. **e** Third and last layer of interrupted sutures

II. Management

1. Positioning

Supine Trendelenburg position.

2. Operative Approach

The standard approach is median transperitoneal laparotomy. When the aneurysm is located very proximally, a left-sided thoraco-abdominal approach may be of advantage (see p. 595). In rare cases, a right retroperitoneal approach is recommended. Both retroperitoneal approaches are similar to the approaches to the left or right renal artery (see p. 613).

When the aneurysm is located at its most common site, the radix mesenterii, a median laparotomy is performed. The entire small bowel is retracted to the right and cranially, the root of the mesentery then being on the right side of the operative field. Usually the aneurysm can be palpated. Then, the proximal trunk of the superior mesenteric artery is dissected and a tape placed around it. Dissection is likewise performed at the distal segment, and then the aneurysm itself is dissected. Since this lesion is usually of mycotic origin, dissection must be performed with great care, so as to avoid perforation. Technically, the most difficult part is to dissect possible jejunal tributaries branching off the aneurysm, to place tapes around them, and to cross-clamp them.

When angiography reveals good collateral flow to the distal vascular system of the superior mesenteric artery, simple ligation of all tributaries of the aneurysm, together with partial resection, is sufficient. Subsequent intraoperative control of the small bowel circulation is important. For this purpose, all tributaries branching off the aneurysm should first be cross-clamped temporarily. By means of Doppler ultrasonography it can be determined whether there is sufficient blood flow in the ileal or jejunal arcade. Where there is doubt, aneurysmorrhaphy, rather than resection, should be performed [6].

III. Aneurysmorrhaphy

Once the aneurysm has been isolated by clamping, it may be opened (Fig. 15.3.6a). The adherent mural thrombi are removed and flushed out. Deeper within the aneurysm, one can usually recognize the course of the original vessel interior, with its normal layer of endothelium (Fig. 15.3.6b). The opening is closed by placing uninterrupted mattress sutures in such a way as to restore the normal circumference of the superior mesenteric artery (Fig. 15.3.6c). Absorbable suture material is recommended. One or two additional layers of mattres sutures are sewn over the first layer in the same fashion (Fig. 15.3.6d, e).

After a drain has been introduced, the peritoneum is closed over the aneurysmorrhaphy.

Now, the viability of each small bowel segment is ascertained. If ischemia is clearly present, partial resection of the small bowel is necessary.

In case of doubt, a second-look operation, 12–24 h later, is required. In this way, the viability of the small bowel can be better judged and possible consequences forseen.

G. Aneurysms of the Pancreaticoduodenal Arcade

I. Prevalence, Pathology

Aneurysms of these arteries are very seldom described. In all of the literature, only about 40 cases are known. Besides arteriosclerosis (the most frequent cause), cases involving fibromuscular dysplasia, trauma, penetrating duodenal ulcer, and recurrent chronic pancreatitis have been described.

II. Management

1. Positioning

Supine position, flexed at the thoracolumbar junction.

2. Operative Approach

Transverse incision in the upper abdomen.

3. Intra-abdominal Approach

For aneurysms localized in the anterior pancreaticoduodenal arcade, the supracolic approach should be chosen (see Fig. 12.6; p. 596). It is desirable to open the gastrocolic ligament on the right medial side. Aneurysms of the gastroduodenal artery can best be approached by opening the lesser sac. For aneurysms of the posterior pancreaticoduodenal arcade, mobilization of the duodenum according to KOCHER is recommended (see Fig. 22.9, p. 598).

Dissection is extremely difficult when the aneurysm is partially or completely embedded in the pancreas. If angiography does not reveal branches of the aneurysm, then simple ligation of efferent and afferent arteries is sufficient. However, if the aneurysm has one or more branches, additional thrombosis must be induced [2].

In all cases extensive dissection within the pancreatic tissue should be avoided. Very often this may cause postoperative pancreatitis or pancreatic fistula. The latter may result in massive bleeding by arrosion of a dissected vessel in that region. Although complete or partial pancreatectomies have been described, we think that these procedures should be limited to extreme situations.

Reconstructions in this region are unnecessary because of the very pronounced collateral flow. The operation is finished by placing a drain in the operative field which will stay until secretion has ceased. It is advisable to check the level of amylase in this fluid, depending on its quality.

H. Aneurysms of the Gastric Artery, the Ileal Arteries, and the Inferior Mesenteric Artery

I. Prevalence, Pathology

Aneurysms in these arteries are extremely rare and are only reported sporadically [5, 14]. In the majority of cases, they are diagnosed accidentally by angiography. Ruptures seldom occur. Concerning the etiology, many of the factors already mentioned may be involved. However, congenital aneurysms may be somewhat more common in this region.

II. Management

These aneurysms are treated adequately by resection and ligation of afferent and efferent arteries. Following exclusion of the aneurysms, it is important to test the viability of organs supplied by the artery involved and to perform a bowel resection, if necessary.

In principle, aneurysms of the inferior mesenteric artery are managed in the same way. In this case, it is important to bear in mind that simultaneous occlusion of the superior mesenteric artery or simultaneous occlusion of both internal iliac arteries may result in a deficient blood supply to the descending and the sigmoid colon.

REFERENCES

1. Beaussier M (1770) Sur un aneurysme de l'artere splenique dont les parios se sont ossifes. J Med (Toulouse) 32:157
2. Van Berge Henegouwen DP, Koning J, Padmos M, Barwegen MGMH, Schwilden ED (1980) Aneurysmen der intestinalen Arterien. Angio 4/2:259–268
3. Boijsen E, Efsing H-O (1969) Aneurysms of the splenic artery. Acta Radiol [Diagn] (Stockh) 8:29–41
4. De Bakey ME, Cooley DA (1953) Successful resection of mycotic aneurysm of superior mesenteric artery: case report and review of literature. Am Surg 19:202
5. Deterling RA Jr (1971) Aneurysms of the visceral arterie. J Cardiovasc Surg 12:309
6. Matas R (1888) Traumatic aneurysm of the left brachial artery: incision and partial excision of sac: recovery. Phila Med News 53:452
7. McNamara MF, Basksi KB (1982) Mesenteric artery aneurysms. In: Bergan JJ, Yao JST (eds) Aneurysms, diagnosis and treatment. Grune and Stratton, New York (pp 385–485)
8. Mreyen FM (1960) Mycotic aneurysm. Arch Chir Neerl 12:180
9. Pernot JHM (1970) A patient with multiple aneurysms of the splenic artery. Arch Chir Neerl 22:165
10. Slors JMF, Taat CW, van Berge Henegouwen DP, Mallonga ET (1982) Rupture of aneurysm of the middle colic artery. Neth J Surg 34:174–177
11. Spanes PK, Kloppedal EA (1974) Aneurysms of the gastroduodenal and pancreaticoduodenal arteries. Am Surg 127:345
12. Spittel JA, Fairbarn JF, Sheps SC et al. (1961) Splentic artery aneurysms. Surg Clin North Am 41:1121–1126
13. Stanley JC, Fry WJ (1974) Pathogenesis and clinical significance of splenic artery aneurysms. Surgery 76:898
14. Stanley JC, Thompson NW, Fry W (1970) Splanchnic artery aneurysms. Arch Surg 101:689
15. Tham G, Ekelund T, Olin et al. (1983) Renal artery aneurysms. Ann Surg 348–352
16. Weaver DH, Flemming RJ, Barnes WA (1968) Aneurysms of the hepatic artery: the value of arteriography in surgical management. Surgery 64:891
17. Westcott JL, Ziter FM (1973) Aneurysms of the splenic artery. SGO 136:541

15.4 Aneurysms of the Abdominal Aorta

F.W. Schildberg and A. Valesky

CONTENTS

A. Unruptured Infrarenal Aortic Aneurysms

I. Anatomy

Between 95% and 98% of all aneurysms of the abdominal aorta develop within the infrarenal portion of the aorta. Aneurysmal enlargement is also commonly found in pelvic vessels. The main cause of aneuryms is arteriosclerosis (over 95% of all cases).

There are several reasons why arteriosclerotic abdominal aortic aneurysms occur primarily in the infrarenal segment (segment V) of the vessel. Evidence of increased collagenolytic activity [5] within the aneurysmal wall and the increased deposition of cholesterol and lipids [4] in the infrarenal aortic segment indicate local metabolic disorders. The angle of the aortic bifurcation also plays a very important role in the development of abdominal aortic aneurysms [15]. Elongation of the aorta, caused by arteriosclerosis, forces both limbs of the bifurcation apart, thereby enlarging the angle. As a result, the pulse waves are more strongly reflected than in an undiseased bifurcation with an acute angle. Another factor is the topographic-anatomic situation of the infrarenal segment of the aorta: it is relatively unsupported by neighboring organs and tissues. The connection here becomes clear from the fact that the aneurysms in question usually extend farther to the left – the direction of least peritoneal resistance – than to the right, where the root of the mesenterium and the inferior vena cava prevent further distention.

The inflammatory abdominal aortic aneurysm is less common. It occurs in about 3%–5% of all arteriosclerotic aneurysms. It remains unknown whether this type of aneurysm is merely a variation of arteriosclerotic disease or has its own etiology. Syphilitic and mycotic aneurysms are rare. The same is true of aneurysms that develop in connection with peripheral arteriovenous fistula. The increased blood flow leads to aneurysmal enlargement of the main vessels, including the abdominal aorta. Such alterations usually do not regress after repair of the peripheral arteriovenous fistula [24].

II. Diagnostic Procedures

The abdominal aortic aneurysm is often identified by inspection and palpation alone. One may assume that the aneurysm is limited to segment V of the aorta if its expansile borders can be palpated entirely below the costal margin. Ultrasound scanning detects aneurysms in over 95% of all cases [16]. Lateral abdominal X-rays have lost their importance for the detection of calcified aneurysms owing to the higher accuracy of ultrasound imaging. Another noninvasive diagnostic procedure is CT, with or without contrast media. It reliably detects an aneurysm and at the same time gives valuable information for planning surgical reconstruction. It precisely determines the extent of the aneurysm and then shows whether or not aneurysmal enlargement has spread to segment IV of the abdominal aorta. Positional anomalies of the inferior vena cava or the left renal vein (retroaortic position) may also be visualized. CT scanning better identifies a retroperitoneal hematoma in symptomatic aneurysms and may assess the degree of possible rupture. Symptomatic aneurysms which show no leakage can then be treated electively after adequate preparation of the patient for surgery; in this way, one avoids emergency operations of considerably higher risk [22]. For example, an inflammatory aneurysm often causes symptoms such as flank or lower back pain without demonstrating rupture. This type of aneurysm can be identified preoperatively on the CT scan. It regularly shows a perianeurysmal layer of tissue several centimeters thick which holds back contrast medium (angio-CT) [23].

Infrarenal aneurysms often extend into the renal arteries. Therefore, preoperative angiograms of this region are mandatory [20]. The simplest method is digital subtraction angiography. Conventional angiography is performed if it is presumed that the patient has occlusive arterial disease of the lower limbs or a horseshoe kidney. The thrombotic coating of the internal wall of the aneurysmal sac often simulates an undiseased aortic lumen. In such a case, absent visualization of the lumbar arteries is enough evidence for the presence of an abdominal aortic aneurysm.

III. Indications for Surgery

The rupture of an aneurysm is the most serious and most common complication. Thrombotic occlusion or embolic dissemination leading to peripheral ischemia are seen less often. Many studies on the prognosis of patients with an abdominal aortic aneurysm show that spontaneous mortality in unoperated patients is two to three times higher than in those who undergo surgery. All aneurysms should be treated operatively because of the risk of rupture. Exceptions are made only in high-risk patients with serious contraindications, such as therapy-resistant congestive heart failure, global pulmonary insufficiency, or progressive neoplastic disease. The danger of rupture increases proportionally with the diameter of the aneurysm. The probability of rupture cannot be reliably predicted since ruptures of small aneurysms also occur [9]. Estimation of this risk is also difficult in age groups of 70 years and more, to which most patients belong today.

Arteriosclerotic lesions of the supra-aortic branches or coronary arteries needing surgical repair should be treated prior to surgery of an abdominal aortic aneurysm. Under certain conditions, simultaneous repair of such lesions may be considered.

IV. Positioning

The surgical approach usually chosen for repair of an infrarenal aneurysm is the transabdominal approach. The patient is placed in a supine position. The upper part of the body is reclined slightly, the point of backward rotation lying between the umbilicus and the xiphoid process. The groin is always regarded as a potential operating area and is therefore prepared accordingly. External rotation of the thigh with slight flexion at the knee facilitates exposure of the inguinal vessels for femoral attachment of a prosthesis, if needed.

V. Surgical Exposure

A long midline incision or a wide transverse incision may be performed to expose the infrarenal aorta (Fig. 15.4.1). A median laparotomy is usually preferred. This incision, extending from the xyphoid process to the symphysis pubis, allows for better visualization of the entire aortoiliac region and is usually carried out more quickly. The transverse laparotomy above or below the umbilicus causes less respiratory dysfunction postoperatively.

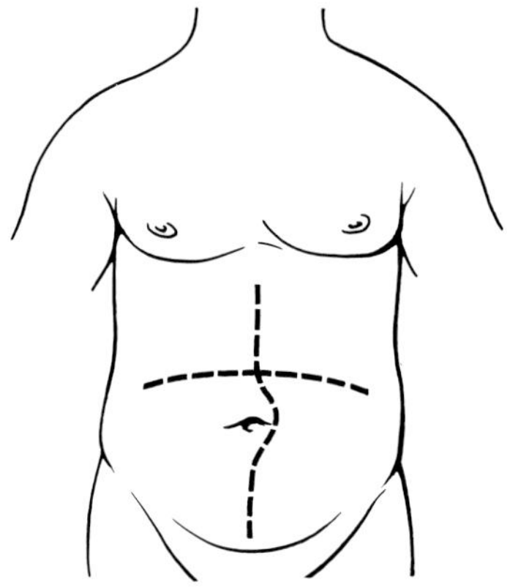

Fig. 15.4.1. Incisions for exposure of an infrarenal aneurysm median or transverse laparotomy

VI. Exposure of the Infrarenal Aortic Aneurysm

1. Surgical Exposure

For the exposure of the aneurysm the small intestine is retracted to the right side of the abdomen or placed outside the cavity to the upper right of the incision. In the latter case heat loss is prevented by protecting the small intestine in a plastic bag. Following mobilization of the duodenojejunal flexure, a broad retractor is placed on the left and right side of the aneurysm and two narrow ones adjacent to the cranial end. This allows good visualization of the entire infrarenal aortic lesion (Fig. 15.4.2a).

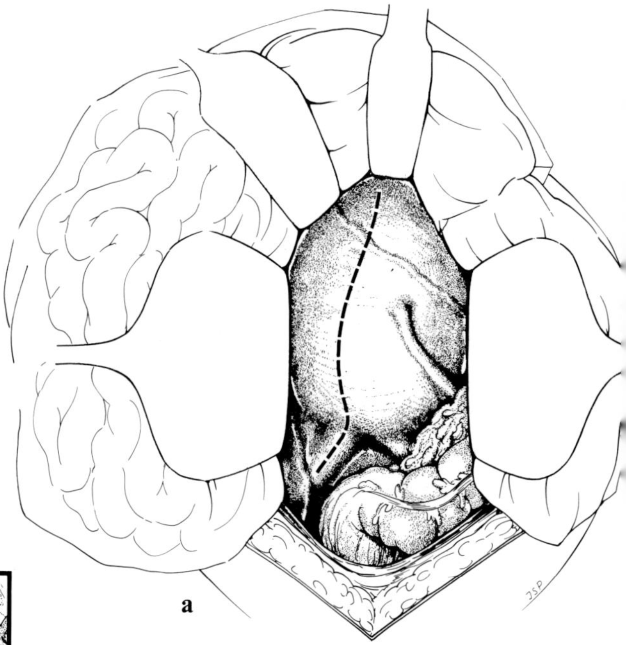

a

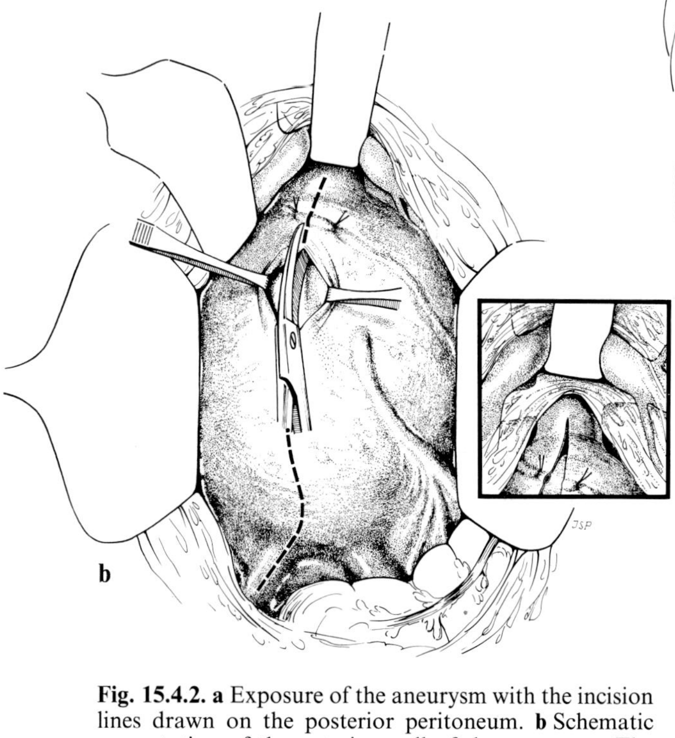

b

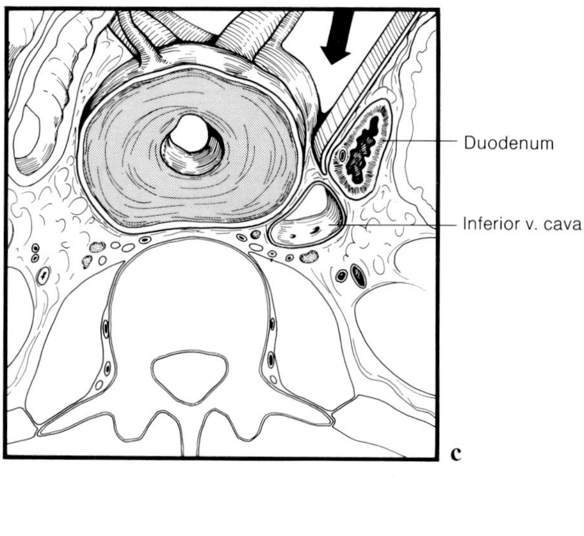

c

Fig. 15.4.2. a Exposure of the aneurysm with the incision lines drawn on the posterior peritoneum. **b** Schematic presentation of the anterior wall of the aneurysm. The inferior mesenteric vein has been divided following ligation. **c** Transverse section of the aneurysm from the surgeon's point of view. Relationships to the duodenum (ascending portion) and inferior vena cava

2. Preparation of the Aneurysm

Peritoneum and periaortic tissue above the aneurysm are incised down to the adventitia of the aneurysmal sac on the right side of the midline to spare the inferior mesenteric artery and the vascular arcade that supplies the left colon (Fig. 15.4.2b). One now has access to a relatively avascular dissection plane that allows blunt and sharp dissection of the anterior aspect of the aneurysm (Fig. 15.4.2c). The incision is lengthened cranially up to the renal vein, which crosses about 1 cm distal to the duodenum. With larger aneurysms, division of the inferior mesenteric vein, which crosses the infrarenal segment of the lesion, may permit better exposure. The incision is extended distally in the direction of the right iliac artery. This spares the vascular arcades of the inferior mesenteric artery essential for proper perfusion of the left colon and preserves the, essential nerve plexus for sexual potency (see p. 180ff). Transverse dissection at the bifurcation should be avoided, if possible.

3. Preparation of the Proximal Aorta ("Aneurysmal Neck")

Exposure of the undiseased infrarenal segment of the aorta, which varies in length, is performed by sharp and blunt dissection as far as the left renal vein. This vein has a retroaortic position in 1%–2%. The elongation of the infrarenal aorta that is typical in such cases levers the neck of the aneurysm away from the spine. This allows the surgeon to dissect bluntly beneath it simply by using a finger (Fig. 15.4.3a). This maneuver prepares a plane for transverse cross-clamping of the proximal aorta, which affords a better view during suturing of the anastomosis than sagittal clamping would. The entire circumference of the aorta should be mobilized only if it can be done with ease. With very large aneurysms extending just beneath the origins of the renal arteries or in the presence of inflammatory changes of the retroperitoneum, sagittal clamping is preferred without complete circumferential mobilization of the aorta. Atypically localized renal arteries must be identified during dissection of the aneurysmal neck. Branches within the undiseased portion of this area can usually be saved without difficulty. Renal arteries having their origins within the aneurysmal wall itself may be excised together with an aneurysmal patch for reimplantation into a prosthesis. Pole arteries should be ligated only if their calibers are small. Otherwise, renal function may be impaired by the loss of too much parenchyma.

4. Preparation of the Distal Aorta and Pelvic Vessels

The preparation of the distal aorta and proximal pelvic vessels is facilitated by a retroperitoneal approach. All tissue lying in front of the aortic bifurcation is mobilized en bloc in the plane of the adventitia and reflected to the left side (Fig. 15.4.3b). This allows for good visualization without injury to nerve plexus that are important for the sexually active male [21]. Circumferential preparation of the distal aorta or common iliac arteries and mobilization of the vessels by placing rubber tubing around them is not necessary in this region. Dissection of two thirds of the anterior aspect of the large pelvic vessels is usually adequate for safe control of hemorrhage distally. In dilating and obliterating vascular lesions of the pelvic vessels, dissection is performed distal to

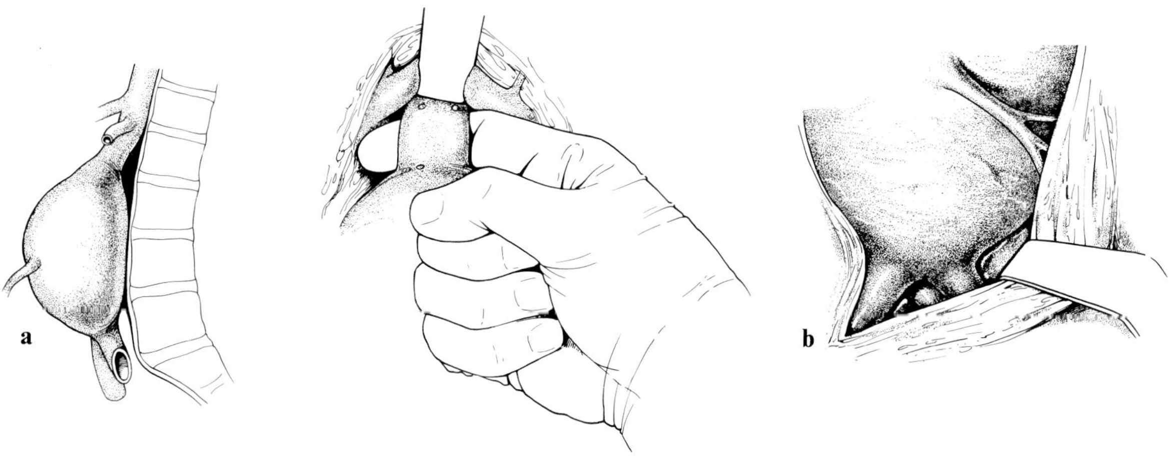

Fig. 15.4.3. a Preparation of the proximal aorta and digital tunneling beneath it. **b** Exposure of the distal aorta and aortic bifurcation

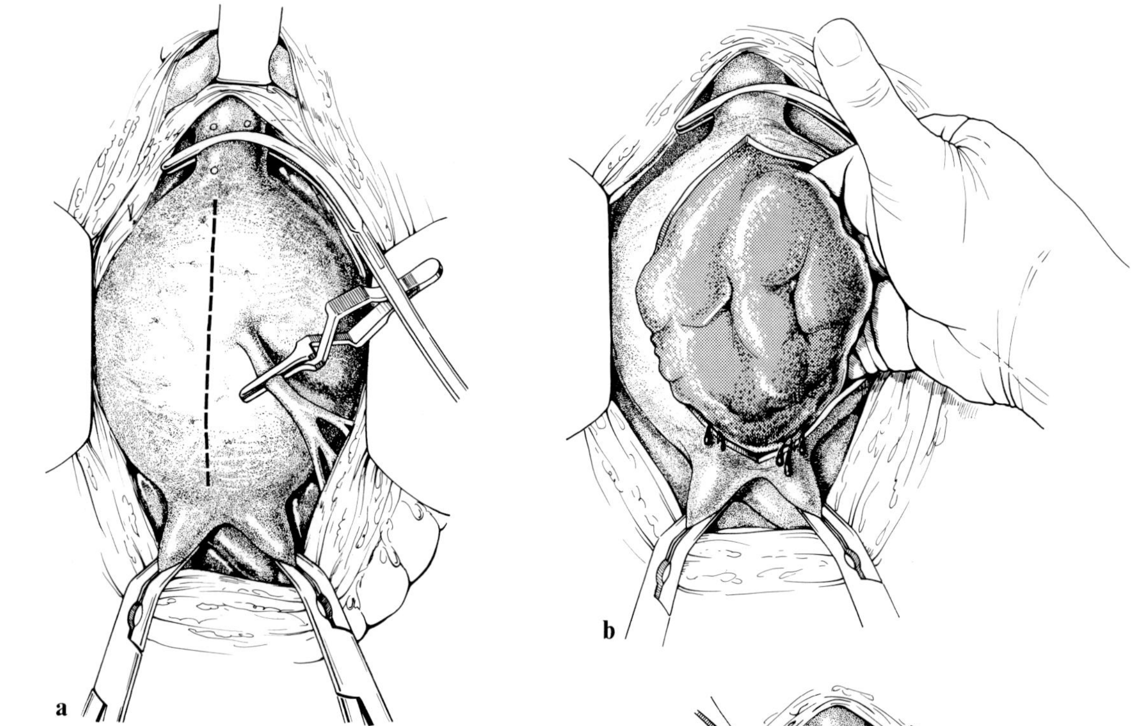

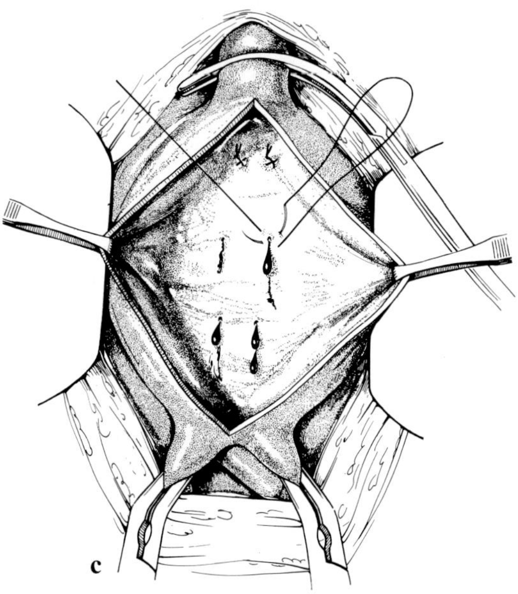

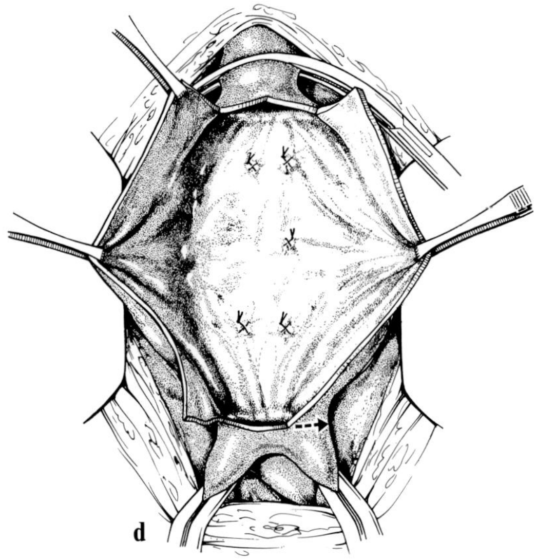

Fig. 15.4.4. a Clamping of the aorta. Line of incision. **b** Removal of thrombotic material. **c** Closing the back-bleeding lumbar arteries with sutures. **d** Semicircular incision of the aorta at the neck of the aneurysm and the level of the bifurcation. Aortic back wall protrudes into the lumen

these diseased segments. Should circumferential mobilization of these vessels be necessary in some cases, preparation is started at the visible right iliac vein. This decreases the risk of intraoperative injury as the plane of dissection between the vein and the artery is very easily found in this area. Dissection distal to the origin of the internal iliac artery is performed through an additional incision of the peritoneum made in the iliac fossa. On the left side this is only possible following mobilization of the sigmoid colon away from the lateral abdominal wall.

VII. Clamping and Division of the Aneurysm

Following preparation, the aneurysmal neck is clamped in either a transverse or sagittal direction, just beneath the origin of both renal arteries. After clamping the inferior mesenteric artery near its origin, the iliac vessels are clamped for control of back bleeding (Fig. 15.4.4a). In lesions limited to the aorta and bifurcation, clamping of the common iliac artery is recommended. Separate clamping of the internal and external iliac arteries is necessary if an additional aneurysm of the common iliac artery is found extending downward to the origin of the internal iliac artery. The aneurysm is opened by a longitudinal incision to the right of the midline, preserving the origin of the inferior mesenteric artery. The thrombotic material is removed en bloc. Back bleeding from the lumbar arteries is controlled by oversewing each bleeding orifice (Fig. 15.4.4b, c). Owing to extensive arteriosclerosis, local disobliteration of the orifice is usually necessary prior to suture ligation. After back bleeding from the lumbar arteries has been brought under control, the proximal aorta is digitally explored and the aortotomy is extended upward until the undiseased infrarenal aortic segment is reached. Usually the distal portion of the incision is lengthened down to the bifurcation. If the iliac arteries also show aneurysmal enlargement, the arteriotomy is continued downward until an arterial segment is reached to which the prosthesis may be connected. Remaining thrombotic material may be removed by extensive flushing locally, peripherally, and proximally.

VIII. Technique of Vascular Reconstruction

1. Synthetic Material

Knitted double velour prostheses made of Dacron have always shown the best long-term results. Tube or bifurcation prostheses are employed, depending on the extent of the aneurysmal and arteriosclerotic lesions at the aorto-iliac bifurcation. Knitted prostheses are usually implanted in unruptured abdominal aortic aneurysms. Woven prostheses are used at the stage of rupture since the risk of dangerous clotting disorders in such a situation is extraordinarily high. Unlike knitted prostheses, woven grafts do not have to be preclotted. Poorer healing of the woven prostheses is one of the acceptable disadvantages of the material in this particular case. Recently, impermeable knitted prostheses that do not have to be preclotted became available. As for PTFE and other newer synthetics, only more clinical experience over a longer period of time can show how well they compare with better-known materials.

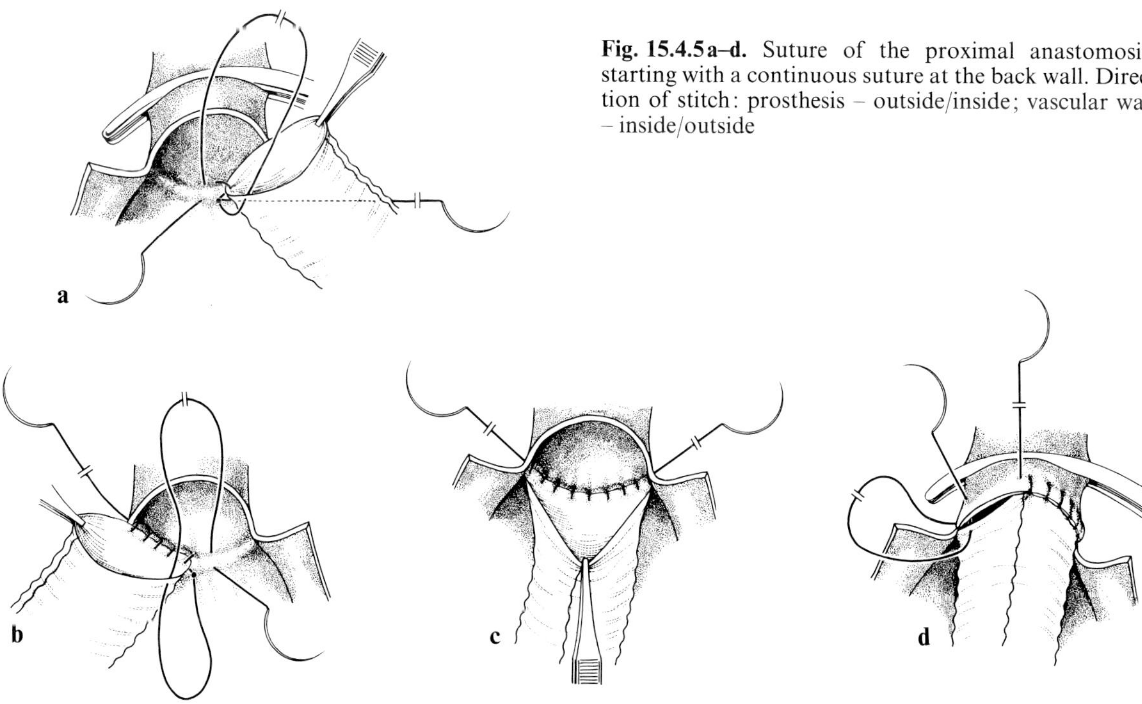

Fig. 15.4.5a–d. Suture of the proximal anastomosis, starting with a continuous suture at the back wall. Direction of stitch: prosthesis – outside/inside; vascular wall – inside/outside

2. Proximal Anastomosis

a) Standard Procedure. The infrarenal aorta is semicircularly incised across its anterior wall at the upper corner of the aortotomy (Fig. 15.4.4d). The back wall usually remains intact. Complete transection of the aorta is recommended only in exceptional cases, for better visualization of the back wall during suture (see Fig. 15.4.2b). The diameter of the prosthesis should be about equal to the size of the proximal aorta. Exact evaluation for appropriate graft selection may be facilitated by using a measuring device. The anastomosis is sutured continuously with 4–0 nonabsorbable monofilament suture material (Fig. 15.4.5). Stronger material with a larger needle is recommended only in vessels showing high grade arteriosclerosis. In such cases, however, suture-hole leakage is much more common. In our experience with this technique, we have not found it necessary to place a Dacron cuff around the upper anastomosis.

b) Suprarenal Clamping. In very large aneurysms, extending up to the renal arteries, the aorta must be clamped above the origin of these arteries. Better exposure can be achieved by thoroughly mobilizing the left renal vein following division of the spermatic or ovarian vein. Division of the left renal vein is only rarely required (Fig. 15.4.6). The maneuver requires careful preservation of all venous branches coming from the gonads and suprarenal glands. Otherwise, venous return from the left kidney would be considerably impaired. Clamping the renal arteries is also recommended to prevent thrombotic material from embolizing into these vessels during suprarenal clamping of the aorta. Clots within the aneurysm often extend all the way up to the orifices of the renal arteries. After the aneurysm has been opened, thrombectomy may be performed under direct vision. The origins of the renal arteries may be checked for back bleeding during this maneuver.

Complete transection of the aorta facilitates suturing of the anastomosis since the back wall of the aorta is fixed to the spine. Complete transection allows the back wall to be entirely mobilized away from the spine, thereby facilitating the precise placement of sutures in close proximity to the renal arteries (Fig. 15.4.6).

3. Distal Anastomosis

a) General Remarks. The frequency of implantation of tube grafts in comparison with bifurcation grafts is reported to be 0%–85% in operative treatment of infrarenal aneurysms. This wide range in preference can be explained by the great differences in the indication for reconstruction. An aneurysm with undiseased iliac arteries is beyond doubt best-suited for the interposition of a tube graft. This situation, however, is only rarely en-

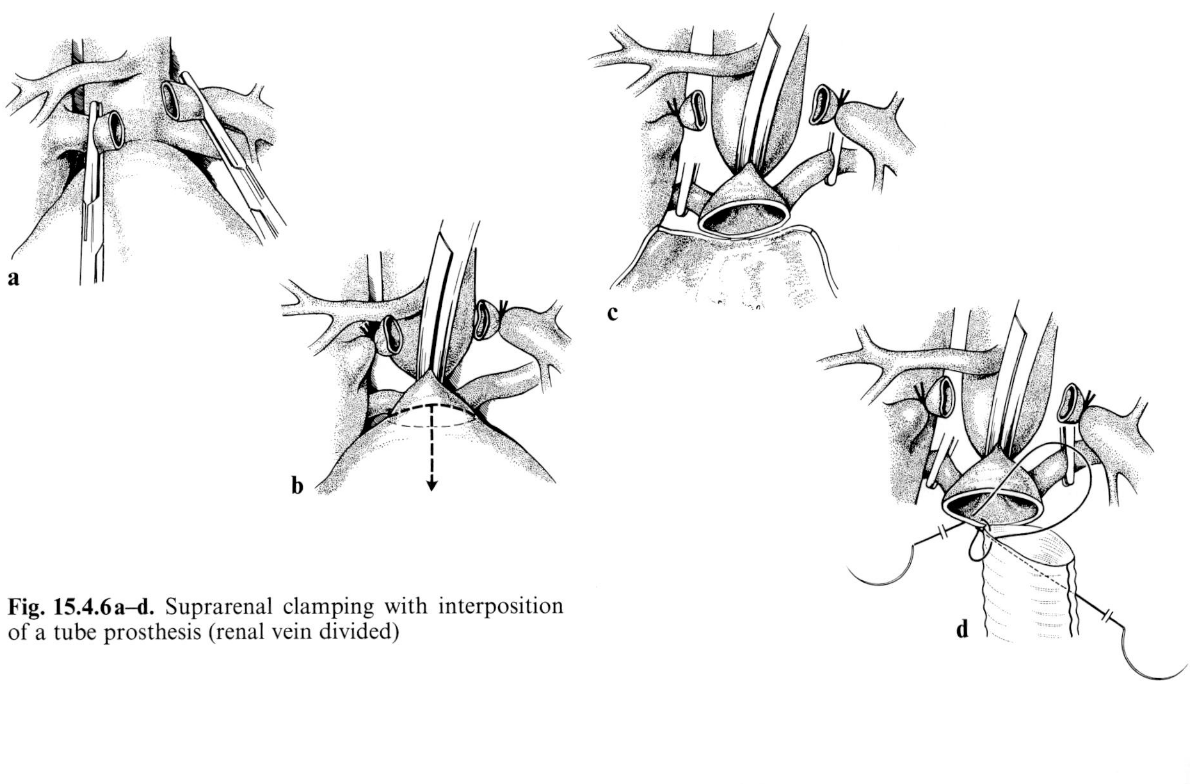

Fig. 15.4.6a–d. Suprarenal clamping with interposition of a tube prosthesis (renal vein divided)

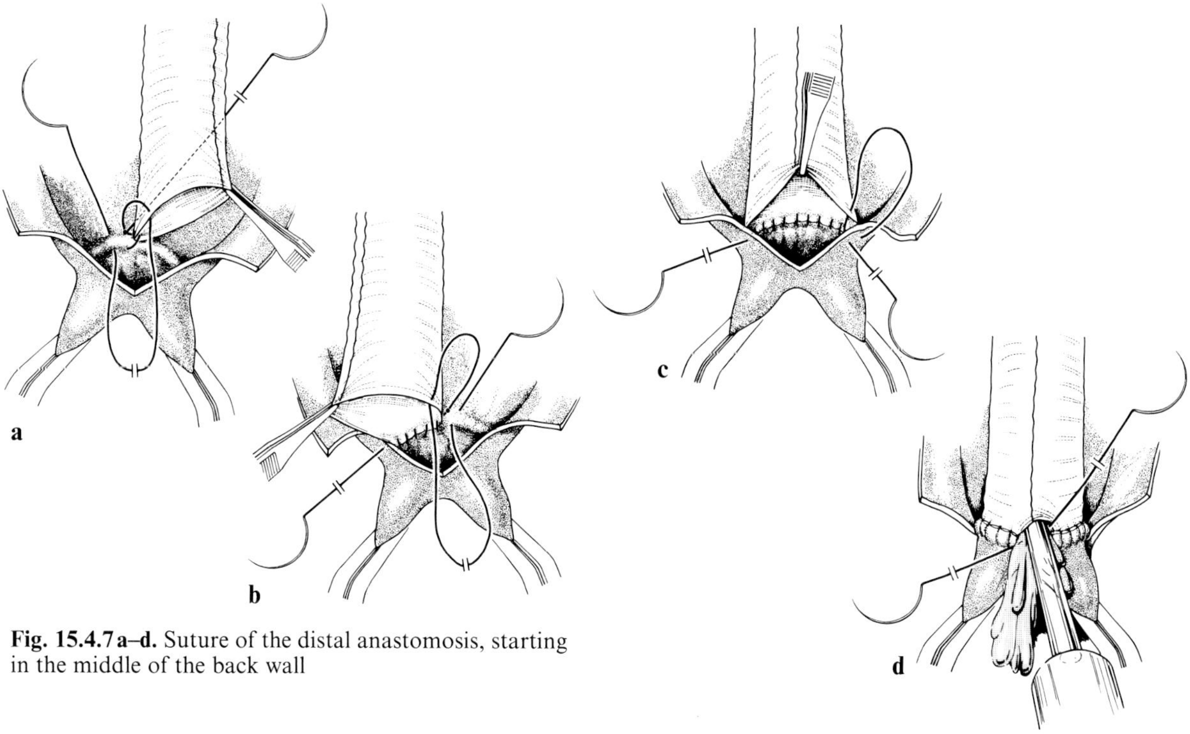

Fig. 15.4.7 a–d. Suture of the distal anastomosis, starting in the middle of the back wall

countered. Additional arteriosclerotic lesions or dilatations of the iliac arteries are often found next to the aneurysm itself. We have observed that the implantation of tube prostheses has a significantly lower mortality as compared with bifurcation grafts. Therefore, if no clinical symptoms of occlusive arterial disease within the iliac arteries are present, we implant a tube graft, even though arteriosclerotic lesions may be found at the aortic bifurcation and in the iliac arteries. Dilatations of the pelvic arteries, except aneurysms, do not contraindicate the interposition of a tube graft. The percentage of tube grafts implanted in our patients was 45%, which is relatively high. The late results ($n = 100$) were good. No second operation had to be performed for occlusive arterial disease of aneurysma formation within the pelvic arteries during a follow-up period of up to 6 years. Yet, aneurysms of the pelvic arteries or clinically manifest occlusive arterial disease of the pelvic type require the implantation of a bifurcation graft.

b) Tube Graft. In aneurysms limited to the distal aorta, the aortotomy ends at the aortic bifurcation. A semicircular incision is made at the distal end of the arteriotomy (see Fig. 15.4.4d). The continuity of the back wall of the aorta is preserved. Larger arteriosclerotic lesions at the aortic bifurcation can be removed by limited disobliteration. Kinking of the prosthesis is avoided if the distal anastomosis is established while the upper part of the body is slightly flexed and the prosthesis is tightly stretched. Suture of the anastomosis is performed in the same manner as in the proximal anastomosis (Fig. 15.4.7).

c) Bifurcation Graft. Prior to implantation, the aortic portion of the graft is shortened so as to measure 2–3 cm from proximal end to bifurcation. This prevents kinking of the iliac limbs of the graft. Additional aneurysms of the common iliac artery make extension of the arteriotomy necessary. It is extended over the aneurysmal sacs, until an undiseased segment of the artery is reached. The peripheral connection is then established at the common iliac artery, iliac bifurcation, or external iliac artery in the form of an end-to-end anastomosis, depending on the condition of these vessels. Continuous suture is performed using a 5–0 monofilament nonabsorbable suture (Fig. 15.4.8a). An aneurysm of the internal iliac artery is treated simply by closing the orifice of the internal iliac artery from the inside of the opened aneurysm (see p. 279). In patients with symptoms of occlusive arterial disease of the pelvic type the distal aortic lumen is closed from within the aneurysmal sac by continuous suture, and both iliac branches are

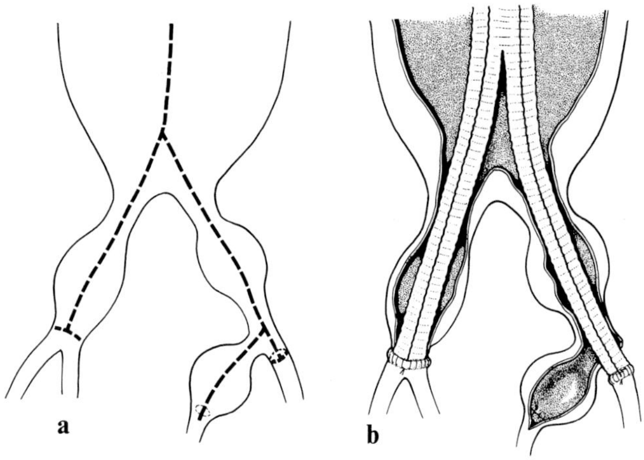

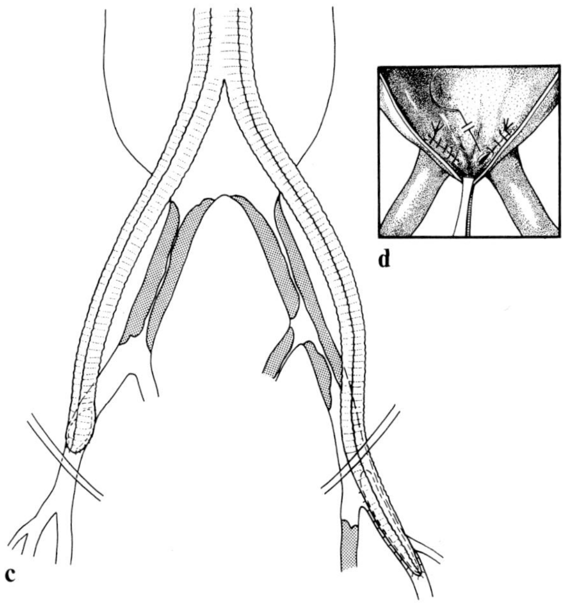

Fig. 15.4.8. a, b Distal connection of the prosthesis to the iliac arteries with aneurysmal enlargement. The left internal iliac artery is closed from the inside. **c, d** Distal connection to the iliofemoral segment in occlusive arterial disease (external iliac artery, femoral artery, and profunda femoris artery)

anastomosed end-to-side to the external iliac artery. An end-to-end anastomosis should be performed only if the internal iliac artery is occluded and cannot be perfused by reversed blood flow. Extensive arteriosclerotic changes within the iliac arteries may necessitate construction of a distal anastomosis within the groin region. In addition, revascularization of the profunda femoris artery may be necessary in cases of occlusive disease of the femoral artery (Fig. 15.4.8c, d). Before finishing the distal anastomosis, peripheral and proximal flow through the prosthesis are checked. Thrombectomy is not necessary if the duration of surgery is not too long and systemic heparinization has been performed prior to reconstruction. Declamping of a tube bifurcation prosthesis may lead to a sudden drop in blood pressure. Maintenance of optimal cardiac performance and prompt therapeutic intervention may avoid such mishaps [27] (see p. 198).

4. Reimplantation of the Inferior Mesenteric Artery (Fig. 15.4.9)

Clinical criteria for reimplantation of the inferior mesenteric artery are a weak back flow in the mesenteric artery or signs of colonic ischemia following clamping of the origin of the inferior mesenteric artery. Objective assessment of colonic circulation is possible by measuring the stump pressure of the mesenteric artery [11]. In most cases, ligation of this artery does not lead to subsequent ischemia of the left colon since it is often occluded by thrombi prior to surgery. The vascular arcades of the sigmoid mesocolon can be saved by ligation near the aorta. If the patient has had large bowel resection in the past, or if aneurysms of the internal iliac artery are present, reimplantation of the inferior mesenteric artery should be performed. The vessel must be patent and wide. It is sutured onto the prosthesis with a wide cuff of the aortic wall attached to it.

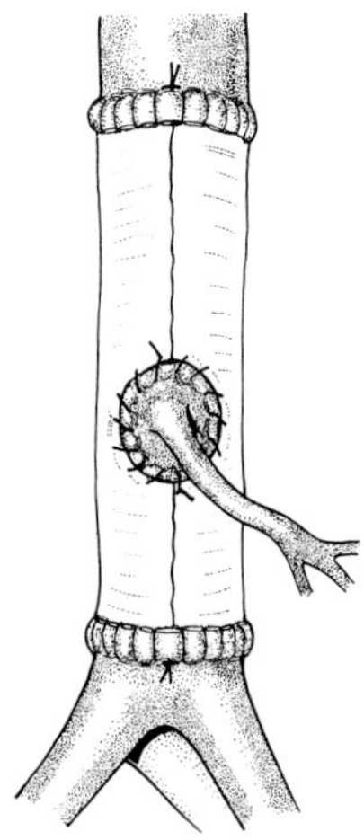

Fig. 15.4.9. Reimplantation of the inferior mesenteric artery

5. Surgical Management of Renal Artery Stenoses

Correction of renal artery stenoses is indicated during elective surgery for an abdominal aortic aneurysm. It lowers postoperative risk, possibly by eliminating the cause of renovascular hypertension or renal insufficiency. Reconstruction of the renal arteries may be achieved by direct thromboendarterectomy with subsequent patch graft angioplasty or bypass. The most favorable surgical procedures are aortorenal vein bypass, grafting from an undiseased segment of the aorta or venous bridging in bilateral renal artery stenoses [20] (see p. 619). These have the best long-term results. Most vascular surgeons do not use the methods just mentioned if an abdominal aortic aneurysm is repaired at the same time. To shorten operating time, a synthetic bypass graft is usually implanted. Usually Dacron double velour prostheses with a diameter of 6 or 7 mm are anastomosed to the aortic prothesis and poststenotic region of the renal artery.

IX. Closure of the Posterior Peritoneum

The residual aneurysmal sac is sutured around the implanted graft (Fig. 15.4.10a) with a continuous suture (Fig. 15.4.10b). In large aneurysms, partial resection of the wall is necessary before suturing of the aneurysmal sac. The cut edges of the sac should be bloodless before closure. Some parts of the graft, especially around the anastomoses, may remain exposed. They should, however, be carefully covered by periaortic tissue. The interposition of a thick layer of tissue, especially at the proximal anastomosis is the best prophylaxis against the formation of an aortoduodenal or aortoenteric fistula. The flexura duodenojejunalis is reattached to its original site of fixation. The posterior peritoneum is closed with a continuous suture (Fig. 15.4.10c). A drain is not necessary.

X. Surgical Management of Special Types of Infrarenal Aortic Aneurysms

1. Mycotic or Bacterial Aneurysm

Mycotic aneurysms account for about 1% of all abdominal aortic aneurysms. Usually staphylococcus and salmonella are found to be the infectious agents. A mycotic aneurysm is best managed by reconstruction in stages. In the first stage, a subclavian-bifemoral prosthetic bypass is constructed, then the infected portion of the aorta is resected in a second session (see p. 539ff). Only very few cases have been reported in which surgical repair was successful.

2. Horseshoe Kidney and Abdominal Aneurysm

a) Anatomy. In a horseshoe kidney the lower poles of the left and right kidneys are fused at the level

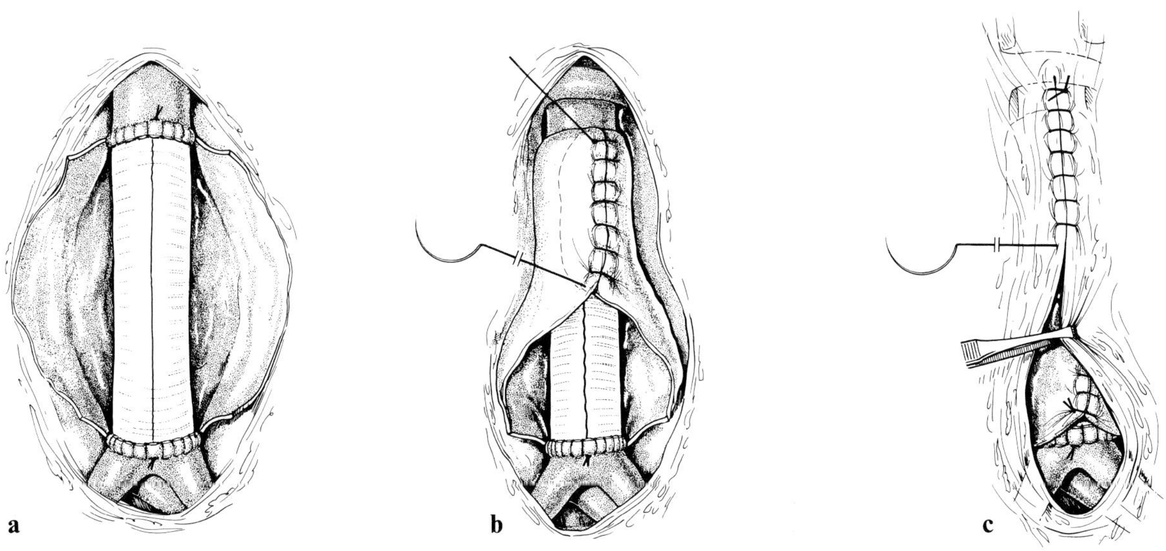

Fig. 15.4.10. a Interposition of a tube graft. **b, c** Covering of the graft with the aneurysmal sac and closure of the retroperitoneum

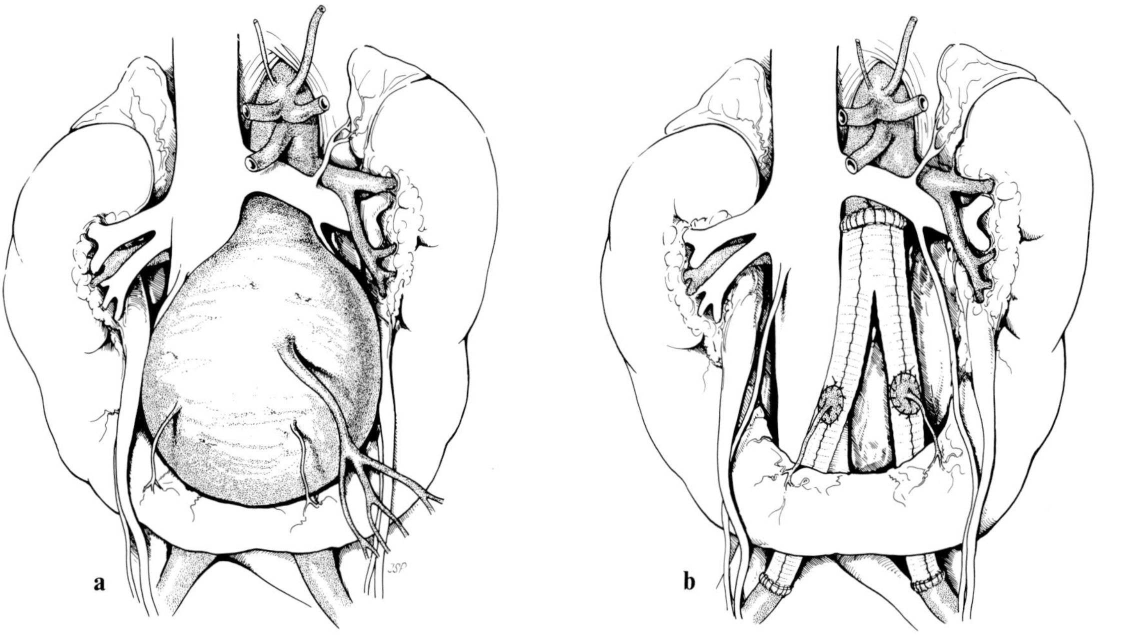

Fig. 15.4.11. a Infrarenal aortic aneurysm and horseshoe kidney. **b** Situation following resection of the infrarenal aortic aneurysm and interposition of a bifurcation prosthesis with reimplantation of the renal arteries

of the fourth lumbar vertebra (Fig. 15.4.11a). The renal tissue usually lies in front of the aorta and vena cava, but it may also lie behind both vessels. The ureters arise in the upper portion of each kidney and run in front of the isthmus. Only about 50% of all horseshoe kidneys have a normal vascular supply. If anomalous arteries are present, there are two patterns of distribution: each half of the kidney is supplied by only a few arteries in 25% of cases, and in 25% multiple renal arteries supply all portions of the renal substance [19]. Most of the anomalous arteries arise directly from the aneurysm.

b) Surgical Procedure. The surgical procedure is adjusted according to the vascular supply of the kidney. If a normal vascular pattern is identified, aortic replacement and reconstruction may be performed after mobilization and elevation of the isthmus. Frequently, the connection between the lower poles is no more than a fibrous band. In such cases, the isthmus may safely by divided in the midline. Arteries arising from the aneurysm, which supply the renal substance connecting both poles, may be cut out with an aortic patch and reimplanted into the prosthesis (Fig. 15.4.11b). This is not necessary if severely arteriosclerotic and stenosed vessels are found which supply only the isthmus or the lower renal poles. When multiple renal arteries supply the bulk of the renal mass, the failure to reimplant several arteries (multiple) may severely impair renal function. This situation represents an inoperable condition. In large, symptomatic, or ruptured aneurysms, there is usually no alternative to the implantation of a synthetic prosthesis. Chronic renal insufficiency may be a consequence and must be taken into account.

3. Inflammatory Aortic Aneurysm

a) Anatomy. An inflammatory abdominal aortic aneurysm is an infrarenal aneurysm surrounded by solid perianeurysmal tissue. This layer may reach a thickness of several centimeters and fill the entire retroperitoneal space, extending from the kidneys down into the small pelvis [26]. Microscopically, this type of tissue proliferation is similar to retroperitoneal fibrosis. Complications may occur due to compression of retroperitoneal structures by this bulky mass. The ureters are commonly involved. In inflammatory aneurysms, the ureters are usually displaced medially, and not laterally as with large aneurysms of other types. Patients complain of severe back pain. This often creates the impression of a contained rupture of an aortic aneurysm. Computed tomography may show the typical, perianeurysmal, homogeneous layer of tissue, which takes up a lot of contrast medium. This characteristic finding easily establishes the preoperative diagnosis [23]. The uptake of contrast medium can be explained by the high degree of vascularization of the fibrotic tissue [23].

b) Indications for Surgery. Reconstruction is always indicated because of the increased risk of rupture and possible obstruction of neighboring structures such as ureters and intestine. The danger of rupture, however, is not as high as with typical arteriosclerotic aneurysms [26]. Conservative treatment with cortisone [7] is still controversial, owing to the possibility of rupture.

c) Surgical Procedure. Surgery is complicated as a result of the very dense fibrotic adhesions by which the aneurysm is attached to the duodenum, left renal vein, and ureters. Injury of the duodenum during preparation may lead to secondary infection of the prosthesis and aortoduodenal fistula. To prevent injury to retroperitoneal structures, such as the duodenum, left renal vein, and ureters, dissection around the aneurysm and its neck should be kept to a minimum. A portion of the fibrotic mass must be left adhering to the duodenum. After opening the aneurysm, the plane of dissection between the aorta and the fibrotic tissue can be found at the neck. This maneuver affords visualization of the aortic wall and the origins of the renal arteries and permits accurate assessment of the proximal and distal extension of the aneurysm. After infra- or suprarenal cross-clamping of the aorta the proximal anastomosis can be sutured. The fate of the in situ fibrotic masses during the postoperative course is still unknown. It is presumed that fibrosis progresses or at least persists. Therefore, if the ureters are obstructed, ureterolysis and intra-abdominal displacement of the ureters is recommended [1].

Recent reports show that retroperitoneal fibrosis recedes following vascular reconstruction and interposition of a prosthesis. Urinary tract obstructions disappear within months after internal splinting of the ureters [1, 23]. Additional cortisone treatment is recommended to accelerate regression of fibrotic tissue. Ureterolysis and intra-abdominal displacement of the ureters should be performed only if the described therapeutic measures have failed.

XI. Alternative Methods of Treatment

Alternative methods have been developed for the treatment of poor-risk patients with very large and symptomatic aneurysms. The introduction of a thin wire into the aneurysm reinforces the aneurysmal wall by rolling up into a coil [13, 17]. But this often leads to thrombosis of the aneurysm. Another method is a staged procedure. First, a subclavian – bifemoral bypass is constructed and then the iliac arteries are ligated; this, too, often leads to thrombosis of the aneurysm. Other methods are embolization of the aneurysm by injecting polymers [6, 12] or thrombin [3] through a catheter. Only a few reports have been published so far on the results of these procedures. They do not completely eliminate the danger of rupture in patients who are inoperable, but they do lower the risk to some degree.

B. Ruptured Infrarenal Aortic Aneurysms

I. Frequency and Localization of Rupture

Aneurysmal rupture is the most frequent and most severe complication of an infrarenal aortic aneurysm. As the diameter of the aneurysm grows, the risk of rupture increases. However, smaller aneu-

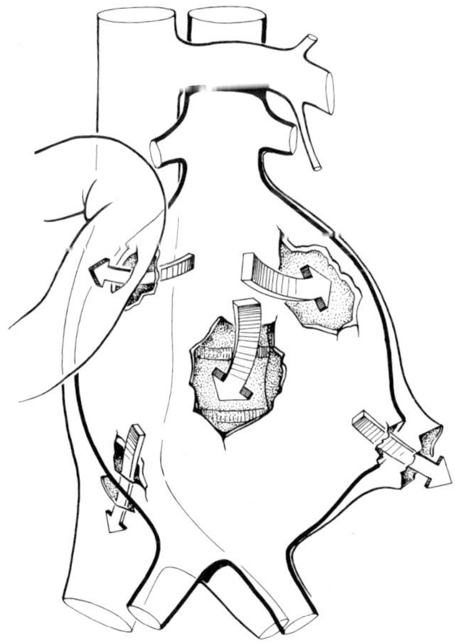

Fig. 15.4.12. Localization of ruptures of infrarenal aortic aneurysms (cumulative statistics from ten published reports)

rysms may also rupture. Autopsy statistics [9] have shown that 17% of ruptured aneurysms not treated surgically had a diameter of less than 4 cm. A summary combining the results of several reports shows that 88% of the aneurysms ($n = 274$) ruptured into the retroperitoneum, 7.3% freely into the abdominal cavity, 2.2% into the duodenum, and another 2.2% into the inferior vena cava (Fig. 15.4.12).

II. Special Diagnostic Procedures

The clinical symptoms are characterized by the classical triad of abdominal pain, pulsating tumor, and shock. Massive gastrointestinal bleeding with shock symptoms or acute congestive cardiac insufficiency accompanied by a machinelike murmur audible over the abdomen indicate rupture into the duodenum or vena cava. The typical symptoms of rupture, such as acute abdominal pain or back pain, pulsating tumor, and shock do not always occur with the same frequency. Therefore, the diagnosis cannot always be confirmed by clinical symptoms alone. Today, the most important diagnostic methods are sonography and computed tomography. These always detect an aneurysm if it is present. If a patient presents with clear symptoms of rupture, an immediate laparotomy should be performed. Diagnostic procedures are less important in such a case. The pulsatile abdominal mass may not be palpable in some patients. Ultrasonography can reliably detect the aneurysm within a few minutes. Rupture cannot be confirmed in all patients by this method. Computed tomography during the rupture stage is still controversial since a delay of about 20–25 min must be expected, even in well-organized hospitals with enough personnel. Therefore, it should be employed only in patients who have stable blood circulation. In these cases CT scanning always leads to correct diagnosis and localization of rupture.

III. Indications for Surgery

Rupture is always an indication for surgery. There is no exception, even for the patient with poor general condition.

Fig. 15.4.14. Subdiaphragmatic clamping of the aorta ▷

IV. Preoperative Hemorrhage Control

The transbrachial or transfemoral introduction of balloon catheters may reduce or completely control bleeding preoperatively [14, 18]. Correct placement of the catheter, however, causes a considerable delay.

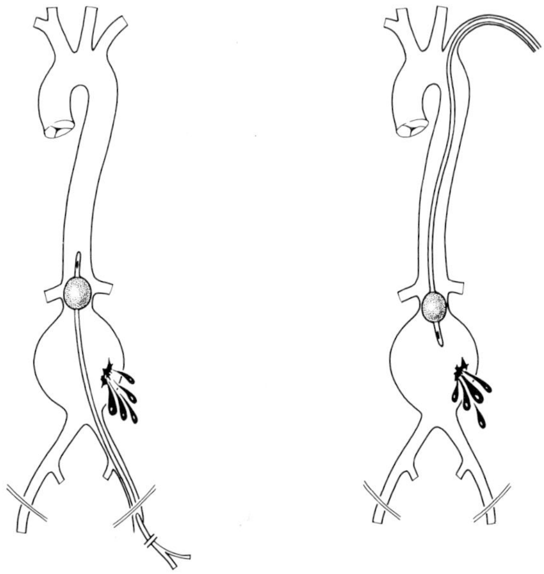

Fig. 15.4.13. Hemorrhage control with balloon catheters introduced transfemorally or transbrachially

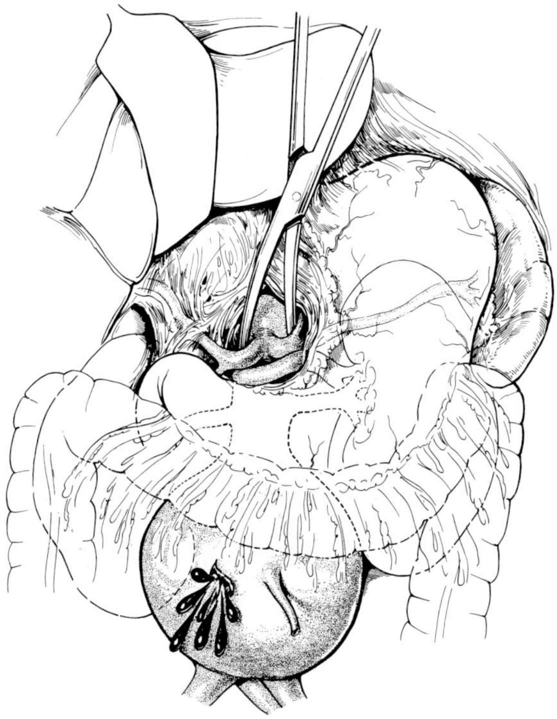

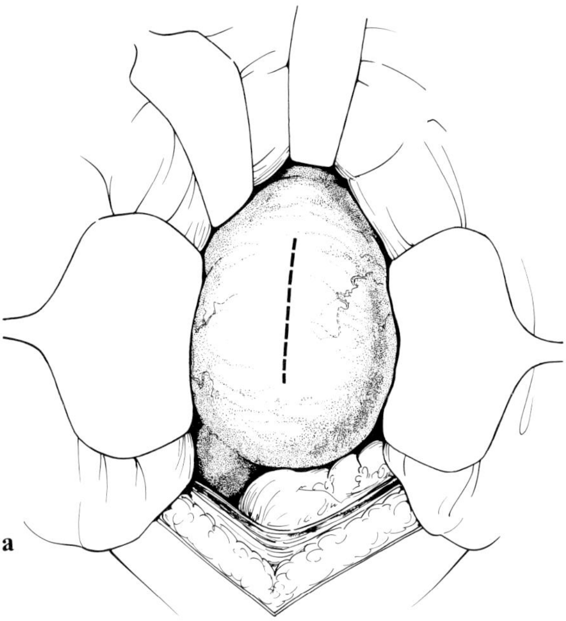

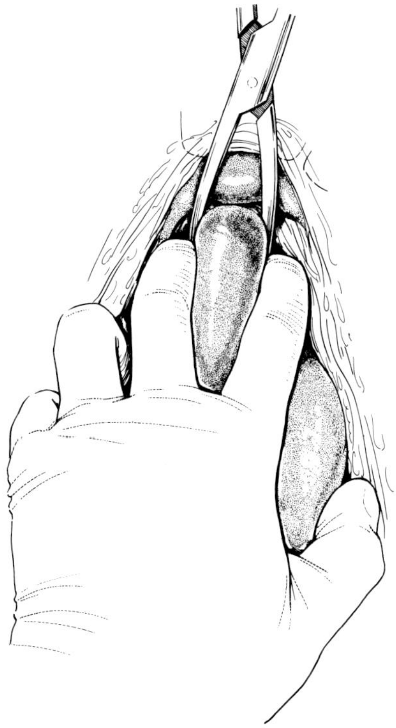

Fig. 15.4.15. **a** Incision line of the posterior peritoneum over a ruptured aneurysm. **b** Finger dissection of a ruptured abdominal aortic aneurysm for exposure of the proximal aorta

V. Surgical Procedure

1. Control of the Proximal Aorta

The most important step in the operation is emergency control of the proximal aorta. There are several ways of accomplishing this.

a) Clamping of the Thoracic Aorta. Today, clamping of the thoracic aorta is not advocated by most surgeons because it extends the procedure by necessitating thoracotomy.

b) Subdiaphragmatic Clamping. Subdiaphragmatic clamping of the aorta is preferred by most surgeons (Fig. 15.4.14). Possible risks during this maneuver are injury of the esophagus and loss of time during preparation.

c) Direct Exposure and Hemorrhage Control. A reliable and commonly used method is direct exposure of the infrarenal aorta. Following division of the posterior peritoneum (Fig. 15.4.15a), the proximal portion of the aorta can be exposed very quickly by blunt finger dissection along the wall of the aneurysm (Fig. 15.4.15b). The hematoma will usually have created the periaortic dissection plane, thereby facilitating access to the normal infrarenal aorta. The danger of injury to the left renal vein is slight. If free rupture occurs during this maneuver, the surgeon can insert the thumb or middle finger of the right hand through the wall defect or arteriotomy after short infracolonic manual compression of the aorta. This controls hemorrhage (Fig. 15.4.16a). In this situation, further dissection to develop an adequate proximal aortic stump can be carried out, followed by clamping of the aorta. The finger may be kept in place during this maneuver; alternatively the proximal aorta can be blocked with a balloon catheter (Fig. 15.4.16b).

d) Instrumental Compression. There are numerous devices for temporary compression of the proximal aorta. Their use may lead to pressure injuries of the pancreas or esophagus.

2. Adjuvant Measures

Control or prevention of clotting disorders and high blood loss is essential for the patient's survival. The risk is lowered by leaving the retroperitoneal hematoma in place and using low- or nonporous prostheses. Furthermore, heparin should not be administered, thrombocyte concentrates should be given early enough, and autotransfusion should

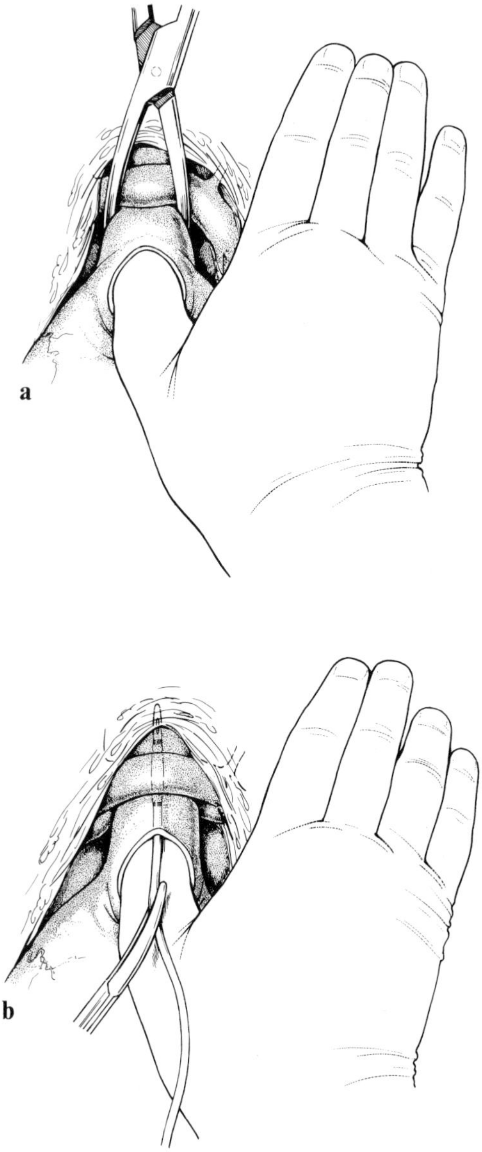

Fig. 15.4.16. **a** Emergency occlusion of the aortic lumen with the thumb and clamping of the proximal aorta. **b** Control of hemorrhage of the proximal aorta with a balloon catheter

be performed. Of course, intraoperative invasive monitoring of cardiac function and blood pressure are essential for correct volume substitution. Improvements in this field have considerably lowered the mortality rate worldwide during the last few years (see p. 198) [8, 27].

VI. Rupture of the Aneurysm into the Gastrointestinal Tract

Rupture into the gastrointestinal tract is most often seen in the fourth *segment* of the duodenum. This portion has a very close anatomic relationship to the abdominal aorta. Because of its retroperitoneal fixation, it is constantly exposed to the strong pulsations of the aneurysm. If adhesions are present, the stomach or deeper parts of the intestine may also be affected in rare cases. The time interval between the onset of hemorrhage and fatal exsanguination is sufficient to save 60% of the patients by early emergency surgery [25]. Subdiaphragmatic clamping of the aorta is recommended. The aortoduodenal fistula and other factors make quick infrarenal dissection difficult. Although only very few patients can be treated successfully in the long run, aortoduodenal rupture of an aneurysm can be treated by primary closure of the fistula in the duodenum, according to the standard technique, followed by implantation of a vascular prosthesis. Among 11 patients who were treated in this manner, not one showed a prosthetic infection in long-term follow up. Thus, treatment of a primary aortoduodenal fistula is different from the surgical management of a secondary aortoduodenal fistula. The lesion must be reconstructed anatomically, and not by closure of the aorta with extra-anatomic bypass for revascularization of the lower limbs. Perioperative administration of antibiotics is necessary.

VII. Rupture of the Aneurysm into the Vena Cava Inferior

This type of rupture is seen in 2% of aneurysmal ruptures. It quickly leads to cardiac decompensation since the arteriovenous fistula lies only a short distance from the heart. Clinical symptoms are back pain and acute abdominal pain, increasing venous congestion of the inferior vena cava, and progressive cardiac insufficiency. In over 80% a typical machinelike murmur is heard during auscultation of the abdomen.

Closure of the fistula is best performed through the opened aneurysmal sac. Bleeding from the vena cava can usually be controlled by digital compression. In large fistulas, the vena cava can be temporarily occluded externally with sponges. The fistula is closed from the aortic lumen by direct suture.

VIII. Postoperative Complications

1. General Complications

Postoperative complications following surgery of an abdominal aortic aneurysm, such as hemorrhage or vascular occlusion, do not differ from those encountered after normal vascular procedures. Severe hemorrhage or vascular occlusion necessitate immediate operative revision. However, occlusions of larger reconstructions are rare.

2. Ischemia of the Left Colon

A relatively rare and severe early complication is ischemia of the left colon. It may start with colitis and end in necrosis of the entire left colon. This complication can almost always be avoided if the vascular supply to the left colon is preserved during aneurysmal resection (see "Sect. A.I"). If it does develop, the colon should be resected before total necrosis with perforation occurs.

3. Aortoduodenal Fistula (see pp. 177, 308)

A rare, very serious late complication is aortoduodenal fistula. Its development is promoted by the very close contact between the prosthesis and intestine. Arrosion of the intestine leads to infection of the prosthesis and disruption of the upper anastomosis. During surgical revision the prosthesis must be resected, the aorta closed by suture, and a subclavian bifemoral bypass constructed to preserve blood flow to the lower parts of the body. If bleeding is not life threatening, a subclavian bifemoral bypass should be constructed during reintervention and not postponed to a second session. Careful coverage of the prosthesis and aneurysmal wall with periaortic tissue during the primary reconstruction is a good prophylactic measure against the development of an aortoduodenal fistula.

REFERENCES

1. Bainbridge BT, Woodward DAK (1982) Inflammatory aneurysms of the abdominal aorta with associated uretic obstruction or medial deviation. Cardiovasc Surg 23:365
2. Baker AG, Roberts B (1970) Long-term survival following abdominal aortic aneurysmectomy. JAMA 212:445
3. Berguer R, Schneider J, Wilner HI (1978) Induced thrombosis of inoperable abdominal aortic aneurysms. Surgery 84:425
4. Bomberger RA, Zarins ChK, Glasgov S (1980) Medial injury and hyperlipidemia in development of aneurysms or atherosclerotic plaques. Amer Coll Surg; Surg Forum XXXI:338
5. Butsuttil RW, Abou-Zamzam AM, Machleder HI (1980) Collegenase activity of the human aorta. Arch Surg 115:1373
6. Carrasco H, Parry CE (1982) Transcatheter embolization of abdominal aortic aneurysms. AJR 138:729
7. Clyne CAC, Abercrombie (1977) Perianeurysmal retroperitoneal fibrosis: Two cases responding to steroids. Br J Urol 49:463
8. Crawford ES, Saleh SA, Babb JW, Glaeser DH, Vaccaro PS, Silvers A (1981) Infrarenal abdominal aortic aneurysm. Factors influencing survival after operation performed over a 25-year period. Ann Surg 193:699
9. Darling RC, Messina CR, Brewster DC, Ottinger LW (1977) Autopsy study of unoperated abdominal aortic aneurysms: the case for early resection. Circulation 56:II-161
10. Daugherty M, Shearer GR, Ernst CB (1979) Primary aortoduodenal fistula: Extra-anatomic vascular reconstruction not required for successful management. Surgery 86:399
11. Ernst CB, Hagihara PF, Daugherty ME, Griffen WO Jr (1978) Inferior mesenteric artery stump pressure: A reliable index for safe IMA ligation during abdominal aortic aneurysmectomy. Ann Surg 187:641
12. Goldman ML, Sarrafizadeh MS, Philip PF, Karmody AM, Leather RP, Parikh N, Powers SR (1980) Bucrylate embolization of abdominal aortic aneurysms: An adjuvant to nonresective therapy. AJR 135:1195
13. Hicks GL, Rob C (1976) Abdominal aortic aneurysm wiring: An alternative method. Am J Surg 131:664
14. Hyde GL, Sullivan DM (1982) Fogarty catheter tamponade of ruptured abdominal aortic aneurysms. Surg Gynecol Obstet 154:197
15. Lallemand RC, Goslings RG, Newman DL (1973) Role of the bifurcation in atheromatosis of the abdominal aorta. Surg Gynecol Obstet 137:987
16. Otto R (1978) Fehldiagnose bei oberflächlichem Verlauf der Aorta. Nachweis mit Ultraschall. Chirurg 49:46
17. Peacock JH, Brown GJA (1968) Wiring in the treatment of aortic aneurysms. Br J Surg 55:344
18. Rendl K-H, Prenner K, Paulowitz H-P (1981) Die atypische Behandlung eines abdominellen Aortenaneurysmas unter speziellen Indikationen. Angio 3:89

19. Sidell PF, Pairolero PC, Payne WS, Bernatz PE, Spittell JA Jr (1979) Horseshoe kidney associated with surgery of the abdominal aorta. Mayo Clin Proc 54:97
20. Schwilden E-D, van Dongen RJAM (1976) Behandlung von abdominellen Aorten-Aneurysmen in Kombination mit ein- oder beidseitigen Nierenarterienstenosen. VASA 5:47
21. Thetter O, v Hochstetter A, van Dongen RJAM (1982) Neurogene Störungen der männlichen Sexualfunktion nach Eingriffen im aorto-iliacalen Bereich und deren Vermeidung durch den retromesenterialen Zugang. Angio 4:171
22. Valesky A, Liepe B, Lütten C (1985) Möglichkeiten zur Verbesserung der Behandlungsergebnisse beim rupturierten infrarenalen Bauchaortenaneurysma. Angio 2:41
23. Valesky A, Liepe B, Gmelin E, Sellin D, Schildberg FW (1984) Neuere Aspekte zur Diagnostik und Therapie des inflammatorischen Bauchaortenaneurysmas. Chirurg 55:464
24. Vollmar J (1960) Zentrale Gefäßektasien bei lange bestehenden arteriovenösen Fisteln. Langenbecks Arch Klin Chir 194:627
25. Voyles WR, Moretz WH (1958) Rupture of aortic aneurysms into gastrointestinal tract. Surgery 43:666
26. Walker DI, Bloor K, Williams G, Gillie (1972) Inflammatory aneurysms of the abdominal aorta. Br J Surg 59:609
27. Whittemore AD, Clowes AW, Hechtman HB, Mannick JA (1980) Aortic aneurysm repair. Reduced operative mortality associated with maintenance of optimal cardiac performance. Ann Surg 192/3:414

15.5 Thoracoabdominal Aneurysms

G. HEBERER and H. STIEGLER

CONTENTS

A. Anatomy

The same knowledge of anatomy is needed for surgical therapy of thoracoabdominal aneurysms as for treatment of other parts of the aorta (thoracic aorta, suprarenal and infrarenal abdominal aorta). The pattern of blood supply to the spinal cord is, however, of special importance. In operations on smaller segments of the thoracic or abdominal aorta, injuries to spinal arteries arising at different levels of the aorta are not as extensive, and spinal cord ischemia is avoided, provided that the longitudinal arterial system is intact. But in thoracoabdominal aortic replacement, arterial blood supply to the spinal cord is always in jeopardy depending on the magnitude of the procedure. Preoperative planning is difficult since the arterial supply to the spinal cord shows many variations. The longitudinal arterial system changes physiologically in certain cord segments, and preoperative angiographic presentation of the spinal cord's arterial system is very difficult. Therefore, it is necessary to be well informed about the arteries of the spinal cord and to carefully assess its functional status

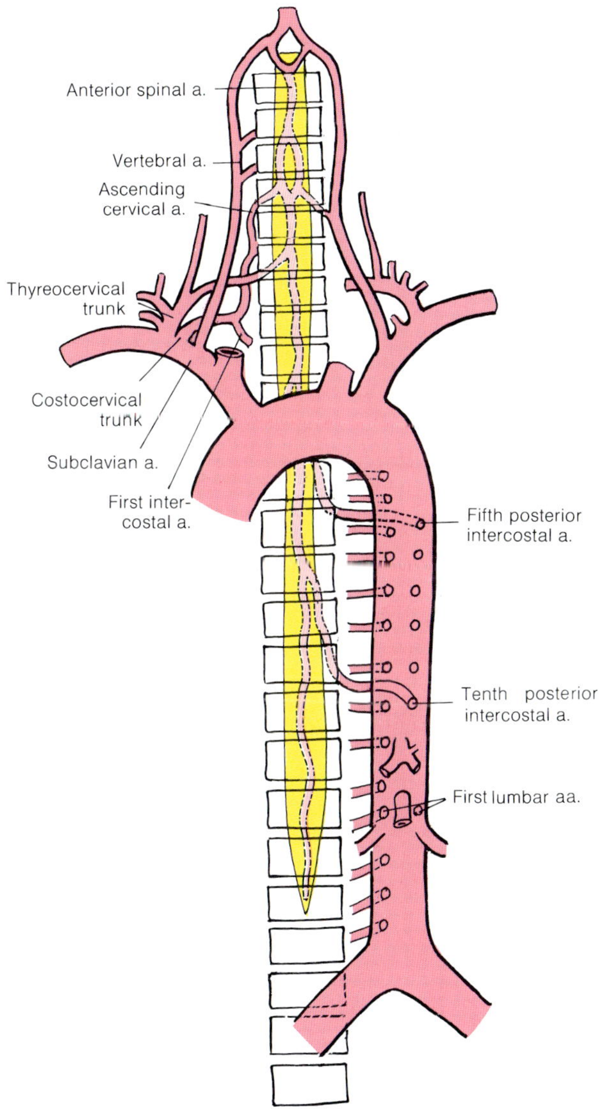

Fig. 15.5.1. Schematic representation of the vascular supply to the spinal cord. (Taken from PISCOL 1972)

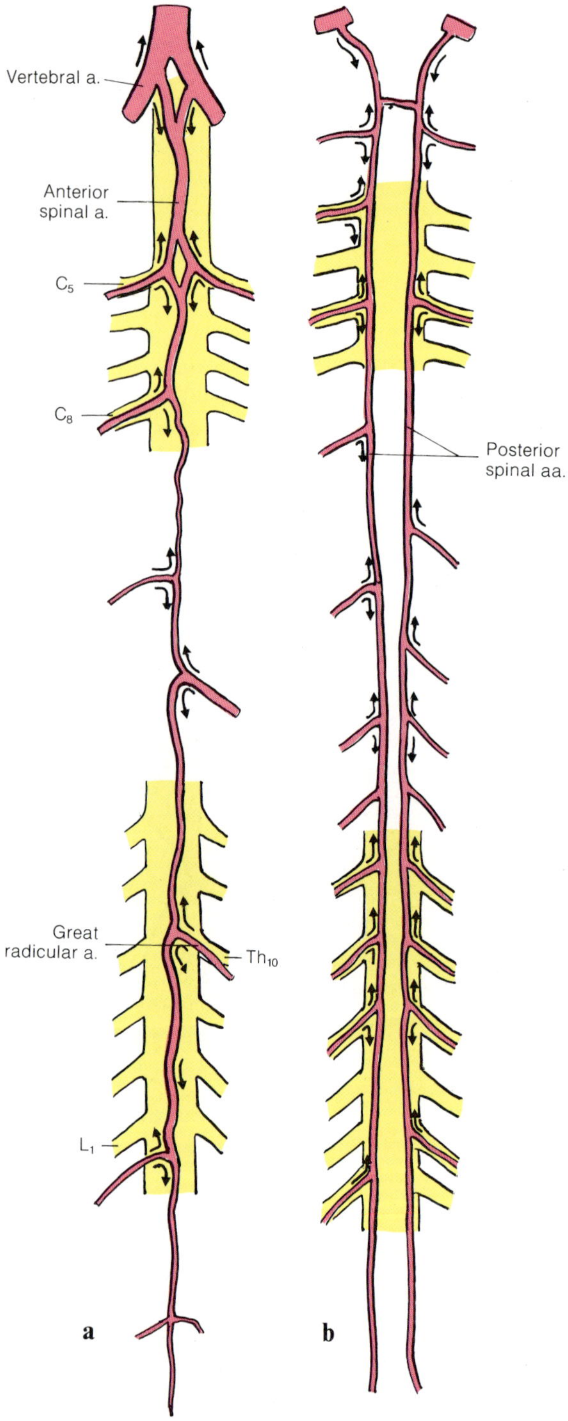

Fig. 15.5.2. The longitudinal arteries of the spinal cord and their branches (**a** ventral, **b** dorsal). Note the changing calibers (JELLINGER and PISCOL 1972)

Fig. 15.5.3. Vascular supply as seen in a cross section ▷ of the spinal cord. The boundary line (*shaded area*) between ventral and dorsal supply is especially vulnerable to ischemia if blood flow is reduced by arteriosclerotic disease (v. LANZ/WACHSMUTH 1982)

preoperatively to be able to estimate the risk of postoperative paraplegia, one of the most serious complications.

The anterior spinal artery is formed by the union of both anterior spinal rami of the vertebral artery at the level of the segments C1–C3. The artery descends in or next to the anterio-median fissure to the filum terminale. Its diameter varies considerably (0.5 mm in the cervical region, 0.34 mm in the thoracic region, and 1 mm in the lumbar region). Short interruptions (up to 5 mm in length) of the artery are described, especially in its cervical portion. Blood flow to this artery is not always reinforced at every level. Therefore, the compensation of a loss of a larger artery is limited. The most important is the great radicular artery, with a diameter of up to 1.2 mm. It is found on the left side in 73% of the cases and may appear between the segments Th6 and L5. In 62% it may be identified at the level Th9–Th12 (12% Th6–Th8, 26% starting from L1 downward). Therefore, it is the most important and lower source of blood flow to the lumbar spine. For the most part, it supplies in most cases only the anterior region of the spinal cord. Blood supply of the posterior region of the spinal cord is better because of the presence of two posterior spinal arteries. These receive a succession of small arterial branches at different segments revealing a good chance of compensating blood flow if one of these vessels becomes occluded (Fig. 15.5.3). Therefore, the anterior region of the spinal cord is more easily damaged by ischemia [8, 9, 11, 13].

The preservation of the great radicular artery is of great importance. The best chance of avoiding

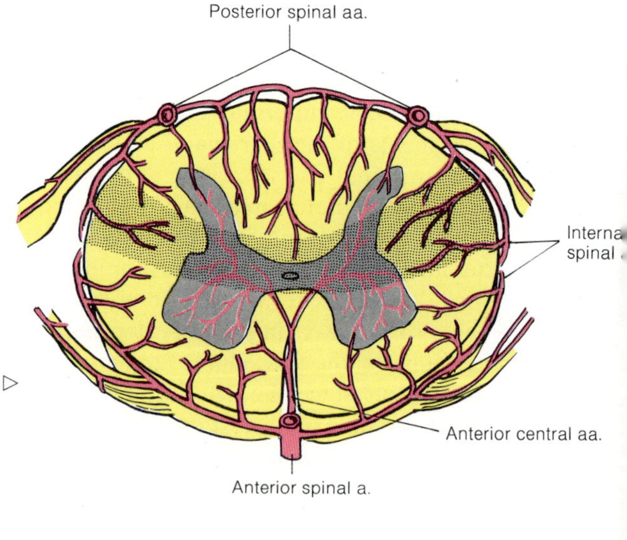

paraplegia is to maintain blood flow to this artery and to segmental arteries by reimplanting aortic spinal branches (CRAWFORD and CRAWFORD 1984; in 313 patients the rate of paraplegia was 2% [3]).

B. Indications for Surgery

The thoracic aorta may be divided into three parts (see p. 331). This differentiation is necessary to plan the surgical strategy correctly. The extension of an aneurysm to the segments I and II would mean that surgery could only be done under hypothermia using extracorporal circulation (see p. 742).

Only aneurysms of the descending aorta, where, moreover, the ascending aorta and the aortal arch are intact, will be discussed here. Furthermore, abdominal suprarenal aneurysms will be presented because the visceral branches of these aneurysms demonstrate the same anatomic characteristics and require the same surgical technique as thoracoabdominal aneurysms.

The prognosis for a thoracoabdominal aneurysm is the same as for aneurysms of each individual aortic segment. Rupture, which is usually preceded by penetration (chest pain, back pain), can occur with any aneurysm (into the pleural cavity, esophagus, duodenum, inferior vena cava, retroperitoneum, intraperitoneal cavity (see p. 333).

Surgery is absolutely necessary in patients with symptoms of imminent rupture, even if several risk factors are present. In an asymptomatic stage, an operation should be considered carefully. When making such a decision, one should determine the risks involved and weigh one against the other. If possible, preoperative improvement should be sought by medical therapy (see p. 100). CRAWFORD reports the following frequencies of risk factors in this large patient group with thoracoabdominal aneurysms [3]:

25% coronary artery disease
18% high blood pressure
22% obstructive lung disease
12% peripheral occlusive arterial disease

The risk factors not only influence the indications for surgery. They are also important factors in limiting the extent of an operation. For example, in a high risk patient with a thoracoabdominal aneurysm with an extension into the infrarenal segment, reconstruction may be limited to the thoracic segment if there was certain evidence of thoracic penetration (symptoms, CT scan), and a reconstruction of all segments was not possible due to high risk. In those cases revealing difficulties in the decision to operate, good interdisciplinary cooperation is necessary. The following aspects of preoperative planning are essential:

Preoperative Measures

1. Assessment of general operability (see p. 191); exercise ECG and pulmonary function tests.

2. Good radiologic documentation of the localization and extent of the aneurysm: (a) conventional angiography with selective visualization of each visceral artery; (b) arterial digital subtraction angiography to save contrast medium, e.g., in patients with elevated creatinine. Venous administration of contrast medium during digital subtraction angiography does not provide adequate picture quality for preoperative planning; (c) CT scans usually performed with contrast medium. If possible, vascular supply to the spinal cord should be visualized, especially the origin of the great radicular artery. Sometimes, this artery cannot be identified in the preoperative CT scan. In such cases, it must be identified intraoperatively as the vessel showing the strongest back bleeding at the thoracolumbar junction. The artery must then be reimplanted into the prosthesis. Anatomic variations and concomitant occlusive arterial disease may be seen in the CT scan (e.g., 20% of all patients with aneurysms in the suprarenal abdominal region, segment IV, have occlusive arterial disease requiring revascularization; additional aneurysms, e.g., of the internal iliac artery, may also be diagnosed preoperatively). This preoperative information greatly influences the choice of surgical technique and surgical strategy.

3. In elective surgery, training with a respirator (e.g., Bird) should begin 2–3 days prior to the operation. In addition to being instructed in the proper breathing technique, the patient should be made aware of how crucial his cooperation will be in the postoperative phase. At the same time, intermittent practice at positive pressure breathing provides an ideal simulation of postoperative weaning from the respirator.

Intraoperative Measures

1. Clamping times can be kept short by reducing the number of anastomoses. Organs should

be reperfused as soon as the prosthesis is in place. The ischemic time tolerated by the liver (with normal liver function, a maximum of 60 min) is difficult to estimate preoperatively because sensitive testing methods are not available.

2. Optimal monitoring (arterial pressure, pressure registration with a Swan-Ganz catheter, blood gas analyses at regular intervals, especially when both sides of the lung are intubated separately and one lung is allowed to collapse). Also the use of a cell saver is mandatory (see p. 197).

Postoperative Measures

Following procedures of this magnitude requires intensive postoperative care by personnel who are highly experienced in the diagnosis and treatment of cardiopulmonary, hepatic, and renal diseases. Correct management of fluids and electrolytes (hyperhydration, polyuria!) and the detection of hepatic insufficiency with the substitution of certain plasma factors (e.g., clotting factors) are necessary.

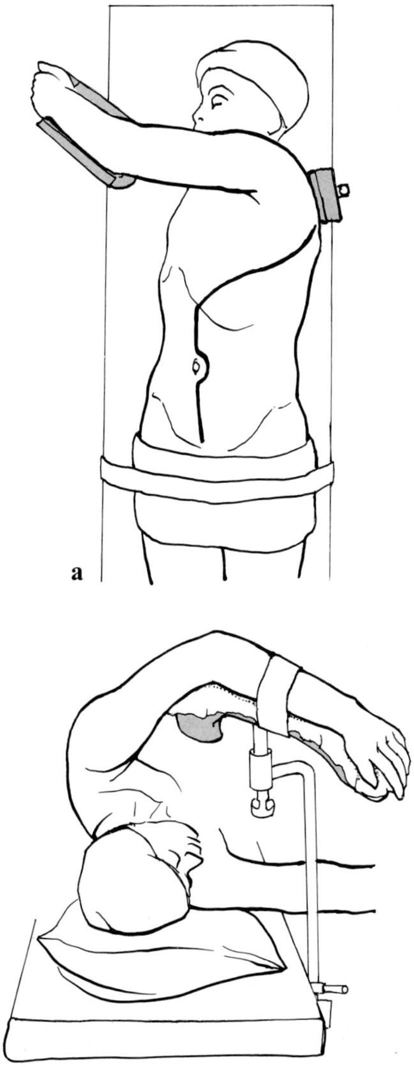

Fig. 15.5.4a, b. Thoracoabdominal right semi-lateral position according to CRAWFORD (thoracic 60° rotation, pelvis in a horizontal plane). The anterolateral thoracotomy runs forward across the left costal margin to the midline of the abdomen and is continued downward as a laparotomy. To prevent the trunk from overtwisting, a half-tilted 60° lateral position is preferable to a 90° lateral position of the thorax

C. Positioning and Surgical Procedure

Surgical management of thoracoabdominal aneurysms depends on their localization and extent

We differentiate:

I. Thoracoabdominal aneurysms
II. Thoracoabdominal aneurysms with intact segment IV
III. Thoracic aneurysms with involvement of the proximal segment IV
IV. Aneurysms of the distal thoracic aorta excluding segment V
V. Aneurysms of segments IV and V
VI. Aneurysms of segment IV
VII. Importance of anatomic variations

I. Thoracoabdominal Aneurysms

1. Positioning and Surgical Approach

A left thoracotomy is performed in a right semilateral position. The thorax should be rotated about 60° to the right (Fig. 15.5.4). *Both hips should lie in a horizontal plane* keeping contact with the surface of the operating table. The abdomen is slightly twisted, allowing good exposure during surgery. Access to both groin regions presents no difficulty. An anterolateral thoracotomy is performed, starting with an incision over the sixth interspace (regular thoracotomies are usually performed one to two interspaces lower). Using the cautery, the intercostal muscles are divided at the upper margin of the rib, and the pleura is opened by an incision of about 1 cm. The lung is held back with a small sponge to prevent injury during division of the pleura. After entering the pleural space, a rib spreader is inserted. The anterolateral thoracotomy is continued to the space between the left medioclavicular line and the middle of the sternum. The incision then crosses the costal margin to the midline of the abdomen. Following division of the costal margin with rib cutters, the diaphragm is divided down to the aortic hiatus. This maneuver must be performed very carefully since the thin, fragile aneurysmal wall may be injured within the hiatus. Hemorrhage as a consequence of injury is very difficult to control.

The splenic flexure of the colon is then mobilized. The left triangular ligament of the liver and the phrenicocolic ligament are divided. The stomach, small and large intestines, liver, spleen, and tail of the pancreas are reflected to the right. The retroperitoneal course of the aorta is exposed distal to the renal arteries. Preparation of the thoracic aorta is easiest with artificial atelectasis of the left lung. This can be accomplished by means of a double-lumen endotracheal tube. Using this technique, blood gas analyses at very short intervals are necessary. If the arteriovenous shunt volume reaches critical values, a straight vascular clamp may be used to occlude the left pulmonary artery, excluding the left lung from perfusion.

2. Resection of the Aneurysm and Reconstruction

The patient should not be heparinized systemically because of the considerable extent of the surgical procedure. Heparin is injected only locally into the clamped vessels (visceral branches, distal abdominal aorta) as a diluted solution (1000 units each).

Following exposure of the thoracic aorta, a small dose of a peripheral vasodilator is administered, and a trial is made by clamping the aorta just below the origin of the left subclavian artery. Pulmonary artery pressure must be observed carefully during this maneuver. Clamping should be done slowly in order to be able to counteract a sudden increase of blood pressure with sodium nitroprusside (see p. 197).

If blood pressure rises too abruptly, the clamps should be opened. A second attempt is made after applying a larger dose of sodium nitroprusside. Then, the distal thoracic aorta is also clamped with a straight vascular clamp, and the aneurysm is divided longitudinally (Fig. 15.5.5a, b). The distal clamp may be replaced by a large, blocking Fogarty catheter allowing retrograde perfusion of the visceral arteries – of course strongly impaired. *Bleeding* from intercostal arteries may be controlled by oversewing them at their origin inside of the aneurysm. Stronger retrograde hemorrhage from intercostal arteries is stopped with small Fogarty catheters. The intensity of bleeding may be an indication of the degree to which certain vessels participate in supplying blood to the spinal cord.

Following proximal anastomosis to the woven Dacron prosthesis (diameter 20–22 mm) (Fig. 15.5.5c), both pairs of dorsal segmental intercostal arteries, which are blocked with catheters, are reimplanted into the prosthesis at those sites where previously an oval patch of synthetic material has been excised (Fig. 15.5.5d). The respective left and right arteries are not isolated from one another during continuous suture of the anastomosis (3–0 Mersilene), but are anastomosed in pairs to the prosthesis. Separation of the arteries might lead to retroaortic vascular injury and would also be too time-consuming. The suture must penetrate the entire thickness of the aortic wall. After venting, blood flow is restored to the intercostal arteries (Fig. 15.5.5f) [3, 4].

If the dorsal wall of the aorta is intact, an oblique proximal anastomosis may be constructed in situ, leaving a long dorsal portion of the aortic wall the intercostal arteries arise from. Such an oblique end-to-end anastomosis may replace thoracic reimplantation of segmental intercostal arteries (Fig. 15.5.5e).

After reconstruction of the thoracic aorta, the visceral arteries are revascularized. Their origins are excised from the aneurysmal wall. Combining the origins of the celiac trunk and superior mesenteric artery reduces the number of anastomoses and saves time (Fig. 15.5.5f). In very large aneurysms, it is often impossible to excise them together; in such cases each artery must be reimplanted separately. Clamping distal to the bifurcation prevents retrograde blood loss. The visceral arteries should not be clamped with traumatic vascular clamps. Instead, they should be blocked with Fogarty catheters following instillation of heparin. Reimplantation is performed in the following order: right renal artery, celiac artery and superior mesenteric artery, left renal artery (Fig. 15.5.5g–k). After each anastomosis is completed, blood flow is restored to the artery. First, the distal clamp is removed. Retrograde blood flow forces the air out of the vessel and flushes out small clots at the same time. Anterograde blood flow can be res-

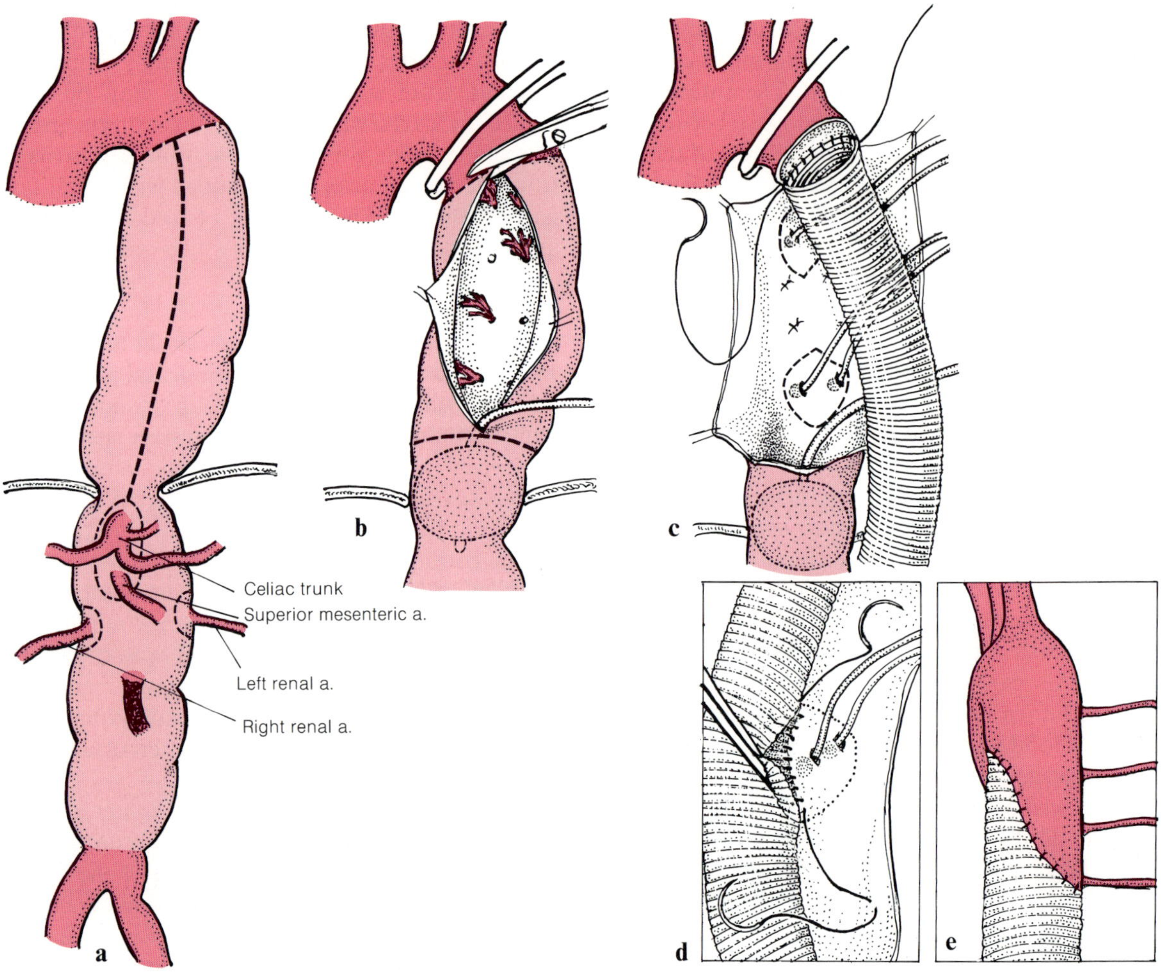

tored. Tangential clamping of the prosthesis during reimplantation of the celiac artery, superior mesenteric artery, and left renal artery provides adequate arterial blood supply to the arteries previously anastomosed to the prosthesis (Fig. 15.5.5g–j). Following completion of the visceral anastomoses, a cranial pair of lumbar arteries is reimplanted to insure supply to the caudal portion of the spinal cord. The pair showing the strongest back bleeding should be reconnected as shown for the thoracic segment of the prosthesis [2, 6, 7].

An alternative technique, introduced by Crawford, may be used instead. In order to apply this method, the aortic wall surrounding the origins of the visceral arteries must be free of severe pathologic change [3, 5]. This is not true for the revascularizing technique described above. It may be performed even in the most severely damaged aortas. One major advantage of the Crawford technique is the reduced number of anastomoses. This is accomplished by modifying the incision and dividing the abdominal aneurysm in a different way. The thoracic incision is directed toward the left and continues downward, passing just behind the left

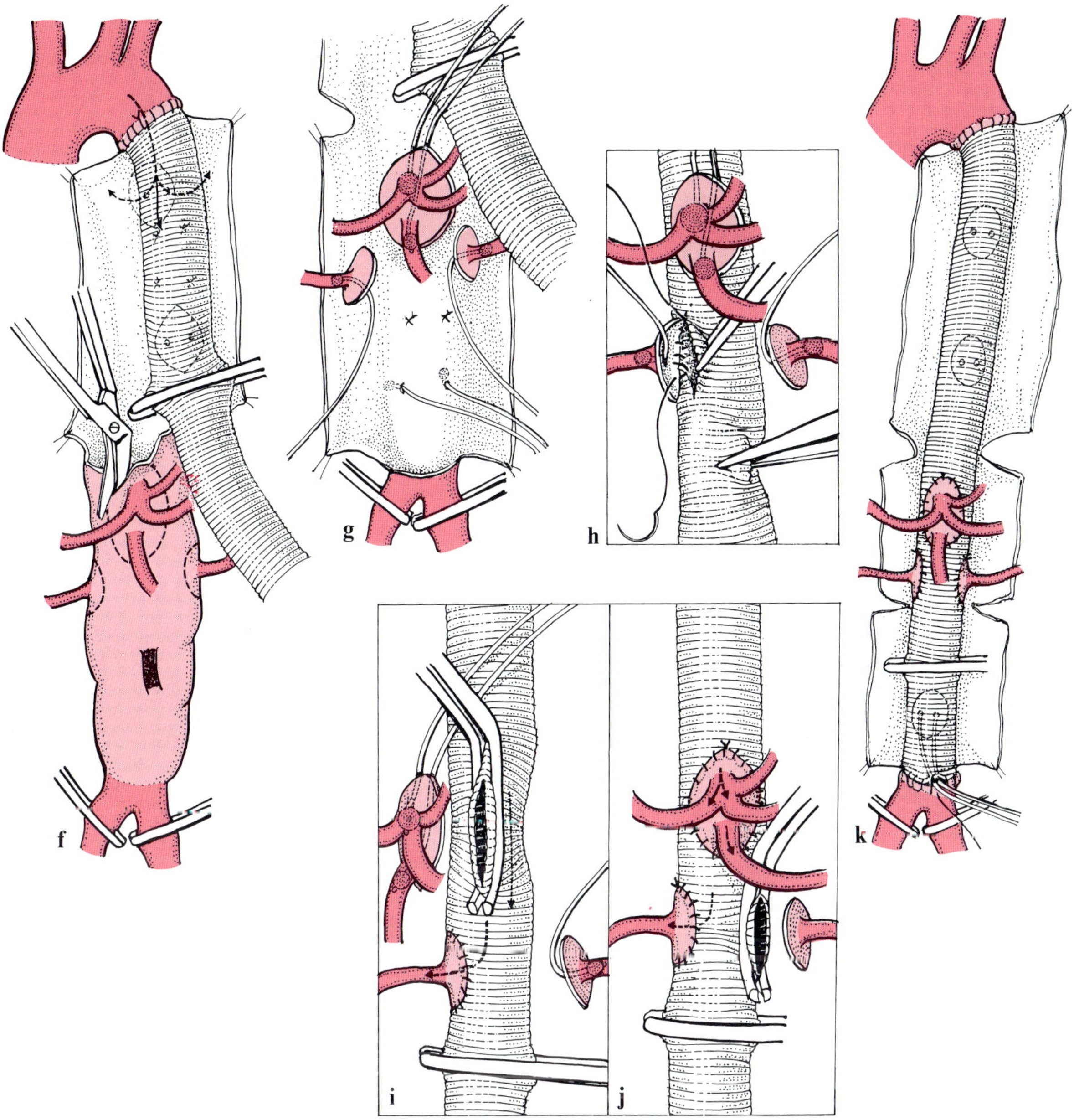

Fig. 15.5.5a–k. Replacement of a thoracoabdominal aneurysm. **a** Full extent of the aneurysm, incision, funnel-shaped excision of the visceral artery orifices. **b** Division of the anterior wall of the thoracic aneurysm. **c** Proximal end-to-end anastomosis. The localization of two thoracic segmental tributaries with the strongest back bleeding is shown. These must be reimplanted into the graft. The other intercostal arteries are closed transaortically with sutures. **d** Anastomosis of the prosthesis to a pair of thoracic intercostal arteries blocked by a Fogarty catheter. **e** As an alternative to **c** and **d**, a beveled end-to-end anastomosis may be attempted, provided the dorsal aortic wall is still intact. **f** Restoration of blood flow to the segmental intercostal arteries. Visceral arteries excised with a funnel-shaped origin. **g** Blood loss reduced by using blocking catheters. **h** Anastomosis of the right renal artery. For anastomosis of the excised origin of the renal artery to the prosthesis an oval patch of synthetic graft material must be cut out of the prosthesis (a simple longitudinal incision of the prosthesis is not adequate!) **i** Restoration of blood flow to the right kidney and anastomosis of the celiac artery and superior mesenteric artery by clamping the prosthesis longitudinally around the excised orifice. **j** Anastomosis of the left renal artery during longitudinal partial clamping of the prosthesis. The oval excision of the prosthesis for the anastomosis must be performed on the lateral aspect of the graft to prevent kinking of the renal artery after its implantation. **k** Anastomosis of the lumbar segmental arteries followed by suture of the distal anastomosis; the blocking Fogarty catheters are removed just before the final sutures of the anastomosis are placed

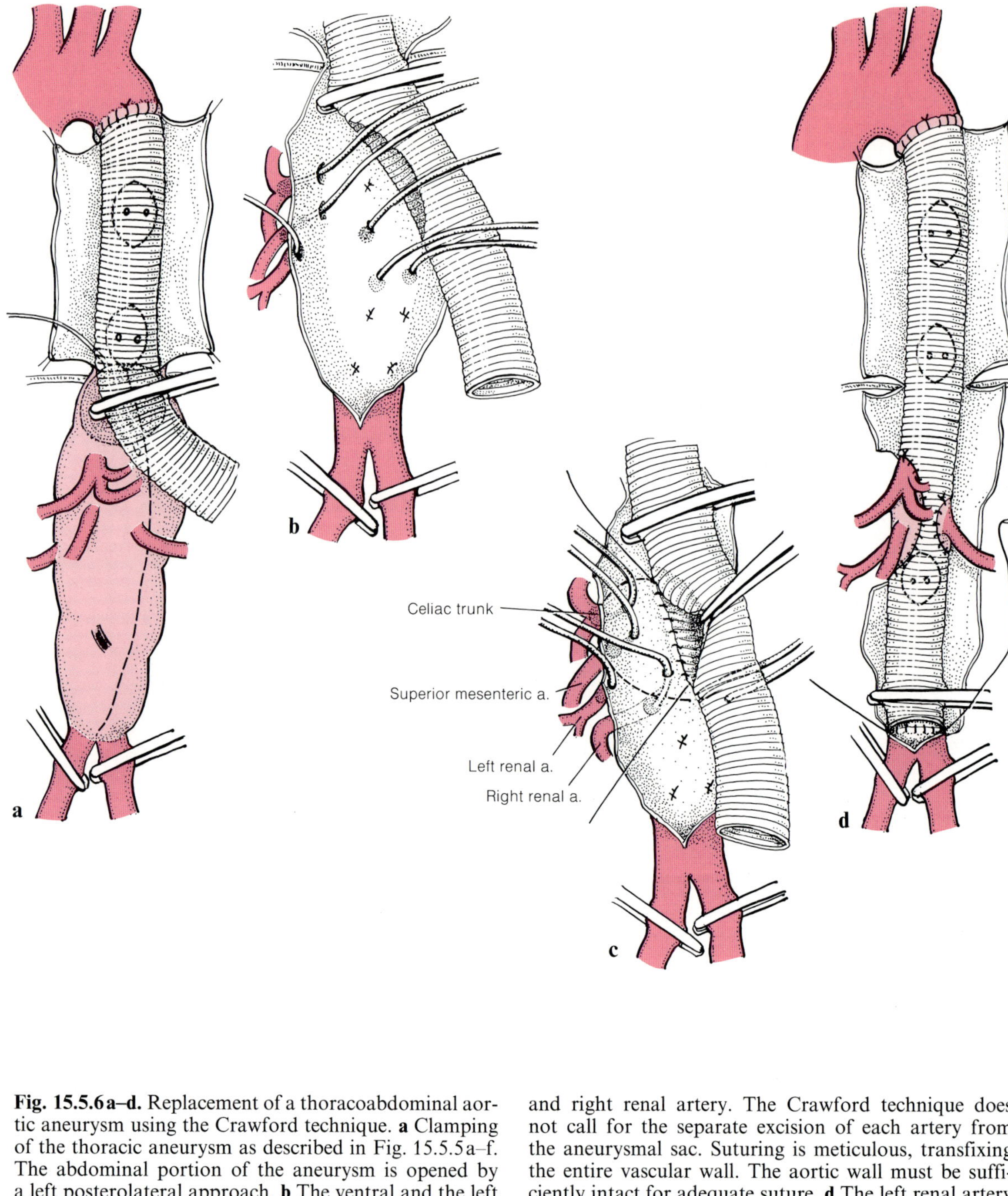

Fig. 15.5.6a–d. Replacement of a thoracoabdominal aortic aneurysm using the Crawford technique. **a** Clamping of the thoracic aneurysm as described in Fig. 15.5.5a–f. The abdominal portion of the aneurysm is opened by a left posterolateral approach. **b** The ventral and the left lateral vascular walls are reflected to the right; retrograde bleeding is blocked by a catheter. **c** Large oval excision of the prosthesis. The anastomosis covers the origin of the celiac artery, superior mesenteric artery, and right renal artery. The Crawford technique does not call for the separate excision of each artery from the aneurysmal sac. Suturing is meticulous, transfixing the entire vascular wall. The aortic wall must be sufficiently intact for adequate suture. **d** The left renal artery is sutured to the prosthesis following generous excision of the prosthesis at the appropriate site. The prosthesis is clamped tangentially. The distal anastomosis is completed after revascularization of the lumbar arteries

renal artery (Fig. 15.5.6a). The left kidney is rotated to the right. The ventral wall is pulled apart and opened in one piece with guide sutures attached to it (Fig. 15.5.6b). All orifices are visualized and checked. Back bleeding is stopped by balloon catheters after heparin instillation (Fig. 15.5.6c). A longitudinal oval patch is excised from the prosthesis. The first abdominal anastomosis between the aortic wall and the prosthesis should contain the celiac, superior mesenteric, and right renal arteries. The anastomosis is completed from within the aneurysm, each stitch transfixing the entire aortic wall. The left renal artery is sutured to a second excised opening in the graft.

There are several ways of connecting the prosthesis distally. The selection of the appropriate method depends on the caudal extension of the aneurysm into the pelvic arteries (see p. 436). One should bear in mind that the spinal cord is also supplied by branches of the internal iliac artery. Great care must therefore be taken in reimplanting these arteries, should it become necessary to do so (see p. 280) (Fig. 15.5.6d).

The distal anastomosis completes aneurysmal reconstruction. Before restoring anterograde blood flow to the graft, the distal clamps are removed and the graft is vented. Blood pressure must be monitored carefully after unclamping the graft proximally. Pressure may drop suddenly, even if the pelvic arteries are unclamped in succession. If hypotension is severe, the prosthesis must be reclamped, and one must wait until sodium nitroprusside has been eliminated.

The aneurysmal sac is then closed over the thoracic portion of the prosthesis, and the pleura is reconstructed. The diaphragm is sutured from the abdomen. Exact reconstruction is necessary to prevent pulmonary complications and diaphragmatic hernias. The lung must be inflated until all atelectatic regions regain their normal contour. The thoracotomy is then closed in layers after inserting two chest tubes. The retroperitoneum is sutured. The mobilized organs are placed back into their original positions.

A matter of great controversy is whether or not a temporary bypass is necessary in this type of reconstruction. Arguments in favor of assisted circulation (e.g., from the left subclavian artery to the right common femoral artery, see p. 320) are that blood flow to the visceral organs and the spinal cord is best maintained under the protection of a bypass. Vascular reconstruction without a bypass is always a race against the clock.

CRAWFORD, who operated on 313 patients without using bypasses, had the highest incidence of paraplegia in the group of thoracoabdominal vascular replacements (aortic segments III, IV, and V). The highest rate was seen in the group with concomitant occlusive arterial disease (of 63 patients, 10% had paraplegia). If a longer thoracic segment did not have to be reconstructed, the incidence of paraplegia sank to 0% (in 84 patients [3]).

Therefore, to reject the temporary bypass technique a priori is not justifiable in our view. It should be applied in cases where aneurysmal reconstruction might lead to considerable impairment of segmental perfusion to the spinal cord. In such cases, however, segmental reimplantation is also mandatory.

3. Surgical Management of Additional Lesions Found at the Origins of the Visceral Arteries

If the aneurysm extends into the orifice of a visceral artery, the aneurysmal segment of the vessel must be resected. Continuity is restored by direct reimplantation of the peripheral stump into the prosthesis. This may also be done by placing an interposition graft between the aortic prosthesis and the visceral artery (Fig. 15.5.7a–c).

A concomitant stenosis may be relieved by direct disobliteration. The whole cutout of the prosthesis for anastomosis of the visceral artery should be tailored in such a way that a tongue of synthetic material remains, protruding into the lumen. The visceral artery is then reimplanted, incorporating this flap into the suture in the manner of a patch graft, thereby preventing constriction at the suture line (Fig. 15.5.7d, e).

Extensive thromboendarterectomy of the aortic wall with desobliteration of the main arteries is also possible. The crucial point in this technique is that the peripheral ends of the thromboendarterectomized segments show projecting ledges of thickened intima. The transition from the thromboendarterectomized proximal segments of the arteries to the untouched distal portions must be smooth. Otherwise, intimal dissection and thrombosis may occur (Fig. 15.5.7f, g).

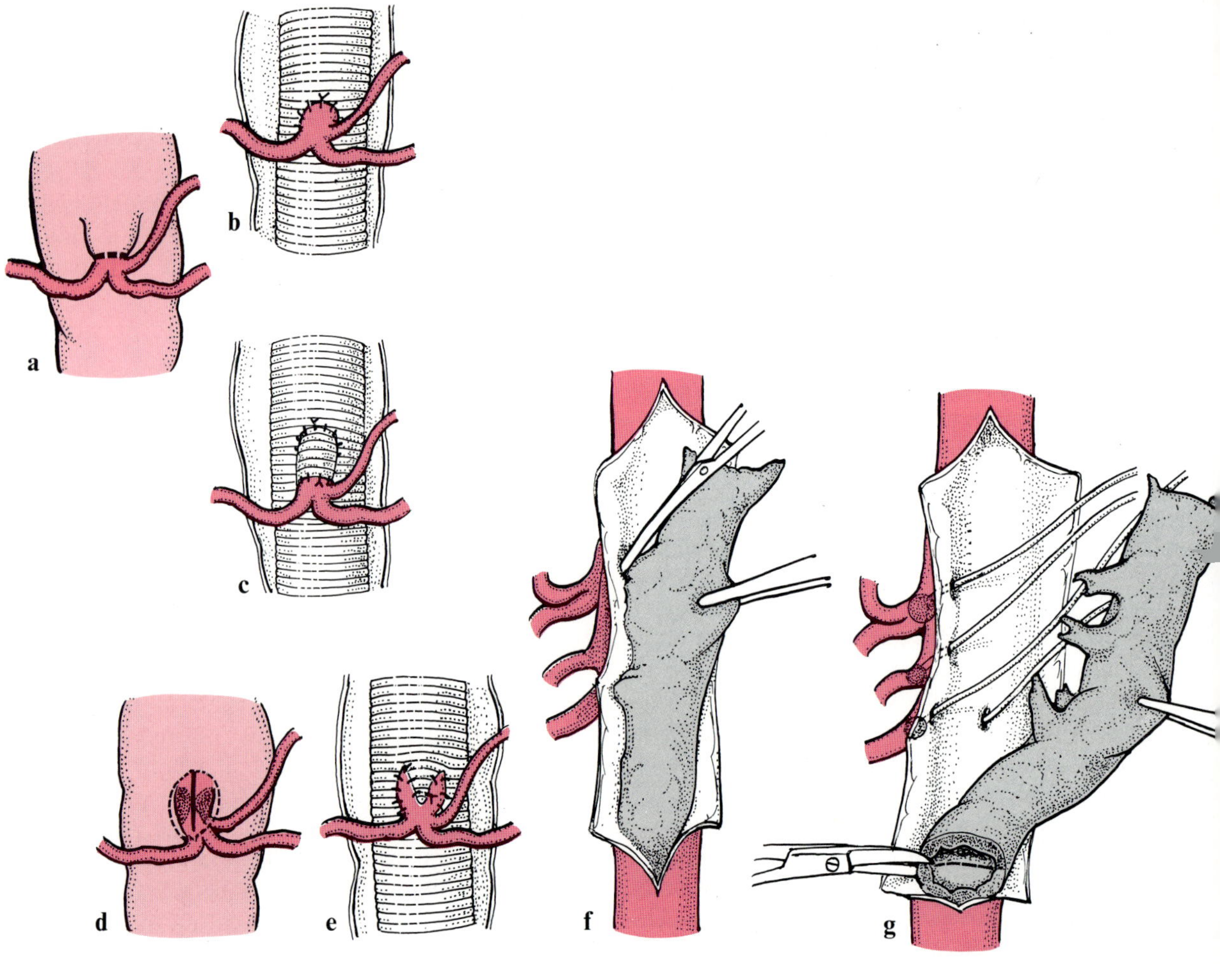

Fig. 15.5.7 a–g. Variations in the origins of the visceral arteries. **a** The aneurysm extends into the orifice of the visceral artery (in this case the celiac artery). **b** The aneurysmal segment near the orifice is resected, and the anastomosis is established directly or **c** via an interposition graft between the aortic prosthesis and the visceral artery. **d** The orifice of the artery is narrowed by arteriosclerotic plaques. **e** If a local thromboendarterectomy is not possible, the vessel is opened longitudinally, disobliterated, and connected to the aortic prosthesis. A small strip of prosthetic material is tailored out of the graft at the site of anastomosis in order to obtain the same widening effect as in patch angioplasty. **f** Severe arteriosclerotic lesions may be removed in toto by applying the Crawford technique. Thromboendarterectomy should not leave an intimal step at its peripheral ends. **g** The inner arteriosclerotic core of the thromboendarterectomized material is divided distally; retrograde blood loss from the visceral arteries is prevented by blocking catheters

4. Temporary Bypass

There are several bypass procedures for maintaining arterial peripheral perfusion during thoracic and visceral reconstructions. They should not prolong operating time and should not hinder reconstruction.

The methods described by SELLE [12] meet these requirements best. He uses a 9-mm Gott shunt for temporary bypass. This shunt is inserted proximally through the left subclavian artery into the aortic arch and not directly into the aorta. The peripheral connection is established via the right common femoral artery. Tourniquets prevent dislocation of the shunt at the introduction sites (Fig. 15.5.8 a).

The distal aorta is perfused retrograde after cross-clamping of the proximal thoracic aorta. Reconstruction is performed in the same manner as described earlier.

If the aneurysm is very large, a heterotopic rather than an orthotopic replacement is chosen. The following techniques are available: The vessels are exposed in the same manner as with the Crawford technique (see p. 314ff). In addition, the vessels in both groins are exposed. A woven Dacron bifurcation prosthesis is anastomosed on the left side to the femoral artery and extended upward by a tube (e.g., 22-mm woven Dacron). The proximal end-to-end anastomosis is then completed. The temporary shunt is removed and blood flow through the interposition graft is restored, keeping the right branch of the prosthesis clamped (Fig. 15.5.8c); the latter is then anastomosed end-to-side to the right common femoral artery. The proximal anastomosis may also be performed end-to-side if the aortic wall just distal to the origin of the left subclavian artery is in fair condition (Fig. 15.5.8b). The clamping technique makes a temporary bypass superfluous. A disadvantage, however, is the unfavorable anastomotic angle, which causes turbulence. Reinsertion of the visceral arteries is performed in the following order:

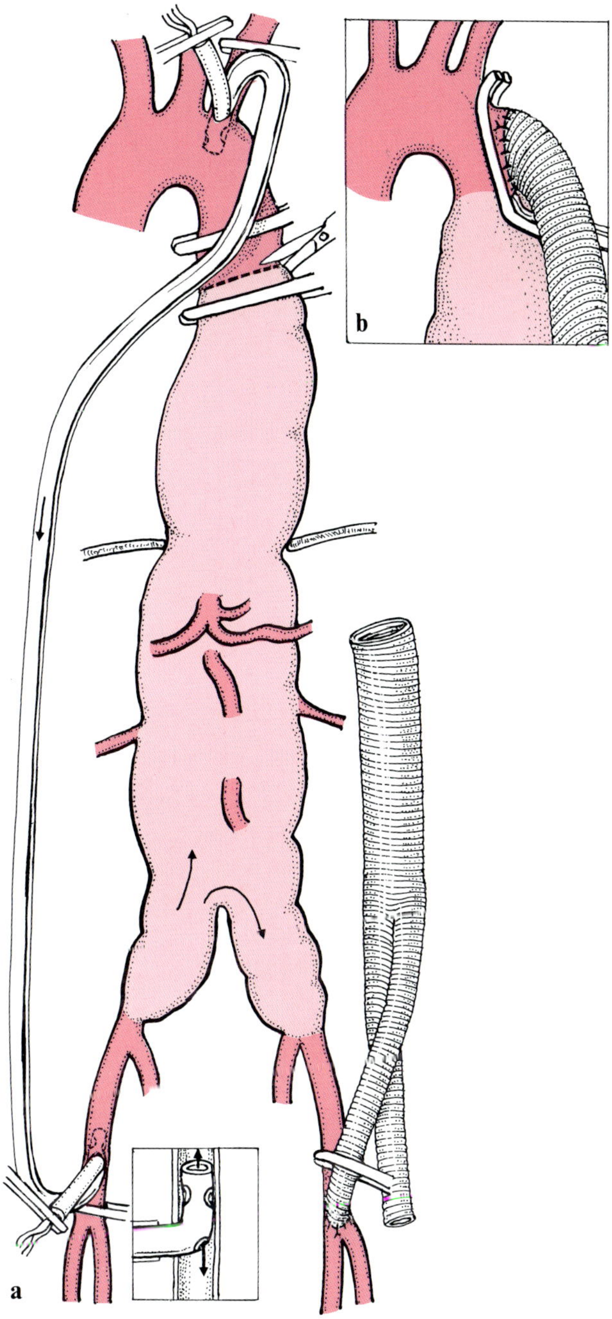

Fig. 15.5.8a, b. (Fig. 15.5.8c–e see p. 322)

Fig. 15.5.8a–e. Bypass of a thoracoabdominal aortic aneurysm and its isolation from systemic circulation. **a** The temporary bypass tube is inserted over the left subclavian artery into the aortic arch and connected to the right common femoral artery. Retrograde perfusion of the abdominal and thoracic segments (spinal cord!) is achieved. The left limb of a bifurcation prosthesis is anastomosed end-to side to the left common femoral artery and clamped. **b** The proximal anastomosis may be performed end-to-side if the thoracic aorta offers enough space for this connection. Temporary bypass is not needed in such a case. If the hemodynamically more favorable proximal end-to-end anastomosis is chosen, the bifurcation prosthesis is implanted first. **c** The bifurcation prothesis is lengthened proximally by two end-to-end anastomoses under protection of a temporary bypass. The temporary bypass is then removed, and the right arm of the prosthesis is clamped. Abdominal and thoracic perfusion is again achieved by retrograde flow through the prosthesis. **d, e** Anastomosis of the right branch of the prosthesis to the right common femoral artery. The visceral arteries are then connected to the prosthesis, sometimes through interposition grafts, using the tangential clamping technique. Order of implantation: (*1*) right renal artery; (*2*) celiac trunk; (*3*) superior mesenteric artery; (*4*) left renal artery. The aortic orifices of these arteries are closed by suture. The aneurysm is finally isolated from systemic circulation by ligation above the origins of the internal iliac arteries. Its proximal end is closed by mattress sutures. A great disadvantage of this type of reconstruction is thrombosis of the aneurysm remaining in situ, with risk of ischemic damage to the spinal cord

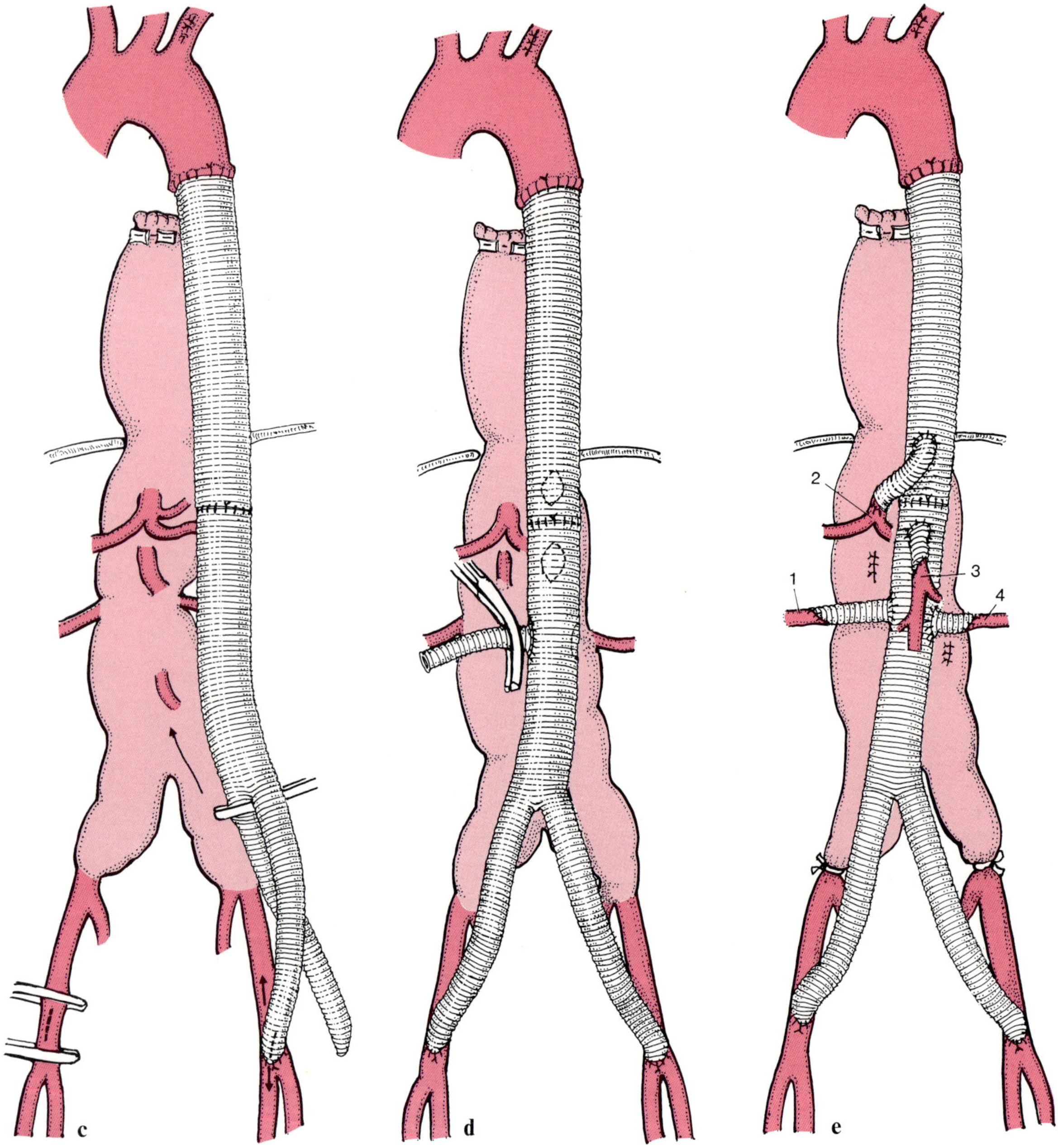

Fig. 15.5.8c–e. Legend see p. 321

right renal artery, celiac trunk, superior mesenteric artery, left renal artery (by separate anastomosis of each artery). Usually several synthetic interposition grafts (Dacron, 8 mm in diameter) are necessary to restore the continuity of the visceral arteries if the aneurysm remains in situ. Ischemic time can be shortened by constructing the primary prosthesis-to-prosthesis anastomosis by the tangential clamping technique (Fig. 15.5.8d). An end-to-end anastomosis is constructed between the stump of the visceral artery and the distal end of the prosthetic interposition graft after beveling both ends (Fig. 15.5.8e). The aneurysmal wall is closed by continuous suture at the sites of the previously excised origins of the visceral arteries. The aneurysm is totally isolated from circulation by ligating the common iliac arteries following completion of all visceral anastomoses. This leads to total thrombosis of the aneurysm. Ischemia of the spinal cord may be a consequence of this process.

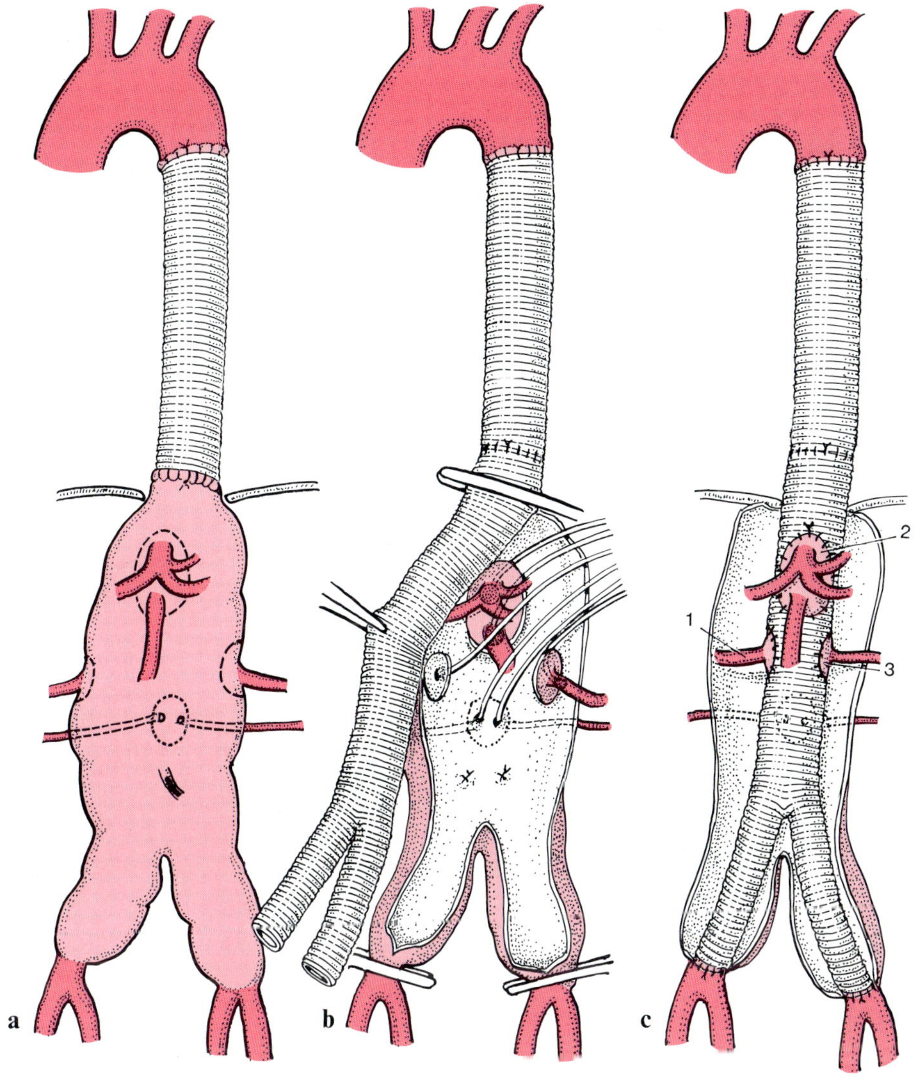

Direct aortic replacement, as accomplished by the modified Crawford technique in combination with temporary bypass, is more favorable since in the thoracic and lumbar regions, at least one pair of segmental arteries can be reanastomosed to the prosthesis.

5. Aneurysms of the Suprarenal and Infrarenal Abdominal Segments Following Earlier Resection of Thoracic Aneurysm

Further progression of aneurysmal disease following previous surgery of a thoracic aneurysm may necessitate operative correction in segments IV and V (Fig. 15.5.9a–c).

This procedure is performed using the same approach, with the patient in the same position, as in the primary thoracoabdominal operation (see

Fig. 15.5.9a–c. Replacement of the aorta in an abdominal aortic aneurysm following previous thoracic vascular replacement. **a** Extension of the aneurysm, funnel-shaped excision of the origins of the visceral arteries. **b** The old distal anastomosis is resected, and the bifurcation prosthesis anastomosed proximally. The origins of the visceral arteries are excised. Blocking catheters prevent retrograde bleeding. **c** Reimplantation of the visceral arteries in the following order: (*1*) right renal artery; (*2*) celiac trunk and superior mesenteric artery; (*3*) left renal artery. One pair of lumbar arteries showing good reflux should be reimplanted since no intercostal arteries were attached to the graft during primary replacement of the thoracic aorta

Fig. 15.5.4). If during the first operation segmental intercostal or lumbar arteries were not reanastomosed to the graft, reimplantation of these arteries is of special importance in reoperation. This is done according to the same principles as those described previously. Here also, two techniques are possible: combined insertion of the visceral arteries following longitudinal excision of the aortic wall surrounding them, as well as the separate anastomosis of each artery to the graft.

During reintervention, care must be taken not to injure lung tissue. Leaks in the parenchyma must be carefully closed by suture to prevent infection of the prosthesis and the development of larger air leaks. The latter complicate mechanical ventilation during the early postoperative period.

II. Thoracoabdominal Aneurysms with Intact Segment IV

Surgical treatment of this type of aneurysm is done with the patient lying in the semilateral Crawford position (Fig. 15.5.4). Following thoracotomy in the sixth intercostal space, the thoracic portion of the aneurysm is exposed. If the aneurysm ends above the diaphragm, it may be clamped at that site. Extension of the incision with division of the costal margin is not necessary in such a case. The procedure may be completed in one step by thoracic implantation of a tube prosthesis (in such a case, two pairs of arteries, one situated proximally and one distally, should be reimplanted). The infrarenal aneurysm is then exposed by a median laparotomy without division of the diaphragm (see p. 296). Reconstruction in this manner is advisable only if the thoracic aneurysm ends proximal to the diaphragm and there is enough space to clamp the aorta securely above the diaphragm (Fig. 15.5.10). If there is any doubt as to the distal extension of the aneurysm, thoracotomy should be extended over the left costal magin to the abdomen, as described earlier (see p. 314). After posterolateral division of the diaphragm in the direction of the aortic hiatus, the proximal segment IV can be identified and the caudal end of the aneurysm exposed. Here again, a temporary bypass is recommended. Distal connection of the prosthesis is performed in accordance with the peripheral extension of the aneurysm, e.g., iliac or femoral attachment.

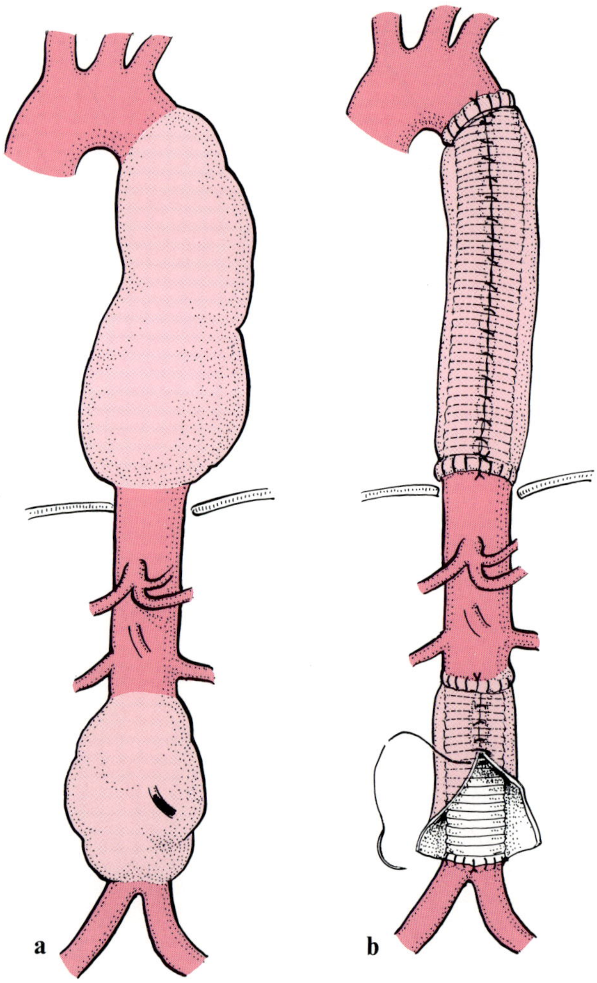

Fig. 15.5.10 a, b. Thoracic and infrarenal aortic aneurysm. **a** Anatomy. **b** Repair with an interposition graft. Covering the prosthesis with the aneurysmal wall

III. Thoracic Aneurysm with Involvement of Proximal Segment IV

This aneurysm ends just above the origin of the celiac trunk. The portion of the aorta lying between the right and left diaphragm is also enlarged. It cannot be reached by a thoracic approach alone. It is reconstructed by the technique of interposition grafting (see Fig. 15.5.10). The patient is placed in a thoracoabdominal position (see Fig. 15.5.4).

Another technique is replacement of the aneurysm with an intraluminal prosthesis. The intraluminal prosthesis is cut according to the extent of aneurysmal involvement and a ring-enforced Dacron prosthesis is sutured to each end of the tube graft. The proximal ring is pulled into the proximal

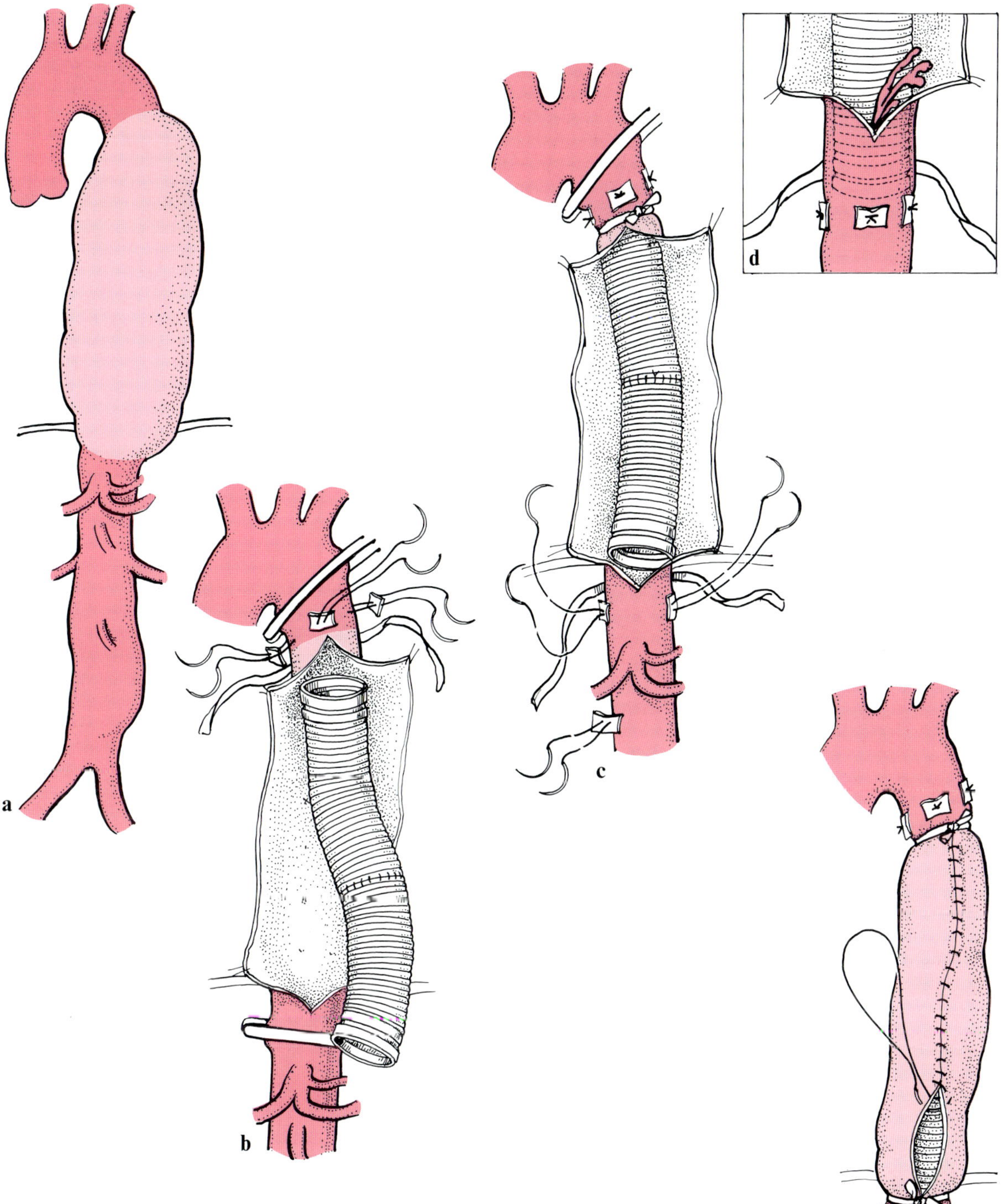

Fig. 15.5.11 a–e. Replacement of a thoracic aneurysm extending into segment IV with an intraluminal prosthesis. **a** Before intervention. **b** An intraluminal prosthesis of the appropriate length is fashioned. Dacron ring prostheses are sutured on proximally and distally, and secured using sutures reinforced with Teflon felts. **c** A broad tape is tied around the groove in the Dacron ring. **d** Before resumption of blood flow the graft is vented distally. **e** The aneurysmal wall is sewn over the prosthesis

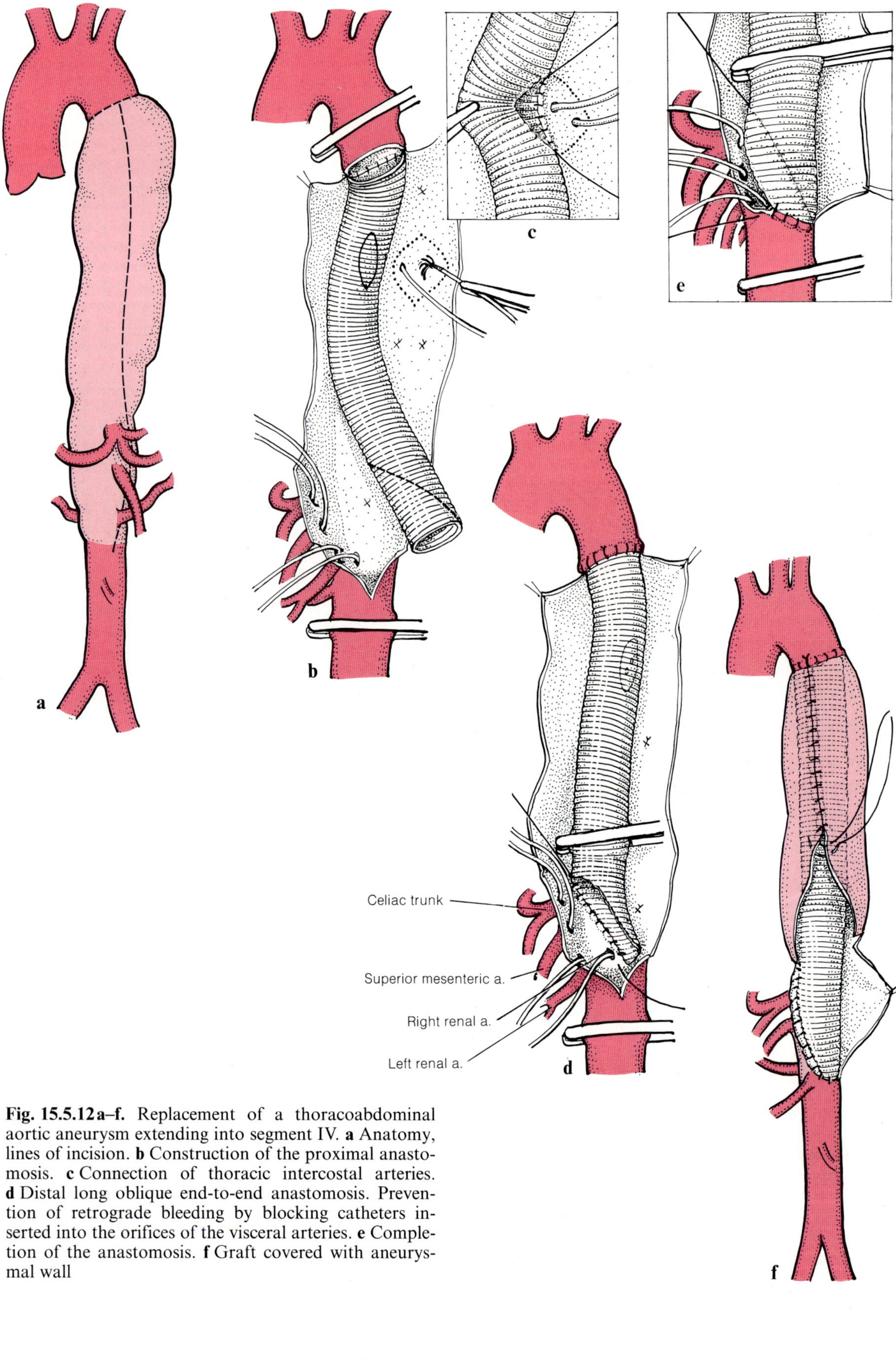

Fig. 15.5.12a–f. Replacement of a thoracoabdominal aortic aneurysm extending into segment IV. **a** Anatomy, lines of incision. **b** Construction of the proximal anastomosis. **c** Connection of thoracic intercostal arteries. **d** Distal long oblique end-to-end anastomosis. Prevention of retrograde bleeding by blocking catheters inserted into the orifices of the visceral arteries. **e** Completion of the anastomosis. **f** Graft covered with aneurysmal wall

aorta telescopically by three sutures reinforced with Teflon felts. The stay sutures are tied, and a broad tape is tied around the aortic wall. This band is securely tightened around a shallow groove beneath the rim of the Dacron ring. The graft is vented at the distal anastomosis before the periaortic ligature is completed (Fig. 15.5.11a–e). An advantage of this technique is the short aortic clamping time. Disadvantages are:

a) Segmental intercostal or lumbar arteries are not reanastomosed to the prosthesis. Careful transluminal suture ligation at the origins of the segmental arteries is mandatory.

b) The prosthesis is anchored proximally at only three sites. The wide periaortic ligature may cut into fragile, thin walls. Blood may gain access to the space between the prosthesis and the old aneurysmal wall (similar to a pseudodissection).

If the aneurysm extends far into segment IV, reconstruction can be accomplished neither by implantation of an intraluminar prosthesis nor by interposition of a graft as shown in Fig. 15.5.10. In such a situation, a modified method is available:

The stomach, spleen, tail of the pancreas, left flexure of the colon, left lobe of the liver, and left kidney are mobilized to the right after exposure by a thoracoabdominal approach. The thoracic aortotomy is lateralized to the left side and passed behind the left renal artery. The anterior portion of the aneurysmal wall can then be pulled back, exposing all origins of the visceral arteries from the inside. After completing the proximal anastomosis (with reimplantation of intercostal arteries), the prosthesis is connected to the aortic wall at its distal end by a long oblique end-to-end suture. A dorsal strip of the graft reaches down below both orifices of the renal arteries. These vessels may not be narrowed by the suture line which runs upward on the right and left sides (Fig. 15.5.12a–f).

One advantage of this technique is that all visceral arteries are reimplanted by means of one anastomosis. Reconstruction cannot be expected to succeed, however, if the distal aortic wall is too severely damaged by aneurysmal disease.

IV. Aneurysms of the Distal Thoracic Aorta Excluding Segment V

If the aneurysm has the same pattern and extension as depicted in Fig. 15.5.13, surgery is done with the patient lying in a thoracoabdominal position, and the thoracotomy is extended downward into the abdomen by dividing the costal margin. The diaphragm is transected until the aneurysm is reached, and the retroperitoneum is exposed from the left side (see p. 595). The other steps of reconstruction are described on p. 315ff. Reimplantation of segmental lumbar arteries may be unnecessary if a large segment of the thoracic aorta is still completely intact. Lumbar arteries showing good evidence of main blood supply to the spinal cord in preoperative angiograms (great radicular artery arising from the lumbar aorta) should be reanastomosed, especially if intercostal arteries in the thoracic region cannot be shown on the angiogram because of extensive arteriosclerosis.

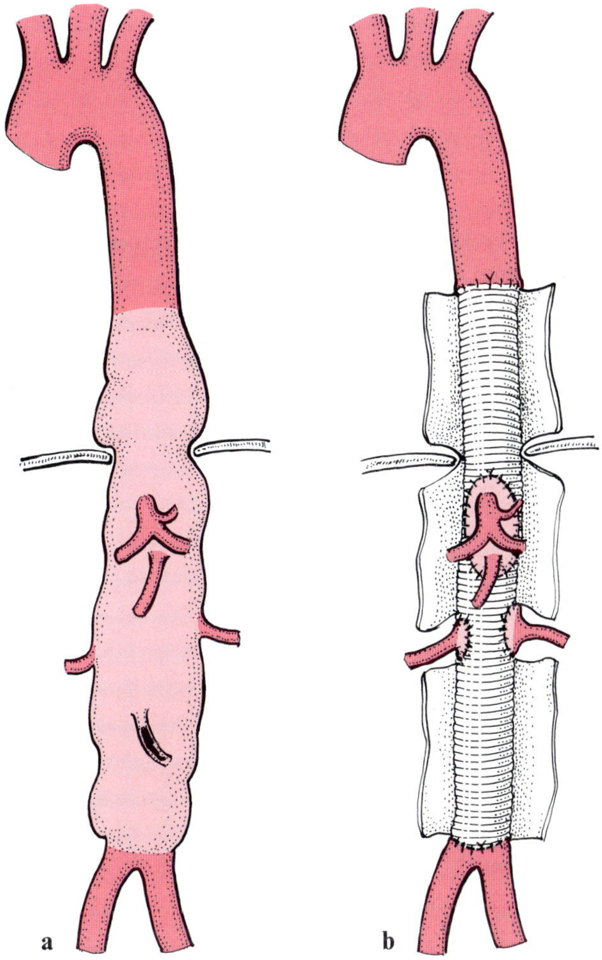

Fig. 15.5.13a, b. Replacement of a thoracoabdominal aortic aneurysm which extends for down to the bifurcation. **a** Anatomy, **b** Completed reconstruction with funnel-shaped excision of the visceral orifices. The Crawford technique may also be applied in such a situation (see Fig. 15.5.6)

One should never attempt to repair the aneurysm by an abdominal approach alone. It is true, of course, that division of the crurae of the diaphragm provides good exposure of a large segment of the thoracic aorta; nevertheless, the aneurysmal wall is always at high risk of tearing during dissection from below, and the massive hemorrhage that follows rupture cannot be controlled using the abdominal approach alone.

V. Aneurysms of Segments IV and V

Exact preoperative evaluation of aneurysmal extension is essential. Exposure may be achieved by laparotomy alone (however, with the patient in a thoracoabdominal position). The retroperitoneal tissue is divided down to the aneurysmal sac. The duodenum is mobilized to the right. The left renal vein is cut between two ligatures, if necessary [1, 10]. The visceral arteries are exposed on the ventral aspect of the aorta. It is advisable to dissect the aorta free at the aortic hiatus and secure it with open clamps positioned around it. The surgeon must then decide whether or not the reconstruction can be performed from below. Resection of the aneurysm and subsequent reconstruction are described in Fig. 15.5.14.

VI. Aneurysms of Segment IV

The rare aneurysms of segment IV are repaired using the technique described in Figs. 15.5.13 and 15.5.14. An exception is presented in Fig. 15.5.15: Since this aneurysm arises from the back wall of the aorta, it does not affect the origins of the visceral arteries (Fig. 15.5.15).

By laparotomy, this aortic segment is exposed. The left kidney, stomach, speen, splenic flexure of the colon, left lobe of the liver, duodenum, and tail of the pancreas are mobilized to the right as described by Crawford. A Dacron patch closes the defect. Dissection in this area may injure mobilized lumbar veins which are difficult to localize in the event of hemorrhage and may bleed postoperatively. Alternatively, the Dacron patch may be incorporated by transaortic fixation.

Fig. 15.5.14a, b. Abdominal aortic aneurysm of segments IV and V. **a** Anatomy. **b** Total reconstruction and reanastomosis of the visceral arteries (see Fig. 15.5.5)

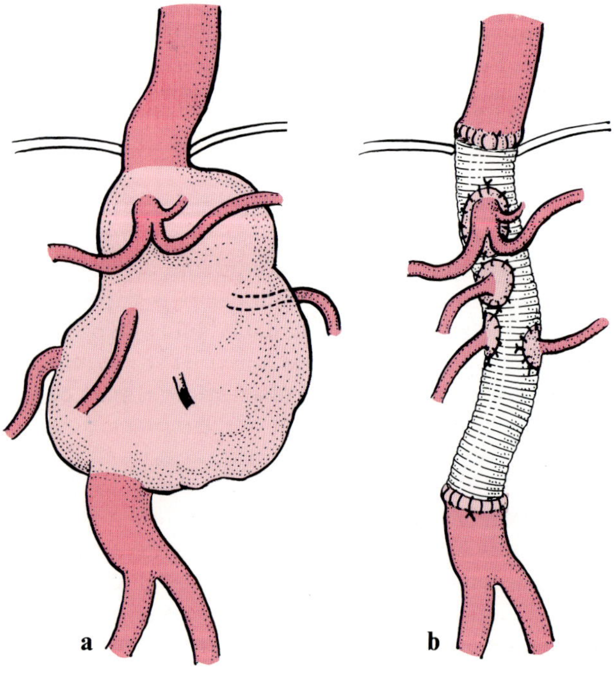

Fig. 15.5.15a, b. Abdominal aortic aneurysm of segment IV. **a** Anatomy. **b** This rare dorsal aneurysm is resected with preservation of the visceral arteries. The defect is closed with a Dacron patch

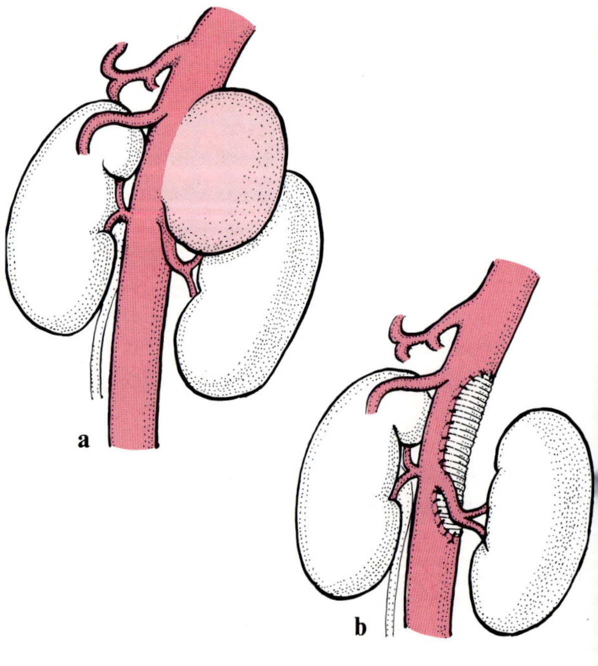

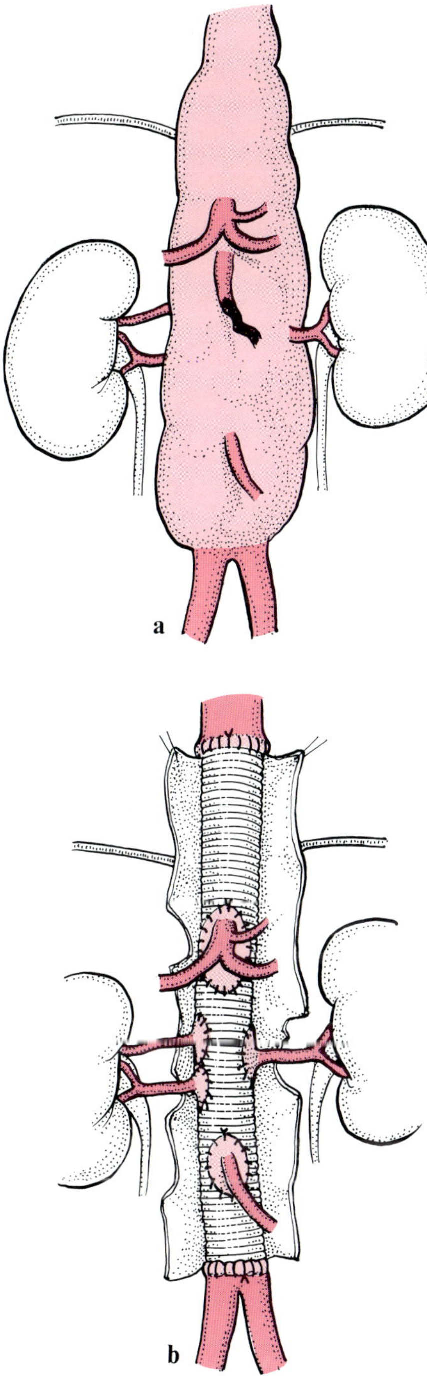

Fig. 15.5.16a, b. Consideration of anatomic variations. An additional pole artery of the kidney must be reimplanted. If the superior mesenteric artery is occluded, reinsertion of the inferior mesenteric artery into the graft is essential (Riolan anastomosis) (see p. 591)

VII. Importance of Anatomic Variations

The visceral arteries may vary considerably in their anatomy. They should be visualized preoperatively by angiography as they are of crucial importance for correct surgical strategy (Fig. 15.5.16).

The following anatomic variations are possible:

a) Supplementary pole arteries of the kidney: They must be dissected free and reimplanted. Ligation leads to partial renal ischemia with subsequent secondary hypertension or renal insufficiency.

b) Occlusive arterial disease may lead to total occlusion of the superior mesenteric artery, making reinsertion of the inferior mesenteric artery mandatory. This is done by performing a Riolan anastomosis to secure adequate blood supply to the small intestine (see p. 591).

c) The common hepatic artery may arise directly from the abdominal aorta. It must be reanastomosed to the graft (for other variations see p. 17).

D. Postoperative Treatment and Complications

The magnitude of these surgical procedures necessitates continuous monitoring (blood pressure, ECG, blood gas analyses) in an intensive care unit. A chest X-ray must be taken immediately following the operation to verify proper ventilation of all pulmonary segments. Intensive respiratory adjunct therapy with higher ventilation pressures should be administered in case of atelactasis. These measures are even more important than the administration of antibiotics to prevent dangerous pneumonia in mechanically ventilated patients following surgery.

Thrombosis of the aortic graft is rare because of the high flow velocities. However, advanced arteriosclerosis may lead to thrombosis in some cases. Low dose heparinization (300 units/h) is recommended. Fluid intake and output should be managed carefully and calculated every 6 h for quick detection of possible disorders of renal function. Polyuria may be a consequence of very long clamping times. It may last for 1–2 days, and renal function may then normalize. Regular laboratory controls of electrolytes and measurements of central venous pressure and pulmonary capillary wedge pressure (by Swan-Ganz catheter) are necessary. Polyuria may, however, end in oliguria which must be treated by hemofiltration or hemodialysis (danger of hyperhydration). One should rule out thrombotic occlusion of the renal artery by angiography (digital subtraction angiography) or renal scan.

Functional disorders of the liver may also occur following long clamping times, especially if the patient has a history of liver disease. One of the cardinal symptoms is jaundice (which may also be a result of massive blood transfusions). The serum values of the specific liver enzymes increase, cholinesterase decreases. Clotting disorders develop, making specific substitution of factors necessary. Liver function is further impaired by hypoxia which may occur, e.g., during weaning from mechanical ventilation.

Postoperative function of the intestine is especially difficult to evaluate. Functional impairment often remains undetected due to sedation of the patient during mechanical ventilation. Evidence of intestinal ischemia is hyperperistalsis followed by ileus. These findings should be evaluated by angiography. If there is uncertainty about the adequacy of intestinal perfusion intraoperatively, a second-look operation must be performed within 48 h. Important complications needing special attention are: myocardial infarction, postoperative hemorrhage, prosthetic infection (rare), and spinal cord paralysis. Paralysis is a very serious complication, which has different rates of occurrence following aortic reconstruction [3]. The patient must be informed preoperatively about both partial and complete forms of this complication.

Thoracoabdominal replacement is one of the greatest challenges in reconstructive vascular surgery. Large series show a mortality of 7% and an incidence of paraplegia of 2%. Correct patient selection coupled with broad experience in surgical management and postoperative treatment of these aneurysms are the main factors on which success is based. Considering how extensive these reconstructive procedures are, the results are good (for further reading on surgery of the ascending aorta and aortic arch see Vol VI/2, Manual of Cardiovascular Surgery).

REFERENCES

1. Cooley DA, Wukasch DC, Lick RF (1980) Gefäßchirurgie: Indikationen und Technik. Schattauer, Stuttgart New York
2. Crawford ES (1973) Thoraco-abdominal and abdominal aortic aneurysms involving renal, superior mesenteric and celiac arteries. Ann Surg 179:763
3. Crawford ES, Crawford JL (1984) Diseases of the aorta. Williams & Wilkins, Baltimore London
4. Crawford ES, Rubio PA (1973) Reappraisal of adjuncts to avoid ischemia in the treatment of aneurysms of descending thoracic aorta. J Thor Cardiovasc Surg 66:693
5. Crawford ES, Snyder DM, Cho GC, Roehm JOF (1978) Progress in treatment of thoracoabdominal and abdominal aortic aneurysms involving celic, superior mesenteric and renal arteries. Ann Surg 188:404
6. DeBakey ME, Creech O Jr, Morris GC (1956) Aneurysm of thoracoabdominal aorta involving celiac, superior mesenteric and renal arteries: Report of four cases treated by resection and homograft replacement. Ann Surg 144:549
7. DeBakey ME, Crawford ES, Garrett HE (1965) Surgical considerations in the treatment of aneurysms of the thoraco-abdominal aorta. Ann Surg 162:650
8. Jellinger K (1966) Zur Orthologie und Pathologie der Rückenmarksdurchblutung. Springer, Vienna New York
9. Richenbacher J, Landolt AM, Theiler K (1982) Rücken. Springer, Berlin Heidelberg New York (Praktische Anatomie, vol 2/part 7)
10. Papadopoulos CD, Manoli A, Sobel A (1971) Surgical-treatment of thoraco-abdominal aneurysms. J Cardiovasc Surg 12:456
11. Piscol K (1972) Die Blutversorgung des Rückenmarkes und ihre klinische Relevanz. Springer, Berlin Heidelberg New York
12. Selle JG, Robicsek F, Daugherty HK, Cook JW (1978) Thoracoabdominal aortic aneurysms. Ann Surg 189:158
13. Spencer FC, Zimmermann JM (1950) The influence of ligation of intercostal arteries on paraplegia in dogs. Surg Forum 9:430

15.6 Aneurysms and Ruptures of the Thoracic Aorta

W.-J. STELTER and G. HEBERER

CONTENTS

A. Anatomy and General Remarks

The thoracic aorta is divided into three segments I–III. This topographic classification is important for surgical strategy and technique since the method of reconstruction used depends on the diseased aortic segment. Lesions of the *ascending aorta* (segment I) can only rarely be repaired without heart-lung bypass, e.g., in saccular aneuryms or traumatic aneurysms which may be resected by simple tangential clamping. They are discussed in the "Manual of Cardiovascular Surgery" (vol. VI/2, p. 575 ff.). The diseases of the *aortic arch* (segment II) are treated by orthotopic aortic arch replacement in hypothermic circulatory arrest by use of the heart – lung machine [3, 4, 14]. Localized lesions of the *distal portion of the aortic arch* may be repaired without the help of the heart – lung machine, using certain modified bypass techniques [9, 17] (Fig. 15.6.3). A prerequisite is an undiseased aortic segment at least 5 cm long above the aortic valve which can be partially clamped. Segment III, the *descending aorta*, includes the origin of the left subclavian artery. This whole segment can be clamped distally and proximally without critical impairment of cerebral blood flow.

The *topography of the aortic arch*, with its transition into Segment III, is of great practical importance when clamping of the aorta is necessary (Fig. 15.6.1d, e). The ascending aorta arises next to the right dorsal aspect of the pulmonary artery. The segment below the origin of the brachiocephalic artery lies within the pericardial sac. The first few centimeters above the valve ring are covered on the right by the right auricle and on the left by a bulge consisting of muscle and epicardial fat tissue and by the pulmonary artery, which can be dissected free down to the level of the orifices of the coronary arteries. In its upward course, the ascending aorta runs somewhat toward the front and slightly to the right. The arch begins just proximal to the cone-shaped take-off of the innominate artery and curves across to the left and somewhat backwards. The convexity of the ascending aorta lies for the most part within the pericardium. It is better exposed by lifting the aorta off the superior vena cava and reflecting it toward the left (Fig. 15.6.3a). This is facilitated by passing a tape around this unvascularized segment after blunt tunneling beneath it. After separation, the ascending aorta may also be partially clamped. Arising from the aortic arch, which runs almost horizontally in a front right to posterior left direction, are its three branches, which can be exposed within the soft tissue of the mediastinum by blunt dissection. The concave surface of the aortic arch sits on top of the right main branch of the pulmonary artery. The pericardium covers the root of the pulmonary artery and of the ascending aorta. A recess is formed at the pericardial fold between the pulmonary artery and the aorta beneath the convexity of the aortic arch. Aneurysms of the descending aorta or of the distal arch may penetrate into this recess. If the recess cannot be held aside when slipping beneath the aortic arch with a curved forceps, the pericardium must be opened at that site, and the back wall of the recess must be penetrated to allow dissection around the aortic arch proximal to the left subclavian artery (Fig. 15.6.1e). The left tracheobronchial angle lies dorsally and to the right of the branching pulmonary artery, close to the proximal portion of the aortic arch at the origin of the innominate artery.

The soft esophagus lies next to the aortic arch to the right of the left subclavian artery. The thoracic duct ascends between the esophagus and the aorta, following the subclavian artery from right to left. The adventitia of the dorsal left curved portion of the descending aorta at the origin of the subclavian artery has fibrous connections to the prevertebral fascia. These fibers must be transected close to the aortic wall at the angle between the subclavian artery and the aorta, which faces the left shoulder (Fig. 15.6.1d, e). Blunt dissection may then be performed close to the aortic wall, giving access to the dorsal and right side of the aortic arch. The thoracic duct, esophagus, and trachea may be retracted. A curved clamp or a finger is inserted under the concavity of the arch from the ventral side and proximal to the ligamentum arteriosum into the pericardial recess (Fig. 15.6.1e). Dissection is continued in this manner until there is a free connection between the ventral and dorsal sides of the aortic arch. Larger arterial branches do not arise from the concavity or dorsal side of the aortic arch.

The bronchial arteries arise from the descending aorta distal to the ligamentum arteriosum. The branches supplying the left main bronchus and the bifurcation branch off ventrally, and the right main bronchus is supplied by vessels coming from the subclavian artery. The first two left intercostal arteries arise from the costocervical trunk, which has its origin at the left subclavian artery. The third intercostal artery branches off some distance away from the origin of the subclavian artery. It runs diagonally in an upward lateral direction, together with the other intercostal arteries, since the aorta does not keep up with the growth of the vertebral segments during its embryonic development [9].

As they branch off from the descending aorta, the intercostal arteries take a more horizontal course. Care must be taken to preserve those branches which are important for adequate blood flow to the vascular network which supplies the spinal artery and shows great variation from individual to individual (see p. 312). A large vein crosses the proximal convexity of the descending aorta from the left side parallel to the arch and connects the ascending hemiazygos vein to the cava system (see p. 16). This branch must be divided and ligated during dissection of the aorta lateral to the left vagus nerve. The respective positions of the left vagus nerve, the recurrent nerve, and the phrenic nerve are of great importance when dissecting on the left side of the aortic arch. The phrenic nerve lies ventrally in front of the pulmonary hilus. It is usually found just beneath the pleura. The vagus nerve curves in a dorsal direction around the aortic arch. It lies dorsolateral to the top portion of the pleura and follows the right anterior margin of the subclavian artery at a deeper level (Fig. 16.5.1d). After the recurrent nerve arises from the vagus nerve, often cranial to the pulmonary hilus, the vagus nerve runs dorsal to the hilum and may be easily identified by lifting the hilus. Its recurrent branch curves around the aorta distal to the ligamentum arteriosum. It can be injured during clamping of the aorta in this region. *The patient should be informed of this possible complication if elective surgery is planned.*

Surgical strategy depends not only on the topographic extent of the aneurysm, but also on its form. One should differentiate between a saccular aneurysm strictly localized to a certain side and a fusiform aneurysm which is usually more extensive. The *saccular type* has an especially high risk of rupture. It can, however, be repaired more easily by partial tangential clamping of the aorta or by bypass grafting if it is located at the aortic arch. In surgery for a *fusiform* aneurysm, complete cross-clamping distally and proximally is necessary for repair of the aortic segment.

The *etiology* of these aneurysms is also of great practical significance. Traumatic and dissecting aneurysms are special. The *traumatic aneurysm* is caused by a localized destruction of the aortic wall (false aneurysm!), owing to a transverse tear just beneath or a few centimeters distal to the origin of the left subclavian artery. The other aortic segments remain unharmed. Patients usually have no symptoms of concomitant arteriosclerotic disease [19]. A *dissecting aneurysm* (see p. 349) results from an acute aortic dissection (primary hemorrhage into the media) leading to dilatation of the remaining mural layers. The dilation may be limited to local aortic segments. The dissection, however, may extend beyond this. During the acute stage of dissection, rupture of the outer wall layer may occur, causing exsanguination. This may happen even before prominent aneurysmal dilatation has developed. The chronic dissecting aneurysm behaves like the fusiform type, e.g., an arteriosclerotic aneurysm. The extension of chronic dissection often remains undiscovered until surgery. It may extend to remote regions of the aorta, and repair may be technically very difficult.

B. Indications for Reconstructive Procedures

The decision whether to perform surgery for reconstruction of a thoracic aortal aneurysm must be made in a timely manner in order to avoid serious complications such as rupture or compression of adjacent structures. Thromboembolic complications are less important in thoracic aneurysms. This fact is probably due to the high flow rate in the aorta. The danger of possible complications must always be weighed against the surgical risk. The surgeon's decision mainly depends on the clinical stage (asymptomatic/symptomatic; penetrating/contained/perforated), the *form* of the aneurysm, and the etiology.

Saccular aneurysms have an especially high risk of rupture. Fusiform arteriosclerotic aneurysms are often seen in elderly patients who have other risk factors. Therefore, the indication for surgery must be considered carefully. As a rule, surgery is indicated only when the aneurysm is very large (at least twice the diameter of the aorta) or has become symptomatic. *False traumatic aneurysms* near the isthmus are always to be corrected, even if they are asymptomatic. Wall calcifications in relatively small traumatic aneurysms and apparent stability in size over a longer observation period should not tempt the surgeon to wait [18, 19]. In an *acute aortic dissection* of the descending aorta, we first recommend conservative therapy with controlled blood pressure reduction and analgesics. If pain cannot be relieved and new clinical or radiologic signs of expansion or penetration develop (chest X-ray, pleural effusion, CT scan), surgery should be performed following exclusion of contraindications [17]. Here, computed tomography using a contrast medium has proven especially valuable as a diagnostic tool; it allows accurate assessment of the enlargement and the extent of penetration.

In *acute dissection* of the thoracic aorta (see p. 351) ischemia of the visceral organs and extremities may develop, owing to obstruction of the true aortic lumen and its arterial branches. In certain circumstances surgery may be urgently indicated; but it is sometimes difficult to decide which method of reconstruction is best: replacement of the thoracic aorta with a prosthesis, establishing a connection between the true and the false lumen at the distal anastomosis, or a fenestration in the abdominal portion of the aorta for the purpose of perfusing both lumina. Abdominal fenestration usually cannot prevent rupture. This operation has therefore become less favored during the last few years. The asymptomatic dissecting aneurysm is treated like an arteriosclerotic aneurym and should be operated on only if rupture is imminent (size) or symptoms (compression) develop (see p. 351).

Traumatic ruptures of the aorta are usually found in the descending aorta at the isthmus, a few centimeters distal to the origin of the left subclavian artery and just below the ligamentum arteriosum (typical location). A high percentage of those patients who experience rare ruptures of the ascending aorta or of the aortic arch die at the scene of the accident and are therefore not encountered in everyday routine trauma management. The transverse rupture of all mural layers produces a pulsating hematoma. If this condition persists for more than 6 weeks, the lesion is called by definition a traumatic aneurysm.

Once traumatic rupture of the aorta has been confirmed, aortic reconstruction is urgently indicated. Fatal rupture into a neighboring hollow organ (pleura, lung, bronchus, esophagus) may happen at any time, even if the patient's condition seems to have stabilized. Signs and symptoms, such as a wide mediastinum, hypertension in the upper limb, and a pressure gradient between the upper and lower extremity, both known as the pseudocoarctation syndrome, must be confirmed by accurate diagnostic methods that have to locate the rupture exactly. In severely traumatized patients with multiple injuries the following priorities of surgical treatment must be considered. Treatment of abdominal and cerebral injuries has priority over reconstruction of the thoracic aorta. Limb injuries may also have priority if vascular trauma with severe hemorrhage or imminent irreversible ischemia is present. The ultimate risk of surgical treatment of a fresh aortic rupture is mainly determined by the severity of concomitant injuries (abdominal and cerebral) [18].

The main risk factor in any procedure done on the descending aorta is beyond doubt coronary heart disease. If there is any evidence of this disease, exact preoperative diagnostic confirmation should be obtained, even if it is necessary to employ coronary angiography. A decision on the necessity of myocardial revascularization must be reached *prior* to reconstruction of the descending aorta as the latter operation sometimes causes considerable strain on the left ventricle. Coronary bypass operations and reconstructions of the descending aorta cannot be performed *in one session* since the surgical approach differs in each procedure. Sometimes, symptomatic aneurysms of the descending aorta that are in great danger of perforation must be repaired before myocardial revascularization can be performed. Cardiopulmonary bypass during coronary surgery otherwise can lead to perforation of such aneurysms (heparinization, retrograde perfusion).

Hemodynamically effective stenoses (Doppler ultrasonography) of the cerebral arteries should be diagnosed and corrected *prior* to the operation on an aneurysm. Aortic surgery often leads to considerable fluctuations in blood pressure during manipulation of the aorta.

C. Positioning

For the left thoracotomy the patient should be in the right lateral position (Fig. 15.6.1a–c). The pelvis is supported posteriorly and a padded belt is tightened around the left hip. In this position, however, neither the femoral nor the iliac artery can be exposed for possible cannulation. If necessary, a different position, such as that for the thoracoabdominal approach must be chosen (see p. 314). The left arm is loosely attached to an arm support (Fig. 15.6.1a, b). If it is placed too high, the elevated left shoulder blade might be in the way. Changing the position of the operating table can lead to overstretching of the muscles or nerves at the shoulder. A small pad is put under the right armpit to prevent compression injuries of the right arm plexus. Another support should be placed behind the neck for better stabilization and to ease tension on the left arm. This is especially recommended if the entire table is rotated to the left.

D. Surgical Approach

The entire descending aorta and the aortic arch are best exposed by a wide thoracotomy in the fourth or fifth left interspace (Fig. 15.6.1c). The skin incision is directed around the caudal margin of the shoulder blade (Fig. 15.6.1a). A short indentation of the latissimus dorsi is performed in its caudal portion, and the serratus anterior is divided as far caudally as possible in order not to impair vascular and nerve supply from above. The intercostal muscles are divided electrically at the upper margin of the rib. To obtain better exposure, both ribs, which are spread apart, can be divided dorsally with rib cutters. If necessary, the lower rib may be divided ventrally at the junction between bone and cartilage. Step-by-step expansion of the rib spreader permits good exposure of the entire thoracic aorta.

For even better visualization of the aorta from the left side, the left lung is cut off from mechanical ventilation and is allowed to become atelectatic. To accomplish this, the patient must be intubated with a double-lumen endotracheal tube prior to surgery. This method of ventilation does not lead to a drop in pO_2 below the critical level which may result from a shunt in the unventilated lung. Should this condition occur, however, the main stem of the pulmonary artery may be temporarily occluded with a straight vascular clamp or a bulldog clamp.

For better exposure of the aortic arch and the descending aorta, a lateral thoracotomy can be extended by means of an upper sternotomy. To perform a modified bypass procedure, it often suffices to clamp the intrapericardially exposed ascending aorta tangentially. A lateral thoracotomy usually allows sufficient exposure for this maneuver as the ascending aorta, curving upward, can be pulled toward the left into the clamp (see Fig. 15.6.3a).

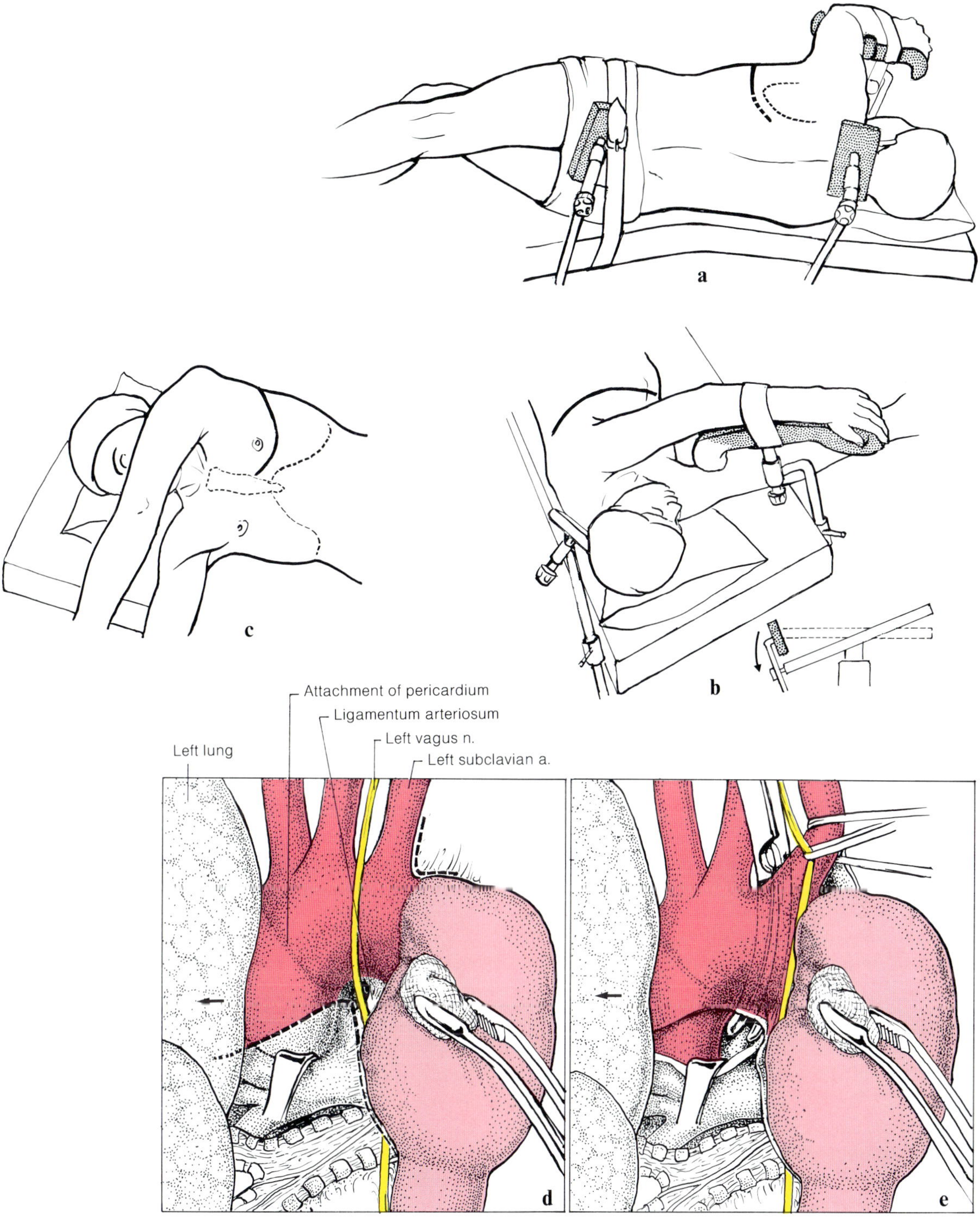

Fig. 15.6.1 a–e. Position and anatomy during repair of an aortic aneurysm located in segment III. **a–c** Patient positioned on the right side. **d–e** Anatomy of an aneurysm located in segment III (typical location). Because the aneurysm lies close to the left subclavian artery, the aorta is dissected free within the segment of the arch

E. Surgical Procedures

I. Exposure of an Aneurysm of the Descending Aorta

The lung is wrapped in a moist towel and reflected downward and to the right without compressing the heart. Exposure of the aorta distal to the aneurysm is usually easy and is therefore done first. Following longitudinal incision of the mediastinal pleura, the aorta is dissected free by blunt circumferential dissection, and tapes are passed around it. The intercostal arteries are identified and temporarily occluded by tourniquets consisting of thick, soaked catgut. Permanent occlusion is achieved by using clips. Both maneuvers are necessary to prevent strong hemorrhage from the tributaries following division of the aneurysm (Fig. 15.6.2a–d). Dissection at the distal portion of the aortic arch proximal to the aneurysm is then begun. This part of the operation may lead to dangerous complications. After passing tapes around the phrenic nerve and the left subclavian artery, the mediastinal pleura is incised above the upper portion of the descending aorta. The communicating branch of the azygos vein is clamped and divided. While staying close to the lung hilum, the aortic arch is approached from below. This exposes the ligamentum arteriosum and the vagus nerve, which lies a little caudad and dorsal to the ligament. The ligamentum arteriosum is carefully transected. Both ends can be sutured. The concave margin of the aortic arch is reached from below, while holding the pericardial recess away from the arch. If this is impossible, owing to penetration of the pericardial recess by the aneurysmal sac, the pericardium is opened at the recess and perforated further proximally between the aortic arch and the pulmonary artery (Fig. 15.6.1e). Then dissection is continued, starting at the angle distal to the origin of the subclavian artery and keeping close to the aortic wall, or one may begin above, between the subclavian artery and the left common carotid artery, and proceed downward and to the right until free passage is possible beneath the aortic arch in a proximal direction (Fig. 15.6.1e). No arterial branches arise in this area. A tape is passed beneath the aortic arch, between the left common carotid artery and the subclavian artery, and then a second tape is placed around the aortic arch distal to the left subclavian artery at the angle between the subclavian artery and the descending aorta. If a lusorial artery exists distal to the left subclavian artery, it is dissected free, and a tape is passed around it. It can then be easily occluded with a vascular clamp.

The same technique of dissection is used with traumatic ruptures of the descending aorta (typical location). The mediastinal pleura covering the aortic defect is left intact as long as possible. Exact identification of the defect is sometimes difficult owing to the large hematoma along the entire aortic wall.

After a short segment of the distal descending aorta has been exposed, so that cross-clamping is possible at any time, a tape should be passed around the left subclavian artery, which can be identified at the uppermost margin of the pleura. From there, the aortic arch is exposed proximally and a tape is also passed around it, as described earlier. This permits clamping in case of free rupture of a pulsating hematoma.

II. Clamping of the Aorta and Opening of the Aneurysm

The tapes passed around the aortic arch make clamping of the aorta easier to accomplish. Clamping may, however, be performed in an emergency without passing tapes around the arch. Strong clamps should be used proximally since high pressures may develop following occlusion. The branches of a clamp may be forced apart by the increased pressure. This may be prevented by applying a second clamp with the same shape as the first one. Clamping should be performed slowly to give the anesthesiologist time to compensate an excessive rise in blood pressure with appropriate vasodilators (see p. 199) [8]. The proximal clamp should be applied distal to the left subclavian artery. If this is not possible, the aortic arch can be clamped temporarily. The clamp should then be repositioned distal to the left subclavian artery as soon as possible, thus restoring perfusion to the collaterals arising from the left subclavian artery. The use of a clamp with only a slight curvature (Fig. 15.6.2a, e, g) does not afford the best view of the back wall of the proximal aortic stump, and, as a result, a wedge-shaped "gusset" may be created there (Fig. 15.6.2g). A right-angled vascular clamp facilitates transverse occlusion and affords better visibility, but it is also more difficult to place. A longitudinal incision is made in the midline of the aneurysm. Material found inside is sucked out, and the internal aneurysmal wall

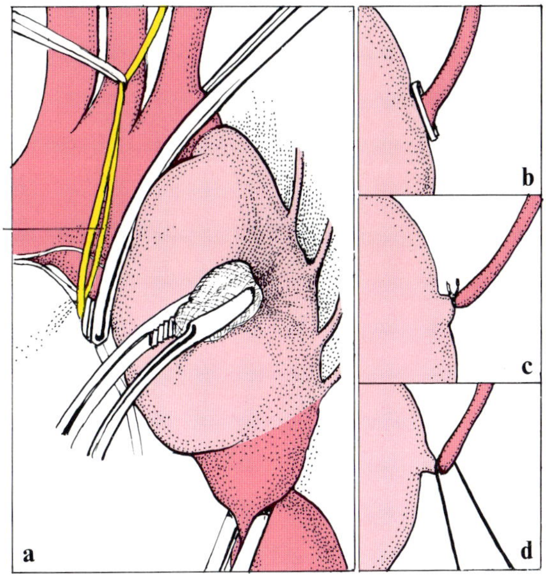

Fig. 15.6.2a–h. Exposure and opening of the aneurysm. **a** Proximal and distal clamping; mobilization of the aneurysm exposes the origin of the intercostal arteries. **b–d** Occlusion of an intercostal artery with a clip, ligature, and tape. **e** Evacuation of material from within the aneurysm; both wings of the incision are depicted. **f** Control of back-bleeding from an intercostal artery by transluminal transfixion suture. **g** Opened aneurysm prior to interposition of a prosthesis. **h** Proximal clamping with a transversely applied right-angled aortic clamp: the clamp is harder to put in place; the view of the back wall of the aorta is better

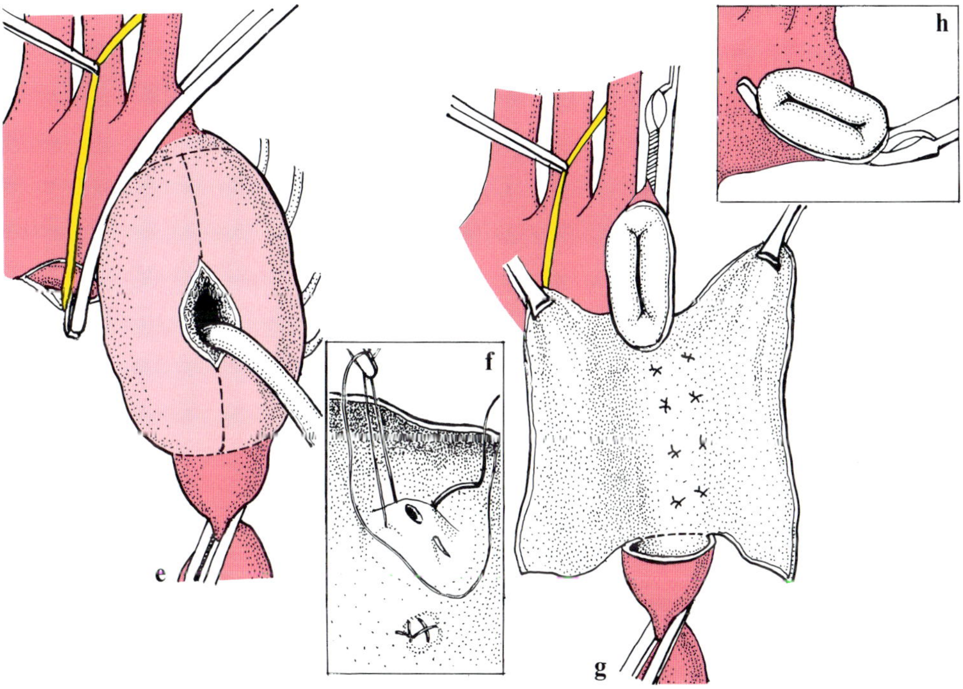

surface is inspected. The aortotomy may be kept small at first in order to evaluate the internal mural surface and to save parts of the wall that could be used for reconstruction (Fig. 15.6.2e). This is especially important in traumatic aneurysms with transverse tears in which the remaining aortic stumps have not been separated too far. The opening is then enlarged under direct vision (Fig. 15.6.2e). Back bleeding from intercostal arteries is controlled by transluminal sutures of 3–0 Mersilene (Fig. 15.6.2f). Blood loss from intercostal arteries during division of large aneurysms may be reduced by identifying these arteries as they run toward the left side of the aortic wall and ligating them at their origins (Fig. 15.6.2b, c, d). One can also place an additional clamp over the aneurysm. The clamp is then moved step-by-step to a more distal portion of the aneurysmal sac following suture of the intercostal orifices along the proximal back wall of the aneurysm. The intercostal arteries,

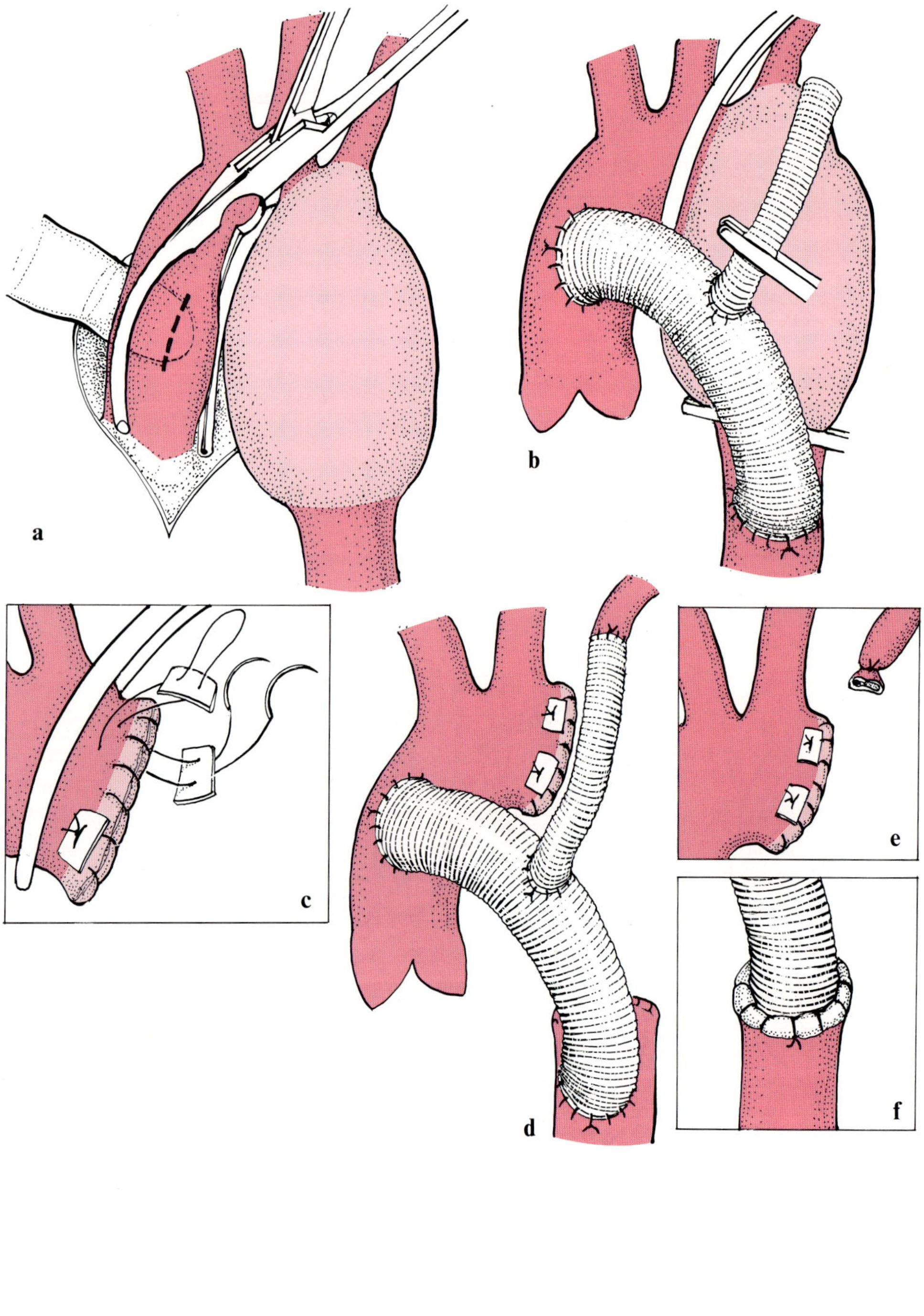

Fig. 15.6.3a–f. Atypical surgical technique in an aneurysm extending far upward. **a** A prosthetic bypass graft is constructed from the ascending aorta to the descending aorta before the aortic arch is occluded. The portion of the ascending aorta lying intrapericardially is slightly lifted forward by a finger inserted behind it and manipulated in between the branches of the clamp. **b** Situation after construction of the ascending-descending bypass; the connection of the left subclavian artery to the graft has been constructed beforehand. **c** Double, firmly anchored suture of the proximal aortic stump, the anastomosis secured by mattress sutures reinforced with Teflon pledgets. **d** Situation following resection of the aneurysm and revascularization of the left subclavian artery. **e** Total ligation of the subclavian artery is a poor alternative. **f** End-to-end suture of the distal anastomosis is possible

which are located deeper, can then also be sutured. Semicircular inicisions are made at the proximal and distal margin of the aortotomy. This produces two aortic stumps which can be anastomosed to both ends of the graft. Enough wall must be left behind to ensure adequate anchorage and tightness of the suture line (Fig. 15.6.2g).

In traumatic rupture of the aorta, the pulsating hematoma should be evacuated through a small stab incision in the adventitia following clamping of the aorta. Dissection of surrounding mediastinal and adventitial tissue should be the minimum necessary to achieve adequate exposure of the torn edges of the aortic wall without inflicting any further disputive damage. In this way, the margins of the tear are carefully preserved for possible direct suture.

F. Intraoperative Measures

Clamping the thoracic aorta only a short distance away from the heart produces strain on the left ventricle and can lead to cardiac failure or to ischemia of the lower half of the body. Renal failure is usually reversible. However, serious spinal cord ischemia occurs in 3%–6% regardless of the methods of protection employed (see p. 361) [2, 5, 6, 8, 10, 11, 15, 17].

I. Simple Clamping

In simple clamping of the thoracic aorta, easily controllable vasodilators are administered to counteract an excessive rise in afterload. Sodium nitroprusside is the best substance for this purpose. Blood pressure proximal to the clamp should be reduced, keeping it above normal values since collateral blood flow passively follows the pressure gradient existing between the proximal and distal portions of the body. *Hypovolemia* must be avoided, though it is difficult to detect during administration of vasodilators. It leads to a reduction in cardiac output, resulting in inadequate perfusion of organs lying distal to the clamp. Cardiac performance is best monitored by a balloon-tipped, flow-directed pulmonary artery catheter with registration of left ventricular filling pressure and cardiac output. With optimal anesthesia and volume input, the cardiac output will even increase during the clamping phase [18].

Regional and systemic heparinization is usually not necessary. Nitroglycerin can lead to a reduction of cardiac output since the doses needed to lower blood pressure are so high that they also lead to a *reduction* in preload. Administration of the vasodilator must be started a few minutes before clamping and stopped at the right time prior to declamping [18].

II. Temporary External Shunt
(Fig. 15.6.4 and 15.6.5)

A frequent alternative to simple clamping is the use of a temporary external shunt made of heparin-covered tubing [11]. Cannulation is performed proximal to the designated clamping site on the ascending aorta or aortic arch, distal descending aorta, iliac artery, or femoral artery. A two-row purse-string suture is constructed at the aorta by superficial, tangential sewing, using 2–0 woven Mersilene suture and an atraumatic needle. Each suture is pulled through a rubber tube (tourniquet). An appropriately large longitudinal stab incision is made in the center of the purse string sutures and held by finger pressure while a cannula is quickly inserted. The tourniquet is pulled tight and held in position with a clamp (Fig. 15.6.4c). The cannula is tied to the tourniquet with one or two ligatures (Fig. 15.6.4a). The tube is vented through a side arm (Fig. 15.6.4a). Systemic heparinization is not necessary. Distal cannulation of the aorta is performed in the same manner or retrograde via the iliac artery or femoral artery. To remove the cannula (Fig. 15.6.4d–f), the aortic wall and the cannula are grasped with a curved vascular clamp. After quick removal of the cannula, the clamp is closed gently to avoid intimal tears or plaque dislodgement. A second clamp with the same curvature should be held in reserve and, if necessary, used to obtain more surface area for closure of the small aortotomy, which is done by continuous over-and-over suture with monofilament 3–0 or 4–0 polypropylene suture material. The suture line may be constructed in two rows, going back and forth. An alternative, which is not safe, however, is to close the arteriotomy by pulling the purse string sutures tight and oversewing the incision with a monofilament suture.

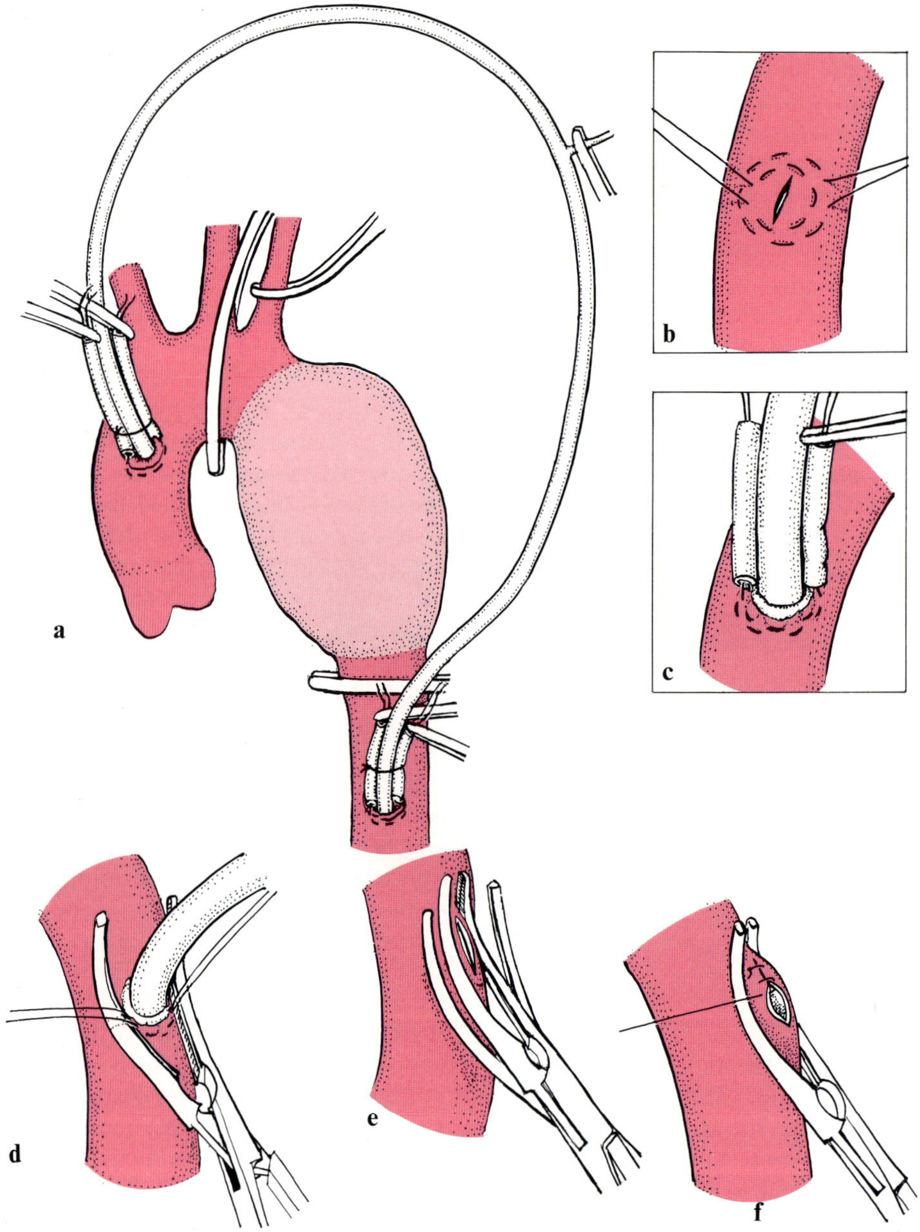

Fig. 15.6.4a–f. Construction of a temporary external shunt. **a** Shunt inserted and aorta clamped. **b** Two-row purse-string suture. **c** Tourniquets prevent leakage after introduction of the shunt. **d** Decannulation of the aorta. **e** If the first clamp slips a little, a second one can be placed beneath it. **f** Closure of the arteriotomy with a continuous suture

III. Temporary Internal Shunt

If an internal shunt of large caliber is used, the vascular prosthesis must be slipped over the cannula. The application of this method is rarely reported. It is a very difficult shunt technique and may lead to embolization near the branches of the aortic arch. Furthermore, the cannula is in the way during construction of the anastomoses. We have not found any advantages in the use of an internal shunt and therefore cannot recommend it.

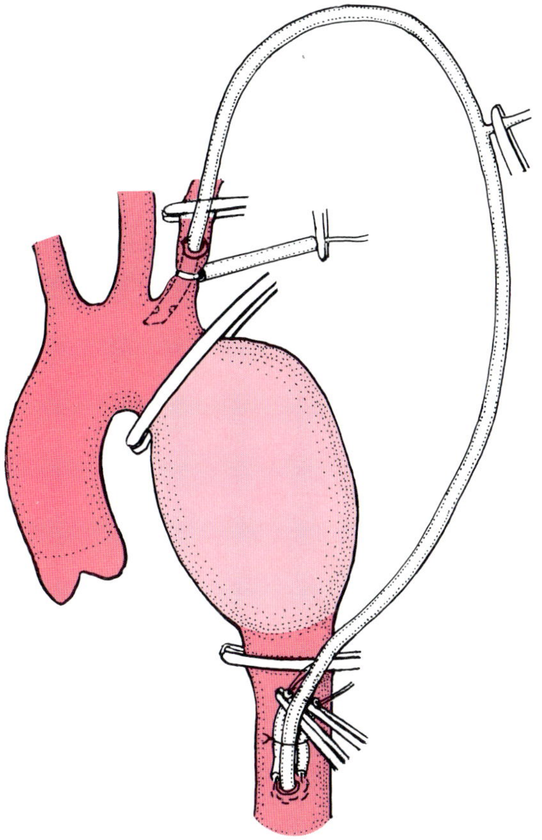

Fig. 15.6.5. A possible alternative: a temporary external shunt from the left subclavian artery to the descending aorta

IV. Left Heart Bypass

A bypass extending from the left atrium to the femoral artery was once the most commonly used method of protection (see "Manual of Cardiovascular Surgery"). An oxygenator positioned in between is not necessary. The patient must be heparinized, and this has several disadvantages (higher rate of bleeding complications, hemorrhage into the lung). The flow rate should be kept at 1–2 l/min. Correct regulation of flow and adaptation to the momentary hemodynamic situation of the patient frequently causes difficulties, even for experienced cardiotechnicians; this is especially true when disturbances of cardiac performance are present [9]. Other types of bypass procedure are also applied successfully, e.g., femorofemoral bypass with or without an oxygenator; however, these procedures will not be discussed here.

Pressure registration in the femoral artery or the evaluation of somatosensory cortical-evoked potentials as a parameter for the functional state of the spinal cord have been used to monitor and maintain adequate blood flow to the clamping site. These procedures have not established themselves as routine in clinical practice and therefore cannot be recommended [2, 5, 10, 15].

Alongside measures employed to guarantee adequate spinal cord perfusion, proven methods for saving donor blood, both in elective and emergency surgery, deserve to be mentioned:

(a) In younger patients without cardiac disease (traumatic aneurysm, aortic rupture), *isovolemic hemodilution* is possible. An experienced anesthesiologist will perform isovolemic hemodilution, especially in emergency situations, until units of whole blood (warm, fresh blood) arrive. Blood units are not taken preoperatively. Blood losses are substituted with up to 1000 ml dextran or hydroxyethyl starch. Afterward, a surplus of albumin and crystalloid solutions are infused. Improvement of microcirculation also intensifies collateral circulation beyond the clamping site.

(b) Constant suction in the operative field removes even clotted blood and transports it to a prepared reservoir, where the blood is recycled in the cell saver to yield high-grade washed erythrocyte concentrates; 80% of all erythrocytes may be returned to the body. Clotting factors must be given separately.

Use of the cell saver is generally recommended, sometimes even in combination with hemodilution. One must always keep within the required limits (coronary reserve). No systemic heparinization is necessary while using the cell saver.

While performing left heart bypass or other forms of pump bypass requiring heparinization, extravasated blood can be transported to a reservoir by separate suction pumps and then returned to the circulatory system.

We no longer use the Bentley pump. Disadvantages are the necessity of full systemic heparinization and the poor quality of retransfused blood.

G. Reconstructive Techniques

I. Direct Suture

Direct suture of the thoracic aorta is possible following resection of a *saccular* aneurysm only if the aorta can be clamped tangentially with an appropriately shaped clamp. The wide margin at the base of the aneurysm should be preserved for firm anchorage of the broad continuous suture. 3–0 monofilament polypropylene is preferred for a double continuous over-and-over suture (Fig. 15.6.4f; oversewing of the aortic cannulation site). *Direct suture* is also possible in traumatic rupture of the aorta even if several days have intervened (Fig. 15.6.6d and 15.6.9). Only seldom can it be performed in a traumatic aneurysm [18].

Direct suture is easier if the aorta has not been disrupted over its entire circumference and the torn edges are therefore not too far apart. If the torn edges are difficult to visualize, one should not hesitate to convert a partial rupture into a complete circumferential rupture by a snip of the scissors (Fig. 15.6.9a). Total transection permits a clear view during suture. But here, the assistant performs a very crucial maneuver: the two aortal stumps, which tend to retract because of their elasticity, must be precisely approximated to one another and thus held in place until the first stitches of the back wall have been placed. 3–0, or in younger patients 4–0 polypropylene suture material is used for continuous over-and-over suture of the defect, which should catch as much of the surrounding adventitial tissue as possible. If these smooth double-needle sutures are used, no initial knot must be tied. The margins of the back wall are sewn first with an over-and-over suture on the inside and then adapted by gently pulling on the elastic suture (Fig. 15.6.9b–d). The entire suture line has only one knot which must be tied five to seven times because of the smoothness of the suture (Fig. 15.6.9e). Before completing the last stiches, retrograde and anterograde flow must be checked, as always (flush). Venting of the suture area is not necessary. Thrombosis is unlikely.

II. Closure with a Prosthetic Patch (Fig. 15.6.6)

If a partial mural defect of the aorta remains following resection of a saccular aneurysm, and it cannot be repaired by direct suture, the defect can be closed with a tailored patch of knitted Dacron velour material. Only saccular aneurysms with a relatively narrow base or traumatic aneurysms with smaller partial circumferential wall tears are repaired in such a way (Fig. 15.6.6a). To obtain a better view of the defect which is too large for direct suture, clamping proximal and distal to the aneurysm is necessary. To prevent leakage and to anchor the patch firmly, its margin should be pulled into the lumen so that it tightly caps off the hole from the inside. The aortic wall bulges over the border of the patch, of which only small bites are taken during each stitch (Fig. 15.6.6b, c). We prefer woven 3–0 Dacron sutures in Dacron prostheses; the sutures guarantee permanent and firm anchorage since they are incorporated into the surrounding tissues. Before completing the suture, retrograde and anterograde flow are checked (flush). Venting of the area is not necessary; thrombosis is unlikely.

Fig. 15.6.6a–d. Reconstruction of the aorta following rupture in segment III (typical location). **a** Exposure of the defect. **b** Suture of the Dacron patch. **c** Situation following closure with a Dacron patch. **d** A fresh rupture can also be repaired by direct suture of the aortic wall

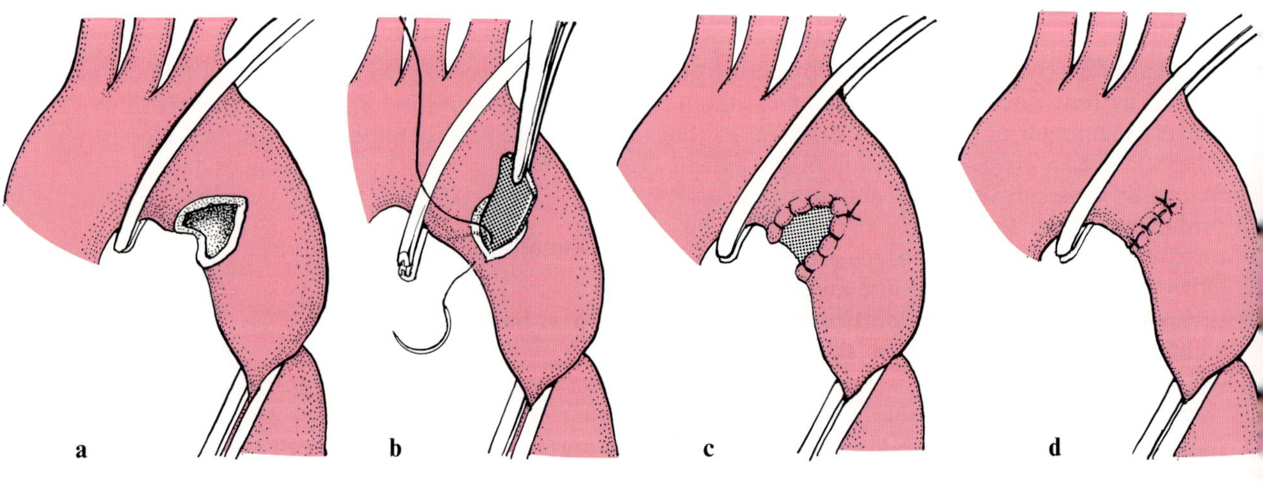

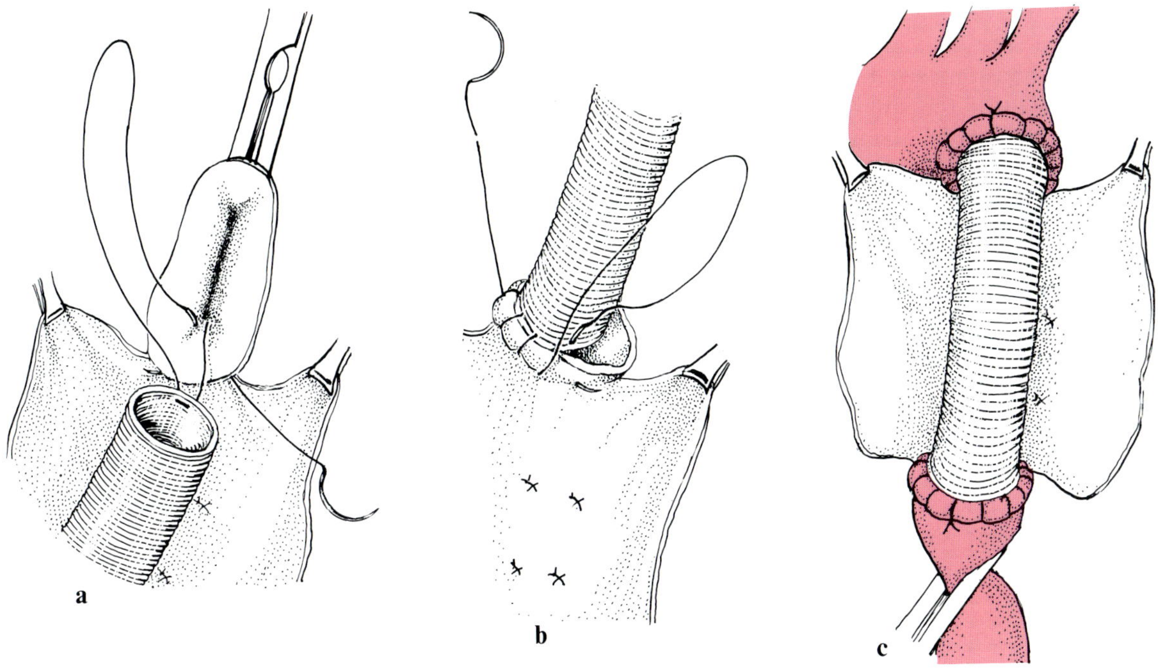

III. Interposition of a Prosthesis (Fig. 15.6.7)

The most common method of reconstruction in fusiform aortic aneurysms is interposition of a prosthesis. A woven Dacron graft is recommended in elderly patients (arteriosclerotic aneurysms) or poor risk patients (aneurysmal rupture, imminent clotting defect). This prosthesis is leak proof from the beginning. The late results are just as good as in porous knitted or knitted velour prostheses since there is always a high flow rate through the graft. We prefer Dacron velour only in younger patients (traumatic aneurysm, aortic rupture) as it quickly becomes impermeable at high flow rates. The caliber of the prosthesis should not be too large, so that it may be slightly pulled into the intact aortic stumps telescopically during suture (Fig. 15.6.7c).

After division of the aneurysmal sac and semicircular transverse incision at both aortic stumps, the sac is tailored. Enough wall material must be left to allow the edges of the aortic stumps to be pulled over the margins of the prosthesis by tightening the carefully placed sutures. The bulging aortic margins thus produced seal the anastomosis and guarantee safer anchorage of the prosthesis (Fig. 15.6.7a, b). In traumatic aneurysms with total circumferential disruption of the aorta, both stumps often retract and recoil into the aneurys-

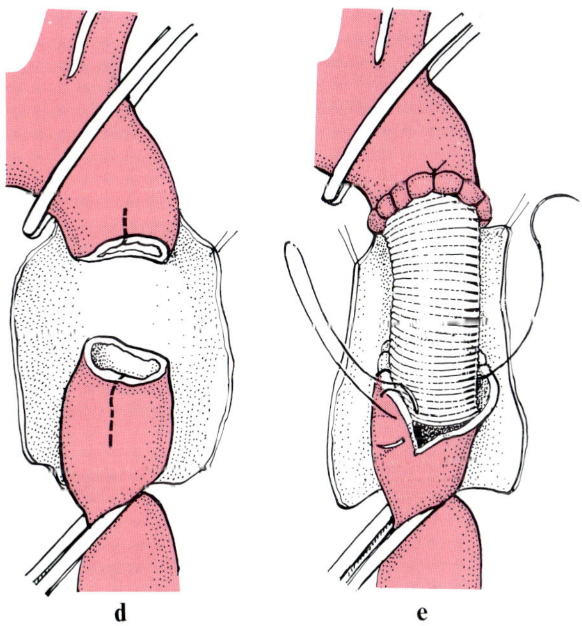

Fig. 15.6.7a–e. Interposition of a tube prosthesis. **a** Proximal end-to-end anastomosis using a double needle. **b** For secure suture of the aortic back wall the distal end of the prosthesis may be elevated. **c** Interposed tube prosthesis; the lateral walls are partially resected and continuously sutured over the prosthesis. **d** If the ruptured margins are retracted, the orifices are enlarged by longitudinal incision of the anterior wall. **e** Suture of the graft

mal sac. To avoid stenosis at the suture line, and to achieve a better view and more space for the telescopic anastomosis, it is advisable to incise the anterior wall of the stumps, spread them apart, and sew the aortic margins over the prosthesis (which can be slightly beveled at its edges) (Fig. 15.6.7d, e). After completing the anastomosis, the prosthesis is clamped, and the suture line is checked for leakage by briefly opening the distal aortic clamp. Especially the back wall of the anastomosis must be examined since it is not accessible later on. If an aneurysm begins just below the subclavian artery and the aorta is clamped just distal to this artery, sometimes only a very narrow aortic margin is available for suturing. Since the suture is supposed to catch large bites of the aortic wall, the clamp must in this case be placed proximal to the subclavian artery while the upper anastomosis is being sutured (Figs. 15.6.1e and 15.6.3b). The subclavian artery must be clamped separately. After completing the proximal anastomosis, the clamp is repositioned distal to the subclavian artery in order to restore blood flow to this vessel, which is important for the perfusion of collaterals supplying the lower half of the body. If a lusorial artery arises distal to the origin of the left subclavian artery, this vessel is often difficult to expose and to clamp behind a large aneurysm. Under such circumstances, the orifice of the artery can be blocked with a balloon catheter (Fogarty catheter) following opening of the aneurysmal sac. Back bleeding can be prevented while the anastomosis just distal to the orifice is being constructed. If necessary, the catheter must be inserted through the lumen of the prosthesis. After checking for leaks, the aortic clamp is transferred to the prosthesis, restoring blood flow to the subclavian artery. While performing the distal anastomosis, the intercostal arteries may be spared by placing the clamp very obliquely or, even better, by using a right-angled aortic clamp, leaving enough of the anterior wall exposed, but occluding the back wall orifices of these arteries. The beveled prosthesis can then be sutured to the opening. A larger portion of the well-preserved back wall remains. We prefer woven 3–0 Dacron sutures which guarantee permanent anchorage by firm incorporation into the surrounding tissues.

IV. Intraluminal Interposition Graft (Fig. 15.6.8)

To make anastomosis of thoracic aneurysms easier, an alternative method has been developed. Tapes are passed around the aorta proximal and distal to the aneurysm. The aorta is then clamped. The aneurysm is opened by a longitudinal incision.

Fig. 15.6.8a–d. Intraluminal interposition of a prosthesis. **a** Aneurysm located further distally in segment III. **b** The prepared intraluminal prosthesis is introduced; tapes have been previously placed around the aorta. **c** The intraluminal prosthesis is placed in the correct position; the tape is tied proximally, sealing off the prosthesis; a tape is put in place for distal attachment of the prosthesis. **d** After typing both tapes, the aneurysmal sac is closed around the prosthesis

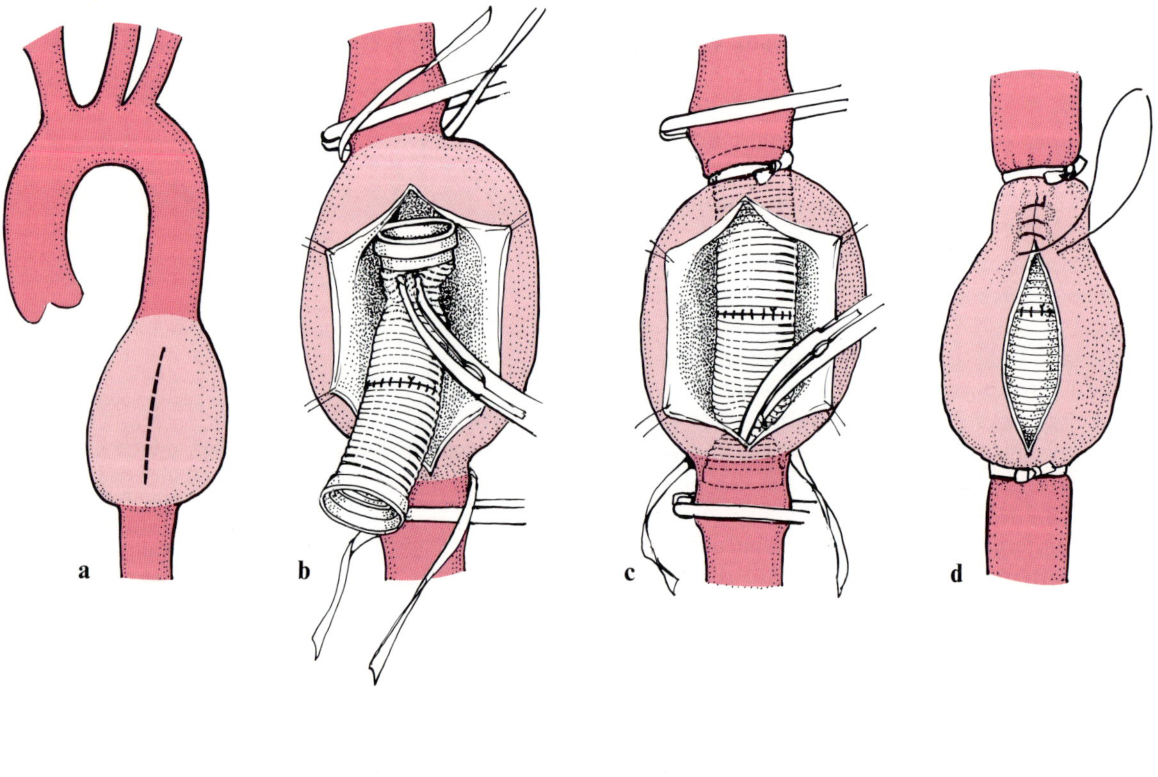

A Dacron prosthesis with Dacron-covered rigid rings at both ends is put in place. The tapes are tied over the rings and tightened around the grooves under the rim of these rings. This seals the anastomosis completely. The aneurysmal sac is then securely sutured over the prosthesis. This technique shows good long-term results, but has not yet gained overall acceptance. It has many advantages in surgical treatment of acute dissection, in which the tissue is very fragile and difficult to sew. A disadvantage is that the anastomosis must be adapted to the preformed manufactured prosthesis. This is very difficult in view of the great variability in the forms of aneurysms (Fig. 15.6.8a–c) [1, 2].

Successful *transfemoral endoluminal implantations* of prostheses have been reported recently. They closely adapt themselves to the healthy aortic wall and securely seal the aneurysmal wall. This very interesting procedure has not yet been tested on a broad clinical scale.

V. Bypass Grafting (Fig. 15.6.3)

If clamping of the aorta and interposition of a prosthesis is not possible or too dangerous, a prosthetic bypass graft may be constructed following partial clamping of the healthy proximal and distal aorta. An end-to-side anastomosis is performed at each end of the graft The aneurysm is then clamped step by step, and a portion of its wall is resected. Aortic stumps are oversewn twice, always taking big bites of the aortic wall. Such closure may be reinforced or sealed even tighter by mattress sutures under which small prosthetic strips are placed to keep the sutures from cutting through the aortic tissue at the suture line (Fig. 15.6.3c, d) [7, 18].

Larger arteries, such as the left subclavian artery, may be implanted into the synthetic bypass graft via prosthetic interpositions (Fig. 15.6.3d). This technique may be modified by constructing a distal end-to-end anastomosis (Fig. 15.6.3d, f). For example, in a large aneurysm situated just distal to the origin of the left subclavian artery, the first step is to anastomose a bypass graft in an end-to-side fashion to the ascending aorta using a left thoracic approach. The descending aorta is clamped just above the diaphragm, divided, and an oblique distal anastomosis performed just as described on p. 336 (Fig. 15.6.3f). The aneurysm is then clamped step by step, starting at its distal end, moving in the direction of the left subclavian artery. This maneuver, which obliterates the aorta, may be extended even proximal to the left subclavian artery, if necessary. The subclavian artery is connected via an interposition graft to the aortic bypass graft (Fig. 15.6.3e, b). The synthetic prosthesis recommended for such reconstructions should be of woven Dacron and have a diameter of 18–22 mm. The suture material usually preferred is 3–0 braided Dacron for the anastomosis and 2–0 Dacron for oversewing of the aorta.

H. Complications

I. Preoperative Complications

1. Compression of the Left Main Bronchus (and of the Trachea)

An aortic aneurysm can cause compression of the bronchial system with recurrent pneumonia. Surgical intervention to eliminate the aneurysm relieves arterial pressure against the bronchial wall and with it, in most cases, the cause of the compression. The affected wall segment of the bronchial system may consolidate. In rare cases, severe chondromalacia may necessitate resection of a portion of the bronchus. If a peripheral lung segment has been destroyed by chronic infection, it should be resected.

2. Perforation of the Aneurysm

Perforation of an aortic aneurysm is fatal unless thrombi temporarily cover the defect and there is enough time to prepare the patient for emergency surgery. Hemorrhage into the mediastinum, pleura, lung, or hollow organs like the trachea, left bronchus, or esophagus may occur. In rare cases, blood coming from a perforated aneurysm in segment III may reach the pericardial recess between the aortic arch and the pulmonary artery and produce cardiac tamponade. The cardinal symptoms (hemothorax, hematemesis, hemoptysis) always dictate further diagnostic evaluation of the patient (endoscopy, angiography, CT). The bleeding site is not always found during these examinations because the site of hemorrhage may be temporarily covered by tissue. Such a finding, however, should not mislead the investigator to underestimate the need for urgent surgical intervention. Under certain circumstances, the surgeon

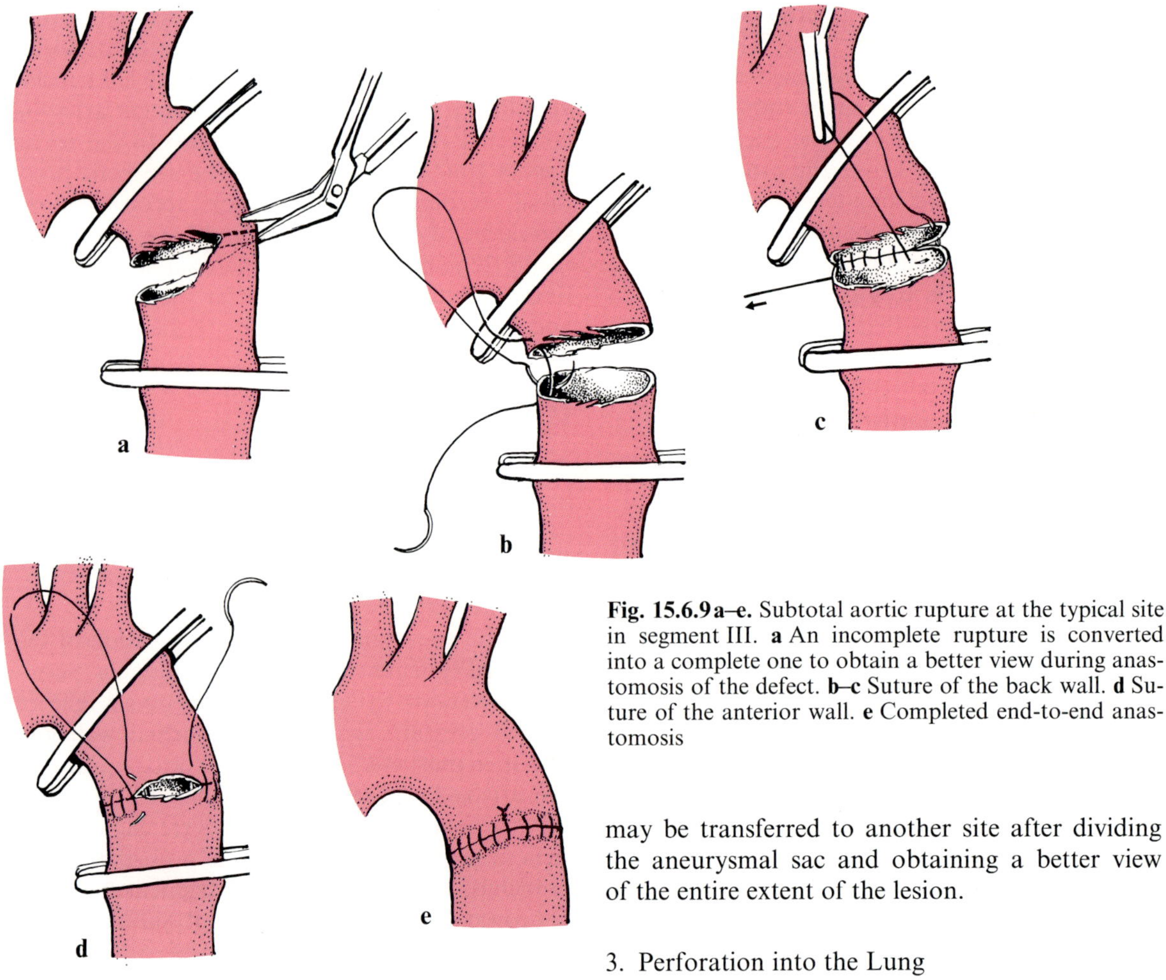

Fig. 15.6.9 a–e. Subtotal aortic rupture at the typical site in segment III. **a** An incomplete rupture is converted into a complete one to obtain a better view during anastomosis of the defect. **b–c** Suture of the back wall. **d** Suture of the anterior wall. **e** Completed end-to-end anastomosis

may have to operate without knowing the exact site of the perforation. If the patient's clinical condition is stable enough, diagnostic measures (angio-CT, angiography) should at least locate the aneurysm and evaluate its dimensions, indicating the most probable site of perforation. This information facilitates the choice of surgical approach. The view of the area surrounding the perforation is often obstructed by the hematoma or by proliferated connective tissue. The aorta should be exposed at a site distant from the perforation so that it can be clamped in an emergency. This can even be done without passing tapes or rubber tubing around the aorta. If a large hematoma surrounds the aorta, lifting the connective tissue off the aortic wall, digital dissection is the quickest and least traumatic method of exposure under such emergency conditions. The aorta is compressed with the fingers and temporarily clamped. Reconstruction is performed as described earlier. The clamps may be transferred to another site after dividing the aneurysmal sac and obtaining a better view of the entire extent of the lesion.

3. Perforation into the Lung

Perforation into the parenchyma of the lung with subsequent hemorrhage may make lung resection necessary (atypical partial resection, lobectomy). Segmental resections are technically more difficult and therefore cannot be recommended in emergency situations.

4. Perforation into a Bronchus

Bronchial defects are excised and closed using absorbable, interrupted, all-layer suture (Dexon or Vicryl, sizes 2–0 or 3–0). If portions of the lung have been destroyed by chronic obstruction and infiltration peripheral to the site of perforation, appropriate resection is recommended [8].

5. Perforation into the Esophagus

Perforations into the esophagus occur in 10% of all fatal ruptures of thoracic aortic aneurysms and are a special challenge for the vascular surgeon.

First of all, it must always be presumed that the wall of the aneurysm is contaminated. Secondly, a two-row suture of the esophageal defect with coverage by a pedicled pleural flap is often unsuccessful. The aneurysmal wall should be totally resected, except its back wall, to prevent retention of infected fluid around the prosthesis. Sometimes, one must even consider removing the esophagus. If the patient is in poor clinical condition, the esophagus is drained at the neck and divided at the cardioesophageal junction. A jejunostomy with insertion of a feeding tube is constructed to preserve the stomach for reconstruction later on. If the patient is in good clinical condition, the stomach may be pulled up and anastomosed to the esophagus above the aortic arch, with preservation of the gastroepiploic vessels, during the same operation. The operative field is flushed several times. Orthotopic reconstruction is preferred during primary surgery, just as in surgery of an aortoduodenal fistula. An extra-anatomic bypass is too complicated. Primary orthotopic reconstruction does not have an increased risk of infection. An extra-anatomic procedure (bypass grafting from the ascending aorta to the abdominal aorta with subsequent removal of the descending aortic prosthesis and closure of the aortic stumps) is reserved for infections that may develop during the postoperative course (see p. 549) [16].

II. Intraoperative Complications

Stenosis at the suture line may occur after repair of a traumatic aneurysm with rolled up, fibrotic aortic margins if the aneurysmal wall is not incised longitudinally at its anterior aspect (Fig. 15.6.7d). Stenosis is recognized by weak pulsation distal to the anastomosis and by a palpable thrill. A slight thrill and systolic gradients of up to 20–30 mmHg may be tolerated. They often disappear during the postoperative course. If higher pressure gradients are encountered, the anastomosis must be made by incising the aorta longitudinally. An alternative is to construct a bypass between the left subclavian artery and the distal aorta using an 8–10 mm prosthetic graft with end-to-side anastomosis at both ends. This method avoids having to cross-clamp the aorta a second time. Formation of thrombi within the aorta distal to the clamp is unlikely. A brief unclamping before completing the last stitches of the anastomosis flushes out thrombi lodged within the aorta.

III. Postoperative Complications

Postoperative hemorrhage requiring surgical reintervention may be recognized by blood constantly coming out of the large chest drainage tubes (Charrier 28–32). If the drains do not indicate blood loss from the chest and hemorrhage is still *suspected* (loss of volume), it is advisable to take a chest X-ray during the first few hours following surgery; this will quickly detect a hemothorax. Immediate reintervention should not be delayed! Bleeding usually comes from injured intercostal arteries, from the plane of dissection around the aneurysm, or from the partially resected aneurysmal wall.

Postoperative thrombotic occlusions need not be feared since there is always a high flow rate in the aorta.

At the end of the operation, the peripheral pulses are checked and the limbs inspected for evidence of thromboembolism; this step is absolutely mandatory.

REFERENCES

1. Berger RL, Romero L, Chaudhry AG, Dobnik DB (1983) Graft replacement of the thoracic aorta with a sutureless technique. Ann Thorac Surg 35:231–239
2. Coles JG, Wilson GJ, Sima AF, Klement P, Tait GA (1982) Intraoperative detection of spinal cord ischemia using somato-sensory cortical evoked potentials during thoracic aortic occlusion. Ann Thorac Surg 34:299–306
3. Crawford ES, Vaccaro PS (1982) Aneurysms of the transverse aortic arch. In: Bergan GJ, Yao JST (eds) Aneurysms, diagnosis and treatment. Grune and Stratton, New York, pp 131–150
4. Crawford ES, Snyder DM (1983) Treatment of aneurysms of the aortic arch. J Thorac Cardiovasc Surg 85:237–246
5. Cummingham JN, Laschinger JC, Merkin HA, Nathan JM, Colvin J, Ransohoff J, Spencer FC (1982) Measurement of spinal cord ischemia during operations upon the thoracic aorta. Initial clinical experience. Ann Surg 196:285–296
6. De Bakey ME, McCollum CH, Graham JM (1978) Surgical treatment of aneurysms of the descending thoracic aorta: long term results in 500 patients. J Cardiovasc Surg 19:571
7. Ergin MA, O'Connor JV, Blanche C, Griepp RB (1983) Use of stapling instruments in surgery for aneurysms of the aorta. Ann Thorac Surg 36:161–166
8. Gelman S, Reves JG, Fowler K, Samuelson PN, Lell WA, Smith LR (1983) Regional blood flow during cross-clamping of the thoracic aorta and infusion of sodium nitroprusside. J Thorac Cardiovasc Surg 85:287–291

9. Heberer G, Rau G, Löhr HH (1966) Aorta und große Arterien. Springer, Berlin Heidelberg New York
10. Laschinger JC, Cummingham JN, Nathan JM, Knopp EA, Cooper MM, Spencer FC (1983) Experimental and clinical assessment of the adequacy of partial bypass in maintenance of spinal cord blood flow during operations on the thoracic aorta. Ann Thorac Surg 36:417–426
11. Lawrence GH, Hessel EA, Sauvage LR, Krause AH (1977) Results of the use of the TDMAC-heparin shunt in the surgery of aneurysms of the descending thoracic aorta. J Thoracic Cardiovasc Surg 73:393–398
12. Lemole GM, Strong MD, Spagna PM, Karmilowicz NP (1982) Improved results for dissecting aneurysms. Intraluminal sutureless prothesis. J Thorac Cardiovasc Surg 83:249–255
13. Lerberg DB, Bahnson HT (1982) Surgical treatment of thoracic aortic aneurysms. In: Bergan JJ, Yao JST (eds) Aneurysms, diagnosis and treatment. Grune and Stratton, New York, pp 119–129
14. Livesay JJ, Cooley DA, Reul GJ, Walker WE, Frazier OH, Duncan JM, Ott DA (1983) Resection of aortic arch aneurysms: a comparison of hypothermic techniques in 60 patients. Ann Thorac Surg 36:19–28
15. Roberts AJ, Michaelis LL (1979) The use of bypass techniques and other forms of organ protection during thoracic aortic cross-clamping. In: Bergan JJ, Yao JST (eds) Surgery of the aorta and its body branches. Grune and Stratton, New York, pp 109–127
16. Snyder DM, Crawford ES (1983) Successful treatment of primary aorto-esophageal fistula resulting from aortic aneurysm. J Thorac Cardiovasc Surg 85:467–463
17. Stelter WJ, Schildberg FW, Imig H (1981) Arterielle Aneurysmen. In: Zencker R, Deucher F, Schink W (eds) Chirurgie der Gegenwart, vol 7. Urban and Schwarzenberg, München Wien Baltimore, pp 1–48
18. Stelter WJ, Becker HM, Heberer G (1983) Rupturen und traumatische Aneurysmen der Aorta. Chirurg 54:135–142
19. Williams TE, Vasko JS, Kakos GS, Cattaneo SM, Meckstroth CV, Kilman JW (1980) Treatment of acute and chronic traumatic rupture of the descending aorta. World J Surg 4:545–552

15.7 Dissecting Aneurysms

H.M. Becker and K.W. Jauch

CONTENTS

A. Anatomy and Classification

Dissecting aortic aneurysms develop from hemorrhage in the region of the vasa vasorum, with the formation of a hematoma and secondary intimal tear. The starting point is the ascending aorta just above the aortic valves in 65% and the descending aorta just distal to the origin of the subclavian artery near Botalli's ligament in about 20%. Dissection originates at the aortic arch in about 15%. In the Marfan syndrome, coarctation of the aorta, and rarely in different forms of aortitis, the aortic wall is predisposed to split up into two layers, with the plane of cleavage running within the media. The most common cause, however, is arteriosclerosis occurring together with hypertension. Following an acute intimal tear, the dissection may continue on into the pelvic arteries, where the dissection lies on the left posterolateral aspect of these vessels. The left renal artery is therefore also involved in this process and is perfused through the false lumen. The dissection reaches the abdominal aorta in about 50%, leading to occlusion and ischemia of the right common iliac artery (see Fig. 15.7.1a). Another possible complication is rupture of the outer layer with acute hemorrhagic shock and development of a hemopericardium or hematothorax if the rupture is localized further proximally. Rupture into the true lumen creates two complete lumina (Fig. 15.7.1c). This "reentry" often leads to an improvement of symptoms of ischemia or penetration. Another complication is thrombosis of the vascular lumen.

Classification of aortic dissections according to their localization is essential for patient selection, operative strategy, and reconstructive technique. The De Bakey classification [8] describes the intimal tearing point with subsequent intramural hemorrhage and its extension distally (Fig. 15.7.1a–c). The caudal extension of dissection varies considerably in types I and III, producing a great variety of clinical symptoms. A disadvantage of this classification is that intimal tears at other sites are not taken into account, and that only dissection in the direction of the bloodstream is considered. Dissections developing in a retrograde direction cannot be classified. The same holds for acute dissections with no clearly localized point of entry. Autopsies show that these directions without known arteries make up about 10% of all cases [9].

These disadvantages have led to a new therapeutic evaluation of dissecting aneurysms: The Stanford classification [7] is becoming more and more accepted. The point of entry is unimportant. Classification is strictly according to the dissected aortic segments. Type A is a dissection of the ascending aorta. Type B is a dissection of the descending aorta, which may involve the distal portion of the aortic arch, even if dissection of this segment occurs in a retrograde direction (Fig. 15.7.2a, b).

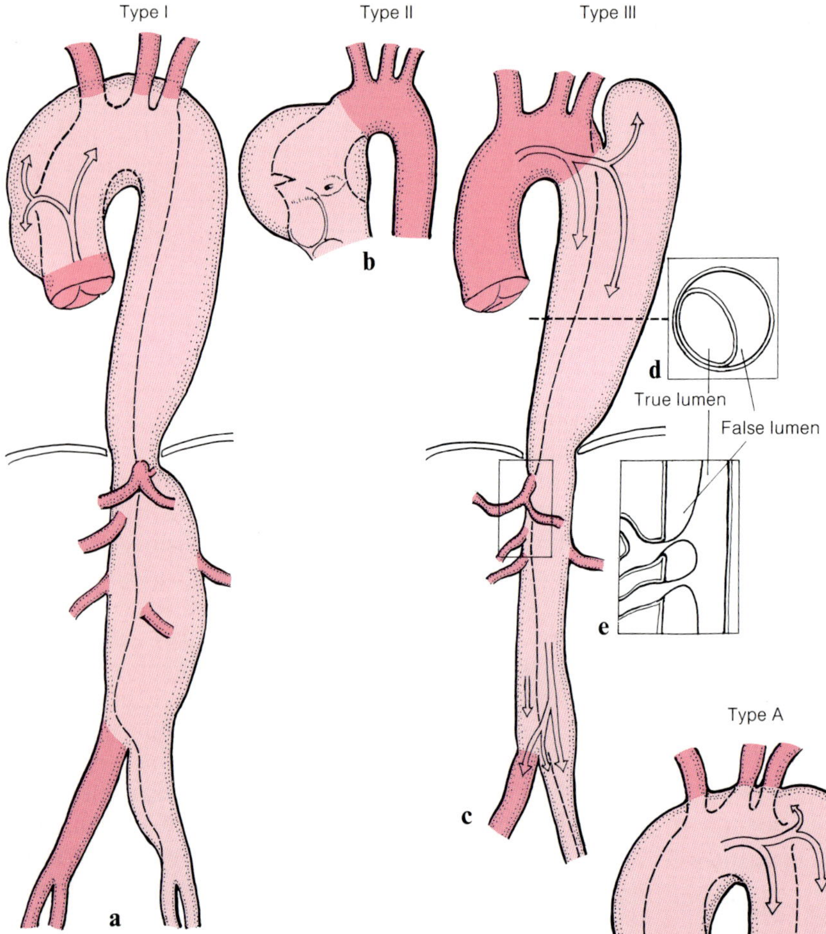

Fig. 15.7.1 a–e. De Bakey classification of aortic dissection into the three types I–III. **a** Type I, showing point of entry with intramural hemorrhage at the ascending aorta. Dissection may extend across the aortic arch down to the thoracic aorta or, as presented in the diagram, to the abdominal aorta and lower. In such a case, obstruction of the common iliac artery can lead to ischemia of the leg. **b** Type II with the same point of entry as in type I, but with limitation of the dissecting aneurysm to the ascending aorta. **c** Type III is characterized by a normal ascending aorta and aortic arch. The intimal tear typically occurs just beyond the origin of the subclavian artery, and dissection may continue on to more distal regions, ending at various levels. Reperforation at the bifurcation prevents limb ischemia, in contrast to **a**. **d** Transverse section at the level of the thoracic aorta, showing the smaller true lumen and the larger false one. **e** Compression and obstruction of the orifices of the visceral artery by the false lumen, depicted in a lateral view

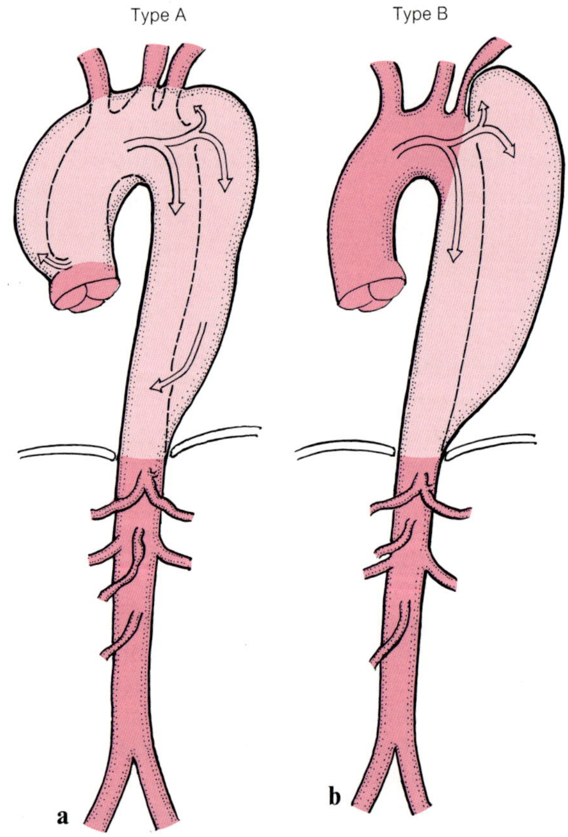

Fig. 15.7.2 a, b. STANFORD classification of aortic dissection into type A and type B [7]. **a** Dissection involving the ascending aorta and aortic arch. The original point of entry (ascending aorta, retrograde dissection from the descending aorta) does not play an important role in the classification. **b** Type B does not involve the ascending aorta. Dissection may be limited to the thoracic aorta, just as in type A, or extend onto the abdominal aorta

B. Indications for Reconstructive and Palliative Procedures

The stage of a dissection is of crucial importance for the surgical indication and the choice of surgical procedure. A dissecting aneurysm is acute from the onset of clinical symptoms to the end of the 2nd week. An aortic dissection is chronic after the 14th day. Sometimes it is called subacute in the 3rd and 4th week [12]. The fresher a stage is, i.e., the more acute the symptoms, the larger the danger of fatal rupture is, even if a false aneurysmal channel does not develop. The danger of rupture of the false channel in a chronic dissection is only present in saccular aneurysms. A chronic dissecting aneurysm behaves like a fusiform or saccular arteriosclerotic aneurysm.

A *type A dissection* with involvement of the ascending aorta almost always necessitates immediate surgical intervention during the acute stage since there is a high risk of aortic insufficiency or cardiac tamponade, and the mortality rate within the first 4 weeks is over 90%. During replacement of the ascending aorta, aortic valve replacement is usually necessary under cardiopulmonary bypass. Therefore, type A is discussed in the Manual of Cardiovascular Surgery (vol. VI/2, p. 576 ff).

Type B aortic dissection may be repaired without having to employ the heart-lung machine. How an acute type B dissection should be treated is still a matter of great controversy worldwide. There are different opinions regarding indications for surgical vs. conservative treatment [3, 6, 7, 12, 14, 15]. Retrospective studies have shown that the prognosis of patients with an undiscovered and untreated type B dissecting aneurysm is considerably better than patients with a type A aneurysm, provided that they survive the acute stage [11, 12]. Some 70%–80% of the conservatively treated patients survive the acute stage in type B dissection without surgery. The survival rate seems to be better if a false lumen cannot be detected by angiography, or only at a later stage. Such findings certainly favor conservative therapy.

A contained or free rupture with development of a hematothorax must be treated by an emergency operation; no alternative treatment exists.

If conservative treatment does not relieve pain and if the dissection progresses and complications develop during conservative therapy, surgery is indicated. Complications such as obstruction of the aortic branches with ischemia of the kidneys, extremities, intestines, or central nervous system (restlessness or somnolence) may occur (Fig. 15.7.1e). Surgery is also indicated if the patient has contraindications to antihypertensive and negative inotropic medication. Between 20%–30% of all patients who had adequate primary conservative therapy develop complications requiring surgery. Recently published favorable results show that there is an increasing tendency to treat these aneurysms surgically in the subacute stage. The great variety of dissections and symptoms make it impossible to formulate strict guidelines for optimal treatment.

In *chronic type B* dissection, surgery is not indicated very often. We perform surgery only if patients develop symptoms that are clearly the result of dissection and if the false channel expands, causing aneurysmal dilatation (Fig. 15.7.1d). In such cases, thoracic or lumbar back pain develops, just as in penetrating arteriosclerotic aneurysms. However, a wide variety of symptoms have been reported which may be associated with the enlargement or penetration of an aneurysmatically dilated false lumen. Especially with saccular aneurysms, where dilatation can exceed 10 cm, rupture becomes imminent. In asymptomatic patients without aneurysmal enlargement of the false channel, there is no risk of rupture; surgery is not indicated except to prevent further retrograde dissection into the aortic arch toward the ascending aorta.

C. Positioning

If aortic dissection is limited to segment III of the thoracic aorta, the patient is placed on the right side for a left thoracotomy (Fig. 15.7.3b). The pelvis is supported dorsally, and a padded belt is fastened around the left hip. The raised left arm is positioned on a padded arm rest. It should, however, not be abducted too far; otherwise, the left shoulder blade is elevated and is in the way during posterolateral thoracotomy. While the arm is in such a position, the cranial portion of the operating table should not be lowered too far as this would overstretch the brachial plexus. The right arm is pulled forward and also placed on an arm rest. A soft pad is placed under the right shoulder. Access to the abdominal and iliac vessels is not possible in the right lateral position. Cannulation of the femoral arteries is also impossible in this position. If such access is necessary in order to repair a dissection extending beyond the thoracic aorta into the abdominal aorta and both iliac arteries, a thoracoabdominal approach should be chosen. The thorax is rotated 45° into a right semilateral position, keeping the pelvis in a horizontal plane (Fig. 15.7.4a). The position is exactly the same as in surgery of a thoracoabdominal aortic aneurysm (see p. 314) and permits a median or left paramedian laparotomy and also an anterolateral to lateral thoracotomy, with possible extension to the posterior axillary line.

D. Surgical Approach

The right lateral position gives access to the descending aorta through a posterolateral thoracotomy at the upper margin of the sixth rib. The incision can be extended anteriorly, if necessary. The latissimus dorsi and the serratus anterior muscles are divided as far caudad as possible to spare the nerves and vessels coming from above. The intercostal muscles are divided at the upper border of the rib with a cautery. The neighboring ribs may be partially divided dorsally using the List rib cutter which leads to fracture at the designated site. The same maneuver may be done ventrally at the costochondral junction of the lower rib. One rib spreader is inserted dorsally and one ventrally. Expansion is performed step by step, allowing for good exposure of the total descending aorta from the distal aortic arch to the diaphragm. If only the distal portion of the aortic arch, i.e., the cranial portion of the descending aorta is to be exposed, anterolateral thoracotomy is performed in the Crawford position (45°, see thoracoabdominal approach) at the upper border of the fourth or fifth rib. This also gives good access to the entire aortic arch and ascending aorta. The serratus anterior muscle is divided over the fourth rib. The latissimus dorsi may be partially transected, but usually remains fully intact. The muscles holding the shoulder blade in place are preserved. This spares the internal thoracic artery and vein. If the pericardium must be opened to obtain access to the ascending aorta, these vessels should then be divided and the thoracotomy extended as far as the sternum. Tapes are then passed around the ascending aorta. This aortic segment is gently pulled forward or to the left side for partial tangential clamping of its wall.

In operations performed on the thoracic descending aorta through a left thoracotomy, it is advisable to intubate both sides of the lungs separately and then isolate the left lung from mechanical ventilation. The collapsed left lung is easily reflected with a retractor. This allows for better exposure of the aorta and reduces the risk of injury to the left lung. Regular blood gas analyses done at short intervals and taken from the radial artery of the right arm are used to check for adequate oxygenation of the blood. If an arteriovenous shunt in the unventilated lung leads to a critical drop in pO_2, the main stem of the pulmonary artery may be temporarily clamped, or the lung inflated from time to time.

Exposure of the abdominal aorta in order to perform a fenestration or reconstruction of the visceral, renal, or pelvic arteries is achieved by a median longitudinal laparatomy in a supine position beginning at the xiphoid process, passing the umbilicus on the left side, and ending at the symphysis pubis. A Rochard retractor may be employed for better exposure of the aorta in the upper abdomen. If the procedure has to be extended to two body cavities (abdominal extension following primary thoracotomy, thoracic extension following primary laparotomy), the thoracoabdominal position should be chosen. Following longitudinal laparotomy and division of the costochondral junctions of the sixth and seventh ribs, an anterolateral thoracotomy is performed at the upper border of the sixth rib. Transdiaphragmatic exposure of the thoracoabdominal aorta using the Crawford technique is possible with this approach (see Fig. 15.7.4a, see p. 314).

E. Surgical Techniques

I. Prosthetic Interposition

Replacement of the descending aorta in a type B dissecting aneurysm is advisable if the dissection is limited almost entirely to the thoracic portion and the false channel is ruptured or in danger of rupturing (Fig. 15.7.3a). To replace the entire diseased segment starting at the proximal side of the intimal tear, prosthetic interposition is the method of choice. Prosthetic interposition with a distal transection suture is also a good method of surgical treatment in more extensive aneurysms of the descending thoracic aorta in which the dissection begins just below the left subclavian artery. The

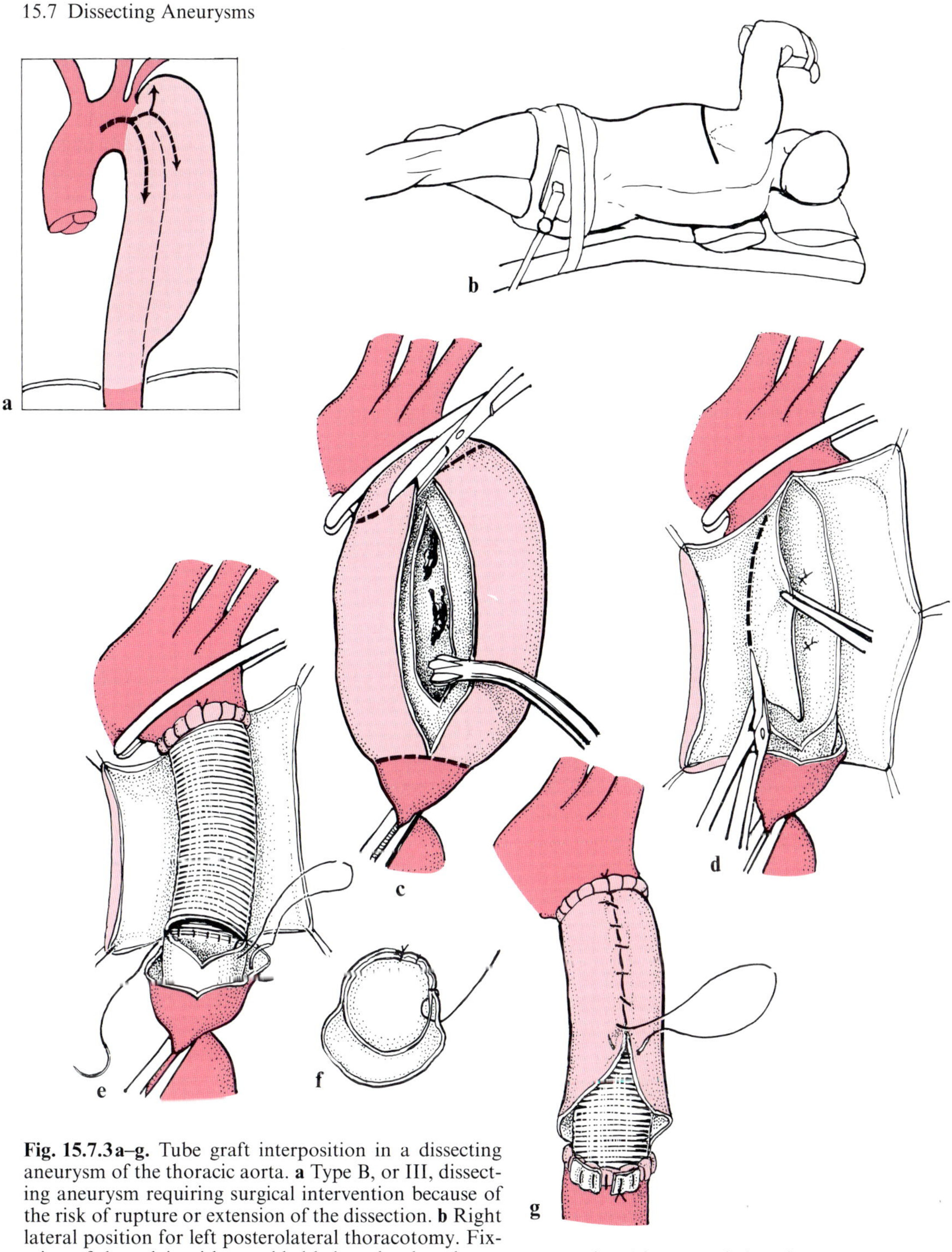

Fig. 15.7.3a–g. Tube graft interposition in a dissecting aneurysm of the thoracic aorta. **a** Type B, or III, dissecting aneurysm requiring surgical intervention because of the risk of rupture or extension of the dissection. **b** Right lateral position for left posterolateral thoracotomy. Fixation of the pelvis with a padded belt and a dorsal support, fixation of the elevated left arm on a cushioned arm rest. **c** Exposure of the diseased aortic segment with proximal and distal clamping of the aorta; division of the false channel and the true lumen. The incision is continued with transverse incisions proximally and distally. Back-bleeding intercostal arteries are closed with transfixion sutures. **d** Resection of overlapping portions of the inside wall to produce the proximal aortic stump. The proximal end-to-end anastomosis is then constructed. **e** After completing the proximal anastomosis, the distal anastomosis is constructed with a continuous over-and-over suture. At the same time, both dissected walls are reattached to one another. If the walls are widely separated from one another, they may be adapted by suture prior to the construction of the anastomosis (**f**). **g** To prevent the sutures from cutting through the aortic tissue at the distal anastomosis Teflon pledgets are placed underneath them for protection. The graft is covered by the aneurysmal sac

danger of rupture and the extension of dissection may be eliminated by this procedure.

Following a left thoracotomy it is advisable, especially in a dissecting aneurysm, to expose the aorta first at the distal aortic arch. Preparation and dissection in this area is performed as previously described in the chapter on thoracic aortic aneurysms (see p. 336). If the aneurysmal dissection extends proximal to the subclavian artery, this vessel must be clamped separately. If necessary, the aorta must also be clamped proximal to the subclavian artery. In contrast to the usual procedure performed for repair of an arteriosclerotic thoracic aortic aneurysm, tapes should not be passed around the distal descending aorta just above the diaphragm. The wall of the false channel may be so friable following acute dissection that preparation in its vicinity or the passage of a tape around it may cause immediate rupture. If the attempt at clamping the aorta leads to further tearing of the false channel, the massive hemorrhage that results cannot be brought under control.

A strong, firm clamp should be used to occlude the distal aortic arch or the beginning of the descending aorta. In the epiphrenic portion of the aorta, a soft clamp suffices for proper occlusion. An intestinal clamp is preferred for this purpose. It adequately occludes the false channel and the true lumen of the aorta without tearing the friable walls of the false channel. After clamping, a longitudinal incision of the false and true lumina is made. Back bleeding from intercostal arteries (identified by continuous suction of blood from these sites) is brought under control by closing the orifices of these vessels with transfixion sutures (Fig. 15.7.3c). Both lumina are incised transversely about 1–2 cm distal to the proximal aortic clamp. The inside wall is resected and the proximal aortic stump visualized (Fig. 15.7.3d). A Dacron prosthesis is connected end-to-end to the proximal aortic stump. The graft must be of the correct size and may consist either of woven or knitted albumin- or collagen-coated Dacron material. The anastomosis is constructed with a continuous over-and-over monofilament suture (polypropylene 3–0). Each stitch should catch both the true and the false wall of the aneurysm. This means that both walls are sutured to the graft and at the same time reconnected to one another. This causes a rather large bulge of the aortic wall at the suture line (Fig. 15.7.3e). Therefore, the proximal anastomosis does not have to be secured using a supplementary suture technique.

The distal anastomosis is performed in the same way. A difficulty often complicating the suture process is that both walls of the true and false lumen are usually widely separated from one another. Sometimes, both walls must first be sutured to one another before the anastomosis can be performed (Fig. 15.7.3f).

Teflon pledgets are placed on the outside of the false wall and also between the false and true walls to prevent the sutures from cutting through the mural layers. Here it is advisable to use interrupted mattress sutures rather than a continuous suture. If the false channel is not very wide, the same anastomotic technique may be employed as for the proximal anastomosis (Fig. 15.7.3e). The anastomotic bulge not only seals off the suture line, but also contributes to its durability. 3–0 Polypropylene or PTFE sutures are recommended. Each stitch must be checked to see whether it is firmly anchored, especially where a distal anastomosis is performed. If one is not sure whether the sutures will cut through the aortic tissue, Teflon pledgets should be used to secure them on the outside (Fig. 15.7.3g). Shortly before completion of the distal anastomosis, backward flow from the abdominal aorta must be checked and any thrombi lodged within it flushed out. The graft should be vented before blood flow is completely restored. Systemic heparinization is usually not necessary when this technique is used. It is, however, advisable to instill a heparinized solution (1000–2000 units) into the distal aorta with a large cannula.

Replacement should be limited to the most severely diseased proximal portion of the aorta so that not too many pairs of intercostal arteries have to be sacrificed (see p. 312). It is important to replace those portions of the aorta in which intimal tears have led to dissection. A distended aneurysmal sac of the false channel which is in danger of rupturing must also be repaired.

The anesthesiologist must be informed in good time before the distal anastomosis is completed so that controlled intraoperative pressure reduction can be interrupted and preparations made to begin volume substitution and administration of catecholamines, which will be needed to deal with the drop in blood pressure following restoration of distal blood flow (see p. 199).

II. Thoracoabdominal Aortic Bypass

If a type B dissection is limited to the thoracic portion of the descending aorta and ends at the diaphragm or just below it, a bypass procedure should be chosen for reconstruction. A disadvantage is that a two-cavity procedure is necessary. The advantage of this method is that the surgeon avoids having to perform a difficult distal anastomosis to the lower portion of the thoracic aorta, where dissection is still present, and instead constructs the easier end-to-side anastomosis to the healthy infrarenal aorta (Fig. 15.7.4c). The CRAWFORD right semilateral position, as with the thoracoabdominal approach, is preferred (see p. 312). (Fig. 15.7.4a). The proximal anastomosis is constructed in the same manner as previously described (see p. 352). Just as in repair of an atypical coarctation of the abdominal aorta, the prosthesis is posteriorly passed through the diaphragm, behind the aorta, close to the anterior surface of the spine. Blunt tunneling in the retroperitoneal space is performed dorsal to the pancreas and the renal vessels. This positions the prosthesis next to the aorta in the middle infrarenal aortic segment.

Sometimes, it is better to place the prosthesis dorsal to the pancreas in the retroperitoneal space and then, when it reaches the root of the mesocolon, to pass it anterior to the renal vessels (also anterior to the left renal vein) into the exposed retroperitoneal space. There, it is obliquely anastomosed end-to-side to the infrarenal aorta. This technique is identical to the surgical treatment of an atypical coarctation of the abdominal aorta (see p. 209). The distal aortic stump of the descending aorta is closed by suture (Fig. 15.7.4d). We prefer double suture ligation as a safeguard and use Teflon pledgets for reinforcement.

To prevent prolonged ischemia of the visceral organs and kidneys, the end-to-side anastomosis to the infrarenal aorta is constructed first. The prosthesis is then passed through the diaphragm

Fig. 15.7.4a–d. Thoracoabdominal aortic bypass. **a** Positioning of the patient for a thoracoabdominal approach according to CRAWFORD, with the pelvis in the horizontal position and the thorax rotated 45° to the right. Extension of the median laparotomy upward for anterolateral thoracotomy in the seventh interspace. **b** Type B, or III, dissecting aneurysm. **c** Situation following completion of the proximal end-to-end anastomosis and distal infrarenal end-to-side anastomosis. The aortic stump in the region of the descending aorta is closed by double suture ligation, using Teflon pledgets for reinforcement (**d**)

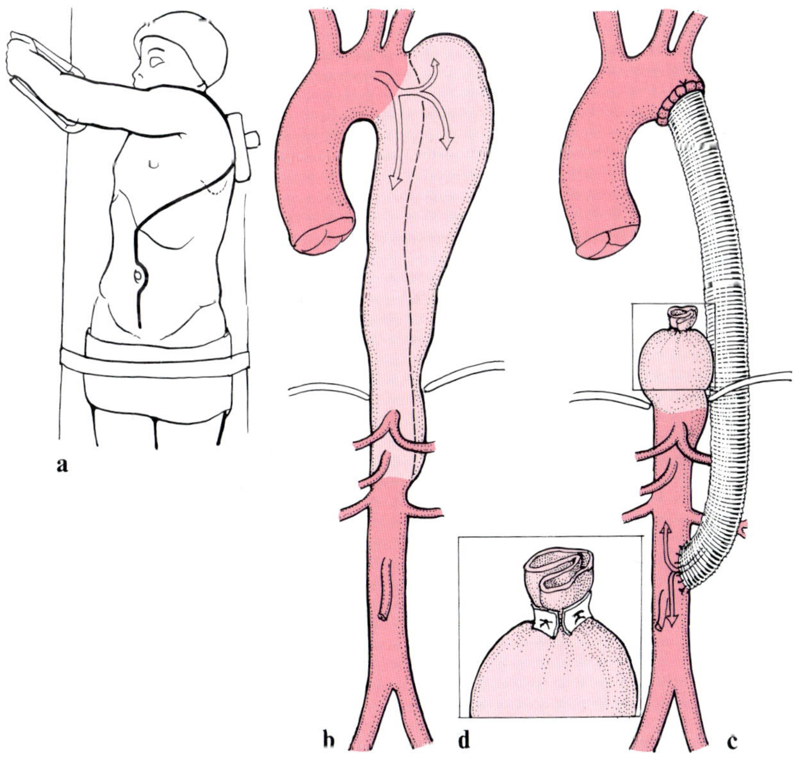

into the thorax and connected circularly end-to-end to the descending aorta at the level of Botalli's ligament. This means that the surgeon decides to perform bypass grafting without knowing beforehand whether or not a thoracic tube interposition graft alone would be sufficient for aortic repair (removal of the rupture site and the dissected segment). This bypass grafting technique must always remain an alternative for those cases where a tube graft cannot achieve aortic reconstruction in the thoracic region.

III. Thoracoabdominal Aortic Replacement Using the Crawford Technique

Thoracoabdominal aortic replacement is indicated in acute or progressive ischemia of the visceral organs and the kidneys and in transdiaphragmatic or subdiaphragmatic retroperitoneal rupture of the false channel (Fig. 15.7.5a). The patient is placed in the thoracoabdominal position with the thorax rotated toward the right side and the pelvis remaining in a horizontal position. Exposure of the aorta is accomplished using the Crawford technique [6] (see Fig. 15.5.4, see p. 314). The median laparotomy is extended upward, followed by the division of the costochondral junctions of the seventh or sixth ribs. The incision ends in a thoracotomy performed at the upper margin of the seventh or sixth rib. The parietal peritoneum is incised on the left lateral side in front of the descending colon. The descending colon and its splenic flexure are reflected medially. The peritoneum is dissected away from the iliopsoas muscle distally, and the abdominal viscera is reflected medially in one piece. This exposes the aortic bifurcation and the common iliac arteries on both sides all the way down to the iliac bifurcations. According to the original description of this method by CRAWFORD, the left kidney remains within the retroperitoneum and is not reflected medially.

CRAWFORD temporarily divides the left renal vein, reconnecting it to the vena cava after completing aortic replacement. The left kidney can also be reflected medially; this however, makes it difficult to reimplant the right renal artery. It is usually not possible to dissect the distal peritoneum completely off the bottom surface of the diaphragm all the way down to the aorta without dividing it. Tearing of the parietal peritoneum does not interfere with preparation as long as the capsule of the spleen remains uninjured. Such injuries of the splenic capsule usually make splenectomy necessary. The diaphragm is divided between clamps step by step, starting at its anterior medial portion, extending upward to the central tendon. Its muscular portion is ligated. It is also possible to start at the central tendon and divide the diaphragm step by step until reaching the aorta. The phrenic nerve, which reaches the diaphragm on the ventral side of the aorta, should be spared. Therefore, both crura of the diaphragm should be divided dorsal to the aorta, if possible. This approach exposes the entire thoracoabdominal aorta, from the origin of the left subclavian artery downward to, and even beyond, the aortic bifurcation.

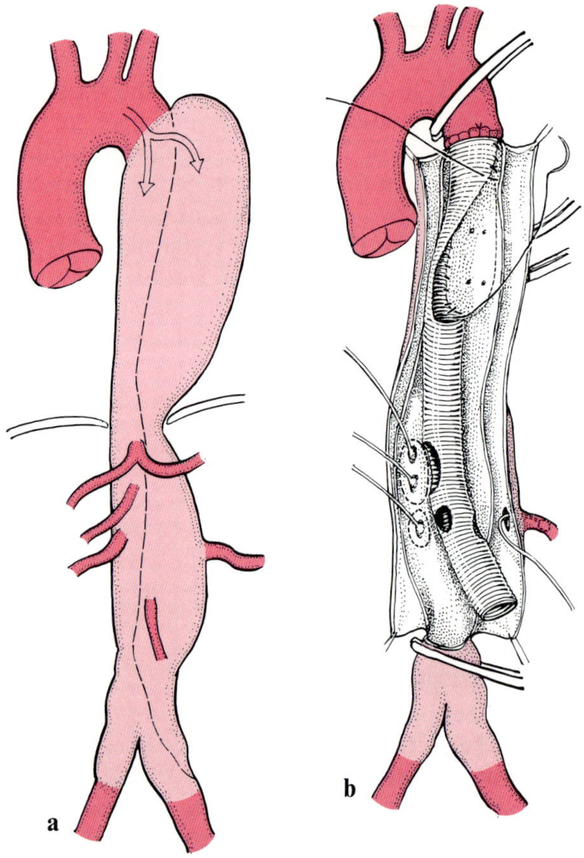

Fig. 15.7.5a, b. Thoracoabdominal aortic replacement using the Crawford technique. **a** Extensive thoracoabdominal dissecting aneurysm. **b** Suture of the proximal, extremely oblique anastomosis. This allows blood flow to be restored first to the clamped thoracic intercostal arteries. The orifices of the main visceral arteries are excised, together with a funnel-shaped patch of aortic wall tissue, and then anastomosed to the graft

Usually, only the thoracoabdominal aortic junction and the abdominal portion of the aorta just distal to it need to be replaced. The distal portion of the descending aorta just above the diaphragm should also be dissected free to permit clamping.

In the original description by CRAWFORD, the proximal anastomosis is performed first (Fig. 15.5.5c). This has the advantage of implanting the major visceral arteries, together with a patch of aortic wall surrounding them, into the graft in rapid succession. It is the same procedure as performed in thoracoabdominal aortic replacement in a nondissecting aneurysm (see p. 317). The anastomotic technique is more difficult in a dissecting aneurysm since the walls of the true and false lumen are usually widely separated from one another. In very acute dissections, it may be advisable to perform a fenestration by cutting out a wedged-shaped portion of the inside wall and then connecting the prosthesis to the wall of the false channel. Suture is performed with a 2–0 or 3–0 monofilament suture reinforced on the outside by Teflon pledgets placed underneath to prevent these sutures from cutting through the aortic wall.

After completing the proximal anastomosis, the main visceral arteries are reimplanted in rapid succession, while the aorta remains clamped. The uneven visceral arteries, celiac artery, and superior mesenteric artery may be reimplanted without sewing the original aortic wall of the true lumen onto the graft, provided that these arteries are supplied by the false lumen. The origins of these arteries may be anastomosed to the prosthesis together with patches of false aortic wall around them. Holes must be cut into the prosthesis adjacent to the arteries (Fig. 15.7.5). No constrictions or stenosing plaques at the orifices should obstruct blood flow to them. If such plaques are present, periorifice thromboendarterectomy should be performed. The distal ends of the arteriosclerotic inner core plugs can usually be removed without leaving behind an intimal ledge at their distal ends (see p. 320; Fig. 15.5.7g). Reimplantation of the funnel- or trumpet-shaped, excised origin of the right renal artery often causes difficulties. According to CRAWFORD the right renal artery should be implanted into the prosthesis first, either by excising its origin separately or together with the superior mesenteric artery and celiac artery as one single large aortic patch containing all three orifices. The excised origin of the left renal artery is reimplanted last. CRAWFORD states that the inferior mesenteric artery need not be reconnected if the superior mesenteric artery and both internal iliac arteries are patent. If there is doubt, however, one should reimplant them in order to avoid ischemia of the sigmoid colon and of the gluteal region. The aortic prosthesis is sutured end-to-end to the distal aortic stump a short distance proximal to the bifurcation. In most cases, however, a bifurcation prosthesis must be implanted, replacing the aortic bifurcation and both common iliac arteries down to the iliac bifurcation on both sides, since dissection usually extends beyond the aortic bifurcation into both iliac arteries. At the iliac bifurcation, both lumina, the false and the true, are easily rejoined, which makes femoral attachment of both arms of the bifurcation prosthesis at the groin unnecessary.

To keep the ischemic time of the visceral organs as short as possible, we perform the distal anastomosis first. After completing the proximal anastomosis between graft and aorta, the visceral arteries are reimplanted in rapid succession. It is often difficult to rotate the aortic prosthesis, which is tensely stretched between the distal and proximal anastomosis, and to clamp it tangentially for implantation of the corresponding artery at the correct side. The method as originally described by CRAWFORD avoids this problem since the prosthesis is not anchored distally before the visceral arteries are reconnected.

If a longer segment of the thoracic aorta has to be replaced, at least one, and preferably several pairs of intercostal arteries arising from the distal portion of the descending aorta should be reimplanted into the prosthesis to avoid postoperative paraplegia (see p. 316).

The great radicular artery (Adamkiewicz) may be distinguished from other intercostal arteries by its rather large caliber and by its relatively strong backward flow following division of the aneurysmal sac. CRAWFORD reimplants this artery last. However, tangential clamping of the prosthesis, which is a necessary maneuver for reconnection of this artery, is very difficult once the graft has been attached elsewhere, so that many authors reimplant this pair of intercostal arteries first and then go on to connect the visceral arteries.

Ischemic times of up to 30–40 min in visceral organs and 40–60 min in kidneys may be tolerated during this procedure. When all visceral and renal arteries have been connected to the graft, the prosthesis should if at all possible be covered with portions of the wall from the false channel. Once the prosthesis lies within the retroperitoneum, it is covered by two layers of tissue, as described elsewhere (see p. 303). The diaphragm is closed with interrupted sutures, and a chest drainage tube is put in place. The descending colon is reattached to the lateral wall of the abdomen. The retroperitoneal space is drained by one or more tubes, and the spleen is put back in place. Chest and abdomen are closed using the standard technique.

IV. Fenestration Operations

Fenestration operations are performed when severe isolated ischemia of organs persists, especially of the kidneys and the lower limbs, and no other method is capable of relieving these complications (Fig. 15.7.6b–d; see p. 370). Fenestration is usually limited to the aortic bifurcation or to one iliac artery.

Laparotomy, extending from the xiphoid process to the symphysis pubis, passing the umbilicus on the left, is performed with the patient in a supine position (Fig. 15.7.6a). After reflecting the small intestine to the right and the mesocolon with the transverse colon upward, the infrarenal abdominal aorta, the aortic bifurcation, and the common iliac artery are exposed on both sides (see p. 378). One should always attempt to dissect the aorta free above the origins of the renal arteries as far upward as possible so that it may be occluded with a clamp. It is not advisable to pass Teflon tapes under the aorta since this maneuver may lead to tearing of the wall of the false channel. Broad, strong clamps should be used which cannot tear the fragile wall of the false channel during clamping. The aorta is then longitudinally incised just above the bifurcation in a cranial direction. If both orifices of the renal arteries require inspection, the incision is extended upward beyond the origin of the renal arteries, while the left renal vein is slightly reflected upward by means of a tape. At least one renal artery usually arises from the true lumen. The other renal artery, which branches off from the false lumen, must be examined in its proximal portion. To reduce back bleeding, an inflatable balloon catheter attached to a three-way

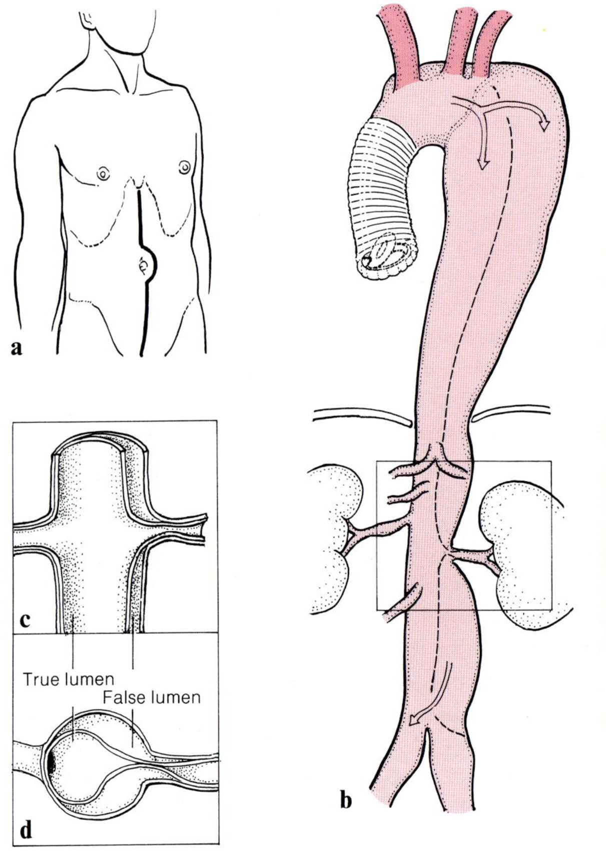

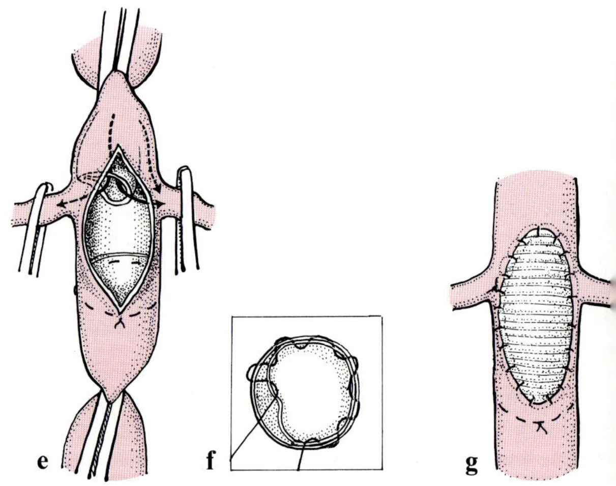

Fig. 15.7.6a–g. Abdominal fenestration in renal ischemia. **a** Supine position for longitudinal laparotomy which passes the umbilicus on the left side. **b** A thoracoabdominal dissecting aneurysm in a patient who had undergone aortic valve replacement and replacement of the ascending aorta. Fenestration was necessary because of renal ischemia. **c**, **d** Ischemia of the left kidney owing to compression of the renal artery as it arises from the true lumen. **e** Following a longitudinal incision of the external wall, the wall of the true lumen is resected near the origins of the renal arteries. Resection must be performed proximal to the renal orifices. The distal intimal ledge is transfixed by an interrupted or continuous mattress suture (**f**). **g** Closure of the longitudinal aortotomy with a synthetic patch of double velour Dacron

stopcock is introduced into the lumen of the renal arteries. The inside wall of the two-walled renal artery is usually removable without leaving an intimal ledge behind. This restores unobstructed blood flow from the false lumen to the kidney. A wedge-shaped resection of the wall of the true lumen is performed at this level. This is also done anteriorly if both orifices of the renal arteries arise from the true lumen. No portions of these walls should act as a blocking valve, sealing off the orifice when blood flow is restored (Fig. 15.7.6e). The wall of the true lumen is totally resected over its entire circumference further distally (Fig. 15.7.6e). The distal intimal ledge is tacked down by an interrupted or continuous mattress suture (Fig. 15.7.6f) or by a continuous over-and-over suture sewn in part from the inside, in part from the outside, and tied on the outside. It is advisable to use monofilament 2–0 to 4–0 suture material. If the suture must be secured on the outside, Teflon pledgets should be used for this purpose. The longitudinal aortotomy is usually closed by direct suture. Only rarely is a patch used for closure. In such cases, a double velour Dacron or Teflon patch (Goretex) is preferred (Fig. 15.7.6g). The patient is systemically heparinized during the operation, making neutralization of the heparin with protamine necessary following restoration of blood flow. Fenestration of the iliac artery is performed in the same way as in obstructions and is described on p. 370. Thrombosis of the iliac arteries is rarely seen after acute dissection. If it does happen, however, and recanalization of the iliac arteries cannot be achieved by thrombectomy, an aortoiliac or aortofemoral bypass must be constructed to normalize leg perfusion. A femorofemoral cross-over bypass would be an alternative in such a case (see p. 545).

V. More Recent Surgical Techniques

To reduce blood loss during anastomosis of a graft to a dissected aorta, several groups [2, 9, 12] have developed ringed intraluminal Dacron prostheses, which are inserted into the true lumen and then tied to it [4, 6]. The tapes are passed around the false lumen and occlude it when they are tied over the ring. This method is especially suited to the surgical management of dissections in the descending aorta (see p. 343, Fig. 15.6.8). Once the long-term results of this therapeutic concept have been studied, its real value as a technique for the surgical management of aortal dissections will be known. About the same average aortic clamping times are necessary in this reconstructive procedure as with the conventional techniques. No final results have yet been reported on graft migration, aortic wall necrosis and erosion, formation of false aneurysms, etc. Recently, reports on methods for external reinforcement of dissecting aneurysms in danger of rupture have been published. Earlier, several different methods were employed with varying results [1]. External reinforcement of the aneurysmal sac seems to be possible with woven or knitted Dacron material. This applies more to the ascending aorta than to the descending aorta since the intercostal arteries arising from the descending aorta must be selectively divided before external coverage with synthetic material can be performed. This may lead to disruption of the false channel in dissecting aneurysms with subsequent uncontrollable hemorrhage. However, progressive dissection cannot be treated by this method, and therefore it should be considered only in exceptional cases.

F. Postoperative Treatment and Complications

Direct postoperative treatment of the patient always begins in the intensive care unit. In addition to constant blood pressure and ECG monitoring, postoperative mechanical ventilation is usually necessary for proper blood oxygenation (see p. 203). Hemorrhage in the thorax or abdomen following surgery must be reexplored early enough. Thrombosis of the prosthetic aortic graft seldom occurs because of the high flow rate through the prosthesis. Renal functional disorders such as anuria or polyuria must be treated carefully. Anuria may be a sign of thrombotic occlusion of the main renal artery which should be confirmed by early angiography or by functional radionuclear tests. Functional disorders of the liver and acute or subacute intestinal ischemia must also be diagnosed in time. Postoperative jaundice is usually caused by hemolysis following multiple blood transfusions. Liver function tests, especially cholinesterase, provide a further evaluation of the possible extent of ischemic liver damage. A specific treatment for this disorder is unfortunately not available at the moment.

Acute thrombotic occlusions of the visceral arteries are rarely detected since the patient requiring mechanical ventilation is sedated. Clinical symptoms such as hyperperistalsis shortly after the operation and paralysis about 5–8 h following surgery should be clarified by angiographic control of intestinal perfusion. An acute postoperative thrombotic occlusion of the superior mesenteric artery, which is fortunately rare, is usually detected when severe abdominal pain develops. The surgeon in charge must then decide whether or not extensive resection of gangrenous bowel improves the patient's prognosis of living a worthwhile life. The surgical mortality rate in dissecting aneurysms of the aorta depends on the type of operative procedure and the stage of aortic dissection. It varies between 0%–10% and 50% (Table 15.7.1). The main causes of death are myocardial ischemia, cerebral ischemia, bleeding complications, and, in recent years, mainly rupture and pericardial tamponade.

Table 15.7.1. Frequency of paraplegia (complete or partial) and operative mortality in 250 surgically treated patients with a dissecting aneurysm of the aorta, as reported by CRAWFORD [5, 6]

	Paraplegia		
	Complete %	Partial %	Mortality %
Replacement of the ascending aorta			
Acute ($n=19$)	0	0	32
Chronic ($n=33$)	0	0	9
Aortic arch replacement			
Acute ($n=7$)	0	0	43
Chronic ($n=21$)	0	0	19
Replacement of the descending aorta			
Acute with shunt ($n=6$)	17	0	50
Acute without shunt ($n=16$)	6	0	50
Thoracoabdominal aortic replacement			
Acute ($n=11$)	18	9	45
Chronic ($n=71$)	6	14	8
Total aortic replacement ($n=3$)	33	33	0
Abdominal aortic replacement ($n=1$)	0	0	0
Total ($n=250$)	11 (4.4)	14 (5.6)	46 (18.4)

Another typical complication is paraplegia, which may be complete or partial, with a frequency that differs according to the various types of aortic reconstructions. Whether or not a temporary shunt is used to maintain peripheral perfusion of the spinal cord seems to have no influence on the incidence of paraplegia (Table 15.7.1).

REFERENCES

1. Abbot DA (1949) Clinical experiences with application of polyethylene cellophane upon aneurysms of thoracic vessels. J Thor Surg 18:435
2. Ablaza SGG, Ghosh SC, Grana VP (1978) Use of a ringed intraluminal graft in the surgical treatment of dissecting aneurysms of the thoracic aorta. J Thorac Cardiovasc Surg 76:390
3. Campbell CD (1981) Aortic dissections. In: Campbell CD (ed) Aortic aneurysms: surgical therapy. Futura, New York
4. Cooley DA, Wukasch DC (1979) Techniques in vascular surgery. Saunders, Philadelphia
5. Crawford ES, Crawford JC, Stowe CL, Safi HJ (1984) Total aortic replacement for chronic aortic dissection in patients with and without Marfan's syndrome. Ann Surg 199:358
6. Crawford ES, Crawford JC (1984/1985) Diseases of the aorta. Williams and Wilkins, Baltimore London
7. Dailey PO, Trueblood HW, Stinson EN, Eurtgrin TF, Shumway NE (1970) Management of acute aortic dissections, Type A and B. Ann Thorac Surg 10:237
8. De Bakey ME, Henley WS, Cooley DA, Morris GC, Crawford ES, Beall AC (1965) Surgical management of dissecting aneurysms of the aorta. J Thorac Cardiovasc Surg 49:130
9. Dureau G, Villard J, George M, Deliry P, Froment JC, Clermont A (1978) New surgical technique for the operative management of acute dissections of the ascending aorta. J Thorac Cardiovasc Surg 76:385
10. Gurin D, Bulmer IW, Derby R (1935) Dissecting aneurysm of the aorta: diagnosis and operative relief of acute arterial occlusion due to this cause. NY State J Med 35:1200
11. Hirst HE, Johns VJ, Kime SW (1958) Dissecting aneurysms of the aorta: A review of 505 cases. Medicine 37:217
12. Miller DC (1983) Surgical management of aortic dissections. In: Doroghazi R, Slater E (eds) Aortic dissections. McGraw-Hill, New York
13. Shaw RS (1955) Acute dissecting aneurysm. Treatment by fenestration of the internal wall of the aneurysm. N Engl J Med 253:331
14. Wheat MW (1973) Treatment of dissecting aneurysms of the aorta: current status. Prog Cardiovasc Dis 16:87
15. Wheat MW (1980) Acute dissecting aneurysms of the aorta: diagnosis and treatment. Am Heart J 99:373

16 Acute Obstructive Disease of the Extremities

H. Denck

CONTENTS

A. General Remarks

I. Causes

Acute arterial obstruction may be caused by embolism of dislodged thrombotic material or by acute arterial thrombosis of an artery with a diseased or injured wall. Other causes of acute arterial obstructions are trauma, posttraumatic changes of the artery, dissecting aneurysms, subintimal hematoma, spastic diseases of the arteries, and several rare conditions. The main source of arterial embolism is the heart, from which 75%–94% of all peripheral emboli originate [21, 23, 26, 28]. Over the last few decades, the main cause of embolism from the heart – rheumatic valve disease and atrial thrombosis with atrial fibrillation – has been replaced by embolism of parietal mural thrombi following myocardial infarction [21]. Rheumatic heart disease has dropped to second place among the causes of embolism.

Although the heart is still the main source of embolism, arterioarterial embolism should not be forgotten [13, 19, 27]; it occurs in at least 10% of all embolic episodes. An atheromatous or aneurysmal aorta or iliac artery may act as a source of embolism. Other origins may be a thoracic outlet syndrome causing embolism of the upper extremity, a popliteal aneurysm, etc.

With the increasing frequency of invasive tests and therapeutic interventions, there has been an increase in the number of iatrogenic injuries leading to embolism. Parts of the Fogarty or other catheters may embolize, and preexisting thrombi at the site of intervention may be dislodged. Emboli originating from malignant tumors are rarely seen. Of these, atrial myxoma is probably the most common cause. In contrast, emboli from lung tumors are extremely rare [26]. Between 50%–75% of all acute arterial embolisms occur in the extremities.

Acute arterial thrombosis in the extremities often develops on the basis of arteriosclerotic, ulcerous, or stenotic arterial wall lesions, aneurysms, posttraumatic arterial wall injuries, subintimal hematoma, intimal tears, etc.

Acute occlusions of the iliac artery are found in 26% of all dissecting aneurysms [18]. Intermittent symptoms of acute arterial occlusion are found in cystic adventitial degeneration, primarily in the popliteal artery (Atkins and Key 1947) [26].

A persistent arterial spasm may also be the cause of an acute arterial obstruction in the extremities. Since 1981, spastic vascular reactions have been reported following the administration of dihydroergotamine – heparin preparations for postoperative (posttraumatic) prophylaxis of thromboembolism. This complication, occurring primarily in trauma patients, usually affects the lower limb in younger persons at an average age of 37.3 years [20].

II. Clinical Findings

Tissue hypoxia becomes manifest distal to every obstructed artery and sooner or later leads to necrosis, depending on the grade of ischemia. The severity of ischemia is, of course, determined by the sensitivity of the affected tissue to hypoxia (1. nerve; 2. muscle; 3. skin), and by the degree of collateral circulation. Sensory impairment of the skin is an alarming clinical sign since the peripheral nerves are most sensitive to hypoxia. As ischemic damage progresses, regional anesthesia develops. Finally, paralysis is the severest ischemic symptom and marks the beginning of tissue necrosis [21].

III. Indications for Surgery

In acute complete ischemia, therapeutic intervention should commence immediately, and everything possible should be done to relieve acute arterial obstruction. One of the first therapeutic measures is the intravenous injection of heparin (5000–10000 units) to prevent the growth of an appositional thrombus. If ischemia is incomplete, one can wait a short while until the patient has been examined and the diagnosis confirmed. These diagnostic procedures should, however, be done under heparinization, analgesia, and shock treatment. We think that incomplete acute ischemia should be treated immediately by recanalizing the obliterated segment. The development of fatal secondary thrombi, especially in shock, is not predictable. Such conditions cause irreversible injury within an extremely short time period.

A general surgeon acquainted with the basics of vascular surgery may treat classic embolism, provided the rules of embolectomy are observed. If an acute arterial thrombosis occurs in a patient with chronic occlusive arterial disease, or if obstruction is caused by other factors, a complicated and difficult operation will be necessary to revascularize the artery. In such a case, a fully trained vascular surgeon should be consulted.

IV. Indications for Other Methods of Treatment

Complete ischemia should be treated by surgical embolectomy or thrombectomy (the quickest procedure in acute arterial obstruction). The more centrally located an obstruction, the more favorable are the conditions for successful surgical treatment. In peripheral locations unsuitable for surgical treatment, local streptokinase therapy is a good alternative in relieving obstruction [17] (see p. 106). In acute spastic diseases, such as ergotism, the medication responsible for these symptoms must be discontinued. Vasoactive drugs and prostaglandins may relieve spasms. If these conservative therapeutic measures fail, semi-invasive transluminal arterial dilatation (PTA) may be successful [20] (see p. 113). An acute sympathectomy is considered only in rare cases. This method rarely relieves symptoms.

Venous thrombectomy is the method of choice in phlegmasia cerulea dolens with spastic occlusion of the arteries. This procedure relieves vasospasms of the venous and arterial systems. If thrombectomy does not lead to success, extensive fasciotomy over the lower limb or thigh muscles (fascia lata) is performed to decompress the endangered arteries [4].

B. Surgical Therapy

I. Choice of Anesthesia

Patients experiencing acute arterial obstruction of the extremities usually have additional cardiac and/or vascular risks. Therefore, methods of anesthesia should be chosen which exert as little strain on the patient as possible. We find local infiltration with a 1% solution of procaine (or lidocaine) the best method of anesthesia for embolectomy. Of course, an intravenous line must always be available for infusion or transfusion. Since making it a rule to use local anesthesia when operating on our poor risk patients with acute obstruction of a limb artery, surgical mortality has dropped remarkably. Lumbar-spinal peridural anesthesia is

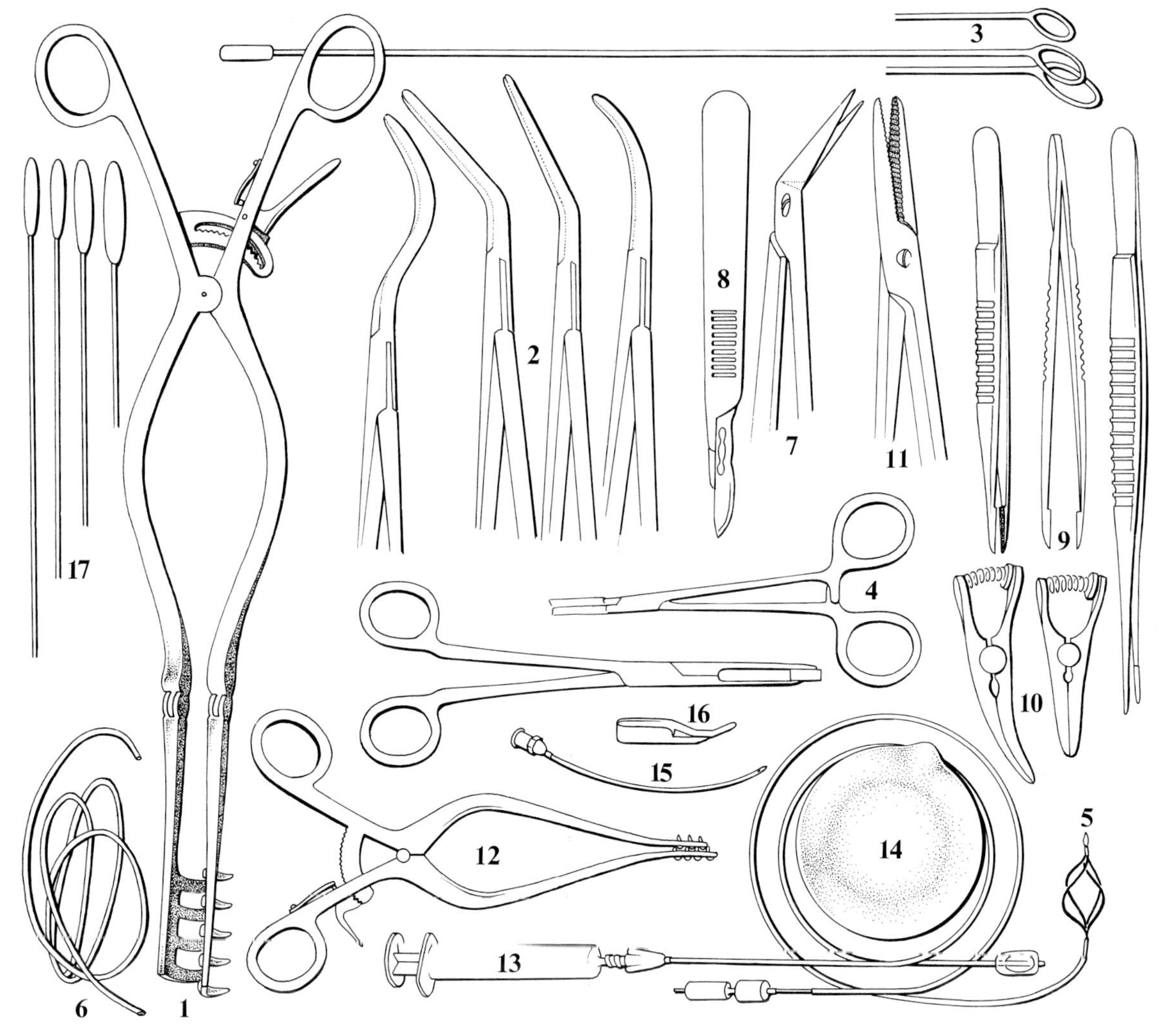

recommended in patients with chronic occlusive arterial disease in whom revascularization cannot be achieved by simple embolectomy, and who instead require extensive thrombectomy or complicated vascular reconstructions (see p. 195).

II. Instruments

The instruments used in vascular surgery are described in detail in the General Section. Figure 16.1. presents the "mini" instruments which each general surgeon needs to manage acute vascular problems such as embolism, acute thrombosis of peripheral vessels, intraoperative vascular injuries.

Fig. 16.1. Emergency vascular surgical instruments for embolectomy of a limb artery. *1*, Large wound retractor; *2*, atraumatic vascular clamps (De Bakey type); *3*, one small set of ring strippers; *4*, rubber-shod Pean forceps used in the clamping of prosthetic material (acute prosthetic occlusion); *5*, Dormia basket; *6*, loops for encircling vessels; *7*, angled vascular scissors; *8*, fine vascular scalpel; *9*, atraumatic vascular forceps; *10*, atraumatic bulldog clamps; *11*, vascular needle holder; *12*, small wound retractor; *13*, Fogarty catheters of different sizes; *14*, porcelain bowl for a heparinized solution (5000 units per 100 ml); *15*, flushing cannula; *16*, mini-bulldog clamps; *17*, one set of olive-shaped vascular dilators and atraumatic monofilament suture material 5–0 and 6–0

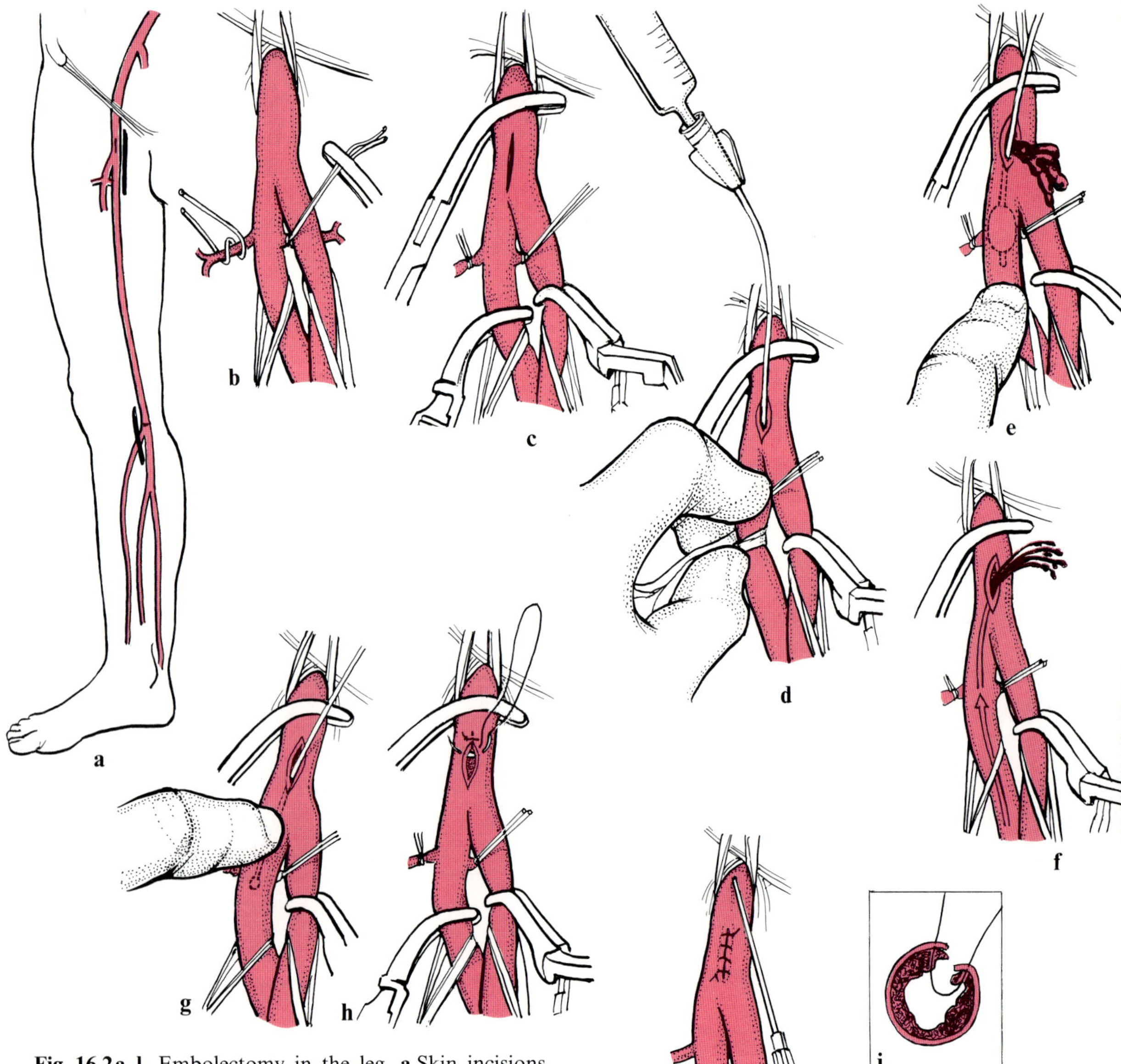

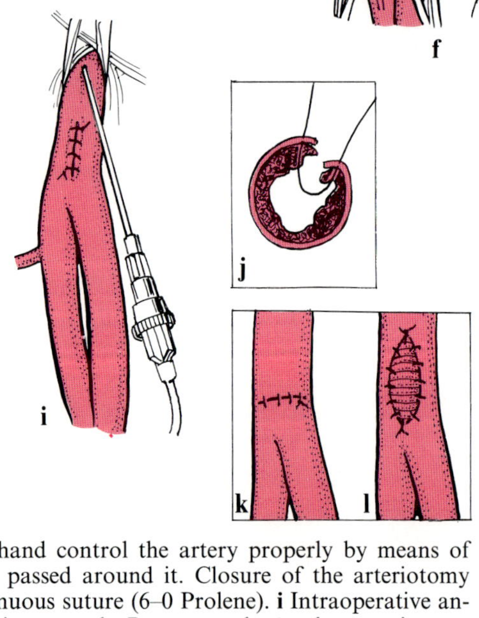

Fig. 16.2 a–l. Embolectomy in the leg. **a** Skin incisions for inguinal and popliteal embolectomy. The sites of arteriotomy are indicated. **b** Tapes are passed around the common femoral artery, profunda femoris, and superficial femoral artery. Smaller vessels are temporarily occluded with fine vessel loops (hemostasis). **c** Clamping, longitudinal arteriotomy above the origin of the profunda femoris artery allowing good exposure of its orifice. **d** Introduction of the Fogarty catheter (the size is chosen according to the caliber of the artery) into the profunda femoris artery. The left hand gently manipulates the artery; the index finger prevents larger blood loss. **e** Retraction of the balloon catheter while gently compressing the arterial wall; thromboembolic material shoots out of the arteriotomy. **f** Checking retrograde flow. **g** Introduction of a flushing cannula and injection of 1000 units heparin (20 ml of diluted solution). **h** The common femoral and the superficial femoral artery are embolectomized in the same way. When anterograde flow in the common femoral artery is checked, it is important that the left hand control the artery properly by means of the tape passed around it. Closure of the arteriotomy by continuous suture (6–0 Prolene). **i** Intraoperative angiographic control. Puncture above the arteriotomy makes assessment of the suture line possible. **j** The needle should transfix the entire wall when suturing arteriosclerotic vessels. **k** Transverse arteriotomy and closure. **l** Closure of a longitudinal arteriotomy with a patch graft, e.g., during surgical reintervention (vein, Dacron)

III. Surgical Approach in Acute Obstructive Disease of the Extremities

Only those incisions are discussed which provide the best access to the obstructed limb arteries. In principle, the surgical approach should always lie distal to the most peripherally palpable pulse. The surgeon will always try to choose a site from which the obstructed vascular segment can be easily reached. Since the development of indirect embolectomy, this is almost always possible [8] (Fig. 16.2a and 16.3a–c).

IV. Surgical Procedures in Acute Obstructive Disease of the Extremities
(Figs. 16.2 and 16.3)

Vascular preparation must be performed as meticulously as possible, according to the basic rules of vascular surgery. Complete hemostasis is necessary since the patient receives anticoagulants following surgery. Preparation, clamping, and hemostasis are performed as usual. Shortly before clamping the artery, 5000 units heparin is injected intravenously (other authors give 10000 units). We perform the arteriotomy longitudinally to obtain a better view of the large collaterals, especially in the groin (e.g., profunda femoris artery), and to be able to embolectomize or thrombectomize these branches without difficulty (Fig. 16.2b–j). A transverse arteriotomy, as shown in Fig. 16.2k, does not visualize the inside of the vessel as well as a longitudinal incision does. Many surgeons do not perform a longitudinal arteriotomy for fear of a stenosis which might develop following closure. However, a transverse incision increases the risk of tearing the arterial wall at its corners during withdrawal of an inflated Fogarty catheter. In some cases, this may lead to total evulsion of delicate arteries, making an end-to-end anastomosis, or even an interposition graft, necessary. Uncontrolled tearing of a longitudinal arteriotomy may be repaired in every case by closing the incision with a patch graft, thereby avoiding narrowing of the vascular lumen (Fig. 16.21).

Fig. 16.3a–c. Embolectomy in the arm. **a** Incisions made in the antecubital fossa and radially. **b** Exposure of the vascular bifurcation (ulnar artery, radial artery) by partially dividing the bicipital aponeurosis. **c** Selective insertion of the catheter into the radial and ulnar artery (further description on p. 365)

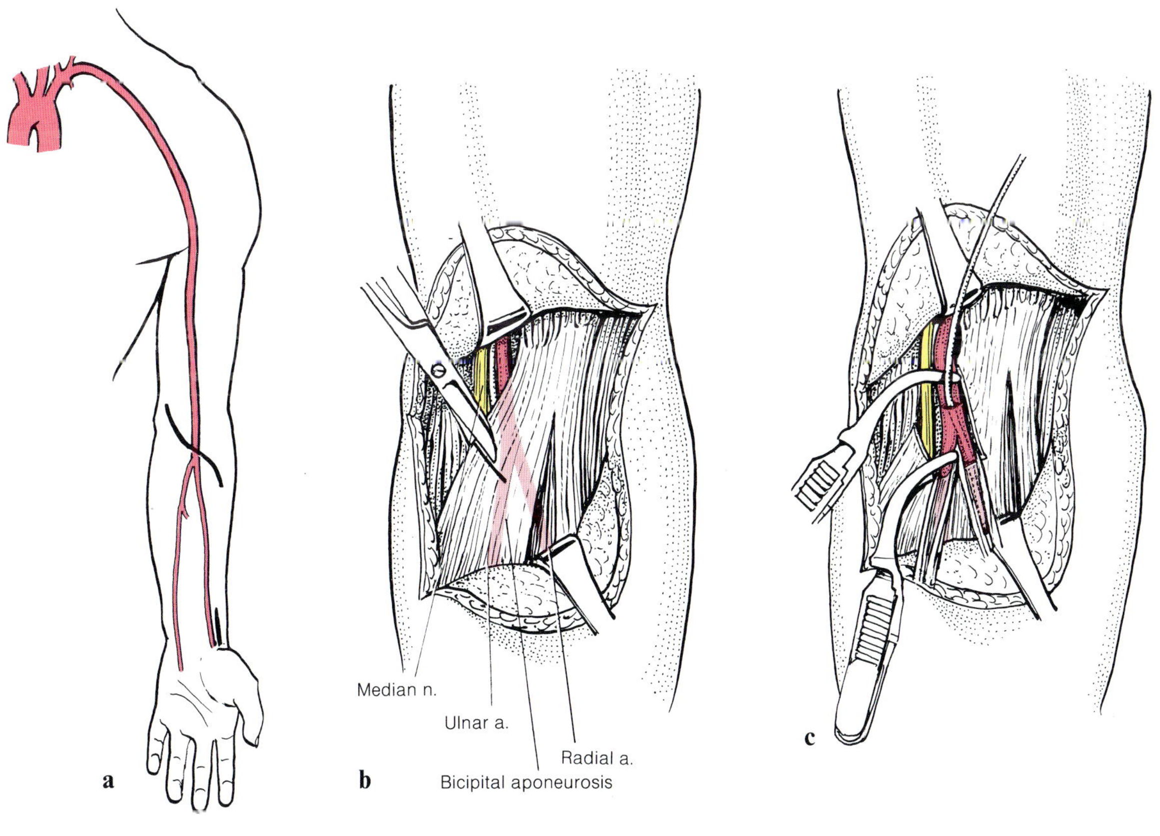

Dangerous suture line stenoses following longitudinal incisions may be avoided by closing the artery with a thin, monofilament nonabsorbable suture (6–0) and taking only very small bites of the wall. It is rarely necessary to close the longitudinal arteriotomy with a patch graft. This may be done sometimes following reinterventions at the same site.

Anterograde and retrograde flow must be precisely monitored, always keeping bleeding under control. The incisions should be flushed locally, preferably in a distal direction with heparinized solutions (5000 units heparin in 100 ml saline). Before closing the wound, a Redon suction drainage tube is introduced.

Because patients experiencing acute arterial obstruction are almost always at increased cardiac and cerebral vascular risk, the most limited procedure possible should be performed. Meticulous dissection technique minimizes blood loss. Vein cannulas must be large enough to provide adequate blood transfusion, if necessary. An anesthesiologist must always be present during operations done under regional anesthesia, to treat shock symptoms and initiate immediate general anesthesia if the patient's condition deteriorates.

After surgery heparin is given continuously by intravenous line. It is regulated according to the prolongation of the partial thrombin time (two–three times the normal value, i.e., 80–120 s).

Between the 3rd and 5th postoperative day coumarin anticoagulation is initiated. The daily heparin dose is slowly reduced with constant monitoring of partial thrombin time and prothrombin time.

Following thrombectomy or embolectomy of limb arteries, the patient is mobilized between the 3rd and 5th day, depending on general clinical condition and wound healing. The sutures are removed from the upper extremities between the 6th and 8th and from the lower extremity between the 8th and 10th day. A Redon suction drainage tube should always be placed within the wound area and not removed until blood or lymph secretion stops.

For correct assessment of one's own results, comparison with other results is necessary. The following figures may help to evaluate surgical success in the treatment of acute arterial obstruction: percentage of full or partial remissions, frequency of amputation, and surgical lethality.

Reviewing the literature of the past few years [7, 25, 26, 28], and considering our own results (3200 patients since 1970), a simple embolectomy performed within a 10-h limit leads to full restitution in more than 70% of surgical patients, to partial remission in 10%, to amputation in 5%, and to lethal complications in 5%. Compared with past results, these are excellent. If the occlusion period is prolonged beyond the 10-h limit, only 50%–60% show full remission, and the amputation and mortality rates increase to 10%–20%. The results for thrombectomy of acute arterial thrombosis are even worse. Total restitution reaches a maximum rate of only 50%, the amputation rate is over 30%, and the mortality rate about 20% or more.

Further improvement of these results can be expected mainly through early detection and early surgical intervention. Increasing the number of extra-anatomic bypass procedures performed in acute arterial thrombosis could lead to substantial improvement of results.

Simple intraoperative quality control is recommended in each case. If surgery is performed under local anesthesia, the subjective comments of the patient during surgery are already a good indication of successful recanalization: the patient no longer experiences pain and can move his toes again. If the patient's limb is draped properly, a nonsterile assistant can simply palpate the peripheral pulses, the presence of which is an indication of success.

Of course, simple measuring devices which can be employed intraoperatively under aseptic conditions are also of great value in evaluating the quality of perfusion. For example, the light plethysmograph developed by Bollinger and Borgis photoelectrically registers the changes in the translucency of body tissues of the hands and feet. These alterations are recorded as typical pulse curves.

Intraoperative angiography is still the best method for evaluating recanalization, especially after thrombectomy. A comparison between pre- and postoperative angiography documents the operation's success. Routine angiography is, however, not absolutely necessary in typical embolic occlusions, but if there is any doubt, it must be recommended.

V. Direct Embolectomy

Before Fogarty introduced the method of indirect embolectomy in 1963 [8, 9, 10] an embolectomy had to be performed through an arteriotomy at

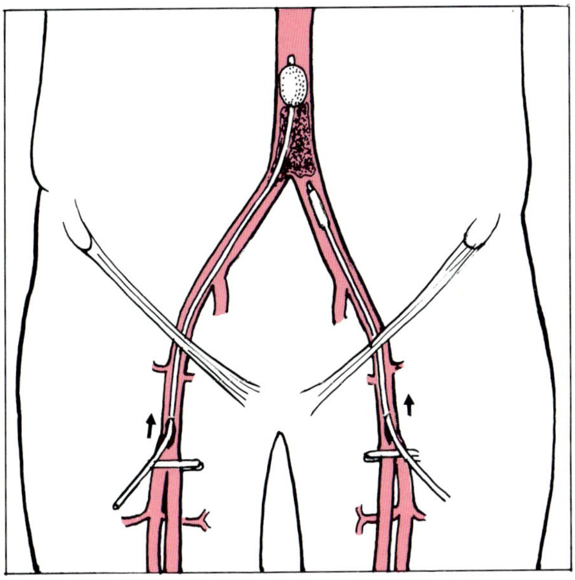

Fig. 16.4. Simultaneous embolectomy of an embolus situated at the aortic bifurcation. The primary decision to operate on both sides simultaneously prevents fragments of the embolus from embolizing into distal arteries. Before the Fogarty catheter was developed, remote embolectomies were sometimes performed with the Dormia basket

the site of the embolus. Today *direct embolectomy* is performed only if the embolus is located at one of the typical sites, e.g., origin of the profunda femoris artery at the groin or cubital artery.

In such cases the embolus is extruded through a simple arteriotomy by digital compression or with a thumb forceps.

Direct embolectomy may also be atraumatically performed with a Fogarty balloon catheter, since this technique prevents fragmentation of the embolus during extraction, removing all secondary thrombi and parts of the primary embolus from the vessel.

If the embolus or a part of it lies in the profunda femoris artery, it may be easily removed with a Fogarty catheter inserted through a groin incision. A good reflux from the profunda femoris artery should be present after removing the embolus. Direct embolectomy of centrally localized emboli in the subclavian artery and in the aortic or iliac bifurcation is attempted only if indirect embolectomy, either by the Fogarty balloon catheter technique or by a ring stripper, does not lead to removal of the embolus (see p. 72). Such problems occur if the embolus is too old or adheres very tightly to the arterial wall.

Anterograde and retrograde flow must be carefully monitored in every case, in order to determine whether or not, in addition to the embolus, a thrombus has formed centrally and distally, which must be completely extracted in an anterograde and retrograde direction with a Fogarty catheter. If anterograde thrombectomy is unsuccessful, retrograde flushing from a peripheral segment can be attempted.

Arterial emboli most often lie at branching points of the arteries (bifurcation, Fig. 16.4), at the origin of the profunda brachii artery, at the division of the brachial artery into the forearm arteries, at the origin of the profunda femoris artery, at the branching of the popliteal artery into the lower leg arteries) and may spontaneously separate into several fragments. In searching for parts of the embolus, the Fogarty catheter must be introduced into all arterial branches at a given branching site, otherwise recanalization of arterial circulation will be incomplete.

VI. Indirect Embolectomy

Until 20 years ago, embolectomy always had to be done directly. This meant that centrally located emboli had to be removed by performing large operations in order to expose the obstructed site. Today, the standard technique is indirect embolectomy as developed by Fogarty. An arteriotomy is performed at a typical site to which the surgeon has easy access. The embolus is removed either by retrograde or anterograde advancement and withdrawal of the balloon catheter.

Figures 16.2, 16.3, and 16.4 show the typical steps in performing indirect embolectomy; sometimes the Dormia basket is still used to reach very peripherally localized tiny emboli. Sometimes, peripheral secondary thrombi adhere to the basket as it is being withdrawn, thus facilitating their removal. If patients present late after an acute event and an attempt to remove the embolus is made using a Fogarty catheter, the embolus may stick to the wall so strongly that it cannot be extracted. This problem may be overcome if in addition the ring stripper is carefully applied.

Although the Fogarty method of embolectomy seems to be very simple, the use of the balloon catheter is always an occasion for the application of precise surgical technique. Incorrect manipulation of the catheter within the artery may lead to vascular wall injury or even iatrogenic dislodge-

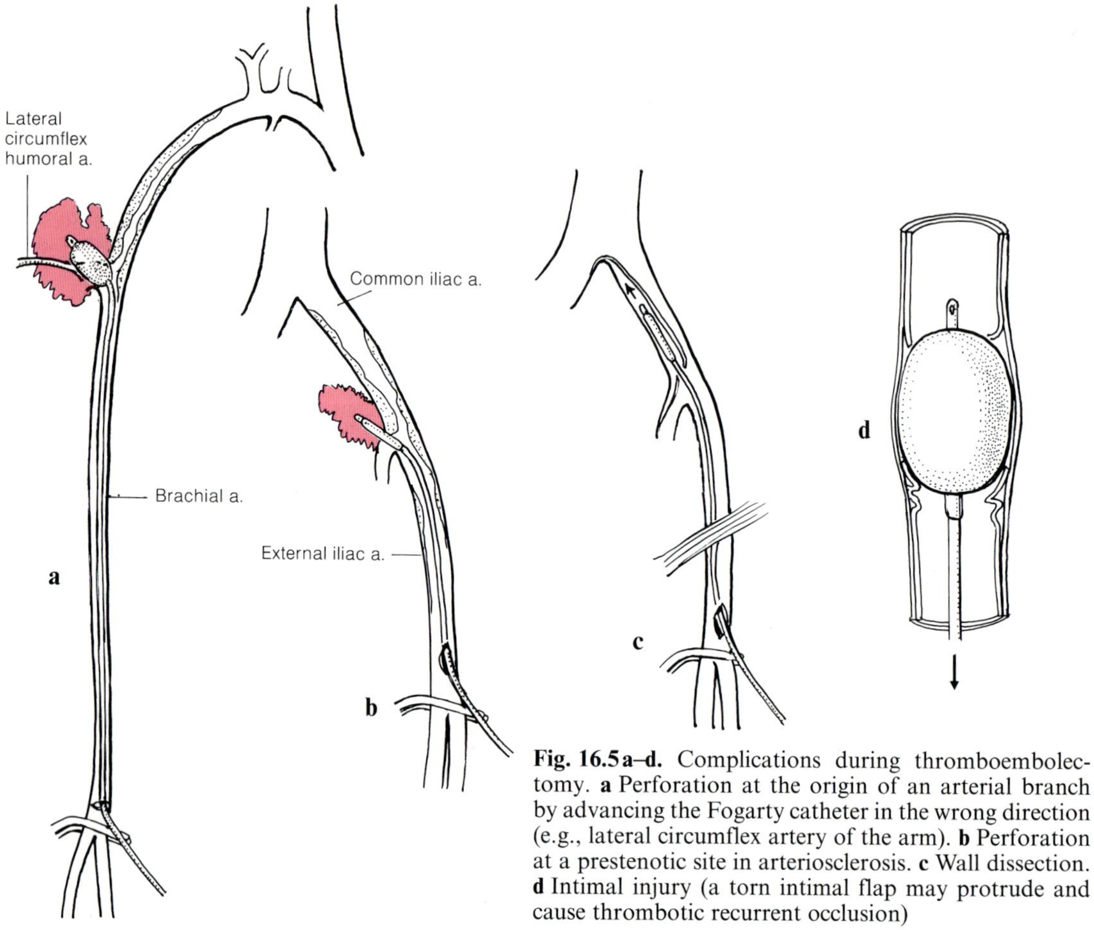

Fig. 16.5a–d. Complications during thromboembolectomy. **a** Perforation at the origin of an arterial branch by advancing the Fogarty catheter in the wrong direction (e.g., lateral circumflex artery of the arm). **b** Perforation at a prestenotic site in arteriosclerosis. **c** Wall dissection. **d** Intimal injury (a torn intimal flap may protrude and cause thrombotic recurrent occlusion)

ment of fragments of the embolus which then may embolize themselves into peripheral vessels. GOLDBERG et al. [2] demonstrated vascular wall injury after rough manipulation with the Fogarty catheter. CHIDI and DEPALMA proved the atherogenic potential of the embolectomy catheter, which was directly proportional to the applied pressures within the balloon [3].

Overinflation of the balloon leads to intimal tears which, of course, cause subsequent dissection and recurrent occlusion (Fig. 16.5a–d). When overinflated, the balloon can disrupt and its remaining fragments embolize into peripheral arteries.

To prevent this complication, the size of the Fogarty catheter should be chosen according to the diameter of the embolectomized vessel. An indirect embolectomy of a proximal vessel is done using a larger sized catheter, in a smaller artery a smaller caliber is used. The surgeon should test the balloon by inflating it before inserting it through the arteriotomy in order to get a feeling for the correct pressure necessary for proper inflation during embolectomy or thrombectomy.

Special care must be taken in the very delicate arteries of children and also in calcified and ulcerated arterial walls in older patients.

VII. Thrombectomy of an Acute Arterial Thrombosis in an Extremity

The surgical procedure in direct and indirect thrombectomy following acute arterial thrombosis in an extremity is equivalent to embolectomy. However, the cause of acute arterial thrombosis is a different one (posttraumatic causes excluded). Thrombosis occurs as a consequence of stenotic, ulcerated, or dilating arteriopathies. If one decides to perform thrombectomy in acute arterial thrombosis, or if an acute occlusion is mistaken for an embolus and it turns out that acute thrombosis

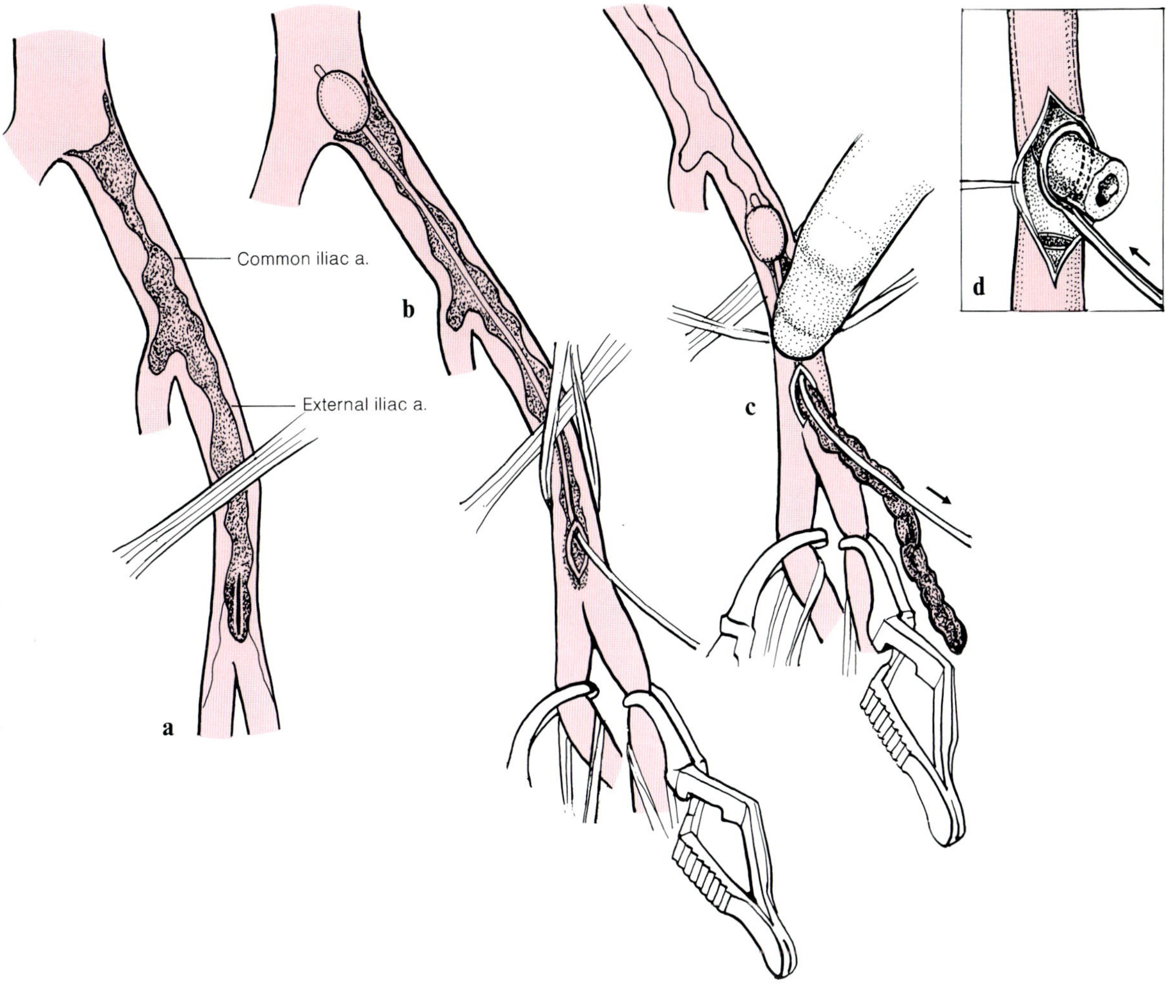

Fig. 16.6a–d. Thrombectomy of the left iliac artery. **a** Thrombosis of the left iliac artery showing severe arteriosclerotic disease. **b**, **c** Thrombectomy using the Fogarty catheter. **d** Thromboendarterectomy using a ring stripper (see p. 381). This additional maneuver is only justified if anterograde flow is inadequate and ultimate preservation of the leg is doubtful. The operative field must be prepared and draped in such a way that quick access to the retroperitoneal space is possible in case of perforation of the iliac arterial wall (insofar as possible, ring stripping should be attempted only in elective procedures following angiography)

has occurred in preexisting arterial wall disease, thrombectomy alone should be performed during the acute stage of ischemic symptoms. Later control angiography can visualize persistent wall lesions which may be corrected in a second operation. The objective of thrombectomy is to save the acutely endangered limb. *On no account* should *thromboendarterectomy* be performed in the acute stage. Such a procedure would lead to irreparable injury of the artery (dissection and disruption) and amputation.

An alternative in acute arterial thrombosis where surgery seems impossible is to bypass the thrombosed segment with an orthotopic or extra-anatomic bypass graft, provided, of course, the distal outflow tract is patent [7, 11].

Thrombectomy is performed in the same manner as an embolectomy, by means of a Fogarty catheter inserted through an arteriotomy at the most advantageous site (Fig. 16.6a–d). If thrombi remain adherent to the wall, the ring stripper may be advanced to dislodge them, followed by the Fogarty catheter for removal of the thrombotic material. Where the ring stripper is employed in acute arterial thrombosis, the smallest resistance encountered during the procedure should not be overcome by force. Otherwise, intimal injuries or perforations may occur. The size of the ring stripper must be chosen carefully so that the ring easily passes through the narrowest segment of the vessel. After saving the limb by thrombectomy, angiography (or even PTA) is performed to plan the necessary reconstructive procedures. Under favorable conditions, immediate reconstruction is possible following intraoperative angiography.

VIII. Acute Arterial Thrombosis in a Peripheral Aneurysm

If during embolectomy or thrombectomy the quantity of thrombotic material being removed seems endless, a thrombosed aneurysm must be suspected.

Poststenotic aneurysms of the subclavian artery (Fig. 16.7a) and the typical arteriosclerotic popliteal aneurysm are some common examples (see p. 281).

If an aneurysm is discovered during an attempted thrombectomy, angiography can clarify the situation. Then, a carefully planned vascular reconstructive procedure can be performed according to the grade of ischemia and the angiographic findings. Immediate surgical management of the aneurysm and bypass grafting with simultaneous, precise peripheral thrombectomy and embolectomy are the methods of choice if the limb is acutely endangered (Fig. 16.7b).

IX. Fenestration in an Acute Arterial Obstruction of an Extremity Caused by a Dissecting Aneurysm or Subintimal Hematoma

The typical dissecting aortic aneurysm and a subintimal hematoma can lead to acute arterial obstruction in an extremity [11, 18, 27]. Such an event is rarely observed in the upper extremity alone. It usually occurs in combination with cerebral ischemia. It is seldom seen in the lower limbs, occurring only if the true inner lumen of the dissecting aneurysm seals off one iliac artery or if dissection extends all the way down to the groin, where it narrows or even occludes the lumen of

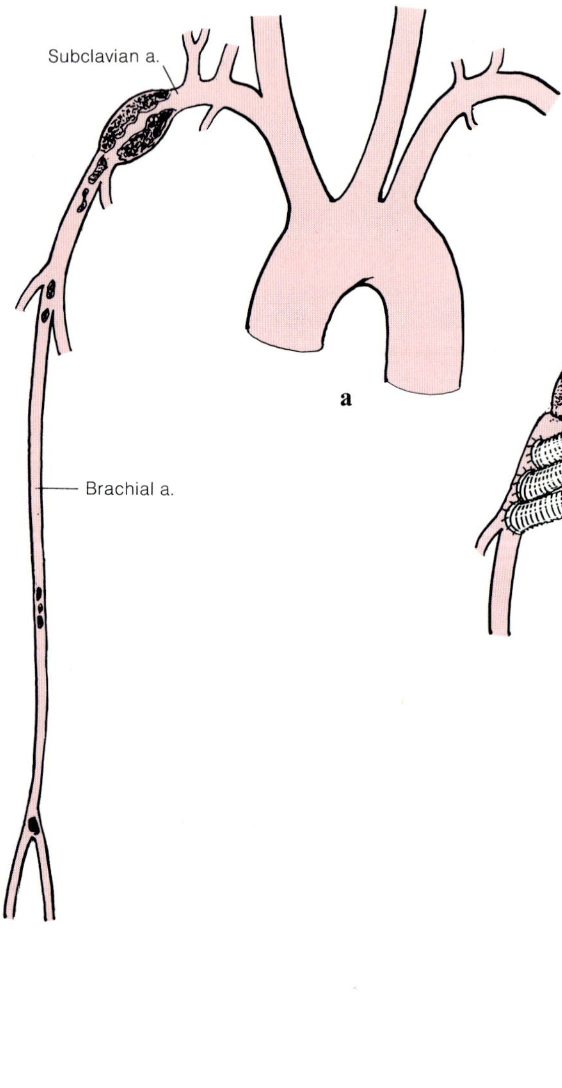

a

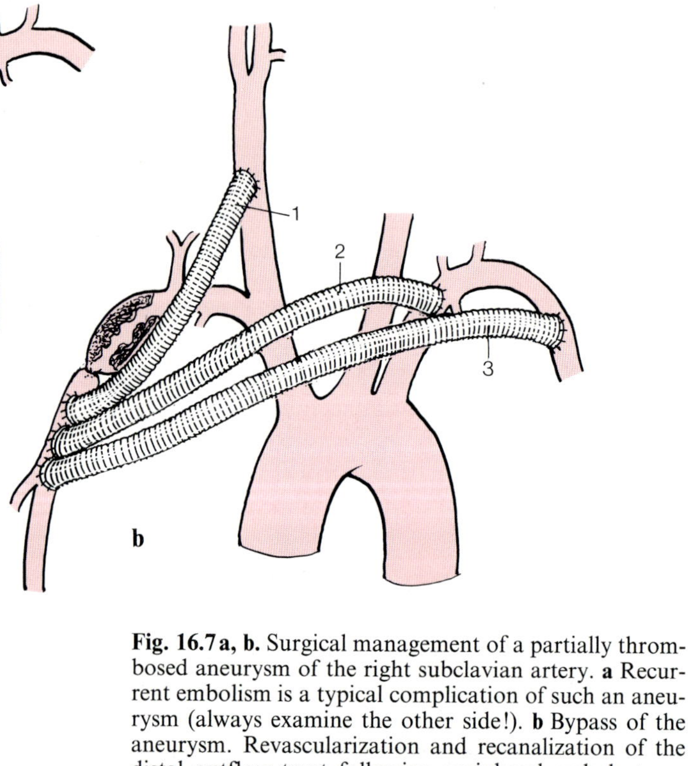

b

Fig. 16.7 a, b. Surgical management of a partially thrombosed aneurysm of the right subclavian artery. **a** Recurrent embolism is a typical complication of such an aneurysm (always examine the other side!). **b** Bypass of the aneurysm. Revascularization and recanalization of the distal outflow tract following peripheral embolectomy and construction of an extra-anatomic, carotid-axillary bypass (*1*). (alternatives: subclavioaxillary bypass (*2*), axilloaxillary bypass (*3*). Material: vein, ring-reinforced PTFE prosthesis the superficial femoral artery or profunda femoris artery (Fig. 16.8a). The case history of the patient and clinical symptoms such as shock, retrosternal, and abdominal pain signify that aortic dissection is responsible for acute arterial obstruction in the limb. However, we have observed cases which presented with an isolated occlusion of a leg artery and were treated as if they had experienced embolism. The knowledge of such peculiarities is important since acute ischemia at least can be relieved immediately by performing a simple fenestration of the inner wall. If the symptoms of dissection progress, elective correction of the aneurysm can be attempted. Figure 16.8b–d shows such an arterial occlusion in the right groin caused by dissection of the vascular wall. Acute relief by fenestration is also demonstrated. We limit therapy to this single procedure, provided the extensive operation of total or partial aortic replacement is not necessitated by increasing shock symptoms or by other arterial occlussions (see pp. 349, 358).

In some patients who were mistakenly treated for acute embolism of the leg, we exposed the femoral artery in the groin region and found a protruding intimal sac beneath which a pulse could be felt (subintimal hematoma). Simple fenestration with fixation of the distal intimal flap usually recanalized the vessel successfully.

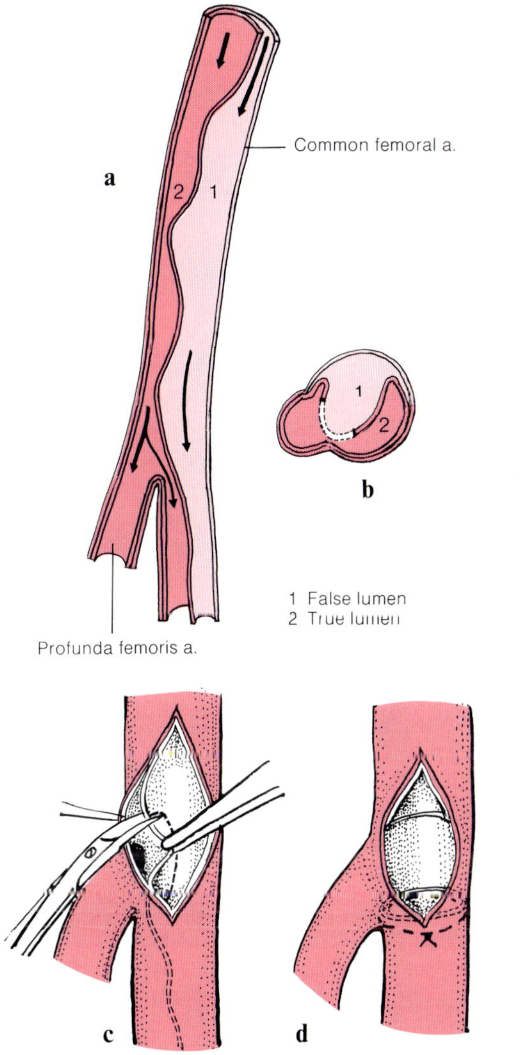

Fig. 16.8a–d. Arterial wall dissection. **a** Schematic representation of an arterial wall dissection in the right inguinal region with partial occlusion of the origin of the profunda femoris artery. **b** Transverse section at the level of the profunda origin. The dissected vascular wall blocks the orifice of the profunda femoris artery. **c**, **d** Following longitudinal arteriotomy, the dissected inner vascular wall is fenestrated (about 2 cm^2). The proximal resection line remains as it is; a distal intimal flap must be fixed to the adventitia

X. Extra-anatomic Bypass in an Acute Arterial Obstruction

Sometimes, a several-day-old or even a week-old acute or subacute arterial obstruction cannot be removed by typical thrombectomy or embolectomy. Occlusions of this kind, lying distal to the axilla or distal to the inguinal ligament, can be revascularized following previous angiography if the peripheral segments of the artery are still patent (see pp. 339ff., 391). In acute situations, extra-anatomic bypass is best suited for this purpose. It can be done quickly under regional anesthesia without too high a risk for the patient (see p. 539ff.). It is especially useful in central occlusions of the subclavian artery, the aortic bifurcation, or the iliac arteries, or in acute obstructions of a bifurcation prosthesis that cannot be lysed or thrombectomized immediately. Only alloplastic material is used for extra-anatomic bypass grafting. PFTE prostheses are best suited since blood loss is minimal with these grafts. The size of the prosthesis is determined by the caliber of the artery involved.

It must be stressed that a peripheral embolectomy or thrombectomy is performed until adequate reflux is restored or an obstruction detected by intraoperative peripheral angiography is removed.

XI. Surgical Management of an Acute Iatrogenic Arterial Thrombosis

With the increasing frequency of diagnostic procedures (angiography) and therapeutic interventions, there has been an increase in the number of iatrogenic peripheral arterial thromboses and also of catheter-induced thromboses or embolisms, with subsequent acute occlusive symptoms. The prognosis of such obstructions is poor since thrombosis often extends all the way into peripheral portions of the artery, and its detection is not always easy (intensive care patients). Furthermore, recanalization requires the employment of all therapeutic tools available without subjecting the patient, who is usually in poor general condition, to excessive stress.

Simple catheter-induced thromboses or embolism are easily removed by immediate exposure of the puncture site, as described previously.

Problems arise when, for example, the entire periphery is obstructed following invasive arterial pressure measurement or incorrect intra-arterial application of a strong irritating substance which injures the intima. Systemic, thrombolytic therapy is usually not possible in these patients (who usually have several contraindications) and usually does not produce the desired effect anyway. Therefore, surgical thrombectomy and localized thrombolytic therapy with adequate irrigation should be combined. FADDEN, OCHSNER and MILES [6] have developed an interesting method which allows the simultaneous application of local thrombolytic substances. They prepared a piece of vein containing one tributary and implanted it as an interposition graft into the artery. A catheter was inserted into the branch of the venous strip and bound to it. Thrombolytics and anticoagulants were continuously infused through the catheter. In extremely difficult cases like this, where negative results frequently lead to court action, it is good to know of such extraordinary measures for saving a limb.

C. Postoperative Treatment of Complications

I. Compartment Syndrome (see p. 638).

If reconstruction or recanalization of an artery is postponed, a postischemic compartment syndrome may develop which absolutely requires treatment (see p. 638).

II. Surgical Management of Recurrent Occlusions

After successful removal of an acute arterial obstruction, accurate postoperative clinical monitoring is necessary. This implies checking the pulse several times a day, Doppler ultrasonographic blood pressure measurement, calculation of the Doppler index, and in some cases pulse curve recordings from the hands or feet. If the postoperative condition of the patient deteriorates and there is clinical evidence of recurrent occlusion presenting the same symptoms as primary occlusion – which may be mitigated if thrombosis develops slowly – the operating area must be reexplored (after angiography).

Causes of recurrent occlusion may be the following:

1. A reembolism, which may occur in the same vessel again and again in the case of arterioarterial emboli, and also cardiogenic emboli under certain hemodynamic conditions
2. Recurrent thromboses as a consequence of technical errors, e.g., thromboses, suture line stenoses, and injudicious application of the Fogarty catheter or ring stripper with subsequent injury to the intima
3. Inadequate anticoagulation

General anesthesia is preferred in reoperation of thrombotic occlusions since the general condition of the patient is usually poor. The operating area is reexposed, the vessel reopened, the obstruction removed using the standard technique, and the results of recanalization evaluated by intraoperative angiography. The rearteriotomy should be closed with a small vein patch to avoid stenosis at the suture line. Another alternative is to construct an orthotopic or extra-anatomic bypass if the occluded segment of the artery cannot be recanalized.

Multiple recurrent embolisms at the same or at different sites should impel the surgeon to look for an embolic source and eliminate it.

III. Elimination of the Embolic Source

In cardiogenic embolisms, a cardiologist or cardiovascular surgeon should be consulted in order to evaluate the possibility of removing the embolic source, which may be an atrial thrombus or a thrombus adhering to an aneurysm of the cardiac wall. If the problem cannot be solved in such a manner, the patient must receive anticoagulants or antiplatelet drugs for the rest of his life.

Proximal aneurysmal or ulcerated arterial wall lesions should, of course, be eliminated. The diagnosis of an abdominal aortic aneurysm can be confirmed by ultrasonography immediately after surgery. Proximal lesions of the aorta are detected by computed tomography and, of course, angiography. Poststenotic aneurysms in the thoracic outlet syndrome or in an arteriosclerotic popliteal aneurysm (comparison with the contralateral side is very important) are diagnosed by angiography. Surgical intervention is indicated in each of these cases.

IV. Wound Infection

The risk of deep wound infection is relatively small since no alloplastic material is used and no large wounds need to be created for removal of an acute arterial obstruction. Infection is rare if the rules of asepsis are observed. No antibiotics are administered prophylactically, except in septic embolisms. If a grade III deep infection does occur (danger of hemorrhage following arterial arrosion), the standard surgical techniques are applied, such as irrigating and drainage systems, coverage with omentum flaps, or extra-anatomic bypass grafting (see p. 167ff.).

V. Amputation

If all attempts at reconstruction of an acute arterial obstruction fail, the only alternative remaining is limb amputation. It is indicated and necessary in the following conditions:

1. Manifest gangrene.
2. If a compartment syndrome is not diagnosed and treated early enough, this complication leads to extensive skin and muscle necroses, even though the artery may have been revascularized properly. Proximal amputation is almost unavoidable in such cases.
3. Agonizing resting pain, without manifest gangrene, following incomplete thrombectomy may become intolerable and make amputation necessary after all secondary reconstructive attempts and conservative treatment have failed (e.g., diabetic microangiopathy).
4. A relative indication for limb amputation may be severe postischemic syndrome with anuria.

Special indications and the technique of amputation are presented on p. 630.

REFERENCES

1. Baue AE, McClerikn WW (1965) A study of shock, acidosis and the declamping phenomenon. Ann Surg 161:40
2. Bywaters EGL (1944) Ischemic muscle necrosis: crushing injury, traumatic edema, the crush syndrome, traumatic anuria, compression syndrome a type of injury seen in air raid casualities following burial beneath debris. JAMA 124:1103
3. Chidi CC, Depalma RG (1983) Atherogenic potential of the embolectomy catheter. Surgery 83/5:549–557
4. Denk W (1934) Zur Behandlung der arteriellen Embolie. MMW 81:437–439
5. Egan TJ, Daly M (1981) Acute upper limb ischemia in the thoracic outlet syndrome: its correction by axillo-axillary bypass grafting. Angiology 32/9:639–641
6. Fadden Mc PM, Ochsner JL, Mills N (1983) Management of thrombotic complications of invasive arterial monitoring of the upper extremity. J Cardiovasc Surg 24:35–39
7. Field T, Littooy FN, Baker WH (1982) Immediate and long-term outcome of acute arterial occlusion of the extremities. The effect of added vascular reconstruction. Arch Surg 117/9:1156–1160
8. Fogarty TJ, Cranley JJ, Krause ES, Strasser S, Hafner CT (1963) A method for extraction of arterial emboli and thrombi. Surg Gynecol Obstet 116:241–244
9. Fogarty TJ (1967) Catheter technique for arterial embolectomy. J Cardiovasc Surg 8:22–28
10. Fogarty TJ, Daily PO, Shumway NE, Krippaehne WW (1971) Experience with ballon catheter technic for arterial embolectomy. Am J Surg 122:231
11. Gautier R, Gordeeff A, Fourquet JQ, Gelas P, Jacquot C, Fauvage B (1982) Dissection auguè de l'aorte de stade III avec ischémie abdominale et jambière. Traitement par pontage aortoiliaque et revascularisations digestives. Chirurgie 108/3:228–233
12. Goldberg EM, Goldberg MC, Chowdhury LN, Gould SA (1983) The effects of embolectomy-thrombectomy-catheters and vascular architecture. J Cardiovasc Surg 24:74–80
13. Hagmüller GW, Denck H, Russe F, Veit F (1982) Die aortoarterielle Embolie als Komplikation atheromatöser und aneurysmatischer Veränderungen der distalen Bauchaorta. Angio Arch 3:75–78
14. Haimovici H (1960) Arterial embolism with acute massive ischemic myopathy and myoglobinuria. Surgery 47:739

15. Haimovici H (1979) Metabolic complications of acute arterial occlusions. J Cardiovasc Surg 20:349–358
16. Haimovici H (1979) Muscular, renal, and metabolic complications of acute arterial occlusions: Myonephropathic-metabolic syndrome. Surgery 85/4:461–468
17. Hess H, Mietaschk A (1983) Fibrinolytische Therapie bei den arteriellen Verschlußkrankheiten. Indikation und Ergebnisse. Hämostaseologie 23: 2
18. Hirst AE Jr, Johns VJ, Kime SW Jr (1958) Dissecting aneurysm of aorta. Review of 505 cases. Medicine 37:217–279
19. Kealy WF (1978) Atheroembolism. J Clin Pathol 31/10:984–989
20. Kniemeyer HW, Sandmann W, Winter J, Kaschner A, Nüllen H, Noack E (1983) Spastische Gefäßreaktion nach Dihydroergotamin-Komplikationen der postoperativen Thromboemboliepropylaxe. Aktuelle Chir 6/18:199–248
21. Lusby RJ, Wylie EJ (1983) Acute lowers limb ischaemia: pathogenesis and management. World J Surg 7:340–346
22. Pratt GH (1954) Cardiovascular Surgery. Kimpton, London
23. Senn A (1963) Die chirurgische Behandlung der akuten und chronischen arteriellen Verschlüsse. Huber, Berlin
24. Shah PM, Clauss RH (1983) Dissecting hematoma presents as acute lower limb ischemia. Diagnostic patient profile and management. J Cardiovasc Surg 24:649–653
25. Sheiner Nm, Zeltzer J, MacIntosh E (1982) Arterial embolectomy in the modern era. Can J Surg 25/4:373–375
26. Vollmar J (1983) Rekonstruktive Chirurgie der Arterien. Thieme, Stuttgart New York
27. Williams GM, Harrington D, Burdick J, White RI (1981) Mural thrombus of the aorta: an important, frequently neglected cause of large peripheral emboli. Ann Surg 194/6:737–744
28. Wuppermann TH. Klinik, Differentialdiagnose und Therapie des akuten Beinarterienverschlusses. Phlebol. Proktol 12:16–20

17 Occlusive Disease in the Lower Extremities

17.1 Aortoiliac Occlusive Disease

M. Trede and H.H. Thiele

CONTENTS

A. Anatomy

The aorta passes through the diaphragm together with the thoracic duct at the level of the 12th thoracic vertebra. It descends in the retroperitoneal space in front of the spine, splitting into the two iliac arteries at the level of the 4th lumbar vertebra, slightly to the left of the midline.

The left renal vein crosses the aorta at the level of the origins of the renal arteries. It rarely passes behind the aorta. Sometimes, it forms a loop which surrounds the aorta entirely (Fig. 17.1).

The abdominal aorta is subdivided into a suprarenal and an infrarenal segment. The suprarenal segment has a diameter of 24 ± 4 mm in men and 21 ± 3 mm in women. The infrarenal segment becomes narrower as it descends, and at the bifurcation it has a diameter of only 19 ± 3 mm in men and 17 ± 2 mm in women.

One must pay special attention to the inferior vena cava during preparation of the infrarenal aorta. It lies directly next to the aorta on the right side and may sometimes, though rarely, present topographical anomalies [7]. It may be doubled, cross the aorta proximally and pass over to the left side, or change its position entirely, as in visceral inversion (see p. 365).

In this region the aorta has several more or less constant branches: four pairs of lumbar arteries arising on its dorsal side, which makes it difficult to control bleeding when these arteries are injured. Also, when dissecting behind the aorta, one must be careful not to injure any of the four left lumbar veins crossing posteriorly. They have very thin walls and are rather large.

The most important uneven branch of this aortic segment is the inferior mesenteric artery, which arises from the lower third of the infrarenal aorta, slightly to the left of the midline, and supplies the left half of the colon. This branch should be preserved whenever possible. Yet, if it is injured, reimplantation is unnecessary as long as Riolan's anastomosis permits adequate collateral blood flow supplied by the superior mesenteric artery [8]. Visible pulsations of the marginal arcades of the sigmoid colon and strong back bleeding from the stump of the accidentally divided inferior mesenteric artery are good evidence of sufficient perfusion of the left colon [9].

The pole arteries, which are accessory renal arteries and may be encountered in some patients,

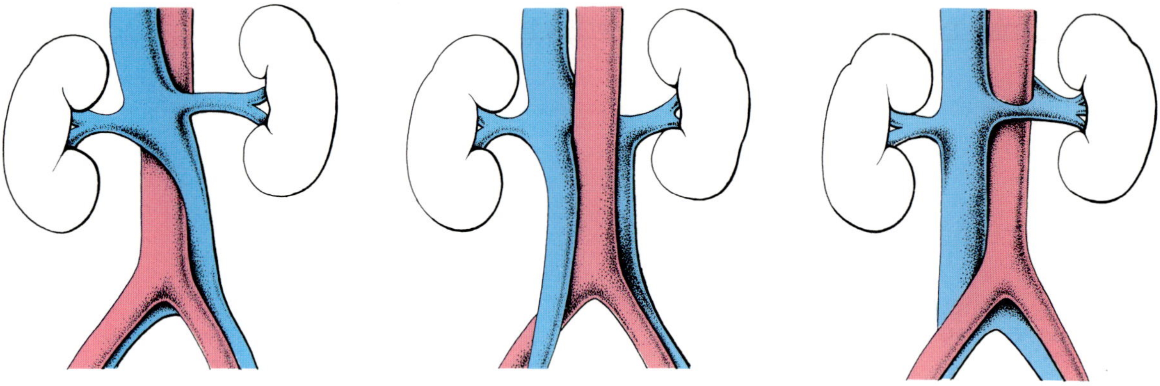

Fig. 17.1.1. Anomalies of the vena cava and the renal veins

are important for supply of renal tissues and therefore must always be preserved. If necessary, they must be reimplanted into the aorta or into a bypass graft. In this context, the horseshoe kidney deserves to be mentioned again. This anatomic variation covers the terminal segment of the aorta down to the bifurcation with its parenchymal isthmus.

Finally, a small variable branch, the presacral artery, arises from the aortic bifurcation.

Both iliac arteries separate into the larger external iliac artery and the smaller internal iliac artery at the level of the iliosacral joint. It is at this point that the ureter crosses these vessels, running along the upper margin of the small pelvis to the bladder. The internal iliac artery gives off parietal and visceral branches. The most important of these branches are the medial hemorrhoidal artery, which supplies the lower portion of the rectum, and the internal pudendal artery, the terminal branches of which supply the corpora of the penis. The external iliac artery runs medial to the iliopsoas muscle, entering the lacuna vasorum under the inguinal ligament, after giving off the inferior epigastric artery and the deep circumflex iliac artery. These vessels and their concomitant veins are easily injured when a synthetic prosthesis is pulled down to the groin (e.g., in an aortofemoral bypass), they can be the source of massive hemorrhage.

The iliac veins enter the inferior vena cava at the level of the aortic bifurcation. The iliac veins run dorsal to the common iliac arteries, remaining in close contact on the right side. During circumferential dissection of these arteries and passage of tapes around them, the danger of injuring the veins is great.

Of special anatomic importance is the sympathetic superior hypogastric plexus which is responsible for ejaculation in the sexually active male. This plexus is formed from two cords meeting at the level of the aortic bifurcation, which themselves arise on both sides of the abdominal aorta from visceral branches of the lumbar sympathetic chains. Its 1-cm-wide network lies over the left common iliac artery and runs across the common iliac vein to the promontorium, and from there to the mesorectum to form the lumbar sympathetic root of the pelvic plexus. The entire plexus forms a membrane, adhering tightly to the peritoneum embedded within the subperitoneal tissue distal to the origin of the inferior mesenteric artery. It can be easily palpated.

B. Indications for Surgery

I. Etiology

Arteriosclerosis is the major cause of occlusive arterial disease within the aortoiliac region in 90% of all cases. Endangiitis obliterans is rarely found. This disease more often affects the distal arteries. Other causes, such as primary idiopathic thrombosis (occurring in familial hyperlipidemia), postembolic occlusion, post-traumatic occlusions, or the extremely rare congenital stenoses and aplasias, are present in only a very small number of cases.

Although arteriosclerosis does not observe any anatomic boundaries, in practice, stenotic lesions are usually limited to the infrarenal aortic segment and the iliac arteries. Arteriosclerotic obstruction usually increases distally. Its main point of concentration lies in the area between the origin of the inferior mesenteric artery and the bifurcation. The proximal portion of the infrarenal segment is usually not so severely diseased and therefore suited for the proximal connection of a bypass graft.

II. Typical Types of Obstruction

Aortoiliac arterial occlusions may be classified morphologically into four different types (Fig. 17.1.2). The most common, type I occlusions, are one- or two-sided segmental occlusions in the iliac arteries or infrarenal aorta. Isolated short stenoses just above the bifurcation are commonly found in women with congenital disorders of lipid metabolism or with small, thin vessels.

In type II disease, multiple stenoses and occlusions are found in both iliac arteries and in the aorta.

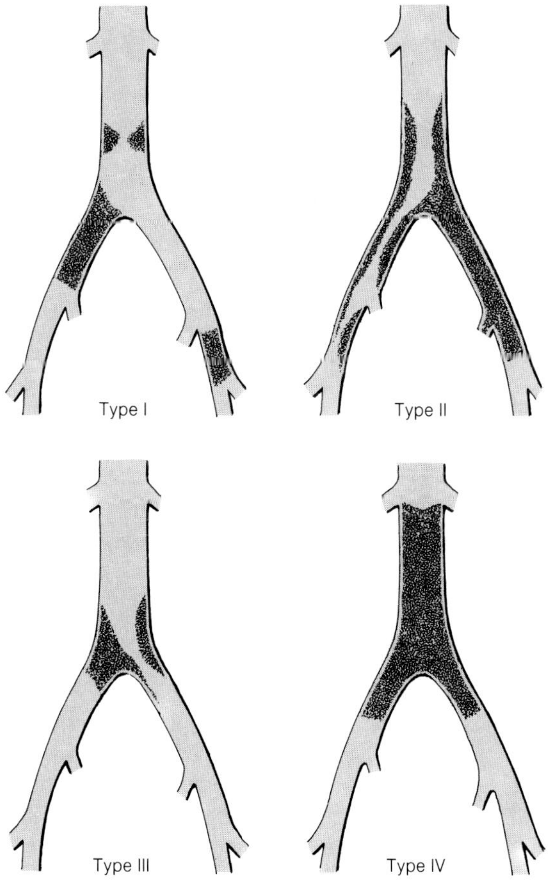

Fig. 17.1.2. Typical forms of aortoiliac occlusive disease

Type III shows lesions limited to the area surrounding the bifurcation.

The "Lériche syndrome" is a complete occlusion of the aortic bifurcation.

Finally, type IV is a proximal aortic occlusion in which the infrarenal segment of the aorta is obstructed all the way up to the renal arteries. This proximal aortic occlusion is usually caused by appositional thrombi forming within this segment just as in the Lériche syndrome.

Type I and type III are best suited for endarterectomy. Type II and type IV should always be revascularized with a bypass graft, for which a bifurcation prosthesis is usually chosen. It must be borne in mind that angiographic presentation of type I and III lesions always gives a more favorable impression of the situation within the diseased arteries, especially if the pictures offer only an anteroposterior view. In reality, the arteriosclerotic segments of the patent vessel frequently turn out to be longer than one might have expected on the basis of preoperative angiograms. Therefore, only a few patients with type I and type III aortoiliac occlusive disease will benefit from endarterectomy alone.

III. Indications and Clinical Stages

The indication for surgery depends on the clinical picture of symptoms, the localization and extension of arterial occlusions, the general condition of the patient, and the accompanying risk factors.

There is only a relative indication for surgery in patients with disease of stage II (according to FONTAINE). Subjective symptoms of the patient and the degree of disability in everyday life must be weighed against eventual risk factors. Once stages III and IV are reached, preservation of the limb has priority. This means that in stage II, optimal surgical conditions can be achieved by intensive preparation of the patient, whereas in stages III and IV, the procedure must be performed in spite of risk factors that are present. In particular, we require that obese patients in stage II undergo drastic weight reduction as a precondition for surgery.

We think that good long-term results (over 80% of all reconstructions are still patent after 10 years) and acceptably low operative mortality (2%–5%) permit more aggressive surgical management of aortoiliac occlusive disease [1, 2, 5]. By contrast, we are much more restrictive in the surgical treatment of femoropopliteal occlusive disease.

In multilevel occlusions, vascular reconstruction is always begun proximally and then continued downward. If stenoses of the aortoiliac segment are present simultaneously with occlusive disease of the femoropopliteal segment, the relevance of these stenoses must be determined by angiographic examinations in two planes, Doppler ultrasonography with calculation of the pulsatility index, and pressure or flow measurements.

Reconstruction of the aortoiliac segment with profunda revascularization often suffices to save the limb [13, 15]. Since 1980, we have been treating short segmental stenoses of the iliac arteries with transluminal dilatation under local anesthesia (see p. 123). If such a stenosis is combined with a femoropopliteal occlusion, simultaneous dilatation (of the iliac artery) and operative reconstruction (of the femoropopliteal segment) have proven to be very successful.

Fig. 17.1.3. Incisions

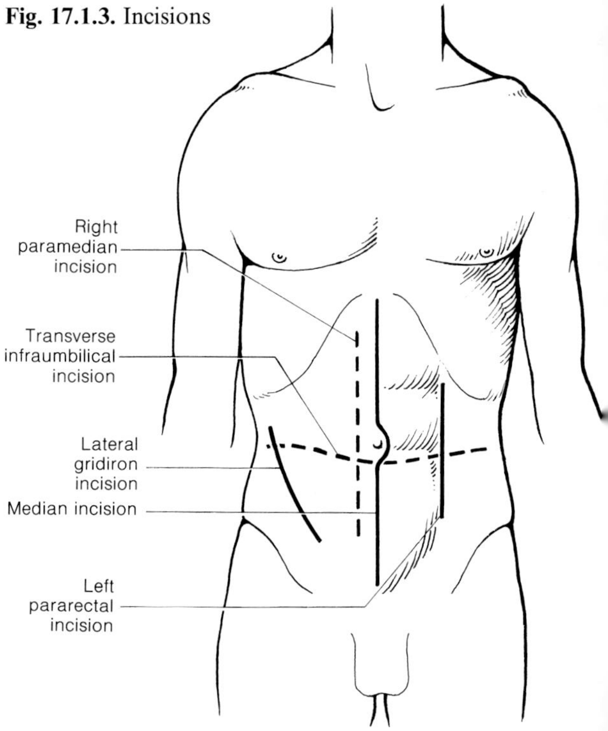

C. Positioning

The patient is placed in a normal supine position with elevation of the pelvis for all reconstructive procedures done on the aortoiliac segment. The operating table may be slightly rotated toward the surgeon on the right side, which permits him to obtain better access to the aorta lying deep within the abdomen. The operative field is prepared and draped from the nipples to the middle of the thigh. In multilevel occlusions with additional reconstruction of the femoral arteries, the corresponding limb must also be prepared and draped down to the ankled joints. A folded towel is placed over the genital region. Towels covering both groins are held in place by a transparent adhesive covering.

D. Surgical Approach

The following incisions can be made in aortoiliac reconstructions:

Transperitoneal approach:

1. Large median incision from the xiphoid process to the symphysis pubis, passing the umbilicus on the left side.
2. Paramedian incision on the left side.
3. Transverse infraumbilical laparotomy of the lower abdomen (especially suited for isolated obstructions at the bifurcation in slim patients) (Fig. 17.1.3).

Extraperitoneal approach:

1. Lateral gridiron incision on the right or left side.
2. Right or left pararectal incision.

If necessary, exposure of the femoral bifurcation is achieved in the standard way, using a longitudinal incision beneath the inguinal ligament, lateral to the main lymphatic vessels. Extension of such an incision upward with division of the inguinal ligament to expose the iliac vessels is an exception.

E. Technique of Exposure

I. Transperitoneal Exposure of the Infrarenal Aorta

After dividing the peritoneum, all abdominal organs are explored to exclude other diseases (e.g., carcinoma of the colon). The transverse colon is reflected upward and the entire small bowel, encased down to its mesenteric root in a moist towel, is mobilized and reflected onto the lateral wall of the abdomen. In very slim patients, the small bow-

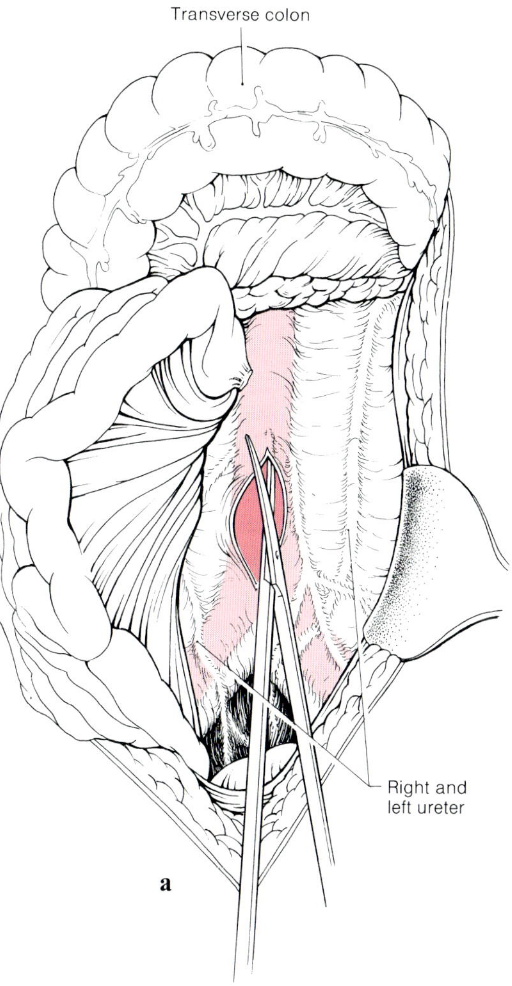

a

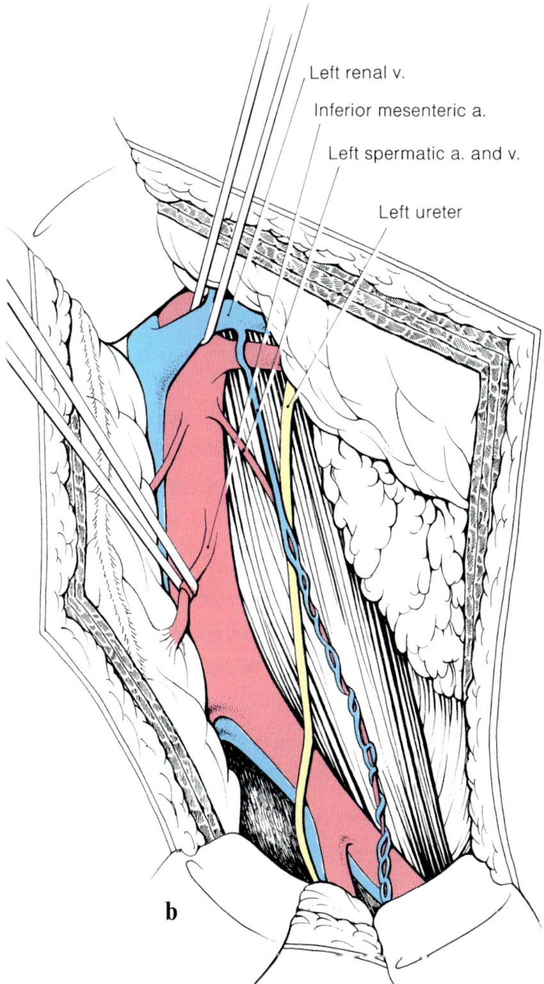

b

Fig. 17.1.4. a Transperitoneal approach to the infrarenal aorta, division of the retroperitoneum. **b** Extraperitoneal approach to the infrarenal aorta and left iliac artery

el may be left in the abdomen and simply pushed over to the right.

We open the retroperitoneum, starting at the duodenojejunal flexure, and extend the incision down the aortic bifurcation. To facilitate later closure of the retroperitoneum, the incision is made at least 1 cm away (left side) from the flexure (Fig. 17.1.4a). The anterior wall of the aorta is exposed by dissecting the preaortic lymph nodes and fat tissue off the front surface. Hemostasis is performed by electrocoagulation.

Further dissection is directed along the left lateral wall of the aorta, keeping just above the adventitia. The origin of the inferior mesenteric artery is visualized and tapes are passed around it. During dissection along the right lateral aortic wall, one must take care not to injure the inferior vena cava lying alongside the aorta in close contact with it. If open disobliteration of the aorta is planned, tapes must also be passed around the lumbar arteries branching off laterally. The lumbar veins accompanying the arteries should not be injured during this maneuver.

We always dissect the aorta free until we reach the crossing left renal vein. Only if the aortic occlusion extends further proximally are tapes placed around the vein. The vessel can then be carefully pulled upward for better access to the aorta. The left suprarenal vein (cranial) and the ovarian or spermatic vein (caudal) must be preserved (Fig. 17.1.4a). The inferior mesenteric vein, which runs further laterally on the left, may sometimes be divided between two ligatures to gain space.

Following preparation of the anterior aortic circumference, blunt Overholt clamps are carefully manipulated beneath the aorta from the right side. Rubber tubing is held between the tips of the clamps and passed around the dorsal wall of the aorta. This maneuver is always done as far proximal as possible, staying just below the renal arteries. If the aortic occlusion extends higher up, suprarenal preparation of the aorta is performed cranial to the crossing left renal vein. We do not pass tapes around the aorta if inflammatory processes impede dissection or if quick control of the aorta is necessary in an aneurysm. Dissection on both sides of the anterior aortic wall beneath the origins of the renal arteries produces enough space to place a strong vascular clamp on the aorta with its tips reaching the spine, thus permitting secure closure even without previous mobilization or placement of tapes.

II. Transperitoneal Exposure of the Iliac Arteries

Access to the right iliac bifurcation is gained after incising the parietal peritoneum and mobilizing the cecum cranially. We incise the peritoneum over the palpable vessels. Tapes are passed around the common iliac artery and external iliac artery. Traction on these tapes exposes the internal iliac artery and permits careful freeing of this vessel from the iliac vein which runs beneath it. Tapes are also passed around the internal iliac artery.

The left iliac bifurcation is also exposed by incising the parietal peritoneum following mobilization of the sigmoid colon and the mesosigmoid. The hypogastric plexus must be preserved when dissection is performed near the left common iliac artery. Of course, on both sides the ureter, which crosses the vessels, must be left unharmed.

III. Extraperitoneal Exposure of the Infrarenal Aorta

A left pararectal incision is best suited for wide extraperitoneal exposure of the infrarenal aorta. A gridiron incision can be used as an alternative approach in slim patients. It causes less trauma to the abdominal wall (Fig. 17.1.4b). The peritoneal sac is mobilized by blunt dissection and reflected medially. Ureter and ovarian vessels must remain attached to the peritoneal sac. After division of the inferior mesenteric artery, the aorta may be exposed by blunt dissection as far as the crossing left renal vein.

This approach, first described by ROB, is supposedly better tolerated by the poor risk patient and is supposedly associated with fewer postoperative complications [18]. We believe that this approach does not permit good exposure of the region, especially of the contralateral (i.e., the right) iliac artery. The situation is even worse in obese patients. Another argument against this approach is that it does not allow exploration of the intra-abdominal organs. In the last few years we have preferred the transperitoneal approach, at least for the construction of bifurcation bypases. Extra-anatomic bypass may be recommended as an alternative in poor-risk patients.

IV. Extraperitoneal Exposure of the Iliac Arteries

Isolated occlusions in the iliac arteries may be repaired by wide extraperitoneal exposure through a right or left pararectal or gridiron incision.

Preparation and mobilization of the peritoneal sac is performed in a cranial to caudal direction by carefully separating it from the transverse fascia. The transverse fascia ends caudad to the semilunar line. This fact must be considered when freeing the peritoneal sac from the transverse fascia in order not to accidentally open the very thin peritoneum below that line. Control and clamping of the aortic bifurcation does not usually cause any difficulties.

V. Retromesenteric Approach to the Aortic Bifurcation

To avoid impotence of a greater or lesser degree in younger patients undergoing surgery on the aortoiliac segment, THETTER has recently recommended the retromesenteric approach to the aortic bifurcation [23] (see p. 187ff.).

Following laparotomy, the sigmoid colon is pulled in a ventrocranial direction exposing the junction between the mesenteric and parietal peritoneum. After division of the peritoneum medial to the left ureter, the superior hypogastric plexus can, by continuous traction on the sigmoid colon, be gradually freed from the underlying tissue in one piece, together with the sigmoid arteries. The neurovascular arch produced in this way forms a bridge between the inferior mesenteric artery and the back wall of the rectum. Dissection may be performed beneath it in a transverse direction from left to right without injuring the plexus. This procedure permits good visualization of the aortic bifurcation.

The superior hypogastric plexus can also be dissected free from the aortic bifurcation in a retroperitoneal approach by carefully pushing the peritoneal sac out of the way. However, this maneuver is technically more difficult and exposes only the junction between the aorta and the iliac artery, since dissection is limited cranially by the lumbar root of the plexus, which runs ventrally [22].

F. Reconstructive Procedures

I. Endarterectomy

In thromboendarterectomy, the arteriosclerotic plug is either removed openly, i.e., under direct vision, using a dissector, or stripped out with a ring stripper in a semiclosed procedure that follows the principle "from bifurcation to bifurcation" (VOLLMAR) [27, 28]. A prerequisite for successful disobliteration, however, is the development of an adequate cleavage plane either between the media and the internal elastic layer or in the outer portion of the media within the external elastic layer. Calcifying arteriosclerotic disease which penetrates all layers of the wall is not suited for this type of revascularization.

The method is preferred in short segmental occlusions in younger patients. The procedure is technically more difficult, more time-consuming, and has more potential complications (early thrombosis!) than a bypass operation. Open thromboendarterectomy is suited for segmental occlusions of the common iliac artery. For good development of the proximal cleavage plane, the aortic bifurcation must be dissected free. We find it especially important to obtain a good view of the origin of the contralateral common iliac artery to avoid dissecting into this vessel. The distal end of the arteriotomy continues on into the external iliac artery to obtain good exposure of the origin of the internal iliac artery and for control of the distal end of the thromboendarterectomized segment, which should show a smooth transition to the non-diseased distal portion of the artery [16, 27, 28].

Occlusions of the internal iliac artery are relieved in younger patients for prevention or treatment of impotence.

We close the arteriotomy with a patch graft. In our opinion, direct suture is justifiable only in very ectatic vessels. If the arteriotomy is extended to the internal iliac artery, a patch must be tailored to fit the Y-shaped incision.

Segmental stenoses and occlusions at the aortic bifurcation (type III, see Fig. 17.1.3) are sometimes also revascularized by open thromboendarterectomy. Some authors (VAN DONGEN) recommend this procedure for primary treatment, especially in younger patients, although it requires more effort and time than bifurcation bypass [26]. This procedure is usually done using a transperitoneal approach. Both common iliac arteries are exposed, with careful preservation of the superior hypogastric plexus, as described earlier. Closure of the arteriotomy is accomplished by sewing a tailored synthetic patch graft, shaped like an inverted Y, to the margins of the incision.

We revascularize occlusions and stenoses of the external iliac artery according to the morphological extension of the occlusion. We often find intraoperatively that the arteriosclerotic lesions are worse than we anticipated from preoperative evaluation of angiograms taken in only one plane. Some operations which began with disobliteration of the artery often ended in construction of a bypass.

Today, we first perform percutaneous transluminal dilatation for short stenoses and occlusions of the external iliac artery. In widespread occlusions which obviously end distal to the iliac bifurcation, we still prefer the retrograde, closed "blind" endarterectomy with the ring stripper. This procedure is performed through an arteriotomy that begins in the common femoral artery and extends to the superficial femoral artery. If there is any doubt about the proximal end of the disobliterated arteriosclerotic core, or if anterograde flow is not fully restored following this maneuver, the iliac bifurcation must then be exposed. An arteriotomy at the iliac bifurcation will visualize the proximal end of the inner core cylinder. Retrograde endarterectomy may then be continued as a semiclosed thromboendarterectomy, which usually achieves satisfactory revascularization.

Because of the constant danger of perforation, retrograde endarterectomy should always be left to an experienced surgeon. As a rule, a large area should always be prepared and draped to allow quick exposure of the aorta and the iliac artery in an emergency. The anesthesiologist must monitor pulse and blood pressure during every phase of the operation (shock symptoms in instrumental perforation!).

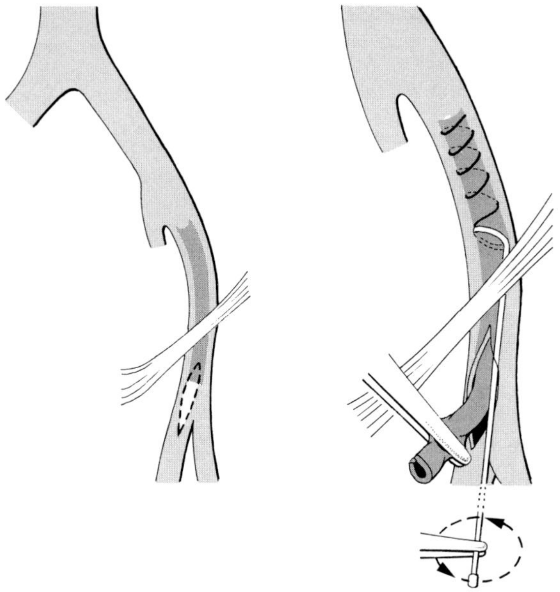

Fig. 17.1.5. Technique of retrograde ring disobliteration of the external iliac artery (schematized). Superficial femoral artery and profunda femoris artery are clamped distally; clamps are not drawn

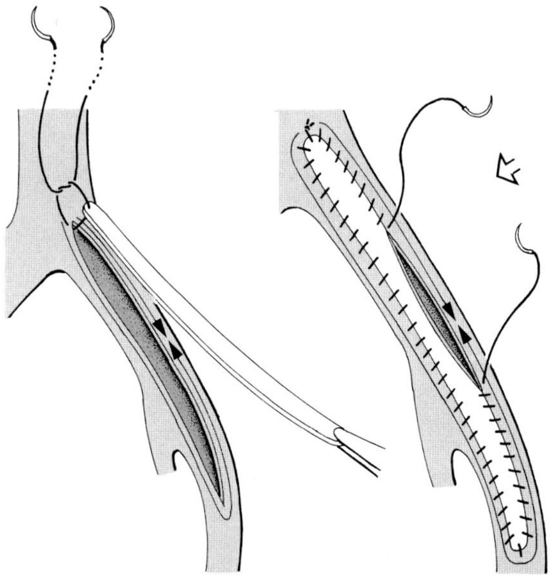

Fig. 17.1.6. Suture technique and position of the thread during sewing of the patch graft onto the artery (schematized); Clamps are placed proximal and distal to the arteriotomy; in order to save space, they are not shown here

In retrograde endarterectomy it is especially important to advance the ring stripper in the upstream direction with constantly rotating spiral movements while simultaneously pulling on the dissected inner core cylinder. If the core does not tear smoothly at the anticipated level, it must be sharply cut with the cutting ring and retrieved by means of a Fogarty catheter (Fig. 17.1.5).

Nevertheless, with this technique an adequate anterograde flow can be restored in most older poor-risk patients without having to open the abdomen or the retroperitoneum. Essential to the success of retrograde disobliteration is an experienced surgeon with a "delicate touch." The stripping procedure should never be forced.

After disobliteration, the arteriotomy is closed with a synthetic patch graft, which should not be too wide. This would cause turbulence that might lead to early thrombosis.

When using an elastic Dacron patch, the material should be sutured to the vessel under tension. This does not pertain to PTFE material, which must be very precisely tailored to the opening.

A double synthetic suture (size 5-0) is used to sew the patch continuously onto the artery. We start at the proximal corner of the arteriotomy and suture the side away from the surgeon first. After reaching the distal corner, the side toward the surgeon is sutured from both ends to the midpoint, where it is tied (Fig. 17.1.6). The assistant must keep the suture taut at all times to prevent dehiscence. The distance between the stitches depends on the size of the bites taken in the patch and the vascular wall. The stitch direction is always from the patch to the vessel.

II. Bypass Grafting

A standardized procedure in occlusions and stenoses of both sides of the aortoiliac segment is bifurcation bypass. In unilateral occlusions, we rarely perform unilateral aortofemoral or iliofemoral bypass instead of disobliteration.

We prefer the transperitoneal approach for the implantation of a bifurcation prosthesis since a wider exposure can be obtained.

The proximal anastomosis should be constructed as high up as possible, i.e., just caudad to the origin of the renal arteries. The anastomosis can either be performed end-to-end or end-to-side. Although hemodynamic considerations and principles favor an end-to-end anastomosis, a lengthy oblique end-to-side anastomosis (at least 4 cm) seems to be better for perfusion of the left colon and for blood supply to the branches of the inter-

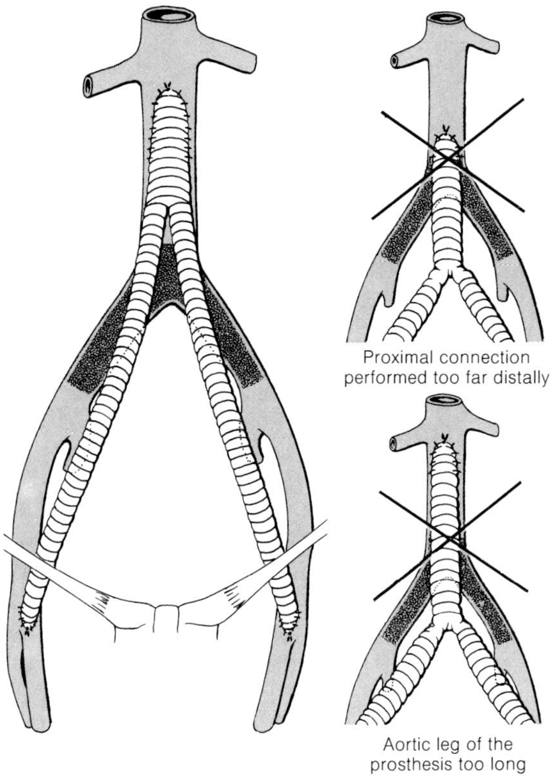

Fig. 17.1.7. Typical errors in implantation of a bifurcation prosthesis

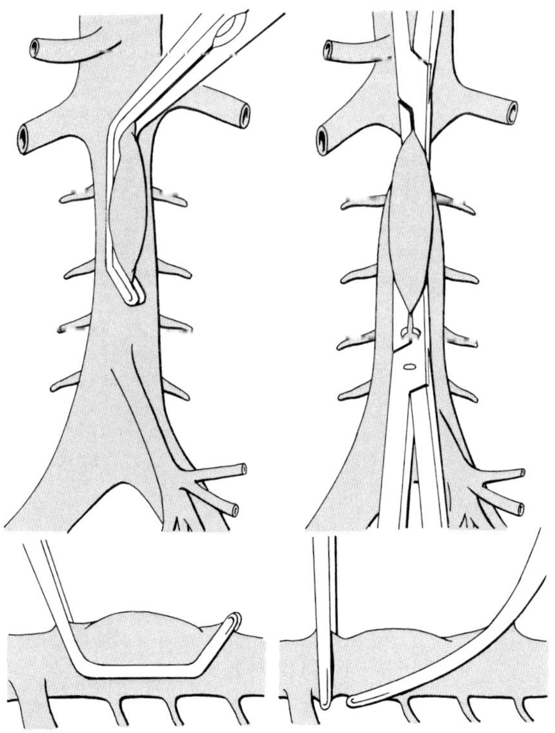

Fig. 17.1.8. Technique of partial and complete aortic clamping

nal iliac artery, which are important for sexual function [17].

It is especially important to keep the proximal portion of the bifurcation prosthesis short. Otherwise, kinks may develop in the arms of the prosthesis, leading to unfavorable hemodynamic flow conditions within the graft (Fig. 17.1.7).

The aorta is clamped proximally following standard exposure. For an end-to-side anastomosis, it suffices to place a straight clamp around the aorta, pointing downward at a slant. Partial clamping of the aorta with a Satinsky clamp is an alternative (Fig. 17.1.8). Prior to total aortic occlusion, 20 ml diluted heparinized saline solution (1:100) is instilled to prevent peripheral thrombosis (Fig. 17.1.10a).

If an end-to-end anastomosis is to be constructed, the distal aortic stump must be closed with a continuous 3-0 suture following transection of the aorta. If the lumbar arteries have been lacerated during transection of the aorta, they must be closed by sutures at their origin on the posterior aortic wall in order to stop back bleeding.

To avoid unnecessary blood loss during clotting of the prosthesis, we draw 20 ml blood directly from the aorta before clamping it. The prosthesis is then preclotted with this blood while the arteriotomy is being performed for the anastomosis (Fig. 17.1.9a, b).

After opening the aorta and perianastomotic disobliteration with a dissecting blade, one must carefully flush the area with a 1:100 diluted heparinized saline solution. This maneuver is done to prevent peripheral embolization. This "disobliteration" should be limited to the removal of appositional thrombi and soft cholesterol particles. Proper endarterectomy is hardly possible if the aorta is clamped tangentially. Moreover, it is dangerous (possible distal dissection!) (Fig. 17.1.10a–c).

After beveling the prosthesis, we perform the proximal anastomosis with a double 4-0 suture, starting at the proximal corner of the arteriotomy. The suture is begun on the side farther away from the surgeon and completed on the nearer side (Fig. 17.1.11).

After completing the proximal anastomosis the prosthesis is flushed by briefly unclamping the aorta. Once the wall of the prosthesis has become blood tight through preclotting and leakage at the anastomosis has stopped, the graft is clamped just distal to the proximal anastomosis, and blood clots are removed from within the prosthesis with a glass suction tube (Fig. 17.1.12).

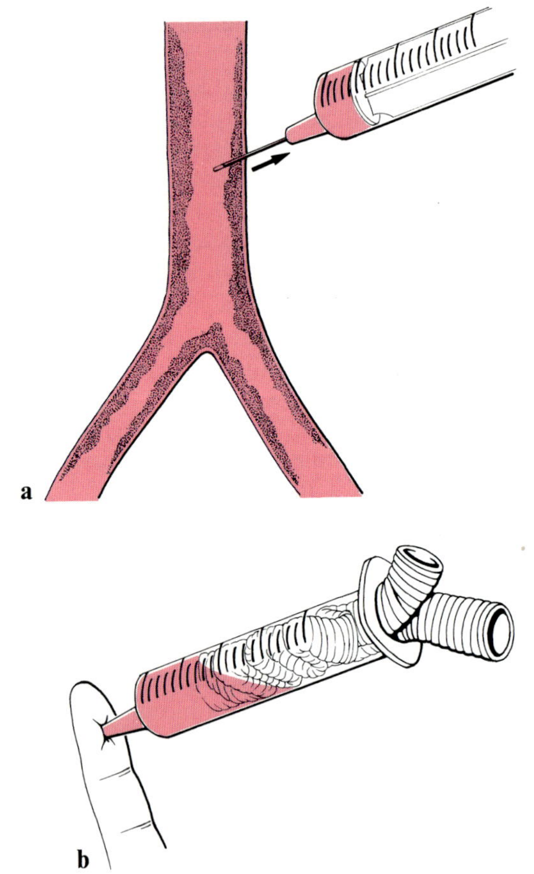

Fig. 17.1.9a, b. Preclotting of the prosthesis in a 20 ml syringe filled with blood

The distal anastomoses may be constructed at the iliac bifurcation or at the femoral bifurcation by separate incisions performed in both groins. The exact site of the distal connection depends on the extension of occlusive arterial disease. VAN DONGEN recommends suprainguinal attachment of the prosthetic limbs. The prosthesis is connected to the distal portion of the iliac arteries directly from the peritoneal cavity or through a separate suprainguinal incision with division of the aponeurosis of the external oblique muscle, parallel to the inguinal ligament. Following transection of the crossing deep circumflex iliac veins and mobilization of the internal oblique abdominal muscle, the suprainguinal portion of the external iliac artery can be exposed.

Access to additional arteriosclerotic lesions (stenotic origin of the profunda femoris artery) may be obtained by separate groin incisions or by distal extension of the incision. Disobliteration may then be performed. VAN DONGEN recommends combining a semiclosed endarterectomy with vein patch graft angioplasty because of the risk of infection (s. p. 440). We prefer bifemoral attachment of the prosthesis to the more extensive method of reconstruction as described by VAN

Fig. 17.1.10a–c. Clamping of the aorta following heparin instillation, longitudinal aortotomy, and tailoring of the prosthesis

▽

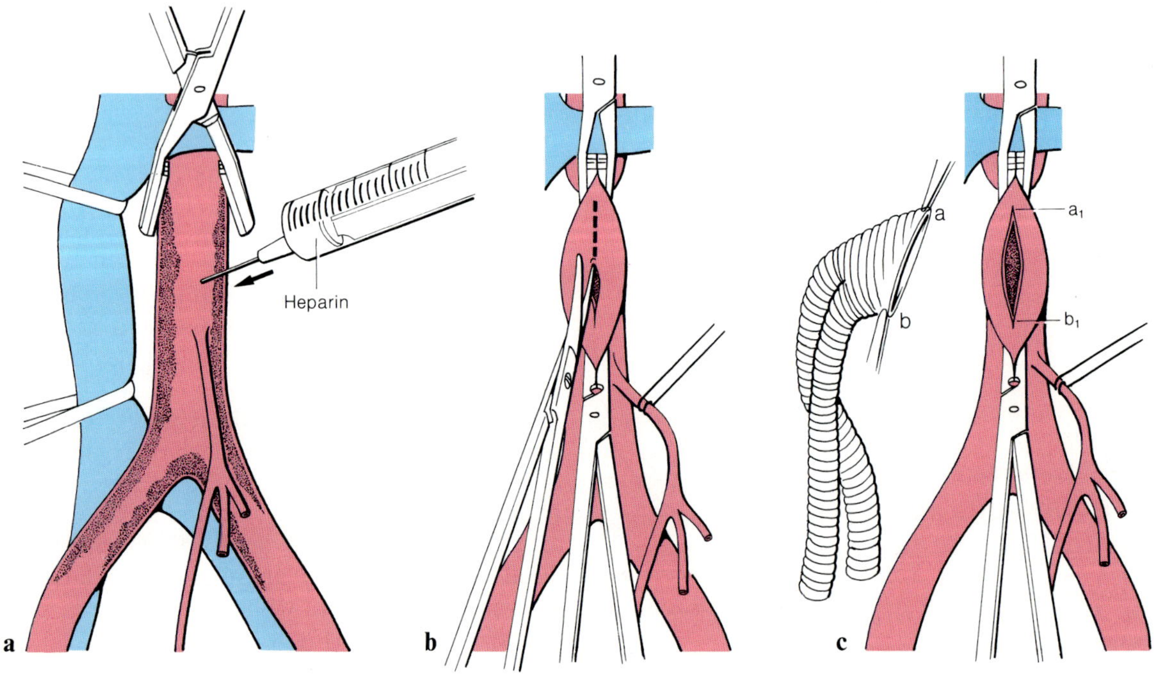

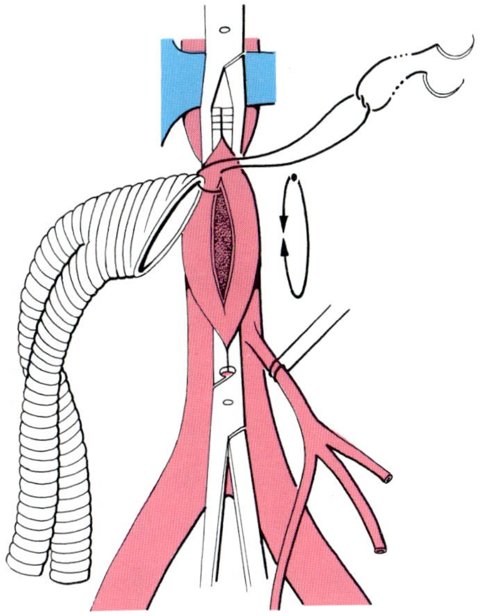

Fig. 17.1.11. Suture technique at the proximal end-to-side anastomosis

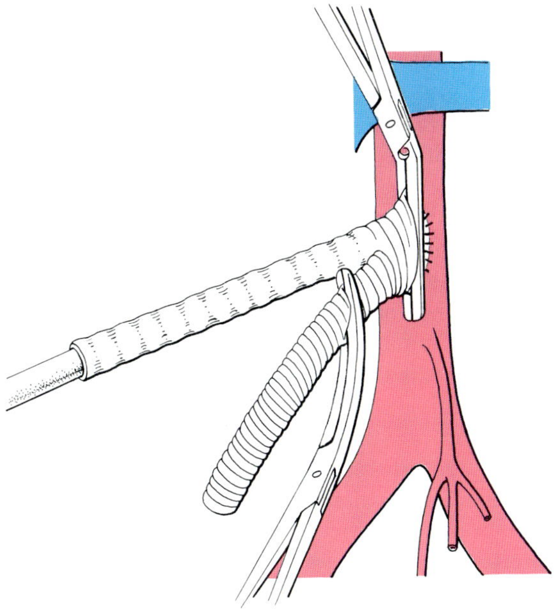

Fig. 17.1.12. Removing blood clots from the prosthesis by suction

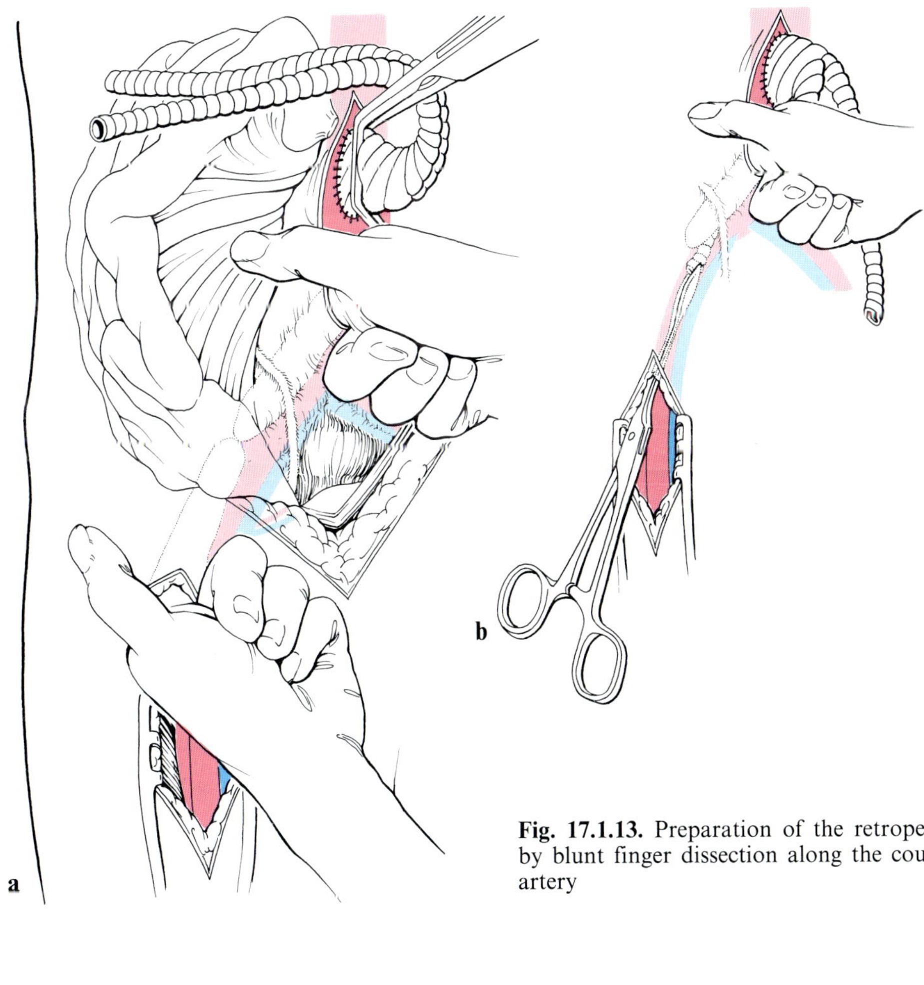

Fig. 17.1.13. Preparation of the retroperitoneal tunnel by blunt finger dissection along the course of the iliac artery

DONGEN. The rate of infection in our own patients remained under 1%.

Pulling the arms of the prosthesis downward into the inguinal region must be done with special care. Tunneling of the retroperitoneum is done by blunt finger dissection from above and below. The dissection is performed in the direction of the axis of the vessels, which are often calcified. Anterolateral dissection along the main stem of the artery avoids injuring the iliac vein which runs medially. The ureter must remain ventral to the arm of the prosthesis. After digital tunneling has been completed, a long forceps is introduced from below. The arm of the prosthesis is then grasped and pulled throughout without twisting it. Markings on the commercially available prostheses may help to align the prosthesis properly (Fig. 17.1.13a, b).

An arteriotomy is then performed on the common femoral artery. We extend the incision down to the origin of the profunda femoris artery so that both main arteries of the thigh are supplied by the limb of the prosthesis. In occlusions of the superficial femoral artery the arteriotomy is extended to the origin of the profunda femoris artery to make patch graft angioplasty of this vessel possible. We do not perform extensive disobliteration of the femoral bifurcation if only a dorsal plaque is present.

After exact tailoring of the prosthesis, we construct the distal anastomosis, on the right side first, in an end-to-side fashion. The suture is started at the upper corner of the arteriotomy on the side farther away from the surgeon and completed in the middle of the nearer side (Fig. 17.1.14).

The proximal and distal corners of the anastomosis are crucial for patency. If the sutures are not correctly placed at these sites, the run-in at the proximal corner may be constricted by the prosthesis. Leakage at this site following suture is very difficult to oversew. Narrowing of the runoff may occur at the distal corner. This may be worsened by supplementary sutures that may have to be added in order to stop leakage at that corner.

Prior to completion of the distal anastomosis the central and right limbs of the prosthesis are flushed (the left limb is, of course, clamped proximally). Retrograde flow through the distal anastomosis is checked by briefly unclamping the superficial femoral artery and the profunda femoris artery.

After completion of the right distal anastomosis the proximal clamp is transferred to the left arm of the prosthesis, restoring blood flow to the right

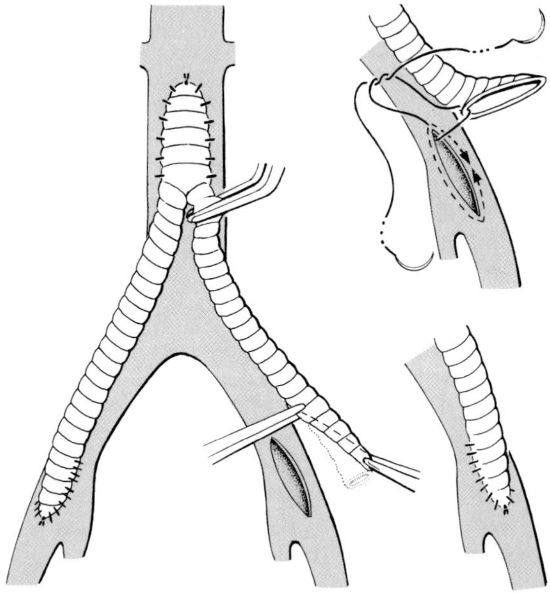

Fig. 17.1.14. Suture technique at the distal end-to-side anastomosis

Table 17.1.1. Steps during implantation of a bifurcation prosthesis

1. Puncture of the aorta to obtain about 20 ml of non-heparinized blood.
2. Temporary tailoring of the prosthesis – shortening of the aortic arm (if this is done under sterile conditions, the rest of the prosthesis can be used again as patch graft material in other procedures).
3. Preclotting of the prosthesis in a 20 ml syringe with the previously drawn blood.
4. Clamping of the aorta.
5. Peripheral heparinization.
6. Aortotomy.
7. Disobliteration of the aorta at the designated site of the anastomosis (being careful of embolization).
8. Exact tailoring of the preclotted prosthesis.
9. Suture of the central anastomosis.
10. Brief flushing of the prosthesis for final clotting of the graft.
11. Clamping of the prosthesis distal to the anastomosis.
12. Clearing the prosthesis of blood clots by suction – verification that prosthesis is completely free of clots.
13. Preparation of the distal anastomoses.
14. Tunneling of the retroperitoneum.
15. Pulling the prosthesis through the tunnel.
16. Preparation of the common femoral artery, final tailoring of the prosthetic arms.
17. Construction of the right distal anastomosis first.
18. Flushing the right arm of the prosthesis and clamping the other.
19. Pulling the left arm of the prosthesis through the tunnel and connecting it to the common femoral artery.

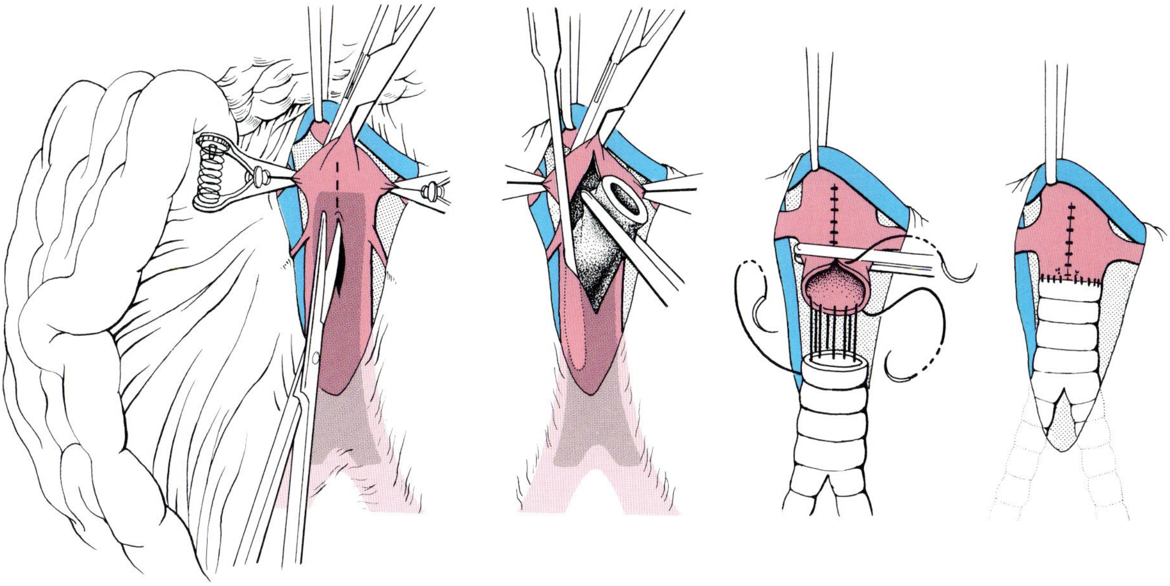

Fig. 17.1.15. Operative procedure in an infrarenal aortic occlusion with temporary clamping of the renal arteries on both sides

prosthetic leg. The left distal connection to the host artery is then established (Fig. 17.1.14).

We cover the proximal anastomosis with a cuff of pedicled greater omentum to guard against anastomotic complications (aortoduodenal fistula, anastomotic aneurysm) [25]. The retroperitoneum is then closed in two layers with a continuous absorbable 3-0 suture.

Table 17.1.1 summarizes each step during implantation of a bifurcation prosthesis.

G. Infrarenal Aortic Occlusion

Surgical management of an infrarenal aortic occlusion (type IV, Fig. 17.1.2) may vary considerably from case to case [4, 6, 19, 31]. Direct revascularization with a bifurcation prosthesis makes preparation of the aorta up to the suprarenal segment necessary. Dissection around the suprarenal aorta is facilitated by passing tapes around the left renal vein. We then also pass tapes around both renal arteries following exposure of the aorta in order to be able to clamp them briefly for proximal disobliteration.

We begin by clamping the suprarenal aorta and both renal arteries and then perform an aortotomy, which is extended upward about 2–3 cm above the origins of the renal arteries. The aorta is locally disobliterated with a dissector and an Overholt clamp. It is usually thrombotic material that is removed. Both orifices of the renal arteries can be viewed directly from the inside, and loose clots obstructing the lumina can be removed.

Following continuous suture of the proximal portion of the aortotomy, the clamps are transferred to the infrarenal aorta. This maneuver restores blood flow to the renal arteries. Then, the end-to-end or end-to-side anastomosis with the bifurcation prosthesis may be constructed according to the standard technique (Fig. 17.1.15).

We recommend direct reconstruction of an infrarenal aortic occlusion only in younger, not too obese patients since exposure of the region is difficult and there is increased risk of renal injury. An extra-anatomic procedure (axillobifemoral bypass) is preferable in older, obese, or poor-risk patients [3].

H. Surgical Reintervention

The type of surgical reintervention depends on the type of primary operation. For example, a transperitoneal approach is recommended in cases where a thromboendarterectomy performed using an extraperitoneal approach is postoperatively complicated by recurrent occlusion.

In unilateral recurrent occlusions with an unoperated contralateral side, disobliteration or bypass grafting of the untouched side can create favorable conditions for crossover revascularization of the reoccluded, previously corrected artery [29].

If the procedure must be done by the same surgical approach, we strongly recommend splinting the ureters with ureteral catheters since the danger of injuring the ureters is especially high in reinterventions at the aortoiliac level.

Basically, one must stress that the surgeon always encounters considerable technical difficulties in these reinterventions. Therefore, extra-anatomic procedures are preferable in doubtful situations (see p. 545).

I. Complications

I. Intraoperative Complications

1. Venous Injury

If hemorrhage occurs from the vena cava or the lumbar veins as the aorta is dissected free, bleeding sites should first be controlled by direct digital compression. Gentle compression (venous pressure is low – fragility of the venous wall high) almost always stops venous hemorrhage. The bleeding site can then be exactly localized and ligated directly with 5-0 or 6-0 sutures. Eager sucking away of blood and blind clamping within a pool of blood very quickly leads to high blood losses. Lacerations of the vena cava may be clamped tangentially without problems. The defect can then be repaired unhurriedly and under direct vision.

Circumferential dissection and mobilization of the common iliac artery may very easily lead to injury of the iliac vein which is in very close contact with the artery. If the maneuvers mentioned do not arrest bleeding, the artery must be transected, dissected free proximally and distally, and the venous defect carefully repaired. The divided artery is then reconnected by direct end-to-end anastomosis.

2. Injuries of the Lumbar Arteries

Circumferential dissection and mobilization of the aorta can lead to injury of the lumbar arteries. Bleeding from these vessels may usually be stopped by suture ligation on the lateral aspect of the aorta. If bleeding continues, the aorta must be temporarily clamped proximally and then completely transected to obtain access to the bleeding sites on the back wall. One may continue the procedure by constructing an end-to-end anastomosis with the aortic limb of the graft and not reconnecting both aortic stumps. However, such bleeding can usually be brought under control by exact suture ligation.

3. Intraoperative Injury to the Intestine

The danger of intraoperative injury to the intestine with opening of the intestinal lumen exists during preparation of the proximal aorta at the duodenojejunal flexure. This complication is very rare. If the small bowel is accidentally opened at that site, the defect must immediately be oversewn in two layers. If the retroperitoneum has been extensively contaminated, an alloplastic prosthesis should not be implanted immediately, but postponed until a later date. In stage III or IV disease, an extra-anatomic bypass may serve as an alternative.

Perioperative antibiotic prophylaxis should always be carried out when alloplastic material is implanted, even without intraoperative intestinal injury [25].

4. Division of the Ureter

If the ureter is accidentally transected, it is reanastomosed end-to-end over an 8 Charrière silicone ureter catheter. An oblique anastomosis is performed with an absorbable 4-0 suture.

5. Complications Due to the Prosthesis

The aortic limb of the prosthesis must be short enough to prevent kinking at the limbs of the prosthesis with resultant impairment of flow to the distal arteries (see Fig. 17.1.9). When the limbs of the prosthesis are placed in the tunnel, special attention must be given to their length; if a limb is too long or too short, there will be tension on the anastomosis. Finally, the twisting of a limb will lead to immediate occlusion; this can generally be avoided by observing the markings on the prosthesis. Should an occlusion occur in this way, a new unilateral bypass must be implanted, or revascularization must be achieved by constructing a crossover bypass from the patent side to the occluded vessel [3, 29].

II. Late Complications

1. Stenoses of the Ureter

Causes of stenoses of the ureters following prosthetic reconstructions at the aortoiliac level include: improper position of the ureter between the vessel and the prosthesis, postoperative hematoma or lymphoma, and prosthetic infections or trophic lesions of the ureteral wall [2, 10, 12, 14, 30]. If the ureter lies between the prosthesis and the vessel, the method of choice is transection of the prosthesis and reanastomosis behind the ureter.

In ureteral lesions with extravasation of urine, infection of the prosthesis usually develops. In such cases, nephrectomy is unavoidable since reanastomosis of the graft is not possible.

Stenoses of a lesser degree may often be relieved by splinting the ureter for a longer period of time. Some authors recommend intraperitonealization of the ureter in widespread retroperitoneal fibrosis.

2. Anastomotic Aneurysms

Anastomotic aneurysms following prosthetic reconstruction at the aortoiliac level are seen in 3% of all cases after 3–15 years. The causes are degenerative changes within the host artery or too extensive local thromboendarterectomy at the site of primary anastomosis. Suture disruption, often discussed in the past, is no longer relevant since the introduction of modern suture materials. Mechanical strain on the prosthesis in the groin is certainly an important pathogenic factor. Local infection may also play an important role in causing pathologic dilatation [11, 24].

Repair of such aneurysms is urgently indicated if they have enlarged considerably in size within a short period of time or if free rupture has occurred. However, ruptures are rather rare. Instead, local thrombosis with symptoms of acute occlusion or with embolization into distal arteries is common.

Surgical exposure of an anastomotic aneurysm is often difficult, owing to the considerable growth of scar tissue within the area. Sometimes, not all branches can be visualized so that Fogarty catheters must be introduced to provide intraluminal blockage for control of hemorrhage. The aneurysm is usually resected and replaced by a new alloplastic interposition graft. Aneurysmorrhaphy is only indicated if the defect is very strictly localized and the suture material clearly shows a flaw (see p. 173).

K. Simultaneous Procedures

In transperitoneal surgery, careful exploration of the abdominal organs is always performed first; if pathological changes are encountered, surgical plans must be modified accordingly. For example, if a stenosing carcinoma of the colon is found in a patient with stage II occlusive arterial disease, we recommend operating on the colon tumor first and postponing vascular reconstruction.

If the patient suffers from gallstones, a cholecystectomy may be performed following vascular reconstruction and secure closure of the retroperitoneum.

We never perform an appendectomy for fear of contamination with intestinal bacteria.

Lesions of the female gonads such as ovarian cysts, should, however, be removed if this is possible without too much effort.

REFERENCES

1. Brewster DC, Darling RC (1978) Optimal methods of aortoiliac reconstruction. Surgery 84:739
2. Carmichael DH, Barnes WF (1979) Obstruction of the ureter due to a false aneurysm. Surgery 86:769
3. Connolly JF, Kwaan JHM, Brownell D, McCart PM, Levine E (1984) Newer developments of extraanatomic bypass. Surg Gynecol Obstet 158:415
4. Corson JD, Brewster DC, Darling RC (1982) The surgical management of infrarenal aorticocclusion. Surg Gynecol Obstet 155:369
5. Crawford ES, Bomberger RA, Glaeser DH, Saleh SA, Russell WL (1981) Aortoiliac occlusive disease: factors influencing survival and function following reconstructive operation over a twenty-five-year period. Surgery 90:1055
6. McCullough JL, Mackey WC, O'Donnell TF, Millan VG, Deterling RA, Callow AD (1983) Infrarenal aortic occlusion: a reassessment of surgical indications. Am J Surg 146:178
7. Davis RA, Milloy FJ, Anson BJ (1958) Lumbar, renal and associated parietal and visceral veins based upon a study of 100 specimens. Surg Gynecol Obstet 107:1
8. Ernst CB, Hagihara PF, Daugherty ME, Griffen WO (1978) Inferior mesenteric artery stump pressure: a reliable index for safe IMA ligation during abdominal aortic aneurysmectomy. Ann Surg 187:641
9. Ernst CB (1983) Prevention of intestinal ischemia following abdominal aortic reconstruction. Surgery 93:102
10. Frusha JD, Porter JA, Batson RC (1982) Hydronephrosis following aorto-femoral bypass grafts. J Cardiovasc Surg 23:371
11. Giessler R (1980) Anastomosen-Aneurysmen nach synthetischem Gefäßersatz. Chirurg 51:14

12. Henry LG, Bernhard VM (1978) Ureteral pathology associated with aortic surgery: a report of three unusual cases. Surgery 83:464
13. Jones AF, Kempczinski RF (1981) Aortofemoral bypass grafting. Arch Surg 116:301
14. Kleinhans G, Leusmann D, Rühland D (1985) Urologische Komplikationen nach gefäßprothetischen Eingriffen im aortofemoralen Bereich. Chirurg 56:1
15. Mulcare RJ, Royster TS, Lynn RA, Conners RB (1978) Long-term results of operative therapy for aortoiliac disease. Arch Surg 113:601
16. Nash T (1979) Aortoiliac occlusive vascular disease: A prospective study of patients treated by endarterectomy and bypass procedures. Aust NZ J Surg 49:223
17. Pierce GE, Turrentine M, Stringfield S, Iliopoulos J, Hardin CA, Hermreck AS, Thomas JH (1982) Evaluation of end-to-side VS end-to-end proximal anastomosis in aortobifemoral bypass. Arch Surg 117:1580
18. Rob CG (1963) Extraperitoneal approach to the abdominal aorta. Surgery 53:87
19. Rückert U, Trede M, Kersting KH (1974) Der „hohe" Aortenverschluß beim Risikopatienten. Thoraxchirurgie, vol 22. Thieme, Stuttgart, p 548
20. Sandmann W, Lerut J (1981) Indikation und Therapie der aortoiliacalen Verschlußerkrankung aus chirurgischer Sicht. Chirurg 52:96
21. Scheele J, März D (1981) Potenzstörungen nach aortobifemoralem Prothesen-Bypass. Chirurg 52:168
22. Taheri SA, Gawronski S, Smith D (1983) Paramedian retroperitoneal approach to the abdominal aorta. J Cardiovasc Surg 24:529
23. Thetter O, v Hochstetter A, van Dongen RJAM (1982) Neurogene Störungen der männlichen Sexualfunktion nach Eingriffen im aorto-iliacalen Bereich und deren Vermeidung durch den retromesenterialen Zugang. Angio 4:171
24. Thiele H, Trede M (1979) Postoperative Komplikationen bei chronischen aorto-iliakalen Verschlüssen. Med Klin 74:667
25. Trede M, Rückert U, Laubach K (1977) Septische Gefäßkomplikationen. Prophylaxe und Therapie. Med Welt 28:838
26. Van Dongen RJAM (1970) Photographic atlas of reconstructive arterial surgery. Springer, Berlin Heidelberg New York
27. Vollmar J (1975) Rekonstruktive Chirurgie der Arterien. Thieme, Stuttgart
28. Vollmar J, Laubach K, Campana JM (1965) Die chirurgische Behandlung der chronischen Arterienverschlüsse im aorto-iliakalen Gefäßabschnitt. Thoraxchirurgie, vol 13. Thieme, Stuttgart, p 453
29. Vollmar J (1980) Reinterventionen wegen Rezidivverschlüssen (Becken- und Beinarterien). Chirurg 51:1
30. Wallijn E, Renders G, Vereecken L (1975) Urological complications following aortofemoral bypass graft. Br J Urol 47:617
31. Zehle A, Diederichs D (1973) Hoher Aortenverschluß. Thoraxchirurgie, vol 21. Thieme, Stuttgart, p 397

17.2 Chronic Occlusive Disease of the Femoropopliteal Artery

F.P. GALL and F. FRANKE

CONTENTS

A. Special Anatomy

I. The Femoropopliteal Segment (Thigh)

The femoropopliteal segment consists of the caudal portion of the external iliac artery, the common femoral artery with its division into the profunda femoris artery and superficial femoral artery, and the popliteal artery down to the trifurcation in the lower leg.

The *external iliac artery* is the continuation of the common iliac artery and runs on the medial side of the greater psoas muscle down to the inguinal ligament. Before entering the lacuna vasorum, it gives off two branches beneath the inguinal ligament: the deep circumflex iliac artery and the inferior epigastric artery curving upward on the inside of the abdominal wall to the crest of ilium.

The *common femoral artery* is the extension of the external iliac artery distal to the inguinal ligament. At first it runs superficially beneath the fascia of the thigh and then passes through the iliopectineal fossa behind the sartorius muscle. Along its 1–6 cm course, until separating into the profunda femoris artery and superficial femoral artery, it gives off three main branches: the superficial circumflex iliac artery and the superficial epigastric artery run to the anterior abdominal wall, the external pudendal artery to the genital region.

The *superficial femoral artery* runs in the groove between the vastus medialis muscle and the adductors, passing under the sartorius muscle into the popliteal fossa. The artery is about 30 cm long and gives off only very small branches. The most important collateral vessel, the descending genicular artery, penetrates the vastoadductor membrane and descends on top of it to the knee joint. The profunda femoris artery has about the same diameter as the superficial femoral artery. The main stem arises on the lateral side of the common femoral artery in 48%, on the dorsal side in 40%, and medially in 10%. Occasionally, it has already branched as it arises from the common femoral artery. In an occlusion of the superficial femoral artery, the profunda femoris artery lines up in the direction of the common femoral artery, leading to enlargement of its diameter. It supplies the thigh muscles and thigh bones (medial and lateral circumflex arteries, perforating arteries I–III) and is the most important collateral vessel for the circumvention of femoral occlusions. The collaterals of the profunda circulation reach the first and second segments of the popliteal artery (recipient segment).

The *popliteal artery* lies on the flexor side of the knee, medial to the vein and nerve, extending down to the soleus arch where it separates into the lower limb arteries. It is usually about 12–18 cm long and gives off various small branches which together form a fine vascular network (vascular network of the knee joint). This collateral circulation is not adequate to maintain perfusion of the lower leg when the popliteal artery is ligated (amputation rate 38%–72.5%).

II. Typical Sites of Occlusion in the Lower Half of the Body

A segmental, short occlusion is found within the distal segment of the superficial femoral artery in the adductor canal in 15%–20% of patients.

A long occlusion of the entire superficial femoral artery from the origin of the profunda femoris artery down to the adductor canal occurs in 40%–65%. It represents an advanced stage of occlusive arterial disease in most patients.

Alternating stenoses and short occlusions are found in the thigh and lower leg arteries in 15%. This type of occlusive disease is typical of diabetic macroangiopathy which terminates distally in microangiopathy.

Some 5% of patients with femoral and lower limb arterial occlusions have segments of the popliteal artery which are patent and to which strong collateralization has developed. This is especially important if revascularization is planned.

The frequency distribution of chronic occlusive arterial lesions in the lower limb is as follows:

Aortoiliac occlusions (inflow tract)	24%
Iliofemoral occlusions	4%
Femoropopliteal occlusions	50%
Isolated popliteal occlusions	5%
Crural occlusions	17%

B. Indications

Indications for reconstructive procedures in the lower half of the body depend only on the clinical symptoms which the patient presents. Stage I according to FONTAINE and LERICHE is not an indication for surgery.

Ischemic stage II is a relative surgical indication if claudication occurs on walking a distance of under 100 m, impeding private and occupational activity, and if there are favorable morphologic conditions with a two-vessel run-off.

Ischemic stage III and IV with rest pain and localized or extensive necroses is an absolute indication for surgery.

Patent arteries proximal and distal to the occlusion are essential for successful revascularization. Run-off is sufficient when two or three patent lower leg arteries, extending all the way down to the foot, can be clearly visualized by angiography.

The run-off is barely sufficient when only one lower leg artery is patent down to the foot. Occlusion of all three lower leg arteries is a very unfavorable constellation. If, in case of an occlusion of the femoral artery, a short segment of the popliteal artery is patent with adequate collateral flow to it, isolated segmental revascularization should be performed only in advanced ischemia. Contraindications against revascularization of vessels in the lower half of the body are severe disorders of coronary, cerebral, and renal function and diseases such as cancer and severe diabetes mellitus. The possibility of arterial revascularization should always be checked prior to any amputation, even if the patient has severe concomitant diseases, as the mortality of limb amputation in patients over 60 years old is 25%–28%.

C. Positioning and Surgical Exposure

Revascularizations in the lower half of the body are always done with the patient in a supine position. The heel and ankle are wrapped in pads to avoid compression and injury. The operated leg is slightly elevated at the hips, abducted, externally rotated, and flexed at the knee joint. Lowering the opposite leg allows for better access to the operative field.

I. Groin

To expose the common femoral artery and its branches, a longitudinal incision is made below the inguinal ligament, midway between the superior anterior iliac spine and the symphysis pubis (Fig. 17.2.1a). One must be careful of the superficial epigastric vessels and the superficial circumflex iliac vessels. The following structures are found in the operative area:

Femoral branch of the genitofemoral nerve
Anterior cutaneous branch of the femoral nerve
Lateral femoral cutaneous nerve
Ilioinguinal nerve and iliohypogastric nerve

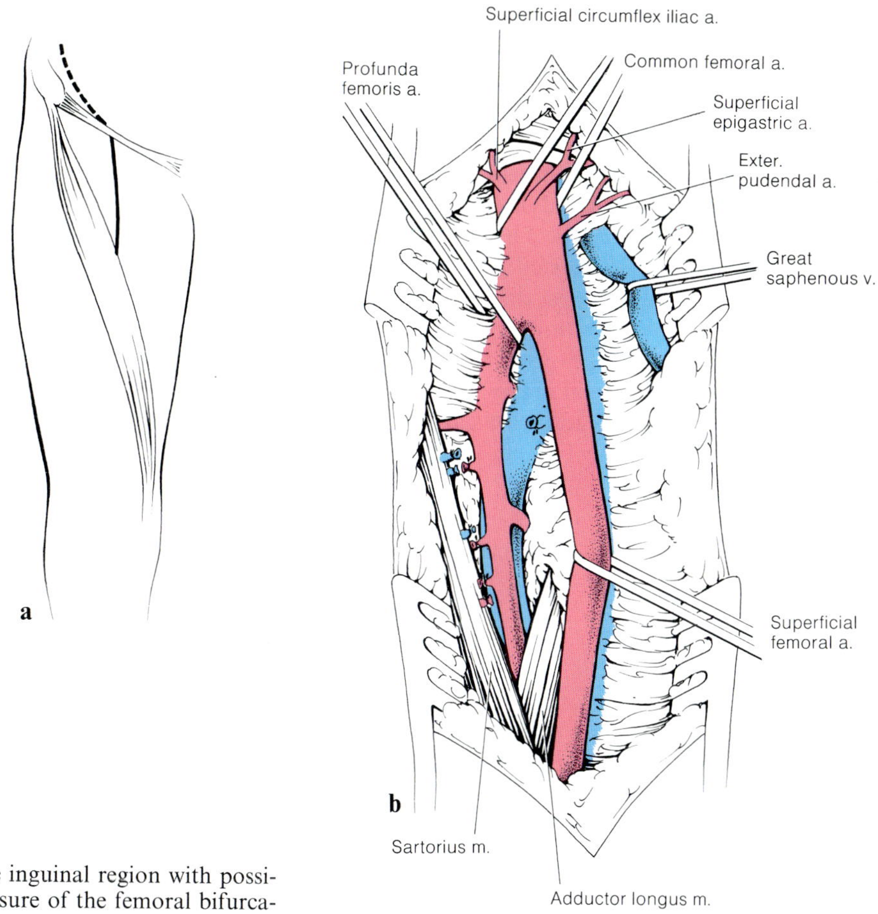

Fig. 17.2.1. a Incision in the inguinal region with possibilities of extension. **b** Exposure of the femoral bifurcation

If the external iliac artery is to be exposed at the same time, an S-shaped, curved incision in the direction of the superior anterior iliac spine is preferred. The incision is extended upward and the aponeurosis of the external oblique abdominal muscle is divided in the direction of its fibers after its detachment from the iliac spine. One must avoid injuring the side branches of the external iliac artery (inferior epigastric artery and deep circumflex iliac artery) and their corresponding veins.

To reach the common femoral artery, it is advisable to divide the subcutaneous tissue laterally, while preserving and retracting the superficial and deep inguinal lymph nodes and lymph vessels. Injured lymph nodes and vessels should be ligated carefully. Electrocoagulation in the groin must be avoided. After dividing the superficial fascia, the femoral artery is easily found. It may also be exposed further distally at the medial border of the sartorius muscle.

The superficial branch of the external pudendal artery must be transected to gain access to the terminal segment of the great saphenous vein and its junction with the femoral vein. The great saphenous vein and the femoral artery can be exposed through the same incision without difficulty, but, in different dissection planes.

A transverse incision in the groin does not expose the vessels as well and cannot be enlarged if necessary.

The division of the common femoral artery into its profunda and superficial branches may be identified by the sudden change in caliber about 1–3 fingerbreadths beneath the inguinal ligament (Fig. 17.2.1b). The profunda femoris artery must be dissected free only down to its first collateral branch. This exposes the artery far enough to allow tapes to be passed around it. Arteriosclerotic plaques usually end at the first collateral branch. If profundaplasty is planned, exposure must be continued downward as fat as the second collateral; this necessitates division of the concomitant veins and the lateral circumflex vein between ligatures.

II. Superficial Femoral Artery

The sartorius muscle serves as a guide muscle in dissection of the superficial femoral artery. The incision runs along the anterior surface of the muscle in continuation of the inguinal incision, down to the readily palpable condyle of the femur at the knee joint (Fig. 17.2.2a). The knee should be flexed about 30° and supported by folded towels. After dividing the thigh fascia, the sartorius muscle is reflected medially and dorsally to expose the artery. At the junction between the distal superficial artery and the popliteal artery, the vessel runs within the 5 – 6-cm-long adductor canal. This canal is bounded medially by the vastus medialis muscle (quadriceps muscle), laterally by the adductors (adductor magnus and longus muscles), and caudally by the tendinous adductorial hiatus (gap at the lower border of the tendinous attachment of the adductor magnus muscle). The roof of the canal is formed by the vastoadductor membrane and the sartorius muscle.

Just before the femoral artery enters the popliteal fossa, the descending genicular artery and the saphenous nerve leave the neurovascular sheath and run superficially in front of the membrane to the knee joint (Fig. 17.2.2b, c). These must be preserved at all costs during dissection. There are many collateral branches in this area and close topographical relationships to the corresponding deep venous system (often doubled).

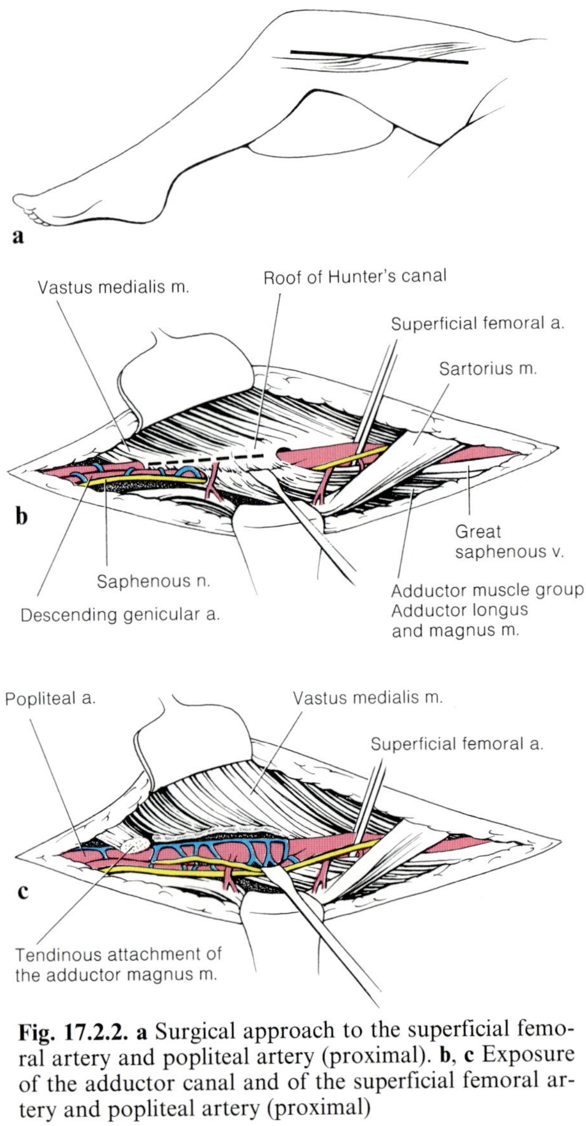

Fig. 17.2.2. a Surgical approach to the superficial femoral artery and popliteal artery (proximal). **b, c** Exposure of the adductor canal and of the superficial femoral artery and popliteal artery (proximal)

III. Popliteal Artery

There are several approaches to the popliteal artery, depending on which segment has to be exposed. An anteromedial approach is usually favored for suprageniculate exposure of the artery (Fig. 17.2.3a). The skin is incised near the dorsal third of the palpable femoral condyle, at the anterior margin of the sartorius muscle. To expose the popliteal artery further, the incision is continued anteromedially to the medial margin of the tibia. Before dissecting deeper, the sartorius muscle is retracted dorsally and medially, and the adductor slit is divided. The proximal third of the popliteal artery is then dissected free. If that portion of the artery is not suited for revascularization, the third popliteal segment (see later) should be exposed first, since this can be done without great difficulty.

To expose the middle third of the popliteal artery, the tendinous attachment of the semimembranosus muscle at the tibial condyle as well as the attachment of the gastrocnemius muscle at the femoral condylus are mobilized and divided. The hamstring muscle group must also be mobilized and divided in the following order: sartorius muscle, gracilis muscle, and semitendinosus muscle (Fig. 17.2.3b, c). The corresponding tendons and muscle attachments should be marked with different sutures for their reconnection later on.

If in an exceptional case isolated exposure of the middle popliteal segment is necessary, a dorsal approach with the patient lying face down is possible (Fig. 17.2.4a, b). To prevent scar contractions, an S-shaped skin incision is made. It starts

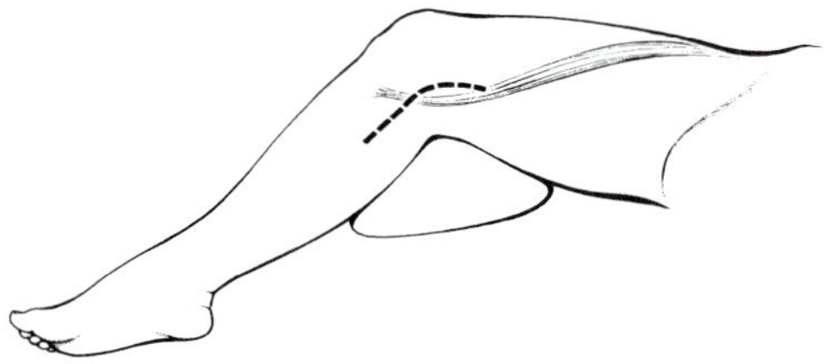
a

Fig. 17.2.3. a Anteromedial approach to the popliteal artery. **b, c** Exposure of the middle third of the popliteal artery with division of the crossing tendons and muscles

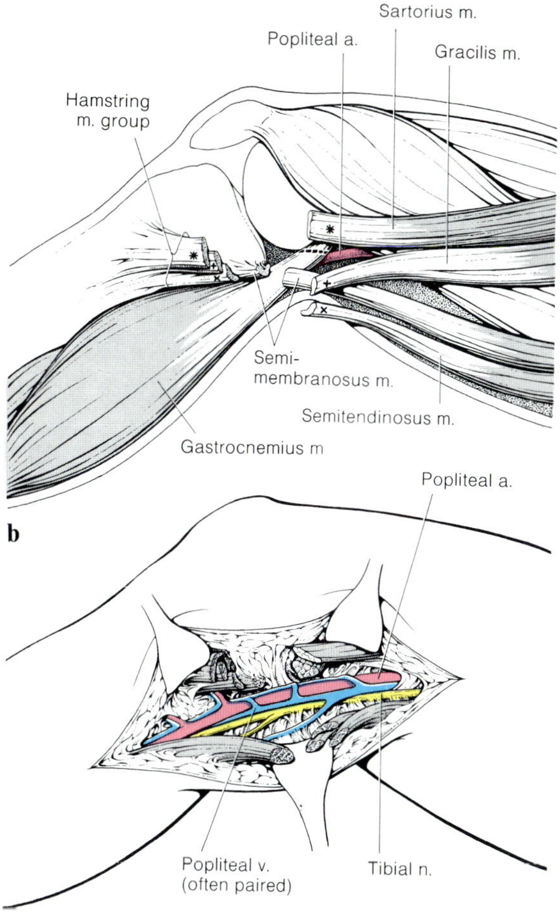

cephalad on the medial side, runs almost completely horizontal in the bend of the knee, continuing downward on the lateral side. Following division of the superficial fascia, the tibial nerve is carefully preserved and retracted laterally. The popliteal artery is then identified in the deeper layer, lying between the biceps femoris muscle and the semimembranosus muscle, usually surrounded by a paired vein.

Exposure of the infrageniculate portion of the popliteal artery for the connection of a bypass graft is preferably achieved using an anteromedial approach (Fig. 17.2.5a). This segment of the vessel is only rarely affected by occlusions and is relatively easy to reach. It gives off only a small branch. The skin incision is made just at the medial margin of the tibia. Following division of the crural fascia as far as the hamstring muscles, the artery can

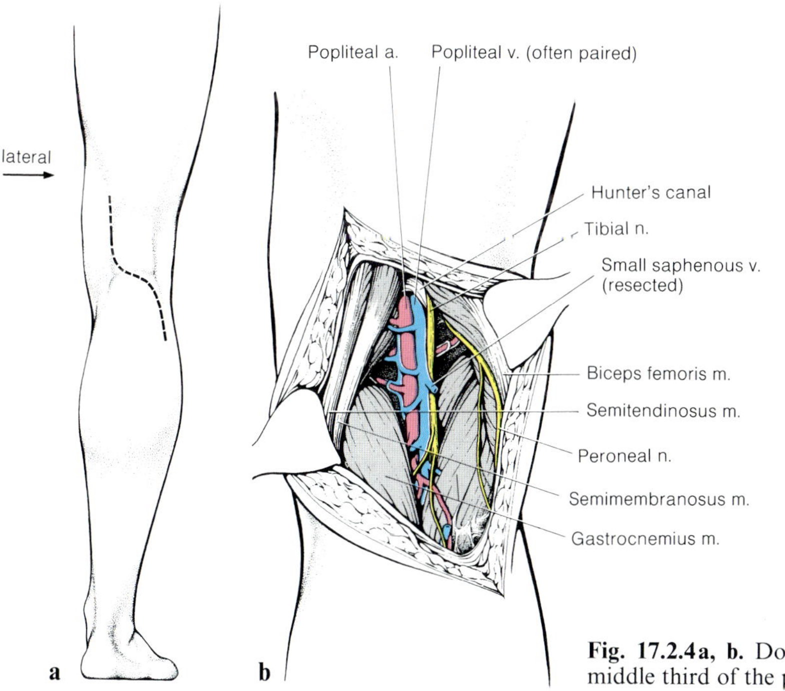

Fig. 17.2.4a, b. Dorsal approach and exposure of the middle third of the popliteal artery

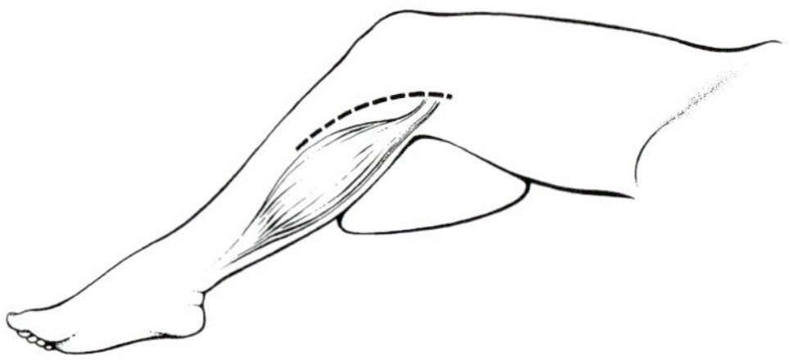

a

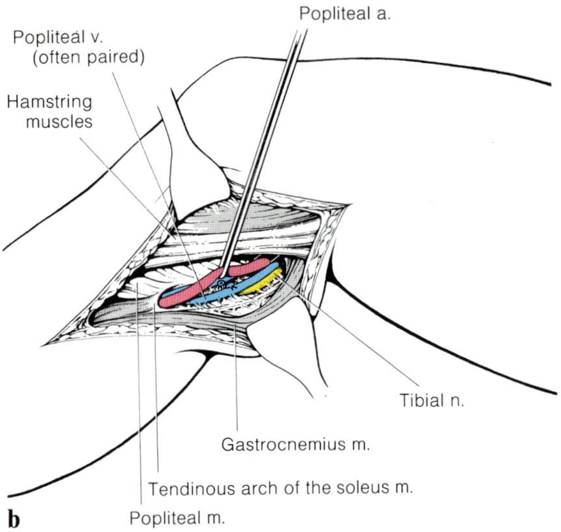

b

Fig. 17.2.5a, b. Anteromedial approach and exposure of the distal third of the popliteal artery and the lower leg trifurcation

be directly exposed by blunt dissection on the anterior side of the medial head of the gastrocnemius muscle. The popliteal artery runs dorsal to the tibial nerve, usually encased by two vein bundles. As soon as the vessel is dissected free circumferentially, tapes are passed around it, and it is pulled slightly forward (Fig. 17.2.5b). This makes further exposure in a proximal and distal direction easier and less dangerous. The crossing anterior tibial veins must be divided between ligatures, especially at the level of the origin of the anterior tibial artery. The tendinous arch of the soleus muscle is identified just distal to this origin. It must be divided for exposure of the lower leg trifurcation.

D. Technique of Revascularization

I. Semiclosed Thromboendarterectomy (TEA)

This technique was introduced in 1946 by J. CID DOS SANTOS and further developed in Germany by VOLLMAR [17]. In the lower limb, it is suitable only for the proximal segment down to the level of the popliteal artery, particularly in short occlusions of the distal portion of the femoral artery. Today, it is seldom used. A few centimeters of the artery are exposed distal to the occluded segment and opened a distance of 2–3 cm (Fig. 17.2.6). The eccentric inner core cylinder is circumferentially isolated with a fine spatula instrument and then divided. A ring stripper of proper size is passed around this core of freed intima and advanced proximally with rotating movements and gentle pressure, keeping traction on the distal end of the cylinder. The proximal end of the intimal core usually tears at the level of the profunda origin. It can then be removed without difficulty. Intraoperative angiography of the thromboendarterectomized artery and its run-off

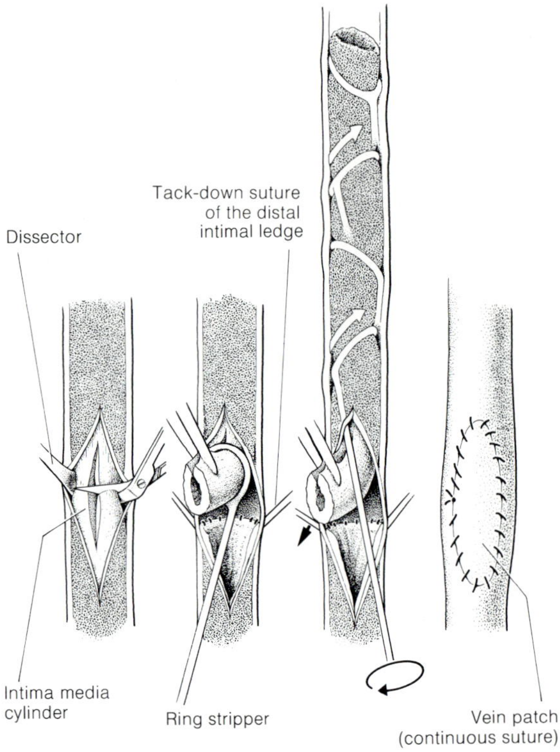

Fig. 17.2.6. Surgical technique of thromboendarterectomy with patch closure

is obligatory. Arterioscopy of the endarterectomized segment may give additional security. The arteriotomy is closed by direct suture or with a vein patch graft.

In lengthy occlusions extending from the profunda origin to the adductor canal, it is advisable to perform an additional proximal arteriotomy at the junction of the common femoral artery and the superficial femoral artery. This also allows direct inspection of the orifice of the profunda femoris artery. The tendon of the adductor magnus muscle should always be divided, since it often initiates the formation of an occlusion.

TEA cannot be performed, or remains incomplete, in 20%–30% of cases. This is especially true in severe calcification of the media and acute inflammatory vascular disease, where the procedure may have to be terminated. The rate of perforation is reported to be 2.7%.

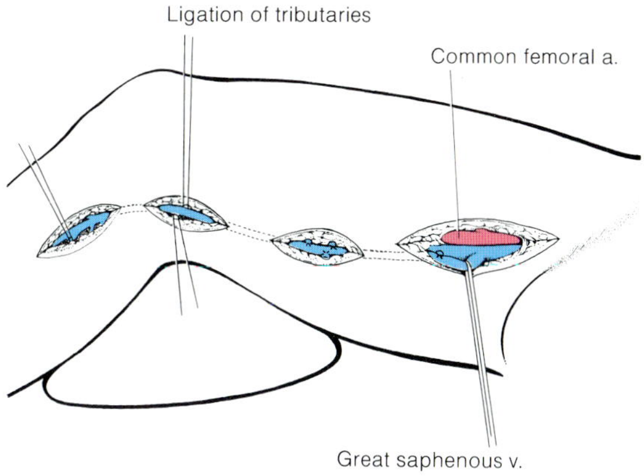

Fig. 17.2.7. Harvest of the great saphenous vein at the thigh and lower leg

II. Bypass Procedures

The first bypass of a vascular occlusion was performed by KUNLIN in 1949. He was the first to use today's standard technique, constructing an autogenous vein bypass. Prior to the operation, the great saphenous vein can be evaluated and marked while the patient is standing. The position of the patient during removal of the vein does not have to be changed for the arterial reconstruction. The incisions for harvesting the great saphenous vein are as a rule the same as for exposure of the artery at the groin and knee joint. The great saphenous vein is easily dissected free step by step, without causing necroses of the skin. The incision on the thigh and lower leg can be either continuous or interrupted by short bridges of skin. The incision is always directed along the course of the vein, which varies from patient to patient. Venous tributaries are carefully divided between two ligatures (4-0). The vein itself should never be grasped with instruments.

Before completing removal of the great saphenous vein, the site of anastomosis to the distal arterial segment should be determined in order to estimate the length of vein necessary for grafting. The distal end of the vein is tied over a beaded cannula. The opposite end is clamped and the vein is distended with heparinized blood. Distention permits the surgeon to assess the caliber of the vein (not below 4 mm, optimal diameter 4–6 mm). Leaking tributaries are atraumatically sutured.

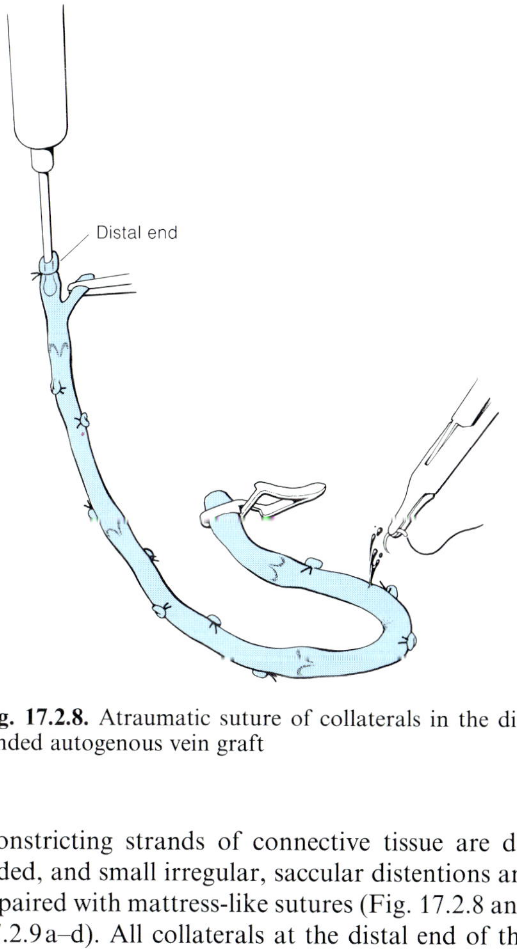

Fig. 17.2.8. Atraumatic suture of collaterals in the distended autogenous vein graft

Constricting strands of connective tissue are divided, and small irregular, saccular distentions are repaired with mattress-like sutures (Fig. 17.2.8 and 17.2.9a–d). All collaterals at the distal end of the vein should be preserved to make it possible to enlarge the transverse diameter for the creation of a wide proximal anastomosis later on (Fig. 17.2.10a–d). The vein graft may be temporarily stored in a blood – heparin solution.

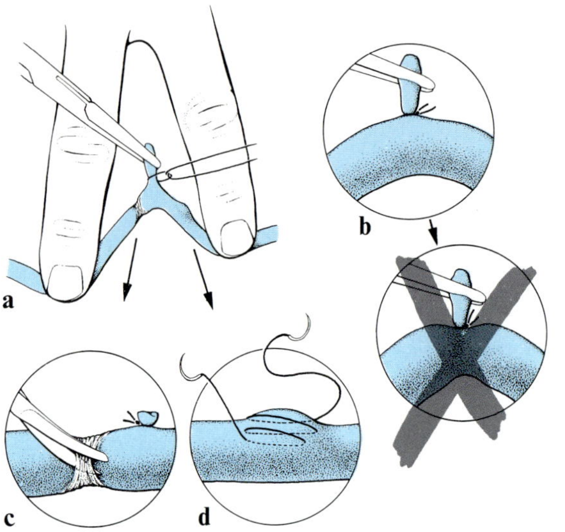

Fig. 17.2.9 a–d. Subsequent corrections performed on the vein graft: ligation of tributaries, division of connective tissue strands, and mattress-like suture of saccular distentions

Fig. 17.2.10 a–d. Storage of the harvested autogenous ▷ vein graft in a blood heparin solution; enlargement of the transverse diameter at the proximal end of the vein graft

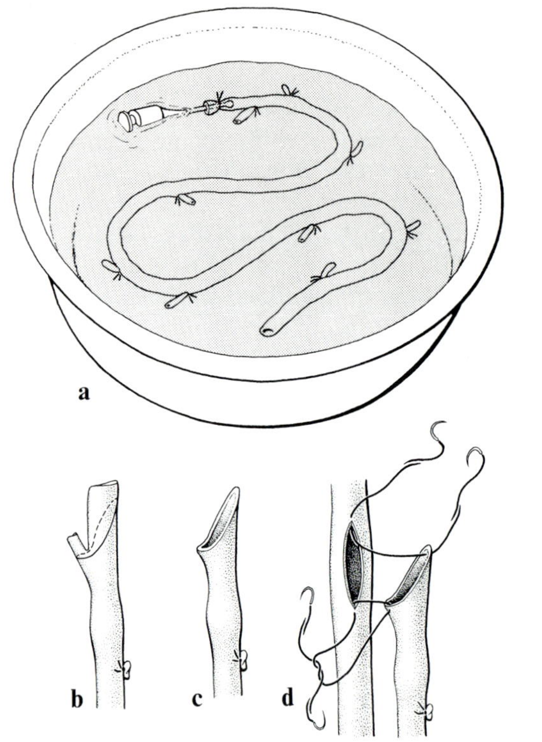

The distended vein is reversed (distal end at the groin). Then, it is pulled through the subcutaneous tunnel with a long forceps and orthotopically placed next to the artery so that both ends lie at the sites of anastomosis to the host artery. It is of the utmost importance to prevent twisting of the graft during this maneuver. The tunnel is prepared by blunt dissection using the fingers of both hands. In order to connect the graft to the proximal popliteal segment, it is passed under the sartorius muscle. If an infragenicular anastomosis has to be constructed, we position the graft beneath the muscle groups that cross the region of the knee joint (gastrocnemius, hamstring muscle group, semimembranosus).

Before the artery is clamped, systemic heparinization is carried out, which does not later require antagonistic measures if the anastomoses show no leakage. We always begin with construction of the bypass at the distal anastomosis. The VAN DONGEN infrageniculate retractor has proven very useful for exposure of the distal popliteal artery. Following a longitudinal incision of the host artery with a pointed scalpel, the arteriotomy is lengthened to 15–20 mm with angled scissors (Potts' scissors). The vascular lumen may be held open by pulling on stay sutures, thus exposing the internal surface

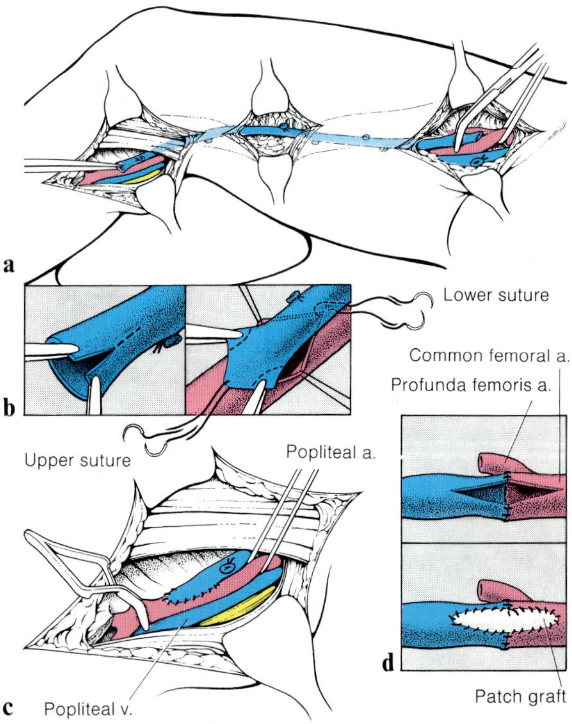

Fig. 17.2.11 a–d. Placement of the graft in the tunnel and construction of the proximal and distal anastomoses (distal end of the graft at the groin; the inset shows the alternative method of a proximal end-to-end anastomosis)

of the artery (Fig. 17.2.11a–d). While inspecting the artery in this manner, one must examine the outflow tract carefully and, if necessary, dilate it using fine Overholt clamps or a vascular dilator. The squeezed end of the vein graft is resected, the graft is longitudinally incised, the corners are cut, and remnants of adventitial tissue are removed at the designated site of anastomosis. Each strand of the doubled corner sutures that are placed at the start is used to complete one quarter of the anastomosis (see inset Fig. 17.2.11). To facilitate precise sewing of the spatulate end of the vein to the artery, a probe can be placed within the distal outflow tract during peripheral anastomosis, and within the vein graft during proximal anastomosis. The stitch direction is always from the wall of the artery to the vein. We prefer to reverse the direction when a synthetic prosthesis is sewn into the arteriotomy. Local endarterectomy cannot be recommended at the distal arteriotomy site. Corrections of stenoses of the profunda femoris orifice may be necessary at the proximal arteriotomy site. Monofilament double sutures (5-0 to 6-0 in size) and a C_1 or BV_1 needle are preferred. Following completion of the distal anastomosis, the vein graft is distended once more and slightly stretched. The preferred site of the proximal anastomosis is the femoral bifurcation. The suture of this anastomosis is a very crucial step in the entire grafting procedure since the caliber of the vein is rather small (see Fig. 17.2.10, enlargement of the transverse diameter). Sewing the vein graft end-to-side to the common femoral artery does not achieve optimal hemodynamic conditions, but restricts blood flow to patent collateral branches. If the superficial femoral artery is totally occluded, the vein graft may be connected proximally in an end-to-end fashion to the proximal stump of the transected superficial femoral artery. Inflow to the graft may be improved through enlargement of the anastomosis by means of a patch graft (see Fig. 17.2.11). This technique has shown good results.

We favor revascularization of an isolated popliteal segment with good collateralization in patients presenting an advanced stage of ischemia. However, reverse blood flow in the arterial segment must be possible.

If run-off is impaired, suitable segments of the artery must be sought further distally to which several additional graft connections may be made (sequential graft, jump graft). This makes revascularization of several vascular regions (anterior tibial artery, posterior tibial artery) possible, at different levels of the lower limb (popliteal artery, posterior tibial artery; Fig. 17.2.12a, b). The additional arterial segment may be connected to the graft using either a sequential bypass in the form of a side-to-side anastomosis or a jump bypass, which is constructed by implanting a second vein graft at the distal end of the primary graft, thus forming a Y-shaped bifurcation.

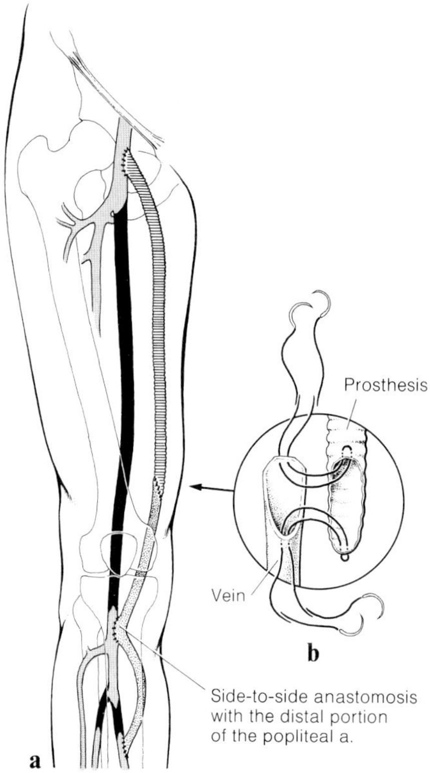

Fig. 17.2.12. a Simultaneous revascularization at several different levels of the arterial system with a sequential graft (popliteal artery and posterior tibial artery). **b** Suture technique in a prosthesis – vein connection (composite graft)

The main problem in peripheral reconstructions is the limited availability of autogenous vein material. Proximal anastomosis is usually performed at the femoral bifurcation. Only in exceptional cases, in vascular injuries at the popliteocrural level, in the outlet syndrome, and in isolated reconstruction of the popliteal segment (cystic adventitial degeneration, entrapment syndrome) can the proximal anastomosis be constructed in the upper third of the popliteal artery, provided that the femoral artery is patent. In such situations, end-to-end connection between vein and artery is preferred because it offers better hemodynamic conditions

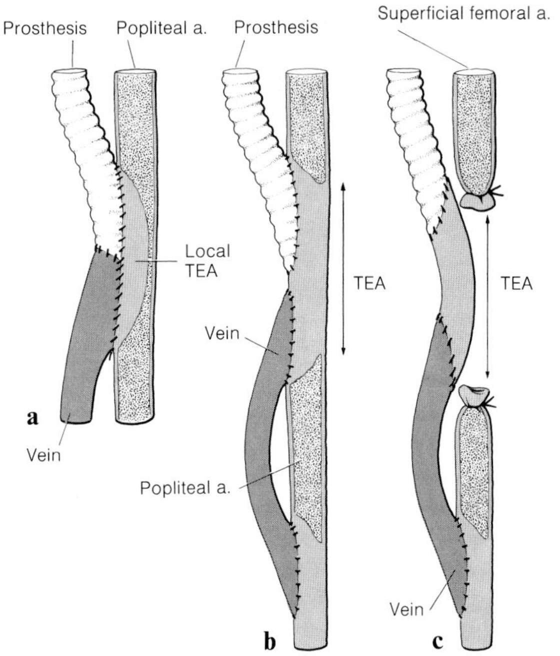

Fig. 17.2.13a–c. Techniques of constructing a hitchhike bypass

without undesirable turbulent flow. Another advantage is that the inflow tract can be widened with a patch graft.

Proximal end-to-side anastomosis is preferred, however, in revascularization of arteriosclerotic occlusions in order to preserve important, peripheral collaterals. Combining lengthy, proximal TEA with above-knee connection of a bypass graft has not shown good results.

If the length of the vein does not suffice (normally 45–50 cm is needed for the femoral segment), several veins may be connected to one another or a composite graft may be constructed between a synthetic prosthesis and an autogenous vein by creating an end-to-end anastomosis (Fig. 17.2.12, see inset). Another alternative is to interpose an endarterectomized arterial segment, forming a hitchhike graft. There are different ways of constructing a hitchhike bypass, depending on the arterial segment involved (Fig. 17.2.13a–c). The thromboendarterectomized arterial segment shown in b and c represent the weakest point of the hitchhike graft since intimal hyperplasia at such a point often leads to circumscribed narrowing over an extended period. The hitchhike bypass is always preferable to the composite graft when the autogenous vein has a small lumen because it does away with the abrupt transition that would result from the end-to-end anatomosis between vein and synthetic prosthesis.

More and more materials are being developed for use in peripheral vascular reconstructions. An autogenous vein is nearly always preferable to foreign materials. In surgical reinterventions where the autogenous vein is unsuitable (20%–30%), alloplastic material is used only for bypass of the femoral artery segment in patients with stage III and IV symptoms. Polytetrafluoroethylene (PTFE) and filamentous, knitted Dacron prostheses have shown satisfactory results. External reinforcement with rings or spirals is necessary in prostheses spanning the knee joint, in order to prevent kinking when the knee is flexed. Such grafts are being used more frequently. The only other graft suitable for crossing the knee joint is the umbilical vein graft (Dardik graft). Heterologous materials are handled in the same manner as described previously for autogenous vein grafts. The anastomoses are performed using the same techniques. The distal anastomosis is constructed first. Large differences in caliber between host artery and synthetic graft are overcome by the use of a 6-mm prosthesis tailored in accordance with the length of the anastomosis.

E. Postoperative Complications, Reinterventions

Suction drains are always left in place for at least 24 h. Immediate surgical revision of the anastomoses is indicated if severe postoperative hemorrhage occurs (see p. 158). Constant postoperative monitoring of blood pressure, pulse, urine output, and replacement of fluid loss and electrolytes must be ensured since the patients have generalized arteriosclerosis with involvement of the coronary arteries, kidneys, and brain. After peripheral, vascular reconstructions, the patient should be mobilized early to reduce postischemic edema. Postoperative dilatation of the peripheral vessels may be achieved by preventing heat loss, e.g., with cotton dressings.

A *compartment syndrome* following peripheral, vascular reconstructions is rare. It may occur if the intraoperative ischemic time is prolonged, leading to serious damage of the muscle and soft connective tissues (see p. 638). Symptoms are increasing loss of sensibility, mobility, and increasing tension of the soft tissues in the anterior, fibular, and tibial compartments. These alarming signs must be relieved by early fasciotomy.

Immediate occlusion always necessitates surgical reintervention, since the cause is invariably a technical one (p. 164). Some of the more frequent causes include: faulty anastomotic technique, incomplete desobliteration or distal intimal flaps, problems with the graft itself, peripheral embolism with subsequent thrombus formation, and incorrect assessment of the inflow, or more often, the outflow tract. Intraoperative angiography (see p.135) following revascularization reduces the rate of immediate occlusions in the femoropopliteal (femorocrural) segment below 5%.

The *patency rates* of peripheral vascular reconstructions depend on the ischemic stage, the number of patent lower leg arteries, the technique of revascularization, and the localization of the distal anastomosis. Good early results may be expected in 82%–100%. The primary amputation rate depends on the operative status of the vessel and the technique of revascularization. Today, it is between 3.1% and 8%.

The *mortality rate* of peripheral vascular reconstructions is reported to be between 0.4% and 4%. Serious complications due to surgical or technical errors are almost completely unknown.

The greatest problem following peripheral vascular reconstructions is deep *wound infection*, occurring in 1.5%–7.2% of all patients, irrespective of the stage of ischemia (see p. 166). If synthetic prostheses have been implanted, all foreign material must be completely removed in order to achieve healing. Extra anatomic bypass can be considered if dangerous ischemia of the limb develops following resection of an infected graft. For example, in groin infections, an obturator bypass with peripheral connection to the popliteal artery is possible. Because a hematogenous etiology of graft infection in the early phase is presently under discussion, perioperative antibiotic prophylaxis is always indicated when foreign materials are used.

Anastomotic aneurysms are of special importance. The cause is leaking along the suture line (see p. 173). The frequency of anastomotic aneurysms depends on the degree of exposure of the suture site and the type of revascularization performed. It is most commonly found in the groin (3%) and less often in distal portions of the reconstructed artery (1.1%). It may always be identified morphologically as a false aneurysm. Graft aneurysms do not belong to this category since they are caused by mechanical weakness of the graft wall, as may be found in varices of saphenous grafts. The clinical picture of anastomotic aneurysms is characterized by a growing, pulsating swelling in the area of a vascular anastomosis or a vascular suture. There is not spontaneous cure. Some 20% present with rupture at the time of surgical reintervention. Therefore, false aneurysms should be diagnosed as early as possible and corrected surgically. The aim of treatment is to resect the aneurysm and restore the continuity of the artery. Often, a portion of the reconstruction must be resected, the graft lengthened, and a new anastomosis constructed. If wound infection is present, only autogenous material may be used. Adjuvant measures such as irrigation-suction-drainage, omentum flaps, and implantation of antibiotic implants containing antibiotics have proven effective.

Patency rates following bypass operations in the femoropopliteal segment as calculated by the life table method vary, depending on the graft material, the grafted segment of the artery, and the preoperative ischemic stage. It has been reported that 72% of all femoropopliteal vein bypass grafts are still patent after 3 years (68%–77%, depending on the stage). The following 3-year patency rates have been calculated according to the type of prosthesis used: 55% with velour prostheses; 65% with PTFE prostheses; and 67% with umbilical vein grafts. The 5-year patency rates for vein bypass grafting procedures are 65% on average for femoropopliteal bypasses; 48% for femorocrural bypasses; and 43% for femoropopliteal prosthetic reconstructions.

REFERENCES

1. Van Dongen RJAM (1970) Photographic atlas of reconstructive arterial surgery. Springer, Berlin Heidelberg New York
2. Friedmann P, De Laurentis DA, Rhee SW (1976) The sequential femoropopliteal bypass graft. Am J Surg 121:452
3. Gall FP (1969) Die Rekonstruktion arterieller Verschlußerkrankungen der Beine durch Transplantation der Vena saphena magna. Materia Medica Nordmark 11:623
4. Heberer G (1979) Aktuelle Fragen der rekonstruktiven Gefäßchirurgie. Straube, Erlangen
5. Heilmann F, Franke F, Gall F (1977) Revascularisation beim Unterschenkelarterienverschluß. Dtsch Med Wochenschr 102:659
6. Imparato AM, Kim GE, Chu DS (1973) Surgical exposure for reconstruction of the proximal part of the tibial artery. Surg Gynecol Obstet 136:453

7. Kahle W, Leonhardt H, Platzer W (1973) Taschenatlas der Anatomie. Thieme, Stuttgart
8. Kunlin J (1949) Le traitment de l'arterite obliterant par le greffe veineuse. Arch Mal Coeur 42:371
9. Leitz KH (1981) Zugangswege in der Gefäßchirurgie. Springer, Berlin Heidelberg New York
10. Linton RR, Wirthlin LS (1973) Femoropopliteal composite Dacron and autogenous vein bypass grafts. Arch Surg 107:748
11. Mehta S (1980) A statistical summary of the results of femoro-popliteal bypass surgery. In: Gore WL (ed) Flagstaff, Arizona
12. Raithel D (1974) Periphere Durchblutungsstörungen. In: Wieck HH (ed) Zerebrale und periphere Durchblutungsstörungen. Aesopus
13. Rühland D, Bünte H, Cramer B (1979) Vorteile modifizierter Polytetrafluoroethylene-Prothesen für den arteriellen Gefäßersatz. Chir Praxis 26:587
14. Schlosser V, Herdter F, Spillner G, Ahmadi A (1977) Neue Transplantat-Materialien in der rekonstruktiven Arterien-Chirurgie. Fortschr Med 95:1012
15. Stockmann U (1982) Der femoro-crurale Bypass. In: Denck H, Hagmüller GW, Brunner U (eds) Arterielle Durchblutungsstörungen der unteren Extremitäten. TM-Verlag, Bad Oeynhausen
16. Vogt B (1981) Gefäßverletzungen mit besonderer Berücksichtigung der peripheren Arterientraumatologie. Huber, Bern Stuttgart Wien
17. Vollmar J (1982) Rekonstruktive Chirurgie der Arterien. Thieme, Stuttgart

17.3 Chronic Occlusive Disease of the Lower Leg Arteries

R.J.A.M. VAN DONGEN and F. FRANKE

CONTENTS

A. Introduction

In recent years the anatomical limits of arterial reconstructive surgery have been pushed farther and farther into the peripheral regions. The most spectacular developments have been in the surgery of leg arteries.

In 1960, PALMA [18] performed the first revascularization of a lower leg artery, the posterior tibial artery. Only by the 1970s, however, had arteriographic and surgical techniques developed to the point where satisfactory results could be achieved with any degree of consistency.

Many factors and new developments led to these advances.

- First, there was an improvement in the quality of arteriographic imaging of the lower leg and foot arteries.
- Second, surgical methods were improved with the aim of reducing peripheral resistance and increasing blood flow through the graft.
- Finally, the development and application of reliable alternative methods to bypass grafting made it possible to treat patients in whom the autogenous great saphenous vein was not suited for total bridging of long femoropopliteocrural obstructions.

B. Anatomy

The topographical anatomy of all three lower leg arteries is described on p. 24–27 and pictured in Fig. 17.3.1a–c.

The popliteal artery separates into the anterior and posterior tibial arteries as it reaches the tendinous arch of the soleus muscle. The anterior tibial artery penetrates the interosseus membrane of the leg or runs anteriorly riding over the superior edge of the membrane and then descends on its anterior surface. It lies between the tibialis ante-

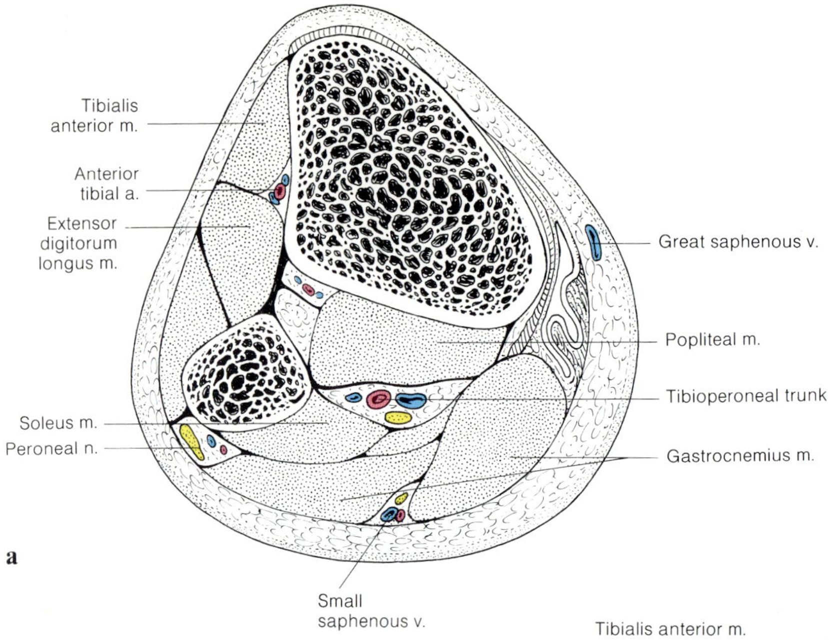

a

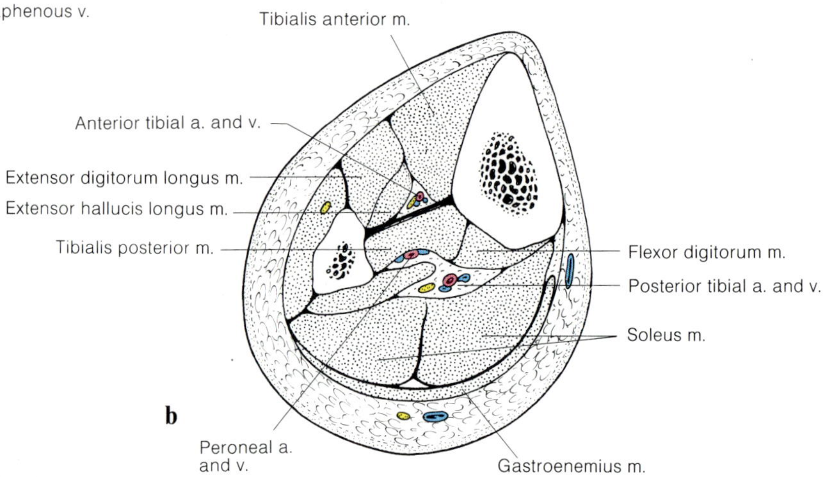

b

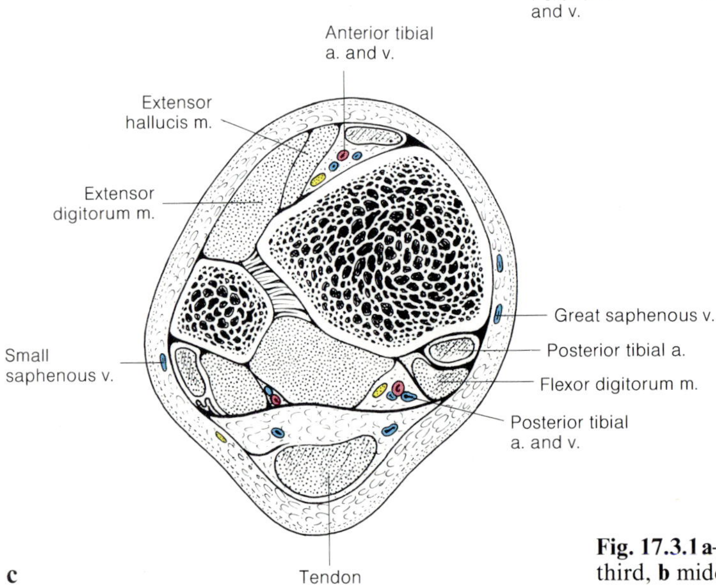

c

Fig. 17.3.1 a–c. Cross sections of the lower leg. **a** Proximal third, **b** middle third, **c** distal third rior muscle and the extensor digitorum longus muscle in its proximal portion, and in its distal portion between the tibialis anterior muscle and the extensor hallucis longus muscle. As it descends, it comes to lie on the anterior surface of the tibia and the capsule of the upper ankle joint. It continues on to the dorsum of the foot as the dorsalis pedis artery. This vessel crosses beneath the tendon of the extensor hallucis longus muscle and the inferior extensor retinaculum and then runs between the extensor hallucis longus and brevis muscles to the distal portion of the foot. The arcuate artery branches off at the level of the proximal ends of the metatarsal bones. The dorsalis pedis artery splits into the deep plantar branch and the first dorsal metatarsal artery between the first and second metatarsal bones.

After the anterior tibial artery branches off, the popliteal artery continues as the posterior tibial artery. The peroneal artery branches off 1–5 cm distal to the origin of the posterior tibial artery. In the literature on vascular surgery, the segment of the posterior tibial artery lying between its origin and the takeoff of the peroneal artery is called the tibioperoneal trunk. Only after the peroneal artery takes off is it called the posterior tibial artery.

The posterior tibial artery descends on the dorsal surface of the tibial posterior muscle between the flexor digitorum longus and flexor hallucis longus muscles, accompanied by the tibial nerve. Further distally, it runs along the medial border of the calcaneal tendon, turning toward the area behind and under the medial malleolus. At that point, it lies between the posterior aspect of the malleolus and the medial edge of the calcaneal tendon. Before reaching both layers of the flexor retinaculum, it splits into the medial and lateral plantar arteries.

The peroneal artery runs on the posterior aspect of the tibialis posterior muscle, then between this muscle and the flexor hallucis longus muscle, close to the fibula, downward. In its distal portion it is located on the posterior surface of the interosseus membrane or the tibia, splitting into its communicating branches, lateral malleolar branches, and calcaneal branches after reaching the posterior aspect of the ankle joint capsule.

C. Indications for Revascularization

Revascularization of the lower leg arteries may be indicated in patients with occlusions of the femoropopliteal artery or the popliteal artery extending into the lower leg arteries. Revascularization of still patent arterial segments is usually considered if severe impairment of blood circulation is present, i.e., in clinical stages III and IV. The stage of intermittent claudication is only rarely an indication for such revascularizing procedures.

If all lower leg arteries are occluded or narrowed by arteriosclerotic plaques, revascularization of the dorsalis pedis artery or of one of the plantar arteries may be considered, but only if the patient has rest pain or gangrene.

D. Angiographic Requirements

Reconstruction of crural arteries should not be attempted without exact arteriographic visualization of the lower leg and foot arteries [2, 3, 13, 17, 21]. Angiography must accurately delineate the pathologic changes of the diseased arteries. Arteriograms should correspond with the actual situation.

First, the arteries must be visualized sharply and with dense contrast. This allows the surgeon to assess to which artery and to which arterial segment the graft should be anastomosed.

Aortography almost never gives a satisfactory visualisation of the lower leg and foot arteries. Aortographic pictures are only suited to judging the state of the inflow tract and determining where the proximal anastomosis of the graft should be made.

Additional arteriography of the femoral artery is absolutely necessary for accurate visualization of the lower leg and foot arteries. The injection of contrast medium should be anterograde, not retrograde. This results in better filling of the distal arteries and therefore greater angiographic contrast.

In this way it is possible to establish whether in the distal portion of an unoccluded artery there are additional stenoses that might be treated in the same operation. Moreover, anterograde arteriography of the femoral artery allows exact assessment of the foot arteries, even if all lower leg arteries are obstructed.

Obtaining all this information is absolutely impossible with digital subtraction angiography. DSA allows one to determine whether or not lower leg arteries are open, but no more than this. It is a screening method. The details necessary for purposes of surgery cannot be seen in DSA pictures.

A second very important point, which must be stressed, is that the series of pictures taken of the lower leg and foot should be continued for a considerable length of time, as the filling of the lower leg arteries is often delayed.

A third precondition is the correct projection. If the legs are externally rotated, the tibia and fibula will be projected superimposed on one another, making correct assessment and identification of the lower leg arteries difficult. The evaluation of the pictures is easier if the lower leg is rotated internally about 20°. The arteries are depicted correctly without the superimposition of bones. Assessment of lower leg arterial patency and the condition of the vessels and their walls is only possible if the leg is rotated internally.

To visualize the posterior tibial artery exclusively, the lower leg must be rotated externally.

The arteries of the foot must always be visualized in two planes.

E. Positioning

To revascularize the posterior tibial artery, the leg is placed in an externally rotated position. The opposite hip is elevated on a pillow. The knee is flexed and supported in that position by means of a wedge-shaped pad. If reconstructive procedures of the anterior tibial artery and the peroneal artery are planned, the leg must be alternately rotated internally and externally. The foot is supported by a padded wedge so that the leg can be rotated freely to the inside and outside. To obtain a better approach to the lateral side of the lower leg, the ipsilateral hip should be slightly elevated on a pillow.

F. Operative Approach

The tibioperoneal trunk and the posterior tibial artery are exposed through a longitudinal incision at the medial margin of the tibia (Fig. 17.3.2a). The proximal segments of the plantar arteries are reached through a curved incision behind the medial malleolus.

The correct exposure of the anterior tibial artery is along a line which joins the point midway between the head of the fibula and the tubercle of the tibia with the point midway between the two malleoli (Fig. 17.3.3a). The dorsalis pedis artery is exposed through an incision along a line connecting the midpoint between the two malleoli with the interdigital space between the first and second toes. The incision lies lateral to the tendon of the extensor hallucis longus muscle.

The lateral approach to the peroneal artery is through an incision over the fibula or just behind it. Medial exposure of the peroneal artery, as with exposure of the posterior tibial artery, is obtained through a longitudinal incision along the medial margin of the tibia.

G. Exposure of the Arteries of the Lower Leg and Foot

[1, 14, 16, 20, 22, 23]

I. Distal Popliteal Artery and Tibioperoneal Trunk

Medial Approach. An incision is made starting 1 cm below and behind the medial condyle of the femur, continuing in a slight curve 1 cm behind the posterior medial margin of the tibia, and descending parallel to this margin about 10 cm. The great saphenous vein is preserved by retracting it posteriorly. The crural fascia is divided longitudinally. The line of dissection should be extended upward as far as possible along the lower margin of the tendon of the semitendinosus muscle. It is not necessary to divide the tendons of the hamstring muscles. These tendons can be easily retracted upward, if the knee is flexed. The medial head of the gastrocnemius muscle is separated from the soleus muscle. The neurovascular bundle can be found at the very bottom of the space between these muscles. The tibial nerve and the popliteal vein are separated from the artery and re-

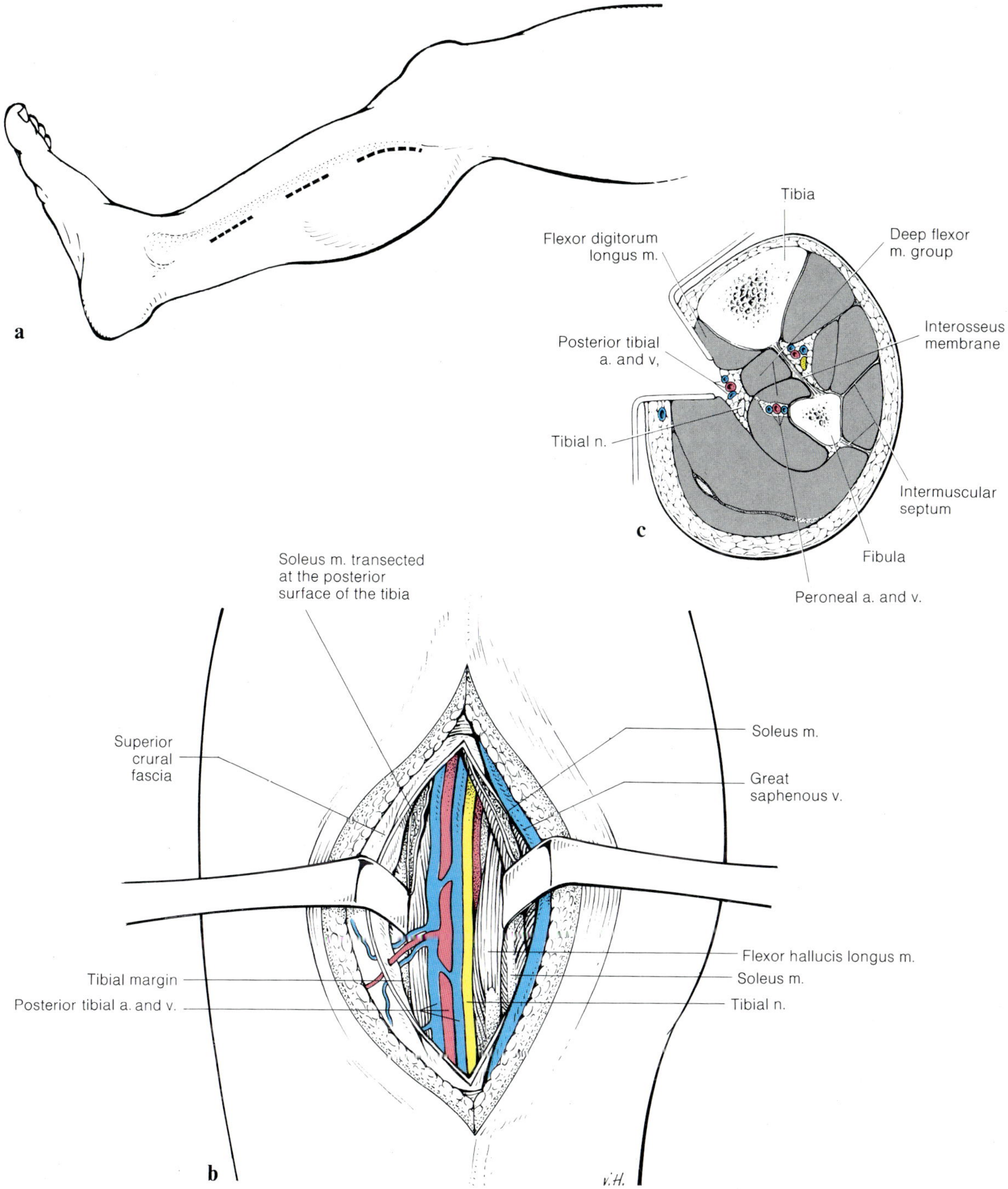

tracted posteriorly. This is facilitated by using the infragenicular retractor designed by van Dongen.

The tibioperoneal trunk begins at the tendinous arch of the soleus muscle and is covered by crossing anterior tibial veins. To reach this segment and the origin of the anterior tibial artery, the soleus muscle must first be separated from the medial margin of the tibia and then from the medial sur-

Fig. 17.3.2. a Line of incision for exposure of the distal popliteal artery and the different segments of the posterior tibial artery. **b** Exposure of the proximal portions of the posterior tibial artery between the soleus and gastrocnemius muscles (dorsal) and flexor digitorum and hallucis longus muscles (ventral). **c** Cross section of the surgical approach to the posterior tibial artery

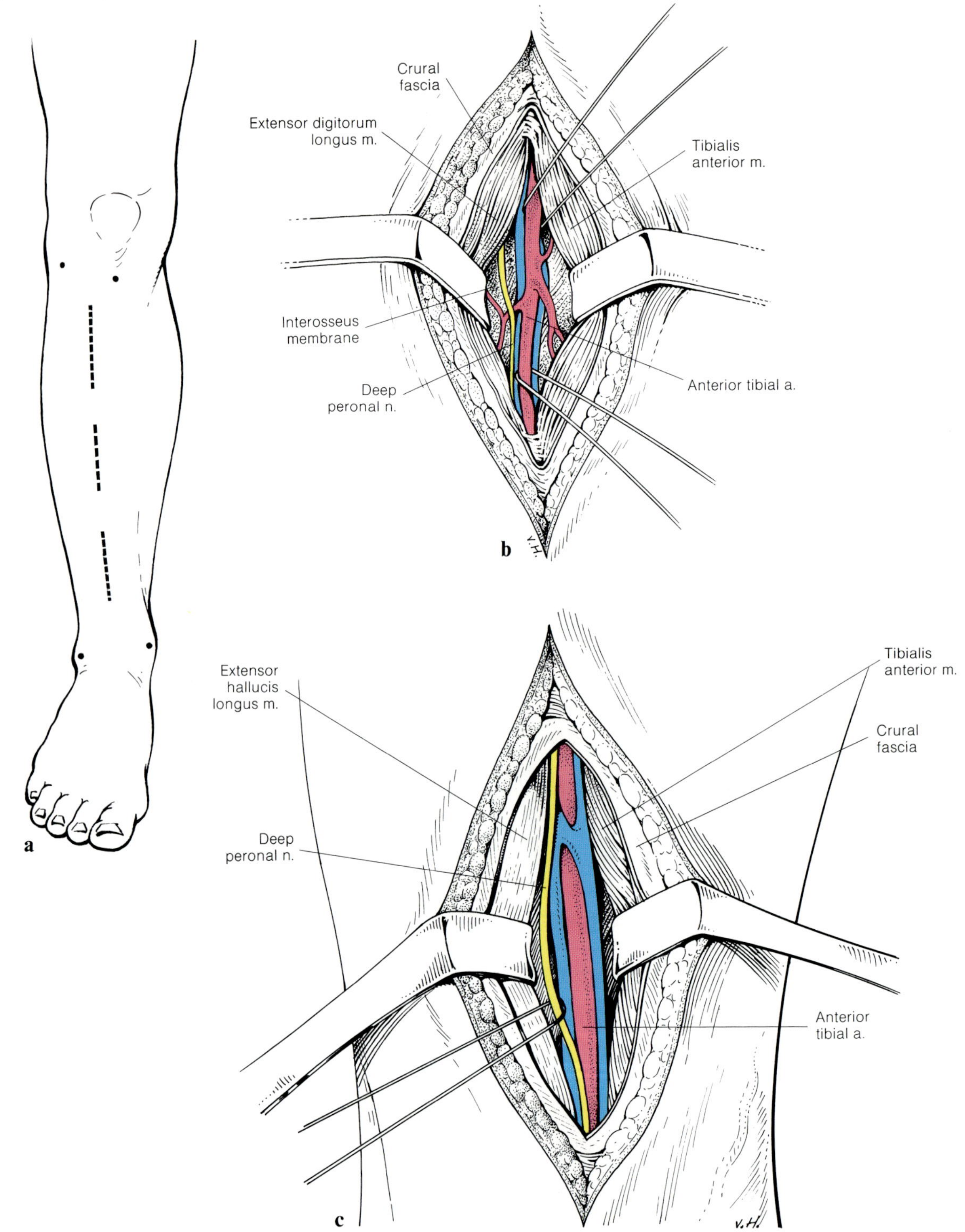

Fig. 17.3.3. a Line of incision for exposure of the anterior tibial artery and dorsalis pedis artery. **b** Exposure of the proximal portion of the anterior tibial artery between the tibialis anterior muscle (in front) and the extensor digitorum longus muscle (behind). **c** Dissection of the distal portion of the anterior tibial artery between the tibialis anterior muscle (in front) and the hallucis longus muscle (behind). **d** Construction of a tunnel between the anterior tibial artery through the interosseus membrane to the infragenicular space

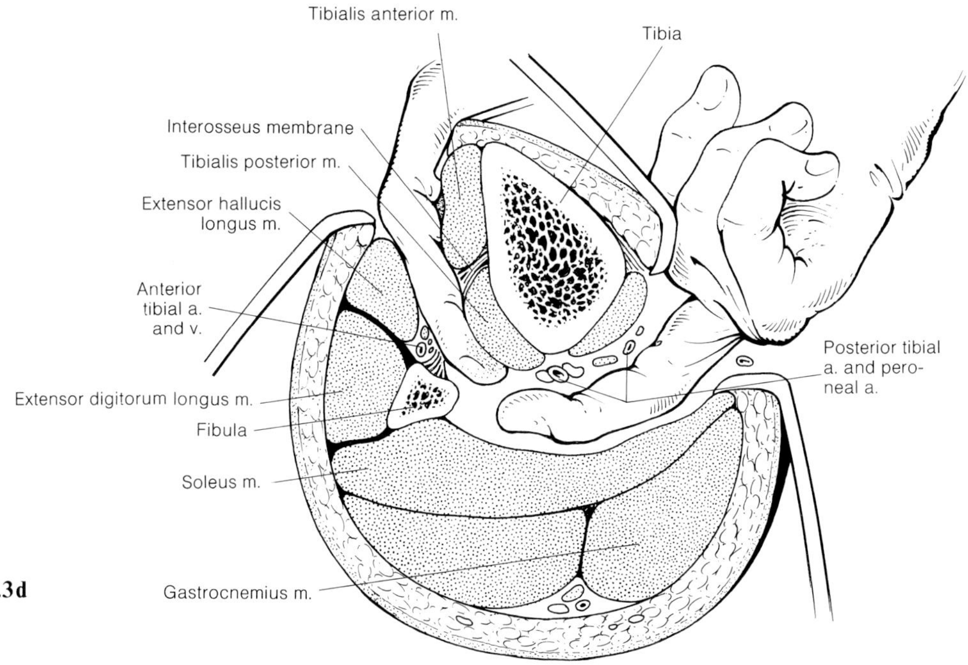

Fig. 17.3.3d

face of the bone. A right-angled curved clamp is passed underneath the tendinous arch and the arch is dissected to expose the crossing anterior tibial veins. These short and vulnerable veins are divided between ligatures. Then, the tibioperoneal trunk and the origin of the anterior tibial artery can be exposed. Dissection may be continued distally which allows for excellent exposure of the proximal portions of the peroneal artery and the posterior tibial artery.

Lateral Approach. The lateral approach to the distal portions of the popliteal artery and to the tibioperoneal trunk is described on p. 412.

II. Posterior Tibial Artery and Proximal Plantar Arteries

To expose the posterior tibial artery in the middle or lower third of the lower leg (following skin incision just behind the medial margin of the tibia, with preservation of the great saphenous vein), the crural fascia is divided, exposing the medial head of the gastrocnemius muscle. Retraction of this muscle visualizes the soleus muscle. The soleus muscle is sharply dissected longitudinally from the posterior surface of the tibia and dorsally retracted together with the gastrocnemius muscle. Between these two muscles and the flexor digitorum longus and hallucis longus muscles dissection is continued deeper until the neurovascular bundle is reached (Fig. 17.3.2b, c). The tibial nerve which lies lateral to the posterior tibial artery should remain untouched.

The distal portion of the posterior tibial artery is easily reached through an incision between the calcaneal tendon and the medial malleolus. Following division of the deep fascia, the neurovascular bundle is exposed, in which the tibial nerve lies dorsally. Dissection may be continued distally until the origins of the plantar branches are reached. Following division of the superficial layer of the flexor retinaculum, and retraction of the tendon of the abductor hallucis muscle distally, the proximal segments of the plantar arteries can be exposed.

III. Anterior Tibial Artery and Dorsalis Pedis Artery

Following skin incision and dissection of the subcutaneous tissue, the dividing line between the tibialis anterior muscle and the extensor digitorum longus muscle is identified. In order to find this line, the ankle joint should be moved. When the foot is pronated, the extensor digitorum longus muscle relaxes, while at the same time the tibialis anterior muscle is stretched. If it is not possible

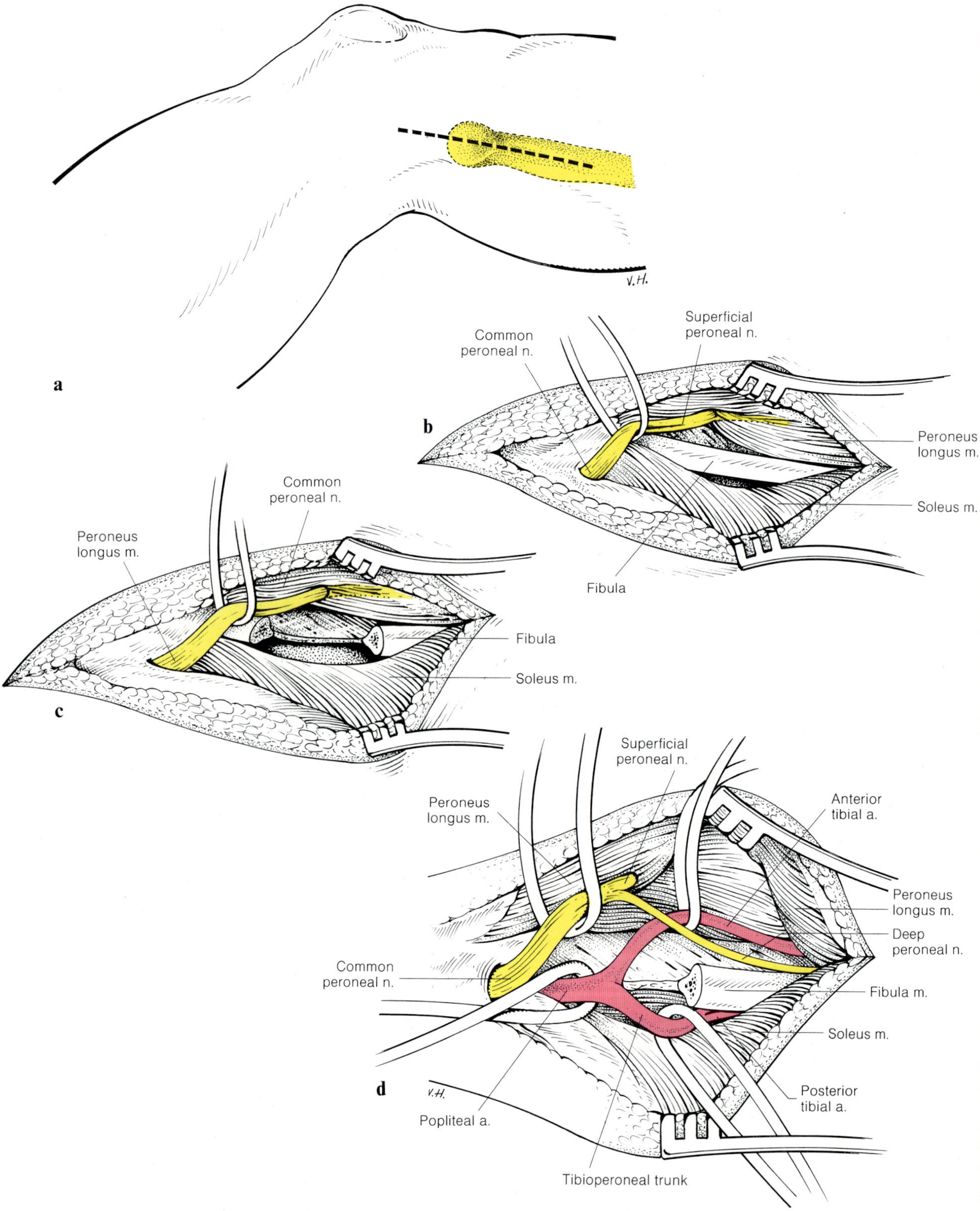

Fig. 17.3.4a–d. Lateral approach to the distal portion of the popliteal artery, tibioperoneal trunk, and proximal segments of the lower leg arteries. **a** Incision over the proximal end of the fibula. **b** Subperiosteal exposure of the proximal fibula. **c** Resection of a segment of the fibula distal to its head. **d** Following dissection of the medial periosteum, the distal portion of the popliteal artery and the trifurcation are exposed

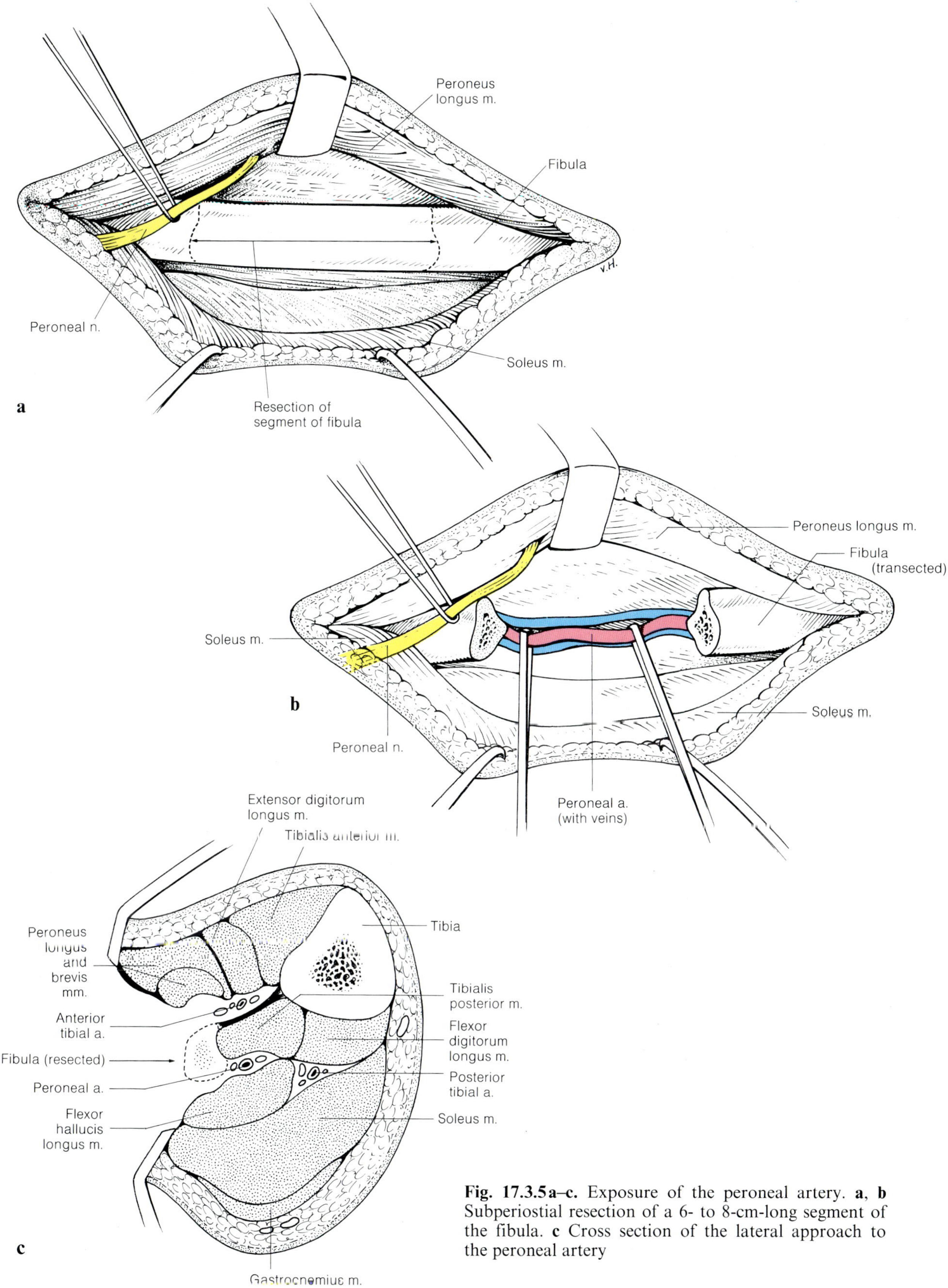

Fig. 17.3.5a–c. Exposure of the peroneal artery. **a**, **b** Subperiostial resection of a 6- to 8-cm-long segment of the fibula. **c** Cross section of the lateral approach to the peroneal artery

to find the dividing line in this way, the fascia should be incised at the lateral margin of the tibialis anterior muscle, which usually lies two fingerbreadths laterally from the tibial margin. The tibialis anterior muscle is retracted medially. Deep dissection is performed on the medial side of the intermuscular fascia, until the neurovascular bundle is reached (Fig. 17.3.3b). The deep peroneal nerve runs lateral to the artery and should remain untouched.

Farther distally, in the lower third of the lower leg, it is easier to find the boundary between the tibialis anterior muscle and the extensor hallucis longus muscle. The anterior tibial artery is reached and exposed in the same manner by deep dissection along the medial side of the intramuscular septum (Fig. 17.3.b).

The dorsalis pedis artery is exposed through a longitudinal incision about 1 cm lateral to the tendon of the extensor hallucis longus muscle. Following division of the fascia, the medial fibers of the extensor digitorum brevis muscle are exposed. These must be retracted laterally in order to reach the dorsalis pedis artery which lies directly on the bony surface.

For exposure of the proximal portion of the anterior tibial artery, the transfibular approach is the best one. A segment of the proximal fibula 6–8 cm long is resected subperiosteally just beneath its head (Fig. 17.3.4a–d). During this maneuver one should be mindful of the peroneal nerve, which may be observed at the upper corner of the incision. Following removal of the fibular segment and incision of the medial periosteum, the distal portion of the popliteal artery and the proximal segment of the anterior tibial artery are exposed. The tibioperoneal trunk may also be well exposed by this approach.

IV. Peroneal Artery

Lateral Approach. There are several possibilities for exposing the peroneal artery. The most common approach is from the lateral side of the leg, with resection of a segment of the fibula [4, 6].

After a longitudinal incision over the fibula, keeping well away from the peroneal nerve, the peroneus longus muscle is retracted anteriorly and the soleus muscle dorsally to permit subperiosteal resection of a 6- to 8-cm-long segment of the fibula (Fig. 17.3.5a–c). Following division of the inner periosteum, the tibialis posterior muscle is exposed. The peroneal artery is situated between this muscle and the flexor hallucis longus muscle.

The anterior tibial artery, which runs down the anterior surface of the interosseus membrane, can also be easily reached by this approach (Fig. 17.3.5c).

It is also possible to expose the peroneal artery without resection of the fibula. The fascia behind the fibula is divided. The peroneus longus muscle is retracted anteriorly and the soleus muscle dorsally. The flexor hallucis longus muscle is dissected sharply from the dorsal surface of the fibula, exposing the peroneal artery. An anastomosis between a vein graft and the peroneal artery can be performed without difficulty. However, this approach does not permit the construction of an arteriovenous anastomosis. Furthermore, the anterior tibial artery cannot be reached by this approach.

Medial Approach. The same approach is used to expose the peroneal artery from the medial side of the lower leg as is used to expose the posterior tibial artery (see p. 409) [11]. In the proximal half of the lower leg the peroneal artery runs parallel to the posterior tibial artery, but lies deeper between the tibialis posterior muscle and soleus muscle. Further distally, the distance between the arteries increases, making exposure of the peroneal artery from the medial side more difficult.

H. Technical Details

A bypass operation is the only procedure that can lead to successful reconstruction of lower leg arteries. A stenotic lower leg artery can be treated by percutaneous transluminal angioplasty, but the results are still unsatisfactory. Endarterectomy of the lower leg arteries is pointless.

A bypass operation can be successful only if the procedure is performed with the utmost care and accuracy.

I. Selection of the Correct Site for Anastomosis

The site for the distal anastomosis of the bypass is chosen according to the preoperative arteriographic findings. Which artery and which segment is chosen depends on the width of the vascular lumen, the smoothness of the vascular wall, the condition of the outflow tract, and the collateral circulation.

If one has the choice between several lower leg arteries, the anterior or posterior tibial artery should be preferred because the peroneal artery has the smallest run-off capacity.

II. Atraumatic Exposure

Exposure of lower leg and pedal arteries should be performed as atraumatically as possible. Because each side branch is important for the run-off capacity, all branches, including the smallest, should be preserved.

Some medial side branches must be sacrificed when a bypass to the anterior tibial artery is planned. The anastomosis must be established between the medial wall of the anterior tibial artery and the graft. This is only possible if the arterial segment is rotated externally by 180° with bulldog clamps or tapes. This rotation can only be accomplished if some side branches are sacrificed.

III. Tunneling

The bypass graft is placed in a tunnel extending from the revascularized lower leg artery to the infragenicular space and from there to the supergenicular region, where it is anastomosed to the popliteal artery, provided the superficial artery is patent. The latter artery is often narrowed, or even occluded, by arteriosclerotic plaques; whenever this is the case, then the superficial femoral artery, too, must be bridged with a bypass graft. All tunnels must be wide enough. Kinking and compression of the bypass graft should be avoided. Connective tissue blocking the way should be removed, and the tunnel walls spread apart by bidigital dissection.

a) Tunnel to the Anterior Tibial Artery. For the construction of a tunnel to the anterior tibial artery, a large window should be cut out of the interosseus membrane, cranial to the designated site of anastomosis. The index finger which is inserted through this window can easily prepare the way dorsally to the tibialis posterior muscle and the tibia, reaching the space between the soleus muscle and deep flexors and, from there, the infragenicular region (Fig. 17.3.4c). The finger should keep close to the tibia.

If an extra-anatomic (lateral) anterior bypass is planned, the tunnel is constructed subcutaneously, lateral to the knee joint.

b) Tunnel to the Posterior Tibial Artery. A tunnel to the posterior tibial artery can be constructed subcutaneously, starting within the infragenicular space or at the junction between the soleus muscle and the flexor digitorum longus muscle. The crural fascia should be divided along the course of the tunnel.

c) Tunnel to the Peroneal Artery. To establish a connection between the peroneal artery and the infragenicular space, the index finger may be used to tunnel a path between the tibialis posterior muscle and tibia, which lie ventrally, and the soleus muscle, which lies dorsally.

IV. Clamping

Thin vessel loops should not be placed around the lower leg arteries. These vessels should only be clamped with very soft bulldog clamps to avoid injuring the arterial wall, particularly the intima. A clamp exerting too much pressure on the vessel may cause an obstruction. Intraluminal occlusion using a small inflatable balloon has proven very reliable.

Clamping should not be performed until precautions have been taken against the formation of thrombi (systemic or local anticoagulation).

V. Bypass Graft Material

The walls of the lower leg arteries are very thin and tender and are easily torn. Only very delicate graft material should be used to revascularize these vessels. Therefore, only vein grafts are suitable for bypasses, or, at the very least, the distal portion of a bypass should consist of vein. Thick, wide, and rigid prostheses and bioprostheses are entirely unsuitable! [8, 21].

It is important that the lumen of the bypass graft have about the same caliber as the diseased lower leg artery. The lower leg arteries have an internal diameter of about 2–3 mm. The internal diameter of the bypass graft may be somewhat larger, but not too large; otherwise, an unfavorable hemodynamic situation with turbulent flow may develop.

VI. Construction of the Anastomosis

Preferably, a long end-to-side anastomosis (with fine suture material) should be constructed between the venous graft and the lower leg artery so that the transition from the graft to the host artery is not abrupt: without widening, narrowing, or kinking, and with no sudden change in caliber. An end-to-side anastomosis is preferable to an end-to-end anastomosis because, in an end-to-side anastomosis, run-off can take place in two directions, which is favorable for the flow within the graft.

VII. Positioning of the Graft

Following completion of the distal anastomosis, blood flow is restored within the host artery. The distal end of the graft is occluded between the fingers. The graft, which is filled with a mixture of blood and heparin, is pulled through the tunnel by means of a long forceps inserted via the infragenicular space. During this maneuver, one must avoid twisting or kinking the graft. The filled graft should lie loosely in the tunnel without tension.

After the graft has been guided through the popliteal fossa and along the sartorius muscle, the knee joint is extended to measure the length of the graft precisely. Then the proximal anastomosis is constructed: a long end-to-side anastomosis with the popliteal artery or with the common femoral artery.

I. Adjuvant Measures to Improve Blood Flow in a Femorocrural Bypass Graft

Many recurrent occlusions following crural bypass surgery are caused by a limited run-off. Therefore, in recent years a number of methods have been developed which aim at improving blood flow through a graft by reducing the peripheral resistance. Such measures to maximize flow through a bypass are clearly indicated in cases where peripheral resistance is high and run-off is poor. Four indications exist:

1. The anterior or posterior tibial arteries are open, but are narrowed or even occluded in their peripheral portions.
2. The anterior or posterior arteries are patent along their entire course, but the run-off is insufficient in the pedal region, because the corresponding foot artery is also occluded or narrowed.
3. In revascularization of the peroneal artery, which has a poor run-off to begin with.
4. In revascularization of a pedal artery – either the dorsalis pedis artery or one of the plantar arteries – in cases where all arteries of the lower leg are occluded.

Several such adjuvant measures are available.

I. Multiple Distal Anastomoses

Considerable improvement of run-off may be achieved by constructing several distal anastomoses at the level of the crural arteries [7, 9, 10, 15].

Different methods can be employed for revascularization of several lower leg arteries.

Sequential Bypass. The basic principle of sequential bypass is that several distal anastomoses are constructed with only one vein graft (Fig. 17.3.6a), e.g., first side-to-side with a still unoccluded segment of the of the anterior tibial artery, and then end-to-side with the peroneal artery. Usually, only two distal anastomoses are performed.

Jump Bypass. In a jump bypass an artificially constructed branch takes off from the distal end of a conventional femoral (popliteocrural) bypass graft (Fig. 17.3.6b) for the purpose of revascularizing a second artery. This is done by connecting a second vein graft end-to-side with the distal portion of the first vein graft. The distal end of the second graft is anastomosed end-to-side to another patent lower leg artery.

Dissection of two crural arteries may be very difficult and time-consuming. The most favorable combination is a graft to the posterior tibial artery with a jump to the peroneal artery. Both arteries can be reached by the same surgical approach on the medial side of the lower leg (see p. 412). Two incisions on the lateral side of the lower leg are needed to combine the anterior tibial artery and the peroneal artery. A solitary transfibular approach is possible only if the most proximal segments of both arteries must be revascularized (see p. 412). Two incisions are needed to combine the anterior tibial artery and the posterior tibial ar-

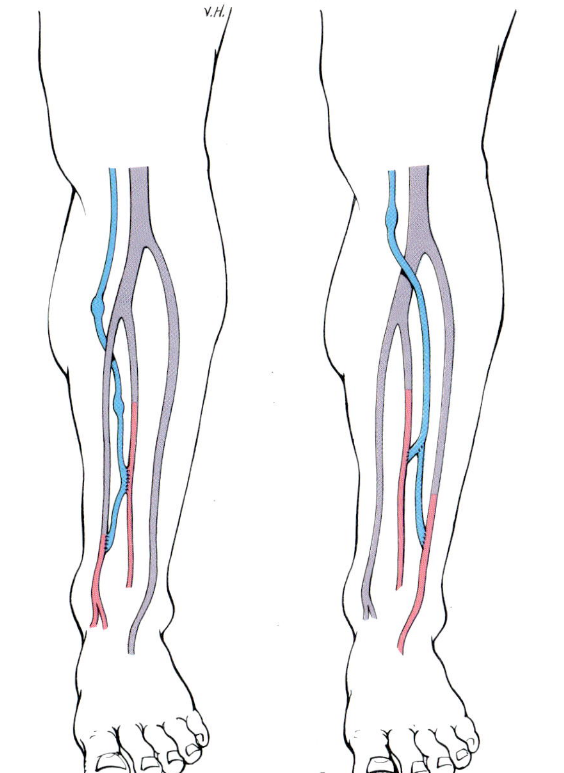

Fig. 17.3.6. a Sequential bypass: first side-to-side anastomosis with the peroneal artery, then end-to-side anastomosis with the distal portion of the posterior tibial artery. **b** Jump bypass. First a femoroperoneal bypass is performed. A second vein graft is anastomosed end to side with the distal part of the first vein bypass graft, serving as a blood conduit to the distal portion of the anterior tibial artery

tery, one on the lateral side and a second on the medial side of the lower leg (see p. 406).

If additional revascularization of the distal portion of the popliteal artery or of the tibioperoneal trunk is necessary, these vessels can be exposed through either a medial (see p. 406) or a lateral incision (see p. 412).

II. Distal Arteriovenous Fistula

In order to construct multiple distal anastomoses, two arterial segments must be patent below the knee joint. If only one segment is patent, or if a sequential or jump bypass is not possible for other reasons, the construction of a distal arteriovenous fistula should be considered [5, 9, 12].

There are several ways of constructing a distal arteriovenous shunt. Figure 17.3.7 shows the methods most often applied. The connection between the host artery and the vein graft must not be too wide.

III. Application of PTA

Finally, there is the possibility of dilating a stenosis in the peripheral portion of the host artery during the operation by PTA, if the length of the available vein graft does not allow the distal anastomosis to be constructed further distally. However, the results of this adjuvant procedure are unsatisfactory.

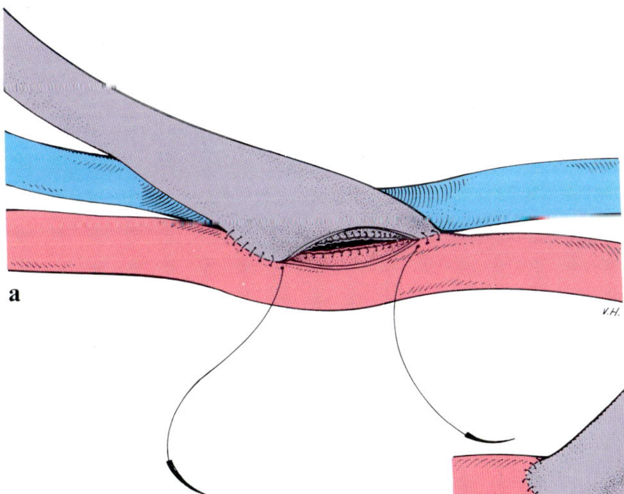

a

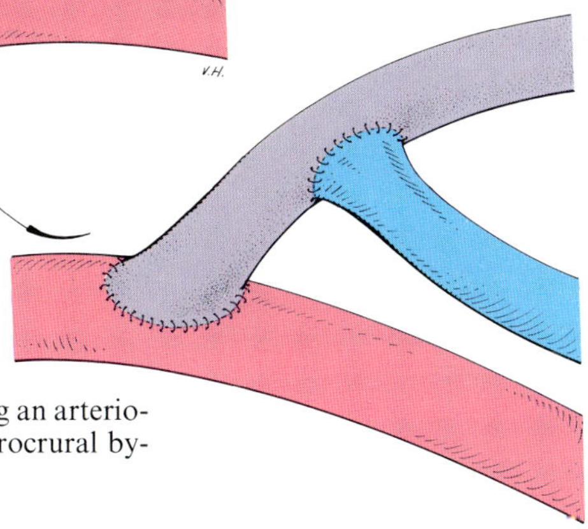

c

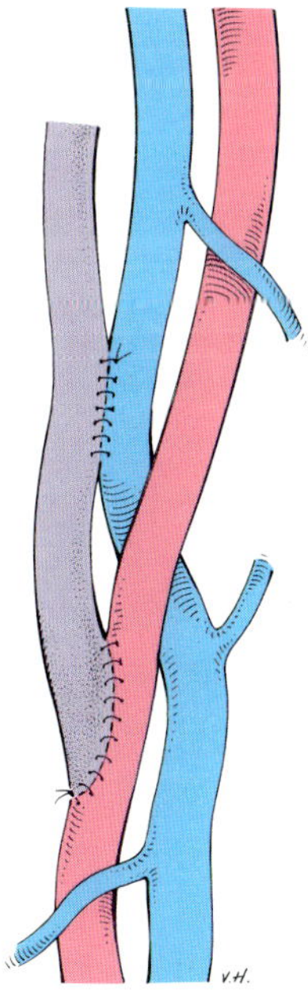

b

Fig. 17.3.7 a–c. Different ways of constructing an arteriovenous fistula at the level of the distal femorocrural bypass anastomosis

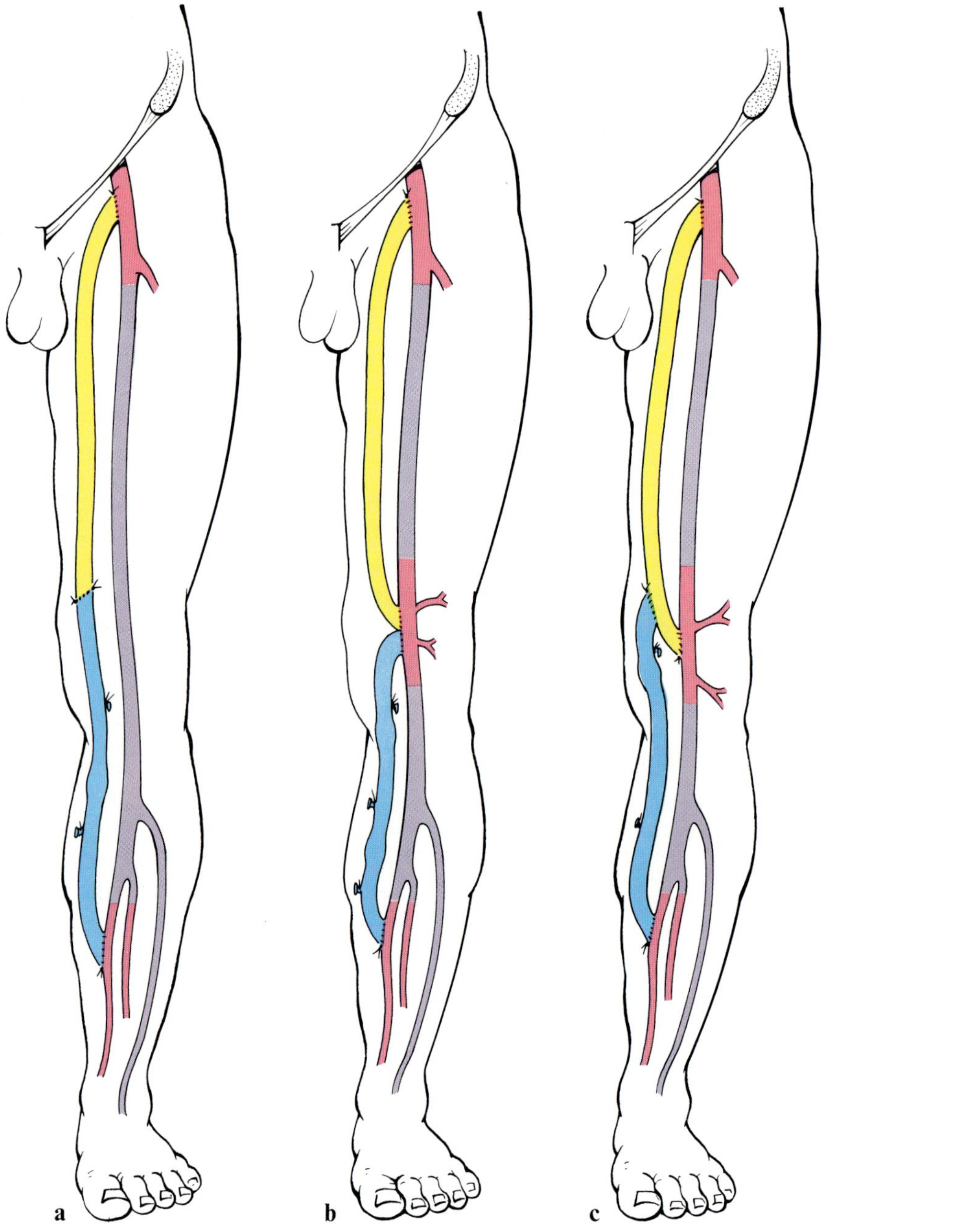

a b c

Fig. 17.3.8a–c. Femoropopliteal bypass alternatives. **a** Composite bypass. **b** Hitchhike bypass. **c** Jump bypass

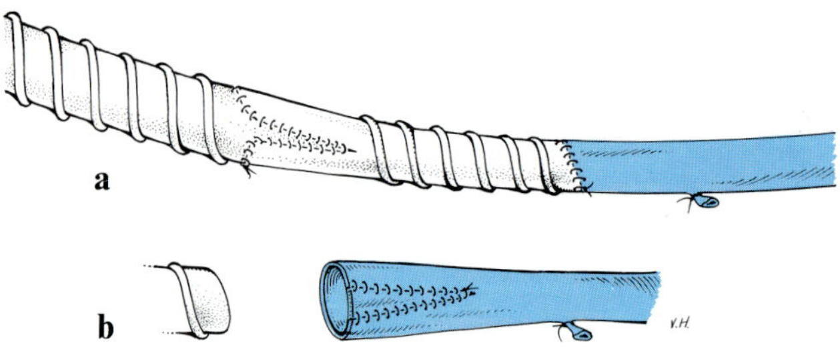

Fig. 17.3.9. a The proximal 6 mm wide prosthesis is anastomosed in a wedge-shaped fashion to a 4 mm wide intermediate tube; oblique anastomosis between the intermediate tube and the vein graft of equal diameter. **b** Widening of the end of the vein graft with a wedge-shaped venous patch. Differences in caliber between the prosthesis and the vein are thus compensated

J. Alternative Femorocrural Bypass Methods

Total bridging with a venous bypass graft is the best method of revascularizing the lower leg and pedal arteries. However, the autogenous great saphenous vein is often too short or unsuitable for total bypass of long femoropopliteocrural occlusions. Synthetic and bioprostheses are inappropriate [19, 21]. They are inferior to venous grafts in every case.

The basic principle of these alternative methods is to bridge the knee joint and construct a distal anastomosis, using only venous graft material [8].

I. Composite Graft (Fig. 17.3.8a)

A composite graft, a synthetic prosthesis lengthened by connecting a vein graft to it, makes it possible to bridge long occluded arterial segments, even if only a short vein graft is available. However, the end-to-end anastomosis between the prosthesis and the vein is a critical point, especially if the vein graft has a small caliber. It is absolutely impossible to construct a reliable direct connection between a 6 mm wide, relatively rigid prosthesis and a narrow thin-walled vein without constriction or kinking.

There are several ways of adjusting differences in caliber between the prosthesis and the vein. Figure 17.3.9a, b shows two of our own methods [8].

II. Hitchhike Bypass (Fig. 17.3.8b)

The hitchhike bypass (a short, disobliterated segment of the popliteal artery used as a connecting conduit between the prosthesis and the vein) is a very successful procedure, especially if the available vein graft is narrow.

The femoral bypass prosthesis is anastomosed to the upper half of the arteriotomy made in the proximal portion of the popliteal artery; the vein graft is anastomosed to the lower half.

A short segment of the popliteal artery is disobliterated within the region of the arteriotomy. This maneuver always opens some collaterals. An advantage of this method is that only a short segment of the great or small saphenous vein or of an arm vein is necessary to bypass the knee joint and perform the distal anastomosis.

III. Jump Bypass (Fig. 17.3.8c)

A variation of the hitchhike bypass is the jump bypass in which a segment of a vein graft is anastomosed end-to-side to the distal portion of a prosthesis.

Using this method, an anastomosis is established directly between the vein graft and the prosthesis. Such a connection is technically and hemodynamically more favorable.

REFERENCES

1. Armour RH (1976) Bypass grafting to the anterior tibial artery. Br J Surg 63:77
2. Auer AI, Hurley JJ, Binnington HB, Nunnelee JD, Hershey FB (1983) Distal tibial vein grafts for limb salvage. Arch Surg 118:593
3. Baird RJ, Tutassaura H, Miyagishima RT (1970) Saphenous vein bypass grafts to the arteries of the ankle and foot. Ann Surg 172:1059
4. Dardik H, Ibrahim IM, Dardik II (1977) Femoral tibial-peroneal bypass. The lateral approach and use of glutaraldehyde-tanned umbilical vein. Am J Surg 134:199
5. Dardik H, Sussman B, Ibrahim IM, Kahn M, Svobada JJ, Mendes D, Dardik II (1983) Distal arteriovenous fistula as an adjunct to maintaining arterial and graft patency for limb salvage. Surgery 94:478
6. Dardik H (1977) Femoroperoneal bypass. Contemp Surg 10
7. Deutsch M, Grabenwöger F, Kalman J, Magometschnigg H (1986) Die komplexe Unterschenkelrekonstruktion. Angio Archiv 11:83–87
8. van Dongen RJAM, Kromhout JG (1986) Femorocrurale and -pedale Rekonstruktionen; alternative Materialien und Methoden. Angio Archiv 11:79–82
9. van Dongen RJAM, Kromhout JG (1986) Hilfsmaßnahmen zur Verbesserung der femoro-cruralen Bypasstransplantatdurchströmung. Angio Archiv 11:60–62
10. Edwards WS, Gerety E, Larkin J, Hoyt TW (1976) Multiple sequential femoral tibial grafting for severe ischemia. Surgery 80:722
11. Grahams JW, Hanel KC (1981) Vein grafts to the peroneal artery. Surgery 89:264
12. Hinshaw DB, Schmidt CA, Simpson JB (1983) Arteriovenous fistula in arterial reconstruction of the ischemic limb. Arch Surg 118:589
13. Imparato AM, Kim GE, Madayag M, Haveson S (1973) Angiographic criteria for successful tibial arterial reconstructions. Surgery 74:830
14. Imparato AM, Kim GE, Chu DS (1973) Surgical exposure for reconstruction of the proximal part of the tibial artery. Surg Gynec Obstet 136:453
15. Jarett F (1978) Sequential femoral-tibial bypass grafting for limb salvage. Ann Surg 188:685
16. Karmody AM, Powers SR, Leather RP (1977) Surgical guidelines for direct anterior tibial bypass. Am J Surg 134:301

17. Kromhout JG, van Dongen RJAM (1986) Femorocrurale Rekonstruktionen; angiographische Voraussetzungen. Angio Archiv 11:9–11
18. Palma EC (1960) Treatment of arteritis of the lower limbs by autogenous vein grafts. Minerva Cardioangiol Europ 8:36
19. Robison JG, Brewster DC, Abbott WM, Darling RC (1983) Femoropopliteal and tibioperoneal artery reconstruction using human umbilical vein. Arch Surg 118:1039
20. Shieber W, Parks CI (1974) Dorsalis pedis artery in bypass grafting. Am J Surg 128:752
21. Thompson JE, Garrett WV (1980) The application of distal bypass operations for limb salvage. Surgery 87:717
22. Tiefenbrun J, Beckerman M, Singer A (1975) Surgical anatomy in bypass of the distal part of the lower limb. Surg Gynec Obstet 141:528
23. Vetra MJ Jr (1982) Pedal artery bypass for limb salvage. Surg Gynec Obstet 155:401

17.4 In Situ Bypass

J.D. GRUSS

CONTENTS

A. Introduction and Historical Background

The basic principle of the in situ bypass technique was introduced with the first grafting operation on a human being. In 1906, in Madrid, GOYANES [3] bridged a defect of the popliteal artery with the popliteal vein, following resection of an aneurysm. The vein remained in situ. The first free transplantation of a vein was performed by LEXER [17] in 1907, following the resection of an aneurysm of the axillary artery. Although many reports on successful reconstruction of femoral arteries [1, 8] were published in German journals, venous grafting did not gain general acceptance until JEAN KUNLIN [12, 13] published his pioneering work in 1949. In the classical vein bypass procedure according to KUNLIN [12, 13], the entire great saphenous vein of the ipsilateral or contralateral leg is resected and orthotopically reimplanted into the arterial system after reversing it. In contrast, the in situ technique leaves the great saphenous vein incorporated in its surrounding connective tissue, and circumferential dissection is performed only at the sites of the proximal and distal anastomoses. The first attempts to bridge an occluded femoral artery with a vein left in situ can be attributed to ROB (1960) [9, 10]. ROB, and later CONNOLLY and STEMMER [2], tried to destroy the venous valves with a stripper by introducing it proximally and advancing it distally. This method was abandoned by ROB in 1962 because of the vascular wall injuries that occurred during this maneuver, particularly at the entries of the venous tributaries. The further development of the in situ technique is practically identical with the advances made in the atraumatic destruction of venous valves and the evolution of instruments necessary for this procedure. Today, the early and late results are still dependent on this decisive maneuver [7].

The basic idea behind the in situ method is logical enough. The wider, proximal portion of the great saphenous vein is anastomosed to the wide common femoral artery and the narrower distal portion of the vein to the popliteal artery, which is about equal in diameter. The conical tapering form of the graft accelerates blood flow within the vein in a distal direction. In contrast to the classical vein bypass method, destruction of the valves allows for the blood to flow dicrotically, which is physiologic. Preservation of the vasa vasorum protects the graft against fibrosis. The almost completely intact endothelium in the vein is the best insurance against immediate or early thrombosis. Because the saphenous vein usually tapers significantly from proximal to distal, the calibers of vein and host artery are practically equal at the distal anastomosis. Consequently, saphenous veins with a distal peripheral diameter

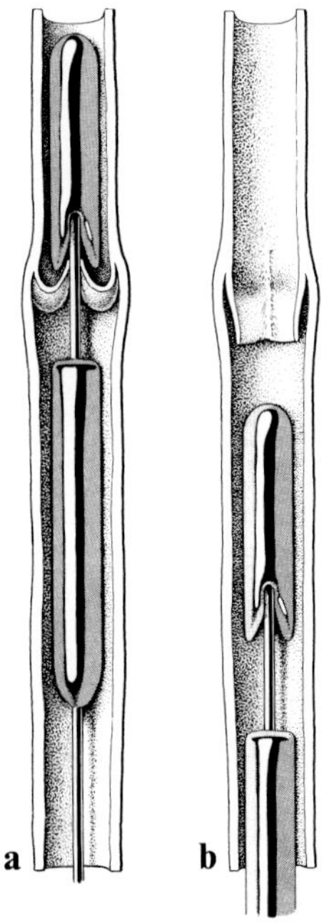

Fig. 17.4.1 a, b. Vein stripper according to Hall. **a** The stripper is introduced in the direction of venous blood flow and withdrawn carefully. The V-shaped base of the upper cylinder catches the leaflets of the valve **b** disrupting them by being withdrawn

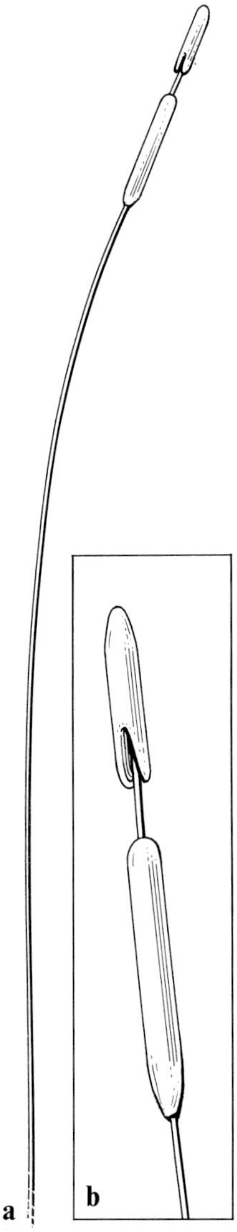

Fig. 17.4.2 a, b. The Hall vein stripper. Modified according to Gruss (Insitucut)

less than 2.5 mm, which would be unsuitable for classic vein bypass grafting, can be successfully anastomosed. K.V. Hall [10] was the first to report on a practical method for destroying the venous valves. From 1961 to 1968, Hall exposed the venous valves through transverse phlebotomies and carefully excised them. The main disadvantage of such a procedure is that it is very time-consuming, particularly if a large number of venous valves are present, as in lengthy femorocrural bypass grafts. Since 1968, Hall has used a vein stripper which he himself developed. The instrument consists of two metal cylinders mounted a short distance apart on a fairly rigid wire. The base of the uppermost cylinder is a negative of a venous valve. The edges are blunt (Fig. 17.4.1). The stripper is introduced distally and passed through the vein in the proximal direction, i.e., the direction of blood flow. As the instrument is withdrawn, the vein is distended and stretched by the first cylinder, so that the second cylinder hooks into the valve leaflets. The in-line arrangement of the two cylinders largely eliminates the problem so common with the older models of getting the stripper caught in the orifices of venous tributaries. Hall's stripper was slightly modified by us in 1983. The tips of both cylinders were molded into a conical form, and a polyfilament wire with a plastic coating was used as a carrier. The conical shape makes advancement and withdrawal of the stripper easier. The flexible metal guide wire gives the stripper enough elasticity to follow the course of the vein through its curves (knee joint, inguinal region) without injuring the endothelium (Fig. 17.4.2). The most important part of the modification is the introduction of a very sharp cutting edge between the two negative forms corresponding to the sinus of the venous valve. So this device is no longer a valve stripper, but a valve cutter (Insitucut R). A technically very complicated system of valve destruction is used by Leather [16]. Incision of the valves is performed while they are closed following flushing of the vein graft from proximal to distal. A specially developed microscissors with a very long handle is introduced into the vein from proximal to distal or inserted through tributaries into the vein. Each obstacle encountered is a closed venous valve with its leaflets aligned parallel to the skin surface. The valves are incised with a single snip of the scissors. Below the knee joint, Leather use a hook-shaped valvotome introduced through tributaries to incise the valves (Fig. 17.4.3). A very atraumatic instrument is the valve cutter developed by Leather, a double olive made of light plastic. The bottom portion

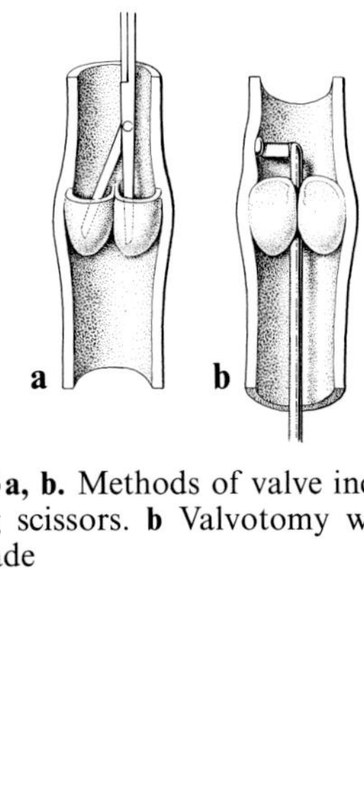

Fig. 17.4.3 a, b. Methods of valve incision. **a** Valve incision using scissors. **b** Valvotomy with a hook-shaped cutting blade

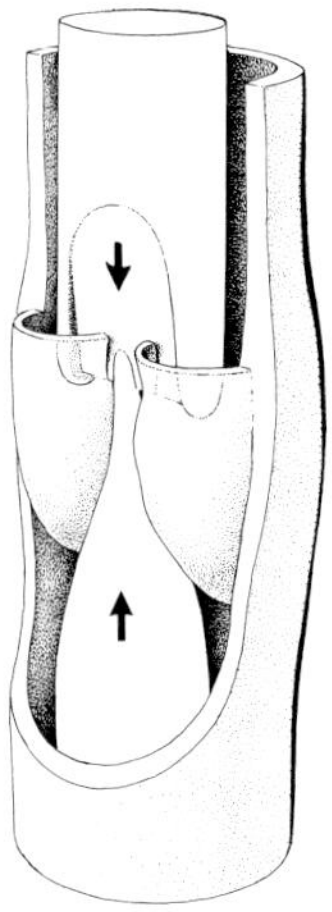

Fig. 17.4.4. Valvotomy catheter according to LEATHER

of the upper olive has an extremely sharp, short cutting blade. The valve cutter is pulled through the great saphenous vein, which has been filled under pressure from proximal to distal with heparinized saline solution (Fig. 17.4.4).

Because the patency rates of 2–5 years following application of the Hall stripper are about the same as with the Leather stripper, long-term results must be evaluated before a conclusive judgment can be made. Furthermore, of course, the long-term results depend on the technique of anastomosis, the intraoperative quality control, the treatment of venous tributaries, and the initial stage of the disease.

B. Indications for Surgery

The indication for in situ bypass is the same as for a classical femoropopliteal or femorocrural vein bypass. Reconstructions of the femoropopliteal and femorocrural segments are usually performed in clinical stages III and IV. The indication for surgery in stage II disease must be accurately and strictly checked and individualized. Reconstruction in this stage may be performed only if the disease has led to considerable physical job disability and serious impairment in everyday living. The following scheme has proven very useful in the surgical decision-making process as it relates to the morphology of occlusive arterial disease.

Thromboendarterectomy is only rarely performed; it is reserved for exceptional cases of highly localized occlusive disease where the short obstructions involved cannot be relieved by percutaneous intraluminal angioplasty. Segmental occlusions between the femoral bifurcation and the adductor canal where the popliteal artery is normal and there is good run-off (i.e., all three lower leg arteries patent) are bridged by orthotopic interposition of a PTFE prosthesis or an umbilical vein graft with a diameter of 6–7 mm.

In situ bypass is indicated in all kinds of femoropopliteal and femorocural occlusive disease, i.e., where the occluded segment of the superficial femoral artery may be of any length and the popliteal artery and/or at least one lower leg artery is diseased.

C. Positioning and Surgical Approach

For in situ bypass, the patient is placed in a supine position. The operating table is slightly tilted toward the surgeon. The leg must be completely free so that during the course of the operation the knee can be flexed or extended, as required. If the peripheral anastomosis is planned at the popliteal artery or the tibioperoneal trunk, the distal part of the lower leg and also the foot are wrapped in sterile towels. If a long femorocrural bypass is planned, then it is better to pull two sterile rubber gloves over the foot. For intraoperative angiography, it must be possible to position the operating table horizontally and to lower it.

The proximal segment of the great saphenous vein and the femoral bifurcation are easily exposed through an S-shaped incision in the groin. The incision should extend from the upper outer part of the inguinal region across the inguinal ligament downward to the medial and anterior side of the thigh. The lymph nodes are retracted laterally (see p. 393).

The distal incision is always made below the knee. If one plans to anastomose the graft to the third popliteal segment or the tibioperoneal trunk, the incision is made just below the knee joint. In other cases, the incision is always made at the level of the designated site of the distal host artery-graft anastomosis and always runs in a longitudinal direction, parallel to the medial margin of the tibia and about one fingerbreadth behind it (see p. 394ff.). Following the skin incison, the great saphenous vein is localized first in order to avoid accidental damage to the graft. Anastomosis of the graft to the proximal peroneal artery is also a medial, longitudinal incision. Only anastomosis to the anterior tibial artery and the distal peroneal artery requires a longitudinal incision on the lateral side of the lower leg, performed in the usual way when exposing this artery.

D. Surgical Technique

I. Dissection of the Vein and Valve Destruction

The first step in the operation is to examine the suitability of the greater saphenous vein for use as a graft. A longitudinal incision is made along the tibia at the level of the designated site of the distal anastomosis, and the greater saphenous vein is exposed. For grafting to the popliteal artery, we find veins up to a diameter of 3 mm suitable, and for anastomosis to peripheral lower leg arteries, veins up to a caliber of 2.5 mm are still adequate. The vein is only inspected and not touched. It is not yet dissected out of its surrounding tissue. Ascending phlebography to test the suitability of the vein for a graft is not performed in order to prevent possible injury to the graft by the contrast medium. If the caliber of the graft is adequate, the host artery is dissected next at the level of the proposed anastomosis, as determined from the preoperative angiogram. The artery must often be exposed peripherally because of vascular wall lesions and calcifications. In the popliteal artery or the tibioperoneal trunk, this is done by dividing the fascia and the hamstring tendons. The host artery is dissected around its entire circumference, and an umbilical tape is passed around it. The next step is to expose the entry of the great saphenous vein into the deep femoral vein through an S-shaped incision in the groin. During this maneuver, it is important to dissect carefully the inferior epigastric vein over a length of about 2–3 cm without dividing it. In addition, a 2- to 3-cm-long portion of a second upper tributary of the great saphenous vein should be saved for intraoperative angiography. Each of the other cranial branches is occluded with two metal clips at the level of their entry and then divided. During dissection, the vein should not be touched with so-called atraumatic instruments. Manipulation of the vein should be done only with a moistened rubber tape. The femoral bifurcation is exposed as usual. Tapes are placed around the superficial common femoral and profunda femoris arteries.

Blood flow is interrupted, and a longitudinal arteriotomy is performed at the site of the distal anastomosis. The length of this arteriotomy should be 2–3 times greater than the diameter of the graft. The vascular wall is inspected and retrograde flow is controlled. The vessel is filled in both directions with heparinized saline solution. To assess the condition of the outflow tract, the distal portion of the vessel is carefully explored with a Fogarty catheter. We perform a trial exposure in the same manner, followed by intraoperative angiography.

Once the level of the distal anastomosis has been determined, the great saphenous vein is dissected circumferentially at the designated site. The branches and peripheral veins are occluded with tantalum clips. The vein is incised transversely, and the anterior wall is marked with a stay suture. After the vein has been flushed with heparinized saline solution, the graft is compressed digitally at the upper corner of the distal incision and slightly dilated by careful injection of heparinized saline solution. An Insitucut with a diameter that just fits through the lumen of the vein without difficulty is introduced distally and advanced proximally in the extended leg. During this maneuver, no resistance whatsoever must be overcome by force. The position of the lower end of the front olive, which has the corresponding negative of a vein valve form can be marked by attaching a Kocher forceps at the end of the stripper. The proximal olive is advanced under digital control through the saphenofemoral junction up into the common femoral vein so that the valve cutter, as it is withdrawn downward, can catch in the terminal valve of the saphenous vein and destroy it. The position of the olive at this site is controlled visually and by palpation. The cutter is withdrawn slowly. The position of the forceps allows for correct orientation of the valve negatives of the cutter in relation to the skin surface. Each venous valve can be identified by a slight resistance or sudden tug. This maneuver is repeated with the same instrument two or three times. The angle which the Kocher forceps makes with the skin surface can be changed slightly. After three passages, it is usually possible to introduce an Insitucut of the next larger size and to repeat the maneuver. Then the vein is flushed once again with heparinized saline solution, and its distal end is occluded with a bulldog clamp.

II. Proximal Anastomosis

Following the interruption of blood flow with common vascular clamps, a longitudinal arteriotomy is performed at the femoral bifurcation. The pelvic arteries, the profunda femoris artery, and any patent proximal portions of the superficial femoral artery are filled with heparinized saline solution. If vascular calcifications or localized stenoses of the common femoral artery or of the profunda femoris artery are found, open thromboendarterectomy at the site of the proximal anastomosis is necessary. The saphenofemoral junction is occluded parallel to the long axis of the great saphenous vein with two large metal clips (Fig. 17.4.5). Using a Potts' scissors, the great saphenous vein is divided tangentially just above the two clips and then pulled toward the femoral artery. In about 80% of our patients, the great saphenous vein is of adequate length, and, following phlebotomy on its posterior side, it can be directly connected to the femoral bifurcation, forming an oblique end-to-side anastomosis. In 20% the great saphenous vein is not long enough. In these patients, a longitudinal phlebotomy is performed on the posterior side of the inferior epigastric vein, starting at the lumen of the great saphenous vein. This maneuver forms a venous strip, extending upward (Fig. 17.4.6). Thus, it is always possible to connect the graft to the common femoral artery. If the inferior epigastric vein is not needed, it is simply ligated at its base with two metal clips and then divided. Prior to anastomosis, the saphenofemoral junction is examined for remnants of the terminal valve or of a proximal valve, which may be carefully excised with a Potts' scissors. The surgeon should be able to flush the graft easily from proximal to distal with heparinized saline solution. If the distal anastomosis is very peripheral, so that only a very small stripper can be used, it may be necessary to excise incompletely destroyed, proximal venous valves locally.

The anastomosis is performed with double monofilament 5-0 sutures. We start at the lower corner and first place five stitches on both sides, between the vein and the artery. Bulldog clamps are then fixed to both ends of the suture to put tension on them. The second suture is started at the upper corner of the incision. The proximal circumference of the great saphenous vein or the rounded-off end of the inferior epigastric vein are fixed to the upper corner of the arteriotomy. The edges are sutured with a continuous over-and-over suture from the vein to the artery, with direction toward the surgeon. The upper sutures on both sides are tied to the lower sutures. After restoration of blood flow, a strong pulse must be palpable at the distal end of the vein.

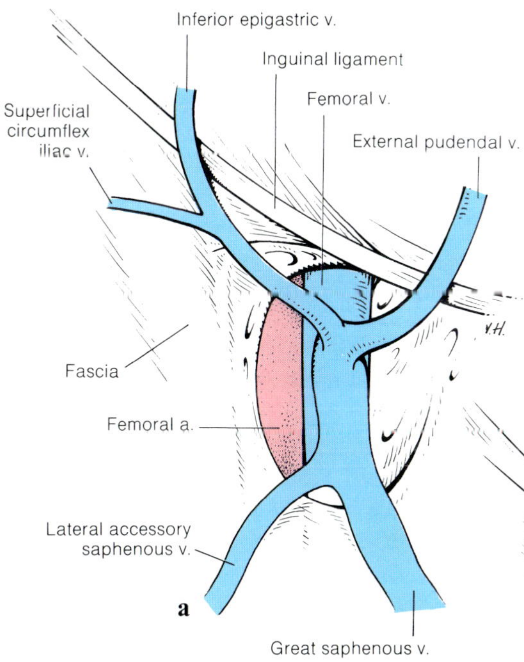

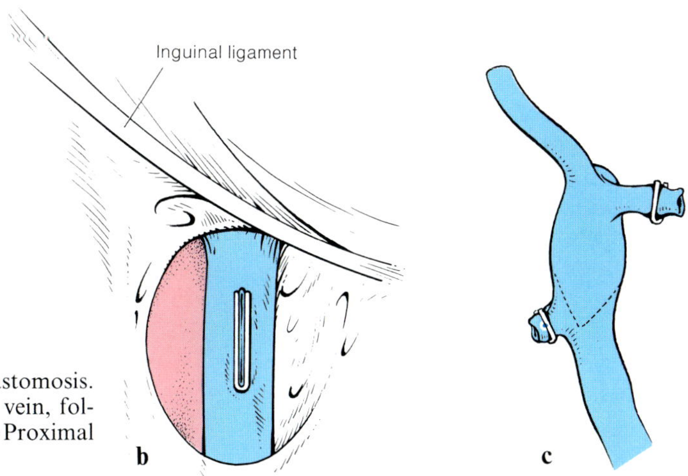

Fig. 17.4.5a–c. Dissection for proximal anastomosis. **a** Anatomy of the inguinal region. **b** Femoral vein, following division of the greater saphenous vein. **c** Proximal portion of the dissected great saphenous vein

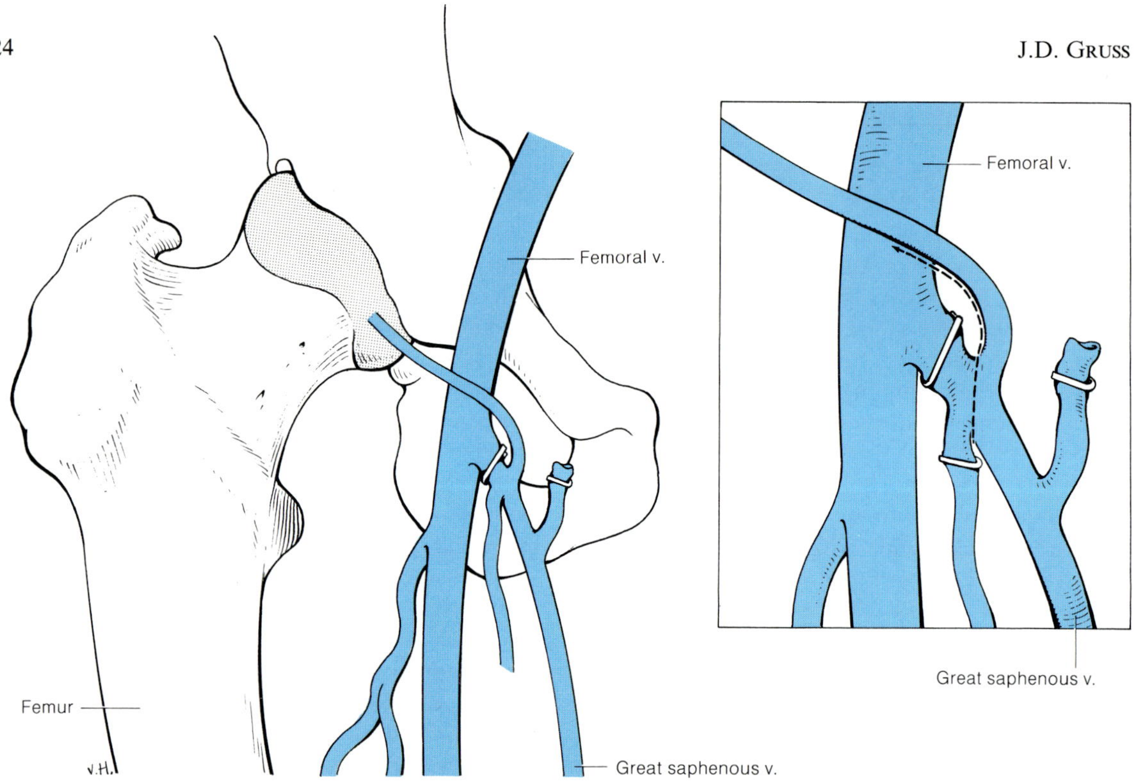

Fig. 17.4.6. Elongation of the graft by incorporation of the inferior epigastric vein. The second unligated venous tributary is necessary for the introduction of the angiographic cannula

In our earliest in situ bypass operations, we performed transverse end-to-end or oblique end-to-end anastomoses of the proximal end of the graft to the superficial femoral artery with and without thromboendarterectomy of the connection site, although the length of the graft was not adequate. Angiographic control of our first 100 in situ bypasses showed filiform stenoses of the superficial femoral segments in 5 of these patients, which had to be relieved by patch angioplasty. The stenoses occurred with and without thromboendarterectomy of the connection site. This observation compelled us to perform the proximal anastomosis only end-to-side at the femoral bifurcation with inclusion of the common femoral artery. In patients who had recurrent occlusions following thromboendarterectomy or who had a bifurcation prosthesis implanted prior to graft surgery, the proximal anastomosis is established with the profunda fermoris artery, bypassing the scarred tissue region [4, 6].

III. Distal Anastomosis

In the popliteal artery (segment III), the anastomosis may be performed either obliquely end-to-side or end-to-end depending on the anatomic situation. An end-to-end, anastomosis seems appropriate if a very proximal popliteal trifurcation causes a sharp angulation of the graft on its course from the subcutaneous tissue to the artery; such angulation, of course, is hemodynamically unfavorable (Fig. 17.4.7).

In such cases, the popliteal artery is occluded as far proximally as possible with two metal clips and divided; its peripheral portion is then approximated to the vein graft. Its periphery is filled with heparinized saline solution. The distal end of the graft is positioned near the artery, and the length of the graft necessary for anastomosis is measured only when the leg is extended. It should not pass the edge of the fascia under tension; otherwise, kinking of the graft will result. The peripheral end of the vein which has been mechanically injured by grasping it with the forceps and by introduction of the stripper is always discarded. The stay suture at this end is needed for orientation, in order to prevent twisting of the graft.

An end-to-end anastomosis is performed with two double monofilament 6-0 sutures, using the rotation technique. The oblique end-to-side anas-

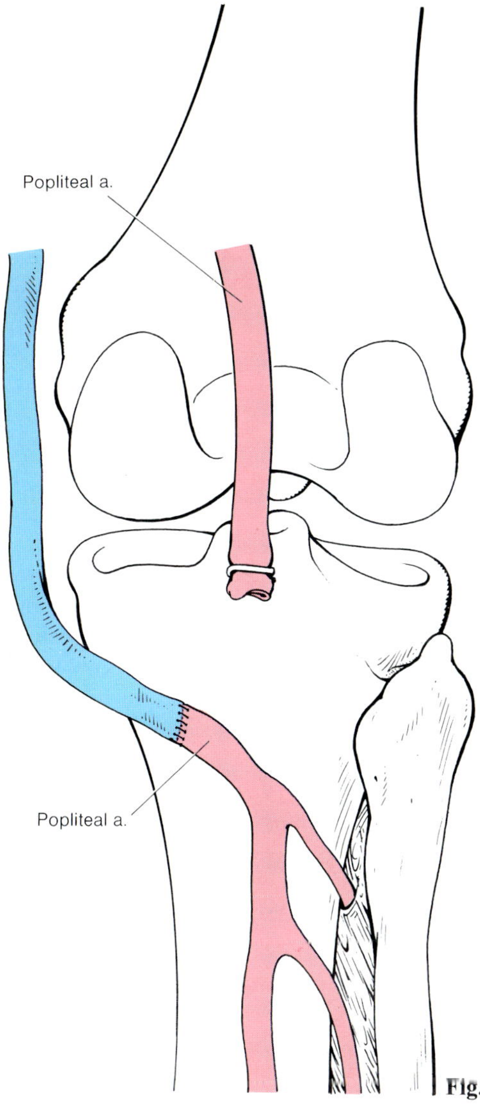

Fig. 17.4.7

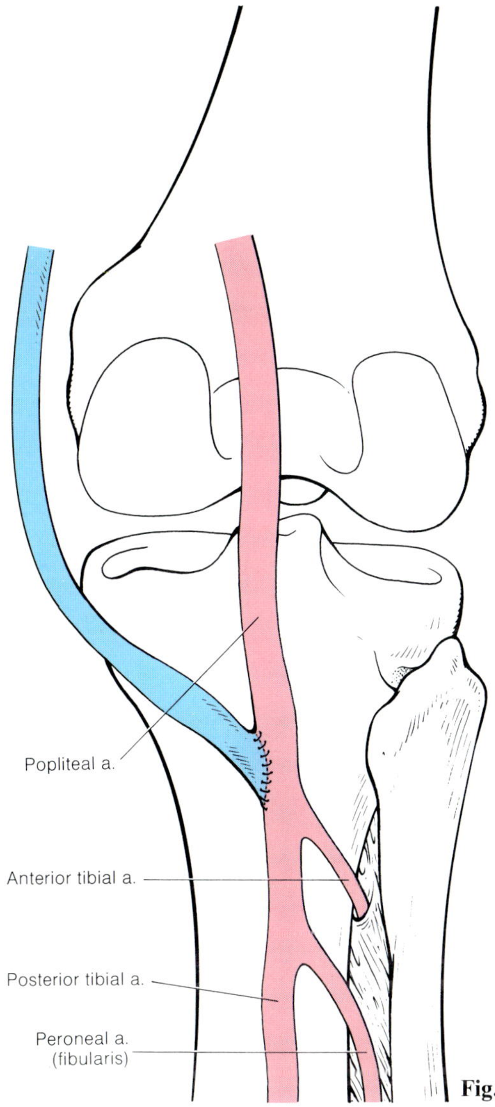

Fig. 17.4.8

Fig. 17.4.7. Distal end-to-end anastomosis

Fig. 17.4.8. Distal end-to-side anastomosis

tomoses at the third popliteal segment, the tibioperoneal trunk, the posterior tibial artery, or the peroneal artery are performed as described earlier for the proximal anastomosis (Fig. 17.4.8). Thromboendarterectomy at the peripheral host artery-graft junction should be avoided, if possible. Additional precautions must be taken when constructing an anastomosis at the anterior tibial artery:

1. A longer portion of the great saphenous vein must be exposed and dissected out of the surrounding tissue.
2. The window in the interosseous membrane must be large enough, and it must lie 2–3 cm above the peripheral anastomosis.
3. Special care must be taken to prevent twisting of the graft and to facilitate its orientation with the stay suture.
4. The distal arteriotomy must be performed on the anterior aspect of the artery by rotating the artery externally, using both vascular clamps to obstruct blood flow.

To construct the anastomosis at the peripheral lower leg arteries, we use magnifying glasses with a magnifying power of $2^1/_2$ times. Technically

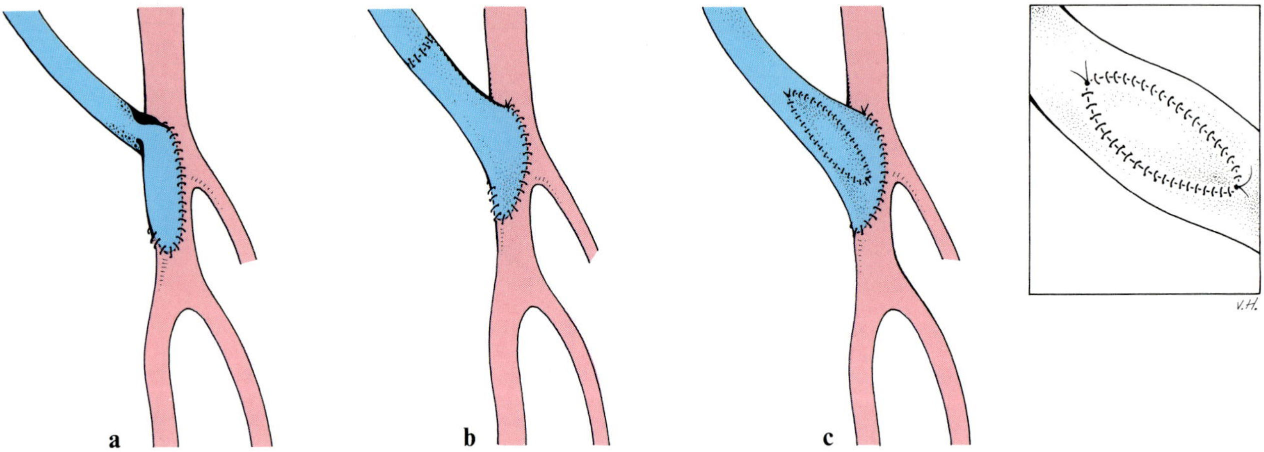

Fig. 17.4.9 a–c. Correction of a stenosis caused by twisting and kinking at the distal anastomosis. **a** Stenosis through kinking and twisting. **b** Transverse phlebotomy, straightening, end-to-end anastomosis. **c** Longitudinal phlebotomy and venous patch angioplasty (with less distortion)

speaking, the most difficult step in the peripheral end-to-side anastomosis are the first stitches at the upper corner of the anastomosis. In order to prevent narrowing at this site, only a very small bite of the venous wall should be taken, and the adventitia at the margins of the phlebotomy must be removed. If, in spite of these precautions, a stenosis is present following the restoration of blood flow, immediate correction by incorporation of a short autogenous vein patch should be performed during the same operation. This patch technique has proven very reliable and effective in eliminating slight twisting and distortion of the graft (Fig. 17.4.9).

IV. Technical Problems

If an obstruction is encountered during destruction of the venous valves, no effort should be made to overcome this obstruction with a smaller or a larger stripper. The great saphenous vein is exposed through a short longitudinal incision at the level of the palpable head of the stripper and inspected. If the tip of the cutter is caught in an orifice of one of the venous branches, this tributary should be occluded with two metal clips and the cutter advanced proximally under direct visual control (rare). If the obstruction is caused by a localized postphlebitic venous lesion, the vein must be dissected in that area for assessment of the extension of the lesion. Sometimes, one is successful in excising a short segment of the vein and restoring its continuity by an oblique end-to-end anastomosis. In other cases, interposition of a peripherally excised venous segment is necessary. A third possible complication is perforation by the cutter, which we observed only once during our first year of experience with the in situ technique and never again thereafter. We were able to correct injury in one case by an end-to-end suture and in two other cases by incorporation of a venous patch [5, 7].

Once the proximal anastomosis has been completed and blood flow is restored, the peripheral portion of the graft should pulsate; if it does not, the cause may lie in an intact, functioning venous valve. In such cases, the venous valve can be destroyed by repeated introduction of an Insitucut of the largest possible size. However, because in most cases a unique anatomic variation is present, this maneuver is not always successful and only direct dissection of the vein at the site of the valve will restore flow to the pulseless part of the graft. One usually finds a venous valve with leaflets that do not originate at the same level within the vein and consequently impede passage of the cutter. The persistent valve is carefully excised with Potts' scissors. Usually, a longitudinal phlebotomy must be performed, which is closed with a venous patch. A third possible cause, spasm of the venous graft, can only be detected by angiography and overcome pharmacologically.

After completion of the peripheral anastomosis, a strong arterial pulse wave can be felt along the corresponding host artery. If the peripheral pulse disappears as soon as the leg is extended for arteri-

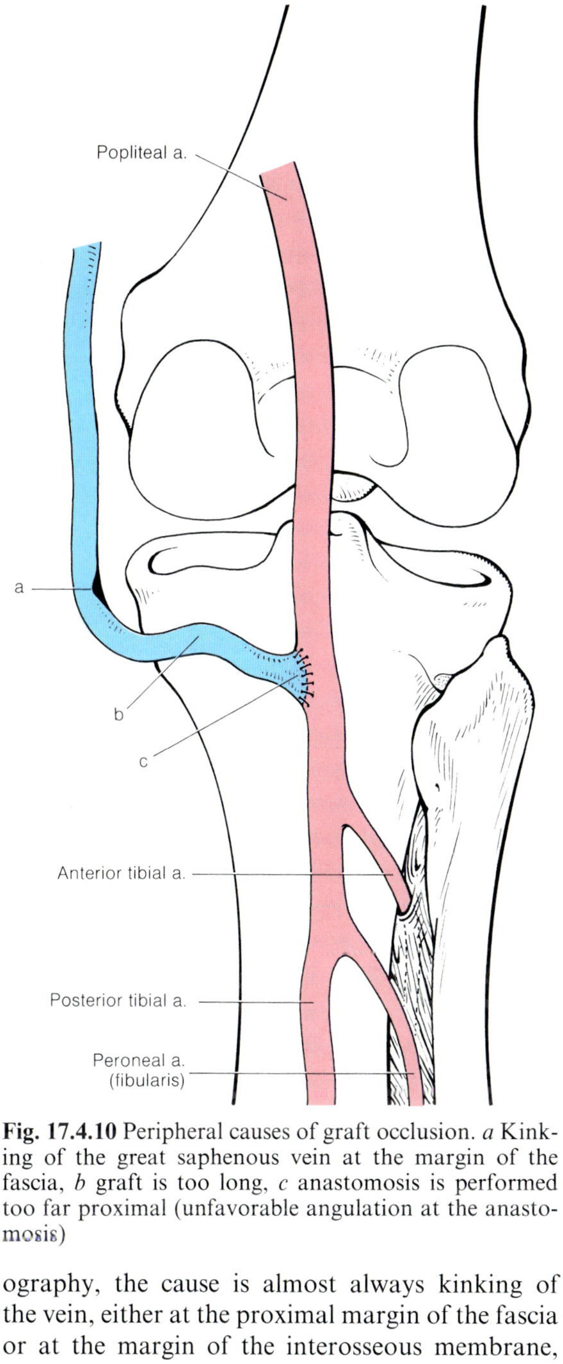

Fig. 17.4.10 Peripheral causes of graft occlusion. *a* Kinking of the great saphenous vein at the margin of the fascia, *b* graft is too long, *c* anastomosis is performed too far proximal (unfavorable angulation at the anastomosis)

ography, the cause is almost always kinking of the vein, either at the proximal margin of the fascia or at the margin of the interosseous membrane, if the window is too small. Both problems are easily solved by a simple snip of the scissors (Fig. 17.4.10).

We think there are only two situations in which it is justifiable to connect an in situ graft to the first popliteal segment above the knee joint:

1. When an isolated segment of the popliteal artery must be revascularized and no peripheral connection is possible.
2. When the distal portion of the great saphenous vein shows postphlebitic changes and a graft long enough for revascularization is therefore not available [4].

In all other cases the bypass is connected below the knee. We have seen high-grade degenerative changes and even occlusions in the second and third popliteal segment develop very quickly when the anastomosis between host artery and graft is performed above the knee. The in situ bypass can be performed with two separate teams working simultaneously, in order to shorten operating time [4, 7, 11].

E. Intraoperative Angiography

Intraoperative angiography is absolutely essential [6]. If the inferior epigastric vein is not needed for construction of the anastomosis, the plastic angiographic cannula is inserted and tied to this vein. Then, 50 ml of warm 60% contrast medium is injected by hand. After removal of the cannula, the venous tributary is closed with two metal clips.

Angiography allows accurate assessment of the course, length, and caliber of the graft. Venous loops, kinking at the margin of the fascia, and technical errors at the distal anastomosis can be discovered. All efferent branches of the great saphenous vein are well filled with contrast medium, whereas the afferent venous branches are only shown as far as the first closed valves. In 22% of cases, intraoperative angiography detects errors that require correction [6, 7]. These are mostly sharp angulations and kinking of the graft at the margin of the fascia, which are simply relieved by notching the fascia. Grafts which are too long, stenoses at the anastomoses, distortions of the graft, or peripheral intimal dissections are corrected immediately (Fig. 17.4.9).

Contrary to the opinion of several French authors [14], we find it necessary to interrupt all larger efferent (perforating) veins and all larger afferent venous branches. The ligation of venous branches is easier if, prior to angiography, mosquito clamps and cannulas are placed alternately along the medial surface of the thigh at intervals of 10 cm. This maneuver allows exact localization of venous branches so that with a palpable graft only short (about 2 cm) additional incisions need be made along the medial side of the thigh and the lower leg in order to identify the branches and ligate them with clips. Thus, complete denudation or circumferential dissection of the great saphenous vein can be avoided. Branches which have been overlooked and left in situ lead to localized painful inflammation over the venous graft during the first postoperative days and cause a loud machinelike murmur. Large arteriovenous fistulas may lead to very painful skin necroses if they are not ligated.

Large perforating veins which are left in situ pose an additional risk in the long run. If the underlying arterial disease progresses, resulting in higher peripheral resistance, these veins can cause a steal phenomenon, whereby arterial blood is shunted directly into the deep venous system. This may lead to distal thrombosis of the graft. Recently, in a few cases with very impaired peripheral run-off, we purposely left one or two peripheral venous branches unligated in order to provide adequate flow through the graft. It is still undetermined whether such peripheral arteriovenous fistulas are effective in limb preservation.

Electromagnetic flow measurements, done in addition to intraoperative angiography, show that flow at the proximal anastomosis is twice as great as at the distal anastomosis in many cases. Blood flow at the proximal anastomosis should be between 340 and 114 ml/min in femoropopliteal bypasses prior to ligation of the venous branches. After ligation, the measured blood flows are almost equal. However, two observations are important:

1. Following ligation of the branches, there is almost always a greater flow in the proximal portion of the graft than in its distal portion.
2. On average, proximal blood flow is almost always slightly reduced following ligation of the branches.

The average flow through a femoropopliteal in situ bypass at the upper anastomosis is 220 ml/min prior to branch ligation and 210 ml/min thereafter. The corresponding values at the lower anastomosis are 160 ml/min and 195 ml/min. Our flow measurements were done with the Nycotron 376 flow meter.

Postoperatively, all patients who have no contraindications are anticoagulated with dicoumarin preparations for a longer period of time. Patients who may not receive this medication are given 0.5 g acetylsalicylic acid daily.

F. Postoperative Complications

I. Immediate Occlusion

Postoperative patency control of an in situ bypass is simple and can be done by the patient or by the nursing personnel; only simple palpation of the graft is required, preferably at the level of the knee joint (on a solid surface). An immediate occlusion on the day of the operation or during the next few days can have three causes:

1. A poor general circulation with long hypotensive periods and external compression of the graft
2. Excessively high resistance to run-off
3. Technical errors

The first two causes are rare because blood flow through in situ transplants is usually maintained, even if blood pressure is severely reduced and the peripheral run-off is extremely limited. In most cases the problem can be traced to surgical technique or to mechanics. To correct the occlusion, the longitudinal incision along the tibia is reopened, the distal anastomosis exposed, and the graft opened by a longitudinal phlebotomy at the anastomosis. A thrombectomy of the bypass using a Fogarty balloon catheter is performed with extreme caution. If the balloon is inflated too much, the intima and the entire venous wall may tear longitudinally. Disobliteration is technically very simple. As soon as pulsatile blood flow is restored, the graft is filled with heparinized saline solution. When the anastomosis is inspected, intimal dissection is one of the most frequent disorders found distal to the anastomosis. This usually develops only after blood flow has been restored for a considerable time and is thus often overlooked during intraoperative angiography. Further causes are stenoses at the anastomoses or slight twisting of the graft which the surgeon did not deem severe enough for correction. If no cause of the occlusion is found, the proximal anastomosis should be checked in every case, even though intimal dissection and graft occlusion are rare at this site. Intraoperative control angiography should always be repeated. Following thrombectomy, it also provides a means of detecting an overlooked functioning venous valve. Some 10% of all bypasses with immediate reocclusion exhibit long-term patency following thrombectomy alone, even though no mechanical cause of the occlusion is found.

II. Arteriovenous Fistula

Between the 2nd and 8th postoperative day, painful inflammation and swelling may occur along the course of the vein graft on the medial side of the thigh and lower leg. In auscultation over these sites, a typical continuous machinelike murmur can be heard, which makes the diagnosis simple. The murmur is produced in afferent vessel branches. These branches escape detection during intraoperative angiography because their valves are at that point still intact; but dilatation then renders the valves insufficient with consequent hemodynamic effects on the arteriovenous blood flow. These tributaries can be localized very precisely by palpation, auscultation, and Doppler ultrasonography. This makes their ligation through short additional incisions easy. Smaller venous branches usually occlude by themselves. The larger ones have a high risk of producing painful skin necrosis with danger of infection.

III. Early Occlusion

Graft occlusions which occur after hospital discharge up until the end of the 6th postoperative month are treated just like immediate occlusions. In addition to the causes already discussed, two more must be added to the list:

1. Progressive impairment and limitation to the run-off (treatment is the same as in chronic recurrent occlusions).
2. A steal phenomenon as a result of an arteriovenous fistula. In this case pulsation is found in the proximal portion of the graft, ending at the site of the fistula. The distal portion is clotted. Following thrombectomy, the venous branch responsible is usually visualized as a large perforating vein in the intraoperative angiogram. Ligation is therefore always possible.

IV. Late Occlusion

Graft occlusions beyond the 6th postoperative month may be classified into acute and chronic forms. An acute graft occlusion usually resembles the clinical picture of a complete ischemic syndrome of the extremity. Angiography should not be performed on admission to hospital, and intramuscular injections should be avoided. The patient immediately undergoes fibrinolytic therapy. If the time between the occlusion and the beginning of treatment is not too long, patency of the graft can be restored in a few hours at the earliest. Detection of an occlusion is by palpation and Doppler ultrasound. Only after these measures should angiography be performed. It usually allows the cause of the occlusion to be discovered, and the type of surgical reconstruction can be determined accordingly. Some of the causes include proximal stenoses of the pelvic arteries, proximal stenoses at the anastomoses, distal stenoses at the anastomoses as well as stenoses and occlusions within the outflow tract. The third step in treatment is the elimination of these irregularities: thromboendarterectomy of a pelvic artery stenosis with patch angioplasty or bypass; vein patch angioplasty of a proximal or distal anastomotic stenosis; or extension of the bypass graft by interposition of short vein segments, most likely an extension from the distal anastomosis to the posterior or anterior tibial artery.

In chronic recurrent occlusion, patients slowly develop a severe ischemic syndrome over weeks or months, sometimes even reaching clinical stage IV. The venous graft, however, remains palpable, and pulsatile flow through the graft remains detectable by Doppler ultrasound. Total occlusion, which may ultimately occur, does not necessarily lead to worsening of clinical symptoms.

Chronic, recurrent occlusion is rarely caused by a slowly increasing steal syndrome through a large perforating vein, as described above, but rather, a progressive restriction of peripheral run-off, culminating in the total occlusion of the distal popliteal artery and the lower leg arteries. Because the patients do not experience recurrent occlusion acutely, fibrinolysis is usually not applied soon enough. Lysis is only successful in every third case. If angiography shows a perforating vein, correction is easy. Yet, most commonly a totally occluded peripheral run-off is found which cannot be recanalized by lysis. Thus, blood flow in the vein bypass fills only the proximal portion of the popliteal artery. Correction is only possible if patent peripheral segments of one of the three lower leg arteries are seen in the arteriograms. In such a situation, the in situ graft can be extended and connected to an open lower leg artery by using the remaining distal portion of the saphenous vein or the small saphenous vein. If this procedure cannot be performed and lysis is unsuccessful, one can try to improve circulation by profundaplasty and lumbar sympathectomy.

V. Rare Complications

The infection of an in situ graft or of an anastomosis in an in situ bypass graft is extremely rare. We have not observed this complication in any of our 500 in situ bypasses. Also, traumatic rupture of an in situ graft is very rare. We observed this complication in only one case. The graft experienced varicose, tortuous degeneration within 6 years after surgery. A very wide great saphenous vein with a proximal diameter of over 6 mm was used in this patient. A sports injury led to rupture of the graft with massive arterial bleeding. A venous diameter of 6 mm should be the upper limit for in situ bypass grafting.

G. Results of Treatment and Comparison with Classical Vein Bypass

We have performed about 500 in situ bypasses. At the end of the first postoperative year, 87% of the grafts were still functioning well. After 2 years, the patency rate was 84% [11], after 5 years 76% [4, 7]. The 2-year patency was examined in every case by angiography. These results are comparable to those of other authors (Table 17.4.1).

Results of 10-year follow-up have been reported only by Hall [20]. Some 50% of his 227 patients died during the follow-up period. Of those who were still alive after 10 years, 55% showed a patent, well-functioning femoropopliteal or femorocrural in situ graft [5, 15].

The patency rates of classical vein bypass seem to lie somewhat below the results achieved with in situ bypass (Table 17.4.2). The 10-year patency rates, which are comparable to the results of Hall, are 54% in femoropopliteal bypass grafts and 42% in femorocrural bypass grafts [7, 18, 19].

A comparison between such follow-up statistics must always remain questionable and should be interpreted with caution. The surgical patient groups differ as to age, severity of clinical symptoms, risk factors, and additional conservative therapeutic measures. In spite of all criticism, the tendency in favor of the in situ bypass is supported by a prospective randomized study done by Leather [16]. In a series of 69 femorocrural vein grafts in limbs with stage IV disease and impending amputation, the cumulative patency rate after 12 and after 30 months was 93% and 91% for in situ bypass and 68% and 63% for the classical reversed vein bypass graft ($p<0.01$). The study was officially discontinued in view of these impressive and overwhelming results.

Table 17.4.1

Author	Year	2-year patency rate
Hall	1979	87% (valve excision)
Rostad	1979	80% (valve stripper)
Leather	1982	85% (valve cutter, valvotomy)
Gruss	1984	84% (Hall stripper)

Table 17.4.2

Author	Year	5-year patency rate
Cutler et al.	1976	72%
Darling et al.	1977	72%
Stevens et al.	1980	57%
Reichle et al.	1980	60% (femoropopliteal)
Reichle et al.	1980	47% (femorocrural)
Müller-Wiefel et al.	1983	68%
Mannick	1983	72%

REFERENCES

1. Bier A (1915) Chirurgie der Gefäßaneurysmen. Beitr Klin Chir 96:556–559
2. Connolly JE, Stemmer EA (1970) The nonreversed saphenous vein bypass for femoro-popliteal occlusive disease. Surgery 68:602–609
3. Goyanes J (1906) Nuevos trabajos de cirurgia vascular substiticion plastica de las venas o arterioplastica venosa, aplicada como nuevo metodo al tratamiento de los aneurismios. Siglo Med 53:546–561
4. Gruss JD, Bartels D, Tsafandakis E, Straubel H, Ohta T, Karadedos C (1981) Bericht über 5 Jahre Erfahrung mit dem in-situ Bypass bei femoro-poplitealen Verschlußprozessen. Angio Archiv 1:97–100
5. Gruss JD, Bartels D, Vargas H, Karadedos C, Schlechtweg B (1982) Arterial reconstruction for disease of the lower extremities by the in-situ vein graft technique. J Cardiovas Surg 23:231–234
6. Gruss JD (1983) Intra- und postoperative Angiografie beim femoropoplitealen Vena saphena magna insitu Bypass. Angio Archiv 5:49–62
7. Gruss JD, Vargas H, Bartels D, Simmenroth HW, Sakurai T (1984) The in situ saphenous vein bypass. Vasa 13:153–158
8. v Haberer H (1916) Kriegsaneurysmen. Arch Klin Chir 107:611–617
9. Hall KV (1962) The great saphenous vein used in-situ as an arterial shunt after extirpation of the vein valves. Surgery 51:492–495

10. Hall KV (1964) The great saphenous vein used in-situ as an arterial shunt after vein valve extirpation. Universitetsforlaget Oslo
11. Karadedos C (1982) Mittelfristige Ergebnisse des femoropoplitealen in-situ Bypass and apparative Untersuchungen zur Modifikation der OP-Indikation und Ergebnisverbesserung. Inauguraldissertation, Marburg
12. Kunlin J (1949) Le traitement de l'artérite oblitérante par la greffe veineuse. Arch Mal Coeur 42:371–374
13. Kunlin J (1951) Le traitement de l'ischémie artéritique par la greffe veineuse longue. Rev Chir 70:206–236
14. Langeron P, Puppinck P (1980) Arterial reconstruction of the lower limb in situ saphenous vein bypass. In: Suy R, Shaw HL (eds) Arterial reconstruction of the lower limb. Medical Education Services, Oxford, pp 79–83
15. Leather RP, Shah DM, Karmody AM (1981) Infrapopliteal arterial bypass for limb salvage: increased patency and utilization of the saphenous vein used in situ. Surgery 190:1000–1008
16. Leather RP, Karmody AM (1982) The in situ saphenous vein for arterial bypass. In: Stanley JC (ed) Biologic and synthetic vascular protheses. Grune and Stratton, New York, pp 351–364
17. Lexer E (1907) Die ideale Operation des arteriellen und arteriovenösen Aneurysmas. Arch Klin Chir 83:459–463
18. Mannick JA (1983) Redo arterial surgery following failure of femoro-popliteal reconstructions. XVI World Congress of the International Society of Cardiovascular Surgery, Rio de Janeiro
19. Reichle FA, Martinson K, Rankin P (1980) Infrapopliteal arterial reconstruction in the severely ischemic lower extremity. Ann Surg 191:59–65
20. Rostad H, Hall KV, Dundas P (1979) The great saphenous vein used in situ after vein valve extirpation. J Cardivasc Surg 20:545–552

17.5 Two-Level Arterial Obstructions

R.J.A.M. van Dongen

CONTENTS

A. Introduction

Two-level arterial obstructions of the lower limb soon lead to high-grade, peripheral impairment of blood flow; the result is a greatly reduced walking distance, rest pain, or ischemic tissue lesions. In most cases, there is an absolute indication for vascular reconstruction as long as advanced gangrene does not necessitate amputation.

Basically, two-level arterial obstructions in the pelvic and femoral regions can be classified into two forms: segmental and continuous.

The segmental form does not pose great problems. If an unoccluded patent segment lies between a pelvic artery obstruction and a femoral artery obstruction, the first operation should be limited to reconstruction of the proximal arterial segment. This often results in an increase in the patient's walking distance, so that surgical treatment of the distal obstruction is not necessary. Of course, if symptoms are still severe and tissue lesions persist, the patient must undergo a second operation for reconstruction of the femoral artery segment.

If one of the two levels is obstructed by a short occlusion or stenosis, percutaneous transluminal angioplasty may be indicated. Preferably, transluminal dilatation of one segment and surgical reconstruction of the other are performed during the same session. If, however, the surgical team does not have the necessary experience, or if the appropriate X-ray equipment is not available, both procedures should be performed separately, with careful consideration of the time interval between them. If PTA is performed a few days prior to surgical reconstruction, the correct surgical approach will be complicated by the presence of an inguinal hematoma and consequently by a higher risk of infection. Postponing surgery until the hematoma is absorbed means a longer period of hospitalization. This is the main reason why PTA and surgery should be done on the same day. That way, a hematoma will not disturb surgery, and the risk of infection is not increased.

More difficulties are encountered in continuous two-level arterial obstructions. In the operative treatment of such extensive occlusive disease, the surgeon, like Odysseus, has to steer a course between Scylla and Charybdis. He either strives for a total and hemodynamically perfect reconstruction of both levels, which may exceed a reasonable surgical risk, or, in view of such a high risk, he limits arterial reconstruction to the pelvic level, which may lead to unsatisfactory results. Our own experience confirms the observations of several authors who have shown in clinical hemodynamic studies that 30–57% of all patients with continuous two-level arterial obstruction had to undergo a second operation at the femoral arterial level [4, 6, 9, 11].

B. Choice of Surgical Procedure – Total Correction Versus Profunda Revascularization

There are two basic methods of reconstruction:

1. Reconstruction of the pelvic arteries alone (profunda revascularization), which is relatively short, technically simple, and has a low rate of reocclusion, but sometimes an uncertain outcome or subjectively unsatisfactory results, and
2. A time-consuming and technically complicated unilateral or bilateral total reconstruction, with a higher risk of reocclusion, but better long-term results, ultimately leading to total elimination of clinical symptoms and complete cure.

In recurrent occlusion, reconstruction should be limited to the pelvic arteries in combination with profundaplasty, especially if in the first operation the great saphenous vein has been used as a graft.

The decision as to which procedure is best is much more difficult in primary surgery.

It is often maintained that reconstruction should always be limited to the pelvic arteries in the correction of a thrombotic obstruction of both pelvic and femoral arterial levels. It is argued that, if the results are unsatisfactory, the distal femoral segment can always be revascularized in a second operation.

There are certainly objections to this opinion. First of all, the percentage of failure following sole reconstruction of the pelvic region is relatively high, 20–57%. All of these patients must undergo surgery a second time. This involves considerable physical and psychological stress for the patient, and also for the surgeon! Such a second operation is very difficult. The risk of infection is higher. And there is the question as to whether there will even be a second operation. One must not forget that in most cases a lack of clinical improvement following reconstruction of the pelvic region is a sign that run-off is inadequate, and this is the most important factor leading to reobliteration of a reconstructed vessel.

A recurrent occlusion is almost always inoperable, mainly because the obstruction usually affects the profunda femoris artery. Furthermore, ischemia of the limb is often so severe that amputation is inevitable. The surgeon should be aware of these complications when deciding whether to perform only a partial correction.

The question as to which method of reconstruction should be applied in primary surgery can best be answered after assessment of the following criteria:

- General condition of the patient
- Severity of symptoms
- Angiographic details
- Preoperative noninvasive, diagnostic measurements

There is also the possibility of predicting the outcome of a reconstructive procedure by intraoperative measurements.

It must be emphasized that the prediction of such results is possible only if all criteria are seen as interrelated and are accordingly weighed against each other.

I. General Condition of the Patient

Surgery for two-level arterial obstructions always imposes a considerable burden on the patient. This is especially true for bilateral total correction, an operation which is only seldom indicated. But even a unilateral reconstruction of the pelvic arteries should be performed only if the coronary, cerebral, pulmonary, and renal condition of the patient does not make the surgical risk unacceptable.

On the other hand, one should remember that a major limb amputation is considerably more dangerous than an extensive vascular operation. The operative mortality of a major amputation is about 25%, and that of an extensive vascular reconstructive procedure 3–10%.

Patients in whom ischemic damage and severe symptoms (rest pain, gangrene) might make amputation necessary, should not be excluded from attempts to preserve the limb, even if their general condition is not the best. However, only that procedure should be performed which has the best chance of being successful, and that is total correction.

II. Severity of Symptoms

Only certain general and basic guidelines exist which aid in assessing this criterion correctly.

Intermittent claudication is only a relative indication for surgery. An operation is advisable only if the walking distance is extremely limited (shorter than 100 m), and the patient feels strongly disabled in private and professional activity, or the walking capability quickly deteriorates in a short time. If the limb is not at risk at the moment, there are no objections to partial correction, especially if all other criteria promise success of sole reconstruction at the pelvic level.

In patients with stage III or IV disease total correction should be preferred.

III. Preoperative Angiogram

Previous publications have stressed the importance of preoperative angiograms for the localization of arterial obstructions and for choosing the best surgical procedure [3, 10]. Table 17.5.1 contains an expanded algorithm showing which reconstructive procedure achieve the best results in certain types of two-level occlusive arterial disease. Four different constellations are considered:

Type A is a two-level obstruction with good patency of the profunda femoris artery and a good collateral system between the profunda branches and the popliteal artery, but with insufficient peripheral circulation. If no gangrene is present and this constellation is found, reconstruction at the pelvic level alone usually achieves good results, so that the procedure may be limited to profunda revascularization. If peripheral gangrene is present, profunda revascularization alone seldom leads to cure of the gangrenous lesions. Total reconstruction should be preferred under these circumstances.

A second form (type B) shows the same constellation: obstruction of the iliac artery and femoral artery with good patency of the profunda femoris artery, but with an insufficient collateral system of the profunda branches or with occlusion of the recipient segments of the popliteal artery.

Independent of the condition of the distal popliteal and lower leg arteries, revascularization of the pelvic arteries alone in such cases usually leads to unsatisfactory results, especially if gangrene is present. This obstructive type does not allow for alternatives in reconstruction. The only successful procedure is total reconstruction in one operation. This means that the profunda femoris artery and the lower leg arteries have to be revascularized.

The third combination (type C) is a continuous two-level obstruction with an occluded or strongly sclerotic profunda femoris artery, poorly developed profunda – popliteal collateral system, but with patent peripheral vessels. Profunda revascularization is not very promising (assuming it is even possible) so that correction of both levels must be preferred.

With the fourth variation (type D) (profunda femoris artery, its collaterals, and the peripheral vessels all patent), there are two alternatives: (1) sole reconstruction at the pelvic level (profunda revascularization) or (2) total reconstruction at both levels (restoration of profunda circulation and reconstruction of the femoropopliteal segment).

The choice between the two operative regimens in this type are principally dependent on the factors listed in Table 17.5.2.

If the greater saphenous vein is not suitable for a bypass graft, the profunda femoris artery is of good quality, and the profunda – popliteal collateral system is well developed, the procedure is limited to definitive revascularization of the profunda

Table 17.5.1. Choice of surgical procedure in obstructions of the pelvic and femoral arteries with reference to angiographic findings

Type of combined obstructions	Iliac artery and femoral artery	Profunda femoris artery	Profunda–popliteal collateral system	Distal popliteal artery lower leg arteries	
A	occluded	patent	sufficient	insufficient	→ without gangrene → profunda revascularization → with gangrene → total correction
B	occluded	patent	insufficient	insignificant	total reconstruction
C	occluded	stenosed or occluded	insufficient	sufficient	total correction
D	occluded	patent	sufficient	patent	→ profunda revascularization or → total reconstruction

Table 17.5.2. Factors which influence the choice of operative regimen in obstructive type D disease

Social environment
Availability of suitable autogenous material for reconstruction
Access to the vascular region
Condition of the profunda femoris artery
Condition of peripheral run-off
Severity of limb ischemia

femoris artery. This is also the operative method of choice for recurrent occlusion and in cases where peripheral run-off is not very good.

Simultaneous total reconstruction of both levels must be preferred: if no significant general risk factors are present; if the great saphenous vein is suitable for use as a bypass; if adequate flow through the profunda femoris artery is doubtful; if the peripheral vessels are patent; if ischemia is severe with strong limitation of walking distance; if resting pain or gangrene exist; if the cure of these clinical symptoms by sole revascularization of the profunda femoris artery would take too long or is doubtful and unrestricted walking ability is necessary or desirable for occupational or social activities.

IV. Preoperative Noninvasive Assessment

Results of examinations in the vascular laboratory help in choosing between profunda revascularization and total correction. Certain tests aim at measuring the hemodynamic effects of occlusive processes in aortoiliac and femoropopliteal arteries. They help to establish which of the two levels dominates the hemodynamic situation. Basically, the question should be answered whether reconstruction of pelvic segments alone is promising or not.

Some of these examinations together with the criteria discussed above can have considerable influence on the surgeon's choice of operative procedure.

If there is doubt that an iliac lesion found during preoperative angiography is of hemodynamic significance for the lower limb, direct invasive measurement of common femoral artery pressure is the most reliable diagnostic means of clarifying this point, especially if the pressure gradient at rest and following reactive hyperemia is determined [5]. Positive findings signify that sole reconstruction of the pelvic arteries will lead to success in over 90% of cases [2].

Segmental blood pressure measurement by Doppler sonography is also recommended for this purpose. In patients with high pressure in the thigh, the hemodynamic effect of iliac lesions is minimal, and therefore positive results cannot be expected in proximal reconstruction. However, the sensitivity of this diagnostic measure in multilevel occlusive disease is too low for practical use [1, 2]. The same holds true for segmental pulse volume registration (PVR), for quantitative analysis of the pulsatility index registered over the common femoral artery during Doppler ultrasound, and for the determination of the profunda popliteal collateral index [2, 7, 8].

V. Intraoperative Measurements

The effect of a reconstruction at the pelvic level may be assessed by certain measuring techniques. A rise in the ankle pressure index of more than 0.1 is a reliable indication that the operative procedure is a clinical success.

Intraoperative improvement of plethysmographic pulse-volume values also signifies a successful reconstruction [2].

Continuous intraoperative temperature measurement may also help to decide whether or not simultaneous reconstruction of the femoral artery is necessary [12].

If one reviews the literature, one can find no method for predicting how an ischemic limb will react to revascularization of the profunda femoris artery, especially in stage IV disease. The results of preoperative and intraoperative noninvasive measurements are significant only if they are interpreted along with the other criteria mentioned.

C. Classification of Two-Level Obstructions – Definitions

The term two-level obstruction should be reserved for arterial occlusive diseases leading to occlusion of the iliac and femoral arteries or significant stenoses of both vessels. Usually, the origin of the profunda femoris artery, and, rarely, the popliteal artery or lower leg arteries are also affected. Even if the latter arteries show arteriosclerotic changes

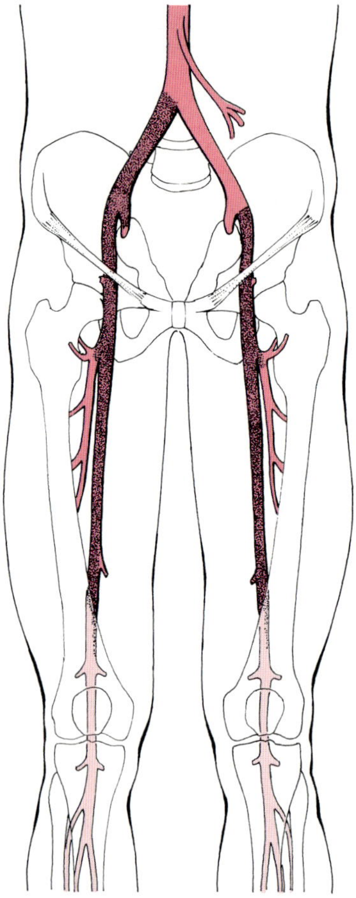

Fig. 17.5.1. Quadruple obstruction with a patent left common iliac artery. Preferential correction of the dominant right side is necessary (surgical risk is reduced by a retroperitoneal approach to the right pelvic area)

or in some cases are obstructed, the term "two-level occlusion" should still be used to describe this situation. One should talk of a three-level occlusion only if the lower leg arteries are also revascularized, in addition to the pelvic and femoral segments.

Because the popliteal artery forms an anatomic unit with the superficial femoral artery, obstructive lesions of the iliac artery and superficial femoral artery should be termed a two-level occlusion, even if the popliteal artery also shows arteriosclerotic stenoses or occlusions.

The classification of two-level occlusions into continuous and segmental forms has already been discussed on pp. 378 and 433.

Two-level occlusions are sometimes present on both sides. In such a case VOLLMAR speaks of a "quadruple obstruction" [13].

In such a quadruple obstruction, it is not always necessary to treat both sides at the same time. Bilateral reconstruction of the pelvic arteries is very stressful for the patient. Therefore, both sides should be treated separately. This is only possible if one of the common iliac arteries is patent and wide enough (Fig. 17.5.1). This situation is common. One should not perform a reconstruction of both sides, e.g., with a bifurcation prosthesis, but should limit the correction to the dominant limb. The other limb may be treated at a later date.

This delayed type of correction has several important advantages. A long, extensive operation of a quadruple obstruction, with laparotomy, incisions in both inguinal regions, and sometimes several incisions on both legs, can be avoided. If only one side is operated on, the procedure may be performed more carefully, making good technical and hemodynamic results probable. Furthermore, a one sided reconstruction of the pelvic arteries can always be carried out by a retroperitoneal approach.

D. Principles and Special Considerations in Two-Level Repair

In synchronous treatment of combined obstructions of the pelvic and femoral type, many techniques and reconstructive methods are applied. Only the most important will be presented.

I. Unilateral Two-Level Repair

In unilateral combined obstructions the pelvic arteries may be treated by thromboendarterectomy or ipsilateral and, sometimes, crossover alloplastic bypass techniques. The femoropopliteal segment is preferably reconstructed with an autogenous vein bypass graft.

1. Thromboendarterectomy of the Pelvic Arterial Segment Combined with Vein Bypass of the Femoropopliteal Segment

This method of revascularization of the pelvic and femoral arteries uses three different reconstructive principles (Fig. 17.5.2a). It is a combination of open endarterectomy with patch angioplasty (of the common iliac artery), semiclosed endarterectomy (of the external iliac artery) and vein bypass

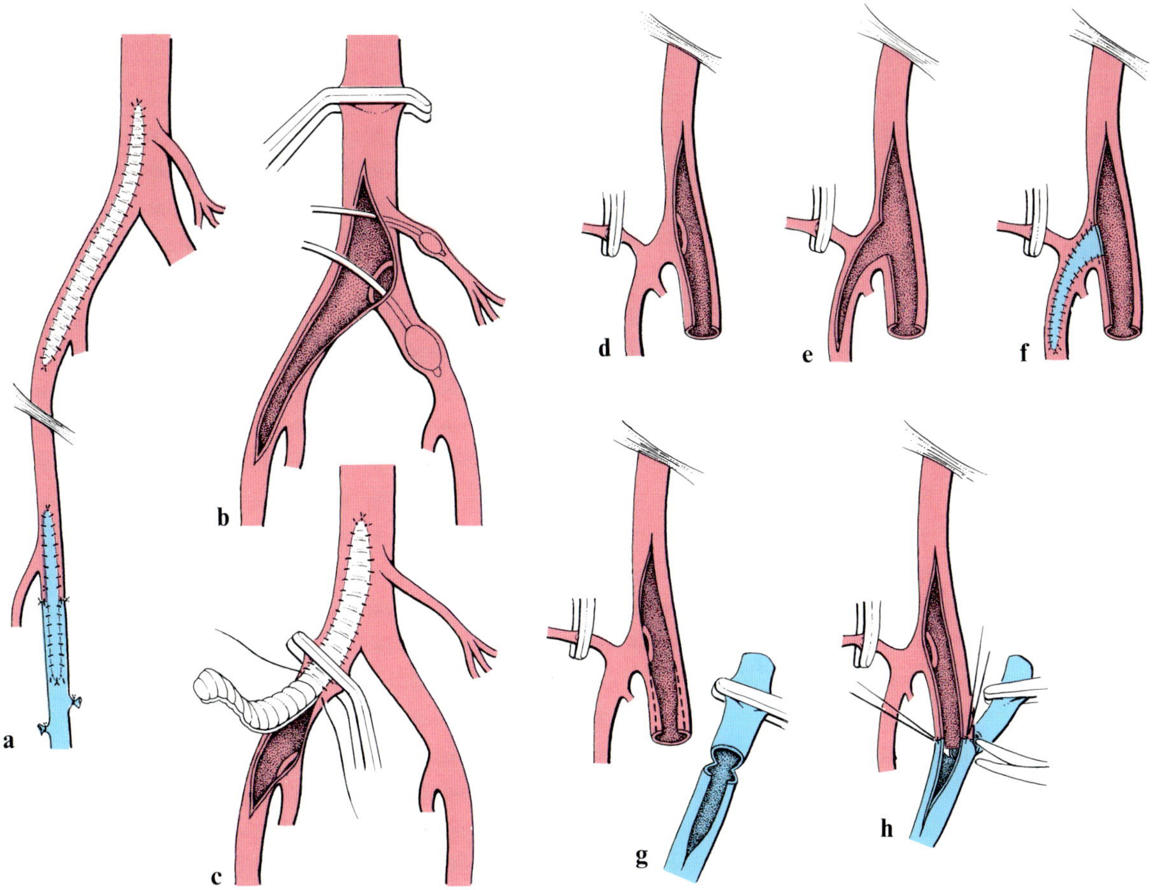

Fig. 17.5.2a–h. Reconstructive procedures following localization of the obstruction. **a** Proposed solution with retroperitoneal Dacron patch, inguinal venous patch, and femoropopliteal vein graft. **b** Incision of the right common iliac artery up into the aorta. Blocking catheter prevents retrograde blood loss. Following disobliteration, an intimal ring remains on the left side (danger of dissection). **c** Suture of the Dacron patch. **d** Disobliteration of the origin of the superficial femoral artery. **e** For disobliteration of the origin of the profunda femoris artery, adequate longitudinal incision of the profunda femoris artery is necessary. **f** Closure of the profunda arteriotomy with a vein patch. **g** Preparation of the vein graft for the proximal anastomosis. **h** Anastomosis of the vein bypass to the superficial femoral artery. Then, suture of the vein patch onto the common femoral artery and the vein graft

graft technique (of the femoropopliteal artery). Semiclosed endarterectomy of the external iliac artery does not have a negative effect upon the short-term or even long-term results. The external iliac artery is the only artery of the lower extremity which is suitable for a semiclosed endarterectomy.

Technique. Following a pararectal incision down to the peritoneum, the distal aorta, the common iliac artery, and the proximal segment of the external iliac artery are exposed retroperitoneally, care being taken not to injure the fibers of the abdominal preaortic plexus and the hypogastric plexus. For the same reason, the common iliac artery on the contralateral side is not dissected free of surrounding tissue. The initial portion of the internal iliac artery, if it is still patent, and the open lumbar arteries are isolated and prepared for clamping. In the inguinal region, dissection of the common femoral artery and its bifurcation is done in the usual manner.

An atraumatic clamp is applied at the proper site on the aorta, above the origin of the inferior mesenteric artery, and, if necessary, the internal iliac artery is occluded with a bulldog clamp; then, the distal aorta and the proximal common iliac artery are opened by a longitudinal arteriotomy on their anterolateral sides. An intravascular occlusion catheter with two lumina is introduced into the common iliac artery of the contralateral side and inflated (Fig. 17.4.2b). If the patient does not receive systemic anticoagulation, thrombosis due to blood stasis within the contralateral iliac artery may be prevented with heparinized saline solution administered under pressure through the second lumen of the catheter, distal to the obstructing balloon. A small intraluminal occlusion catheter is introduced through the arteriotomy into the inferior mesenteric artery. The arteriotomy is then extended distally into the wall of the external iliac artery over a length of about 2 cm.

The patency of the contralateral common iliac artery is checked by inserting a right-angled curved clamp through the proximal portion of the arteriotomy and calibrating the common iliac artery with olive-shaped dilators.

Open disobliteration of the ipsilateral common iliac artery is then performed, leaving an intimal ring at the orifice of the contralateral iliac artery so that no dissection of the intima of the contralateral common iliac artery may occur (Fig. 17.5.2b).

If an occlusion or a stenosis of the internal iliac artery is present, an attempt is made to disobliterate the vessel using an oval ring stripper. Usually such attempts are successful in restoring patency to the internal iliac artery.

The arteriotomy is closed with a synthetic patch, starting at the aortic portion of the incision. As soon as the patch is sutured halfway onto the common iliac artery, both intraluminal occlusion catheters are removed. Immediately thereafter, the common iliac artery is clamped in its proximal portion with a transversely applied atraumatic clamp (Fig. 17.5.2c). The aortic clamp is removed, restoring blood flow to the contralateral limb. Suture of the synthetic patch to the artery is continued to a point just above the origin of the internal iliac artery.

The external iliac artery and common femoral artery are then reconstructed. The obstructed superficial femoral artery is transected about 2 cm distal to the origin of the profunda femoris artery. The anterior wall of the superficial femoral artery stump is incised longitudinally up to the common femoral artery (Fig. 17.5.2d). The distal portion of the common femoral artery and the femoral stump are then disobliterated, care being taken that an intimal ring remains, surrounding the ostium of the profunda femoris artery.

The profunda femoris artery should never be treated by antegrade disobliteration. A slight stenosis at its mouth may be dilated with olive-shaped dilators. If a high-grade stenosis or an occlusion of the proximal portion of the profunda artery is present, open endarterectomy of these segments should be performed after the vascular wall has been incised downward into the undiseased portion of the profunda femoris artery (Fig. 17.5.2e). Following restricted dissection of obliterative material the arteriotomy is closed with a vein patch ending proximally at the lateral edge of the incision of the common femoral artery (Fig. 17.5.2f).

Now the oval ring stripper is used for retrograde disobliteration of the proximal half of the common femoral artery and the entire length of the external iliac artery. Proximally, the intima is trimmed flat just below the takeoff of the internal iliac artery.

Then, the suturing of the synthetic patch into the arteriotomy of the iliac artery is continued downward (Fig. 17.5.2a). The external iliac artery is clamped in its proximal portion, but distal to the synthetic patch, with a soft bulldog clamp. The proximal clamp on the common iliac artery is removed, restoring blood flow to the internal iliac artery.

The next step is the reconstruction of the occluded femoropopliteal segment. The great saphenous vein, resected at the very beginning of the operation, is anastomosed obliquely end-to-side to an intact arterial segment above or below the knee joint, distal to the obstructed segment. The graft is pulled through a tunnel posterior to the sartorius muscle up to the groin incision. There, the graft is filled under slight pressure with a blood–heparin solution and stretched after extending the leg.

At the level of the proposed proximal anastomosis, half of the vein's circumference is transected. Starting at this transverse incision, a T-shaped 1.5 mm longitudinal incision is made distally (17.5.2g). The corners of artery and vein are attached to one another with interrupted sutures. Differences in length between the two vessels, the femoral artery usually being wider, are compensated by a wedge-shaped excision at the edges of the arteriotomy.

Then, because twisting of the proximal portion of the vein is impossible, the remaining part of the graft may be cut off at the level of the anastomosis (Fig. 17.5.2b).

With the help of the corner sutures the arteriovenous junction is rotated, bringing the posterior wall around to the front. This is only possible if the distal end of the artery is completely mobilized posteriorly.

The semicircular anastomosis between the femoral artery and the vein graft is completed using either a continuous suture or interrupted sutures. Then, the anastomosis is brought back into its initial position by rotation.

The anterior gap of the anastomosis is closed with a narrow vein patch constructed from the remaining graft material (Fig. 17.5.2a). In the meantime, despite anticoagulation therapy, thrombi may have formed within the disobliterated external iliac artery. Therefore, the proximal artery segment is cleaned with a Fogarty catheter shortly before the vein patch is completely sutured into the arteriotomy.

When the patch has been completed, the clamp on the proximal external iliac artery is removed, and blood flow to the limb is restored.

This combined method has four important advantages:

1. Only a strip of synthetic material is needed.
2. There is no synthetic material in the inguinal region.
3. It is a simple matter to extend the operation to restore patency of the internal iliac and profunda femoris arteries, thereby effecting a truly total correction.
4. The junction between artery and vein graft is arranged in a straight line without turbulence. Thus, the hemodynamic conditions of this reconstructive technique are quite favorable.

2. Reconstruction of the Pelvic Vessels with a Synthetic Bypass and the Femoropopliteal Segment with a Vein Graft

The simplest method of treating a two-level obstruction is by combining an aortofemoral synthetic bypass with a femoropopliteal vein bypass. The junction between the synthetic prosthesis and the vein graft can be constructed in several different ways.

The common femoral artery and the profunda femoris artery are sometimes occluded by a thrombus, which can be easily removed through an arteriotomy of the common femoral artery. In such a case, the distal end of the prosthesis can be anastomosed to the upper half of the arteriotomy and the proximal end of the vein graft to the lower half (Fig. 17.5.3b). Sometimes the end of the prosthesis can be connected to the entire arteriotomy and the vein to the distal portion of the prosthesis (Fig. 17.5.3c).

However, it is usually necessary to endarterectomize the common femoral artery and the proximal portion of the profunda femoris artery. Then, it is possible to suture a bevel of the prosthesis into the wall of the profunda femoris artery, and to anastomose the vein graft to the distal portion of the prosthesis (Fig. 17.5.3d).

Enlargement of the profunda femoris artery using a distal bevel of the prosthesis is not at all reliable. Preferably, the arteriotomy in the profunda femoris artery should be closed with a vein patch. This should continue up to the arteriotomy in the common femoral artery. The prosthesis should be anastomosed to the common femoral artery only (Fig. 17.5.3e).

To avoid the placement of alloplastic material into the inguinal region, the distal end of the prosthesis may be anastomosed to the distal portion of the external iliac artery above the inguinal ligament. The arterial segment behind the inguinal ligament must then undergo semiclosed endarterectomy (Fig. 17.5.3a).

This method has several important advantages. Not only is the risk of infection reduced, but anastomotic aneurysms occur less frequently after suprainguinal anastomosis than after conventional anastomosis of the artery in the inguinal region.

The proximal end-to-end anastomosis of the vein bypass graft, as well as the suprainguinal connection of the prosthesis, are important improvements in the technique of bypass grafting of two-level obstructions and will therefore be discussed in detail (Fig. 17.5.3a, f, g, h).

Technique. Following pararectal incision the infrarenal aorta is exposed extraperitoneally. Patent lumbar arteries are prepared for clamping.

The inguinal incision is extended a few centimeters further upward than usual. The fascia of the external oblique muscle is divided parallel to its fibers at the upper margin of the inguinal ligament. The ligament is mobilized, encircled with a tape, and pulled downward. The internal oblique muscle is separated from the inside of the inguinal ligament and displaced cranially. The deep circumflex iliac vein crossing the anterior wall of the artery is transected between two ligatures (Fig. 17.5.3f). The tissue in front of the external iliac artery is pushed aside with the index finger. After elevating the abdominal wall muscles with two Langenbeck retractors, the entire length of the external iliac artery is exposed (Fig. 17.5.3g).

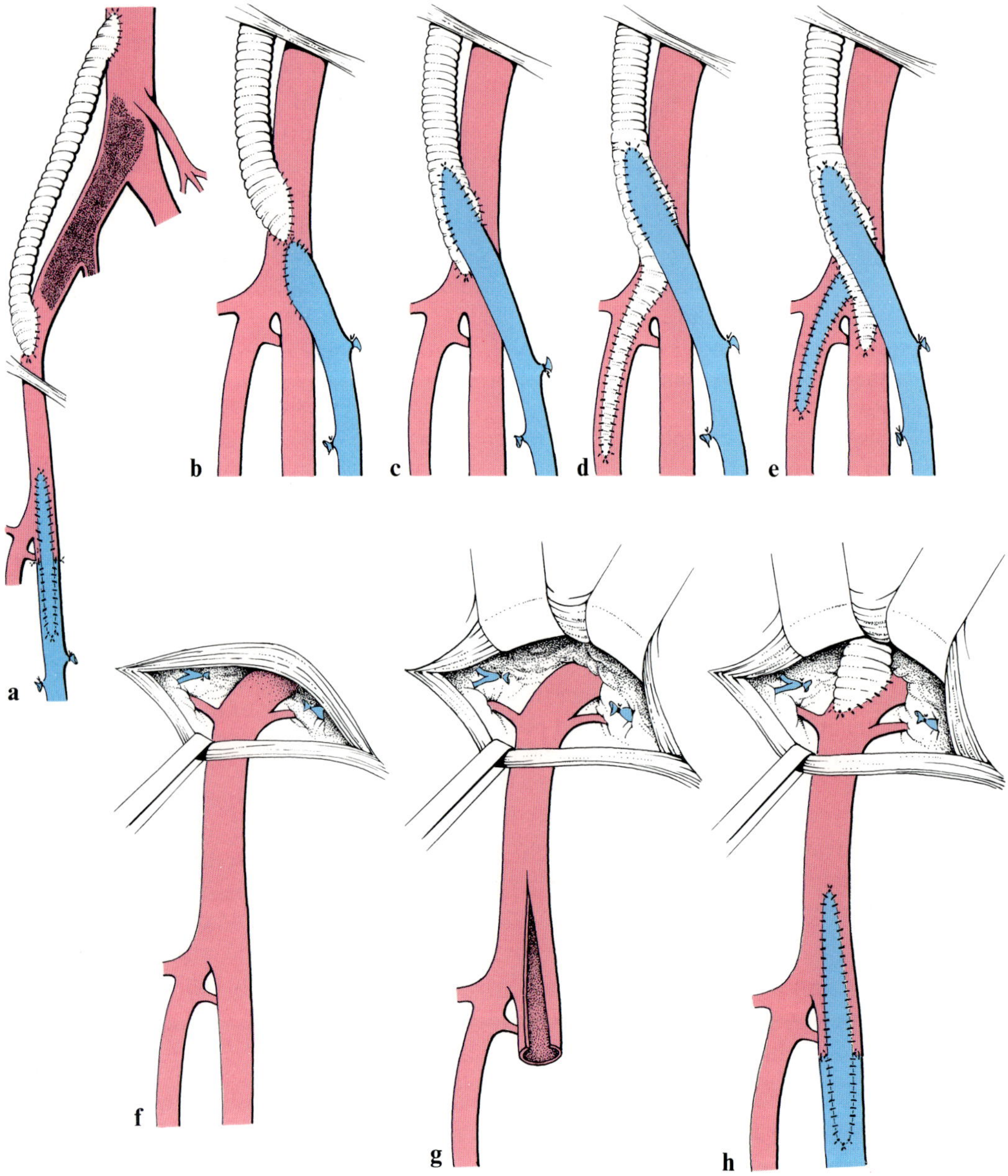

Fig. 17.5.3 a–h. Dacron bypass of the pelvic segment in a two-level obstruction. **a** Proposed solution; **b** separate anastomoses in the inguinal region; **c** integrated anastomoses in the inguinal region; **d** integrated anastomoses in the inguinal region with patch angioplasty of the profunda femoris artery using a distal tongue of the prosthesis; **e** integrated anastomoses in the inguinal region with separate profundaplasty; **f–h** approach to the suprainguinal bypass anastomosis

A suitable aortic segment is clamped at both ends, and a longitudinal oval window is excised from the aortic wall; then a prosthesis 8 mm in diameter is anastomosed obliquely end-to-side to the aorta. Following anastomosis, the prosthesis is clamped proximally, and the aorta is declamped.

The next step is reconstruction of the femoropopliteal segment. The vein bypass graft is connected distally to an undiseased segment of the popliteal artery lying beyond the obstruction and pulled up through the tunnel behind the sartorius muscle to the groin incision.

In the inguinal region, the femoral artery bifurcation is prepared as described on p. 438 (Fig. 17.5.3g). Through the arteriotomy in the anterior wall, the common femoral artery, the segment behind the inguinal ligament, and the external iliac artery are revascularized by upward retrograde disobliteration using an oval ring stripper.

During the next step, the external iliac artery is incised longitudinally as far as possible from the inguinal ligament. The obliquely cut end of the prosthesis can then be easily anastomosed to this arteriotomy (Fig. 17.5.3h).

A semicircular anastomosis is performed between the venous graft and the stump of the femoral artery. A venous patch is sutured onto the anterior gap of the anastomosis. By removing the clamp on the proximal part of the bypass, blood flow is restored through the prosthesis and vein graft (Fig. 17.5.3h).

An additional obstruction at the takeoff of the profunda femoris artery is treated as described on p. 438 (see also Fig. 17.5.2e, f).

The technique of suprainguinal anastomosis described here is no more time-consuming or complicated than the usual anastomosis between the prosthesis and the common femoral artery. However, the decisive advantage is that no alloplastic material is located in the inguinal region.

A disadvantage of this type of bypass grafting is that an obstruction of the internal iliac artery cannot be treated.

3. Reconstruction of the Pelvic Arteries Using a Crossover Synthetic Bypass Graft and of the Femoropopliteal Segment Using a Vein Graft

If the general condition of the patient does not allow an abdominal operation to be performed (nor an extraperitoneal procedure), it is possible to use the contralateral iliac artery as a donor for perfusion of the endangered limb. There is only one precondition: the contralateral iliac artery must be perfectly patent. A crossover synthetic bypass prosthesis between both common femoral arteries may be constructed. Better hemodynamic conditions are achieved if both anastomoses are done at the level of the external iliac arteries, i.e., above the inguinal ligament. This has the great advantage that alloplastic material is not implanted in the inguinal region (Fig. 17.5.4a).

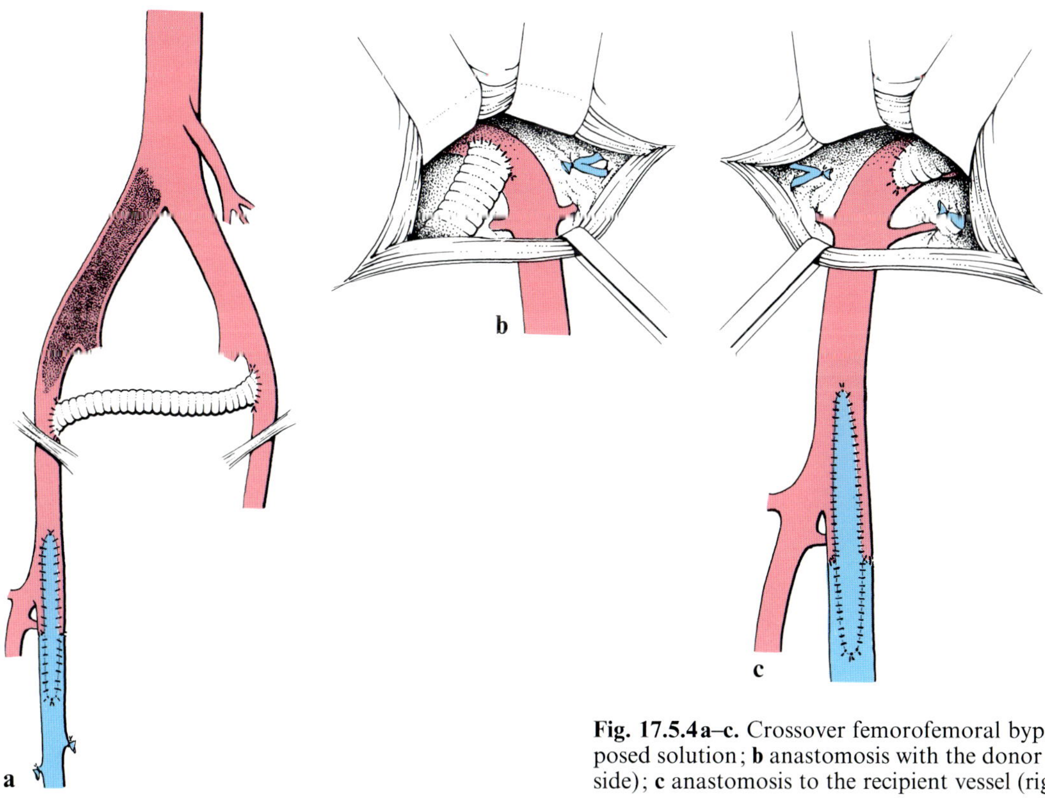

Fig. 17.5.4a–c. Crossover femorofemoral bypass. **a** Proposed solution; **b** anastomosis with the donor vessel (left side); **c** anastomosis to the recipient vessel (right side)

Technique. A small oblique incision is made above the inguinal ligament to expose the distal external iliac artery on the contralateral side. Following the division of the fascia of the external oblique muscle just above the inguinal ligament, the distal external iliac artery is reached (see p. 439).

On the occluded side, the common femoral artery, its bifurcation, and the distal external iliac artery are exposed and prepared (see p. 439).

Reconstruction starts with anastomosis of the prosthesis (8 mm diameter, obliquely end-to-side) to a clamped segment of the distal external iliac artery on the opposite side. This produces a hemodynamically favorable flow angle (Fig. 17.5.4b). After completion of the anastomosis, the prosthesis is clamped near the anastomosis, and the clamps on the external iliac artery are removed.

Using one finger of each hand, a tunnel is formed between both distal external iliac arteries, either through the subcutaneous tissue above the pubic bone in front of the rectus muscles or, preferably, through the prevesicle space.

On the occluded side, one proceeds in the same manner as described on p. 440. Following retrograde endarterectomy, the prosthesis is pulled through the tunnel and then anastomosed end-to-side to the distal external iliac artery. One should try to construct a hemodynamically favorable flow angle. The femoral artery is then bypassed with a vein graft (Fig. 17.5.4c).

II. Bilateral Two-Level Repair

In bilateral combined obstructions of the pelvic and femoral arteries (quadruple obstruction), total correction of both sides produces considerable surgical stress on the patient. Total reconstruction of both sides during one operation is only necessary if the profunda arteries or their run-offs are insufficient and both limbs are threatened by amputation. If, however, patency of the profunda femoris artery is good, the profunda–popliteal collateral circulation is well developed, and the preoperative and intraoperative measurements indicate that sole reconstruction of the pelvic arteries will be successful clinically, reconstruction should be limited to bilateral profunda revascularization with a bifurcation prosthesis in combination with resectional profundaplasty on both sides.

Technique. The infrarenal aorta is exposed through a median laparotomy. The common femoral arteries and their bifurcations are prepared on both

Fig. 17.5.5a–d. Connection of one limb of the aortic bifurcation prosthesis. **a** Anastomosis to the common femoral artery with widening of the profunda femoris artery (not recommended). **b, c** Widening of the profunda femoris artery using a vein patch, anastomosis of the Dacron prosthesis to the common femoral artery. **d** Suprainguinal connection of the prosthesis

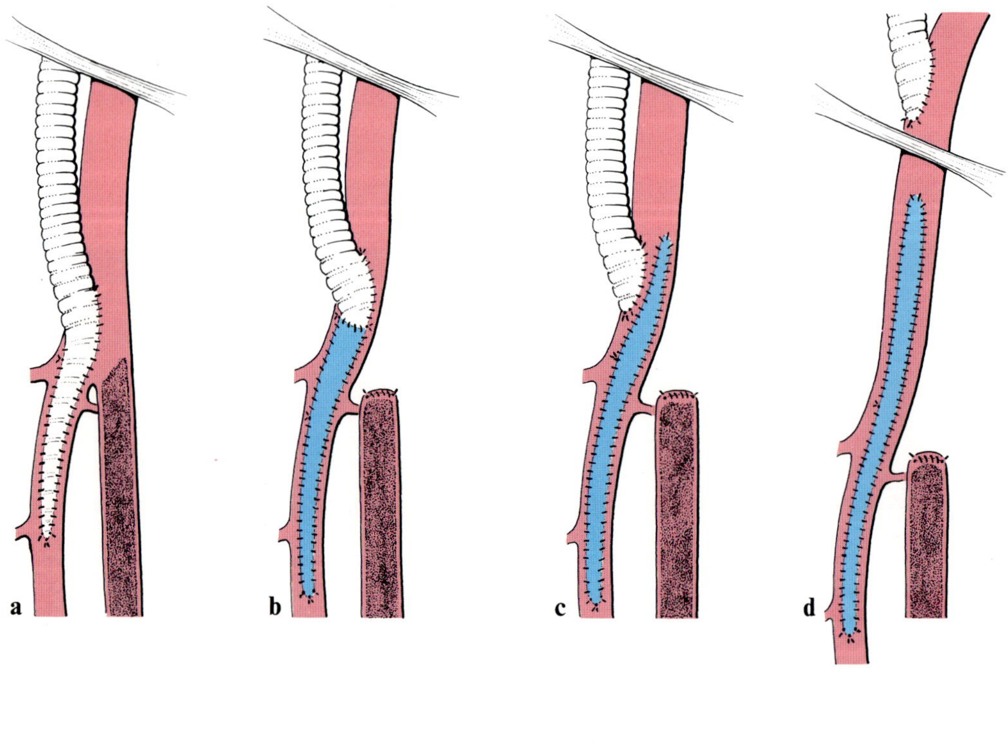

sides, and dissection of the profunda femoris artery is extended distally until a fully patent segment is exposed.

First, the aortic portion of the bifurcation prosthesis is anastomosed end-to-side to the infrarenal aorta. After clamping the prosthesis near the anastomosis, aortic blood flow is restored. Both arms of the prosthesis are pulled down retroperitoneally to the groin incisions.

As already mentioned, it is not advisable to anastomose the prosthetic limb to the common femoral artery and to widen the profunda femoris artery with a bevel of the prosthesis as shown in Fig. 17.5.5a. There are several alternatives which can be considered.

If an inguinal connection of the prosthesis is preferred, anastomosis of the prosthesis to the common femoral artery may be performed following completion of profundaplasty with resection of the origin of the superficial artery. The connection with the common femoral artery is best done lateral to the patch graft (Fig. 17.5.5c). The prosthesis may also be connected to the proximal portion of the arteriotomy. The vein patch is then sutured to the edge of the prosthesis (Fig. 17.5.5b).

If a suprainguinal connection is chosen, anastomosis can easily be performed as described on p. 439 following completion of profundaplasty and retrograde disobliteration of the proximal vessel segment (Fig. 17.5.5d).

If the femoropopliteal segment must be bypassed with an autogenous vein graft on either one or both sides, the proximal anastomosis of the graft should be performed at the distal portion of the graft if the limbs of the prosthesis are connected to the common femoral arteries, as this will save time. If suprainguinal connection of both arms of the prosthesis is chosen, the vein graft is anastomosed end-to-side to the common femoral artery.

In the treatment of patients with multilevel occlusions, two points must be considered:

1. Attempts should be made not only to reconstruct the obstructed arterial segment morphologically, but also to achieve good hemodynamic conditions. Furthermore, reconstructive procedures which show unsatisfactory results should be avoided. For example, if one tries to save operating time by endarterectomizing the femoral artery using the semiclosed method, the results, especially the long-term results, will be unsatisfactory. Reocclusions occur which are usually not operable.

2. Of course, in the discussion of the correct choice of operative procedures in patients with multilevel obstructions, no rigid concept can be established. Instead, one should carefully consider which method of treatment will be best for each patient. And in every case, many factors will have to be considered before that decision can be made.

REFERENCES

1. Bone GE, Hayes AC, Slaymaker EE (1976) Value of segmental limb blood pressures in predicting results of aortofemoral bypass. Am J Surg 132:733–738
2. Brewster DC, Perler BA, Robinson JC, Darling RC (1953) Aortofemoral graft for multilevel occlusive disease. Predictors of success and need for distal bypass. Arch Surg 117:1593–1600
3. Dongen RJAM van (1979) Operationstaktik bei Verschlüssen der Becken- und Oberschenkelarterien. Angio 1:10–16
4. Edwards WH, Wright RS (1973) A technique for combined aorto-femoral-popliteal arterial reconstruction. Ann Surg 179:572–578
5. Flanigan DP, Ryan TJ, Williams LR (1984) Aortofemoral or femoropopliteal revascularization? A prospective evaluation of the papaverine test. J Vasc Surg 1:215–223
6. Galland RB, Hill DA, Gustave R (1980) The functional results of aortoiliac reconstruction. Br J Surg 67:344–346
7. Noer I (1978) Preoperative estimation of run-off in patients with multiple level arterial obstructions as a guide to partial reconstructive surgery. Ann Surg 188:663–670
8. O'Donnell TF Jr, Lahey SJ, Kelly JJ (1979) A prospective study of Doppler pressures and segmental plethysmography before and following aortofemoral bypass. Surgery 86:120–128
9. Royster TS, Lynn R, Mulcare RJ (1976) Combined aortoiliac and femoro-popliteal occlusive disease. Surg Gynecol Obstet 143:249–252
10. Schwilden E-D, Dongen RJAM van (1979) Zur operativen Taktik beim Zwei-Etagen-Verschluss. Langenbecks Arch Chir 348:87–91
11. Summer DS, Strandness DE Jr (1978) Aortoiliac reconstruction in patients with combined iliac and superficial femoral arterial occlusion. Surgery 84:348–355
12. Trusheim H, Sperling M, Winter G (1979) Über die Behandlung der Zweietagenverschlüsse; Ergebnisse aus den Jahren 1967 bis 1977. Angio 1:32–37
13. Vollmar J (1975) Rekonstruktive Chirurgie der Arterien. Thieme, Stuttgart

17.6 Surgery of the Profunda Femoris Artery

E.-D. Schwilden and R.J.A.M. van Dongen

CONTENTS

A. Anatomy

The profunda femoris artery is one of two terminal branches of the common femoral artery, which separates into the superficial femoral artery and the profunda femoris artery below the inguinal ligament. This branching site usually lies between 1.5 and 5 cm below the inguinal ligament. In rare cases, it may lie at the level of the inguinal ligament or as far as 10 cm distal to the ligament. The profunda femoris artery takes off in a dorsolateral direction in about 50% of cases and it is located strictly dorsal in about 40%. A medial origin of the profunda femoris artery is encountered in 10% of cases [8, 9]. Duplication of the artery in a medial and a lateral course is extremely rare. The profunda femoris artery and its branches supply the ventral region of the hip, the deeper layers of the buttocks and the thigh (Fig. 17.6.1). The first branches of the profunda femoris artery are the medial and lateral circumflex arteries. The origin

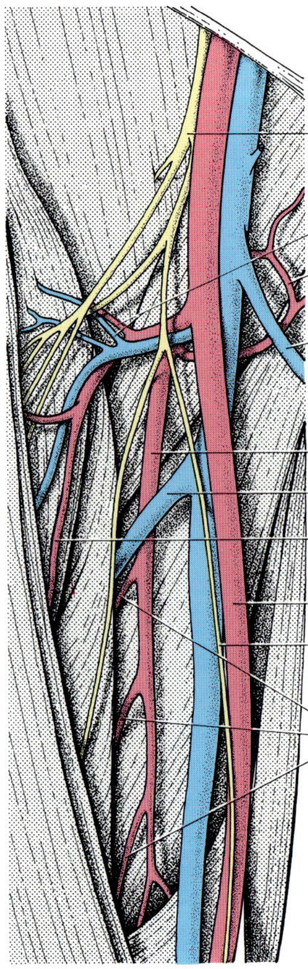

Fig. 17.6.1. Anatomy of the femoral bifurcation and the profunda femoris artery with its branches

of both arteries from the profunda femoris artery in the form of a profunda–circumflex trunk (Fig. 17.6.2a) is seen in about 50%. In this variation, a combined origin of the lateral and medial circumflex arteries with subsequent separation may occur (Fig. 17.6.2b). In particular, the origin of the medial circumflex artery varies considerably. In 30–40% it branches off at the common femoral artery, usually on its dorsal side (Fig. 17.6.2c), and in 2%–3% it is localized at the proximal portion of the superficial femoral artery

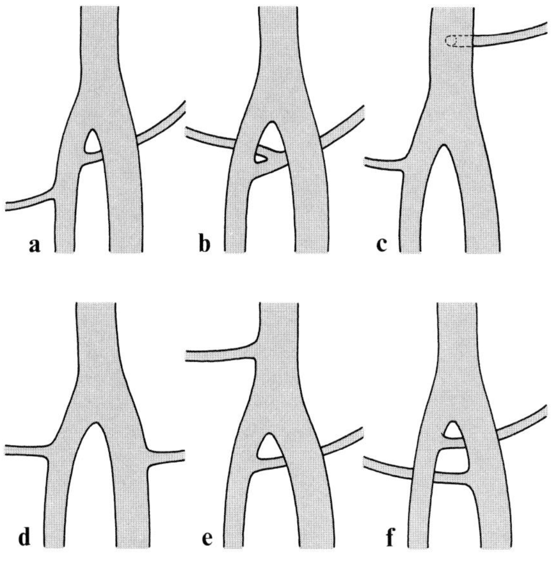

Fig. 17.6.2. Normal anatomy (**a**) and variations (**b–f**) of the origins of the medial and lateral circumflex arteries

(Fig. 17.6.2d) [19]. After it branches off, this tributary runs behind the superficial femoral artery in a medial direction, between the adductors. It is the main arterial supply of these muscles. It has a connection running upward to the obturator artery.

The lateral circumflex artery branches off at the profunda femoris artery in 80%–90% of cases. In 5%–15% it originates from the common femoral artery (Fig. 17.6.2e) and in 1%–6% from the proximal superficial femoral artery (Fig. 17.6.2f) [19]. It runs dorsal to the rectus femoris muscle and sartorius muscle toward the lateral side of the thigh and soon separates into an ascending, a horizontal, and a descending branch. The ascending branch supplies the sartorius muscle, the gluteus medius muscle, and the tensor fasciae latae muscle. The horizontal branch runs to the greater trochanter. Both branches have connections with the gluteal arteries and the terminal branches of the medial circumflex artery.

The large descending branch is of great importance because it can serve as a collateral to compensate for occlusions in the superficial femoral artery. It runs beneath the rectus femoris muscle downward, supplies the vastus muscles and gives off branches to the network of the knee. If the lateral circumflex artery arises atypically from the common femoral artery or superficial femoral artery, its descending branch cannot act as a collateral in the event of an obstruction. A common origin of the profunda femoris artery and both circumflex arteries is extremely rare.

As it continues distally between the the vastus medialis muscle and the adductor muscle group, lateral to the superficial femoral artery, the profunda femoris artery gives off from 3 to 5 perforating arteries which enter the adductor muscles near the linea aspera of the femur. There they give off several branches, which supply the flexor group. They have connections to one another and have additional anastomoses proximally with the gluteal arteries, the obturator artery, the medial circumflex artery, and, distally, with muscular branches of the popliteal artery and recurrent tributaries of the lower leg arteries. In this way the profunda femoris artery and its branches form a vascular bridge, which parallels the superficial femoral artery and connects the iliac arteries with the popliteal artery and the arteries of the lower leg [11, 12].

The femoral nerve accompanying the common femoral artery passes through the lacuna musculorum together with the iliopsoas muscle and, covered by the iliopectineal fascia, lies lateral to the artery. Beneath the inguinal ligament, it soon splits into its branches, with sensory innervation of the skin on the anterior side of the thigh and motor fibers to the pectineus, sartorius, and quadriceps femoris muscles. Its terminal branch, the saphenous nerve, containing only sensory fibers, runs together with the superficial femoral artery downward (Fig. 17.6.1) and innervates the skin on the tibial side of the lower leg and at the tibial margin of the foot.

B. Hemodynamic Aspects

Except in its proximal portion, the profunda femoris artery usually does not show advanced arteriosclerosis, even though other arteries in the body may be severely diseased. Therefore, it is one of the most important collateral vessels in maintaining blood flow to the lower leg and foot following femoropopliteal occlusions. One exception is diabetes mellitus of long duration. The collateral circulation through the profunda femoris artery has three potentially weak points which follow each other in series (Fig. 17.6.3). Their hemodynamic resistances are added together and therefore determine the compensating capacity of collateral flow through this artery.

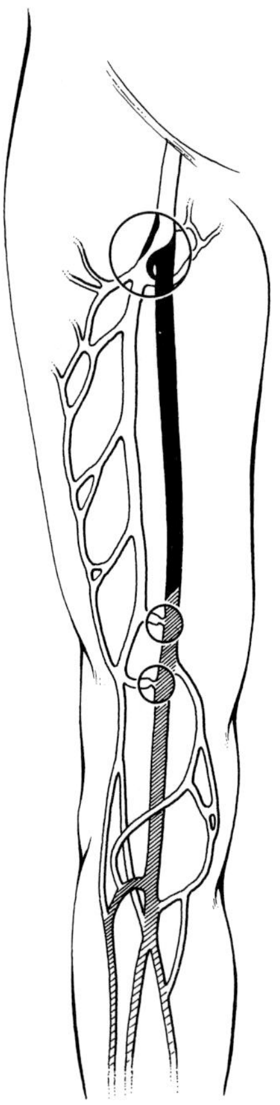

Fig. 17.6.3. Schematic representation of the collateral compensation of a femoropopliteal occlusion via the profunda femoris artery and the weak points (◯ proximal stenosis of the profunda femoris artery; ○ stenoses at the entry of dilated profunda collaterals; /// occluded recipient artery of profunda collaterals)

The *first* weak point is the origin and proximal portion of the profunda femoris artery. The sharp curve formed by the dorsolateral takeoff of the profunda femoris artery causes considerable loss of kinetic energy and therefore poor hemodynamic conditions at the bifurcation. Furthermore, this part of the profunda femoris artery, in contrast to its other segments, often shows arteriosclerotic disease, especially in femoropopliteal obstructions. In such cases there is usually a plaque on the posterior wall of the common femoral artery which extends into the profunda femoris artery for a short distance, causing narrowing of the lumen. For many years, operative removal of these localized stenotic lesions, usually by endarterectomy over a short distance with dilatation of the orifice, was thought to be sufficient for restoration of impaired flow through the profunda femoris artery. However, investigations and geometric analyses by Berguer [1] found additional new hemodynamic aspects which must be taken into account in revascularization of the profunda femoris artery (Fig. 17.6.4).

In the area of any great vascular bifurcation, including the femoral bifurcation, the total diameter of the branches is usually greater than that of the arterial trunk (Fig. 17.6.4a). In an occlusion of the superficial femoral artery, the flow tract undergoes an abrupt reduction in caliber at the origin of the profunda femoris artery. Thus, independently of existing wall lesions within the profunda femoris artery, the origin of the vessel itself represents an anatomic stenosis which is relieved at the next later branch in accordance with the same geometric principle (Fig. 17.6.4b). Arteriosclerotic plaque in the profunda femoris artery further increases the degree of stenosis, and of course this in turn has a significant negative influence on hemodynamic conditions (Fig. 17.6.4c). Consequently, surgical enlargement of the profunda femoris artery will not bring about hemodynamic improvement merely by removal of the arteriosclerotic material; the anatomic stenosis resulting from the obstruction of the superficial femoral ar-

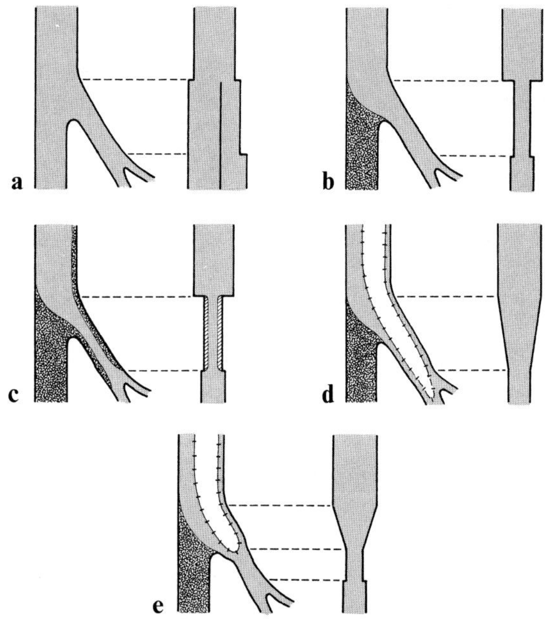

Fig. 17.6.4. Schematic representation of vascular geometry at the femoral bifurcation under normal conditions (**a**) and in the case of femoropopliteal occlusion with an intact proximal profunda femoris artery (**b**), with a pathologically altered profunda segment (**c**), following profundaplasty (**d**), and following widening of the orifice of the profunda femoris artery over a short distance (**e**) (modified according to Berguer et al. [1])

tery must also be relieved, i.e., the enlargement procedure must include branching of the profunda femoris artery that is extensive enough to meet the geometric requirements (Fig. 17.6.4d). Depending on vascular anatomy and morphology, this enhancement of total arterial diameter can be effected at the proximal branches, the origins of the perforating arteries, or even at the most distal branch [4, 7, 17]. Limiting the enlargement procedure to the orifice of the profunda femoris artery or to the diseased region alone, without inclusion of the geometrically most significant branch, is inadequate from the point of view of hemodynamics; it merely lessens, but does not relieve, the preexisting anatomic stenosis (Fig. 17.6.4e).

The *second* limiting factor in adequate collateral circulation through the profunda femoris system is stenoses at the entry of dilated profunda branches into the collateral recipient segment of the popliteal artery [20]. The cause is not only arteriosclerotic lesions but also the inability of the terminal portions of these to dilate properly owing to their peculiar intraluminal mural structure.

The *third*, and commonly decisive, morphological factor influencing the efficiency of collateral circulation through the profunda femoris system is the existence or nonexistence of patent recipient segments along the course of the popliteal artery and lower leg arteries, to which the collaterals may conduct blood.

C. Definition

The only portion of the collateral circulation which is accessible to surgical treatment is the profunda femoris artery itself. The other two factors which might limit the efficiency of this collateral system, stenoses at the entries of the dilated profunda collaterals and a poor run-off, cannot be corrected. Operative procedures performed on the profunda femoris artery are called "profundaplasties", "profunda reconstructions", and "profunda revascularizations". The confusing terminology in this field makes necessary a clear definition of the different operative procedures.

The term "profundaplasty" should be reserved for those procedures which relieve the anatomic stenosis at the mouth of the profunda femoris artery by enlarging the caliber of the orifice and also of the main trunk over the hemodynamically necessary distance (see Sect. B). In addition, a localized organic stenosis due to atheromatous plaques is treated by open endarterectomy.

"Profunda reconstructions" should be defined as procedures by which a diseased profunda femoris artery is replaced with an interposition graft or bridged with a bypass graft.

"Profunda revascularizations" are procedures which improve or normalize a reduced or absent blood flow to the profunda femoris artery and therefore do not involve reconstruction of the profunda femoris artery itself but rather the proximal inflow tract, consisting of the iliac arteries. A profunda revascularization is especially considered in two-level arterial obstructions of the aortoiliac and femoropopliteal segments and aims at improving circulation through the profunda femoris artery by reconstruction of the proximal aortoiliac segment, thus attempting to compensate a femoropopliteal occlusion by increasing flow through the collateral system of this artery. In such cases, the profunda femoris artery functions as the sole outflow tract of the iliac artery reconstruction. To maximize run-off conditions, a profunda revascularization should always be combined with a profundaplasty.

D. Indications

Surgical procedures on the profunda femoris artery in the form of profundaplasty or a profunda reconstruction aim at compensating the occluded femoropopliteal artery via the collateral system of the thigh. The effectiveness of these operations is dependent not only on the technical and hemodynamic perfection of the procedure, but also to a great extent on the caliber and number of preexisting distal collateral vessels and their entry sites. Finally, the quality of the distal collateral recipient segments of the popliteal artery and lower leg arteries is also very important [3, 16]. Alternative methods are a femoropopliteal or femorocrural bypass.

If the conditions for profundaplasty are ideal – absence of gangrenous lesions, preexistent wide and numerous profunda collaterals, an undiseased or only slightly arteriosclerotic recipient segment of the distal femoropopliteal artery – a significant improvement in ischemic symptoms can be expected [15]. Because of the relatively short operating time required, the technical simplicity of the procedure, and the favorable long-term prognosis,

Table 17.6.1. Criteria for choosing between profundaplasty and femoropopliteal or femorocrural bypass

1. General risk factors
2. Available reconstructive material
3. Access to the operating area (repeat operation)
4. Severity of ischemia in the limb
5. Quality of the profunda collaterals and their entry segments
6. Quality of run-off

profundaplasty should be preferred to femoropopliteal bypass under these conditions. Only the social consideration of unrestricted walking capability favors a distal bypass graft. In cases of insufficient collateral circulation of the profunda femoris artery caused by entry stenoses of the collateral vessels and significantly diseased collateral recipient arteries, profundaplasty or reconstruction must be expected to be less effective, and the cure of preexistent gangrenous lesions must be questionable [18]. This unfavorable constellation is found especially in occlusions of the distal popliteal artery and its trifurcation. In these cases compensation of femoropopliteal occlusion via the collateral system of the profunda femoris artery is unlikely because of missing recipient segments for these collaterals. If under these circumstances angiography indicates that a femoropopliteal bypass is also possible, the decision as to which reconstruction procedure is preferable should depend on the factors listed in Table 17.6.1. If the general surgical risk is acceptable, if proper venous reconstructive material is available, and if the peripheral run-off is of adequate quality for distal bypass anastomosis, a femoropopliteal or femorocrural bypass graft is the procedure of choice. An ideal solution is the simultaneous combination with profundaplasty (see p. 456). If there exist any serious general risk factors, if there is a lack of venous reconstructive material, and if conditions for a distal bypass anastomosis are poor owing to impaired run-off or to technical difficulties in repeat surgery, a profundaplasty is preferable. In such cases, however, this should be extended as far as possible to the most distal branches of the profunda femoris artery. If the goal of curing gangrene is not reached, it is still possible, even under very unfavorable conditions, to shift the border of amputation from the thigh region to an area below the knee. Profunda reconstructions must be considered if arteriosclerotic lesions extend all the way into the peripheral parts of the profunda femoris artery and the risk of a very time-consuming profundaplasty extending into the most distal branches is not acceptable. They are also indicated where it is feared that endarterectomy would involve local technical difficulties owing to extreme calcification or transition problems at the distal end of the segment to be endarterectomized. If repeat surgery is performed on the profunda femoris artery and dissection of the artery is difficult, profunda reconstruction should be attempted by exposing the artery through two separate incisions over the still patent proximal and distal arterial segments to which bypass grafts can be connected. However, a preliminary condition for such procedures is that the morphological state of the profunda femoris collateral system will guarantee patency of the bypass after implantation.

E. Positioning

Operations on the profunda femoris artery are done in a supine position. Abduction and external rotation of the thigh exposes the groin region and allows for better access. This effect is reinforced by placing a soft pillow under the hip of the other side and flexing the knee (Fig. 17.6.5). To prevent ischemic decubital necroses during the operation, the foot should be wrapped in cotton dressing, or the heel raised on a pad. A means for protecting the very sensitive inguinal region from infection is to cover the penis and scrotum with gauze pads and fix them to the opposite thigh with an adhesive bandage. Following this the anal and genital re-

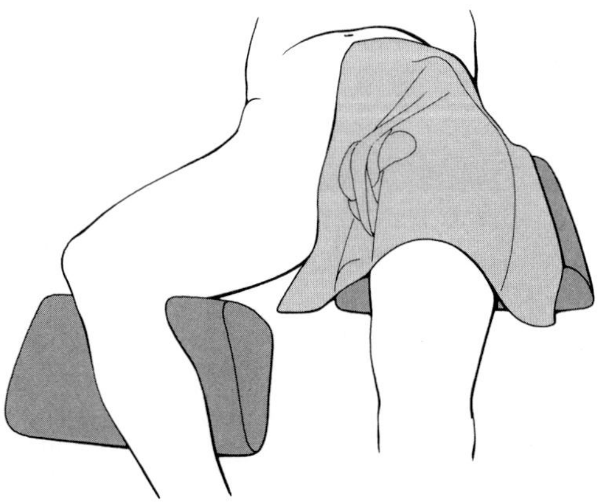

Fig. 17.6.5. Position of the patient and draping of the scrotum and genital region prior to reconstructive procedures on the profunda femoris artery

gion is draped with a large abdominal towel. Only after these preliminary precautions may the operating area be draped as usual from the lower abdomen to the knee or, if additional proximal or distal reconstructions are planned, over a large area.

When draping the area, one must always consider the possibility that a vein graft may have to be resected. Venous material for patch grafts should under no circumstances be taken from the great saphenous vein of the inguinal region. If blood circulation in the contralateral leg is intact, the necessary venous segment should be resected from the great saphenous vein at the medial malleolus. Resection in the ipsilateral leg may lead to impaired wound healing at the donor site if ischemia is severe. In reconstructions with bypass grafts or venous interpositions, resections of the usually great saphenous vein are performed in the thigh area through an inguinal incision and, if necessary, a second short distal incision. If its caliber is large enough, a lower leg saphenous segment may also be used for reconstruction. This can preserve the proximal great saphenous vein.

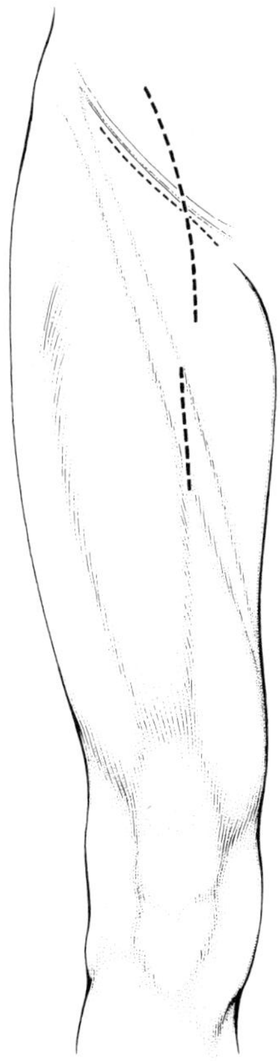

Fig. 17.6.6. Skin incisions to expose the proximal and distal portions of the profunda femoris artery

F. Incisions

An oblique inguinal incision in the groin or a longitudinal incision midway between the anterior iliac spine and the pubis, with a slightly curved course, exposes the femoral bifurcation and the proximal portion of the profunda femoris artery (Fig. 17.6.6). The advantage of the oblique incision is the much lower rate of wound healing impairment, particularly necrosis of the wound margin. A disadvantage is the limited exposure and the difficulty of extending the incision distally or proximally, if this is necessary. It usually suffices if the patients are not too obese and profundaplasty is not too extensive. On the other hand, a longitudinal incision across the groin may be extended without difficulty. It exposes the whole course of the profunda femoris artery down to its most distal branches. It should be employed if there is still uncertainty about which type of reconstructive procedure to perform and how extensive it may be.

A longitudinal incision over the medial third of the thigh, across the sartorius muscle, exposes the distal portion of the profunda femoris artery (Fig. 17.6.6). Such an additional exposure of the profunda femoris artery is advisable for distal anastomoses in profunda reconstructions (distal connection of a bypass graft or venous interposition) and necessary in profunda revascularizations in which the groin must be bypassed for special reasons, such as infections, previous operations in this area, or radiation therapy.

G. Method of Exposure

Following division of the skin and subcutaneous tissue the medial margin of the sartorius muscle is located, and, starting from there, all fat tissue, together with the entrapped lymph nodes, is dissected and retracted medially (Fig. 17.6.7a). This maneuver avoids dividing the lymphatic vessels coming from the medial side of the leg. Opened lymphatic vessels are carefully ligated or sutured with ultrafine material. These precautions help prevent a highly intractable postoperative lymphatic fistula, which may lead to secondary infection in some cases. The next step is the exposure of the femoral bifurcation. The perivascular sheath over the palpable common femoral artery is in-

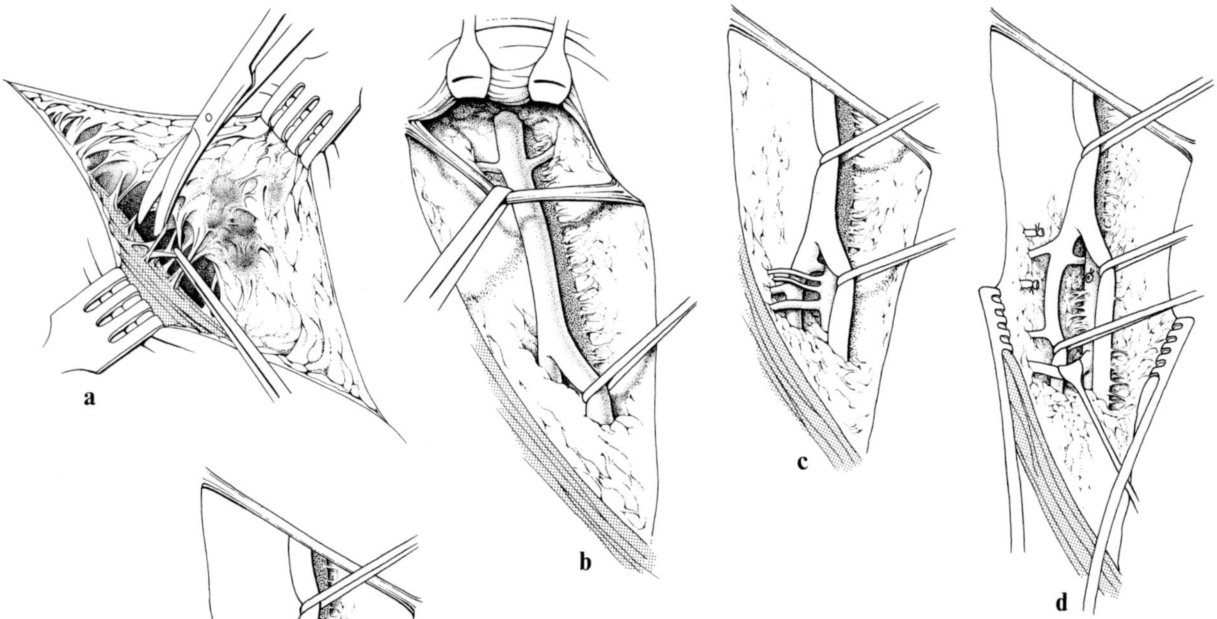

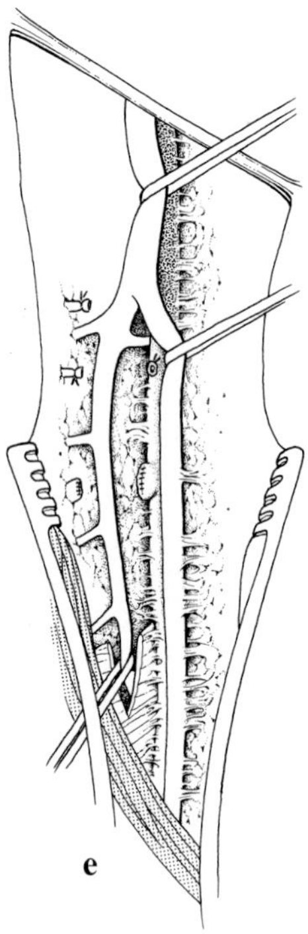

Fig. 17.6.7 a–e. Method of exposure of the femoral bifurcation and profunda femoris artery

cised longitudinally, and the anterior surface of the common femoral artery is dissected free. This preparation is usually performed up to the level of the inguinal ligament. If a more proximal exposure above the inguinal ligament is desired, blunt retractors may be placed beneath the inguinal ligament and the tissue retracted upward, allowing visualization of 2–3 cm of the artery. The distal portion of the external iliac artery can be exposed more simply by dissecting the inguinal ligament free of muscular tissue, separating it from the inguinal canal, and retracting it distally.

Following the division of the circumflex iliac veins that cross the distal portion of the external iliac artery, the abdominal muscles can easily be pulled upward with a long Langenbeck retractor, exposing the external iliac artery almost up to the origin of the internal iliac artery (Fig. 17.6.7b). In lateral dissection of the common femoral artery, care must be taken not to overlook possible variant arterial side branches; these must be preserved at all costs because of their collateral function (see p. 445). Unintentional severing of these vessels, especially of the back wall of the common femoral artery, may lead to awkward hemorrhage. The localization of the origin of the profunda femoris artery and the preparation of its proximal segment is easier if a tape is passed around the proximal portion of the superficial femoral artery, which is identified by an absent pulse or an abrupt change in caliber. With slight tension on the tapes holding the common and the superficial femoral artery, the profunda femoris artery is identified, and the tissue covering it is dissected. First, one or two thin venae comitantes are encountered, running in front of the profunda femoris artery. Then, somewhat deeper, the lateral circumflex vein can be visualized (Fig. 17.6.7c). These veins are divided and a stitch is placed through each stump for secure ligation. In about 3% of cases, they lie behind the profunda femoris artery and can be injured unintentionally during dissection on the lateral side of the artery. Next, the first branches of the profunda femoris artery, the lateral and medial circumflex arteries are exposed; these are important for collateral circulation. The space between the femoral vessels on the medial side and the sartorius muscle on the lateral side is spread apart, and the profunda femoris artery is dissected further distally in the deeper layers. At this point, the very large profunda femoris vein crosses over the artery to the femoral vein. It can be retracted downward with a small vein retractor exposing the profunda femoris artery more distally (Fig. 17.6.7d). During the downward dissection of the profunda femoris artery, the profunda femoris vein can be ligated and divided if venous run-off is normal. The stumps are oversewn atraumatically. The perforating arteries branching off along the downward course of the profunda femoris artery are carefully identified and preserved. Finally, the profunda femoris artery disappears behind the adductor longus muscle, which must be partially divided (Fig. 17.6.7e). During dissection of the profunda femoris artery, the femoral nerve with its branches should be preserved.

The isolated distal exposure of the profunda femoris artery through a separate incision corresponds with the last step of the preparation described above. Following division of the subcutis, dissection is continued between the sartorius muscle and the superficial femoral vessels. The profunda femoris artery is identified embedded in fat tissue in the deeper layers. The upper margin of the tendinous sheath of the adductor longus muscle may serve as a marker during this maneuver.

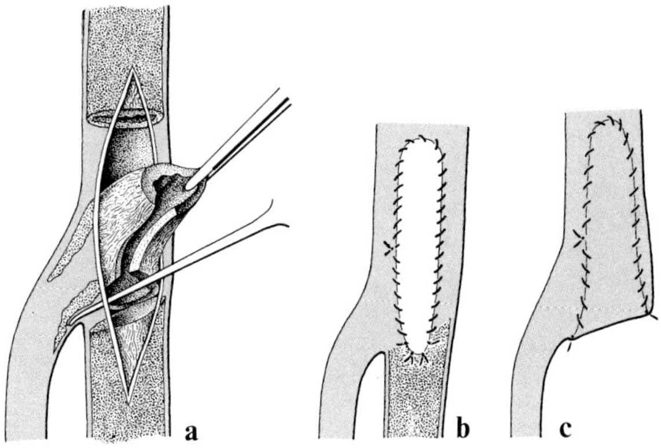

Fig. 17.6.8. Method of anterograde disobliteration of the ostium of the profunda femoris artery (**a**) and closure of the arteriotomy with a venous patch (**b**) or an endarterectomized superficial femoral artery flap (**c**)

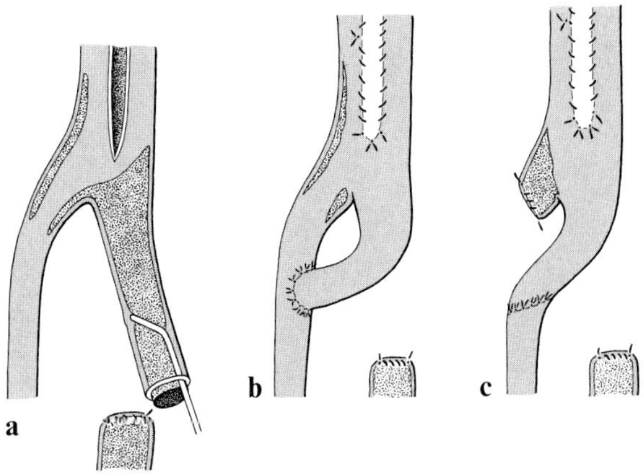

Fig. 17.6.9. Technique of autogenous superficial femoral artery bypass with semiclosed endarterectomy of the proximal superficial femoral artery (**a**) and end-to-side (**b**) or end-to-end anastomosis (**c**) to the poststenotic or postocclusive portion of the profunda femoris artery

H. Operative Procedures

I. Profundaplasties

This procedure is defined as the surgical correction of an anatomic stenosis developing as a consequence of a superficial femoral artery occlusion and also as the correction of an organic stenosis of the profunda femoris artery due to atheromatous lesions. Its purpose is to improve the collateral compensation of a femoropopliteal occlusion. Under these circumstances, manipulations at the orifice of the profunda femoris artery, e.g., anterograde disobliteration of a sclerotic plaque extending into the initial segment of the artery through an arteriotomy in the common femoral artery (Fig. 17.6.8a), are inadequate for successful profundaplasty. Furthermore, the closure of the arteriotomy in the common femoral artery with a vein patch (Fig. 17.6.8b) or a pedicled endarterectomized superficial femoral artery flap reflected upward (Fig. 17.6.8c) increases the degree of the anatomic profunda stenosis by local enlargement of the artery in the region of the patch graft, thereby creating an even poorer hemodynamic situation at the arterial junction. A short extension of the common femoral arteriotomy into the orifice of the profunda femoris artery, with local endarterectomy and patch enlargement, must also be rejected because by this procedure only the organic stenosis is eliminated; the anatomic stenosis is merely reduced (see p. 446). Autogenous bypass constructions with an endarterectomized proximal superficial femoral artery (Fig. 17.6.9a–c) are also unac-

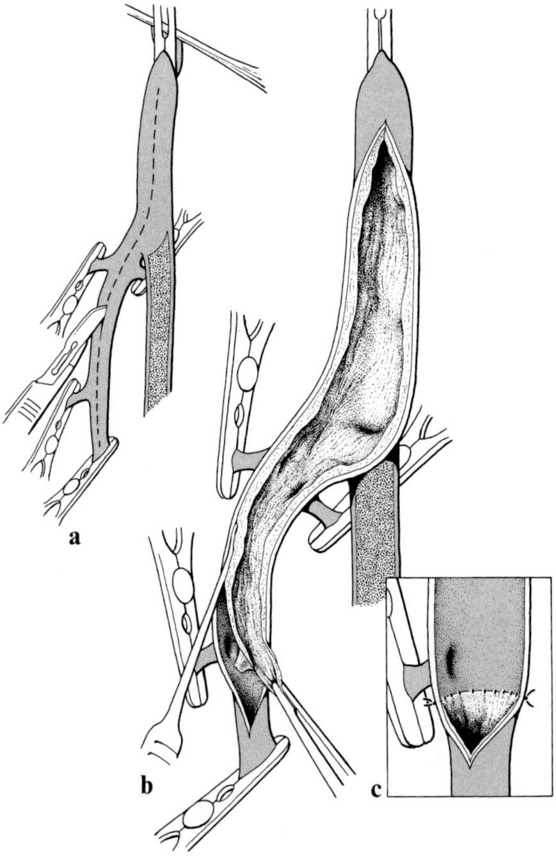

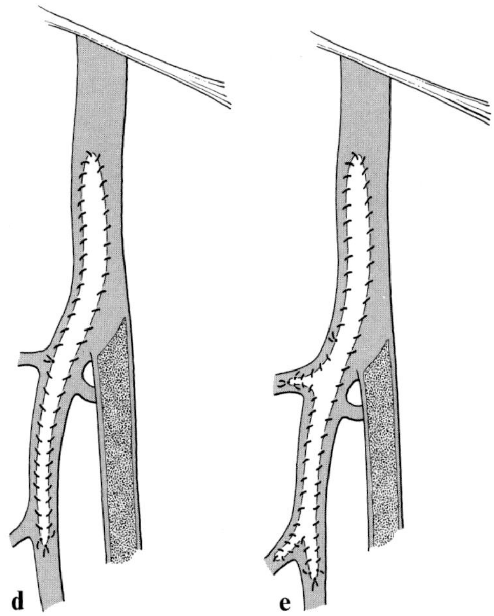

Fig. 17.6.10a–e. Technique of patch graft profundaplasty

ceptable for hemodynamic reasons and have therefore become obsolete [2, 4, 21]. The only reconstructions that meet the hemodynamic requirements of profundaplasty are those patch graft enlargements which include the entire anatomic stenosis of the profunda femoris artery. These may be combined with open endarterectomy, depending on the condition of the vascular wall.

1. Isolated Profundaplasties

a) Patch Graft Angioplasty. Following preparation of the femoral bifurcation and adequate exposure of the profunda femoris artery in a distal direction, the segment to be reconstructed is clamped on both sides. Because every side branch is of great importance for collateral perfusion, it should not be injured. For this purpose, extremely soft bulldog clamps that exert very gentle pressure on the vascular wall are preferable to so-called tourniquets, which do not offer the possibility of dosed pressure control. The profunda femoris artery is then opened by a stab incision of the anterior wall, and the arteriotomy is extended proximally up into the common femoral artery, using Potts scissors, until the proximal clamp just beneath the inguinal ligament is reached. The profunda femoris artery is opened distally in the same manner (Fig. 17.6.10a[1]). This incision should not be made too near the branches or the origin of the superficial femoral artery. To prevent clot formation due to blood stasis, the profunda femoris artery is continuously perfused with heparinized saline solution through an inserted thin catheter.

Starting distally, the atheromatous plug is loosened in the cleavage plain by means of a sharp spoon or dissector and removed at the proximal end of the arteriotomy. If the orifices of the tributaries are also narrowed by arteriosclerotic debris, everything should be done to normalize blood flow through these openings. Normally, anterograde removal of the sclerotic lesion, which usually extends only a few millimeters into the branches, is facilitated by careful eversion of the side branch into the lumen of the profunda femoris artery

---

[1] In order to simplify presentation of the different procedures, the origin of the first perforating artery is assumed to be the geometrically relevant bifurcation in profundaplasty.

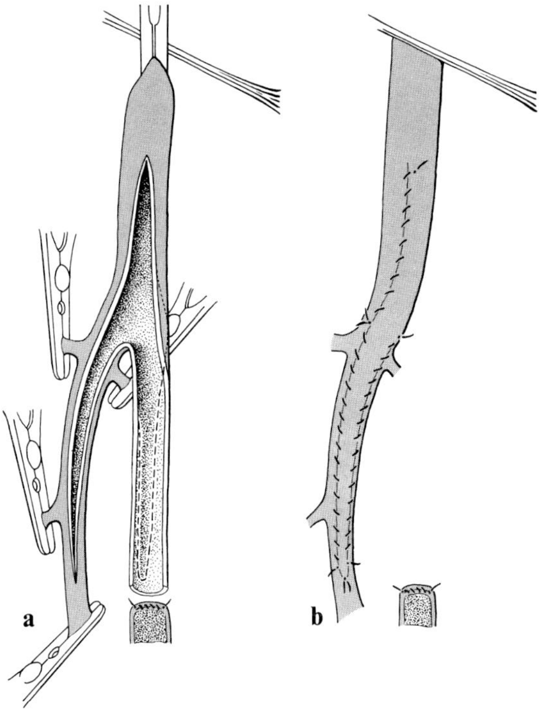

Fig. 17.6.11 a, b. Construction of a "beak patch"

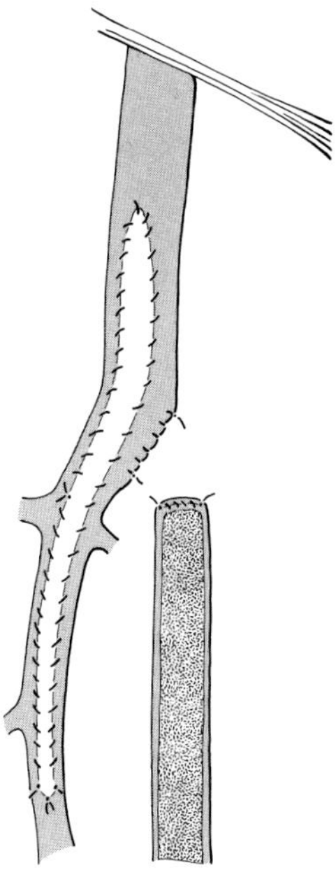

Fig. 17.6.12. Method of close division of the superficial femoral artery at the femoral bifurcation

(Fig. 17.6.10b). If these anterograde disobliterations fail or if the plug tears within the branch, leaving an intimal flap or ledge behind, a Y-shaped arteriotomy at the mouth of the tributary should be performed (particularly if it is a branch of large caliber) and an open endarterectomy done under direct vision.

When an artery shows sclerotic lesions throughout its entire course, so that proper dissection through the arteriotomy is impossible, it is best, if the intima is relatively smooth, to avoid endarterectomy completely. An alternative is to cut the lesion obliquely in a distal direction with a scalpel at the most suitable point. The remaining distal intimal protrusion is fixed to the wall with tack-down stitches. The subsequent patch graft should overlap this site distally by about 0.5–1 cm (Fig. 17.6.10c). The closure of the arteriotomy is done with a vein patch (Fig. 17.6.10d); where side-branch arteriotomies are required, the patch must be appropriately tailored to cover those arteriotomies as well (Fig. 17.6.10e). The venous material is taken from a segment of the great saphenous vein in the region of the ankle joint. If venous material is lacking, an arterial patch may be taken from a resected and endarterectomized segment of the obstructed proximal superficial femoral artery. Patch angioplasty with a pedicled endarterectomized, proximal superficial femoral artery flap is called a "beak patch" (Fig. 17.6.11a, b). It is technically much more difficult and usually offers no advantage. It may be considered in infections in order to avoid using foreign materials. Synthetic patches should not be used because of the small caliber and the wall structure of the profunda femoris artery (particularly after endarterectomy) and also because of the high susceptibility of the groin to infection.

A hemodynamic weak point of patch graft angioplasties performed on the profunda femoris artery is the origin of the superficial femoral artery. It sustains the hemodynamically unfavorable, sharply bending dorsolateral takeoff of the profunda femoris artery and often complicates open endarterectomy, which is normally very simple. If an arteriosclerotic intimal lesion continuing into the superficial femoral artery is divided directly at the origin of this artery, the remaining end of the intima may dissect and lead to local thrombosis. If the lesion is endarterectomized into the origin, the result is either dead space, which causes turbulence in the blood stream, or a thrombus with possible extension into the lumen of the common femoral artery. Attempts have been made to prevent this hemodynamic complication by proximal division of the superficial femoral artery at the bifurcation and suture of the remaining stump (Fig. 17.6.12). Today, this technique is obsolete. Because of its sometimes poor hemodynamic results, vein patch angioplasty of the profunda femoris artery is indicated only if the superficial femoral artery is still patent in its proximal portion and the preservation of potential collaterals branching off along the artery seems necessary for the compensation of a distal femoropopliteal occlusion.

b) Resectional Profundaplasties. These procedures differ from the usual vein patch graft in that local problems originating at the femoral bifurcation, e.g., dorsolateral kinking, intimal dissection, or local thrombosis, are eliminated by excising the superficial femoral artery or profunda femoris artery. This additional maneuver creates superior hemodynamic conditions [5].

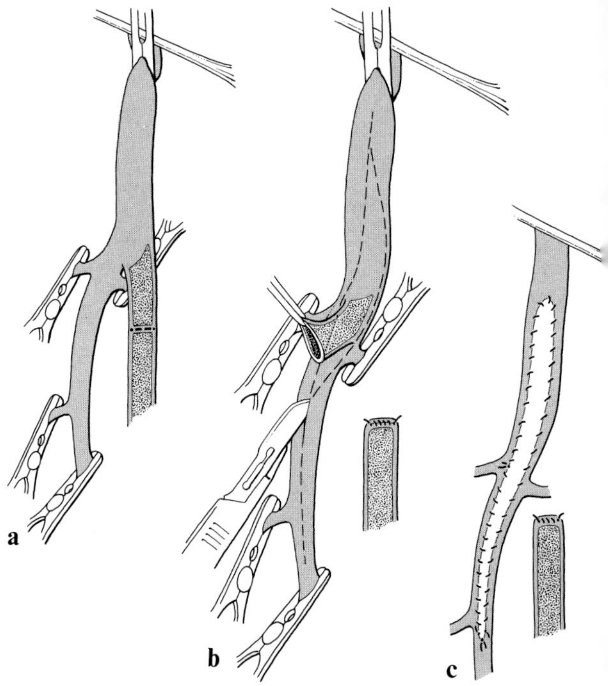

Fig. 17.6.13a–c. Profundaplasty with resection of the origin of the superficial femoral artery

c) Profundaplasty with Resection of the Origin of the Superficial Femoral Artery (Fig. 17.6.13). Dissection and clamping of the arterial segment to be reconstructed are the same as in vein patch profundaplasty. First, the superficial femoral artery is transected about 1 cm distal to the femoral bifurcation (Fig. 17.6.13a). In the event of backbleeding, the distal stump is sutured atraumatically. The completely mobilized proximal stump of the superficial femoral artery, branching off in a ventromedial direction, is rotated anteriorly with a clamp or forceps and then the profunda femoris artery is opened by a stab incision about 1–1.5 cm distal to the bifurcation. The entire stump of the superficial femoral artery is ovally excised and the incision extended into the common femoral artery. During the excision the incision line must not be extended too far laterally on either side. Otherwise, the back wall of the common femoral artery will be narrowed too much. The arteriotomy is extended distally beyond the geometrically relevant tributary of the profunda femoris artery (Fig. 17.6.13b). As in the vein patch technique, this is followed by an open endarterectomy. A vein patch is used for closure of the anterior wall defect (Fig. 17.6.13c). It must be appropriately tailored, narrowing distally. This creates a conical transition from the common femoral artery to the distal profunda femoris artery, thus adapting the calibers of the vessels to one another. The longer the vein patch, the smoother is the adjustment between the lumina.

d) Profundaplasty with Resection of the Origin of the Profunda Femoris Artery (Fig. 17.6.14). This technically rather extensive procedure is rarely indicated, and that is when, during dissection of the femoral bifurcation, the origin of the profunda femoris artery is injured at its back wall, leading to technical difficulties in accurate repair. Following dissection and clamping, the profunda femoris artery is transversely divided below the bifurcation. The level of division depends on the exact location of the lesion, the branches which must be preserved, and the distal spread of the atheromatous debris. Then the superficial femoral artery is transected somewhat distal to the profunda femoris artery in order to allow subsequent adaptation of the corresponding stumps without tension (Fig. 17.6.14a). Starting at the distal end of the obliterated stump of the superficial femoral artery, a portion of the ventrolateral wall of this artery and the entire stump of the profunda femoris artery are removed by a lengthened oval excision,

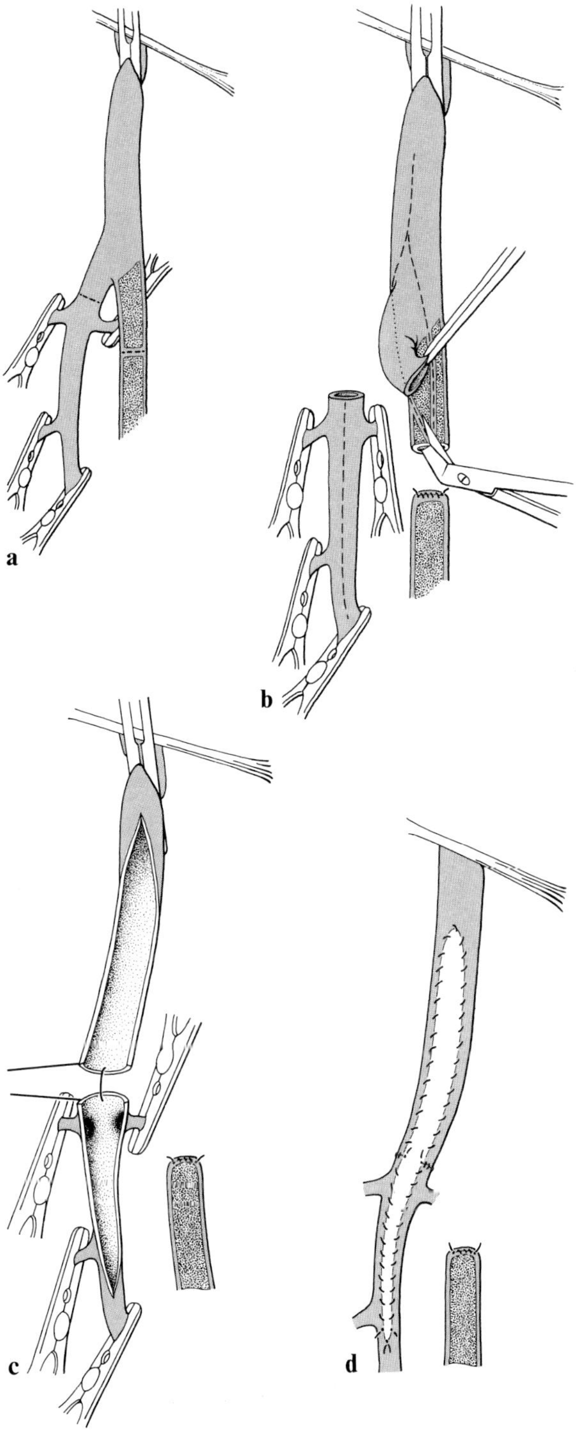

Fig. 17.6.14a–d. Profundaplasty with resection of the origin of the profunda femoris artery

and the common femoral artery is opened proximally, ending just below the inguinal ligament. Correspondingly, the profunda femoris artery is also incised distally as far as necessary to achieve a geometrically and anatomically correct reconstruction (Fig. 17.6.14b). Then, the superficial femoral stump, the common femoral artery, and if necessary the opened portion of the profunda femoris artery are endarterectomized. The stump of the profunda femoris artery and the completely mobilized superficial femoral stump are approximated and sutured at the back wall with interrupted sutures (Fig. 17.6.14c). Different-sized lumina are tailored to fit one another by cutting small tissue wedges out of the proximal edge of the larger artery. The remaining defect in the anterior wall across the anastomosis is then closed with a vein patch graft. Narrowing of the patch creates a smooth conical transition from the common femoral artery to the distal profunda femoris artery (Fig. 17.6.14d).

2. Combined Profundaplasties

a) Profundaplasty and Proximal Superficial Femoral Artery Reconstruction. Combining profundaplasty with reconstruction of a proximal superficial femoral artery stenosis is usually done by first performing an open endarterectomy with subsequent vein patch angioplasty. Following exposure of the femoral bifurcation and adequate distal dissection around the branches to be reconstructed, a Y-shaped incision is made at the femoral bifurcation (Fig. 17.6.15a). The subsequent open endarterectomy of the profunda femoris artery is usually not difficult. However, at the distal edge of the arteriotomy in the superficial femoral artery, it is necessary to cut the arteriosclerotic plug which ex-

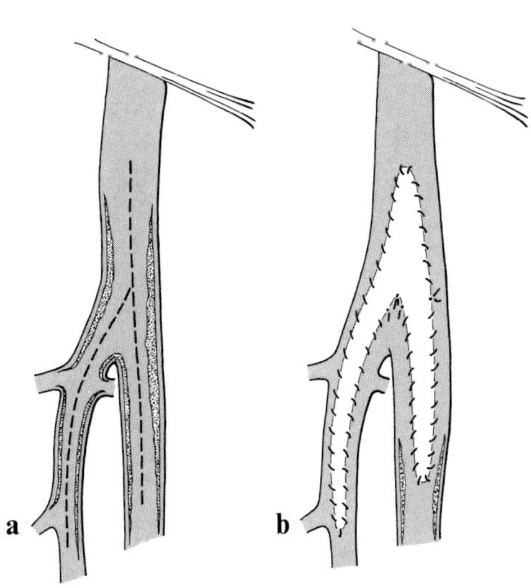

Fig. 17.6.15a, b. Open endarterectomy of the femoral ▷ bifurcation and its proximal branches with a Y-shaped vein patch graft

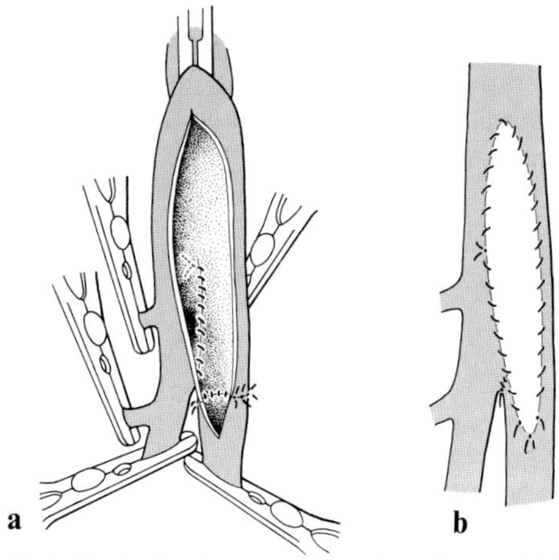

Fig. 17.6.16a, b. Endarterectomy of the femoral bifurcation and its proximal tributaries with distal displacement of the bifurcation by a back-wall suture and vein patch graft

tends further distally, and to fix it to the vascular wall by tack-down stitches. The arteriotomy is closed with a Y-shaped vein patch, overlapping the site of intimal fixation distally by about 0.5–1 cm (Fig. 17.6.15b).

An alternative method to the Y-shaped vein patch graft is distal transposition of the femoral bifurcation [13]. Following a Y-shaped arteriotomy and subsequent endarterectomy, the medial walls of the profunda femoris artery and superficial femoral artery are joined, and the existing anterior wall defect is closed with a long oval vein patch (Fig. 17.6.16a, b).

b) Profundaplasty and Femoropopliteal Bypass. The first variation, combining a femoropopliteal or femorocrural bypass with profundaplasty, is a proximal end-to-end anastomosis between bypass and proximal superficial femoral stump, with Y-shaped patch angioplasty of the anterior wall of the anastomosis and of the profunda femoris artery. After distal connection of the graft and good exposure of the femoral bifurcation, the superficial femoral artery is transected 1 cm below the bifurcation. If back-bleeding occurs, the distal stump is sutured. Starting at the open end of the superficial femoral artery, the common femoral artery and profunda femoris artery are incised in a Y-shaped fashion and then, if necessary, endarterectomized. The bypass graft which is pulled upward to the groin is shortened to the level of the proximal superficial femoral stump, and its anterior wall is incised longitudinally, the incision running downward for a distance of 1.5–2 cm

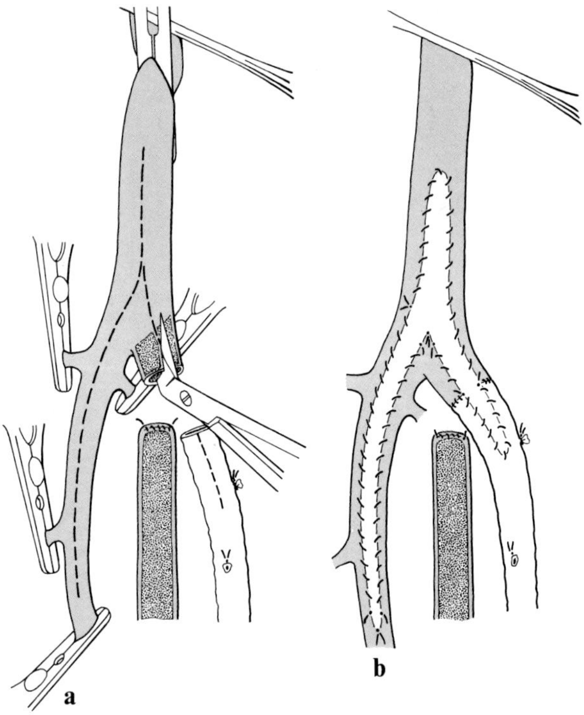

Fig. 17.6.17a, b. Profundaplasty with femoropopliteal graft anastomosis to the proximal superficial femoral artery

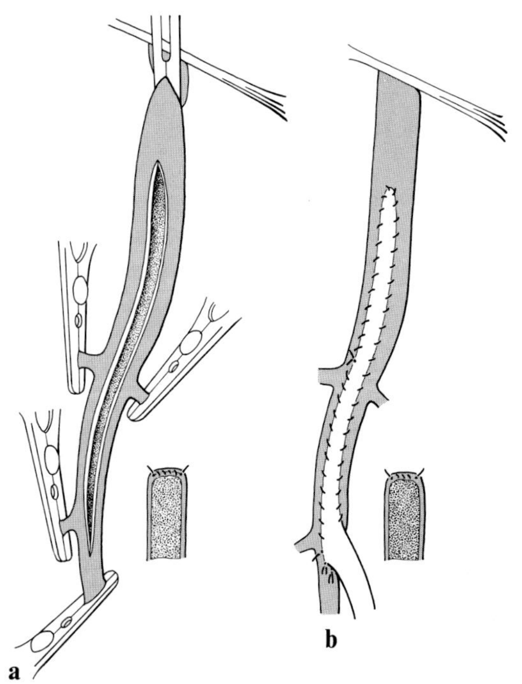

Fig. 17.6.18a, b. Profundaplasty with excision of the origin of the superficial femoral artery and enlargement of the proximal segment of the profunda femoris artery by a long end-to-side anastomosis to the femoropopliteal bypass graft

(Fig. 17.6.17a). The graft is then anastomosed semicircularly to the superficial femoral stump with interrupted sutures. The rotation method (see p. 61.) may be employed during anastomosis. Different-sized lumina are adapted by a wedge-shaped excision at the margin of the arteriotomy. The remaining defect in the anterior wall of the bifurcation is finally closed with a Y-shaped vein patch graft (Fig. 17.6.17b). If the available venous material does not allow Y-shaped tailoring, two separate patches may be used instead to close the arteriotomy.

The second method of reconstruction is to combine profundaplasty with excision of the superficial femoral stump and subsequent enlargement of the proximal segment of the profunda femoris artery by means of an end-to-side anastomosis of the bypass. Apart from the incorporation of the vein patch graft, the surgical procedure in the groin is identical to profundaplasty with resection of the superficial femoral artery (see p. 454). The remaining anterior wall defect (Fig. 17.6.18a) is closed by end-to-side anastomosis of the graft to the edges of the arteriotomy. After distal anastomosis of the bypass, it is pulled up to the groin and tailored to fit the distal end of the profunda arteriotomy; the result is a long end-to-side anastomosis (Fig. 17.6.18b). A small venous tributary may be used to complete the anastomosis at the uppermost corner, forming a "boot-shaped" end-to-side anastomosis (see p. 66). This improves the hemodynamics in this area of the distally transposed bifurcation.

c) Profundaplasty and Aortoiliac Reconstruction ("Profunda Revascularization"). The particular techniques of profundaplasty used during profunda revascularization depend largely on the methods of iliac artery reconstruction being employed. In endarterectomy of the iliac arteries that includes portions of the common femoral arteries, profundaplasty with resection of the superficial femoral stump is preferred as being technically the simplest and hemodynamically the most favorable method (see p. 454). If the iliac arteries are bridged with a bypass graft (anatomically or extra-anatomically), the extension of the common femoral artery incision into the profunda femoris artery and its closure with a short tongue of the prosthesis (Fig. 17.6.19a) are often not adequate to meet the hemodynamic requirements of profundaplasty.

Extension of the profunda arteriotomy beyond the geometrically relevant branch bifurcation and

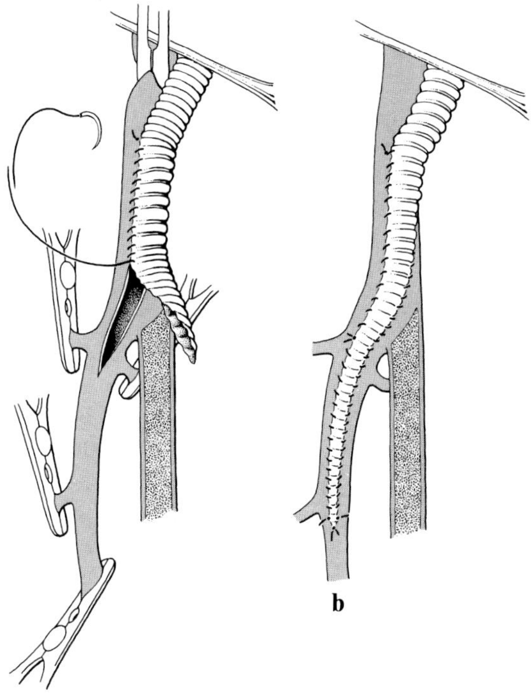

Fig. 17.6.19. Hemodynamically inadequate enlargement of the orifice by extending the distal connection of the prosthesis only into the origin of the profunda femoris artery (**a**) and enlargement of the profunda femoris artery with a long tongue-shaped prosthetic flap (**b**)

use of a prosthetic patch graft with a long tongue-shaped flap (Fig. 17.6.19b) relieves the anatomic stenosis of the profunda femoris artery, as in classical profundaplasty, but has the disadvantage that a long patch of synthetic material must be sutured to an artery whose wall structure is more compatible with venous reconstructive material. Figure 17.6.20a shows one way of solving this problem by connecting the prosthesis to the proximal femoral artery and closing the profunda arteriotomy with a vein patch graft extending upward to join the distal end of the prosthesis. Simultaneous resection of the superficial femoral artery at the bifurcation helps to improve run-off conditions in this type of reconstruction. If no synthetic material is wanted in the groin, the synthetic prosthesis is anastomosed to the distal external iliac artery after mobilization of the inguinal ligament and retraction of the abdominal wall muscles cranially (see p. 450). The vein patch graft is extended proximally to reach the end of the prosthesis (Fig. 17.6.20b). If the common femoral artery shows only slight arteriosclerotic changes, vein patch graft angioplasty and distal anastomosis of the prosthesis may be performed in a discontin-

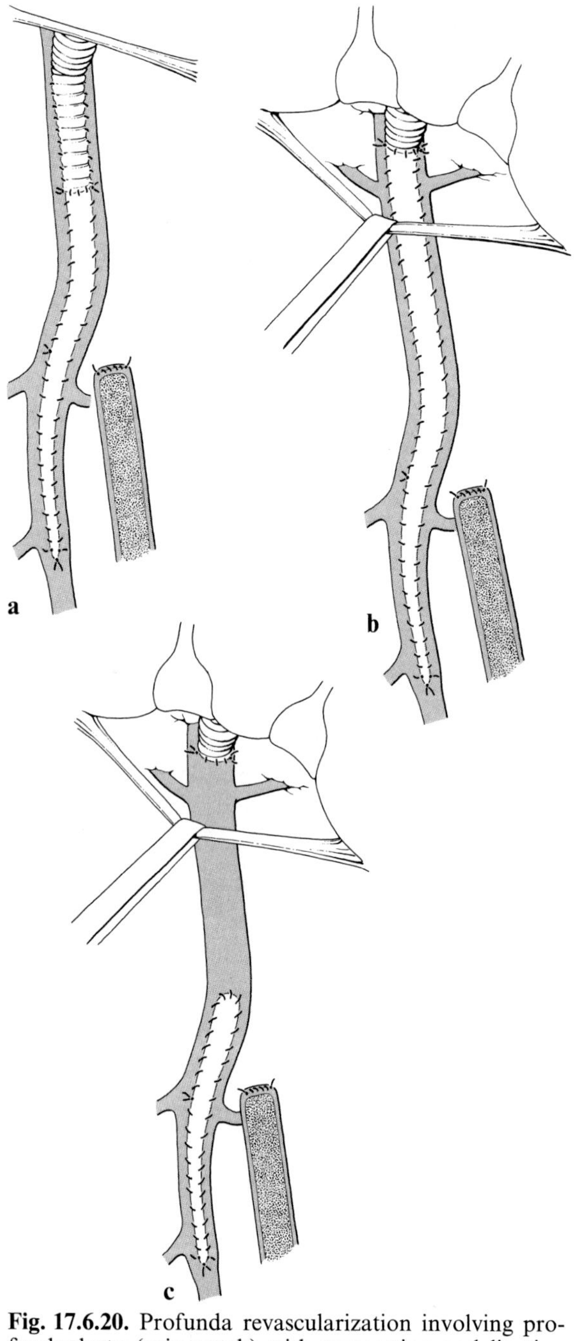

Fig. 17.6.20. Profunda revascularization involving profundaplasty (vein patch) with transection and ligation of the superficial femoral artery and continuous inguinal (**a**), suprainguinal (**b**) and discontinuous suprainguinal (**c**) connection of the prosthesis

uous manner (Fig. 17.6.20c). The same reconstructive alternative exists after semiclosed endarterectomy of the common femoral artery segment between the vein patch graft and distal anastomosis of the prosthesis.

II. Profunda Reconstructions

Reconstructions of the profunda femoris artery either bridge or replace diseased profunda segments.

1. Femoroprofundal Bypass

The simplest method, technically speaking, is a femoroprofundal bypass with proximal and distal end-to-side anastomosis (Fig. 17.6.21). Both connection sites are exposed either by an extensive longitudinal incision or by two separate incisions, one obliquely in the groin and the other a smaller, longitudinal one in the middle of the thigh (see p. 449). Only venous material should be used for grafting. In a relatively short bypass graft, the valves should be resected with the vein turned inside out, because then the proximal and distal ends of the vein segment correspond much better in size with the host artery, and this is hemodynamically more favorable than reversing the graft end-for-end before connecting it. First, the distal end-to-side anastomosis is performed. If the distal connecting segment of the graft is thin, with spastic constrictions, it is carefully distended with heparinized saline solution between two bulldog clamps before opening it. The anastomosis itself should be stretched in order to achieve a shallow angle of entry for the bypass graft at the distal profunda femoris artery. The advantage of this distal end-to-side anastomosis compared with distal transection and an oblique or semicircular end-to-end anastomosis, is that differences in caliber or a back-wall plaque extending beyond the anastomosis can be ignored, and, in addition, retrograde blood flow in the proximal profundal segments perfuses the profundal side branches. The proximal connection of the vein graft, which reaches the groin either through the open wound or through a tunnel, is performed end-to-side with the common femoral artery. The hemodynamic disadvantage of this simple technique is that the geometric aspects of the femoral bifurcation are not taken into account.

2. Profundoprofundal Bypass (Fig. 17.6.22)

Much better hemodynamic conditions are achieved by a profundoprofundal bypass graft with a proximal end-to-end anastomosis between the graft and the profundal stump. The profunda femoris artery and superficial femoral artery are transected about 1 cm distal to the bifurcation. If the circumflex arteries are still patent, the profun-

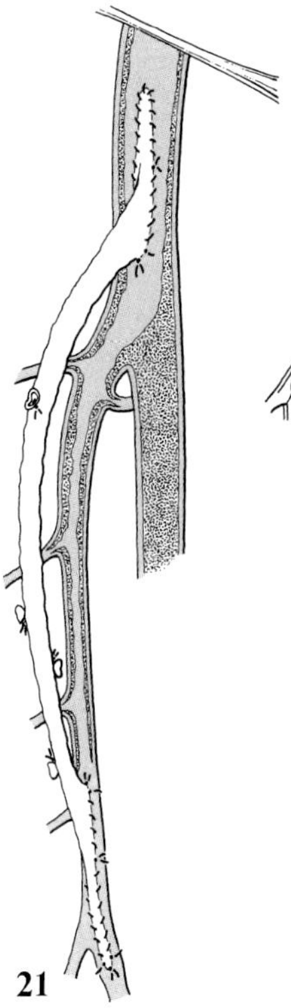

21

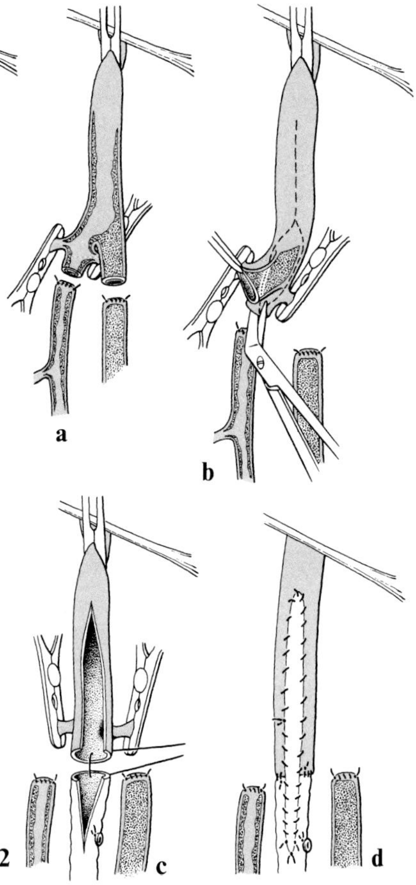

22

Fig. 17.6.21. Femoroprofundal bypass

Fig. 17.6.22 a–d. Profundoprofundal bypass

da femoris artery is divided distal to these open vessels (Fig. 17.6.22a). If backbleeding occurs, the openings of the distal stumps are sutured atraumatically. Starting at the lumen of the proximal profundal stump, the superficial femoral stump is excised from the bifurcation by a long oval incision, and the arteriotomy is extended upward into the common femoral artery (Fig. 17.6.22b). Then, the profundal stump and the common femoral artery are endarterectomized in the correct cleavage plain. The length of the venous segment, which is already anastomosed distally, is first tailored according to the position of the profundal stump, and its anterior wall incised distally for a distance of about 1.5–2 cm. The profundal and venous stumps are then anastomosed semicircularly using interrupted sutures (Fig. 17.6.22c). The anterior wall defect over the anastomosis is closed with a vein patch graft (Fig. 17.6.22d). Narrowing of the patch allows for a smooth transition from the common femoral artery to the vein bypass graft.

REFERENCES

1. Berguer R, Higgins RF, Cotton LT (1975) Geometry, blood flow, and reconstruction of the deep femoral artery. Am J Surg 130:68
2. Bernhard VM, Millitello JM, Geringer AM (1974) Repair of the profunda femoris artery. Am J Surg 127:676
3. Boren CH, Towne JB, Bernhard VM, Salles-Cunha S (1980) Profundapopliteal collateral index. Arch Surg 115:1366
4. Cohn HL, Trueblood W, Crawley LG (1971) Profunda femoris reconstruction in the treatment of femoropopliteal occlusive disease. Arch Surg 103:475
5. Dongen van RJAM, Schwilden ED (1974) Die Profundarevaskularisation; alte und neue Methoden. Folia Angiologica 22:222
6. Hersaey FB, Auer A (1974) Extended surgical approach to the profunda femoris artery. Surg Gynecol Obstet 138:88
7. Lawson DW, Gallico GG, Patton AS (1983) Limb salvage by extended profundaplasty of occluded deep femoral arteries. Am J Surg 145:458
8. Lengua F, Pajot A, Fernandez R, Kunlin J (1980) Plaidoyer pour une meilleure terminologie de la chirurgie de l'artère fémorale profonde. J Chir 117:37
9. Lippert H, Pabst R (1985) Arterial variations in man. Bergmann, Munich
10. Martin P, Renwick S, Stephenson C (1968) On the surgery of the profunda femoris artery. Br J Surg 55:7
11. Martin P, Frawley JE, Barabas AP, Rosengarten DS (1972) On the surgery of atherosclerosis of the profunda femoris artery. Surgery 71:182
12. Martin P, Jamieson C (1974) The rationale for and measurement after profundaplasty. Surg Clin North Am 54:95
13. Menzoian JO (1982) Simultaneous correction of stenosis at the origins of the superficial femoral and deep femoral arteries. Surgery 155:732
14. Morris CG, Edwards W, Woley PA (1961) Surgical importance of the profunda femoris artery. Arch Surg 82:32
15. Myhre HO (1977) The place of profundaplasty in surgical treatment of lower limb atherosclerosis. Acta Chir Scand 143:105
16. Strandness DE (1970) Functional results after revascularisation of the profunda femoris artery. Am J Surg 119:240
17. Taylor LM, Baur GM, Eidemiller LR, Porter JM (1981) Extended profundaplasty. Am J Surg 141:539
18. Towne JB, Bernhard VM, Rollins DL, Baum PL (1981) Profundaplasty in perspective: limitations in the long-term management of limb ischemia. Surgery 90:1037
19. Vaas F (1975) Some considerations concerning the deep femoral artery. Arch Chir Neerl 27:25
20. Vollmar JF, Heyden B, Voss EU (1982) Für und Wider der Profundaplastik. Zentralbl Chir 107:440
21. Waibel PP (1966) Autogenous reconstruction of the deep femoral artery. J Thorac Cardiovasc Surg 7:179

17.7 Service Operations on the Limb Arteries

U. Brunner

CONTENTS

A. Indications, Techniques, and Results

"Service operations" are localized corrective procedures to relieve stenoses due to hyaline or connective tissue proliferation in a vein bypass graft, or endarterectomy [2, 3]. Performed promptly, these operations can recanalize vessels totally occluded by thrombosis and preserve the function of autologous blood conduits as long as possible. They are therefore an alternative to the implantation of synthetic prostheses. Extensive or polytopic hyperplasias must be bridged with a bypass during a second operation. However, if these myointimal proliferations are localized, they may be excised. Figures 17.7.1a–17.7.4a schematically represent the arteriographic images of such stenoses. At short intervals between the primary operation and the service operation (less than 3 months), macroscopic ring-shaped ridges consisting of mural thrombi or mesenchymal connective tissue are found. In this initial stage of development, they may still be treated by PTA. After a longer interval (more than 3 months), these ridges form stenoses consisting of solid, collagenous connective tissue that must be removed sharply with a scalpel. Blunt dissectors are not suited for this purpose, as they do not penetrate the indurated tissue. Stenoses within a venous bypass graft consist of concentrically arranged fibrotic tissue. The predominant

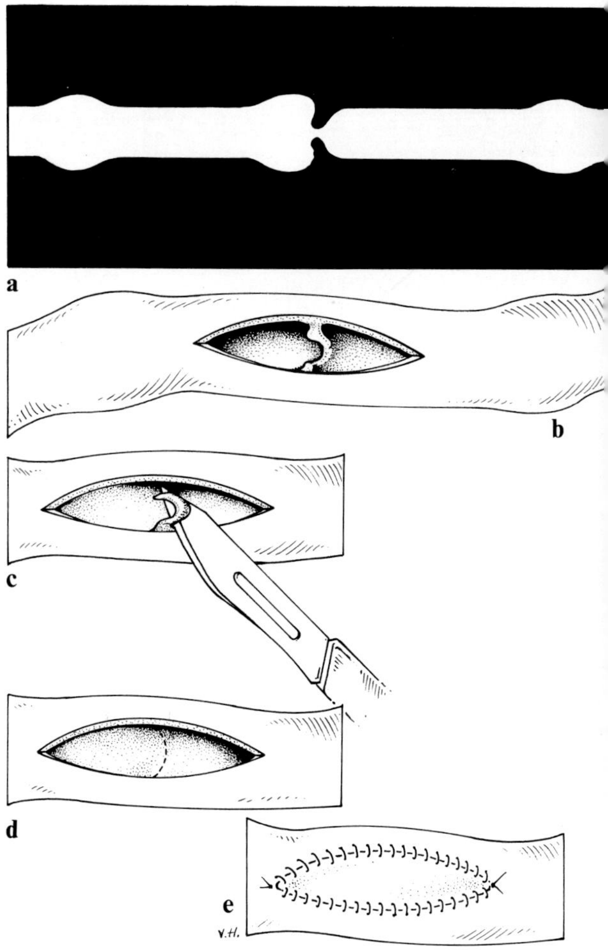

Fig. 17.7.1a–e. Service operation to relieve a recurrent stenosis within an autologous vein bypass graft. **a** Arteriographic picture of a recurrent stenosis. **b** Exposure of the recurrent stenosis. **c** Removal of the myointimal proliferation. **d** Smoothing of the internal surface without tack-down sutures. **e** Patch graft angioplasty with autologous vein graft

sites of these lesions are the indurated rings of the previous valve leaflet attachments (Fig. 17.7.1 b). Stenoses located at proximal or distal anastomoses are not caused by shrinking, but mostly by extension of arteriosclerotic lesions into the vascular connections (Figs. 17.7.2b, 17.7.3b). Following the removal of hypertrophic connective tissue from endarterectomized segments, the stimulated proliferation of the myointimal tissue does not necessarily continue, especially if the tendency of the "internal wound" toward scar formation has receded. Long-term analyses show that service operations on vein bypass grafts achieve a longer period of patency than the same procedures done on endarterectomized arterial segments [1].

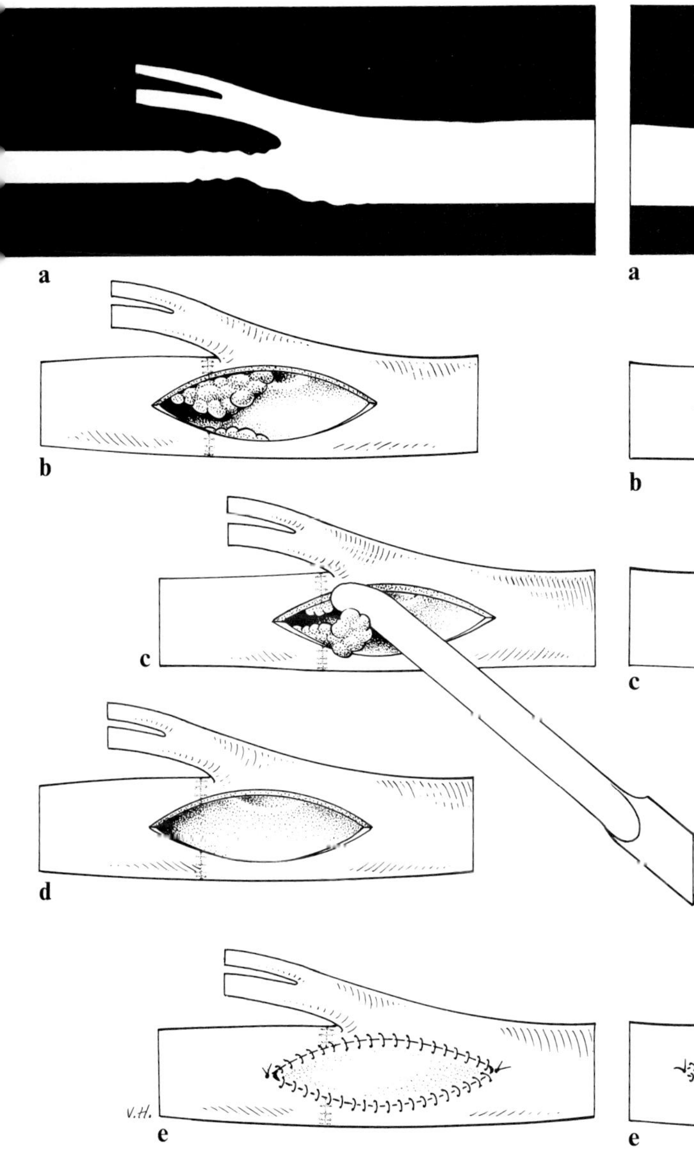

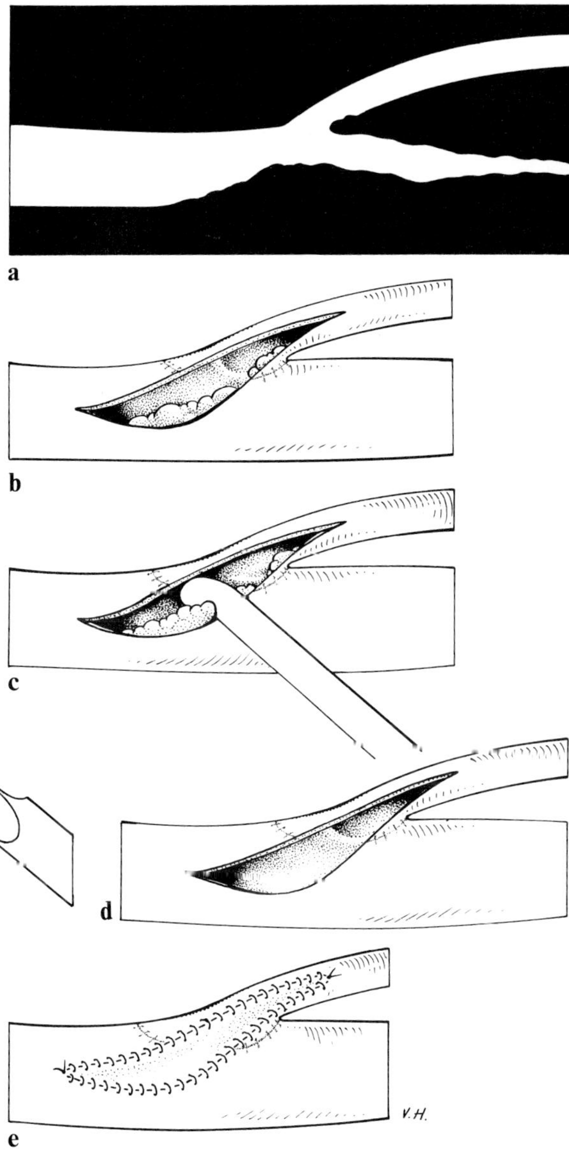

Fig. 17.7.2 a–e. Service operation for removal of a recurrent stenosis near the proximal end-to-end anastomosis of a vein bypass graft. **a–e** As in Fig. 17.7.1

Fig. 17.7.3 a–e. Service operation for removal of a recurrent stenosis near the distal end-to-side anastomosis of a vein bypass graft. **a–e** As in Fig. 17.7.1

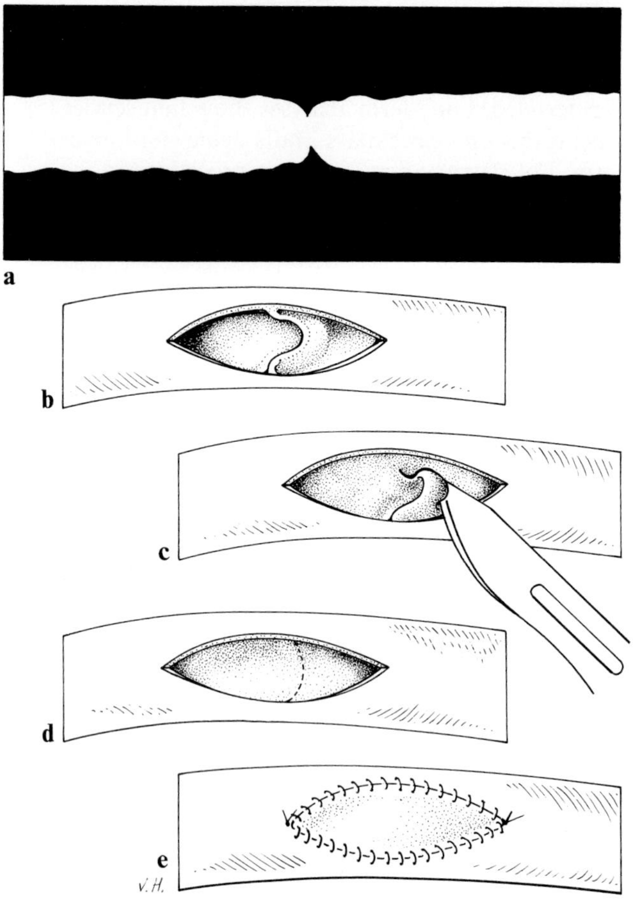

Fig. 17.7.4a–e. Service operation for removal of a recurrent stenosis in an endarterectomized segment of an artery. a–e As in Fig. 17.7.1

B. Basic Technique for Indications and Localizations

A recurrent stenosis within a vein bypass graft or an endarterectomized segment of an artery is exposed by a longitudinal arteriotomy (Fig. 17.7.1b–17.7.4b) and removed with a scalpel (Fig. 17.7.1c–17.7.4c). Fixation of intimal flaps or protrusions is not necessary, due to the adherence of the connective tissue. Only its margins must be smoothed by applying slight pressure (Figs. 17.7.1d–17.7.4d). The arteriotomy is closed with an autologous vein graft (Fig. 17.7.1e–17.7.4e).

Following surgery, medication must be administered as a prophylaxis against recurrences of such proliferations: anticoagulants should be administered in vein bypass grafts and anti-platelet drugs in endarterectomies.

REFERENCES

1. Brunner U, Leu HJ, Ricklin F (1984) Postrekonstruktive Service-Operationen: Resultat über 4 Jahre. Angio Archiv 6:175
2. Leu HJ, Brunner U (1973) Zur Pathogenese der degenerativen Veränderungen an autologen Venentransplantaten. Dtsch Med Wochenschr 98:2433
3. Leu HJ, Brunner U, Stamm F (1979) Zur Morphologie der Neointima nach Endarteriektomie. In: Wagner O, Kubiena K (eds) Der Rezidivverschluß nach Gefäßrekonstruktion an der unteren Extremität. Egermann, Vienna, p 63

18 Occlusions of the Supra-aortic Branches

18.1 Occlusions of the Carotid Arteries

G. CARSTENSEN and K. BALZER

CONTENTS

A. Anatomy (see also p. 13)

The branching point of the common carotid artery, the carotid bifurcation, may be found at different levels, anywhere between C2 and C5/C6. It is most commonly found at the level of C4, (Fig. 18.1.1). The level of the carotid bifurcation has an influence on the angle between the two arteries originating at this point: a caudal division leads to an acute angle and a more cranial division to a more archlike bifurcation [18]. The internal carotid artery usually lies on the lateral side and in 8% of cases on the medial side. A medial location may make exposure of this artery difficult. The carotid arteries are almost always very straight and tightly stretched as they run up through the neck. However, sometimes they may show marked elongation, especially the internal carotid artery. There are congenital elongations, which are found in children, and acquired elongations due to arteriosclerotic lesions. Elongations are more often found in eldery patients, and may be C- or S-shaped with or without a kinking stenosis. Some may even have a sigmoid shape and,

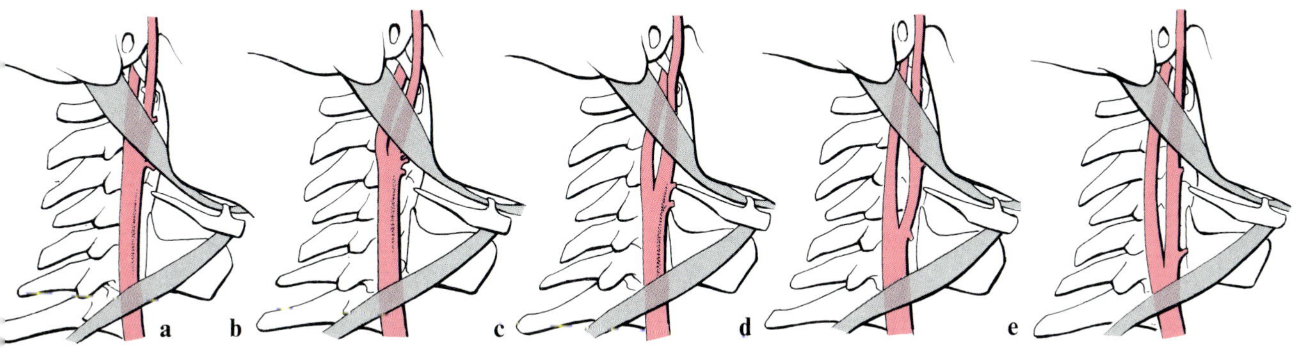

Fig. 18.1.1 a–e. Different levels and locations of the carotid bifurcation (according to VON LANZ and WACHSMUTH) [17]. Besides the differences in location depicted here, many other variations may occur: medial position of the internal carotid artery, variations in the course of the external carotid artery, as well as the very rare aplasia of the internal carotid artery

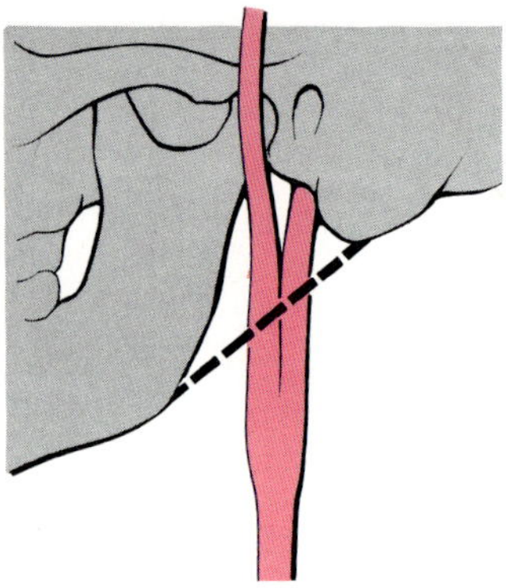

Fig. 18.1.2. The line drawn between the mastoid process and the angle of the jaw, as described by BLAISDELL [4], represents the boundary for operable lesions in the carotid artery. Additional dissection may be performed above this line to expose the distal portion of the artery; however, preparation is very extensive and difficult

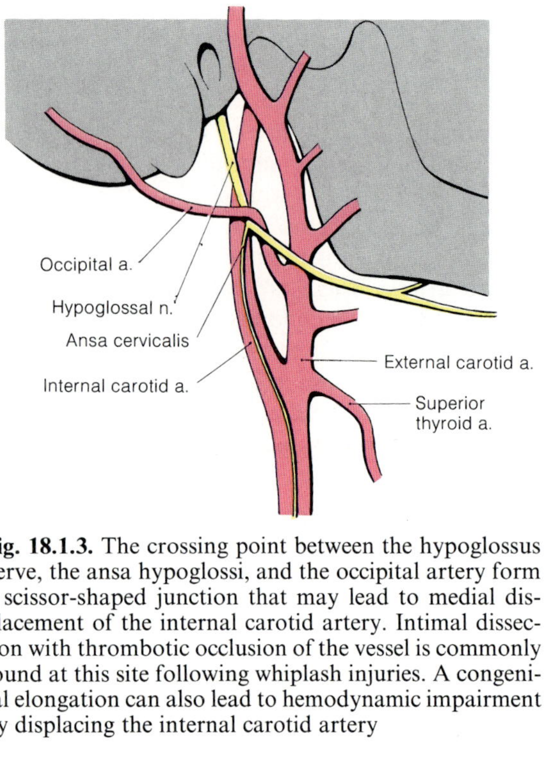

Fig. 18.1.3. The crossing point between the hypoglossus nerve, the ansa hypoglossi, and the occipital artery form a scissor-shaped junction that may lead to medial displacement of the internal carotid artery. Intimal dissection with thrombotic occlusion of the vessel is commonly found at this site following whiplash injuries. A congenital elongation can also lead to hemodynamic impairment by displacing the internal carotid artery

in extreme cases, loop formations. One should also bear in mind the occurrence of fibromuscular dysplasia of the internal carotid artery, which may considerably limit the possibility of reconstruction.

No access to the carotid bifurcation and the internal carotid artery can be obtained in the regions cranial to a line drawn between the mastoid process and the angle of the jaw (Fig. 18.1.2) [2]. Dissection a few centimeters above this line is possible in some cases; however, exposure of the internal carotid artery beneath the base of the skull is technically very difficult and also quite risky. In case a carotid lesion is located far up under the skull, an extra-intracranial bypass may be considered as an alternative (see p. 488). Aplasia of the internal carotid artery is very rare.

The origins of the branches of the external carotid artery show great anatomic variability. The superior thyroid artery may arise from the common carotid artery or from the external carotid artery. The occipital artery usually originates at the external carotid artery and crosses the internal carotid artery. In less than 0.1% of cases it arises from the internal carotid artery. The auricular artery is found above the occipital artery. The hypoglossal nerve is most commonly situated at the level of the occipital artery. The point at which it gives off the descending branch to form the ansa hypoglossi, at the same time passing beneath the occipital artery, forms a scissor-shaped junction that may lead to medial displacement of the internal carotid artery. This is why intimal dissections following whiplash injuries are found at this site (Fig. 18.1.3).

The carotid triangle is bordered cephalad by both parts of the digastric muscle and the jaw, laterally by the sternocleidomastoid muscle, medially by the midline of the anterior surface of the neck, and caudad by the omohyoid muscle [8].

B. Indications

Reconstruction of the carotid bifurcation, including the internal carotid artery and external carotid artery, is indicated in stenoses, occlusions, or elongations of the vessels where blood flow is impaired. In our own patients, 85% of all operable lesions of the supra-aortic branches are found in this region. Postmortem statistics show that two thirds of all cerebral insults have extracranial causes [12]. Therefore, early diagnosis and selection of patients for reconstruction are of special importance.

A classification into clinical stages, analogous to Fontaine's system for classifying symptoms in the lower extremity, has been established, although it has been treated with much skepticism.

Clinical stage I characterizes the asymptomatic stage, in which an operation can be seen purely as a prophylactic measure. Examinations have shown that, at this stage, the risk of a cerebral insult is present only in very high grade stenoses; narrowings of lesser degree should be taken as signs of underlying arteriosclerotic disease, with the danger of coronary heart disease. Surgery should be performed in stage I patients only if the degree of stenosis is 80% or more [6, 13, 23]. However, this stage gains in importance if the patient has to undergo surgery for a different reason and there is a risk that a hypotensive episode may occur during that operation. In such cases, it is advisable to search for asymptomatic carotid stenoses and to relieve them if they are high grade lesions.

Clinical stage II is a stage in which the patient experiences intermittent cerebral insufficiency with transitory ischemic attacks in the form of amaurosis fugax, syncopal episodes, or other symptoms that may be interpreted as signs of an existing carotid stenosis. If the TIA is not fully reversible within 24 h (stage IIa), it can be classified as a prolonged reversible ischemic neurologic deficit (PRIND, stage IIb). It can only be differentiated from a definitive cerebral insult if cerebral ischemia is found during computed tomography. Usually, one may correctly locate the side on which the degenerative process has developed, but sometimes this is not possible in patients who present with global signs of cerebral insufficiency, e.g., vertigo, syncopal attack, forgetfulness, or abnormal psychological behavior. In such cases it can be very difficult to associate the clinical symptoms with an extracranial stenosis of the carotid arteries. Thoroughgoing, comprehensive differential diagnosis is necessary in order to rule out other possible causes, in particular an ischemic eye disease, which often goes undetected or is misdiagnosed. In occlusions of the contralateral side, an intracerebral steal effect should always be considered.

If, however, typical focal ischemic neurologic symptoms and temporary contralateral pareses or amaurosis fugax are present, the indication for surgery in a high grade stenosis is absolute. In a stenosis of lesser severity, the decision to operate depends on the type of arteriosclerotic wall lesion. Lesions constantly emitting emboli into the brain must be removed by surgery [28].

Clinical stage III ("progressive stroke") is the transition between functional and structural impairment. In this clinical stage, it is therefore very difficult to know whether surgery would benefit the patient; in fact, the only sure indication for operative intervention in this stage is an acute occlusion of the internal carotid artery. Sometimes, however, a very high grade stenosis, in other words, a subtotal occlusion, can be an indication for surgery [22]. The surgeon must be sure that the neurologic deficit has an extracranial cause and is not a result of repeated emboli spreading from ulcerated plaques in other vascular regions. During reconstruction, there is always the danger of converting an anemic infarction into a hemorrhagic one.

Clinical stage V represents complete and permanent stroke. Here, surgery can have only palliative value and is only feasible following absorption and organization of the infarcted area with scar tissue. Depending on the neurologic defects, it may be possible, even in this clinical stage, to prevent another CVA and thereby limit the neurologic deficit.

In cases where a clearly defined high-grade stenosis is present, together with unmistakable clinical symptoms, diagnostic measures may be limited to ultrasonic Doppler examinations without angiography, provided that clear evidence of ischemic brain damage or other brain disease has been demonstrated by computed tomography [1]. Experience shows that some patients with a carotid stenosis may have additional lesions, such as a brain tumor or heart disease.

Doppler ultrasound has proven extremely helpful as a screening method [21]. It has become the diagnostic method of choice alongside clinical examination, which includes auscultation and neurologic examinations, and it often allows the final diagnosis to be made [25].

Computed tomography is not always necessary in an asymptomatic, accidentally discovered carotid stenosis that is correctable prior to a more extensive surgical procedure. If computed tomography is done on a patient who has experienced a TIA with complete neurologic reversibility of symptoms, small, infarcted areas may be found, which are usually not a contraindication for surgery. In stage III, CT scanning during the first 6–8 h after the onset of symptoms may not contribute substantial information as to whether or not surgery should be attempted. More important are the patient's degree of consciousness and the time interval since the onset of acute symptoms. Full consciousness and reasoning ability may favor surgery. Not more than 6–8 h should have passed since the onset of symptoms [29]. Surgery is contraindicated if the patient is unconscious or stuporous. An operation may be attempted in exceptional cases, but only following computed tomography [7]. In stage IV of cerebral insufficiency the size of the defect or the number of small defects may help to decide whether or not vascular reconstruction will be of any benefit to the patient. If very large areas of the brain are locally or diffusely impaired, one must be very cautious in deciding whether to operate. Revascularization can lead to an overcompensated perfusion of the brain, which might not be tolerated in every case.

Angiography is still the most reliable diagnostic tool in selecting patients for surgery. All doubtful cases must undergo angiographic clarification, which allows adequate assessment of wall conditions in two planes. This requirement is met by classic carotid angiography with two projections. Digital subtraction angiography of the supra-aortic branches can be employed only as a screening method. Even if the contrast medium is injected intra-arterially, DSA may not always allow adequate delineation of the carotid bifurcation or more cranially localized loops with kinking stenoses. It is a great mistake to try to interpret blurred pictures of the carotid artery. In such cases, ultrasonic Doppler examinations or B-mode ultrasonography should additionally be utilized [19]. It is even better to repeat angiography, using the conventional method in two projections.

Angiography allows for classification of vascular wall lesions in most cases. Especially dangerous are mural atheroma or atheromatous plaques and debris from which microemboli tend to dislodge. Smooth, high-grade carotid stenoses must always be seen as precursors of an obstruction. Therefore, they should always be treated surgically during the asymptomatic stage I [22, 23].

If displastic vascular processes are suspected, X-rays should be obtained. Fibromuscular dysplasia or a kinking stenosis cannot be reliably assessed except by angiography. For this purpose, conventional angiography in two projection planes is better suited than digital subtraction angiography. While conventional angiography does of course involve a certain risk that can never be completely eliminated, the risk is very low in the hands of an experienced radiologist. Angiography should be performed if it is important for the further course of treatment, i.e., only if the patient consents to a possible operative correction and meets the requirements for general operability.

Finally, one must consider if the patient is taking certain drugs, especially anticoagulants or antiplatelet medication [5]. The risk of perioperative hemorrhage is undoubtedly higher in such patients. If surgery must be performed in spite of such medication, careful hemostasis is of the utmost importance. Laboratory examinations of the clotting system, including the thrombin time, are mandatory. Blood samples for type and crossmatching should be sent. Usually, blood units do not have to be available in routine reconstructions of the carotid arteries [9, 10].

C. Anesthesia (see also p. 201)

The fact that many patients are elderly means that additional risk factors pertaining to anesthesia and the operation itself are present. Besides metabolic and pulmonary disorders, coronary heart disease, myocardial infarction, and hypertension with concomitant arrhythmias are undoubtedly the most important risk factors. Preoperative antihypertensive therapy should be continued or extended, and beta-blocker therapy should not be discontinued. Preoperative digitalization should not be interrupted. Starting digitalis therapy before surgery cannot be recommended; instead, positive inotropic drugs should be administered intraoperatively. In untreated hypertension and coronary heart disease with one or two previous episodes of infarction, a Swan-Ganz catheter should be inserted for correct and reliable treatment of hypertensive episodes. As a rule, arterial pressure measurement should be done in addition to ECG monitoring (see pp. 195ff., 201).

Anesthesia should have only slight cardiodepressive side effects. Inhaled anesthetics such as halothane and isoflurane are preferred. A strong tendency toward hypertensive episodes during anesthesia makes it necessary to administer antihypertensive drugs in 30% of cases (see p. 195).

Arterial pressure measurement in combination with a Swan-Ganz catheter makes it easier to achieve a balance between preload-reducing drugs such as trinitrosan and afterload medications such as nifedipine (Adalat) and sodium nitroprusside for the prevention of left heart failure.

A large fall in systemic blood pressure may be expected during induction of anesthesia and is quickly reversible. Increasing the systolic pressure during occlusion of the internal carotid artery for improvement of cerebral perfusion is ineffective and carries the additional risk of provoking cardiac arrhythmias and a hypertensive crisis. During the surgical procedure, slight hyperventilation of the patient with constant checking of blood gas measurements is preferred, maintaining arterial pO_2 around values of 150 mmHg. Starting osmotic therapy intraoperatively just before the common carotid artery is occluded, as prophylaxis against cerebral edema, is controversial. Diffuse cerebral injury due to clamping is rare. Localized defects with perifocal edema cannot be treated by osmotic therapy.

The patient should recover from anesthesia after leaving the operating room. To prevent postoperative hypertensive episodes, adequate analgesia must be achieved. Prophylactic ventilation without hyperventilation must be continued under blood gas control until the patient is totally awake.

Postoperative hypertensive episodes must be treated immediately. Another cause of a hypertensive crisis, besides respiratory and cardiac disorders, may be a distended urinary bladder.

Hypertensive crises are often precursors of neurologic deficits. If neurologic deficits are present almost immediately after surgery, osmotic treatment should be started and artificial ventilation continued under careful control of blood pressure values. Without ventilation, there is a tendency toward cardiac decompensation and acute respiratory insufficiency. The patient's head should be raised on a pillow for adequate drainage following surgery. Also, adequate sedation is necessary. The patient should always remain in the intensive care unit for the first 24 h, as hemorrhage with immense tissue swelling may occur, leading to acute obstruction of the airways. Usually, adjustment of hypertensive treatment is also necessary postoperatively.

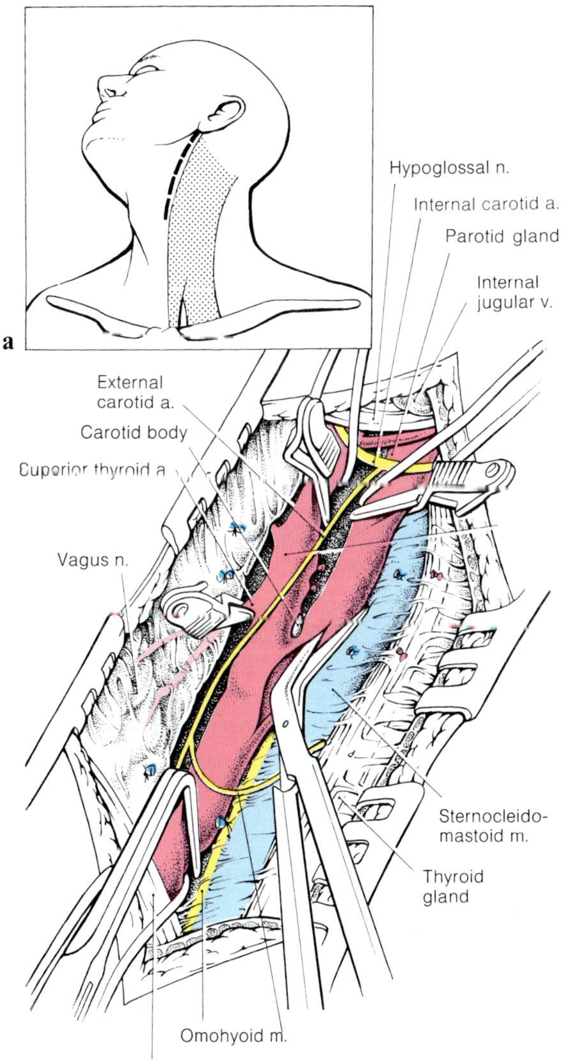

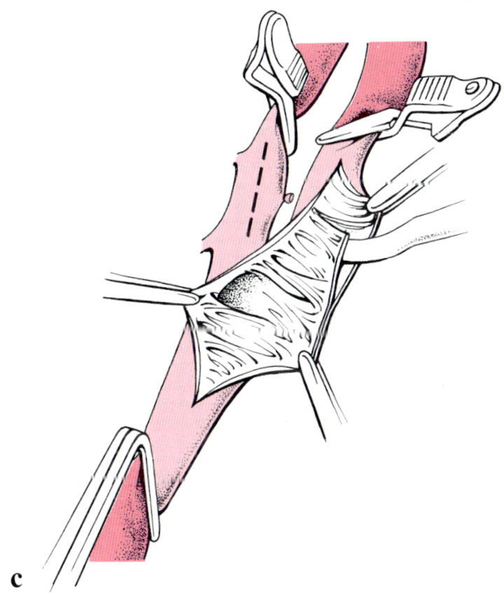

Fig. 18.1.4. a Incision along the anterior margin of the sternocleidomastoid muscle. Other types of incisions for exposure of the carotid artery are obsolete. **b** After opening the neurovascular sheath the hypoglossal nerve, together with its ansa, is exposed, and the vessel is incised following adequate exposure of the artery. **c** The incision must be extended over the arteriosclerotic plaques until an undiseased segment of the internal carotid artery and of the common carotid artery is reached. One should always watch out for lesions within the external carotid artery (*broken line*). If necessary, they should be removed by a separate arteriotomy

D. Positioning

The patient is placed in a supine position, with the head bent back slightly and turned toward the opposite side. Sometimes, the half upright position, as in a goiter operation, is recommended, usually by advocates of local anesthesia. This position is, however, not preferred by most surgeons. Dangerous hypotensive episodes may result if the thorax is kept upright while the legs remain lowered. The operating area to be disinfected includes the entire side of the neck, as well as the lower jaw and earlobe, and extends below the clavicle. When draping, the earlobe should remain uncovered in order to serve as an orientation point (Fig. 18.1.4a).

E. Surgical Approach

The surgical approach must allow for good exposure of the arterial region in question. This is best done by an incision made at the anterior margin of the sternocleidomastoid muscle (Fig. 18.1.4a). Anatomic variations must be considered, particularly the level of the carotid bifurcation. The internal carotid artery must be adequately exposed. The incision is extended upward to the lower margin of the earlobe. It should not be made ventral to the earlobe because of the greater chance of injuring the facial nerve. Transection of the transverse nerve of the neck cannot be avoided. The great auricular nerve, however, should be preserved. Sensory impairment near the ear is often found to be very disturbing postoperatively. After dividing the platysma and the anterior fascia of the neck, the sternocleidomastoid muscle is retracted dorsolaterally, and the common facial vein is transected. Dissection is performed medial to the jugular vein (Fig. 18.1.4b). The lymph nodes are displaced laterally. The descending branch of the ansa hypoglossi runs on the medial side of the jugular vein and should be preserved; however, if exposure is difficult, it may be divided without sequelae. One should always watch for the vagus nerve lying in the posterior portion of the neurovascular sheath. Its position, however, may vary: sometimes, it lies more in front, and in rare cases, it crosses the common carotid artery. If the vagus nerve is accidentally caught during proximal clamping of the carotid artery, postoperative paresis of the recurrent nerve will result.

Following dissection around the common carotid artery, the carotid bulb is exposed. Unnecessary manipulation should be avoided during this maneuver in order not to dislodge possible emboli. If an atheroma is expected at this site, early clamping of the common carotid artery may prevent embolic spread. However, oxygen supply to the corresponding hemispheres is thereby reduced. Therefore, this maneuver should be reserved for cases with a high risk of embolism.

F. Technique of Exposure

The hypoglossal nerve crosses the internal carotid artery in a lateral to medial direction. It courses one fingerbreadth beneath the anterior part of the digastric muscle and should be preserved. In a lower carotid bifurcation, exposure of the artery up to this nerve is sufficient. If the bifurcation lies higher, the hypoglossal nerve must be mobilized and retracted medially; often, the ansa hypoglossi must be divided first. Sometimes, the occipital artery, which crosses at this point, must also be transected (Fig. 18.1.3).

Dissection of the internal carotid artery may be easier if an umbilical tape is passed around the external carotid artery just distal to the bifurcation. Good exposure of the carotid bulb can be achieved by this maneuver. This also facilitates dissection of the internal carotid artery, which takes off medially. Adequate exposure of the external carotid artery is always of great value and should extend upward to the origins of the first branches. Separate origins of the superior thyroid artery, lingual artery, and facial artery are found in 80% of cases, trunk formation in 20% [16]. All three arteries arise from the external carotid artery in 50% of cases. The superior thyroid artery originates at the branching point of the common carotid artery in 20% and arises from the common carotid artery in 10%. This variation is more often found on the left side than on the right and in women more frequently than in men.

Cranial Exposure of the Internal Carotid Artery

Sometimes, lesions within the internal carotid artery reach all the way up to the base of the skull. If these findings are known preoperatively an elective procedure should be planned in a specialized medical center, as the exposure of the internal carotid artery beneath the skull is very difficult.

In emergency operations a high exposure is sometimes necessary, especially in tearing of an intimal ridge, rupture of a vessel caused by a faulty suture technique, or in repeat operations, e.g., after infection of a patched artery.

In this procedure, the anterior part of the digastric muscle must be divided. The jaw is pulled forward. Mobilization of the jaw joint is not usually necessary. During dissection further upward the stylohyoid muscle is encountered, on which the glossopharyngeal nerve decends. It must be carefully preserved. This exposure allows meticulous dissection of the internal carotid artery over a length of about 3–4 cm. Usually, dissection up to the base of the skull is possible. Chiseling away the mastoid process is not necessary. However, removal of the stylohyoid process may be advantageous. Sewing at the entry site of the internal carotid artery into the bone canal is difficult because of poor visualization. A vein interposition graft, however, can be anastomosed to the artery. The sutures may be anchored in the periosteal covering of the carotid canal. The proximal anastomosis is performed according to the usual technique.

G. Intraoperative Diagnostic Procedures

Intra-arterial pressure measurement in the internal carotid artery following clamping of the common carotid artery and the external carotid artery may give a good evaluation of the quality of collateral circulation. This helps one to decide whether or not an intraluminal shunt should be employed [20]. If retrograde flow pressure is more than 50 mmHg, it is not likely that clamping will cause an ischemic deficit. If retrograde flow pressure is under 50 mmHg or is less than one third of the mean systemic pressure, and if abnormalities in the EEG with changes in the evoked potentials are found, the insertion of an intraluminal shunt is advisable since perfusion over the circle of Willis may not be sufficient, especially if the contralateral carotid artery is obstructed.

Flow measurement does not play an important role in a routine operation. The results before and after reconstruction are flawed by reactive cerebral hyperemia. In the presence of a high grade stenosis or a dysplastic vascular system, the effect of reconstruction may be estimated and registered by flow measurements.

The routine application of EEG during the operation is controversial. In our own patients, the intraoperative EEG has never shown the development of a postoperative neurologic deficit with or without clamping or insertion of a shunt. Therefore, we have abandoned routine application of EEG. Evoked potentials may make a better analysis possible in the future and help answer questions concerning insertion of a shunt or duration of the clamping phase during surgery. Furthermore, electronic evaluation of the EEG may also yield helpful information.

Ultrasonic Doppler examination can provide a good postoperative assessment of the results of reconstruction. After putting on sterile rubber gloves, one can hold the probe over the wound area without difficulty, following the application of contact gel. SANDMANN [26] has recommended the use of a pulsed Doppler signal for registration of postoperative turbulence. Surgical results can be assessed with this method, and if errors are found, they can be corrected. This method of perturbation measurement is more sensitive than intraoperative control angiography. A static picture in only one projection allows gross assessment of surgical results. Peripheral vascular changes and, above all, distal stenoses of the internal carotid artery should be known to the surgeon preoperatively; therefore, intraoperative angiography for examination of peripheral intracranial vessels is indicated only in exceptional cases. The risk of contrast medium injection must be considered. Neurologic complications due to intraoperative angiography have been seen in several cases. If angiography is absolutely necessary, only small amounts of contrast medium should be injected into the common carotid artery and X-ray pictures taken immediately thereafter. A repeat injection using the same small amount of contrast medium may be given after a few minutes if the first attempt fails.

H. Reconstructive Techniques

I. Endarterectomy of the Internal Carotid Artery

Progress in the development of surgical techniques for reconstruction of the carotid bifurcation has always been tempered by uncertainty surrounding the question: how long can blood flow to the brain be interrupted without damage to cerebral tissue?

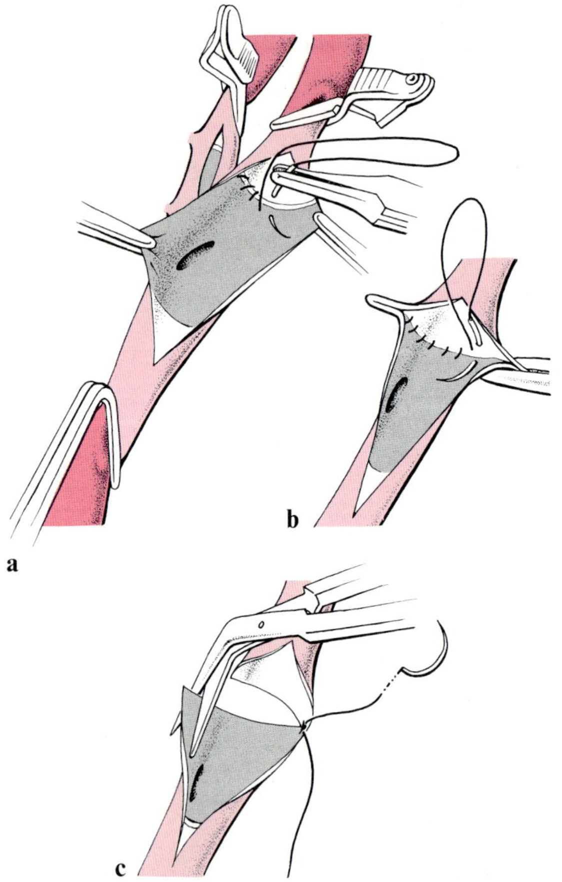

Fig. 18.1.5a–c. The arteriosclerotic plaque does not always tear at its upper circumference without leaving a ledge (**a**). In such cases the plaque should be transversely divided and the intimal ledge fixed by a continuous atraumatic suture. At the same time, the flaccid vascular wall can be plicated with an everting suture, eliminating possible elongation of the vessel (**b**). This technique is not sufficient in larger elongations with kinking stenoses or loop formations. In these cases, resection of elongated vascular segments and end-to-end reanastomosis of the vascular stumps is recommended (**c**)

Even though much knowledge and experience has been gained in the attempt to answer this question, the discussion is not over yet.

The systemic application of 5000 units of heparin is recommended before clamping. However, some investigators feel that heparinazation is not necessary. Following adequate dissection, the internal carotid artery is clamped as far cranially as possible, i.e., in a segment that is free of arteriosclerotic lesions. Blood flow in the external carotid artery and common carotid artery is then interrupted. Clamping of the common carotid artery is done last to prevent the dislodgement of blood clots or atheromatous debris [24]. A short arteriotomy is made to open the common carotid artery and is extended into the internal carotid artery until an undiseased segment of the artery is reached and the stenotic plug can be visualized in its entirety. The incision should extend approximately 1–2 fingerbreadths below the bifurcation. The local arteriosclerotic narrowings often begin at the level of the carotid bulb. Sometimes, it is necessary to lengthen the incision for a certain distance into the common carotid artery. The intraluminal shunt may now be inserted. Disobliteration without a shunt is easier.

The surgical risk is not increased if the shunt is inserted after disobliteration. Endarterectomy is accomplished by dissecting the atheromatous plug with a dissector (Fig. 18.1.4c). The correct cleavage plane lies between the media and adventitia. Sometimes, cleavage may be difficult in patients who have taken antiplatelet drugs. In about 50% of cases, the atheromatous plug may be disconnected cranially without leaving an intimal edge behind. In about as many cases, this is not possible, and a flap remains which must be tacked down to the underlying layers to prevent detachment and embolization (Fig. 18.1.5a). Disobliteration often leads to distinct elongation of the vessel if cleavage has taken place between the outer layer of the media and the adventitia. This must be corrected in every case. The firm, straight course of the vessel must be restored, either by internal plication of the back wall [14] or by resection of an entire segment of the vascular wall (Fig. 18.1.5b). Plication has the disadvantage that it leads to fold formation which protrudes into the vascular lumen, and this may encourage the development of an early occlusion. A segmental resection with reanastomosis of the vascular stumps after continuous over-and-over suture of the back wall may achieve better hemodynamic conditions (Fig. 18.1.5c). The vascular stumps must be adapted in size, which may make a longitudinal resection of a segment of the common carotid artery necessary. An arteriosclerotic plaque which continues into the distal portion of the internal carotid artery can usually be removed without leaving an intimal ledge [27].

II. Endarterectomy of the Common Carotid Artery

Endarterectomy of the internal carotid artery is continued into the common carotid artery. If the atheromatous plug with an inner core containing intima and media does not taper off at its proximal end, it must be sharply divided, leaving a small ledge behind. Because it lies in the direction of blood flow, it does not have to be tacked down. Retrograde application of the ring stripper may be unsafe and hazardous and will not remove the thickened intima without leaving a ledge or injuring the artery at its origin.

Now, the intraluminal shunt can be inserted, which is basically a polyethylene tube with a suture attached to it. Tapes are then placed around the artery proximally and distally and closed tightly. This is a simple, inexpensive, and reliable method of adapting the vessel lumen to the shunt. Other shunt models are discussed elsewhere (see p. 51). The wide variety of shunts on the market indicates that no ideal solution has been found yet. No clots should develop inside or around the shunt. It does not matter whether the shunt is first introduced proximally or distally. The following sequence of insertion is recommended: introduction of the shunt distally, fixation, retrograde flushing, flushing of the common carotid artery, careful insertion of the shunt into the common carotid artery without scuffing an atheroma, and finally, unclamping. Great care should be taken not to inflict any injury when inserting the shunt. This is especially important if the vascular walls are quite fragile, as in dysplasia. In such a case, a shunt should not be used [24]. The tapes used to hold the shunt in place should not be pulled too tightly; otherwise, the intima may be injured (Fig. 18.1.6a–d).

Fig. 18.1.6a–d. An intraluminal shunt should be inserted wherever it is necessary. It is first introduced distally and then flushed before its insertion into the proximal end of the arteriotomy to ensure that no blood clots or atheromatous debris are present that might embolize into the brain. The arteriotomy of the internal carotid artery is closed with a vein patch graft. The external carotid artery may be sutured directly (**b**). **c** Before finishing the suture of the vein patch to the artery, the intraluminal shunt is removed. **d** A vein patch graft should neither widen nor constrict the artery

III. Endarterectomy of the External Carotid Artery

The origin of the external carotid artery is exposed after the arteriosclerotic material has been removed from the internal carotid and common carotid arteries. A shunt may or may not be inserted. The external carotid artery must be freed of all atheromatous debris. The arteriosclerotic cylinder can sometimes be removed without leaving a ledge at the origin; in other cases, such a ledge may extend into the internal carotid artery. In the latter case, the ledge can be extracted using an elevator, or perhaps a ring stripper. Blind disobliteration is dangerous and should not be attempted. There is a high probability of thrombotic occlusion of the external carotid artery if endarterectomy is not done with the utmost care and if debris is not completely removed. If occluded, the artery cannot

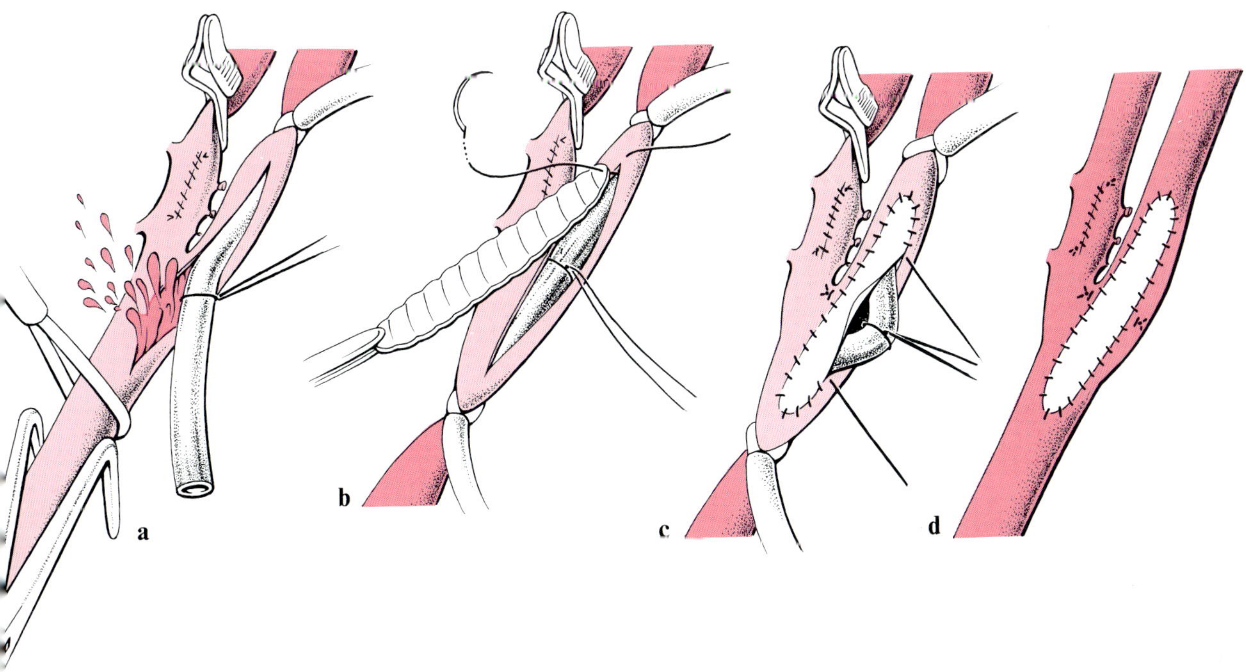

act as a collateral vessel. This leads to hemodynamically unfavorable conditions in the internal carotid artery, owing to the unequal blood flow in the common and internal carotid arteries. And these conditions in turn can facilitate thrombosis. A thrombosis of the external carotid artery may extend into the internal carotid artery. Therefore, the inner core of the arteriosclerotic intimal surface must be removed without leaving an edge or intimal flap within the external carotid artery. If there is doubt as to whether the distal end points of the arteriotomy contain such remaining edges, an additional longitudinal incision of the anterior wall of this artery must be performed. Under direct visualization, the thickened internal layer is sharply divided, and a continuous suture is used to tack down the end point. Usually, the incision in the external carotid artery can be closed by primary suture. A patch graft is recommended only if a transverse internal ledge or flap remains at the origins of the branches. The external carotid artery is patent if a pulse is felt in the temporal artery (Fig. 18.1.3).

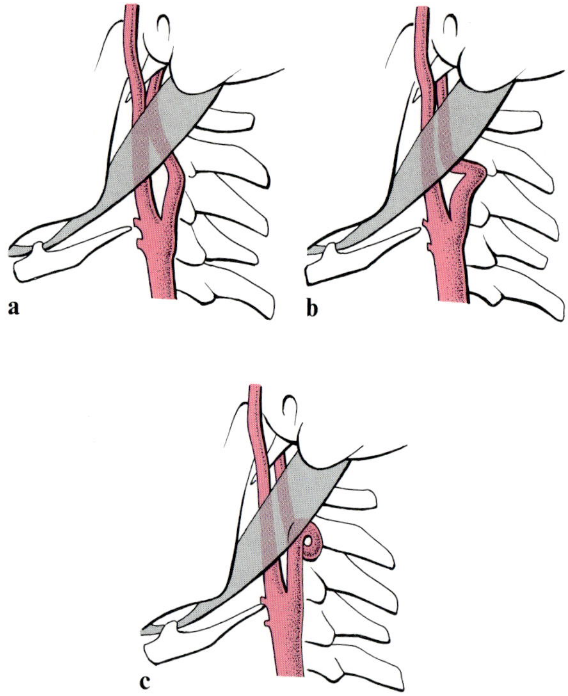

Fig. 18.1.7 a–c. Different types of elongations. **a** C-type elongation without kinking; **b** elongation without a stenotic kink; **c** elongation with coiling

IV. Surgical Management of an Elongated Internal Carotid Artery

Elongations of the internal carotid artery may require surgical correction. Kinking can cause stenoses with impairment of blood flow in certain head positions. Aneurysms and acute thromboses of elongated tortuosities have been observed. An everting suture [14] may shorten the artery by about 1.0–1.5 cm. This technique, however, can be recommended only in some cases because it creates a shelf within the artery. The resection of an elongated portion of the vessel with removal of the tortuous wall parts is preferred. The same is done in stenotic kinks and loop formations. Intimal cushions often develop within kinks. The back wall is closed with a continuous over-and-over 6-0 or 7-0 suture. Small differences in caliber may be compensated by the suture. If the differences are larger, the diameters of the vessel stumps must be adapted before suture. A shunt may be used in this operation. However, manipulations at the peripheral vascular stump may lead to injury of the intima. The shunt, if used at all, should be inserted only after the artery has been shortened. The anterior arteriotomy of both stumps is closed with a patch graft (Figs. 18.1.7 and 18.1.8).

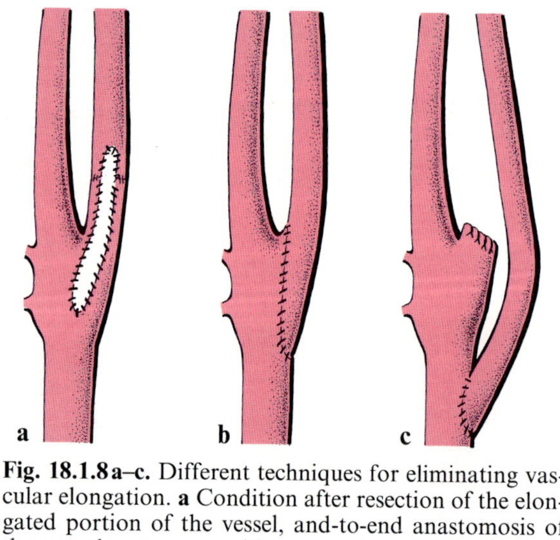

Fig. 18.1.8 a–c. Different techniques for eliminating vascular elongation. **a** Condition after resection of the elongated portion of the vessel, and-to-end anastomosis of the vascular stumps and incorporation of a patch graft. This surgical technique is always applicable. **b** After shortening, the stump of the internal carotid artery is tailored obliquely at the carotid bifurcation and reinserted end-to-end. **c** After transection of the internal carotid artery it is anastomosed obliquely end-to-side, proximal to its primary location. This technique is recommended only in exceptional cases

V. Surgical Management of an Elongated Common Carotid Artery

If all three arteries, internal, external, and common carotid, are greatly elongated, a segmental resection of the common carotid is advocated just beneath the carotid bifurcation. This allows for adequate straightening of the internal and external carotid arteries. If a stenosis at the origin of the internal carotid must be corrected at the same time, this artery is incised, starting at the bifurcation. Stenosis and elongation of the internal carotid are treated as described earlier. The back wall is sewn with a continuous over-and-over suture after segmental resection of the common carotid artery (Fig. 18.1.8).

VI. Closure of the Arteriotomy

The closure of the arteriotomy is usually done with a patch graft. Either an autogenous vein, harvested from the great saphenous vein above the medial malleolus, or a synthetic patch may be used. The patch is tailored to fit the caliber of the vessel. The suture should not constrict or widen the artery. The incision of the internal carotid artery may, of course, be closed by direct suture. However, the danger of immediate or late construction must be considered. A vein patch increases surgical security. Probes and shunts can be helpful [24, 25] during direct suture of the arteriotomy and to prevent narrowing of the lumen. However, their usefulness should not be overestimated.

The patch graft is held in place with a horizontal mattress suture at each corner of the arteriotomy. Back and front walls are sutured, starting at both corners. The intraluminal shunt is checked for patency before finishing the suture. Both arterial stumps are examined by opening the clamps briefly. The suture is then completed. The external carotid artery is unclamped first. Then, the clamp on the internal carotid artery is removed. During unclamping of the common carotid artery the origin of the internal carotid artery should be occluded. This maneuver directs dislodged embolic material into the external carotid artery circulation; it is a precaution to prevent debris from embolizing into the distal portion of the internal carotid artery. Bleeding from the stitches usually ceases spontaneously. Hemorrhage and small tears may occur in dysplastic or very thin vascular walls. In such cases, hemostasis may be achieved by applying fibrin glue to the sites. Supplementary sutures may worsen injury to the vascular wall. Following restoration of blood flow, the caliber of the internal carotid artery exceeds preoperative values. If the artery does not dilate, a Fogarty catheter should be introduced following a stab incision at the patch graft to widen distal segments of the artery. This maneuver eliminates incongruities in caliber which provoke thrombosis. The Fogarty catheter may also be employed in small vessels or spastic narrowings. This maneuver always leads to some injury of the endothelium. Therefore, dilatation should not be performed in vessels of normal caliber. A Redon drain is positioned within the wound area, and the neurovascular sheath is closed by continuous suture. However, this is not absolutely necessary. Continuous suture of the subcutis and platysma usually suffices. A continuous over-and-over backward suture with atraumatic 3-0 suture material should be used for the skin because of the danger of postoperative bleeding.

VII. Angioplasty of the External Carotid Artery

In occlusions of the internal carotid artery, revascularization of the external carotid artery may lead to improvement. A positive effect of this reconstructive procedure may be expected if retrograde flow in a collateral of the ophthalmic artery is found directed toward the circle of Willis. Revascularization is also indicated if an extra-intracranial bypass is planned. If a previously undiagnosed internal carotid occlusion is found after surgical exposure of the carotid bifurcation, angioplasty of the external carotid artery may be performed instead.

The occluded origin of the external carotid artery should be excised in a manner similar to profundaplasty at the femoral bifurcation. This is accomplished by ligating the internal carotid artery distally and transecting it.The incision is extended into the external carotid artery. Remnant portions of the vascular wall are resected. If necessary, local endarterectomy is performed. In such a case, the arteriotomy must be extended beyond the first branch arising from the external carotid artery (just as in profundaplasty). At the end of this procedure, a venous or a synthetic patch is sewn onto the artery. Sometimes, a portion of the resected internal carotid artery can be used as a patch graft following endarterectomy. The transition between the rather wide common carotid artery and the narrow external carotid artery should be as smooth and gradual as possible.

I. Postoperative Complications
(see also p. 157ff.)

I. Hemorrhage

The most common complication in a reconstruction of the carotid artery is hemorrhage. Because of the rich vascularization in the neck area and the common occurrence of postoperative hypertensive crises, most of the blood comes from transected skin vessels. Sometimes, vascular sutures may start to bleed again. This makes intensive postoperative care necessary. Massive hemorrhage may lead to mechanical obstruction of the airways, owing to displacement of the soft connective tissue in the neck. In such a case, reintubation may be very difficult and sometimes impossible. Therefore, the patient should be reintubated early if bleeding is suspected. Once the patient is intubated and spontaneous breathing is restored, it is justifiable in some situations to wait until the bleeding stops. However, in massive hemorrhage, the patient should be reintubated immediately and transported to the operating room with the wound under compression. Then, the skin sutures are quickly opened. Hemostasis is carried out using the standard procedures. Bleeding near the revascularized segment is stopped by suture ligation or application of fibrin glue. Reintervention has a high risk of infection. Therefore, during the postoperative course, the possiblity of septic arrosion must always be considered (see p. 167).

II. Nerve Injuries

Injuries of the recurrent nerve are the most common among those found postoperatively, occurring in 1% of our own patients. These are not direct injuries to the recurrent nerve. Instead, they are caused by accidentally catching the vagus nerve during clamping of the common carotid or internal carotid arteries. In some cases, direct puncture of the common carotid artery during angiography leads to bleeding from the puncture site. The hematoma leads to massive fibrosis around the carotid artery, thereby changing the anatomic position of the vagus nerve. Careful dissection around the common carotid artery and the vagus nerve is a sure way to avoid nerve damage [24].

Damage to the clearly visible hypoglossal nerve is rare. Accidental division of this nerve is avoidable. If this happens on one side, not much harm is done; it only leads to deviation of the tongue. However, division on both sides is a very severe complication, making spontaneous breathing almost impossible.

To avoid this extremely serious complication, a two-sided carotid stenosis is never corrected in one session. This is not, however, the strongest argument against simultaneous reconstruction. It is presently not possible to assess the effects on cerebral circulation if construction on both sides is attempted during the same session.

Injury to the ansa hypoglossi remains without sequelae. Also, division of the transverse cervical nerve does no harm. Numbness experienced after injury of the great auricular nerve is sometimes disturbing, but harmless. Patients sometimes complain about neuralgia within the innervated areas of the transected nerves. These can be relieved by scar revision or transection of the nerves at the punctum nervosum.

Temporary nerve injury may be caused by the retractor, which sometimes compresses the oral branch of the facial nerve. The same may happen to the hypoglossal nerve. These disorders due to retraction during surgery usually disappear within 3 months. In some cases it may take 6 months. Paresis of the facial nerve may develop if the incision is directed too near the angle of the jaw, leading to transection of the nerve. Therefore, the incision should always be made dorsal to the earlobe.

Injury to the accessory nerve is rarely seen. The sequelae are always severe. The nerve is damaged by excess compression during retraction of the deep tissue, which can be avoided.

Injury to the carotid body or the carotid sinus nerves has no postoperative sequelae. Manipulation near the carotid body during surgery can lead to circulatory depression and severe bradycardia. This complication may be eliminated immediately during surgery by infiltrating the carotid sinus nerves and carotid body with a local anesthetic.

III. Infection

Infection of a carotid reconstruction is very rare. The incidence in our own patients was 2–3 per

1000. An infected synthetic patch may be replaced by a vein patch, provided the carotid wall can be sutured. A vein graft within an infected area is also prone to rupture. For safety reasons, the infected vascular segment is sometimes resected and reconstructed with a vein graft harvested from the great saphenous vein. Oblique end-to-end anastomoses are performed. If possible, the external carotid artery should be reconnected.

Infection is a very serious complication. There is always danger of hemorrhage. One should not wait until it heals spontaneously. This allows massive fibrosis to develop around the reconstructed artery and makes reoperation more difficult. Hemorrhage can lead to acute respiratory distress by displacing connective tissue. Compression of the internal carotid artery may generate cerebral ischemia with a neurologic deficit.

IV. Cerebral Deficit

The most dreaded complication in carotid surgery is postoperative neurologic deficit. Copious statistics show the frequency of this complication to lie between 1% and 3% [1, 4, 6, 11, 19]. Although many investigations have been performed, the causes are not known exactly. Dissection at the carotid bifurcation may have caused embolization of arteriosclerotic debris. Another reason may be ischemic injury due to prolonged clamping. Ischemic brain damage is probably less common than microembolisms. At present, it is not known whether a neurologic deficit can be caused by distributive circulatory disorders due to peripheral stenoses. Furthermore, it is still a matter of controversy whether hyperemia after reconstruction may potentiate injury to preoperatively impaired cerebral tissue.

If a neurologic deficit occurs immediately after surgery, a technical error must first be assumed. In such a case, the patency of the vascular reconstruction is checked. This can be done by Doppler ultrasonography alone. If doubt remains, angiography is indicated. Immediate exposure without further diagnostic measures to test the patency of the vessel is justified if an occlusion is suspected. A technical error which has led to thrombotic occlusion must be corrected. The thrombus must be totally extruded until strong back bleeding occurs. However, a thrombotic occlusion which is immediately diagnosed and removed often leads to a neurologic deficit. Most likely, intracerebral vessels are in some way affected when thrombosis occurs. Therefore, local thrombolysis by streptokinase administration in the distal cerebral arteries is recommended. This procedure has a high risk and is only acceptable if structural metabolism has not been damaged. Routine administration of streptokinase is not justified in postoperative occlusions of the internal carotid artery.

According to large scale studies, half of all cerebral deficits end in cerebral coma, leading to an apallic syndrome or death. The other half involve larger or smaller neurologic defects which may be reversible to some degree. The number of postoperative cerebral deficits should not exceed those occurring spontaneously. An upper limit of 3% can be postulated. The risk of a cerebral deficit is greater in a contralateral occlusion of the carotid artery than in a one-sided carotid stenosis. The opinion of a neurosurgeon should be sought before deciding whether a protective extra-intracranial bypass is preferable to reconstruction of the contralateral stenosis in a patient with a symptomatically occluded internal carotid artery on one side and an asymptomatic stenosis on the other.

Other complications may be lymph fistula or injuries to veins or to the parotid gland. These were not observed in our own patients. Indurations of the lymph nodes may occur occasionally.

J. Reinterventions

Depending on the author, recurrent stenoses are reported as developing in 3%–18% of all patients within 1–5 years postoperatively. They are usually asymptomatic. The development of such recurrences correspond to the character of the underlying disease. High grade and hemodynamically effective recurrent stenosis is an indication for surgery. Reoperation is not different from the primary procedure. Dissection is more difficult, owing to scar tissue formation, and therefore the surgical risk is increased. It is a great advantage to free the proximal common carotid artery first. Reconstruction of the recurrent stenosis is not always possible. In such a case, the whole area of the endarterectomized vessel must be resected. Interposition of a vein or synthetic graft is necessary. It must be ascertained whether the proximal and distal stumps can be anastomosed to the interposition graft. The external carotid artery cannot be preserved in every case. If a long portion of the internal carotid artery is greatly narrowed, it is better not to reattach the internal carotid and instead to perfuse the external carotid artery.

Reoperation is also sometimes necessary in anastomotic aneurysms or aneurysms of the incorporated venous patch graft.

REFERENCES

1. Balzer K, Carstensen G (1985) Rekonstruktionen an der A. carotis. Ökonomie der Diagnostik und Ergebnisse. DMW 110:510–512
2. Blaisdell FW, Hall AD, Thomas AN (1966) Surgical treatment of chronic internal carotid artery occlusion by saline endarterectomy. Ann Surg 163:103–111
3. Breslau PJ, Strandness DE (1984) Rezidivstenose nach karotischer Endarteriekomie. Langenbecks Arch Chir 364:474–475
4. Brott T, Thalinger K (1984) The practice of carotid endarterectomy in a large metropolitan area. Stroke 15:950–955
5. Canadian Cooperative Stroke Study Group (1978) A randomized trial of aspirin and sulfinpyrazone in threatened stroke. N Engl J Med 299:53–59
6. Chambers BR, Norris JW (1984) The case against surgery for asymptomatic carotid stenosis. Stroke 15:964–967
7. Courbier R (1985) Basis for a classification of cerebral arterial diseases. Current Clinical Practice 22, Excerpta Medica, Amsterdam
8. Eastcott HHG (1984) Colour atlas of carotid surgery. Single surgical procedures no. 12. Reuter Verlag, Berlin New York
9. Fein J (1984) A history of surgery of cerebrovascular disease. In: Smith R (ed) Strokes and the extracranial arteries. Raven, New York
10. Fein JM, Flamm ES (1985) Cerebrovascular surgery, vol II. Springer, Berlin Heidelberg New York
11. Fields WS, Lemak NA (1976) Joint study of extracranial arterial occlusion. X. Internal carotid artery occlusion. JAMA 235:2734–2738
12. Gottstein U (1976) Zur Pathogenese der Hirnischämie unter besonderer Berücksichtigung der Risikofaktoren. Internist 17:1
13. Hennerici M, Rautenberg W, Mohr S (1982) Stroke risk from symptomless extracranial artery disease. Lancet II:1180
14. Imperato AM, Linn JPT (1967) Vertebral-arterial-reconstruction: internal plication and vein-patch-angioplasty. Ann Surg 166:213
15. Kortmann H, Krämling HJ, Utz F, Becker HM (1986) Chirurgie der zerebrovaskulären Insuffizienz. Ergebnisse 5 Jahre nach Desobliteration der A. carotis. Münch Med Wschr 128:21–24
16. Lang J (1979) Gehirn- und Augenschädel. In: von Lanz T, Wachsmuth W (eds) Kopf. Springer, Berlin Heidelberg New York (Praktische Anatomie, vol I, part 1B)
17. von Lanz T, Wachsmuth W (eds) (1955); Hals. Springer, Berlin Göttingen Heidelberg, p 147 (Praktische Anatomie, vol I, part 2)
18. Lippert H (1967) Arterienvarietäten. Klinische Tabellen 1–3, 51, Med. Klinik 14, 18, 19 und 21. Urban & Schwarzenberg, München Berlin Wien
19. Matsumoto GH, Rumwell CB (1983) Screening of carotid arteries by noninvasive duplex scanning. Am J Surg 145:609–610
20. Moore WS, Hall AD (1969) Carotid artery back pressure. A test of cerebral tolerance to temporary carotid occlusion. Arch Sur 99:702–709
21. Neuerburg-Heusler D (1984) Dopplersonographische Diagnostik der extracraniellen Verschlußkrankheit. VASA [Suppl] 12:59–70
22. Ringelstein EB, Zeumer H (1984) Die sogen. arteriosklerotische Pseudoocclusion der A. carotis interna: Pathogenetische Aspekte, Diagnostik und Therapie. Angio 6:11–18
23. Roederer GO, Langlois YE, Jäger KA, Primozich JF, Beach KW, Phillips DJ, Strandness E (1984) The natural history of carotid arterial disease in asymptomatic patients with cervical bruits. Stroke 15:605–613
24. Sandmann W (1983) Supraaortische Rekonstruktiven. In: Carstensen G (eds) Intra- und postoperative Komplikationen. Springer, Berlin Heidelberg New York, pp 80–88
25. Sandmann W (1985) Rekonstruktive Chirurgie der supraaortischen Arterien: Fortschritte und Kontroversen. In: Sperling M (eds) Gefäßrekonstruktion und Gefäßersatz im Wandel der letzten 25 Jahre. TM-Verlag, Hameln
26. Sandmann W, Peronneau P, Kremer K (1980) Carotischirurgie und Pertubationsmessung. Der Einfluß einer neuen, hämodynamischen, intraoperativen Kontrollmethode auf das Rekonstruktionsgebiet. Angio 2:277
27. Thompson JE, Talkington CM (1982) Carotid endarterectomy. In: Warlow C, Morris PJ (eds) Transient ischemic attacks. Marcel Dekker, New York, pp 253–282
28. van Dongen RJAM (1984) Angiographische Pathomorphologie der A. carotis aus chirurgischer Sicht. In: Mahler F, Nachbuhr B (eds) Zerebrale Ischämie. Huber, Bern, pp 125–129
29. Vollmar J (1983) Rekonstruktive Chirurgie der Arterien, 3rd edn. Thieme, Stuttgart

18.2 Occlusions of the Vertebral Artery

G. CARSTENSEN and K. BALZER

CONTENTS

A. General Remarks

The vertebral artery is the first branch of the subclavian artery. It is an important collateral vessel to the ipsilateral arm in occlusions or high grade stenoses of the proximal subclavian artery. The most common circulatory disorder in this artery is not stenosis or occlusion of the vertebral artery itself, but rather a compromised and reversed blood flow through the vessel, owing to occlusions or stenoses at the origin of the subclavian artery. This disorder is called the "subclavian steal syndrome" and is described in Chap. 18.4 [11, 12].

B. Anatomy

The vertebral artery arises on both sides from the ascending subclavian artery, proximal to the origin of the thyrocervical trunk in 90% of cases. The frequency of atypical origins is equal on both sides. However, the right vertebral artery has a tendency to branch off more laterally, and the left one more medially. The following percentages verify these observations: in 4% the right vertebral artery arises from the subclavian artery distal to the thyrocervical trunk; on the left side this is the case in less than 0.1%. The right artery originates directly at the aortic arch in less than 0.1%, and the left one in 4%. On the right side, the artery arises more than 2 cm proximal to the thyrocervical trunk – and often from the bifurcation of the innominate artery – in 4% of cases; for the left side, the frequency is 3%.

Less significant are the following percentages: origin of the vertebral artery together with the thyrocervical trunk on the right in less than 1%, on the left 2%; origin at the common carotid artery on the right less than 1%, on the left 0%; double origin from the aorta and subclavian artery or accessory vertebral arteries and from the thyrocervical trunk, on the right less than 1%, on the

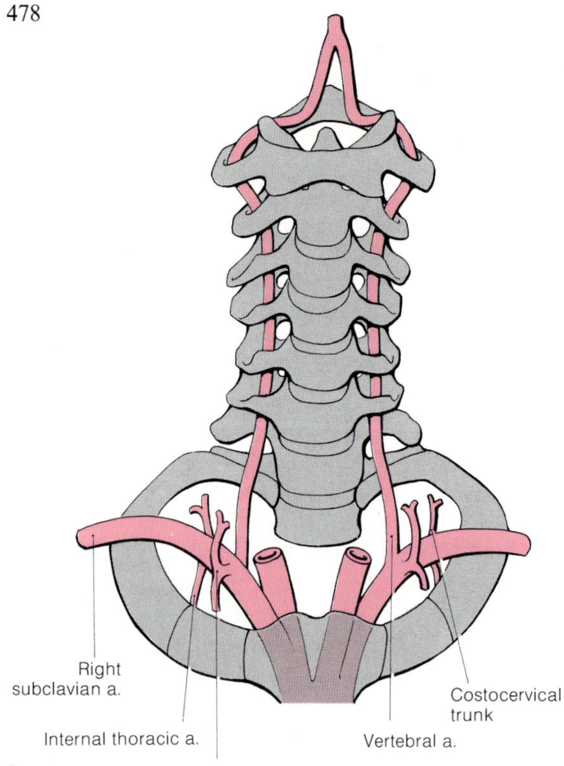

1

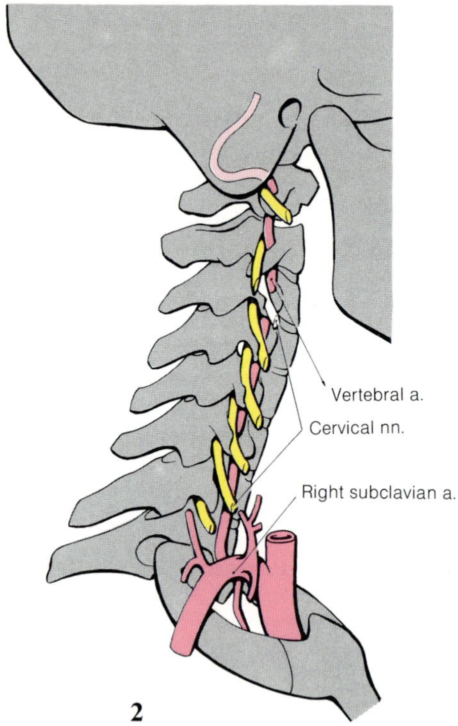

2

Figs. 18.2.1 and 18.2.2. Front (**Fig. 1**) and side (**Fig. 2**) view of the vertebral artery [2]

Figs. 18.2.3 and 18.2.4. Looping of the vertebral artery on the cranial aspect of the atlas. Notice the topographical relationship to the spinal nerve

left 1%. The right vertebral artery shares a common course with the thyrocervical trunk, inferior thyroid artery, and costocervical trunk in less than 1%. The left artery is a direct branch of the aortic arch in 4%, branching off proximal to the subclavian artery in 3%, and distal to it in 1% [7].

It is not known whether unilateral or bilateral aplasia of the vertebral artery exists. If it does, it is very rare. Sometimes, anatomic variation may be mistaken for aplasia. From the surgical standpoint it is important that the vertebral artery usually arises dorsally. The vertebral artery reaches the vertebral canal through the foramen of the transverse process of the sixth cervical vertebra in 90% of cases. On the left side it enters more often into a different foramen: C_5 in 5%, C_4 in 2%, C_7 in 2% and C_3 in 1%. The topographic-anatomic relationship of the vertebral artery to its neighboring regions is important for exposure. The subclavian artery lies anteriorly. On the left side, the thoracic duct joins the venous angle. The sympathetic chain, with its third cervical ganglion, lies behind the artery. The vertebral artery is well protected against injuries after it enters the foramen of the transverse process. It is, however, sensitive to mechanical strain, which is present to a higher degree at this point.

Both vertebral arteries curve forward at the level of the atlas and join to form the basilar artery, which passes along the underside of the brain stem and supplies the circle of Willis, together with both carotid arteries. This is a unique communicating arterial system which easily compensates carotid occlusions by diversion of flow to undersupplied regions. In the same way, vertebral occlusions may be compensated by the carotid circulation. Whether this intricately balanced arterial system will react properly when one of the four inflow arteries is occluded cannot be predicted in each individual case. For example, a thrombosis of both vertebral arteries may, on the one hand, lead to basilar artery occlusion with brain stem infarction and death or may, on the other hand, remain unnoticed. The manifestation of a neurologic deficit varies between these two extremes (Figs. 18.2.1–18.2.4).

3

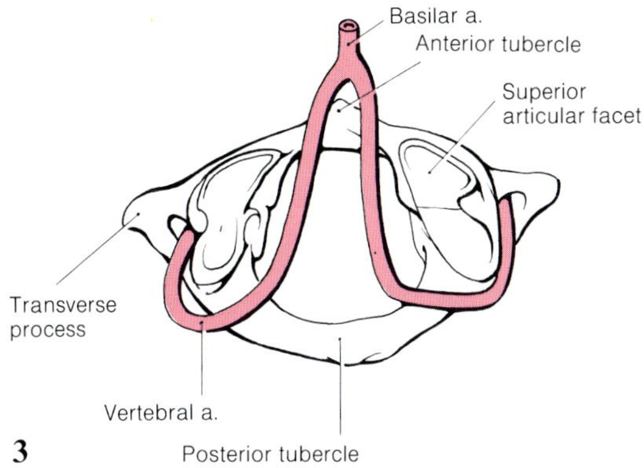

4

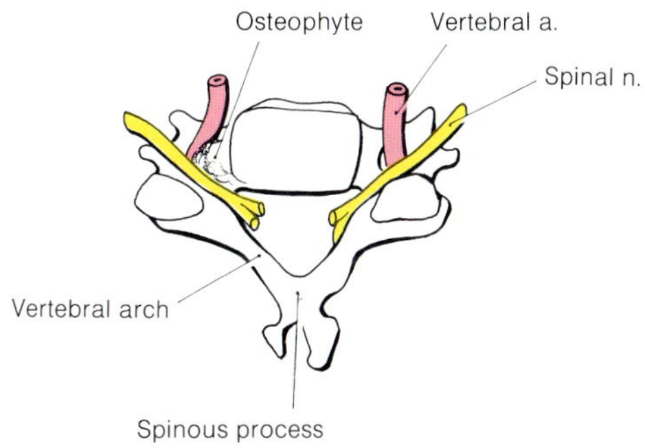

C. Indication for Reconstruction

Vertebrobasilar insufficiency is much less common than carotid insufficiency and is clinically less remarkable [1]. Obscure neurologic symptoms such as vertigo or vaguely defined visual disorders cannot be exactly classified as symptoms of vascular disease since they can also occur in other neurologic disorders. Degenerative lesions of the cervical spine lead most commonly to symptoms of vertebrobasilar insufficiency. Therefore, careful differential diagnosis is absolutely essential for correct patient selection. Vascular reconstruction may be considered only after the full spectrum of differential diagnosis has been covered.

But this does not mean that the vertebro-basilar insufficiency syndrome can be neglected. The "subclavian steal syndrome" is easy to recognize, and its treatment is clearly defined. The assessment and treatment of isolated vertebral lesions is much more difficult [5].

One well-developed vertebral artery supplies enough blood to the basilar circulation. Therefore, vascular surgery is indicated only when there are lesions on both sides or a total occlusion on one side and a high grade stenosis on the other. Of course, the situation must be assessed differently if collateral flow through the carotid arteries is insufficient.

Most lesions are found at the origin of the vertebral artery. They are usually arteriosclerotic stenoses or, rarely, hemodynamically significant elongations with kinks. Along its course through the bony vertebral canal, osteoarthritic lesions may impinge on the vertebral artery and cause compression. At this location, access to the vertebral artery is difficult. Therefore, bypass operations to the atlantal loop are becoming more important.

Preoperative angiography is a mandatory diagnostic procedure in lesions of the vertebral artery. The numerous anatomic variations and the complicated course of this artery justify this requirement. Furthermore, computed tomography should be used for differential diagnosis, e.g., to exclude tumorous processes in the cerebellum or extensive infarct zones.

Among the symptoms of vertebrobasilar insufficiency are postural or rotatory vertigo, so-called drop attacks, that is, sudden unavoidable drops with or without short unconsciousness [9, 10], double vision, transitory paresis of ocular muscles, scotomas, and even blindness. Often, the neurologic deficits are caused by head and neck movements.

D. Positioning

The patient should be in the same position as for a carotid operation. The head is turned away from the operating area and slightly reclined. It is important to let the ipsilateral shoulder hang freely. This may be facilitated by putting a padded wedge between the shoulders. The arms are pulled downward and fixed close to the patient's body. In this position, adequate exposure of the vertebral artery by a supraclavicular approach is usually possible. The entire area of the thorax, including the sternum and the side of the neck, should be prepared and disinfected. This is a precaution in case the incision has to be extended quickly. The incision may be lengthened in the direction of a median sternotomy or by dividing the clavicle (Fig. 18.2.5a).

The same position is necessary to expose the vertebral artery at the level of the atlantal loop [2]. The head must be shaved along a line extending from the corner of the eye across the ear to

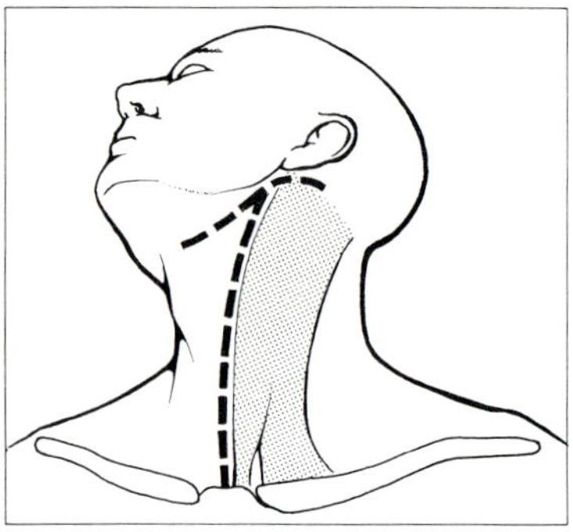

a

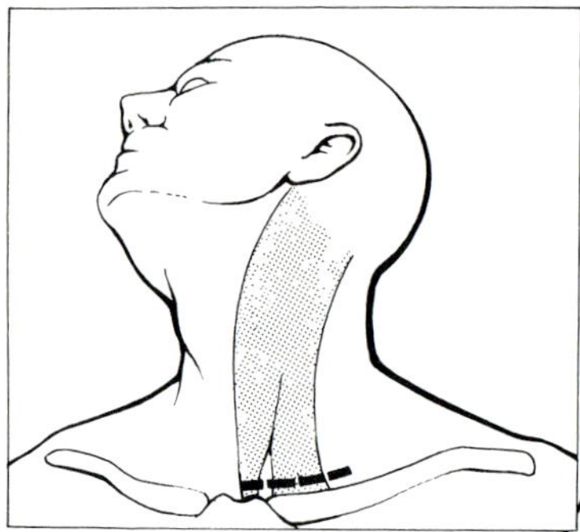

b

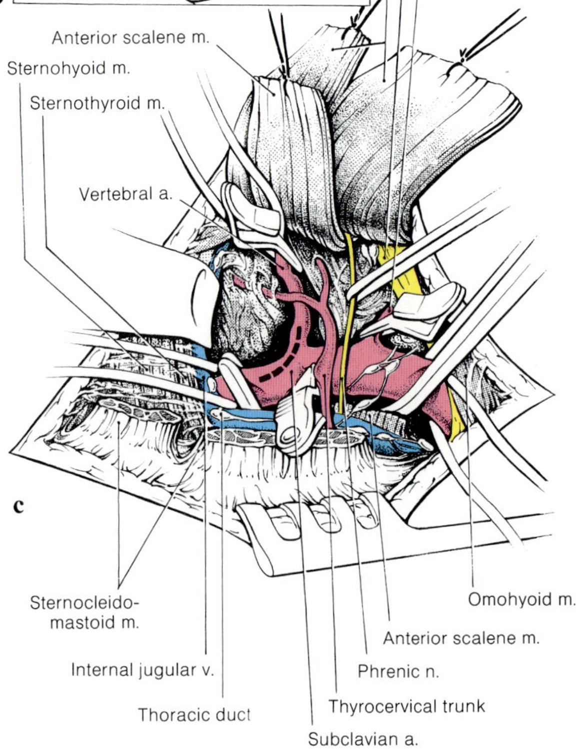

c

Fig. 18.2.5. a Exposure of the vertebral artery in the region of the atlantal loop may be achieved by an antero-lateral or anterior approach in the region of the atlantal loop. The anterior approach allows for simultaneous exposure of the carotid artery and gives a better visualization of the area. The anterolateral approach exposes the proximal carotid artery or the subclavian artery and the origin of the vertebral artery. **b** The supraclavicular approach is recommended for the exposure of the vertebral artery at its origin and the anterior approach for visualization of the vertebral artery at its atlantal loop. **c** Supraclavicular approach following division of the skin and sternocleidomastoid muscle. Notice the phrenic nerve running downward on the scalene muscle. After division of the anterior scalene muscle, the subclavian artery is visualized. The vertebral artery is exposed in its proximal portion

the dorsal midline of the head. In this case, the entire side of the neck, including the supraclavicular triangle, must be disinfected since this approach must also provide access to the donor arteries (Fig. 18.2.5b).

E. Technique of Exposure (Supraclavicular Approach)

The incision is started one fingerbreadth above the clavicle at the sternoclavicular joint and is extended about 10–12 cm laterally. The clavicular portion of the sternocleidomastoid muscle is divided. The veins crossing this area must be ligated. The muscle is transected at its clavicular origin. Blunt as well as sharp dissection of the subcutaneous tissue and lymph nodes is performed until the anterior scalene muscle appears, lateral to the jugular vein. The brachial plexus, running just beside the anterior scalene muscle, must not be injured. The phrenic nerve lies at the anterior margin of the anterior scalene muscle or, rarely, on the midportion or lateral edge of this muscle. It is a very fragile nerve which must be preserved at all costs. There may be two phrenic nerves (accessory phrenic nerve) on one side, but this is very rare. The thoracic duct must not be injured as the lymph nodes are dissected medially. If lymphatic secretion occurs, suture ligation of the leaking lymphatic vessels must be performed. An injured thoracic duct can be ligated without harm. This is recommended if there is doubt. A lymph fistula of the thoracic duct only rarely closes spontaneously. The jugular vein is mobilized laterally. An umbilical tape need not be put around it. If, however, tapes are necessary to retract the vein, one should be careful not to injure the thoracic duct entering at the venous angle or the vagus nerve running within the neurovascular sheath (Fig. 18.2.5c).

The next step is to divide the anterior scalene muscle. The subclavian artery runs just beneath this muscle. The brachial plexus descends alongside it and must be carefully reflected when the muscle is divided. In anatomic anomalies such as a cervical rib, dissection is carried out in the same manner. The origin of the anterior scalene muscle is divided at the first rib. The subclavian artery can then be seen arching forward and, under it, the pleura, which must not be injured when passing an umbilical tape around the artery. The thyrocervical trunk and the costocervical trunk should be visualized. Hemorrhage within the operating area may lead to serious complications because of the limited view of all structures. Hemostasis may be difficult to achieve by clamping vessels. Tapes are passed around the subclavian artery, and the vessel is followed along its proximal portion. The origin of the vertebral artery may vary (see p. 13). The branching point of this artery may be exactly identified in the angiogram if the vertebral artery arises directly from the aortic arch. It should be ligated proximally, divided, and reimplanted at a more favorable site. The thyrocervical trunk is especially suited for this purpose. The concomitant vertebral vein, which often surrounds the artery in the form of a venous plexus, should be handled carefully since hemorrhage of this vessel is very difficult to control. The subclavian artery is adequately exposed proximal and distal to the origin of the vertebral artery. This provides enough space for applying arterial clamps on both sides.

F. Intraoperative Diagnostic Procedures

As with surgery of the carotid artery, intraoperative measurement of blood pressure and flow is also possible in the vertebral artery. These measurements, however, are not obligatory in this case. EEG registration does not provide any valuable information during reconstructions of the vertebral artery and is therefore not indicated. An intraluminal shunt is never needed. Such a maneuver would, moreover, be technically difficult. In rare cases of carotid occlusions on both sides with only one patent vertebral artery, insertion of an intraluminal shunt may be considered. The technique of shunting is the same as described for the carotid artery (see p. 471).

G. Reconstructive Techniques

I. Endarterectomy of the Origin of the Vertebral Artery

After clamping the subclavian artery (as far proximally as possible) and the vertebral artery, a stab incision is made at the origin of the vertebral artery and extended into the subclavian artery in the proximal direction and also into the vertebral artery. An arteriosclerotic plaque can easily be dissected free with an elevator in the correct cleavage plane. An edge or flap is hardly ever left because the further course of the vertebral artery is almost always free of arteriosclerotic stenoses. Only rarely does an atheromatous plug extend further distally. However, should a shelf or flap remain, it is anchored to the wall by sutures. A ring stripper should not be used; otherwise, intimal flaps or edges might develop at sites which cannot be reached for fixation. Dilatation of the peripheral portions of the artery with a balloon catheter seems inadvisable in view of the avoidable injury this would cause to the endothelium.

If in addition the subclavian artery is narrowed at the vertebral origin, disobliteration or patch angioplasty is indicated. While disobliterating the vessel, care must be taken not to dissect in a plane that is too close to the adventitia. This may result in injury to the vascular wall with a resultant dissection that continues distally or may even lead to rupture of the vessel. The subclavian artery is a very delicate vessel. The procedure is completed by suturing a venous or synthetic patch graft onto the arteriotomy.

II. Surgical Management of an Elongation of the Vertebral Artery

Elongations of the proximal segment of the vertebral artery may lead to kinks that affect blood flow. They are corrected according to the same principles as described for the carotid artery. The elongated vascular segment containing the kink is resected or shortened by an everting suture plication of the back wall. In this way, one avoids performing the suture in flimsy, friable vascular tissue, which holds sutures poorly. The vascular wall gains firmness and stability by plication. If a friable vascular wall is directly sutured, it may exhibit significant leakage after blood flow is restored. Such a complication is difficult to control. Of course, the everting suture plication of the back wall does lead to rigidity of the wall, with shelf formation; this narrows the lumen to some extent. The arteriotomy is closed with a patch graft.

III. Transposition of the Vertebral Artery

If the vertebral artery arises further medially, e.g., from the aortic arch or the proximal portion of the subclavian artery, it is easier to transpose the vertebral artery to a larger vessel of the thyrocervical trunk or directly to its main stem. The vertebral artery stump is closed with a transfixion ligature as far proximally as possible. The thyrocervical trunk is visualized. The inferior thyroid artery is exposed, ligated distally, and divided. The anterior wall of the stump of the thyroid artery is incised longitudinally, and the vertebral artery is then implanted end-to-end in the usual fashion. Patch angioplasty of the anterior wall is performed in addition. Any stenosis of the origin of the thyrocervical trunk must be corrected.

IV. Bypass Methods for Stenosis or Elongation

Vein bypass grafting may be the method of choice if very unfavorable conditions at the origin of the vertebral artery make other reconstructive procedures too difficult to perform [2]. The vein graft may be connected proximally to a segment of the subclavian artery or to the common carotid artery if better conditions are found in this vessel. Distal attachment is performed on the front or lateral side of the vertebral artery. This procedure must be individualized according to local conditions. Synthetic grafts should not be used since the calibers of the vessels are very small.

V. Surgical Transposition of the Vertebral Artery

To compensate elongations with kinks, NEUGEBAUER [8] has recommended transection and antefixation of the thyrocervical trunk, with slight forward twisting of the subclavian artery and simultaneous shifting of this vessel into a different position. The advantage of this method is that the vertebral artery is not traumatized. Kinking of the vertebral artery may be corrected by this method in a few cases. However, more extensive elongations of the vessel cannot be compensated. Furthermore, a healthy undiseased vessel is transected during this procedure, and the subclavian artery is transposed from its anatomic position without compelling reasons for doing so.

H. Closure of the Arteriotomy

In exceptional cases, such as a transposition, an oblique end-to-end anastomosis may be performed. Patch graft angioplasty is always the method of choice in all other reconstructions. This creates a smooth and gradual transition from the subclavian artery to the vertebral artery. The suture technique must be meticulous for adaptation of the very delicate arterial walls, especially following disobliteration of the vertebral artery. Hemostasis is desirable. If hemostasis has not been achieved after completion of the suture, full blood flow from the subclavian artery should not be restored, as this could lead to tearing at the stitches. It is necessary to wait a few minutes after covering the suture line with a gelatin net, collagen pad, or hot gauze. If hemorrhage from small stitches continues, reclamping the vessel and applying fibrin glue to the holes could be successful.

After hemostasis is achieved at the anastomosis, the wound area is checked for insufficient lymphatic vessels. Secreting lymph vessels are closed with sutures. Fibrin glue may also help to control lymph secretion and to avoid postoperative complications. After placing a Redon drain within the wound area, the sternocleidomastoid muscle is reattached to its origin. The wound is closed layer by layer.

I. Special Considerations in Surgery of the Right Vertebral Artery

Because of possible anatomic differences between the right and left side, the surgical approach and procedure must be adapted accordingly. Exposure of the right vertebral artery is easier, owing to the fact that the thoracic duct is missing and the takeoff of the vertebral artery lies farther distally. Exposure of the vertebral artery without division of the anterior scalene muscle is possible by a direct approach, lateral to the jugular vein.

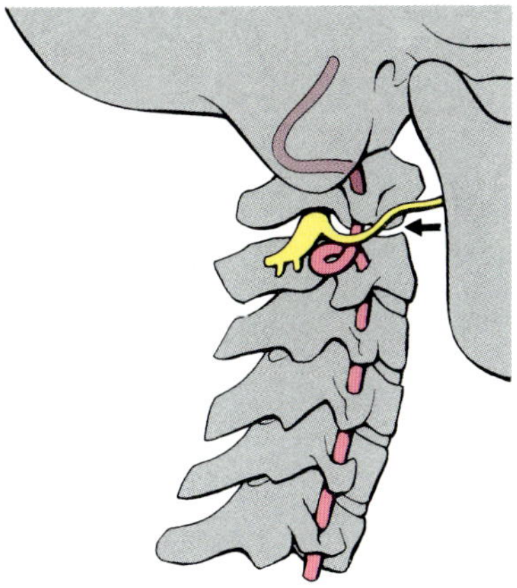

Fig. 18.2.6. The orientation point for exposure of the vertebral artery at its atlantal loop is the atlantoaxial joint. It lies anterior and medial to the vertebral artery and the transverse process

J. Exposure of the Vertebral Artery in Its Bony Canal

A reconstructive procedure in this region is done in only a few patients in whom external compression or narrowing of the vertebral artery within its bony canal is shown by angiography. Possible causes are osteoarthritic lesions or prolapse of portions of the vessel into the intervertebral space. Direct access to this region is achieved by an incision made at the posterior border of the sternocleidomastoid muscle. The accessory nerve is carefully preserved and the longus colli muscle dissected free. The transverse processes of the cervical vertebrae are exposed. The bony canal is opened over the affected segment, and the vertebral artery is dissected free. Usually, relief of compression by the bone restores blood flow completely. Sometimes surgical shortening of the artery or patch angioplasty may be necessary. The entire procedure is technically difficult and should be performed in only the most carefully selected cases (Fig. 18.2.6).

K. Reconstruction of the Distal Vertebral Artery

Reconstruction of the distal portion of the vertebral artery is indicated where there are obstructive lesions in the uppermost segment or multiple stenoses in the lower and middle segments, or where the vertebral origin is inoperable. Furthermore, reinterventions to eliminate arteriovenous fistula along the course of the artery or damage to the artery at the level of the axis caused by whiplash injuries are also indications [2].

I. Anatomy

The vertebral artery is accessible for surgical correction in its atlantal loop portion alone. Before the two vertebral arteries join to form the basilar artery, they leave the bony canal on their way across the transverse process of the atlas to the great foramen.

II. Exposure

Exposure of the distal portion of the vertebral artery can be achieved by an anterolateral or anterior approach. If an anterolateral approach is chosen, the incision is extended dorsally with division of the sternocleidomastoid muscle at the mastoid process. This allows for exposure of the vertebral artery distal to the transverse process of the atlas and the lateral articulation between atlas and axis.

In the anterior approach, the incision is lengthened anteriorly, passing in front of the ear. It may also be extended all the way to the base of the skull. Mobilization of the lower jaw facilitates exposure of the distal vertebral artery, anterior surface of the spine, and the portion of the internal carotid artery just beneath the base of the skull. The anterior approach to the distal vertebral artery is more advisable. In both incisions, the great auricular nerve must be transected. The incisions also lie very close to the accessory nerve.

The most prominent marker is the atlantoaxial articulation which lies in front of and medial to the vertebral artery and the transverse process [2]. The origins of the capitis longus muscle and the medial scalene muscle are divided at the transverse process of the first, second, and third cervical vertebrae. The upper cervical ganglion is dissected free laterally and retracted medially. The anterior branch of cervical nerve II is divided. This exposes the lateral corner of the atlantal loop and allows connection of the vein bypass to the distal portion of the vertebral artery without having to dissect too much tissue. This is important because exposing the medial corner of the vertebral artery at

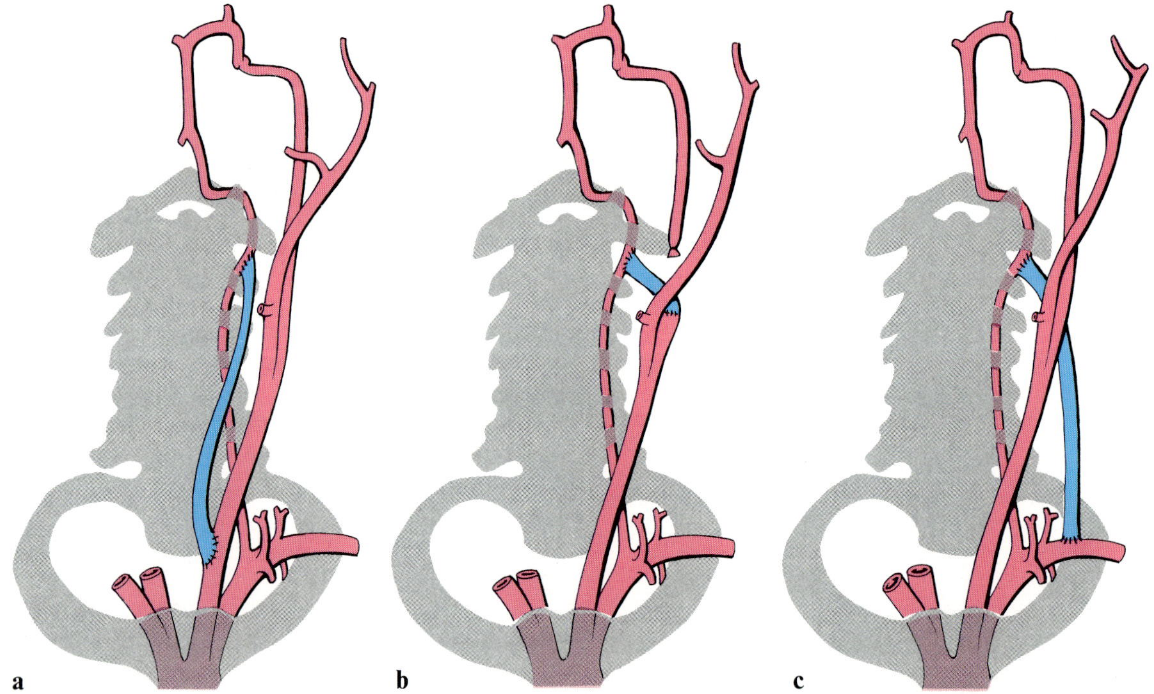

Fig. 18.2.7. **a** Vein bypass grafting from the common carotid artery to the atlantal loop in multiple stenoses along the course of the vertebral artery. **b** Bypass of an occluded internal carotid artery to the atlantal loop of the vertebral artery. **c** Vein bypass from the subclavian artery to the atlantal loop of the vertebral artery (modified according to CARNEY [2])

this point can lead to dangerous complications. The dural sac lies very close to this site, covered by a large venous plexus. Damage to this plexus may lead to considerable blood loss. Hemostasis in this region is only possible by simple compression and is therefore very risky.

III. Resection of the Vertebral Artery and End-to-End Anastomosis

Kinks in the distal portion of the vertebral artery can be resected. An end-to-end anastomosis of the stumps is then performed. This method may suffice to straighten a kink; however, bypass grafting is usually necessary since mobilization of the artery in this area is difficult and the danger of hemorrhage is great [2].

IV. Bypass to the Distal Vertebral Artery

The anterior approach allows simultaneous exposure of the internal carotid artery from the carotid bifurcation nearly all the way up to the base of the skull. The external carotid or internal carotid artery may be used as inflow vessels for the bypass procedure, provided there is adequate flow within them. An autogenous vein should be used for grafting. In exceptional cases the vertebral artery itself may be employed for grafting if, after the opening of the bony canal, the artery has been mobilized proximally and divided in its midportion. The extension of this procedure can lead to serious complications and should not be attempted without extensive knowledge of vertebral surgery. The vertebral artery itself may even serve as an inflow vessel for a vertebral-carotid bypass when the internal carotid artery is to be ligated just beneath the base of the skull and blood flow to it must be restored. Such a maneuver may be considered in tumorous lesions of the neck, inaccessible arteriovenous fistula, or in occlusions of the common carotid artery. In such cases, it may happen that an external-internal bypass cannot be constructed because the donating inflow artery, i.e., the external carotid artery, is occluded and the only possibility of reconstruction is an extra-anatomic bypass from the subclavian artery. Therefore, it should be borne in mind that a bypass graft may be attached to the distal segment of the vertebral artery, provided the vascular surgeon has the necessary experience to perform this operation (Fig. 18.2.7a–c).

V. Closure of the Incision

The sternocleidomastoid muscle is reattached to the mastoid process. Care must be taken to ensure the vein graft has enough space for small movements and is not held back by any structures. If necessary, parts of the muscle may be resected, or its origin displaced. Redon drains are then put in position, and the wound is closed with subcutaneous and skin sutures.

L. Postoperative Complications

(see also p. 157ff.)

Reconstructions of the vertebral artery are difficult. This is true not only for the proximal portion, but especially for the distal one as well. Surgical experience in this field helps to avoid complications.

I. Hemorrhage

Bleeding after vertebral reconstruction does not usually occur from the anastomosis, but from vessels in the immediate vicinity or in the skin. Hemorrhage from these sites is harmless. Wound revision with adequate drainage brings the situation under control. However, bleeding from the reconstructed vascular segment is dangerous since adequate visualization during a repeat operation is very difficult to obtain. Therefore, it must be stressed again that the most important step in this operation is to construct a safe and secure anastomosis. It is better not to perform the procedure than to do it under unsatisfactory conditions. The particular delicacy of the vessels in this region cannot be emphasized enough.

If the fatal situation of a disrupted vertebral anastomosis or a ruptured patch graft does occur, the incision must be extended on a large scale by median sternotomy or division of the clavicle as described earlier. This exposes the entire course of the artery in this region. A defect is repaired by reconstruction of the anastomosis or bypass grafting.

Hemorrhage following reconstructions of the distal portion of the vertebral artery is usually caused by the venous plexus. This complication can be relieved only by compression and tamponade. Bleeding from the stitches or reconstructed arterial segment can be reliably stopped by applying fibrin glue. The delicate vessels can rarely be reanastomosed.

II. Lymph Fistula

A lymph fistula is the most common postoperative complication, especially when the proximal portion of the left vertebral artery is exposed as a result of an injury to the thoracic duct that went unnoticed. Following vertebral reconstruction, there is a constant flow of lymph through the Redon drain. Even if a great amount of lymph is thus discharged, it is advisable to wait for about 3 days. Large lymph fistulas often close spontaneously. If this does not happen, revision is indicated. Pinpointing the severed lymphatic vessel may be difficult or impossible. Following suture ligation, the additional application of fibrin glue is recommended.

III. Nerve Injuries

The nerve most commonly injured during operations on the proximal portion of the vertebral artery is the phrenic nerve. This nerve is not usually damaged by transection. Rather, compression, caused either by retraction or by passing tapes around the arteries, is most often to blame [1]. The nerve almost always recovers completely within 3–6 months after surgery. Complete division of the phrenic nerve can be compensated only if an accessory phrenic nerve is present. Transection does not lead to considerable impairment of respiratory function at rest. However, respiratory insufficiency during exercise is always a result of paresis of the phrenic nerve. Neurosurgical reconstruction of this nerve has only a small chance of success.

The brachial plexus is also in danger of being injured during proximal exposure of the vertebral artery. Pulling the plexus causes reversible impairment, but sensory disorders may continue for a long period of time. Pain is often experienced. If the brachial plexus is divided, immediate reconstruction must be carried out by an experienced surgeon. It is important that no time be lost.

After vertebral reconstructions Horner's syndrome is sometimes observed, owing to intraoperative injury of cervical ganglion III of the sympathetic chain. Recovery is usually complete. In 1%, Horner's syndrome remains. Therefore, one should inform the patient preoperatively about this possible complication.

A severe complication is transection of the accessory nerve during exposure of the distal portion of the vertebral artery. Immediate neurosurgical reconstruction must be initiated. The sequelae can be so serious that they may lead to total work disability. Transection of sensory nerves such as the great auricular nerve is unimportant. However, the patient should be informed preoperatively about sensory impairment resulting from such nerve injury. Damage to the first cervical ganglion of the sympathetic chain does not usually lead to defects of any kind.

IV. Infection

An infection following vertebral reconstruction is rare and is limited to the subcutaneous tissue. We have never observed an infection that extended to the anastomosis. The main danger of infection is possible hemorrhage. Treatment follows the basic principles mentioned earlier. We have never observed a secondary infection within the area of a reconstructed vertebral artery that required surgical reintervention. We have never found reports of such a complication in the literature.

V. Cerebral Deficit

An acute occlusion of the vertebral artery, e.g., during a whiplash injury, may lead to serious neurologic defects with tetraplegia, cerebral coma, and brain death in the young patient. In contrast, postoperative occlusion of an arteriosclerotic vertebral artery does not at first lead to neurologic impairment. The preoperative symptoms that necessitated surgery recur during exercise. The extent of neurologic complications depends on collateral blood flow. If blood flow through the internal carotid artery is impaired on both sides, and the vertebral artery represents the most important cerebral vessel in such a situation, postoperative occlusion will, of course, lead to serious defects. We did not experience such a complication. In over 160 operations on the vertebral artery, only 1 patient died after reconstruction. Postmortem examination of the patient showed a glioma of the brain stem which had not been diagnosed [1]. We did not observe a postoperative CVA or embolism.

M. Reintervention

Surgical reintervention at the origin of the vertebral artery is not only technically very difficult, but also extremely risky. Reintervention in this area cannot be recommended. In reocclusions, bypass grafting is preferable. For example, a bypass from the carotid artery to the distal segment of the vertebral artery may be an alternative. Extra-intracranial bypass may be considered if the patient presents with severe neurologic impairment.

However, an anastomotic aneurysm must be corrected at all costs. The proximal and distal stump of the subclavian artery are adequately exposed. The aneurysmal portion of the vessel is totally resected and replaced with a synthetic prosthesis. Relief of an impending rupture of the subclavian artery has priority over revascularization of the vertebral artery. In such a case, bypass grafting may be performed in a second operation since no suitable vascular stump is usually available for reconstruction.

REFERENCES

1. Balzer K, Stöveken HJ, Carstensen G (1982) Die Anzeigestellung zur Operation an der Arteria vertebralis. Langenbecks Arch Chir 356:243–249
2. Carney LA (1981) Vertebral artery surgery: historical development, basic concepts of brain hemodynamics and clinical experience of 102 cases. In: Carney AL, Anderson EM (eds) Diagnosis and treatment of brain ischemia. Raven, New York, pp 249–282 (Advances in neurology, vol 30)
3. Carstensen G (1978) Die chirurgische Behandlung der vertebrobasilären Insuffizienz. Röntgen-Bl 31:272–275
4. Carstensen G (1980) Reconstructive surgery on the vertebral artery. Neurosurg Rev 3:113–117
5. De Bakey ME, Crawford ES, Morris GC, Cooley DA (1961) Surgical considerations of occlusive disease of the innominate, carotid, subclavian and vertebral arteries. Ann Surg 154:698–725
6. Imperato AM, Linn JPT (1967) Vertebral-arterial reconstruction: internal plication and vein-patch angioplasty. Ann Surg 166:213
7. Lippert H (1967) Arterienvarietäten. Klinische Tabellen 1–3, 51, Med Klinik 14, 18, 19 und 21. Urban & Schwarzenberg, München Berlin Wien

8. Neugebauer J, Stimmel F (1983) Die operative Beseitigung von Knickbildungen der A. vertebralis. VASA 12:55–58
9. Rieben FW (1973) Zur Orthologie und Pathologie der Arteria vertebralis. Sitzungsberichte der Heidelberger Akademie der Wissenschaften, Mathematisch-naturwissenschaftliche Klasse. Springer-Verlag, Berlin Heidelberg New York
10. Rieben FW (1980) Vertebrobasiläre Insuffizienz. Dtsch Med Wochenschr 105:1302–1303
11. Wylie EJ, Effeney DJ (1979) Surgery of the aortic arch branches and vertebral arteries. Surg Clin North Am 59:669–680
12. Wylie EJ, Stoney RJ, Ehrenfeld WK (1980) Manual of vascular surgery, vol I. Springer, Berlin Heidelberg New York

18.3 Extra-intracranial Anastomoses

H.M. MEHDORN

CONTENTS

A. Introduction

Thanks to the development of microsurgical techniques and their use in neurosurgery [30], C.M. FISCHER's idea (1951) of successfully bypassing an occluded cervical artery has become a reality. This operation, the extra-intracranial arterial bypass operation (also called extra-intracranial anastomosis, abbreviated here as EIAB) has gained increasing popularity in the last few years, following the first operation by YASARGIL in 1967. The patency rates of extra-intracranial anastomosis are approximately 95%. The extracranial donor artery, initially having a flow of only about 20 ml/min may be significantly dilated postoperatively and provide a flow of more than 150 ml/min into the intracranial vascular system.

B. Indications for Extra-intracranial Bypass Operations (EIAB)

There are two large groups of indications for EIAB: on the one hand a sort of *prophylactic indication* when occlusions of the internal carotid artery are required therapeutically in cases of giant aneurysms at the base of the skull and carotid cavernosus sinus fistulas, or in cases of tumors constricting the middle cerebral artery [26]. The sequence of the various therapeutic measures is not discussed in detail here.

Also included previously in the group of patients with "prophylactic indication" were all those in whom an EIAB was performed to reduce the risk of recurrent stroke following an ischemic attack or the risk of a stroke following a series of transient ischemic attacks [19, 31]. On the basis of worldwide neurosurgical experience, EIAB usually seemed to be indicated in cases of angiographically proven occlusions and stenoses of supra-aortic arteries that were no longer accessible to vascular surgery (Fig. 18.3.1).

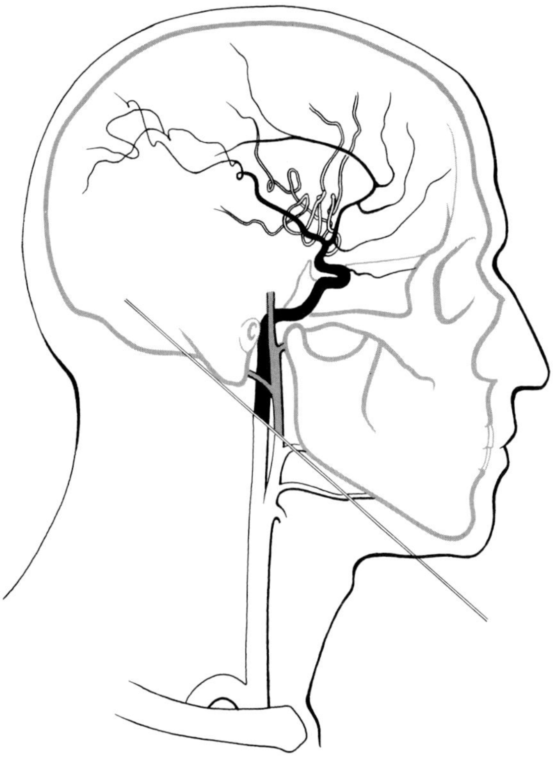

Fig. 18.3.1. Neurosurgical region of cerebral revascularization located above the borderline of the vascular area, between the mastoidal and the mandibular angle

On the basis of this very general indication, the data show that in large series, patients with occlusion of the internal carotid artery constitute about 40%, those with stenoses (mostly of the siphon), 20%. The remainder consists of patients with stenoses or occlusions of the middle cerebral artery as well as multiple vascular stenoses or occlusions [18].

A special group is comprised of patients with symptoms of impaired circulation in the vertebrobasilar vascular system. Patients whose neurologic symptoms cannot be attributed to angiographically proven stenoses or occlusions are considered to be candidates for EIAB only when the symptoms can be attributed to a (mostly interhemispheric, more seldom retinal) "steal phenomenon" [13, 17].

EIAB is mainly considered as a *prophylactic measure*, analogous to vascular indications for revascularizations of the supra-aortic arteries. Therefore, the most favorable candidates for EIAB are those who have suffered only transient ischemic attacks or perhaps a mild ischemic stroke with a definite risk of recurrence. Thus, patients who had suffered a mild stroke as a result of an occlusion of the internal carotid artery were considered to be good candidates for EIAB whenever the combined risk of mortality and morbidity following cerebral angiography and operation in the hands of a particular surgeon was less than the risk of an ischemic stroke following conservative therapy or during the spontaneous course, i.e., less than 4%.

However, in the meantime, an international cooperative study [6] has shown that, considering a combined operative mortality and stroke morbidity of 3.1%, EIAB in the *anterior circulation* offers no significant improvement as regards risk of stroke when compared with a simple medication containing platelet aggregation inhibitors. Naturally, this statement is valid only for the group of patients who were included in the study on the basis of comprehensive criteria. The object of current investigations is to determine how, in cases of ischemic disturbances of the cerebral functions, the selection of patients for prophylactic surgery can be made with greater certainty and with more clearly defined limitations than is the case in the cooperative study. Ischemia of the *posterior circulation* as an indication for prophylactic surgery is not included in the delimitation since it was not dealt with in the study.

The second group of indications is based on the clinically attested fact that in some patients postoperative neurologic deficits disappear. The therapeutic value of EIAB, however, is difficult to judge preoperatively in an individual patient because there are no reliable criteria to determine the viability and functional capacity of brain tissue. Therefore, one should be cautious regarding an exclusively therapeutic indication for EIAB. This is why, in patients with severe ischemic stroke, EIAB is indicated only in exceptional cases. One exception is ischemic ophthalmopathy, especially in the form of ischemic retinopathy, when it is not yet so far advanced that the loss of vision is irreversible.

C. Preoperative Diagnosis

Special preoperative diagnostic measures include *cranial computed tomography* as a noninvasive investigation following the clinical examination (especially for exclusion of an active cardiac source of emboli). This is absolutely essential for obtaining the following information:

- Localization and extent of the ischemic injury to cerebral tissue
- Stage of recovery and scarring of the infarction
- Differential diagnosis of the acute neurologic deficit:
  · Hemorrhagic stroke
  · Hemorrhagic infarction
  · Brain tumor
  · Intracranial extra- and intracerebral bleeding

Cerebral panangiography (at least three-vessel angiography, usually by the Seldinger technique) is required to visualize the following vascular findings:

- Occlusions and stenoses of extra- and intracranial vessels
- Extent of formation of collaterals

Repeat angiography should be performed prior to the operation where there is suspicion of a stenosis or an occlusion that may resolve spontaneously, as indicated by angiography or by Doppler ultrasonography, or where the interval between angiography and the operation is more than 6 weeks.

Even after the international study [6], the assumed advantage of EIAB is improvement of the functional reserve capacity of cerebral circulation. Therefore, it is mandatory to identify this parameter better than is possible by angiography. Additional investigations of the cerebral blood flow using the 133 Xe inhalation method or I-amphetamine single-photon emission tomography are recommended. For the investigation of brain metabolism, positron emission tomography may be used. Unfortunately, none of these methods is yet in routine use owing to a lack of apparatus and personnel; they are restricted to a few centers. Another less expensive method for determining the functional reserve capacity of the cerebral circulation is transcranial Doppler ultrasonography with a CO_2 load. Using these investigative techniques, it should be possible to improve selection of patients who may benefit from EIAB.

D. Anesthesia

Anesthesia for EIAB has to take account of the increased cardiovascular risk. Spiral tube, central-venous, and arterial catheters are routine. In contrast to the common technique of anesthesia in neurosurgery, the aim of which is to reduce intracranial volume and pressure, normal ventilation – even hypoventilation – is attempted during EIAB in order to achieve vascular dilation and consequently increased cerebral blood flow. The intracranial volume should not be reduced too much; otherwise the brain may recede and make it more difficult to perform the anastomosis.

Exceptions are anastomoses in the posterior cranial fossa, where revascularization of the rostral segments of the basilar artery is performed by a subtemporal approach. For this operation, retraction of the temporal lobe is required, which is better tolerated by the dehydrated brain.

Neuroleptic analgesia is most beneficial. In some hospitals, barbiturates and steroids are administered intraoperatively to improve cerebral ischemic tolerance.

E. Microsurgical Anastomoses

The usual anastomosis when performing EIAB is a microsurgical end-to-side anastomosis, joining the extracranial artery to the cortical artery at different angles.

As end-to-side anastomoses are described in detail in the chapter on microsurgical anastomoses (see p. 92), only a few of their peculiarities are mentioned here.

I. Preparation of the Arteries to Be Anastomosed

When performing an end-to-side anastomosis as part of EIAB, one faces the problem of having to join two arteries of different caliber and wall structure. One must be careful that the cortical artery with its weak wall is not twisted or kinked by the rigid extracranial donor artery. Therefore, special care must be taken to place the arteries so that they may be anastomosed without difficulty.

For the anastomosis, the adventitia of the extracranial artery must be dissected off until it no longer impairs the suture and cannot be dragged into the anastomosis (Fig. 18.3.2a). The cortical arteries have no adventitia. However, care must be taken for the same reason to make the incision in the arachnoidea sufficiently long and to dissect it off the cortical artery. Additionally, the fibers

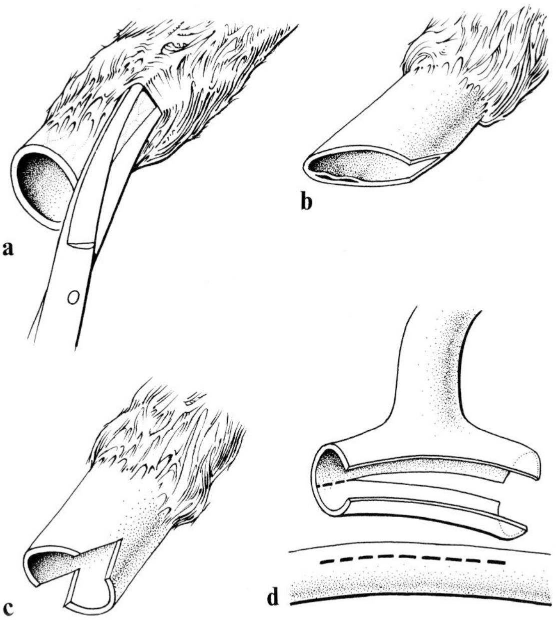

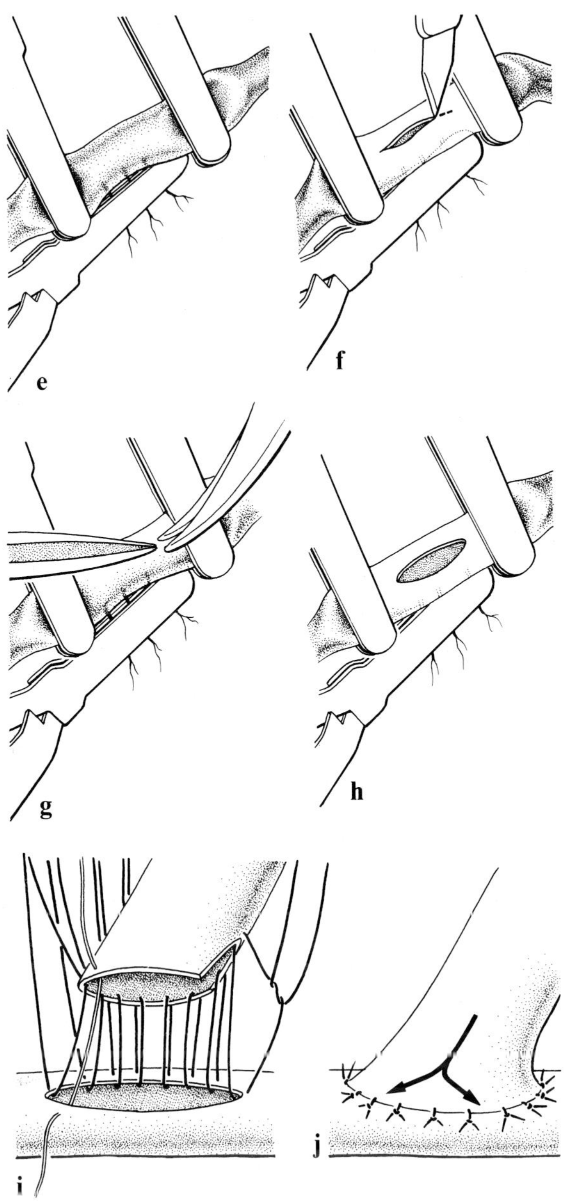

Fig. 18.3.2a–j. Preparation of both arteries involved in the end-to-side anastomosis between the superficial temporal artery and the cortical branch of the middle cerebral artery. **a** Preparation of the stump of the temporal artery: dissecting off the adventitia over a distance of 2–3 mm. **b** Enlargement of the diameter of the anastomosis by beveling the stump of the temporal artery. Note: dissection of the intima. **c**, **d** Enlargement of the diameter of the anastomosis by a fishmouth incision or a dichotomous bifurcation of the temporal artery (cf. 15). **e** Placement of microvascular clips on the cortical artery as well as another clip on the perforating branches. **f** For opening the cortical artery, the vessel is grasped, slightly drawn up, and incised longitudinally with a diamond knife, to provide a sufficiently long slit-like opening, **g** or opened with microscissors, **h** achieving an elliptical opening. Suture technique: either stepwise placement of interrupted sutures, or **i** placement of several sutures which are tied afterward. **j** Result using technique of Fig. 18.3.2b

of the arachnoidea must be dissected off the cortical artery until it is mobilized over a distance of a few millimeters.

Both arteries to be anastomosed show a tendency to dilate if the bypass functions well. First of all, therefore, the diameter of the anastomosis must be tailored appropriately. Various techniques have been described. Probably the most commonly used technique is to bevel the end of the extracranial donor artery (Fig. 18.3.2b). This presumes, however, that the rather rigid donor artery is easily placed in such a manner that, following completion of the anastomosis, the end points proximally. Otherwise, significant turbulence may occur at the anastomosis, with the risk of increased formation of myointimal hyperplasia.

Other techniques for extending the anastomotic diameter are the fishmouth technique (Fig. 18.3.2c) and, occasionally possible, the anastomosis of a dichotomous bifurcation of the extracranial donor artery to the cortical artery (Fig. 18.3.2d).

The cortical arteries, especially those close to the origin of the Sylvian fissure have many perforating branches which should be preserved because a great proportion serve as end arteries. When planning to perform the anastomosis precisely in that region of the cortical artery where several branches originate, one should try to place a narrow temporary clip on these branches – this in addition to the two microvascular clips that occlude the cortical artery over a distance of 3–5 mm – in order to avoid increased bleeding in the operative field (Fig. 18.3.2e).

The incision of the cortical artery (Fig. 18.3.2f–h) is one of the most difficult steps in the procedure, and at the same time one of the most important factors affecting the quality of the anastomosis. Especially in cases of thin cortical arteries a simple, straight longitudinal incision is indicated in order to avoid a stenosing of the recipient artery by the anastomosis. For this purpose, a diamond knife is very suitable. However, it may be somewhat difficult to separate the anterior from the posterior wall of the donor artery, as they are closely attached. In order to avoid this problem, it has been recommended that one makes an elliptical opening in the cortical artery [21]. The length of the incision depends on the diameter of the extracranial artery and should measure approximately 1.5 times the diameter. When the stump of the donor artery is markedly beveled, a greater factor may be chosen.

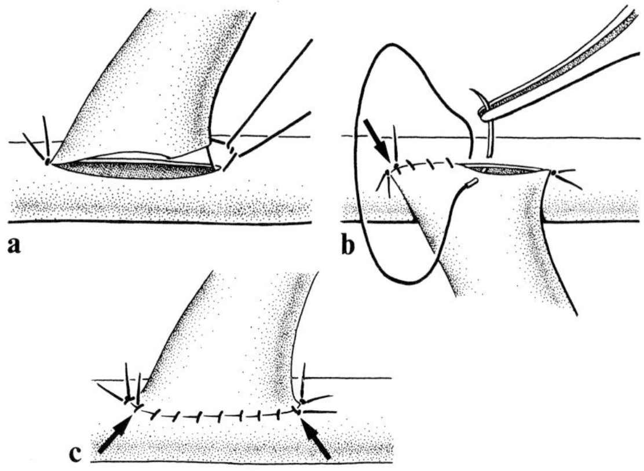

Fig. 18.3.3a–c. Continuous suture of the end-to-side anastomosis. **a** Placement of the corner sutures. **b** Suture of the posterior wall, starting from a new corner suture (*arrow*). **c** Suture of the posterior wall, also starting from a new corner suture (*arrow*), completion of the suture of the anterior wall by a corner suture which is independent of the distal corner suture (*arrow*)

II. Suture Technique

Usually, end-to-side anastomoses are performed using interrupted sutures in order to:

- Exclude the risk of continuous suture rupture with catastrophic sequelae.
- Avoid a "purse string effect" which may occur after the suture is tightened and knotted.
- Avoid the risk of a delayed purse string effect. The anastomosed extracranial artery tends to dilate when bypass function is good, thereby causing a stenosis at the anastomosis.

When suturing, the needle must be placed so that any intima dissected off the media of the temporal artery (see Fig. 18.3.2b) is refixed by the suture. Otherwise, thrombogenic pouches in the vessel wall may occur. In order to achieve a better view of both vessel walls, the stitches may initially be placed along a greater segment of the circumference *before* being knotted (Fig. 18.3.2i, k).

Usually, the posterior wall of the anastomosis is sutured first. However, it may be useful to suture the anterior wall first, or at least that part which is close to the corner. This will provide sufficient stability of the anastomosis before the posterior wall is sutured. This is especially important when the cortical artery must be twisted before the posterior wall can be sutured (in cases where the temporal artery is just long enough).

The number of interrupted sutures largely depends on the caliber of the arteries; usually 15–20 sutures are sufficient. In our experience, the arterial clip on the cortical artery must be in place for 15–25 min before such a conventional anastomosis is completed. This time is well tolerated by the brain because of good collateral circulation. Using fewer sutures may shorten the clamping time, and therefore the time during which the affected portion of the vascular system is undersupplied. However, it may also increase the risk of anastomotic aneurysms and thrombus formation at the site of the anastomosis.

Various methods have been described (Fig. 18.3.3a–c) for avoiding the purse string effect of the almost completely continuous suture [18, 22]. Essentially, these techniques involve a combination of a continuous and an interrupted suture. According to the authors in question, clamping time is reduced by one half.

III. Fibrin Seal of the Anastomosis

Likewise with a view toward saving time and reducing clamping time by 50%, a variation of the anastomotic technique has been developed which

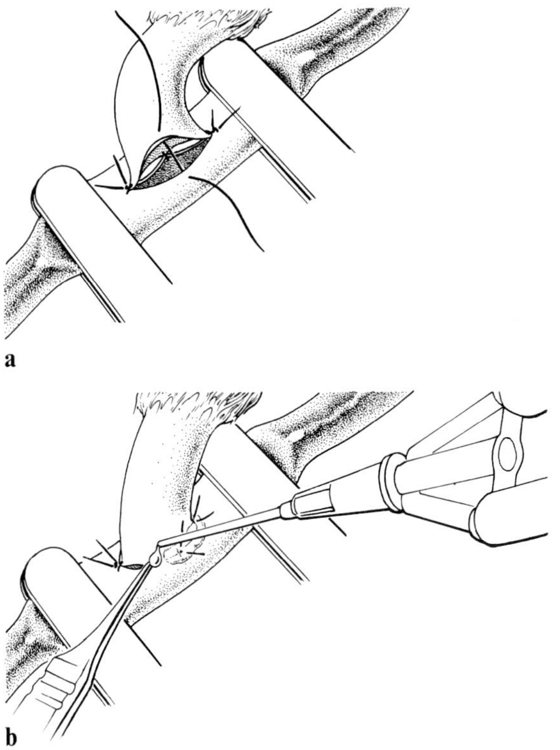

a

b

Fig. 18.3.4a, b. End-to-side anastomosis with fibrin glue. a Placement of at least four sutures (two corner sutures as well as at least one suture in each wall). b Adaptation of the vascular edges in the interspaces between the sutures, and application of fibrin glue

makes use of fibrin sealant [15, 16]. With this technique, corner sutures and two to four additional interrupted sutures are placed in the circumference. Then, fibrin glue is applied in the interspaces (Fig. 18.3.4). With this technique, of course, one must adapt the edges of the arteries to one another with great care, using a microforceps. This is done to prevent development of anastomotic aneurysms that may result in fatal intracranial bleeding.

IV. Laser Seal of the Anastomosis

The anastomosis of arteries by laser technique is currently in its developmental stage and so far has been applied only in the end-to-end anastomosis. Perhaps this technique will be developed further and become a useful part of the microsurgical repertoire.

One thing seems certain: improvements in the lasers are needed in order to achieve the temperature required for fusing the arterial edges over a sufficient distance.

F. Operative Technique of Revascularization of Cerebral Hemispheres – EIAB from the Superficial Temporal Artery to the Cortical Branch of the Middle Cerebral Artery

The most commonly used extra-intracranial anastomosis is that between the superficial temporal artery to the cortical branch of the middle cerebral artery. This operation may be performed under acetylsalicylic acid to increase the protection from thrombosis. However, especially meticulous hemostasis in all layers is required, usually by bipolar coagulation.

I. Conventional Technique

The head is placed in a doughnut or a head holder to get the temporal area in a horizontal position. Usually the patient is in an oblique position, except when turning the head may cause stenosis of elongated arteries of the neck. In such cases, the trunk should also be positioned on the side.

Following the usual preparation, a curvilinear incision is made over the ear (Fig. 18.3.5) starting at the temporal hairline, having its vertex at the cross-section of the angiographically distinguishable posterior branch of the temporal artery, and terminating 1–2 fingerbreadths behind the ear [19]. The base runs just over the ear. Creating such a flap achieves:

- A sufficiently long segment of the posterior branch of the temporal artery, which is especially suitable for anastomosis.

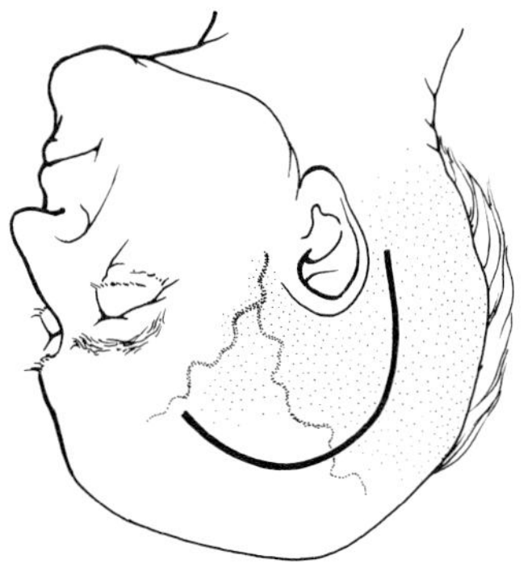

Fig. 18.3.5. Conventional incision for EIAB to expose the carotid circulation, as viewed by the surgeon: broad-based skin flap with the vertex over the temporal artery

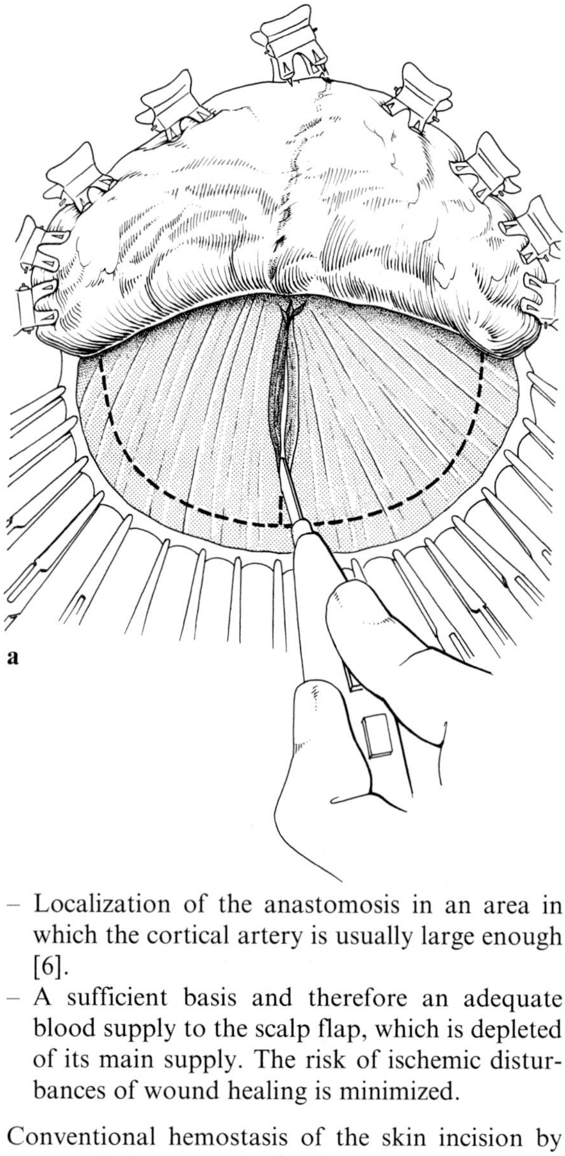

a

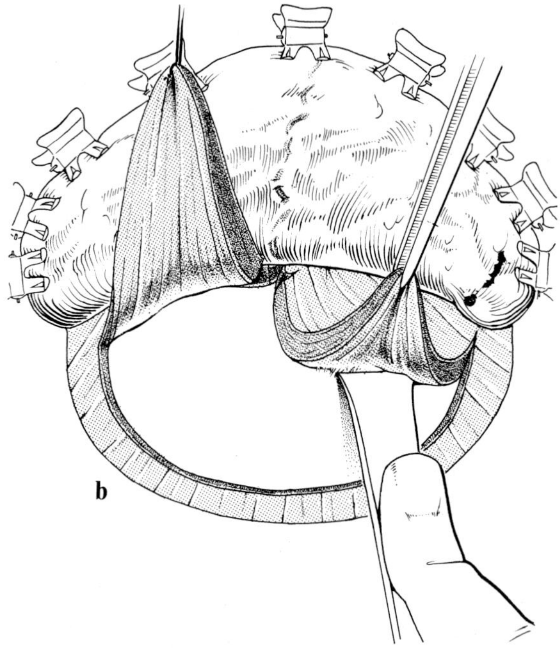

b

Fig. 18.3.6a, b. Operative field following reflection of the skin flap. **a** The temporal muscle is incised, directing the middle incision toward the temporal artery. **b** Reflecting and fixing the temporal muscle

- Localization of the anastomosis in an area in which the cortical artery is usually large enough [6].
- A sufficient basis and therefore an adequate blood supply to the scalp flap, which is depleted of its main supply. The risk of ischemic disturbances of wound healing is minimized.

Conventional hemostasis of the skin incision by means of clamps and other instruments is supplemented with bipolar coagulation of the distal end of the temporal artery.

When the scalp flap is turned down (Fig. 18.3.6a), the pulse of the temporal artery can be palpated or outlined using a Doppler ultrasonographic probe. The temporal muscle is incised along the muscle fibers. The incision is enlarged in a T-shaped fashion, slitting the muscle about 1 cm away from the muscle-periost border, parallel to the skin incision. This step facilitates closure later on. Both muscle flaps are dissected off the temporal bone, fixed with stay sutures, and reflected (Fig. 18.3.6b).

With a spatula held so as to protect the skin flap, which contains the artery, a bur hole is made in the area toward the base of the skull; proceeding from this bur hole, a bone plate 3 cm in diameter is cut out (Fig. 18.3.7). Then, three small holes are drilled for the stay sutures that will later hold the bone plate in place. Afterward strips of hemostyptics are placed between the dura and the bone, followed by a crisscross incision of the dura and placement of stay sutures (Fig. 18.3.8).

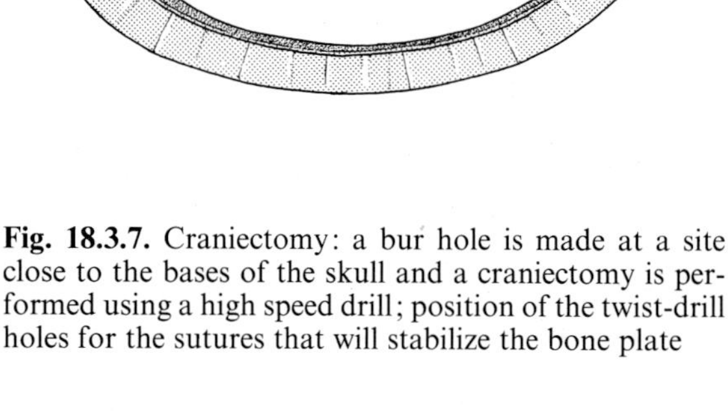

Fig. 18.3.7. Craniectomy: a bur hole is made at a site close to the bases of the skull and a craniectomy is performed using a high speed drill; position of the twist-drill holes for the sutures that will stabilize the bone plate

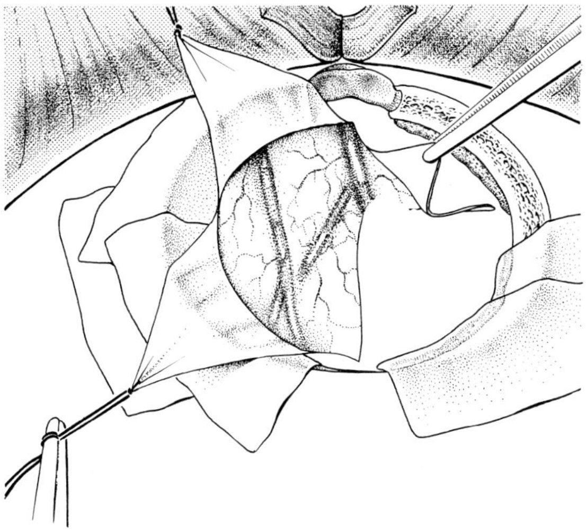

Fig. 18.3.8. Crisscross incision of the dura, followed by lifting and stay-suturing the flaps after strips soaked with fibrin foam have been placed beneath the bone and the area of craniectomy surrounded by cotton pledgets

Now, the microscope is used. A cortical artery of sufficient caliber, i.e., at least 1 mm diameter, is identified, examined to disclose eventual arteriosclerotic plaques, and the branches covered with a papaverine-soaked cotton pledget. The arachnoidea should not yet be opened, so as not to provoke loss of cerebrospinal fluid, causing the surface of the brain (especially in patients with enlargements of the inner and outer subarachnoid space) to fall below the initial level.

The dissection of the temporal artery (Fig. 18.3.9) is performed most easily by starting close to the reflection of the skin flap because there the artery is most often palpated. The fascia above the artery has to be divided for mobilization because the artery is attached between both sheets of the temporal fascia or between the temporal fascia and the parietotemporal and epicranial muscles. When the fascia has been incised over a sufficient distance, the temporal artery may be mobilized completely step by step. Often this may be difficult, owing to significant adhesions with the fascia and/or extensive coiling of the artery. In most cases, the tributaries arise at the convex side of the loops and are coagulated at a safe distance from the main trunk by bipolar coagulation. When the branches are too large to be coagulated without thermal injury to the temporal artery, they are divided following double ligature with 8-0 suture material (Fig. 18.3.9c).

Some authors recommend ligation of the anterior branch of the temporal artery with the aim of bypassing the total blood volume from the temporal artery into the intracranial vascular system. However, this should not be attempted because the anastomosed branch of the temporal artery will enlarge quite well even if the other branch is still contributing to the collateral blood supply. Furthermore, natural collaterals via the ophthalmic artery would be interrupted, and, of course, later anastomosis (additional or as replacement) would no longer be possible.

When the mobilization of the artery is complete, it is ligated distally with a microclip and divided peripherally (Fig. 18.3.9d). A short distal end of the temporal artery should remain protected by the fascia and be coagulated. This technique provides faultless closure of the wound. Fur-

Fig. 18.3.9a–d. Dissection of the temporal artery. **a** Incision of the temporal fascia, followed by **b** mobilization of the temporal artery from the fatty tissue. **c** Double ligation of a large branch which is finally divided. **d** The temporal artery is dissected sufficiently far to the periphery and clipped at its distal end

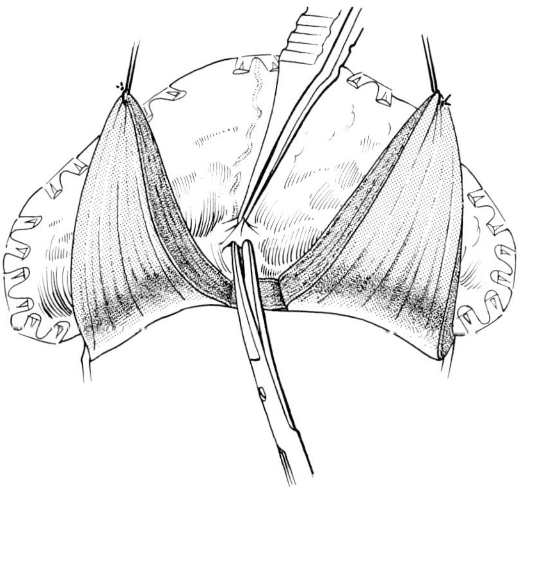

a

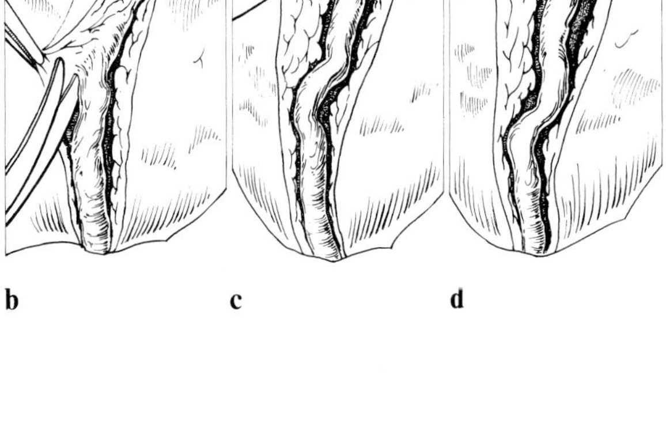

b **c** **d**

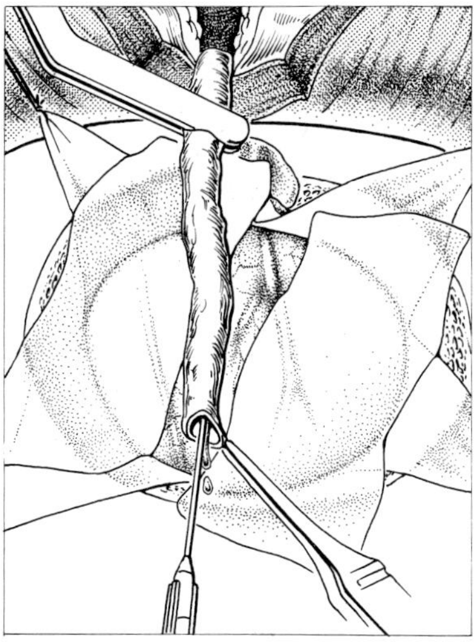

Fig. 18.3.10. Preparation of the temporal artery for the anastomosis: relocation of the clip from a peripheral to a central position and flushing the artery with heparinized solution. Afterwards, dissection of the adventitia for the last few millimeters and beveling of the stump

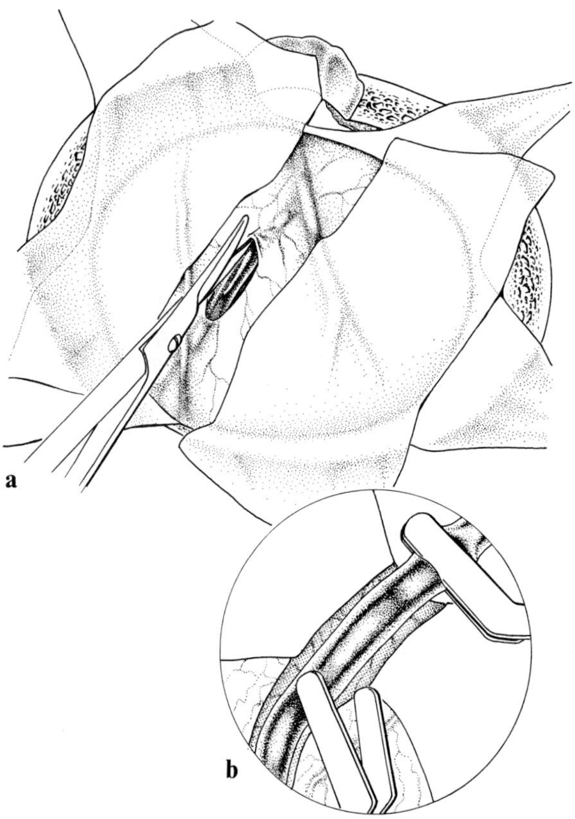

Fig. 18.3.11 a, b. Protection of the brain surface by rubber strips and cotton pledgets and preparation of the cortical artery for the anastomosis. **a** Dissection of the arachnoidea over a distance of a few millimeters. **b** Placement of microclips (see also Fig. 18.3.2d)

thermore, necrosis of the wound margin along the former course of the temporal artery is avoided.

The temporal artery is now prepared for the anastomosis itself (Fig. 18.3.10). When judging the length of the superficial temporal artery, it should be borne in mind that, on the one hand, a short superficial temporal artery has a lower flow resistance than a longer one, which is also more likely to develop a kink, but that, on the other hand, a long superficial temporal artery is more easily anastomosed because it can be rotated more easily for suture of the posterior wall, especially when the surface of the brain has given way, owing to loss of cerebrospinal fluid.

Following determination of the length of the superficial temporal artery, the adventitia is dissected off the last few millimeters, and the stump is beveled as described above (Sect. E.I.). The clip initially placed on the distal end is now repositioned proximally. Finally, the lumen of the artery is cannulated with a blunt cannula and flushed with heparinized solution to remove as many thrombi as possible.

In order to facilitate the anastomosis, the cerebral surface is covered with a cotton pledget and the area close to the anastomosis is covered with strips tailored from rubber gloves (Fig. 18.3.11a). This protects the cerebral surface from mechanical injury and also makes it easier to manipulate needle and suture.

When the cortical artery has been prepared for the anastomosis (following incision of the arachnoidea and mobilization over a sufficient length), the temporary microclips, exerting an occlusion pressure of 15–20 g, are placed. In order to achieve complete filling of the cortical artery, the distal microclip is placed before the proximal microclip (Fig. 18.3.11b).

Once the anastomosis has been completed as described in Sect. E.II (Fig. 18.3.12), the clips on the cortical artery are removed in the sequence in which they were placed. The anastomosis is functioning well when:

- The cortical artery is free of stenosis
- The temporal artery is filled immediately in a retrograde direction
- No major bleeding occurs at the anastomosis

If one of these criteria is not fulfilled, the anastomosis should be inspected, including inspection from inside, to prevent reocclusion or rebleeding. Depending on the situation, the anastomosis may

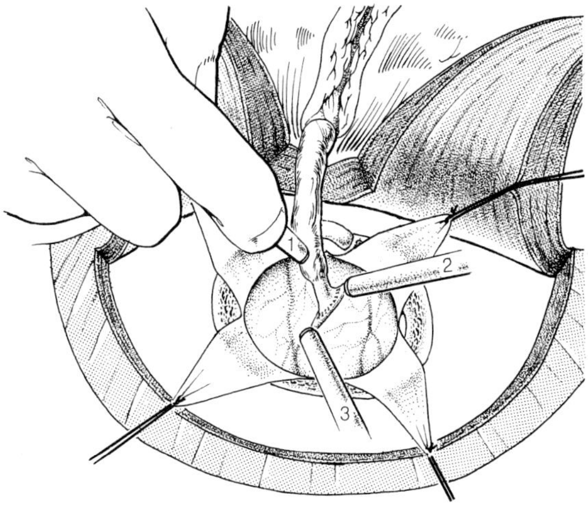

Fig. 18.3.12. Completed anastomosis. Operative field and Doppler ultrasonography of the temporal artery to judge the function of the anastomosis (the *numbers* represent the recommended sequence of investigation by the Doppler probe)

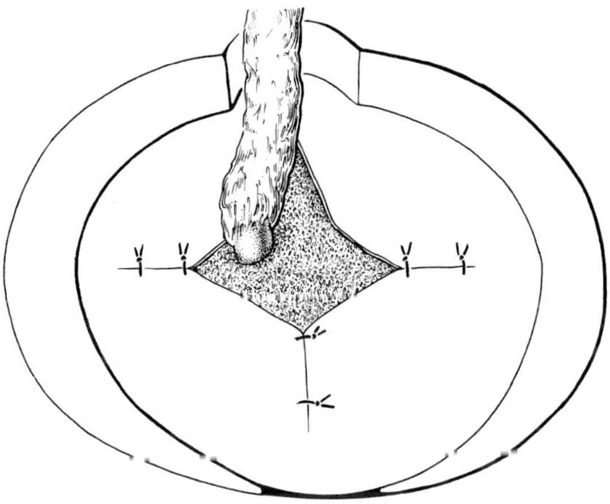

Fig. 18.3.13. Covering the anastomosis with fibrin foam and loose closure of the dura

have to be revised immediately or a suture inserted.

If the anastomosis has been performed correctly, the remaining microclip occluding the temporal artery can be removed and anastomosis function demonstrated by Doppler ultrasonography (Fig. 18.3.12). With the use of Doppler microprobes, it is now possible to investigate the small cortical arteries separately to determine the precise intracranial distribution of the blood flowing through the anastomosis as well as turbulence in the anastomosis, etc. [8].

If the anastomosis is patent, it is covered with fibrin foam and soaked with moxaverine to avoid local vasospasm (Fig. 18.3.13).

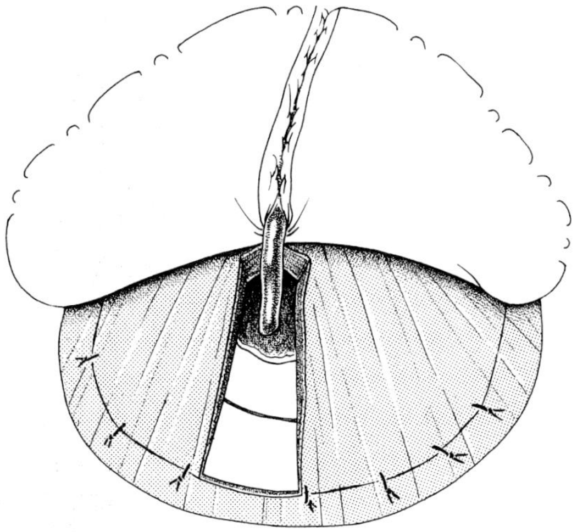

Fig. 18.3.14. Closure of the wound layer by layer: fitting in the bone plate, part of which has been removed in order to provide an opening for the temporal artery and enough room for the anastomosis. Adaptation of the muscle, leaving a slot for the passage of the temporal artery

Afterwards the wound is closed layer by layer (Fig. 18.3.14): the dura is closed as far as the location of the anastomosis allows, and the bone plate is inserted and fastened with sutures. Prior to this, the plate has been slotted to avoid the risk of occlusion of the temporal artery by compression.

The muscle wound is then closed. Here, an opening must be left so that the artery passes through the fascial without kinking or stenosis.

Following placement of a Hemovac drain and control of hemostasis at the anastomosis, the skin flap is turned back, care being taken to insure that the temporal artery passes without kinking. Percutaneous Doppler ultrasonography allows one to check for correct function of the anastomosis [8, 10].

II. Variant I: Incision Over the Temporal Artery (Fig. 18.3.15)

The previously used incisions, creating a skin flap with a narrow base, often caused ischemic disturbances of wound healing. Therefore, another operative technique has been developed and described [21]. The incision is made directly over the temporal artery – detected percutaneously by Doppler ultrasonography – or in its immediate vicinity (Fig. 18.3.15a).

Special care must be taken not to injure the temporal artery while dissecting (Fig. 18.3.15b).

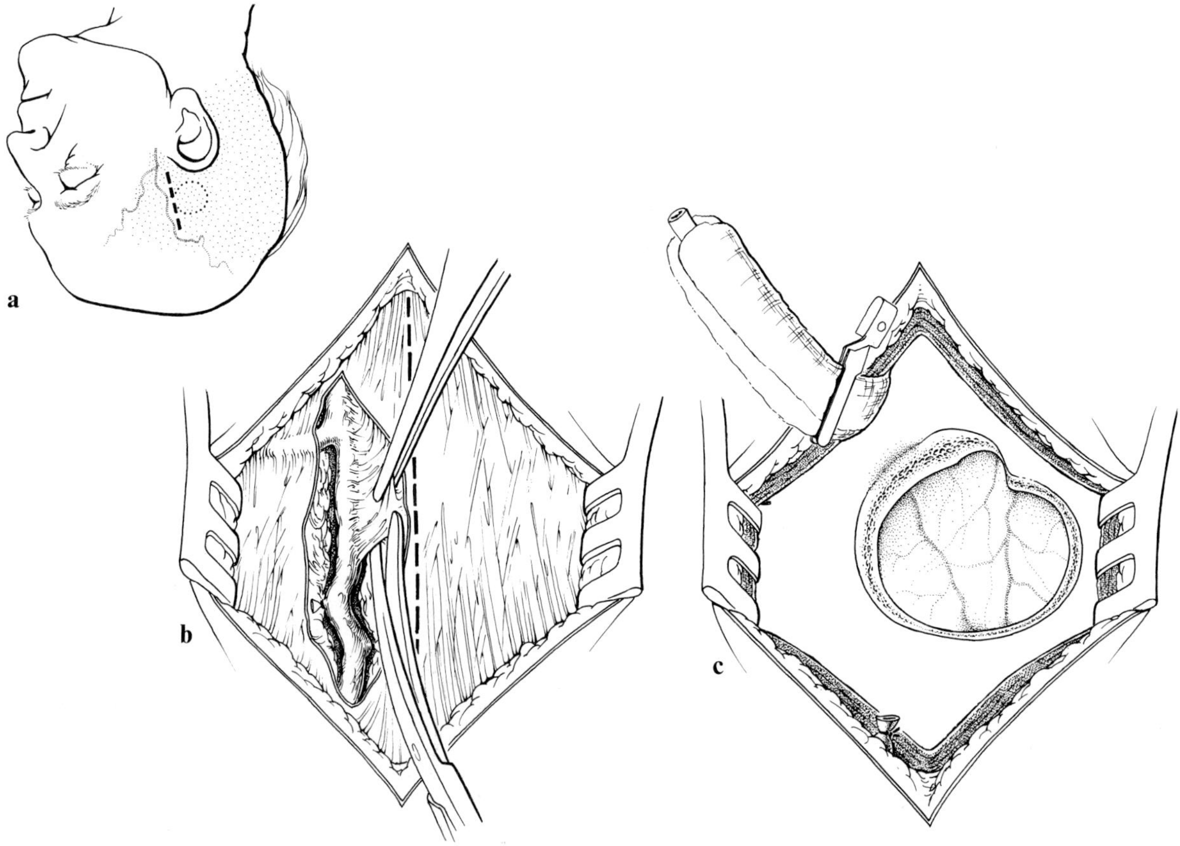

Fig. 18.3.15a–c. Variant I of EIAB: incision over the temporal artery. **a** Line of incision as seen by the surgeon, with reference to the course of the temporal artery. **b** Dissection of the temporal artery from the temporal fascia. **c** Situation following ligation of the temporal artery, incision of the temporal muscle and craniotomy

Without being ligated distally, the artery is wrapped in a moxaverine-soaked cotton pledget following sufficient mobilization and is retracted, allowing incision and retraction of the temporal muscle. Self-retaining retractors or fishhooks allow one to retract the skin, the temporal artery, and the muscle while craniectomy is performed. Following incision of the dura, a cortical artery is identified to serve as the recipient artery. When it has been chosen, the temporal artery is clamped at its distal end and the distal stump ligated or coagulated with bipolar coagulation (Fig. 18.3.15c). Afterwards, the anastomosis is carried out as previously described.

The closure of the wound is done in the usual fashion. Here, too, care must be taken to provide an adequate slot for the passage of the temporal artery through the muscle and the skull.

III. Variant II: Anastomosis Close to the Main Stem of the Middle Cerebral Artery
(Fig. 18.3.16)

The conventional EIAB causes "unphysiologic" circulatory conditions in the recipient artery, because in this case the direction of blood flow is the reverse of normal until the middle cerebral artery divides into its branches. Beyond this point, blood from the remaining cortical arteries will flow in the anterograde direction. In order to avoid possible disadvantages for the function of EIAB, an end-to-side anastomosis may be constructed close to, or on, the main stem of the middle cerebral artery. In this case, it is necessary to dissect the temporal artery over a longer distance than usual and, following temporofrontal or pterional craniotomy, to open the lateral sulcus of the cerebrum (Fig. 18.3.16a) far enough to provide access to the major branch of the middle cerebral artery. Self-retaining retractors are required to retract the frontal (and temporal) lobes. Furthermore, because of the depth of the anastomosis, the instruments used must be longer than usual (Fig. 18.3.16b, c).

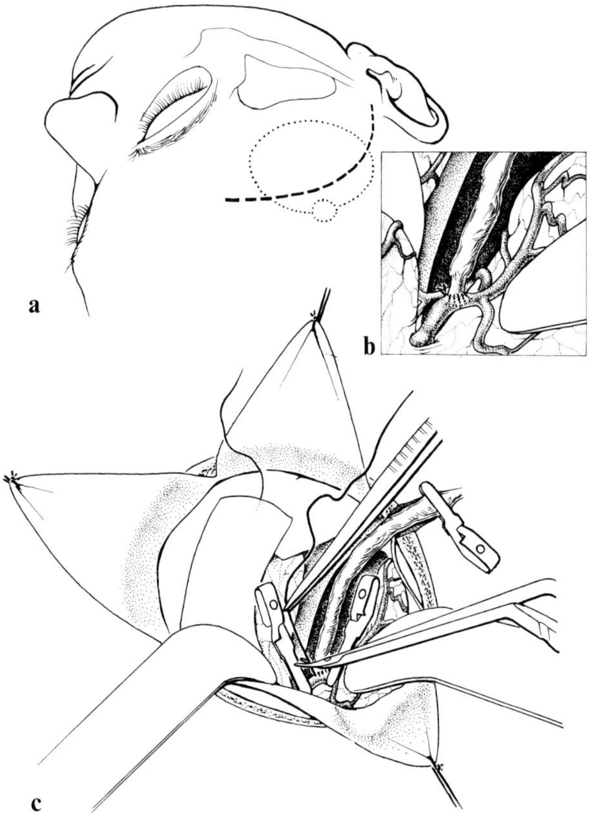

Fig. 18.3.16a–c. Variant II of EIAB: anastomosis close to the major branch of the middle cerebral artery. **a** Incision for pterional craniotomy, preserving the anterior branch of the temporal artery. **b** Anastomosis deep in the lateral sulcus of the cerebrum. **c** Completed anastomosis

IV. Variant III: Other Donor Arteries (Fig. 18.3.17)

Occasionally the posterior branch of the temporal artery will not be large enough to serve as donor artery for EIAB. In this case one has to consider the extent to which the use of the anterior branch would interrupt natural, preformed collaterals; or, one may consider using the occipital artery as a donor artery [24]. The latter may be used as the extracranial artery for EIAB if it is of sufficient caliber distal to the protuberantia occipitalis externa over a distance of 10 cm. The artery must be exposed through a parieto-occipital skin flap and anastomosed to a cortical artery in the angularis region.

For exposure of the anterior branch of the temporal artery the incision is either extended toward

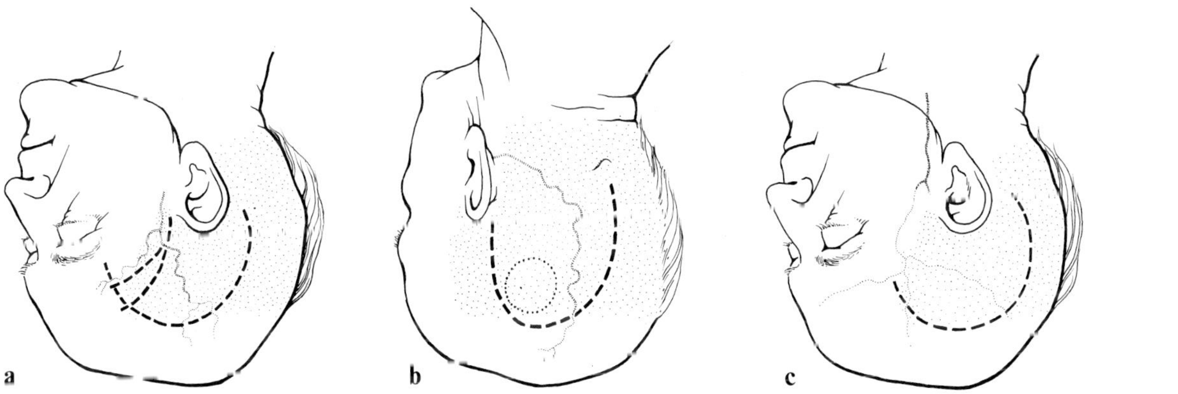

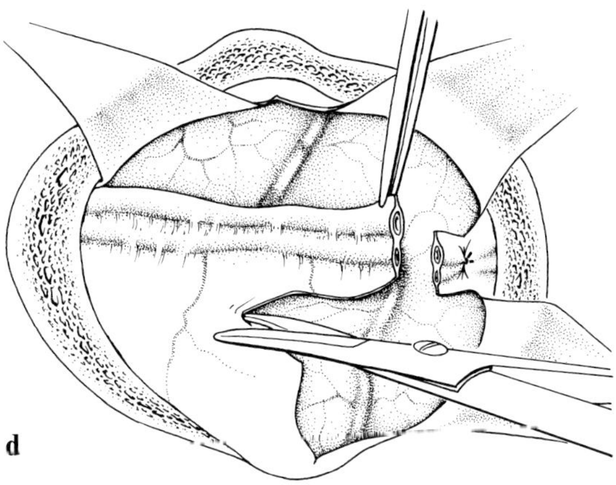

Fig. 18.3.17a–d. Variant III of EIAB: alternative donor arteries. **a** Incision using the anterior branch of the temporal artery. **b** Incision and area of craniotomy using the occipital artery; EIAB for the carotid circulation with anastomosis between occipital artery and angularis artery. **c** EIAB using the middle meningeal artery as extracranial donor artery. **d** Dissecting the meningeal artery and vein off the dura

the forehead or made over the artery, which is often located in the forehead and temporal area and is therefore cosmetically unfavorable (Fig. 18.3.17a).

The technique for dissecting the occipital artery (Fig. 18.3.17b) is essentially the same as for the temporal artery. However, dissecting the artery off the fascia may be more difficult as the fascia in this area is significantly firmer. The pulse of the occipital artery is rarely palpated at the duplication of the skin flap owing to the tightness of the fascia. Therefore, dissection usually starts at a site where the artery (or its major branch) crosses the skin incision. Dissection is continued, following the artery proximally, in which direction its caliber increases significantly. For supratentorial revascularization, the artery is mobilized only as far as the external occipital protuberance.

In the region of the angularis artery, one should not expect to find a sufficiently large cortical artery within the – usually small – craniotomy. Therefore, it is advisable to excise a bone plate almost the size of the palm of the hand in order to insure a sufficient selection of cortical arteries.

Occasionally, a retroauricular artery is found in the temporoparietal region behind the ear instead of the temporal artery. The dissection of this artery, however, does not require variation of the conventional anastomosis.

For the sake of completeness another variant of the anastomosis is mentioned, where the medial meningeal artery is used as the donor artery (Fig. 18.3.17c, d). This is indicated, for instance, in case of a meningioma located at the convexity when a branch of the middle cerebral artery must be ligated in order to remove the tumor, and the meningeal artery and the artery supplying the tumor are sufficiently longer than normal. Then, mobilization of the meningeal artery alone, together with a strip of dura, is required.

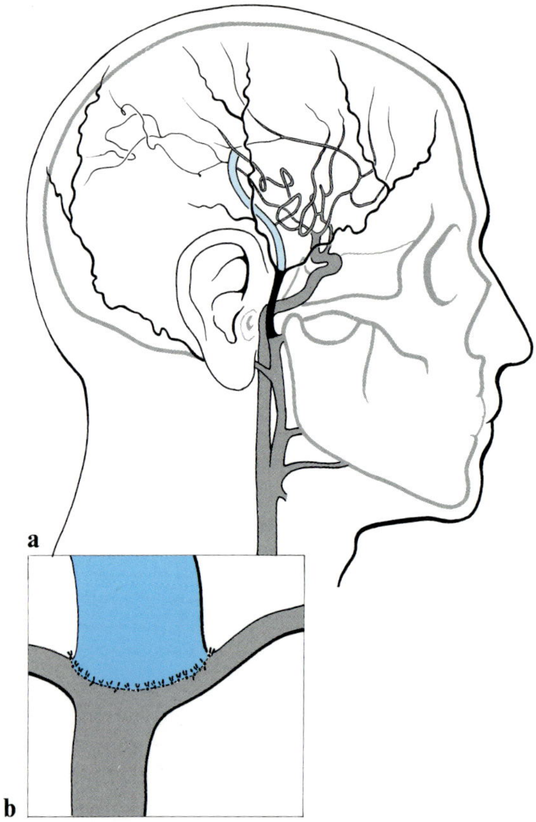

Fig. 18.3.18a, b. Variant IV of EIAB: interposition of short venous segments. **a** Overview: course of the vein graft between temporal artery and cortical artery. **b** Side-to-end anastomosis of the temporal artery to the vein at the dichotomy of the temporal artery, in order to achieve the greatest possible anastomotic diameter

V. Variant IV: Vein Interposition
(Fig. 18.3.18)

When the distal segments of the extracranial donor arteries are no longer sufficiently large, or not suitable for other reasons, one may consider interposition of a short segment, e.g., of the small saphenous vein, between the stump of the temporal artery in front of the ear and the cortical artery, the anastomosis with the temporal artery being either side-to-end or end-to-end. This interposition of short veins provides a greater initial flow than conventional EIAB and provides significantly greater possibilities for choosing the recipient cortical artery. One may even make an anastomosis in the territory of the anterior cerebral artery. The alternative of short vein interposition should be considered before planning large extra-anatomic bypasses (see Sect. H).

The technique does not differ significantly from conventional EIAB. It requires only an additional side-to-end or end-to-end anastomosis between either the temporal artery (in front of the ear) or the occipital artery (behind the ear) and the vein. The anastomosis is performed using 9-0 monofilament suture material. A continuous suture is used for the posterior portion of the anastomosis and interrupted sutures for the anterior portion.

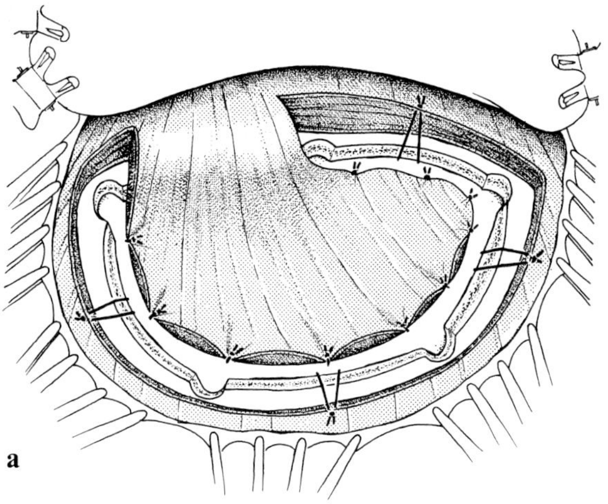

a

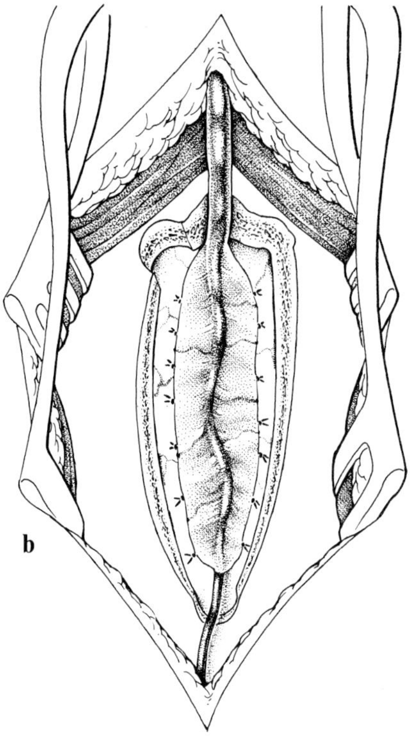

b

Fig. 18.3.19 a, b. Variant V of EIAB: encephalomyosynangiosis (EMS). **a** Conventional EMS, where the temporal muscle is placed on the cerebral surface and sutured to the dura. **b** EMS, where the patent temporal artery is placed on the cerebral surface and the temporal fascia is fixed to the dura

VI. Variant V: Encephalomyosynangiosis
(Fig. 18.3.19)

Especially in patients with moyamoya disease, it may be difficult to find a cortical artery of sufficient caliber to provide a convenient anastomosis [11, 12]. In these cases, one may use the original indirect technique of cerebral revascularization, encephalomyosynangiosis (EMS, i.e., placement of the temporal muscle on the cerebral surface), or variants of this technique.

Some months after an EMS operation, small arteries grow from the muscle on the cerebral surface into the layers underneath, in a manner similar to the development of transdural arterial anastomosis, of the sort known as a "rete mirabile," following conventional craniotomy.

For EMS the dura is opened wide, the temporal muscle is placed on the cerebral surface following careful hemostasis, and its edges are fixed to the edges of the dura (Fig. 18.3.19a). In order to improve the growth of arteries on the cerebral surface, some surgeons have recommended slitting the arachnoidea as far as possible, or removing it.

In a variation of EMS, the temporal artery is dissected free as described in Sect. F.II, but with preservation of its continuity, and the artery, either by itself or with the edge of the remaining fascia, is fixed to the edge of the dura (Fig. 18.3.19b). With this technique, the growth of arteries on the cerebral surface may be improved, as compared with conventional EMS.

Other techniques that have been recommended for revascularization of ischemic brain areas involve the use of the greater omentum. Omentum, in the form of a free graft containing a vascular pedicle, can be transplanted to the cerebral surface by anastomosing the gastroepiploic artery and vein side-to-end with the superficial temporal artery and vein in front of the ear [12]; or, intact pedicled omentum can be mobilized to pass through a subcutaneous tunnel in front of the thorax and behind the ear, to be placed on the cerebral surface [9]. In both operations, the omentum is fixed to the edges of the dura.

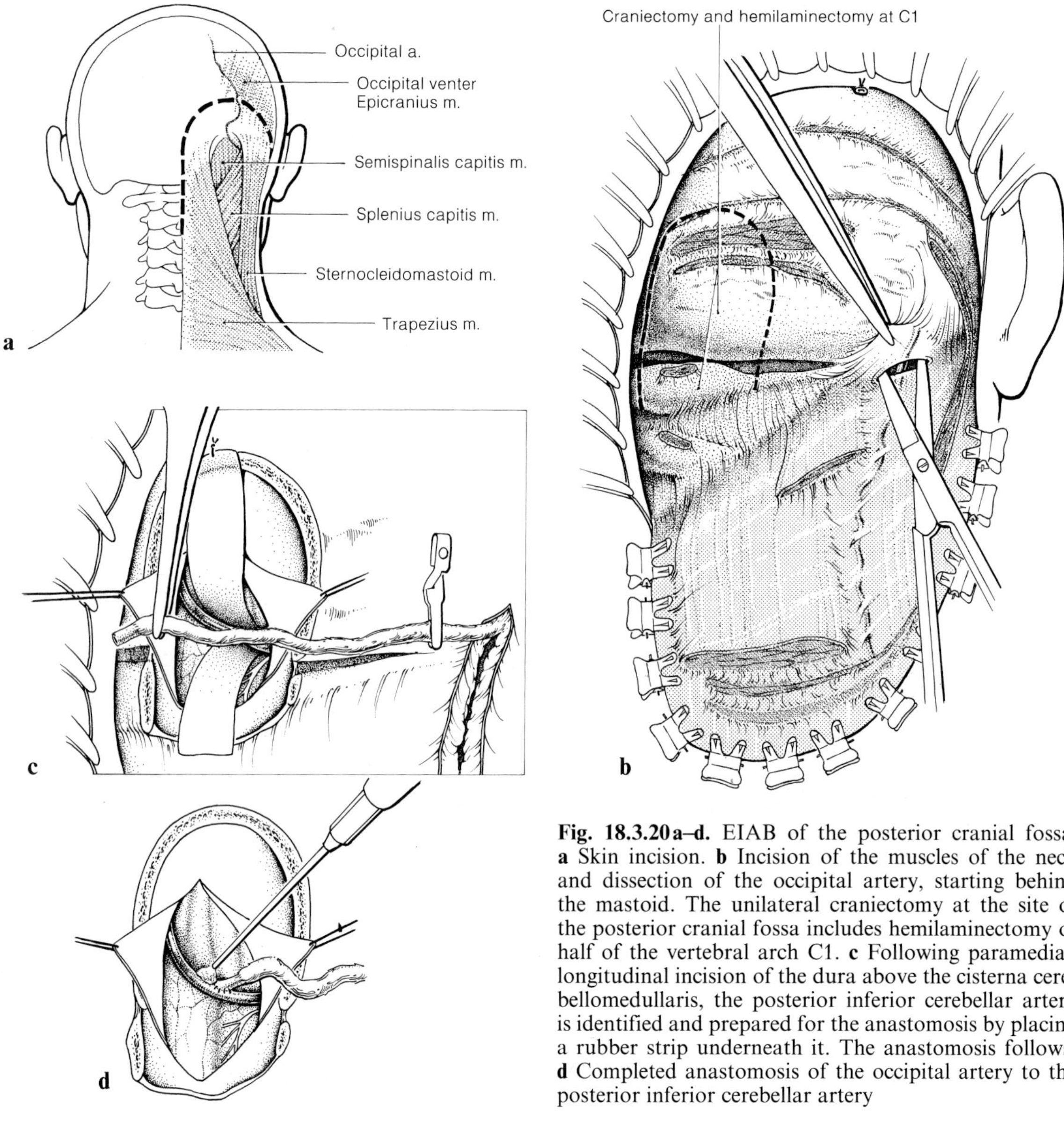

Fig. 18.3.20a–d. EIAB of the posterior cranial fossa. **a** Skin incision. **b** Incision of the muscles of the neck and dissection of the occipital artery, starting behind the mastoid. The unilateral craniectomy at the site of the posterior cranial fossa includes hemilaminectomy of half of the vertebral arch C1. **c** Following paramedian longitudinal incision of the dura above the cisterna cerebellomedullaris, the posterior inferior cerebellar artery is identified and prepared for the anastomosis by placing a rubber strip underneath it. The anastomosis follows. **d** Completed anastomosis of the occipital artery to the posterior inferior cerebellar artery

G. Revascularization of the Posterior Cranial Fossa – EIAB from the Occipital Artery to the Posterior Inferior Cerebellar Artery

(Fig. 18.3.20)

For EIAB of the posterior cranial fossa [14, 27, 28] the patient is put in a semirecumbent position with the head pronated, slightly turned, and fixed by a headholder. Another possibility is a lateral position with the head slightly turned and facing the floor.

Using an inverted-J incision (Fig. 18.3.20a), the dissection is carried out deeply in the avascular midline; the muscles are severed from vertebral arch C1 on one side and from the occiput. The ascending branch of the occipital artery can be palpated deep and medial to the mastoid; it is dissected as far distally as possible (Fig. 18.3.20b). Afterwards a small unilateral suboccipital craniectomy, including resection of half of the vertebral arch C1, is performed. The dura is opened paramedially, and the medullary loop of the posterior inferior cerebellar artery is identified in its course to the vermis. It is mobilized and a rubber dam

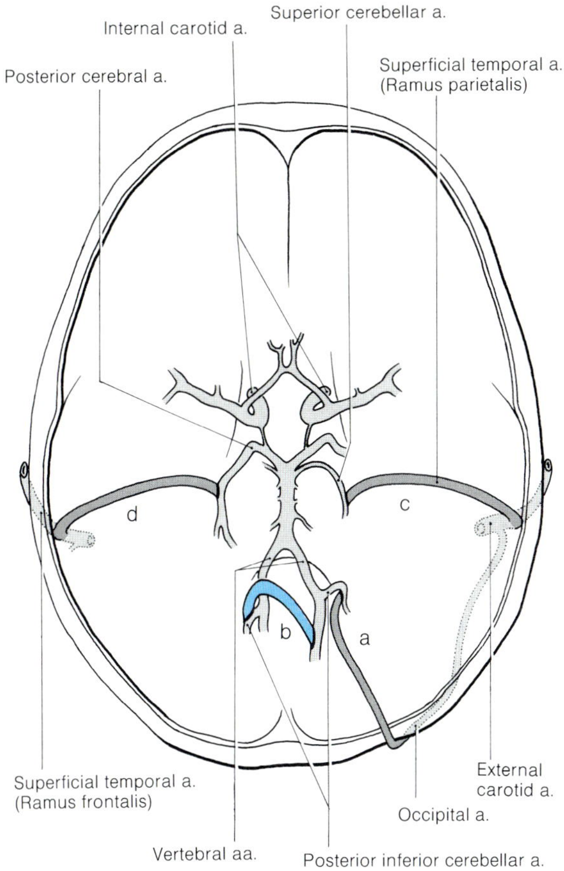

Fig. 18.3.21. Schematic drawing of possible revascularizations of the posterior cranial fossa. **a** From occipital artery to posterior inferior cerebellar artery; **b** from vertebral artery to posterior inferior cerebellar artery (with vein graft); **c** from superficial temporal artery to superior cerebellar artery; **d** from superficial temporal artery to posterior cerebral artery

placed underneath it (Fig. 18.3.20c). After adaptation of the length of the occipital artery to the recipient site and preparation of the arterial stump, the posterior inferior cerebellar artery is occluded with two microclips. A longitudinal incision is made between the clips. An end-to-side anastomosis of the occipital artery to the posterior inferior cerebellar artery is performed using interrupted sutures of 9-0 monofilament material. As described earlier, the anastomosis is inspected upon completion and, following removal of the clips, fibrin foam is placed around it. While closing the wound layer by layer, care must be taken to assure enough space for the occipital artery without endangering secure closure of the dura. Several variants (Fig. 18.3.21) of the revascularization of the posterior cranial fossa have been described, some as case reports [1, 2, 3, 4, 28]. All evidence would therefore seem to indicate that it is possible to bypass all stenoses or occlusions of the greater arteries of the vertebrobasilar circulation. Depending on the localization of stenoses and occlusions, the occipital artery or the vertebral artery can be used for revascularization of the caudal portions of the brain stem (posterior inferior cerebellar artery), using vascular interposition grafts, if necessary. The superficial temporal artery may be used for revascularization of the rostral portions of the brain stem (anterior cerebellar artery, superior cerebellar artery, or posterior cerebellar artery). Although the main technical problems of this very difficult operative procedure seem to be solved, many questions concerning patient selection remain open.

H. Extra-anatomic Bypass Procedures
(Figs. 18.3.22, 18.3.23)

As mentioned earlier, an essential prerequisite for conventional EIAB is an extracranial donor artery with an internal diameter of at least 1 mm in the segment to be anastomosed. Owing to a variety of factors, this precondition might not be fulfilled:

- Extensive arteriosclerosis of the carotid bifurcation with involvement of the external carotid artery
- Injury of the temporal artery, possibly by previous operations, e.g., for aneurysms
- "Arteriospasm" of the temporal artery, especially in young females

If other donor arteries (see Sect. F.III,IV) are not suitable, one has to consider the possibility of vascular grafts. Autogenous saphenous vein has proven to be the best graft material, although numerous other materials have been used (radial artery, denatured human umbilical cord prosthesis, expanded PTFE prosthesis). Autogenous vein had already been used by Woringer and Kunlin [29], prior to the introduction of microsurgery, to perform a bypass from the common carotid artery to the intracranial segment of the internal carotid artery. However, the anastomosis of the vein to the intracranial segment of the internal carotid artery is technically difficult and requires extensive manipulation of the brain. Today, therefore, one usually performs a distal anastomosis to a cortical branch of the middle cerebral artery, usually to

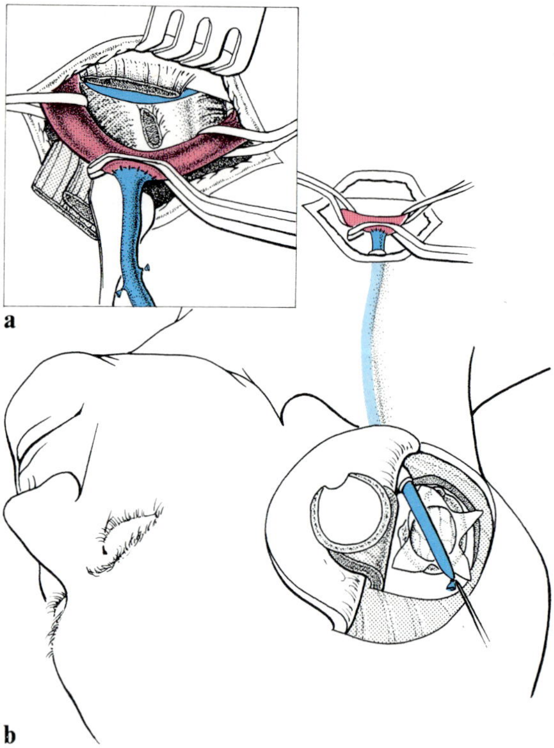

Fig. 18.3.22 a, b. Extra-anatomic bypass from subclavian artery to angularis artery. **a** Exposure of the subclavian artery by a supraclavicular approach and proximal side-to-end anastomosis. **b** Exposure of the cortical artery by skin incision and course of the vein graft

its major branch in the region of the angularis artery; here, the branch has an inner diameter of 1.5–2 mm. For the extracranial anastomosis, the external carotid artery and the common carotid artery were chosen in the early days. However, it has been shown [24] that it is better to connect the prosthesis to the subclavian artery. That way, the prosthesis is straight and therefore subject to less tension when the head is turned.

This operation (Fig. 18.3.22), properly enough, is a cooperative effort between the vascular surgeon and the neurosurgeon: while the craniectomy is being performed (following a parieto-occipital skin incision), the greater saphenous vein is harvested, starting the dissection distally and continuing upward to the knee, where the vein narrows slightly, thereby presenting an obvious advantage for the distal anastomosis. The tributaries are ligated, except for a proximal branch in which a blunt cannula is inserted to flush the vessel with heparinized saline to disclose leaks. Afterwards, the vein is kept in this solution or in heparinized blood until implantation. The direction of the subsequent arterial blood flow in the vein is indicated.

The typical supraclavicular approach to the subclavian artery is made through a skin incision parallel to the clavicle. The subclavian artery is exposed, two tapes are passed around it, and a Satinsky clamp is applied. The vein is then prepared for the proximal anastomosis; this involves dissecting off the perivascular tissue and beveling the stump slightly. Following systemic administration of 5000 I.U. heparin and clamping of the subclavian artery, an oval incision is made, and a side-to-end anastomosis of the subclavian artery to the distal end of the saphenous vein is performed using 6-0 suture material. Following completion of the anastomosis and control of hemostasis, a retroauricular subcutaneous tunnel is created from the craniectomy in the direction of the proximal anastomosis. An essential step is sharp dissection of the adhesions of the cranial fascia off the skull, carefully avoiding compression of the vein graft between the skin and the skull. The vein is passed through the subcutaneous tunnel by means of a 20-gauge trocar; here, one must be careful not to kink or twist the vein. The length of the vein graft is determined by the site of the distal anastomosis; the stump of the vein is beveled to achieve the widest possible anastomosis. The arachnoidea is incised for a sufficient distance over the cortical artery chosen to serve as recipient artery, and the artery is mobilized. After placing rubber dams around the artery, its smaller branches are occluded by long, narrow temporary microclips. Afterwards, the cortical artery is incised longitudinally between two clips placed 1 cm apart, using a diamond knife. Following placement of the two corner sutures, the anastomosis is performed using closely spaced interrupted sutures or a combination of interrupted and continuous sutures with 10-0 suture material. The occlusion time for the cortical artery will be between 25 min (for a continuous suture) and 45 min (for interrupted sutures), according to our experience.

In order to shorten the time required for the anastomosis, the sutures can be placed at somewhat larger intervals and additionally sealed with fibrin glue. Postoperative patency of the vein bypass may easily be ascertained by palpation or percutaneous Doppler ultrasonography.

Variants of cerebral revascularization using vein grafts include: the combination of a vein bypass from the subclavian artery to the external carotid artery and conventional EIAB for bypass-

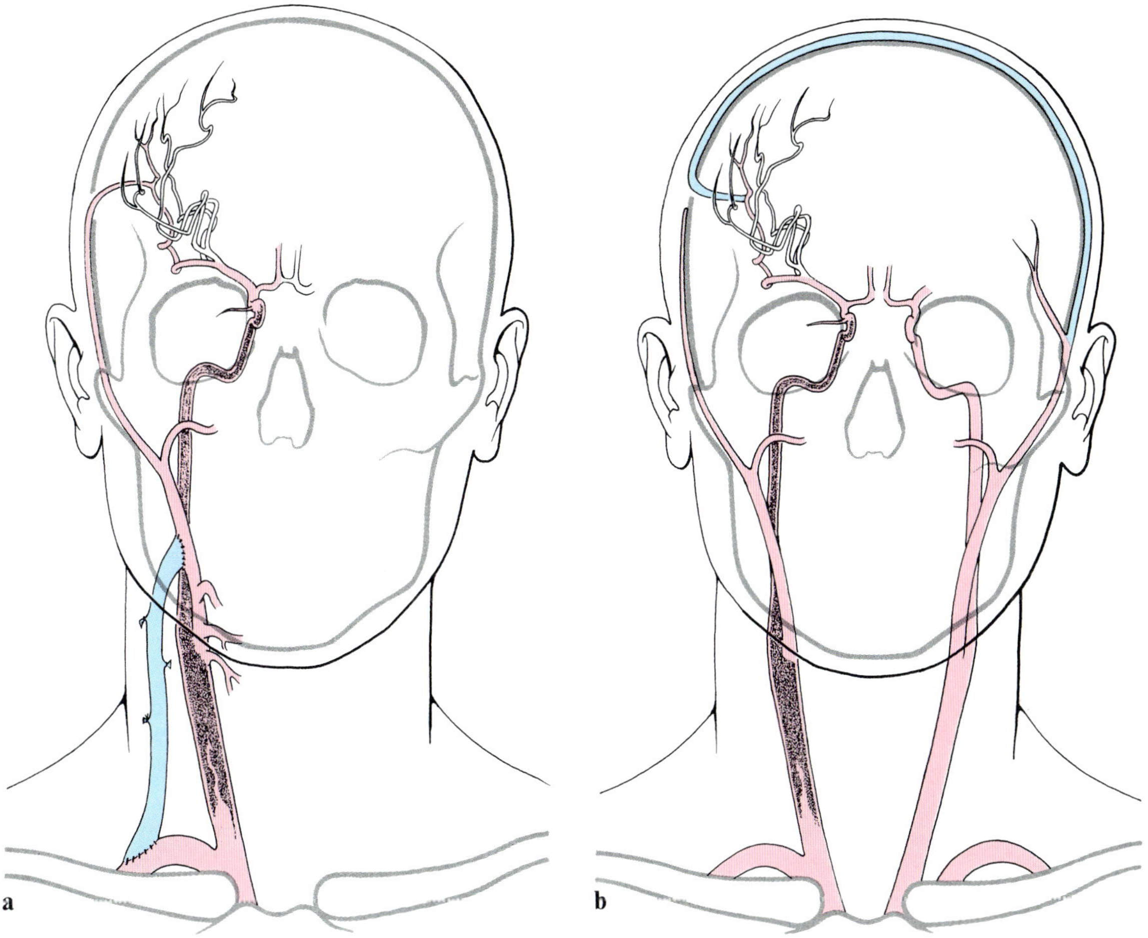

Fig. 18.3.23a, b. Variants of extra-anatomic bypass procedures. **a** In the case of occlusion of the common carotid artery: vein bypass from subclavian artery to external carotid artery followed by conventional EIAB. **b** Bonnet bypass in the case of occlusion of the common carotid and external carotid arteries on one side in the absence of a donor artery on the same side: vein bypass from the contralateral superficial temporal artery to a cortical artery of the occluded side, crossing the midline

ing an occlusion of the common carotid artery, and the bonnet bypass from a temporal artery to the contralateral cortical artery (Fig. 18.3.23a, b).

I. Embolectomy of the Middle Cerebral Artery (Fig. 18.3.24)

The middle cerebral artery, being a terminal branch of the internal carotid artery, represents the "embolism artery." Often, emboli dissolve spontaneously; therefore, some embolic strokes may not require revascularization. However, in rare cases, it is possible [23] to remove an angiographically demonstrated embolus from the middle cerebral artery within a short interval of 4–6 h. This interval, during which computed tomography and angiography must be performed, can be extended if necessary by early administration of barbiturates.

For the embolectomy, a small frontotemporal craniectomy is performed, the Sylvian fissure opened, and the main stem of the middle cerebral artery (or branch of the artery) exposed, showing the thrombus, which can be recognized as a dark segment. The dissection of the main stem may be impaired or even rendered impossible by massive swelling of the brain. Following temporary ligation of the main artery and the distal branches by clips, a branch just distal to the thrombus is incised and the thrombus extruded slowly. Following early removal of the proximal clip, the blood will flush out the rest of the thrombus from a prox-

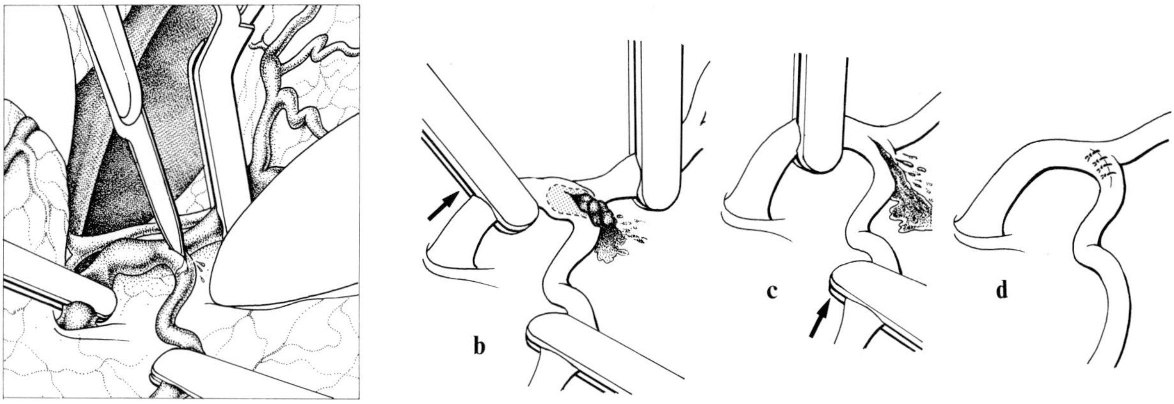

Fig. 18.3.24a–d. Embolectomy in the case of embolism in the middle cerebral artery. **a** Embolism in the major trunk of the middle cerebral artery; application of temporary clips proximal and distal to the embolus, incision of the artery, and flushing or extrusion of the embolus. **b**, **c** Retrograde flushing of the remnants of the embolus by alternately releasing the clips (*arrows*). **d** Interrupted suture of the arteriotomy and removal of the clips

imal direction. Afterwards, the distal clips are opened temporarily step by step to flush out the distal portions of the thrombus. Following flushing with heparinized solution, the arteriotomy is closed with interrupted sutures (7-0 to 10-0).

K. Postoperative Monitoring and Follow-up

After surgery and anesthesia, the patient is kept in the intensive care unit for 1 day for control of possible postoperative hypertensive crisis or hypotensive regulatory disturbances. Afterwards, the patient can be mobilized quickly as EIAB (routinely taking 2 h) does not subject the patient to great stress. (The operation time for EIAB of the posterior cranial fossa is about 4–5 h, somewhat less for the larger extra-anatomic bypasses). Early mobilization is especially recommended from the surgical standpoint; for, if the closure of the dura has been incomplete, too much cerebrospinal fluid may leak into the temporal muscle, resulting in local headache.

Immediately following surgery, the administration of platelet aggregation inhibitors, e.g., acetylsalicylic acid, is resumed, at first intravenously, and on the next day orally. In most cases no further postoperative medical therapy is required. In patients with stenosis of the internal carotid or the middle cerebral artery operated on by EIAB, administration of heparin 3×5000 I.U. is recommended to prevent a stenosis from becoming occluded, which may occur as a result of the postoperatively altered pre-/poststenotic pressure gradient. This medication may be reduced after a few days and terminated when the patient is discharged, i.e., when the stitches are removed, usually on the 7th postoperative day.

For follow-up control, only noninvasive examinations are required. The essential examination for assessment of function is percutaneous Doppler ultrasonography [8, 10], which allows semiquantitative determination of the amount of blood being supplied to the brain via the EIAB. Angiography is only required when new symptoms of cerebral ischemia occur, indicating further surgical therapy. Complications of EIAB, other than cardiac ones derived from the underlying arteriosclerosis, are impairment of wound healing and new temporary or permanent neurologic deficits caused intraoperatively either by ischemia or intracerebral bleeding. The latter complication is found especially in patients whose blood pressure is not well monitored or in cases where EIAB is performed within the first 4 weeks after an ischemic stroke. Although some authors report a mortality of 0% in partial series, the mortality in larger series is 1.5%–2% [19, 31]. The morbidity is about 2.2%.

During follow-up, new ischemic damage of the contralateral side or in the region of the vertebrobasilar circulation may become manifest. Also, a significant proportion of postoperative mortality is caused by myocardial infarction. This indicates that arteriosclerosis is the basic underlying process, which neurosurgery cannot cure. But even though neurosurgical therapy may not increase life expectancy, it may well prevent or ameliorate life-threatening symptoms and thereby improve the quality of life.

REFERENCES

1. Ausman JI, Nicoloff DM, Chou SN (1978) Posterior fossa revascularization: Anastomosis of vertebral artery to PICA with interposed radial artery graft. Surg Neurol 9:281–286
2. Ausman JI, Lee MC, Chater NL, Latchaw RE (1979) Superficial temporal artery to superior cerebellar artery anastomosis for distal basilar artery stenosis. Surg Neurol 12:277–282
3. Ausman JI, Diaz FG, de los Reyes RA, Pak H, Patel S, Boulos R (1981) Anastomosis of occipital artery to anterior inferior cerebellar artery for vertebrobasilar junction stenosis. Surg Neurol 16:99–102
4. Ausman JI, Diaz FG, de los Reyes RA, Pak H, Patel S, Boulos R (1981) Superficial temporal to proximal superior cerebellar artery anastomosis for basilar artery stenosis. Neurosurgery 9:56–66
5. Chater NL, Spetzler RF, Tonnemacher K, Wilson CB (1976) Microvascular bypass surgery. Part 1: Anatomical studies. J Neurosurg 44:712–714
6. EC/IC Bypass Study Group (1985) Failure of extracranial-intracranial arterial bypass to reduce the risk of ischemic stroke. N Engl J Med 313:1191–1200
7. Fisher CM (1951) Occlusion of the internal carotid artery. Arch Neurol Psych 65:346–377
8. Gilsbach JM (1983) Intraoperative Doppler sonography in neurosurgery. Springer, Wien New York
9. Goldsmith HS, Chen WF, Duckett SW (1973) Brain vascularization by intact omentum. Arch Surg 106:695–698
10. Jamjoom ZA, Mehdorn HM, Nahser HC (1983) Comparative study of Doppler sonography and angiography in extracranial-intracranial anastomosis. Adv Neurosurg 11:375–383
11. Karasawa J, Kikuchi H, Furuse S, Kawamura J, Sakaki T (1978) Treatment of moyamoya disease with STA-MCA anastomosis. J Neurosurg 49:679–688
12. Karasawa J, Kikuchi H, Kawamura J, Sakaki T (1980) Intracranial transplantation of the omentum for cerebrovascular moyamoya disease: A two-year follow-up study. Surg Neurol 14:444–449
13. Kearns TP, Siekert RG, Sundt TM Jr (1978) The ocular aspects of carotid artery bypass surgery. Trans Am Ophthalmol Soc 76:247–265
14. Khodadad G, Singh RS, Olinger CP (1977) Possible prevention of stroke by microvascular anastomosis in the vertebral basilar system. Stroke 8:316–321
15. Kletter G (1979) The extra-intracranial bypass operation for prevention and treatment of stroke. Springer, Wien New York
16. Kletter G, Matras H, Dinges HP (1978) Zur partiellen Klebung von Mikrogefäßanastomosen im intrakraniellen Bereich. Wien Klin Wochenschr 90:415–419
17. Laurent JP, Lawner PM, O'Connor M (1982) Reversal of intracerebral steal by STA-MCA anastomosis. J Neurosurg 57:629–632
18. Little JR, Salerno TA (1978) Continuous suturing for microvascular anastomosis. Technical note. J Neurosurg 48:1042–1045
19. Mehdorn HM, Hoffman WF, Chater NL (1979) Microvascular neurosurgical arterial bypass for cerebral ischemia. A decade of development. World J Surg 3:197–206
20. Mehdorn HM (1980) Mikroneurochirurgische Therapie der zerebralen Ischämie. Z Allg Med 56:1731–1737
21. Peerless SJ (1975) Techniques of cerebral revascularization. Clin Neurosurg 23:258–269
22. Peerless SJ, Gamache FW Jr, Hunter IG (1981) Continuous suture method for microvascular anastomosis. Technical note. Neurosurgery 8:695–698
23. Piepgras DG, Sundt TM Jr (1982) Operative management of intracranial arterial occlusions and acute ischemic stroke. In: Youmans JR (ed) Neurological surgery, vol 3. Saunders, Philadelphia London Toronto Mexico City Tokyo, pp 1619–1626
24. Spetzler R, Chater N (1974) Occipital artery-middle cerebral artery anastomosis for cerebral artery occlusive disease. Surg Neurol 2:235–238
25. Spetzler RF, Rhodes RS, Roski RA, Likavec MJ (1980) Subclavian to middle cerebral artery saphenous vein bypass graft. J Neurosurg 53:465–469
26. Spetzler RF, Schuster H, Roski RA (1980) Elective extracranial-intracranial artery bypass in the treatment of inoperable giant aneurysms of the internal carotid artery. J Neurosurg 53:22–27
27. Sundt TM Jr, Piepgras DG (1978) Occipital artery to posterior inferior cerebellar artery bypass surgery. J Neurosurg 48:916–928
28. Sundt TM Jr, Piepgras DG, Houser OW, Campbell JK (1982) Interposition saphenous vein grafts for advanced occlusive disease and large aneurysm in the posterior circulation. J Neurosurg 56:205–215
29. Woringer E, Kunlin J (1963) Anastomose entre la carotide primitive et la carotide intracranienne ou la sylvienne par greffon selon la technique de la suture suspendue. Neurochirurgie 9:181–188
30. Yasargil MG (1969) Microsurgery applied to neurosurgery. Thieme, Stuttgart. Academic, New York
31. Yasargil MG, Yonekawa Y (1977) Results of microsurgical extra-intracranial arterial bypass in the treatment of cerebral ischemia. Neurosurgery 1:22–24

18.4 Reconstructive Surgery in Intrathoracic Supra-aortic Occlusive Disease

O. Thetter and R.J.A.M. van Dongen

CONTENTS

A. Introduction

Occlusive disease of the large branches of the aortic arch and its operative treatment have assumed increasing significance within the last few years as angiologic and angiographic investigations have revealed that approximately 20%–30% of patients with manifest clinical arterial occlusive disease of the cerebrum also have occlusive disease in extracranial segments of the supra-aortic vessels. While approximately 56% of the occlusions are located in the region of the carotid sinus, more than 40% of patients present with hemodynamically effective vascular changes in the proximal segments of the aortic arch branches (innominate artery, common carotid arteries, and subclavian arteries) [1]. Another indication of the frequency of this disease is that among patients suffering from manifest disturbances of the peripheral circulation, 30% also show additional vascular changes in the region of the supra-aortic branches. The significance of cerebrovascular disease is seen from the fact that it occupies third place in the mortality statistics, following cardiovascular disease and malignant tumors.

In the vast majority of cases, arteriosclerosis is the cause of occlusive disease. Stenotic lesions at the origins of the supra-aortic branches owing to inflammatory processes, such as the Takayasu syndrome, are rare.

Occlusions or stenoses of supra-aortic branches are either localized at their origin on the aortic arch (without narrowing the lumen of the aorta) or in their initial segment. The distal involvement is variable, however, rarely extending farther than the takeoff of the first branch.

Occlusive processes most commonly occur at or near the origin of the left subclavian artery. In second place is the innominate artery; less commonly involved are the common carotid arteries.

In most cases, circulatory obstructions in the primary branches of the aorta are not solitary but multiple. Therefore, precise, detailed angiographic visualization of all aortic branches, and of the vertebral arteries as well, is extremely important for the planning of appropriate surgical therapy.

B. Anatomy

The ascending aorta originates from the left ventricle, dorsal and to the right of the pulmonary artery and left of the superior vena cava at the level of the third interspace. Its anterior surface is covered by pericardium up to about 1 cm below the origin of the innominate artery and in adults is hidden by the retrosternal fatty tissue. The ascending aorta, together with the aortic arch, is part of a spiral, ascending in front of the trachea toward the right first interspace and crossing the trachea on its left side. The apex of the aortic arch lies at the level of the manubrium sterni. The aortic arch then turns to the left, passing the trachea, continues dorsally, and reaches the vertebral column at the left circumference of the fourth thoracic vertebra, becoming the thoracic aorta (Fig. 18.4.1).

The arch, being convex toward the cranial side, rides on the left main bronchus. The pulmonary trunk is attached to the concavity of the aortic arch by Botallo's ligament. The right pulmonary artery passes behind the ascending aorta, the left pulmonary artery in front of the descending aorta to the appropriate lobe of the lung. The pulmonary arteries cross both major bronchi ventrally. The right and left innominate veins enter the thorax anterolateral to the artery (Fig. 18.4.2). The longer innominate vein passes from the left sternoclavicular joint on the posterior surface of the manubrium sterni medially to the sternal end of the first interspace, there to join the right innominate vein, creating the superior vena cava. Ventrally, it crosses the origins of the three supra-aortic branches, the left subclavian artery, the left common carotid artery, and the innominate artery. Owing to the almost sagittal position of the arch within the thorax, the origins of the innominate artery and of the left common carotid artery are more superficial than the origin of the left subclavian artery. The origin of the innominate artery is at the level of the sternal end of the second right rib cartilage. The trunk, which is about 2 cm long, passes upward obliquely and to the right, over the anterior and right circumference of the trachea toward the upper thoracic opening. It branches into the right subclavian artery and the

Fig. 18.4.1. Anatomy of the supra-aortic arteries

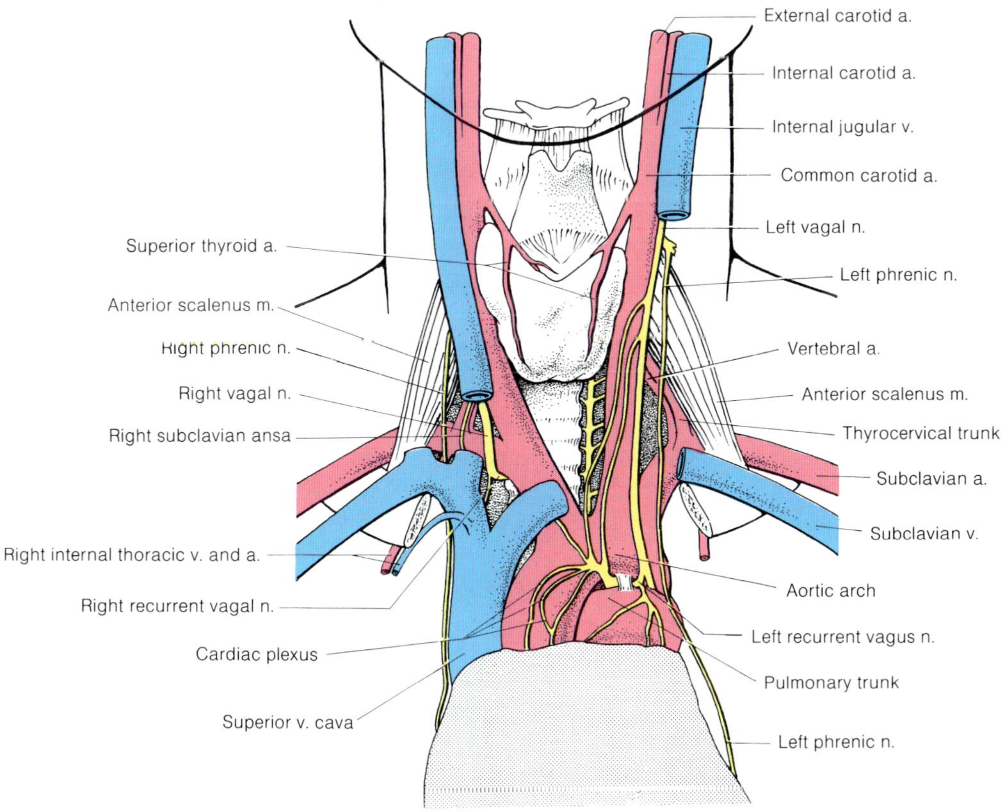

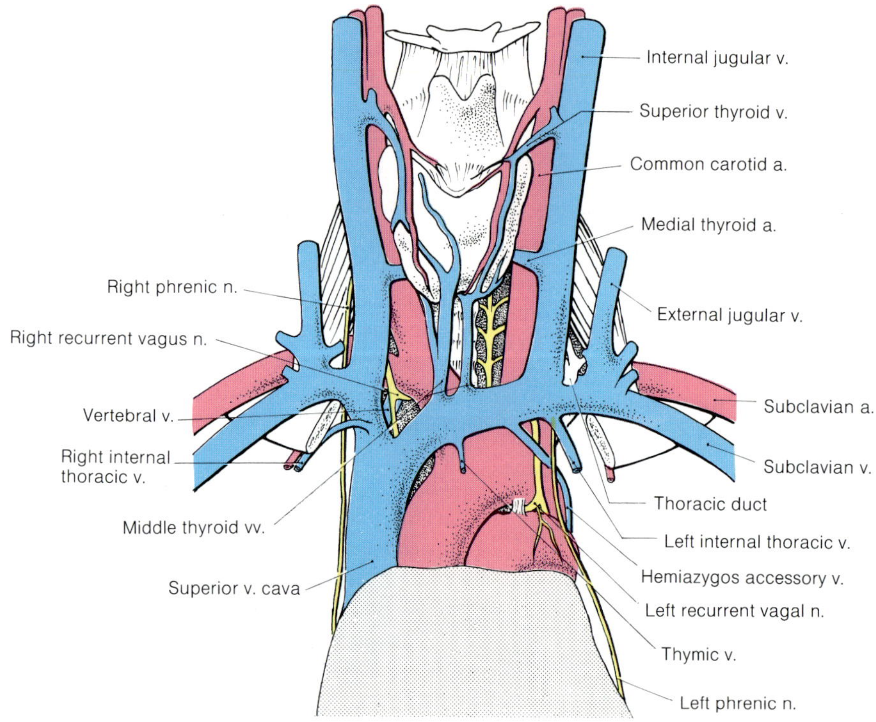

Fig. 18.4.2. Anatomy of the vena cava and its afferent branches

right common carotid artery behind the right sternoclavicular joint. The carotid artery continues in the direction of the innominate artery. In contrast, the right subclavian artery passes curvilinearly across the apex of the pleura to the posterior scalenus space and to the supraclavicular fossa. The right common carotid artery ascends at the lateral aspect of the trachea and the esophagus, covered by the sternocleidomastoid muscle, to the fossa carotica, branching there into two tributaries.

Just after the innominate artery, the left common carotid artery branches off the aortic arch. It turns to the left across the anterior circumference of the trachea and ascends left of the trachea and the esophagus through the upper thoracic opening to the neck.

The left subclavian artery is usually the last and the most dorsal branch of the arch, ascending vertically and finally curvilinearly across the left apex of the pleura to the posterior scalenus space and the fossa supraclavicularis.

For the vascular surgeon, it has been proved to be of advantage to divide the subclavian artery into four segments [4, 5] (Fig. 18.4.3).

The *first segment* extends from the origin of the subclavian artery to the origin of the vertebral artery and the internal thoracic artery.

From the *second segment*, the vertebral artery and the internal thoracic artery branch off.

The third supraclavicular segment is located between the origin of the thyrocervical trunk and the costoclavicular space.

The *fourth costoclavicular segment* is located in the space between the clavicle and the first rib.

The *vagus nerve* and the *phrenic nerve*, as well as the *thoracic duct* are in close contact with the large vessels and are therefore easily injured during dissection. The vagal nerves (Fig. 18.4.1) enter the thorax between the common carotid artery and the internal jugular vein. The right vagus nerve crosses the subclavian artery immediately after branching off from the innominate artery on the anterior surface. The recurrent nerve passes around the vessel from below and ascends cranially into the esophagotracheal groove. The left vagus nerve crosses the aortic arch on its anterior circumference. There, the recurrent nerve branches off, passing around the concavity of the arch to the left of Botallo's duct and ascends into the groove between the trachea and the esophagus up to the larynx.

The *phrenic nerves* (Fig. 18.4.1) are located on both sides on the anterior aspect of the anterior

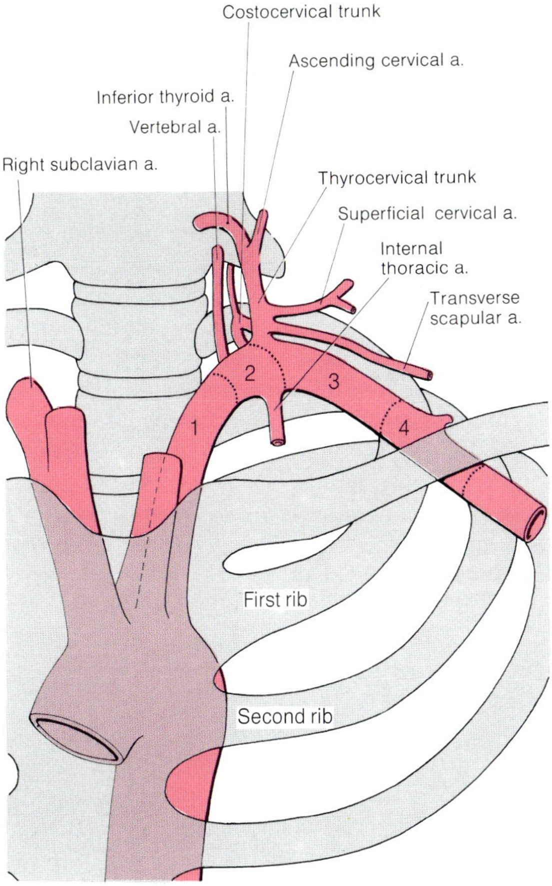

Fig. 18.4.3. Segments of the subclavian artery

scalenus muscles in the upper fascia. They enter the thorax between the subclavian artery and vein and cross the subclavian artery ventrally just before entering the posterior scalenus space. Here, they are located lateral to the vagal nerves. The right phrenic nerve crosses the internal thoracic artery from lateral to ventral to become located lateral to the innominate vein and the superior vena cava. Finally, it descends in front of the hilus of the lung, between the fibrous pericardium and the mediastinal pleura, to the diaphragm. The left phrenic nerve also crosses the internal thoracic artery lateroventrally and passes beneath the mediastinal pleura across the aortic arch to the left border of the heart.

The *ansa subclavia* (*ansa of Vieussens*) must not be injured; otherwise, a Horner's syndrome may result postoperatively. The ansa (Fig. 18.4.1) originates from the medial cervical ganglion of the sympathetic trunk and has two portions. The ventral portion passes the subclavian artery lateral to the origin of the vertebral artery and, like the dorsal portion, reaches the inferior cervical ganglion. This ganglion usually joins the first thoracic ganglion to form the ganglion stellatum and is located in front of the head of the first rib.

The *thoracic duct* is of surgical interest at various locations during its course because of its high susceptibility to injury during dissection of the left subclavian artery [16]. In the angle between the aortic arch and the origin of the left subclavian artery (Fig. 18.4.4), the thoracic duct passes underneath the pleura in the sheath of the esophageal fascia, through the opening of the thorax into the base of the neck. It then passes ventrally between the left common carotid artery and the subclavian artery to the left venous angle, entering there (Figs. 18.4.2–18.4.4). The apex of the arch of the thoracic duct, before it enters the vein, may extend far into the neck and is located medial to the thyrocervical trunk and the anterior scalenus muscle, in whose fascia the phrenic nerve is embedded. Before entering, the thoracic duct usually receives the jugular, subclavian, and bronchomediastinal trunks, which are interrupted by lymph nodes. Some 40% of all iatrogenic injuries to the thoracic duct occur in the left upper mediastinum. In the aortosubclavian angle, the duct is easily injured during dissection of the subclavian artery. This

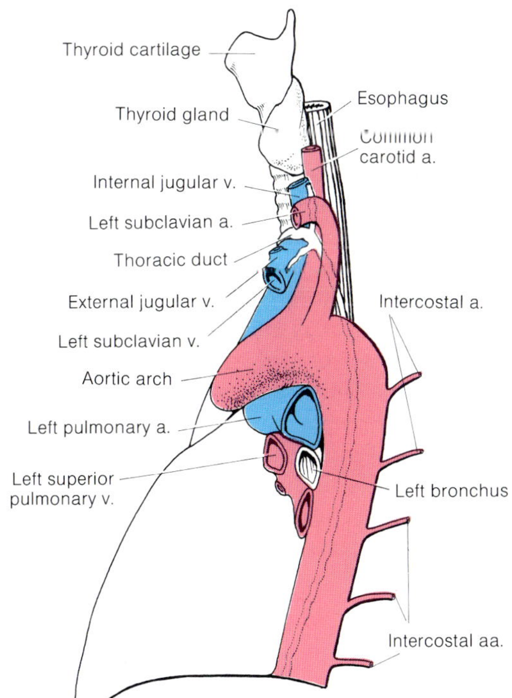

Fig. 18.4.4. Course of the thoracic duct

mainly occurs when one fails to stay close to the arterial wall after division of the parietal pleura and dissects roughly into the depths of the mediastinum.

Another area where injury to the thoracic duct can occur is in the region of the lateral triangle of the neck (Figs. 18.4.12, 18.4.13). With the supraclavicular approach to the subclavian artery, injuries to the terminal thoracic duct (and the phrenic nerve) are likely. Therefore, one must be on guard against injuring the thoracic duct not only when dissecting in the region of the supraclavicular fossa, but also when retracting the venous angle for exposure of the artery.

Also in operations on the right subclavian artery, one must be careful to preserve the integrity of the greater lymph vessels (right lymphatic trunk), and especially the anterior bronchomediastinal trunk, which enters the venous angle there. Because of collateral connections with the thoracic duct, chylus may leak out of the left system in a retrograde direction when the right lymphatic trunk is opened, resulting in a chylothorax.

C. Clinical Manifestation

The clinical symptoms of occlusive disease of the supra-aortic branches depend on the type, the localization, and the extent and multiplicity of the vascular obstruction, but may also depend on the condition of the collateral circulation. Correspondingly, temporary or permanent ischemia may occur in the vascular system of the subclavian artery, the carotid artery, and the vertebral artery. In cases of occlusion of the innominate artery, besides symptoms of carotid artery insufficiency, signs of vertebrobasilar insufficiency and of brachial insufficiency may also be noticed. Occlusions or severe stenoses of the origin of the subclavian artery or of the innominate artery proximal to the origin of the vertebral artery lead to a change in the direction of blood flow in the vertebral artery and consequently to a subclavian steal syndrome, especially during exercise of the upper extremity.

Usually, the physician is consulted either because of ischemic symptoms in the region of the upper extremity or because of neurologic symptoms.

D. Indication for Operation

Surgical intervention to correct an occlusion of the subclavian artery is indicated above all when a vertebrobasilar insufficiency is clinically relevant and reproducible by provocation tests. An isolated occlusion of the subclavian artery resulting in reduced blood flow to the arm during exercise is also an indication for surgery. However, asymptomatic occlusions in this region, even though they are demonstrated angiographically, should not be treated surgically.

Vascular lesions of the innominate artery and the common carotid artery, producing intermittent neurologic symptoms, are always urgent indications for surgery because one never knows whether the next ischemic attack will cause an irreversible neurologic deficit. In particular, it must be stressed that atheromatous plaques that are hemodynamically ineffective, but ulcerated, threaten the patient's life. They serve as a constant source of emboli and consequently as the cause of transient ischemic attacks.

When chosing an operative procedure for the reconstruction of occlusive lesions in the supra-aortic region, considerations of operative morbidity and mortality play a major role. Reports published in the literature over the last few years show that the postoperative results with an extrathoracic approach are not superior to the more invasive transthoracic approach, which also has a higher mortality. This is due to more stringent criteria for patient selection and also to improvements in prostheses, suture materials, and operative techniques. On the basis of our clinical experience, which confirms the experimental data of LORD and EHRENFELD [11], we feel it is sound procedure to divert the blood flow of a healthy artery extrathoracically without the risk of producing a new steal syndrome.

The reconstructive procedure is attempted not only in cases of arteriosclerotic occlusions, but also in Takayasu's disease. The bypass should extend far into the healthy vascular segment because in these patients, who are mostly young, the disease can be expected to progress. It is not advisable to divert blood from the aortic arch, even if a second branch of the aortic arch is already involved. Involvement of a third branch is an extreme rarity. Therefore, it is possible to use the healthy artery to supply the occluded vascular system.

An exact angiogram of all branches of the aortic arch is of decisive significance in planning the operative approach. Incomplete opacification may lead to a faulty assessment of the situation and consequently to an inappropriate choice of reconstructive procedure. Any vessel that is considered as a possible donor artery for extra-anatomic bypass must be free of hemodynamically significant lesions, as proven angiographically and by Doppler ultrasonography. This condition holds not only for the segments proximal to the shunt, but of course for the distal segment as well.

In the future, it is expected that patient selection will be based exclusively on noninvasive investigations. At the moment, however, it is not yet possible to abandon morphological evaluation of the vascular condition. Along with catheter angiography, digital subtraction angiography has also been gaining in importance. In addition to visualization of the blood vessels, this technique also provides a semiquantitative measurement of the blood flow through a stenosed vascular segment (regions of interest).

E. Operative Techniques

Because occlusive processes of the supra-aortic arteries involve lesions distributed segmentally in vessels of large diameter [2], they are usually amenable to management by vascular surgery. Provided there is good run-off in the periphery, in most cases complete operative restoration of the vascular system can be achieved. Concerning the operative approach, especially the question whether a transthoracic or extrathoracic approach is preferred, opinions still differ [6, 7, 8, 10, 12, 14, 17].

The transthoracic procedure became the predominant reconstructive principle in the early 1960s. Nevertheless, in the ensuing years, thoracotomy and sternotomy were not deemed necessary if disease-free, patent arteries were available in the extrathoracic region that could serve as donor arteries for an extrathoracic bypass. Within the last 10 years there has been a growing tendency toward extrathoracic bypass because it avoids the large intervention and the potential complications of thoracotomy or sternotomy and also because it is more feasible for older, high-risk patients with cardiorespiratory insufficiency [17].

In the discussion of these various procedures, the concern has often been expressed that a carotid steal effect may result, for instance, from a carotid subclavian bypass in patients suffering from subclavian steal syndrome. However, this objection was laid to rest by the experimental studies of LORD and EHRENFELD [11] measuring an increase of flow in the carotid artery proximal to the diversion [17]. Of course, it is essential that the donor artery is free of hemodynamically significant proximal and distal stenoses.

In a collective review of the world literature in 1978 GRUSS [9] found that in 931 reconstructions for subclavian steal syndrome the mortality of 3.7% with the transthoracic approach was reduced to 0.7% using the extrathoracic approach. The same review, however, shows significantly better clinical and hemodynamic results with the transthoracic approach. To what extent these postoperative results from the years 1960–1970 are still valid cannot be known without a collective review of recent years. However, in view of the great advances that have since been made in prostheses and suture material as well as operative technique, it is possible to believe reports of recent years showing that the two procedures produce similar postoperative results, except for the persistent difference in mortality [17]. The Department of Surgery of the University of Amsterdam [15] reports that, except for less favorable hemodynamics, the clinical and morphological long-term results obtained using the extrathoracic procedure were as good as those obtained with the transthoracic one.

F. Operative Approaches and Technique of Vascular Exposure

I. Transthoracic Approach

For the transthoracic procedure, essentially two operative approaches, median sternotomy and left posterolateral thoracotomy, are used.

1. Median Sternotomy

The ascending aorta, the innominate artery, the proximal segment of the right subclavian artery, and the intrathoracic segments of both carotid arteries are best exposed by a median total sternotomy.

The patient is placed in a supine position on the operating table with a surgeon on the right side of the patient. If transparent plastic drapes are used, care must be taken to insure access to

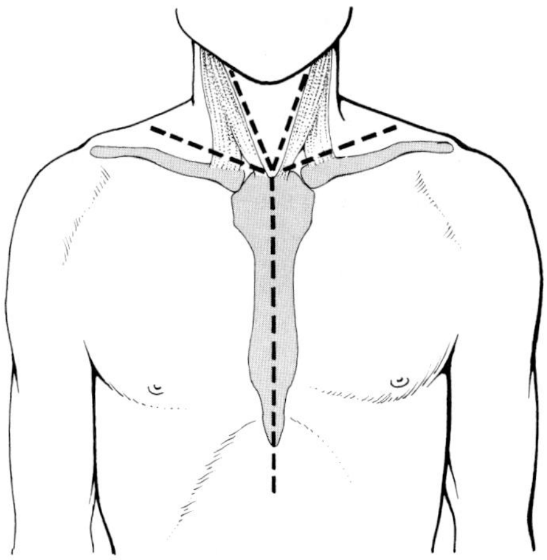

Fig. 18.4.5. Median sternotomy. Skin incision allowing extension in the supraclavicular fossa or along the sternocleidomastoid muscle

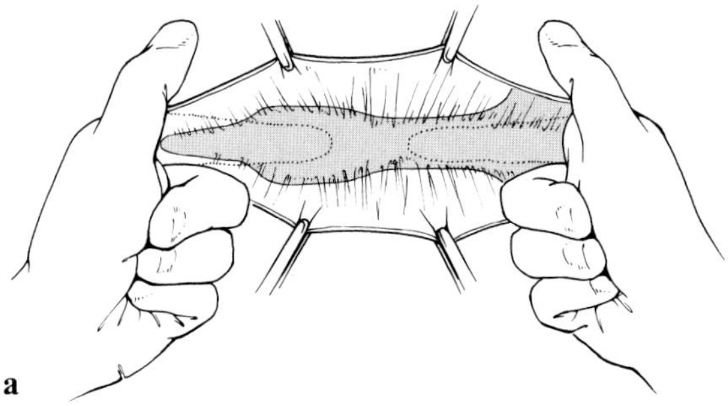

a

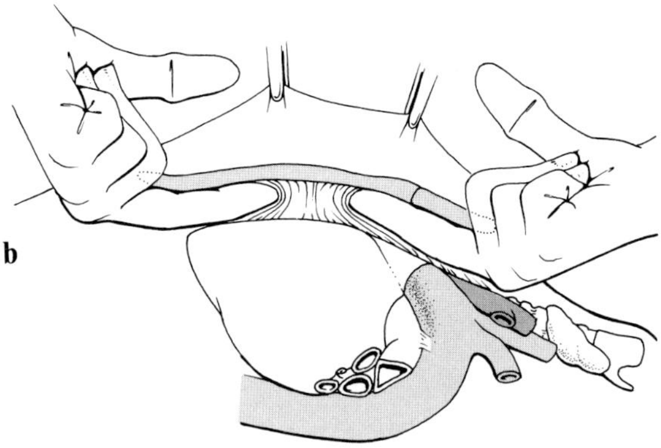

b

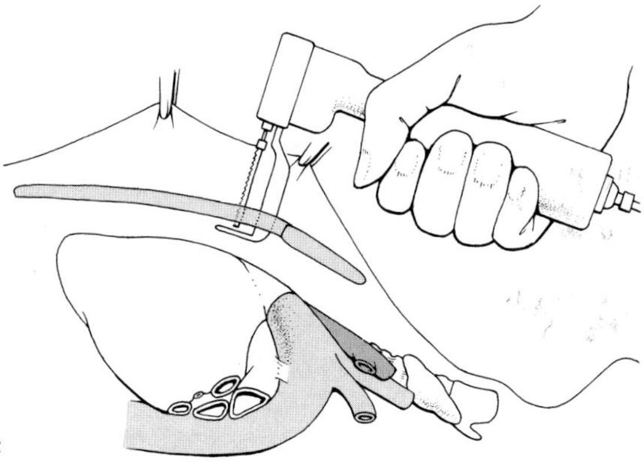

c

Fig. 18.4.6. a, b Blunt digital dissection of the retrosternal space. **c** Division of the sternum using a saw

the anterior part of the neck up as far as the border of the mandible and posteriorly as far as the mandibular angle; the supraclavicular fossa must also remain accessible. The skin incision (Fig. 18.4.5) is made in the midline from the jugulum downward to just below the xiphoid process. If required, the incision can be extended to the right or left in the supraclavicular fossa or along the medial margin of the sternocleidomastoid muscle. The subcutaneous tissue and the periost of the sternum is divided by electrocoagulation. Afterwards, the linea alba is incised over a short distance and the xiphoid process split longitudinally or resected with a large scissors. In the fossa jugularis, the interclavicular ligament is divided and the mediastinal tissue dissected off the posterior aspect of the manubrium sterni, using the left index finger (Fig. 18.4.6a, b). The precordial tissue is dissected off the posterior aspect of the sternum in a similar way, using the finger or a cotton applicator. In this way injuries are avoided while transecting the sternum. Longitudinal splitting of the sternum is best performed with a sternum saw or an oscillating saw (Fig. 18.4.6c). The cut edges of the sternum are covered with wax to prevent bleeding from the bone marrow. Bleeding from the periost of the anterior or posterior surface of the sternum may be stopped by applying the ball-shaped tip of the cautery.

With a thoracic retractor, both parts of the sternum are retracted and both duplications of the pleura are carefully bluntly dissected off the pericardium to avoid opening the pleural cavities. In case of rupture of the pleura, the pleural cavity must be drained upon completion of the procedure.

Now, the fatty thymus tissue covering the pericardium and the great vessels is resected or divided between clamps. Care must be taken of the left innominate vein which crosses the operative field transversely and is therefore easily injured. The vein should never be divided and ligated. In cases of bleeding, the bleeding sites must be closed with a fine suture (Prolene 6–0). As this vein covers the origin of the innominate artery and the left common carotid artery, it must be sufficiently mobilized and retracted with a tape to allow free access to the aortic arch and the aortic branches (Fig. 18.4.7).

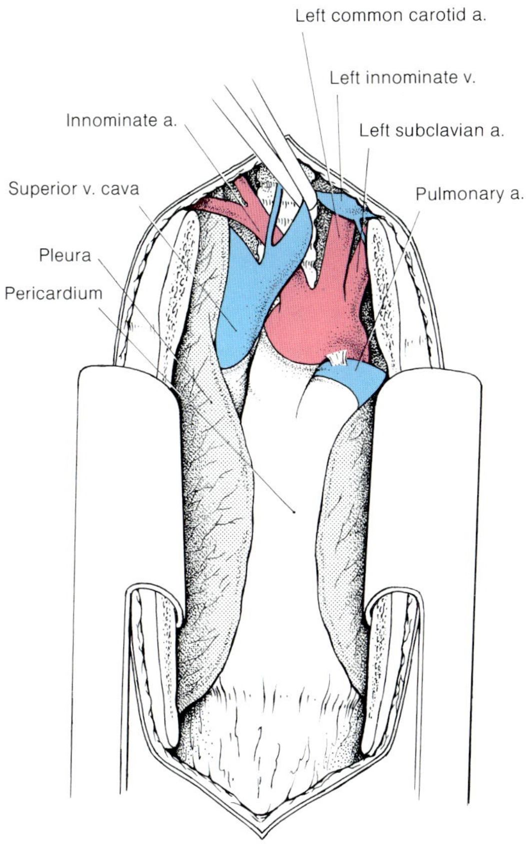

Fig. 18.4.7. Vessels exposed by sternotomy

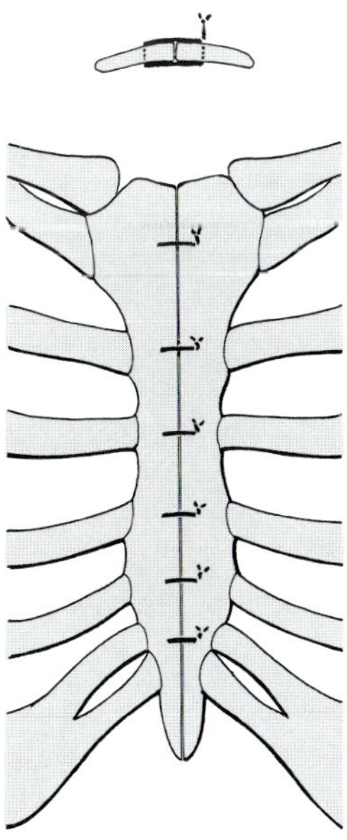

Fig. 18.4.8. Sternum wire suture

If the ascending aorta must be exposed, the upper portion of the pericardium is divided longitudinally. The aorta is then bluntly dissected circumferentially and a tape is placed around it in view of the possibility of injury to the right pulmonary artery, which passes behind the aorta. If the distal segments of the subclavian artery must also be exposed, median sternotomy is extended by a skin incision to the right or to the left into the supraclavicular fossa (Fig. 18.4.5).

In cases of insufficient exposure of the upper segment of the innominate artery by median sternotomy or when the upper segments of the common carotid artery within the neck must be exposed additionally, the incision along the medial border of the sternocleidomastoid muscle is extended upward. It is usually necessary to divide the sternal insertion of the sternocleidomastoid muscle as well as the longitudinal musculature of the neck in order to expose the bifurcation of the innominate artery clearly.

However, the common carotid artery and both its branches may also be exposed by an additional separate incision along the anterior border of the sternocleidomastoid muscle. If the whole length of the common carotid artery from the aorta up to the bifurcation must be dissected, the sternotomy incision along the medial margin of the sternocleidomastoid muscle is extended upward to the thyroid cartilage. After the subcutaneous tissue and the platysma have been divided, the sternal insertion of the sternocleidomastoid muscle, the sternothyroid muscle, and the omohyoid muscle, which crosses the common carotid artery, must be divided. Medial to the internal jugular vein, the common carotid artery is found and dissected as far as the bifurcation.

When dissecting at the origin of the branches of the aortic arch and along their further course, one must be very careful not to injure the phrenic and vagal nerves and the thoracic duct. The left phrenic nerve, the left vagus nerve, and the recurrent nerve are particularly susceptible to injury at the aortic arch. When exposing and dividing the insertion of the sternocleidomastoid muscle on the left side, one must be mindful of the junction of the thoracic duct with the venous angle. The duct, emerging from a caudal and dorsal direction, arches over the subclavian artery (Figs. 18.4.2, 18.4.4, 18.4.14).

The median sternotomy is closed with wire suture or tapes (Fig. 18.4.8).

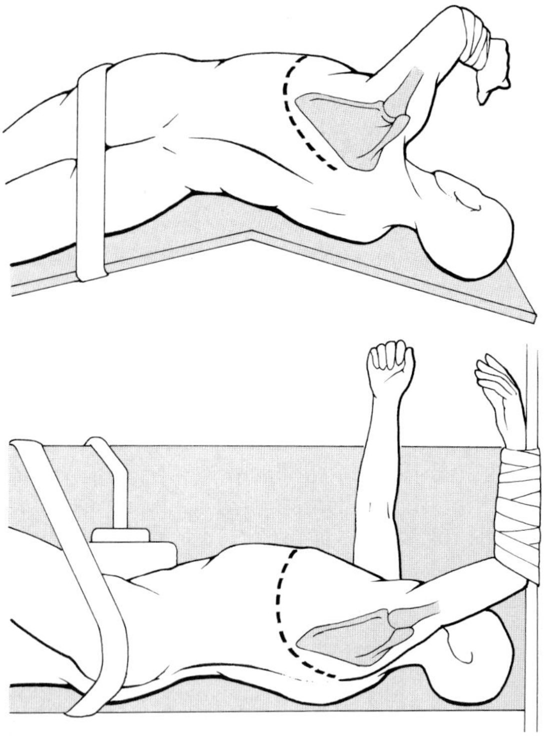

Fig. 18.4.9. Posterolateral thoracotomy, positioning and incision

Fig. 18.4.10. a Division of the latissimus dorsi muscle. ▷ b Anterior serratus muscle divided, latissimus dorsi muscle incised; incision of the periost of the rib with an electric knife

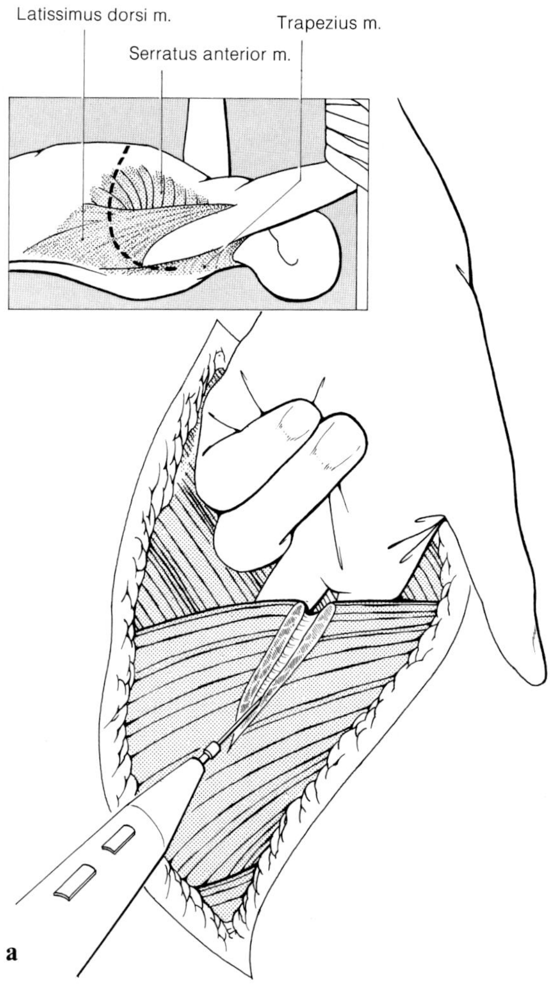

a

2. Left Posterolateral Thoracotomy

The upper portion of the descending aorta and the intrathoracic segment of the left subclavian artery, i.e., segment 1, [3, 4, 5] are best approached through a posterolateral thoracotomy in the bed of the fourth rib. Using this approach, the proximal segment of the left common carotid artery can also be exposed.

The patient is positioned on the right side (Fig. 18.4.9). The right leg is pulled up somewhat, the hip and the knee joint being flexed. The left leg is extended and cushions are placed beneath it. The hip is fixed on the table with a circular belt. Stabilization is achieved by holders hooked to the table. A cushion or a pneumatic roll is placed under the right side of the thorax at the level of the incision to achieve overextension of the hemithorax that is to be operated on. Prior to closure of the thorax, the cushion is removed

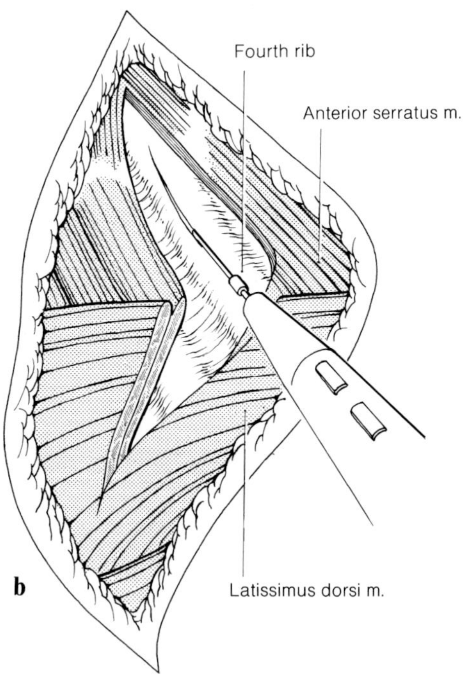

b

or the roll deflated. The right arm is positioned perpendicular to the body axis on an arm holder, providing access to the arm for the anesthesiologist. The left arm is abducted to shoulder level and fixed ventrally to the holder.

The skin incision starts in the midclavicular line, passing beneath the breast in a downward convex curve. In women, this incision should be made in the inframammary fold. The incision is continued dorsally in the axillary line to make a curve around the tip of the scapula at a distance of about 5 cm. Between the vertebral column and the margo vertebralis scapulae, the incision is extended cranially. After the gland is dissected off the fascia of the major pectoralis muscle, the thoracic insertion of the major pectoralis muscle is divided at the level of the fourth rib. Laterally, the anterior serratus muscle is separated in the direction of its fibers and the anterior border of the latissimus dorsi muscle is exposed (Fig. 18.4.10a). Vessels passing there must be divided between ligatures. Afterwards, the muscle is divided by an electric knife over a wooden probe. Sometimes, it may become necessary to incise the trapezius and rhomboid muscle as well.

The scapula is drawn up cranially, and the hand is passed upward between the thoracic wall and the scapula to determine the level of the thoracotomy by counting the ribs. (The first palpable rib is the second.) The fourth rib is now exposed over a sufficient distance, and the periost is incised at the anterior aspect of the rib (Fig. 18.4.10b). The periost and the intercostal muscles are then dissected off the rib with a raspatory. Next, the pleural cavity in the bed of the fourth rib is opened, and one or two retractors are inserted. The thoracotomy may also be performed following division of the intercostal muscles in the third interspace.

The lung is reflected ventrally to expose the aortic isthmus, and the parietal pleura is incised over the aorta and the left subclavian artery. The vessels are now easily dissected, and tapes are placed around them. As already mentioned, in this region one must be careful not to injure the vagal, recurrent, and phrenic nerves or the thoracic duct (Figs. 18.4.2 and 18.4.4).

II. Extrathoracic Approach

If a thoracotomy seems to be impossible because of the advanced age or general condition of the patient, an extrathoracic bypass may be considered, provided there is at least one patent donor artery in the region of the neck or the shoulder. This procedure, though hemodynamically somewhat less favorable, has the advantage of being less stressful. The operative approach depends on the operative method chosen. The literature of the last few years describes a great variety of extrathoracic bypasses. Besides the most commonly used carotid-subclavian bypass employing an ipsilateral or contralateral prosthesis or venous graft [14], a direct side-to-side anastomosis between the subclavian and the carotid artery may also be performed (using a supraclavicular approach) [6]. Another successful method has been proposed by Mehigan et al. [12]. Through a supraclavicular incision, the subclavian artery is divided distal to the occlusion and proximal to the origin of the vertebral artery and anastomosed end-to-side to the common carotid artery.

1. The Supraclavicular Exposure of the Subclavian Artery and the Common Carotid Artery

Using a supraclavicular approach, it is possible to expose the common carotid artery as well as the subclavian artery with its extrathoracic segments. The intrathoracic segment, segment 1, of the subclavian artery may also be exposed by careful dissection, allowing cross-clamping and division proximal to the origin of the vertebral artery. This is done more easily on the right side than on the left because the origin of the innominate artery is located higher on the right side. The pa-

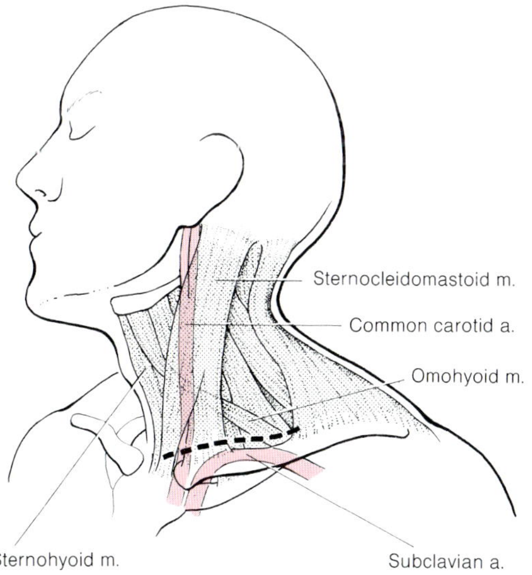

Fig. 18.4.11. Anatomy of the lateral triangle of the neck and skin incision for the supraclavicular approach

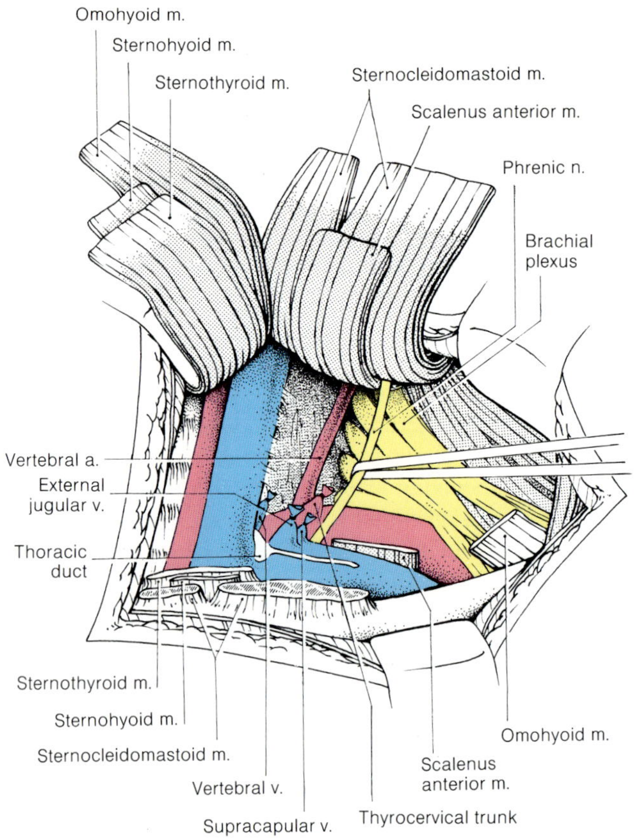

Fig. 18.4.12. Supraclavicular exposure of the subclavian and carotid arteries

tient is placed in a supine position with the head turned to the side. A cushion is placed underneath the ipsilateral shoulder. The incision is made 1 cm cranial and parallel to the clavicle, extending from the sternocleidomastoid muscle down to the anterior border of the trapezius muscle (Fig. 18.4.11). Following division of the subcutaneous tissue and the platysma, the external jugular vein is divided in the lateral triangle of the neck. The clavicular portion, and sometimes also the sternal portion of the sternocleidomastoid muscle, is divided as well as the sternothyroid and sternohyoid muscle, and laterally the omohyoid muscle. In order to avoid postoperative lymph fistulas, care must be taken not to injure the thoracic duct where it enters the left venous angle (Figs. 18.4.12 and 18.4.13). If the exposure is insufficient, it is better to ligate the duct. Following careful dissection of the supraclavicular fossa and retraction of prescalenic fatty tissue, the phrenic nerve is exposed on the anterior aspect to the scalenous anterior muscle. The nerve is retracted with a small cotton applicator. The muscle is then divided at the insertion

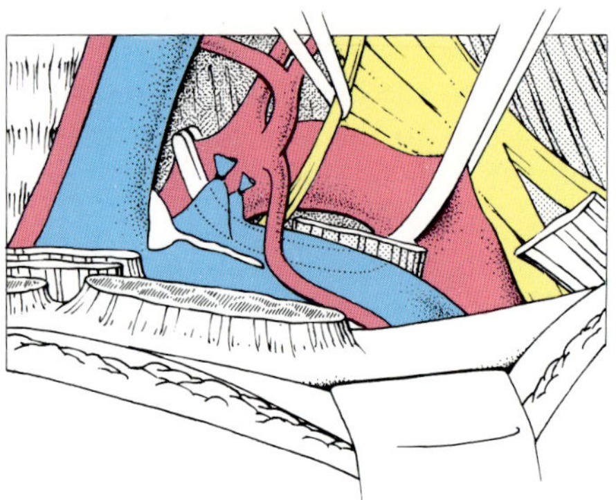

Fig. 18.4.13. Clamping of the subclavian artery

of the first rib with an electric knife over a wooden probe, exposing the subclavian artery with its branches, the thyrocervical artery, and the internal thoracic artery. These branches, as well as the vertebral vein, which crosses ventrally, and the thyrocervical vein must be ligated and divided to allow sufficient mobilization of the subclavian artery together with the vertebral artery. Tapes are placed around them. A tape is also placed around the internal jugular vein, ascending in the medial corner of the wound, and it is retracted laterally. This provides exposure of the common carotid artery, which lies medially; it also preserves the recurrent nerve (Fig. 18.4.12).

The extensive division of muscle tissue and vessels, although not always necessary, provides access to the subclavian artery far behind the sternoclavicular joint, and this allows cross-clamping of the subclavian artery in its first segment. However, it is necessary to draw up the subclavian artery slightly with a tape. The clamp occluding the vessel must be placed securely so that it cannot slip off (Fig. 18.4.13).

Exposure and mobilization of the extrathoracic subclavian segments is above all mandatory for

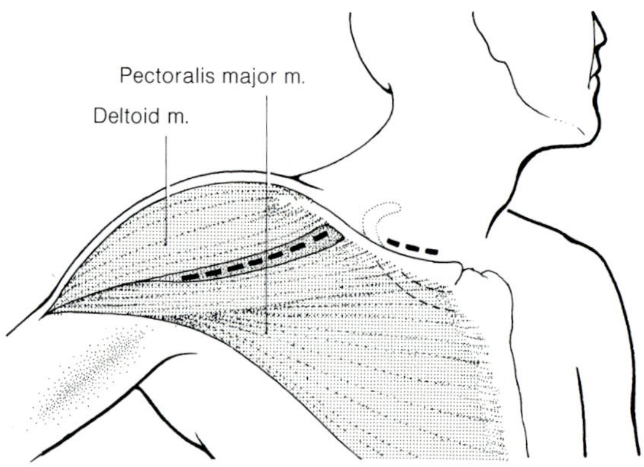

Fig. 18.4.14. Skin incision for carotid-axillary bypass

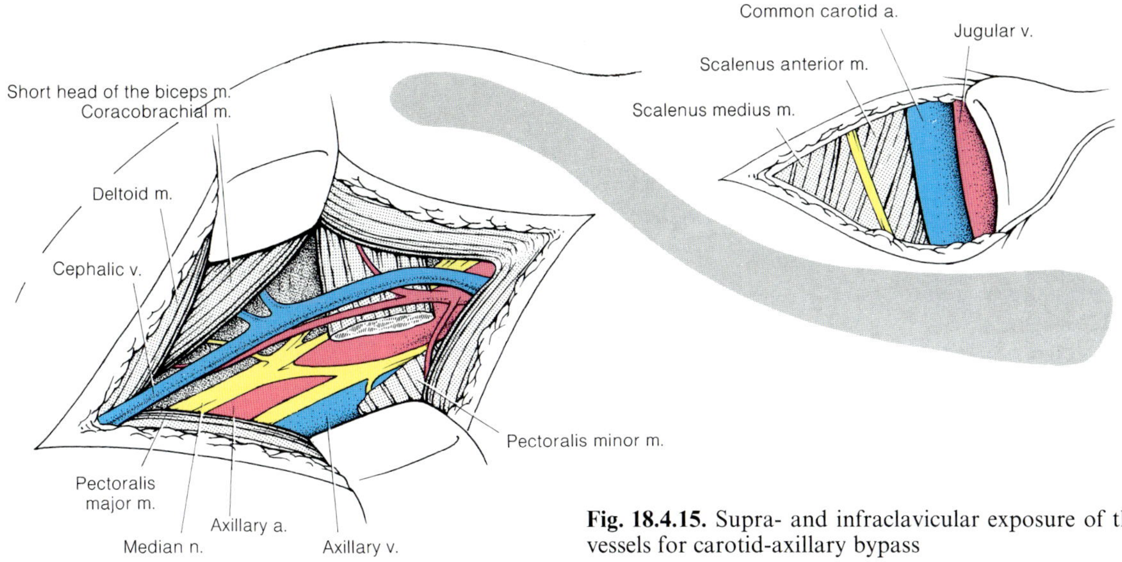

Fig. 18.4.15. Supra- and infraclavicular exposure of the vessels for carotid-axillary bypass

reimplantation (transposition) of the subclavian artery into the common carotid artery [12]. However, for a carotid-subclavian bypass or a side-to-side anastomosis of the common carotid and subclavian arteries using the method of EDWARDS and WRIGHT [6], division of anatomic structures does not have to be so extensive.

The subclavian – subclavian bypass [8] requires supraclavicular exposure of the subclavian artery on both sides. The graft is passed subcutaneously or submuscularly to the contralateral side.

2. The Infraclavicular Approach to the Axillary Artery

The carotid-axillary bypass [13] as well as the axillo-axillary bypass [10] require exposure of the axillary artery in the infraclavicular region.

The patient is placed in a supine position with the arm slightly abducted and rotated outward. The skin incision is made in the trigonum deltoideopectorale from the clavicle along the medial border of the deltoid muscle down to the border of the pectoralis major muscle, i.e., the anterior axillary fold (Figs. 18.4.14 and 18.4.15). The cephalic vein is located within the subcutaneous tissue between the deltoid and pectoralis muscles. It is preserved and serves as a guideline to the axillary vein, which lies deeper. Both muscles are retracted bluntly. The deep pectoralis minor muscle is exposed and divided close to its insertion at the processus coracoideus. Underneath the fatty tissue, the second segment of the axillary artery is exposed, preserving its branch, the acromioclavicular artery. The axillary vein is located medial to the artery and lateral to the brachial plexus. When dissecting the more distal arterial segment, one must be careful not to injure the brachial plexus, branching off into three fasciculi surrounding the artery.

The carotid-axillary bypass requires, in addition to the infraclavicular exposure of the axillary artery, a small supraclavicular incision over the lateral insertion of the sternocleidomastoid muscle, which is divided. The common carotid artery can now be dissected medial to the jugular vein without division of the scalenus anterior muscle. The vascular prosthesis crosses the clavicle in the subcutaneous tissue; this sometimes causes problems in slim patients.

For an axillo-axillary bypass [10] the axillary artery is exposed on both sides in the trigonum deltoideopectorale. The bypass is passed underneath the pectoralis muscle to the contralateral side. Finally, the femoroaxillary bypass should be mentioned. It is used in patients with bad general condition when no patent supra-aortic donor artery is available. Inguinal as well as infraclavicular exposure of the donor and recipient artery is required. The graft is interposed subcutaneously along the anterior axillary line and passed down to the groin.

3. Transaxillary Exposure of the Third and Fourth Segment of the Subclavian Artery

See p. 565ff.

G. Possibilities for Reconstruction

The reader is referred to pp. 47ff. and 71ff. for details of suture and anastomotic technique as well as selection of synthetic prostheses.

Generally, four operative procedures may be used for occlusions of the proximal segment of the supra-aortic arteries:

1. Transthoracic endarterectomy with or without patch graft
2. Transthoracic bypass or patch graft
3. Extrathoracic bypass
4. Extrathoracic reimplantation

The choice of reconstructive procedure to be used for the correction of stenoses or occlusions depends on various factors.

1. Prevailing clinical symptoms:
   a) Carotid insufficiency or transient ischemic attacks
   b) Vertebrobasilar insufficiency
   c) Insufficient perfusion of the brachial artery
2. Localization, extent, and multiplicity of stenoses and occlusive disease
3. Pathogenesis: degenerative (arteriosclerosis) or inflammatory processes (Takayasu's disease)
4. Patency of the adjacent or efferent vessel serving as donor artery
5. Morbidity and mortality of the operative procedure
6. General and cardiorespiratory condition of the patient

Depending on the localization of the occlusion, several reconstructive procedures may be used.

I. Occlusion of the Origin of the Left Subclavian Artery

For occlusions at this location transthoracic as well as extrathoracic procedures may be considered:

1. Transthoracic Procedure (Fig. 18.4.16)

1. Endarterectomy with or without patch graft angioplasty using a synthetic patch. This patch should extend into the descending aorta and beyond the origin of the vertebral artery (Fig. 18.4.16a).

2. Resection of the occluded segment and replacement with a synthetic prosthesis. Differences in the lumen of prosthesis and vessel are overcome by using a tongue-shaped configuration for the anastomosis. Additionally, the first rib should be resected to avoid constriction or kinking of the bypass (Fig. 18.4.16b).

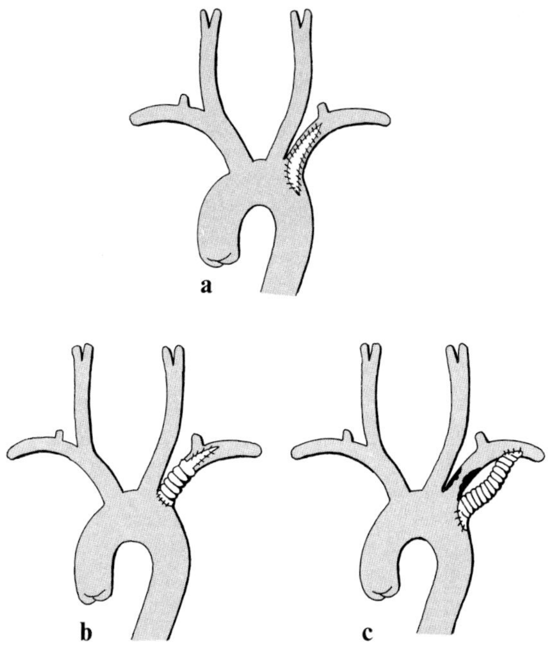

Fig. 18.4.16a–c. Transthoracic reconstructions of an occluded left subclavian artery

3. Synthetic bypass graft from the descending aorta to the left poststenotic subclavian artery. In this case also, resection of the first rib is recommended (Fig. 18.4.16c).

Note: During all these reconstructive procedures, one should be aware of the possibility of injury to the thoracic duct as well as the recurrent nerve in the left upper mediastinum [16] (Figs. 18.4.1, 18.4.2, 18.4.4).

2. Extrathoracic Procedure (Fig. 18.4.17)

1. Synthetic bypass graft from the left common carotid artery to the left subclavian artery. Today, the carotid-subclavian bypass is certainly the most commonly used method (Fig. 18.4.17a). Atheromatous lesions of the proximal segment are not treated using this procedure.

If it is necessary to dissect the atheromatous lesions of the initial subclavian artery segment because peripheral embolization has already occurred, the following two methods are indicated:

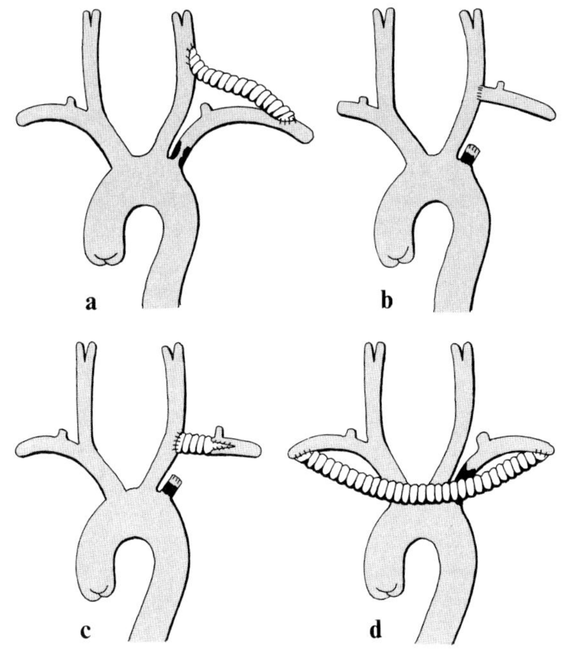

Fig. 18.4.17 a–d. Extrathoracic reconstructions of an occluded left subclavian artery

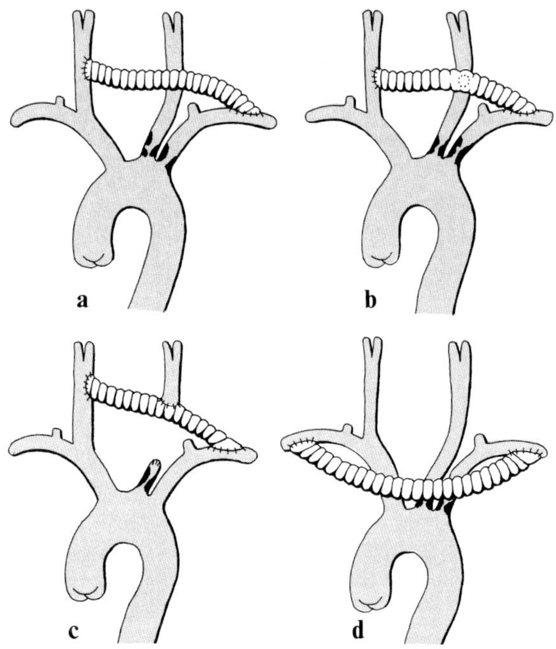

Fig. 18.4.18 a–d. Extrathoracic reconstructions of occlusions in both the left subclavian and left common carotid arteries

2. Reimplantation of the left subclavian artery into the left common carotid artery without graft interposition (Fig. 18.4.17b).

3. Reimplantation of the left subclavian artery into the left common carotid artery with graft interposition (Fig. 18.4.17c). Here again, the distal anastomosis is constructed in a tongue-shaped configuration in order to overcome the luminal discrepancy between prosthesis and artery.

Interposition of a vascular prosthesis is always necessary when lesions extend into the segment II or III of the subclavian artery. Then, the vessel is often too short for implantation. Vascular lesions at the origin of the vertebral artery may be treated by additional endarterectomy.

4. Synthetic bypass graft from the right subclavian artery or axillary artery to the left subclavian or axillary artery (Fig. 18.4.17d).

These methods are seldom indicated because there is almost always the possibility of a short bypass procedure. The results with longer prosthetic bypasses are not as good as with short ones, primarily for hemodynamic reasons.

Note: Because it lies adjacent to the left subclavian artery, the thoracic duct is in danger while the artery is being dissected at its origin at the aortic arch and also along its further course until it emerges from the thoracic outlet. This also has to be taken into consideration when using a supraclavicular approach to the subclavian artery [16].

II. Occlusion of the Origin of the Left Subclavian Artery Combined with a Stenosis of the Left Common Carotid Artery

In this case, the left common carotid artery cannot be used as the donor artery.

1. Transthoracic Procedure

In cases of occlusion of the initial segment of the left subclavian artery, together with a stenosis of the initial segment of the left common carotid artery, all intrathoracic procedures, such as thromboendarterectomy of both arteries, bifurcation prosthesis, or implantation of branching vascular grafts, have been superceded by the extrathoracic approach, which is significantly simplier and shows better results.

2. Extrathoracic Procedure (Fig. 18.4.18)

The following extrathoracic reconstructions for these occlusions are possible:

1. Synthetic bypass graft from the right common carotid artery to the left subclavian artery (Fig. 18.4.18a). This procedure serves only for the treatment of the subclavian steal syndrome. The stenosed carotid artery is not treated by this type of reconstruction, which is justified only if there is no carotid insufficiency of hemodynamic origin and there are no reports of transient ischemic attacks deriving from a source of emboli in the common carotid artery.

2. Synthetic bypass graft from the right common carotid artery, as donor artery, to the left subclavian artery and side-to-side anastomosis to the left common carotid artery (Fig. 18.4.18b). If intraoperative pressure and flow measurement reveals a significant reduction of blood supply in the left carotid artery, then, in addition to the operative procedure described above under (1), a side-to-side anastomosis to the left common carotid artery is required. This procedure is also used in patients with mixed symptoms of subclavian steal syndrome and cerebral vascular insufficiency of the carotid type. It is not recommended, however, if the patient has already suffered from recurrent transient ischemic attacks.

3. When there are additional transient ischemic attacks due to microembolisms, as revealed by the patient's history, then the common carotid artery must be divided distal to the atheromatous lesions and the peripheral segment of the common carotid artery implanted into the prosthesis in order to exclude the source of embolism (Fig. 18.4.18c).

4. Synthetic bypass graft from the right to the left subclavian artery or from the right to the left axillary artery (Fig. 18.4.18d). In this case also, only the subclavian steal syndrome is treated. The inferior results of this bypass have already been mentioned.

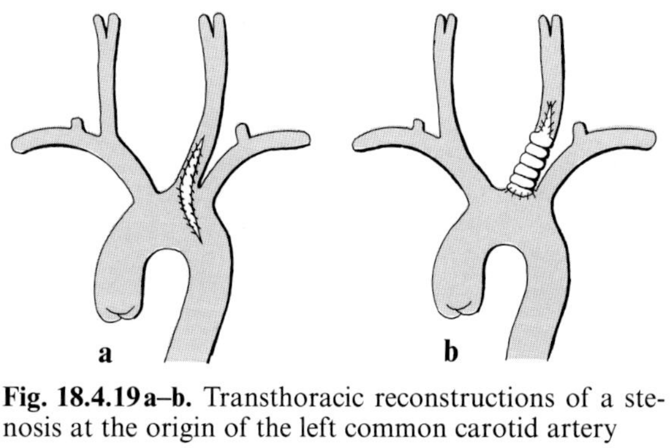

Fig. 18.4.19a–b. Transthoracic reconstructions of a stenosis at the origin of the left common carotid artery

III. Stenosis of the Origin of the Left Common Carotid Artery

1. Transthoracic Procedure (Fig. 18.4.19)

1. Endarterectomy of the stenosed segment (Fig. 18.4.19a). Following thromboendarterectomy the arteriotomy should always be closed with a patch graft extending into the aortic arch and into the healthy segment of the carotid artery. The indication for this procedure is severe stenosis causing insufficient perfusion of the carotid artery or the localization of the source of embolism in this segment. If the occlusion is caused by Takayasu's disease, thromboendarterectomy should never be attempted because one cannot find a dissection plane with this inflammatory disease.

2. Resection of the occluded segment and replacement with a graft (Fig. 18.4.19b). In cases of inflammatory disease not allowing endarterectomy

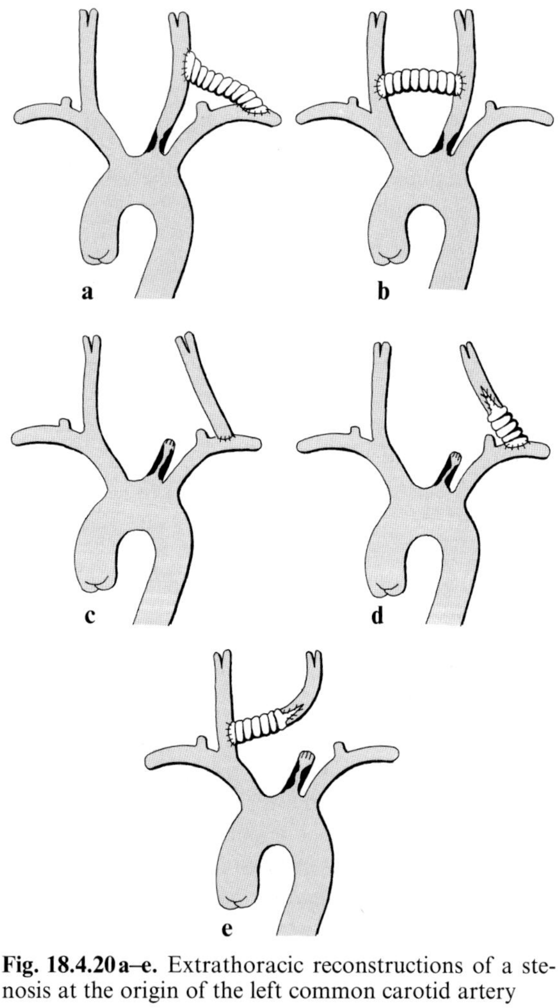

Fig. 18.4.20a–e. Extrathoracic reconstructions of a stenosis at the origin of the left common carotid artery

(Takayasu's disease), the occluded segment should be resected and replaced with an interposition graft. Here, too, differences in the lumina may be overcome by means of a tongue-shaped anastomosis.

2. Extrathoracic Procedure (Fig. 18.4.20)

It is simplier and of lower risk to use one of the following extrathoracic procedures rather than a transthoracic reconstruction. In the first place one of the two adjacent arteries, the left subclavian artery or the right carotid artery, may serve as the donor artery.

1. Synthetic bypass graft from the left subclavian artery to the left common carotid artery (Fig. 18.4.20a).

2. Synthetic bypass graft from the right to the left common carotid artery (Fig. 18.4.20b). This is the simplest procedure. However, it can only be performed when the right common carotid artery is completely patent.

3. Reimplantation of the left common carotid artery into the left subclavian artery (Fig. 18.4.20c). If the patient is suffering from transient ischemic attacks, the vessel should be divided and implanted into the left subclavian artery in order to exclude the source of embolism.

4. Reimplantation technique with interposition of vein or synthetic graft (Fig. 18.4.20d). If the arteriosclerotic lesions involve too long a segment of the common carotid artery, the left common carotid artery can be implanted into the left subclavian artery only after interposition of a vein or prosthetic graft.

5. Reimplantation of the left common carotid artery into the right common carotid artery (Fig. 18.4.20e). Reimplantation of the left common carotid artery into the right common carotid artery is also performed for the most part with interposition of a synthetic (or venous) graft. This procedure also serves to exclude the source of embolism in cases of transient ischemic attacks. This bypass is used especially when the left subclavian artery also shows degeneration and cannot be regarded as completely patent.

IV. Occlusion of the Initial Segment of the Right Subclavian Artery

Occlusions of the proximal right subclavian artery may also be treated using a transthoracic as well as an extrathoracic procedure.

1. Transthoracic Procedure (Fig. 18.4.21)

1. Endarterectomy with or without a patch graft (Fig. 18.4.21a). The patch should extend into the innominate artery and beyond the origin of the vertebral artery.

2. Synthetic bypass from the ascending aorta to the right subclavian artery (Fig. 18.4.21b). This procedure is somewhat more complicated than the left aortosubclavian bypass because the superior vena cava narrows the exposure of the operative field.

2. Extrathoracic Procedure (Fig. 18.4.22)

3. Prosthetic bypass from the right common carotid artery to the right subclavian artery (Fig. 18.4.23).

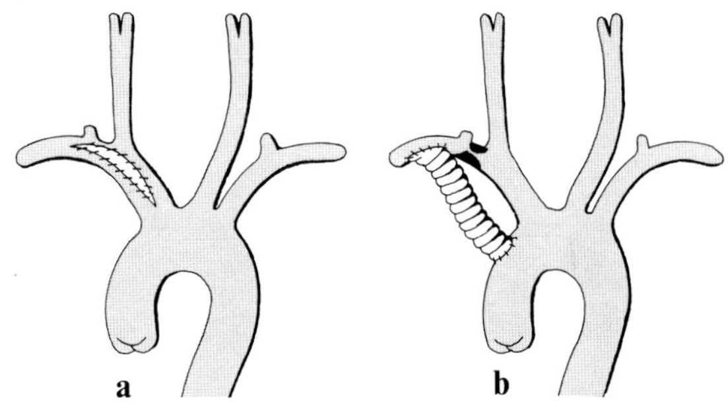

Fig. 18.4.21a, b. Transthoracic reconstructions of an occlusion of the right subclavian artery

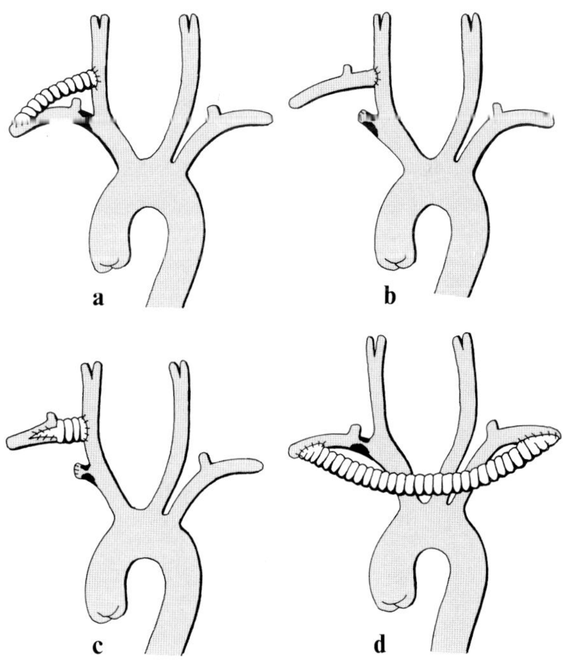

Fig. 18.4.22a–d. Extrathoracic reconstructions of an occlusion of the right subclavian artery

This carotid-subclavian bypass – like the corresponding procedure on the left side – represents the simplest and the most commonly used procedure.

4. Reimplantation of the right subclavian artery into the right common carotid artery (Fig. 18.4.22d). This approach is highly recommended because it avoids the use of synthetic material.

5. Reimplantation of the right subclavian artery into the right common carotid artery with graft interposition (Fig. 18.4.22c). When a direct implantation of the right subclavian artery into the right common carotid artery is impossible because the stump is too short owing to advanced arteriosclerotic lesions, it may be necessary to interpose a graft that has been trimmed so as to achieve a tongue-shaped anastomosis.

6. The subclavian-subclavian or axillo-axillary bypass should be restricted to exceptional cases because of inferior results related to the length of the graft and because of the unfavorable hemodynamics (Fig. 18.4.22d).

V. Occlusion of the Innominate Artery

When there are no contraindications, the transthoracic approach should be preferred.

1. Transthoracic Procedure (Fig. 18.4.23)

1. Endarterectomy with patch graft (Fig. 18.4.23a). Following dissection of the thrombus, a patch graft should always be employed, extending proximally into the aortic arch and distally either into the common carotid artery or into the subclavian artery, or Y-shaped into both arteries.

2. Resection and graft interposition (Fig. 18.4.23b). In cases of extensive arteriosclerotic lesions or chronic occlusion of the innominate artery, the occluded segment may be resected and replaced with a graft. The distal end of the anastomosis, which should be tongue shaped, can extend into either the common carotid or the subclavian artery or, using a Y-configuration, into both arteries.

3. Synthetic bypass graft from the ascending aorta to the right subclavian artery or to the right common carotid artery (Fig. 18.4.23c, d).

All three methods mentioned are used in patients with subclavian steal syndrome or insufficient blood supply to the arm. Using the first and second method, i.e., endarterectomy and resection of the occluded segment, a possible source of embolism is also excluded.

When using the first two methods, as well as methods described in Sect. IV.1, one must cross-

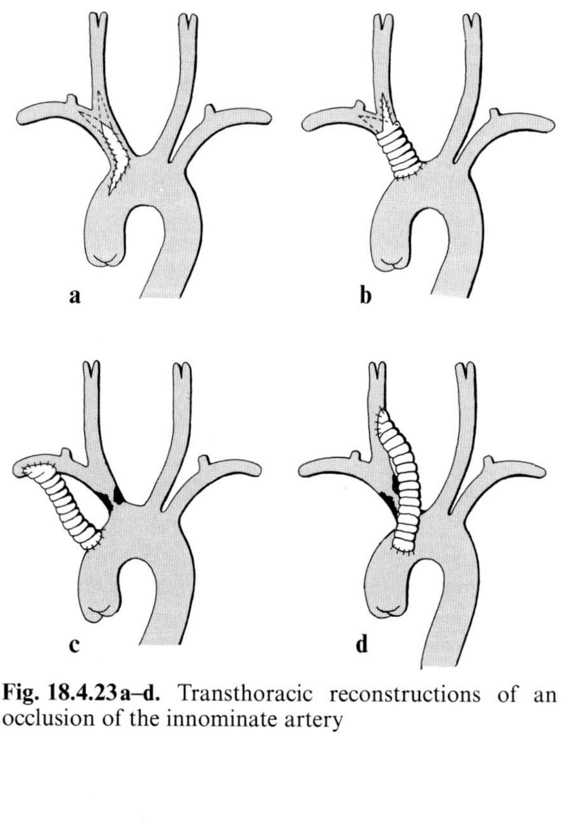

Fig. 18.4.23a–d. Transthoracic reconstructions of an occlusion of the innominate artery

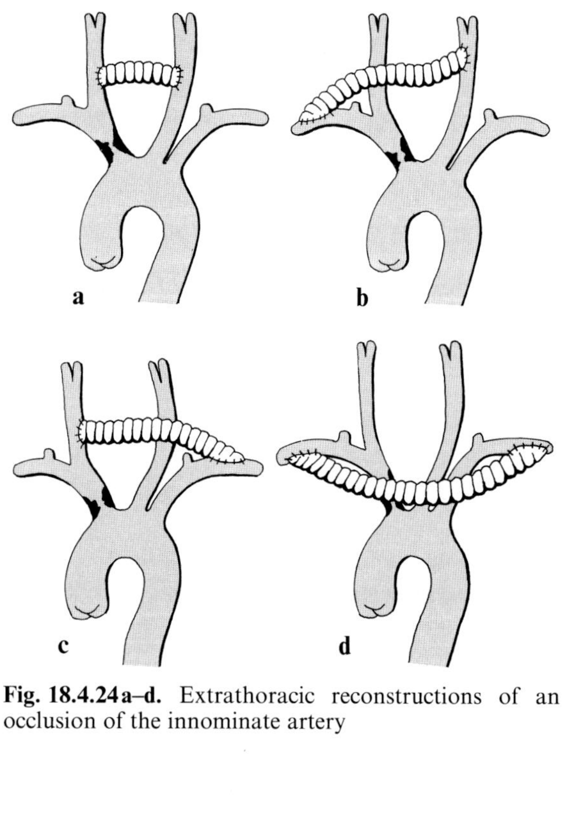

Fig. 18.4.24a–d. Extrathoracic reconstructions of an occlusion of the innominate artery

clamp not only the innominate artery, but also the right carotid and subclavian arteries, and the right vertebral artery as well. Therefore, it is advisable to use an intraluminal shunt in order to avoid insufficient perfusion of the brain intraoperatively.

2. Extrathoracic Procedure (Fig. 18.4.24)

In patients in whom a sternotomy is contraindicated, one of the following extrathoracic operative procedures may be used. First, two methods tapping the left common carotid artery:

4. Prosthetic bypass from the left common carotid artery to the right common carotid artery (Fig. 18.4.24a).

5. Prosthetic bypass from the left common carotid artery to the right subclavian artery (Fig. 18.4.24b).

The left subclavian artery may also be used as donor artery.

6. Prosthetic bypass from the left subclavian artery to the right common carotid artery (Fig. 18.4.24c).

7. Prosthetic bypass from the left subclavian artery to the right subclavian artery – with the poor results already mentioned (Fig. 18.4.24d).

The last two methods are used only when the left common carotid artery is not completely patent and therefore cannot be tapped.

VI. Multiple Occlusions in the Region of the Supra-aortic Branches

In cases of multiple occlusions, a single patent aortic branch may serve as the donor artery. From this patent branch, those occluded vessels showing a high pressure gradient are anastomosed using a bridge graft (Fig. 18.4.25). However, in the literature there is controversy as to how great the pressure gradient must be before a bridge graft is indicated.

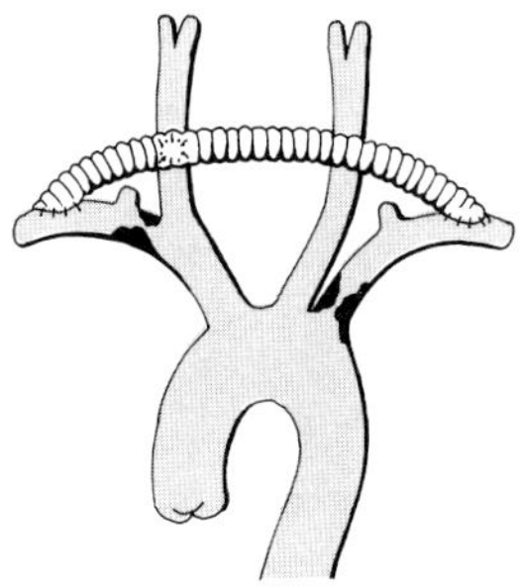

Fig. 18.4.25. Bilateral subclavian artery stenosis. Saphenous vein bridge graft, tapping the right carotid artery

If all supra-aortic arteries are stenosed or occluded, the femoral artery may serve as the donor artery. Here, the supply is established in the form of a femoroaxillary prosthetic bypass.

H. Complications

Bleeding is the predominant intraoperative complication. The most frequent causes are coagulation disturbances, porous prostheses, bleeding from suture canals, or leaking sutures on the posterior wall of the anastomosis, which can be difficult to reach. Especially with the supraclavicular approach to the subclavian artery, one must be sure to cross-clamp the initial segments securely. Otherwise, division of the artery may produce a life-threatening hemorrhage deep in the thorax, which would necessitate an immediate emergency thoracotomy.

Postoperative bleeding should also be mentioned as well as paresis of the recurrent and phrenic nerves. If the thoracic duct has been injured, the postoperative chylothorax must be treated by means of a chest tube with continuous suction. If a lymph fistula does not close spontaneously within 10 days, there is no other choice but to operate.

I. Reintervention

Reintervention is necessary if there is bleeding in the operative field or early or late occlusion of the reconstructed vascular segment. If the occlusion is not clearly demonstrated by palpation, auscultation, or Doppler ultrasonography, an angiogram of the region in question is absolutely necessary.

During revision of the operating field, not only should thrombectomy of the occluded vessel or of the prosthesis be performed, but one should also look for the causes, including operative errors, which absolutely must be corrected.

K. Summary

The therapeutic concept presented has evolved over the last several years through the continuing analysis of clinical and morphological results. Naturally, a pat solution is not possible for each angiologically proven lesion of the vascular system. However, the principles outlined here may serve as a helpful guide in patient selection and in the choice of the optimal reconstructive procedure.

REFERENCES

1. Crawford ES, De Bakey ME, Morris GC, Howell JF (1969) Surgical treatment of occlusion of the innominate, common carotid, and subclavian arteries: A 10 year experience. Surg 65:17–31
2. De Bakey ME, Morris GC, Jordan GL, Cooley DA (1958) Segmental thrombo-obliterative disease of branches of aortic arch. JAMA 166:988
3. van Dongen RJAM (1972) Chronische Verschlüsse der oberen Extremitäten. Langenbecks Arch Chir 332:325–331
4. van Dongen RJAM, Barwegen MGMH, Koning J (1980) Rekonstruktive Chirurgie der Art. subclavia; transaxillärer Zugang. Angio 2(2):93–98
5. van Dongen RJAM (1979) Lesions of the subclavian artery: Reconstructive procedures. In: Greep JM, Lemmens HAS, Roos DB, Urschel HC (eds) Pain in shoulder and arm: an integrated view. Martinus Nijhoff Publishers, The Hague Boston London
6. Edwards WH, Wright RS (1972) Current concepts in the management of arteriosclerotic lesions of the subclavian and vertebral arteries. Ann Surg 175:975
7. Eisenhardt HJ, Zehle A, Pichlmaier H (1980) Indikationsstellung und operationstechnisches Vorgehen bei chronischen Verschlüssen des Truncus brachiocephalicus und der A. subclavia im Abschnitt I. Langenbecks Arch Chir 35:161–169
8. Forestner JE, Ghosh SK, Bergan JJ, Conn J (1972) Subclavian-subclavian bypass for correction of the subclavian steal syndrome. Surg 71:136
9. Gruss JD, Karadedos C, Kawai S (1978) Long-term results after surgical treatment of the subclavian-steal-syndrome. Report of 931 cases. 27th International Congress of European Society of Cardiovascular Surgery. Lyon 28.6.–1.7.1978
10. Lamis PA, Stanton PE, Hyland L (1976) The axillo-axillary bypass graft. Further experience. Arch Surg 111(12):1353
11. Lord RSA, Ehrenfeld WK (1969) Carotid-subclavian bypass; a hemodynamic study. Surg 66:521–526
12. Mehigan JT, Buch WS, Pipkin RD, Fogarty TJ (1978) Subclavian-carotid transposition for the subclavian steal syndrome. Am J Surg 136(1):15–20
13. Shumacker HB (1973) Carotid axillary bypass grafts for occlusion of the proximal portion of the subclavian artery. Surg Gynec Obstet 136:447–448
14. Stimmel F, Belian C (1978) Zur Operationstechnik beim karotido-subklavialen Bypass. Zbl Chir 103:1561–1564
15. Thetter O, van Dongen RJAM (1981) Possibilités de reconstruction dans divers processus obstructifs des artères supraaortiques. Med et Hyg 39:4237–4242
16. Thetter O, von Hochstetter A (1980) Der postoperative Chylothorax, eine Komplikation der rekonstruktiven Chirurgie der A. subclavia. Angio 2(2):109–114
17. Wylie EJ, Ehrenfeld WK (1970) Extracranial occlusive cerebrovascular disease. Diagnosis and management. Saunders, Philadelphia

19 Chronic Occlusions of Upper Extremity Arteries

H. LOEPRECHT

CONTENTS

A. Anatomy

The arteries of the upper extremities are only intermittently located near the surface and are therefore, generally speaking, not easily accessed for reconstruction. In particular, the clavicle and the greater and smaller pectoral muscles offer very considerable protection to the underlying artery. But all too often they are also an extravasal factor in arteriosclerotic occlusions. In addition there is the close proximity to the fascicles of the brachial plexus, of which the ulnar and median nerves accompany the artery. By contrast, the brachial artery, which is accompanied only by the median nerve and crosses it in a medial-to-lateral direction, is easily accessed over its entire length in the medial bicipital sulcus. For anatomic details the reader is referred to the earlier chapters.

B. Indications for Reconstruction of Chronic Occlusions of Upper Extremity Arteries

Chronic occlusions of the upper extremity represent only a small spectrum within the whole complex of arterial occlusive disease. Only 10% of all arteriosclerotic occlusions are located in the upper extremity; 70% of these are located in the distal forearm and the finger arteries, only 27% in the region of the subclavian and axillary artery, and 2.4% in the region of the brachial artery [1]. Occlusions in these arteries are predominantly short. An important factor in the localization of lesions is compression by surrounding anatomic features (e.g., in the costoclavicular segment, see p. 552). Nondegenerative inflammatory angiopathies are often the cause of brachial occlusion. Stress ischemia may also be caused by an unnoticed blunt injury of the artery following trauma to the shoulder or elbow joint [6].

Usually, there are excellent collaterals bypassing such occlusions of the upper extremity, owing to the axillary network and the network of the elbow joint, so that surgery is indicated only in selected cases. The indication is especially strong in patients in whom the upper extremity is extremely stressed by manual work or in whom additional acral occlusions are present [3]. Also, microembolism deriving from stenosed and ulcerated vascular segments may necessitate an operation, even without symptoms of chronic ischemia. In addition to the clinical picture, the indication for surgery depends on the extent of the occlusion as demonstrated angiographically. Precise analysis of the pre- and postocclusion vascular bed is of decisive significance for planning an operative procedure. Nowadays, this is achieved by transfemoral catheter angiography of the upper extremity arteries, which is without doubt the simplest procedure [7]. A significant supplementation and simplification is represented by digital subtraction angiography (DSA), which provides a sufficiently exact analysis of details, at least of the central segment of the brachial artery in many cases. Furthermore, it is much less troublesome for the patient. Usually reconstructive procedures of the subclavian, axillary, and brachial arteries require time-consuming dissection and multiple incisions, so that it is usually best to perform the procedure under intubation anesthesia. Only for reconstructions of the distal brachial artery is regional anesthesia sensible and adequate.

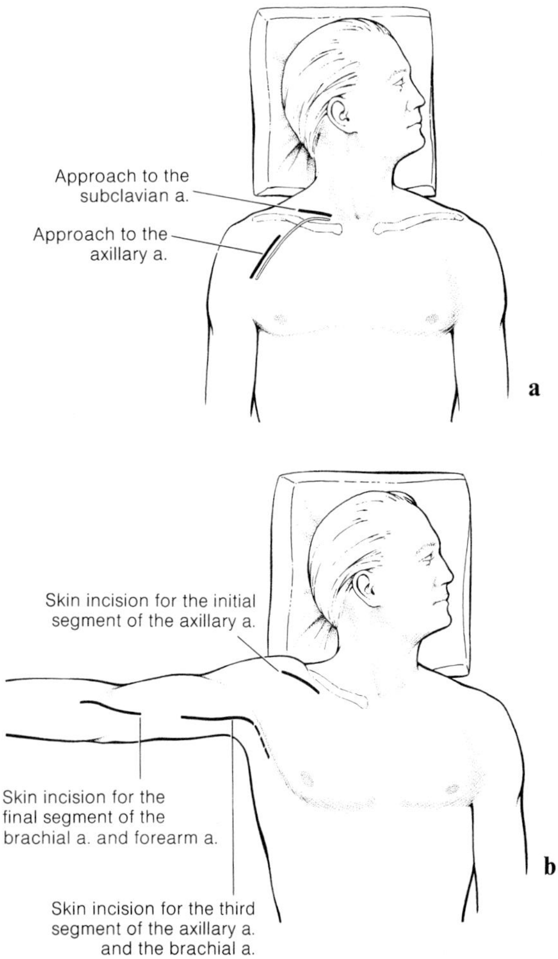

Fig. 19.1. **a** Positioning and skin incision for the approach to the subclavian and axillary arteries. **b** Positioning and skin incision for the approach to the brachial artery

C. Operative Procedures for Distal Subclavian Occlusions

I. Positioning and Draping

For reconstructions of distal subclavian artery occlusions in the costoclavicular space, supraclavicular and infraclavicular incisions are routinely required. Therefore, the patient is in a supine position, the upper part of the body being slightly elevated, the head hyperextended and turned to the opposite side (Fig. 19.1 a). This provides broad access to the supraclavicular fossa [4, 5]. The skin in the area of the mammary region, axillary region, and the lateral triangle of the neck is disinfected widely and covered with a sterile drape, the caudal end of the drape being at the level of the axillary fold. The median border is represented by the sternum and the jugulum. A drape is placed above as far as the acromion and so as to leave access to the supraclavicular fossa; from the acromion the drape runs downward following the contour of the shoulder. It has been found beneficial to place plastic incisional drape over the carefully dried skin.

Alternatively, a transaxillary approach may be used, as described on p. 559. This approach has the advantage of simultaneous resection of the first rib.

II. Exposure of the Subclavian Artery

The skin incision is made in the supraclavicular fossa, parallel to the clavicle, from the lateral border of the sternocleidomastoid muscle for a distance of 6 m (Fig. 19.1 b; see p. 518). For the reconstruction of the distal subclavian artery, however, it is not necessary to divide the anterior scalene muscle, because the arteries can be mobilized over a sufficient length to allow an anastomosis.

III. Exposure of the Axillary Artery in Mohrenheim's Fossa

An oblique incision is made according to the course of Mohrenheim's fossa (Fig. 19.2 a). Following division of the skin and the subcutaneous tissue, dissection is most easily performed following the cephalic vein as a guideline into the depths of the fossa. The cephalic vein is retracted ventrally and all lateral tributaries are divided. Following

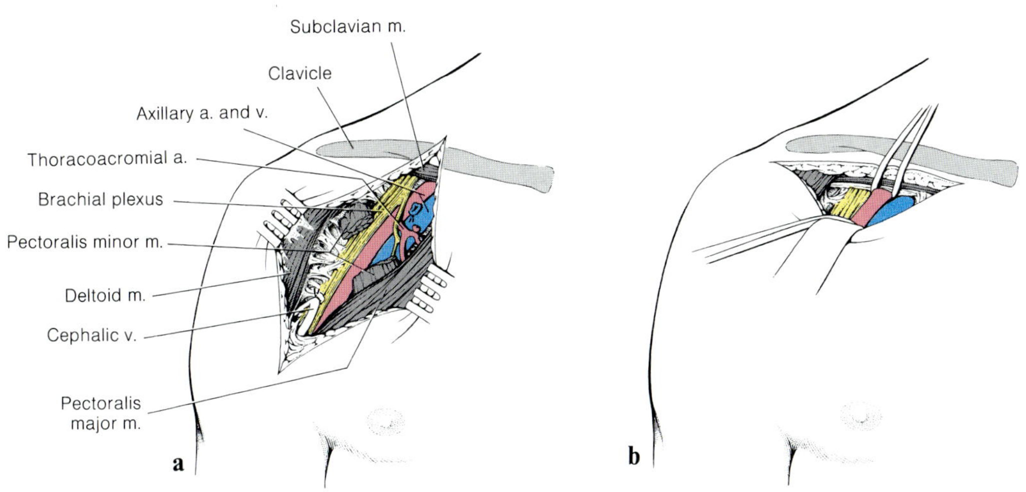

Fig. 19.2 a, b. Approaches to the initial segment of the axillary artery [5, 8]. **a** Deltoideopectoral approach to the axillary artery. **b** Subclavicular approach to the axillary artery

insertion of a retractor between the deltoid and the pectoralis major muscle, the artery is usually found without difficulty in the soft tissue caudal to the clavicle. Special care must be taken not to injure the portion of the brachial plexus passing lateral to the artery. The artery is dissected off the periadventitial tissue, and a tape is placed around it. In order to expose a segment of the axillary artery sufficiently long for anastomosis, it is usually necessary to incise or to divide the pectoralis minor muscle along the course of the artery. Usually, no clinically relevant functional disorders result from this myotomy. Following incision or division of the pectoralis minor muscle, access to the infragenicular segment of the axillary artery is achieved over a distance of 5 cm. Special care should be taken not to injure the thoracoacromial artery, which branches off ventromedially from the axillary artery in this region (Fig. 19.2a).

IV. Osteotomy of the Clavicle [2]

The junction of the subclavian artery and axillary artery is usually best approached in a supra- and infraclavicular incision. The segment in between can be bridged without difficulty using this approach. Only in exceptional cases, e.g., in a thrombosed aneurysm with significant fibrous reaction in the surroundings, it may be necessary to dissect the whole length of the axillary and subclavian artery. In this case, the skin incision is made from the supraclavicular fossa in a curve over the clavicle into Mohrenheim's space (Fig. 19.1a). As described before, the subclavian artery is exposed first in the supraclavicular region and a tape is placed around it. Afterwards, the axillary artery is exposed in Mohrenheim's space. In the region of the clavicle, the subcutaneous tissue is divided down to the periost. The clavicular head of the pectoralis major muscle is incised and the subclavian muscle divided (Fig. 19.5a). Special care should be taken to dissect the dorsal circumference of the clavicle, or it should be digitally dissected off the vessels. The subclavian vein is in special danger during this maneuver. Using an oscillating drill, the clavicle is divided transversely at the level of the subclavian artery, which crosses behind it. Remaining tissue bands are divided with scissors. The median and lateral portions of the clavicle are retracted with two sharp hooks, and a self-retractor is inserted. Following this dissection, the subclavian or axillary arteries are exposed from the scalene space to Mohrenheim's fossa.

Following reconstruction of the subclavian artery, both portions of the clavicle are approximated and fixed in an anatomically correct position by means of a plate conforming to the ventral contour of the clavicle and fixed in place with traction screws (Fig. 19.5d).

V. Thromboendarterectomy of the Subclavian Artery

The dissection of the arteriosclerotic thrombus occluding the vessel may be performed either as an open or as a semiclosed endarterectomy with a

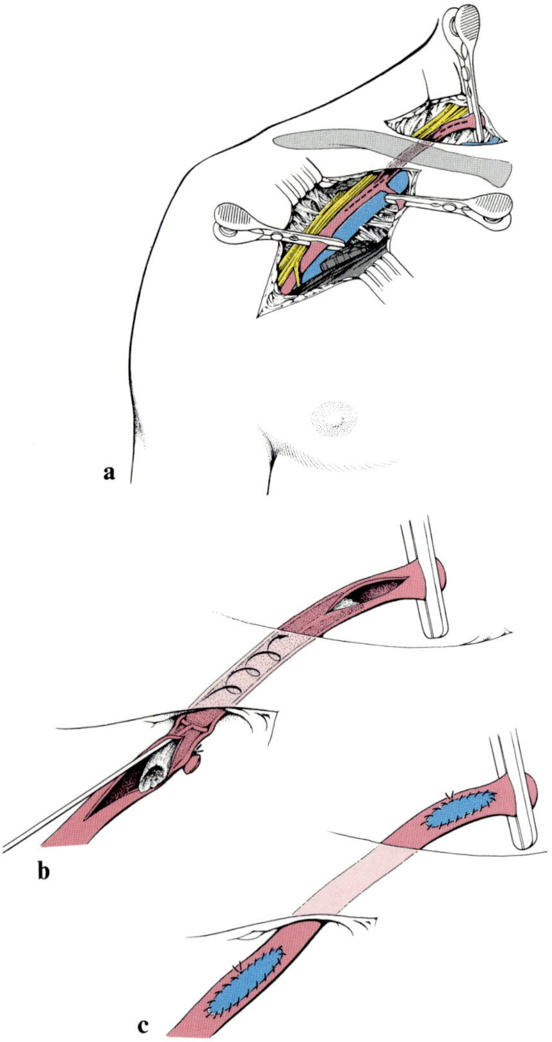

Fig. 19.3 a–c. Semiclosed endarterectomy of the distal subclavian artery. **a** Supra- and infraclavicular incision. **b** Technique for endarterectomy of the subclavian artery using a ring stripper. **c** Following endarterectomy, closure of the arteriotomy with a vein patch

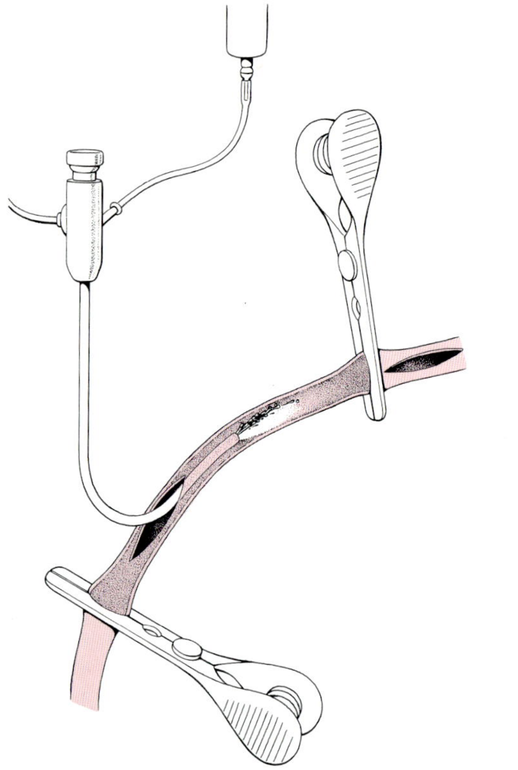

Fig. 19.4. Principle of vascular endoscopy with a flexible endoscope and simultaneous flushing [9]

ring stripper [9]. Prior to the *semiclosed endarterectomy*, the subclavian artery is cross-clamped proximally in the scalene space with an atraumatic clamp, and the axillary artery is similarly clamped in the region of Mohrenheim's fossa. In the region of the axillary artery (the infraclavicular segment) a ventral longitudinal incision is made over a distance of 1.5–2 cm following additional cross-clamping of the thoracoacromial artery (Fig. 19.3a). A similar incision is made at the ventral circumference of the subclavian artery in the supraclavicular fossa. The thrombus is carefully detached with a spatula, and an adequate outer cleavage plane is established. A ring stripper is inserted and the thrombus is dissected by pushing the stripper in spirals and with slight pressure up to the central incision. In the region of the central incision, the arteriosclerotic lesion will become free at a point where it is thin, leaving a smooth tapering end point. Since the free edge of the intima lies in the direction of the bloodstream, it is not necessary to tack it down with interrupted sutures. It is of course extremely important that the results of a semiclosed endarterectomy are assessed intraoperatively. This can be done by inspecting the thrombus and carefully noting any ledges in the dissection plane. Today, however, intraluminal evaluation, using a flexible endoscope [9], is considered more reliable; with this technique, the arterial wall can be inspected to determine whether any intimal flaps remain (Fig. 19.4). The arteriotomy is closed with a small venous patch, using a continuous over-and-over suture. Prior to completion of the suture line the proximal and distal clamps are alternately released for a brief time in order to flush out any thrombi that may have formed (Fig. 19.3b). Following stepwise removal

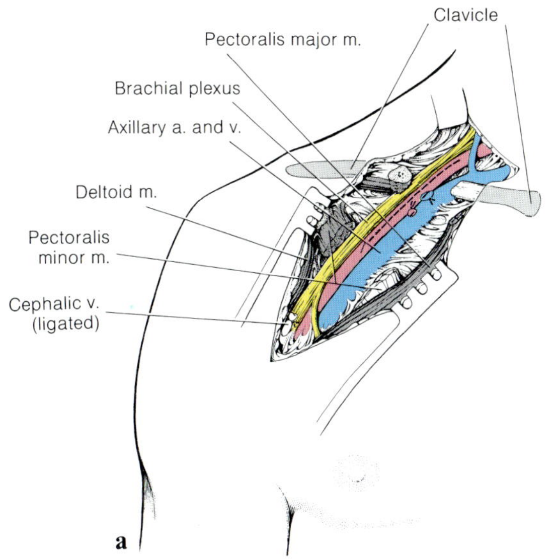

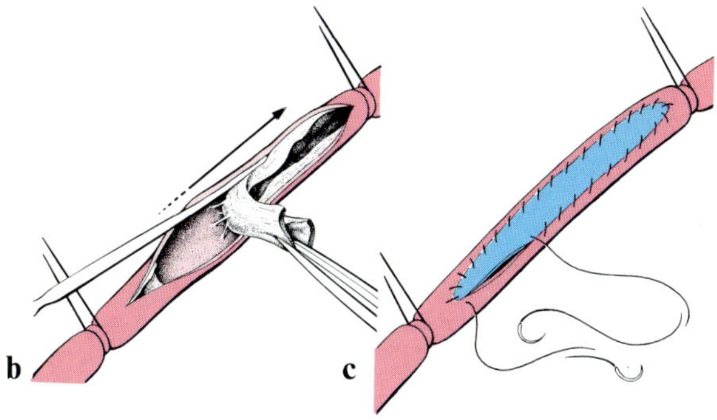

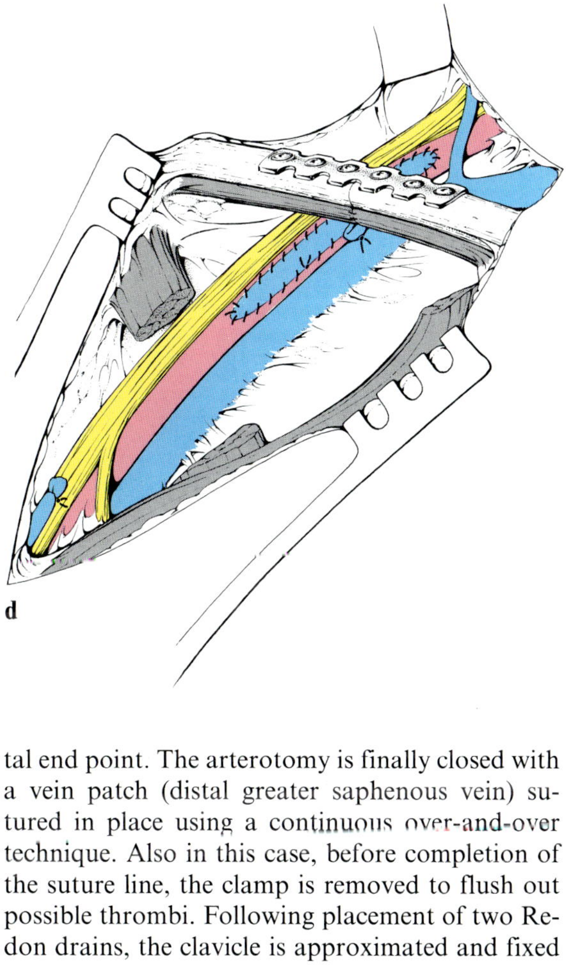

Fig. 19.5a–d. Open endarterectomy of the distal subclavian artery. **a** Exposure of the subclavian and axillary artery and osteotomy of the clavicle [4, 5, 8]. **b** Open endarterectomy of the subclavian artery. **c** Closure of the arterotomy with a vein patch. **d** Osteosynthesis of the clavicle

of the clamps, Redon drains are placed in the supra- and infraclavicular regions. The wound is closed in the supraclavicular region by suture of the platysma and the subcutis as well as the skin. In the infraclavicular region, the partially incised pectoralis major muscle is approximated by interrupted sutures. Afterwards, the subcutaneous tissue and the skin are closed (Fig. 19.3c).

To perform an *open thromboendarterectomy* one must follow the approach mentioned above (see p. 529), including osteotomy of the clavicle (Fig. 19.5a). Then, the subclavian artery is exposed over its whole length, from the scalene space to the axillary artery. Following proximal and distal cross-clamping, a longitudinal incision is made at the ventral circumference of the occluded arterial segment. The thrombus is dissected with a spatula.

Care should be taken not leave floating intimal flaps following dissection (Fig. 19.5b). The incision must extend beyond the intimal shelf proximally as well as distally to prevent a free edge of the intima from being rolled up, resulting in a thrombosis. This may occur especially at the distal end point. The arterotomy is finally closed with a vein patch (distal greater saphenous vein) sutured in place using a continuous over-and-over technique. Also in this case, before completion of the suture line, the clamp is removed to flush out possible thrombi. Following placement of two Redon drains, the clavicle is approximated and fixed by means of a plate (Fig. 19.5c, d). The wound is then closed according to the approach for separate incisions.

VI. Bypass

Endarterectomy is a very demanding procedure, involving precise intraoperative control of the results of disobliteration. From the technical standpoint, bypassing the occluded segment is significantly simpler and is therefore preferred over thromboendarterectomy in the majority of cases. The approach is through a supra- and infraclavicular incision (Fig. 19.6). Following exposure of the axillary and subclavian artery distally in the costoclavicular space, a tunnel is formed dorsal to the clavicle for later pull-through of the graft. If the costoclavicular space is sufficient, the graft can be pulled through without difficulty. However, if the costoclavicular space is relatively narrow, it is sensible to resect this segment of the artery after proximal and distal cross-clamping to provide enough space for the graft. The lumen of the subclavian or axillary artery largely determines the graft material. When the subclavian artery is 6 mm or more in diameter, a double-velour Dacron prosthesis or a PTFE prosthesis may be used. When the diameter is 5 mm or less, a vein graft is strongly recommended.

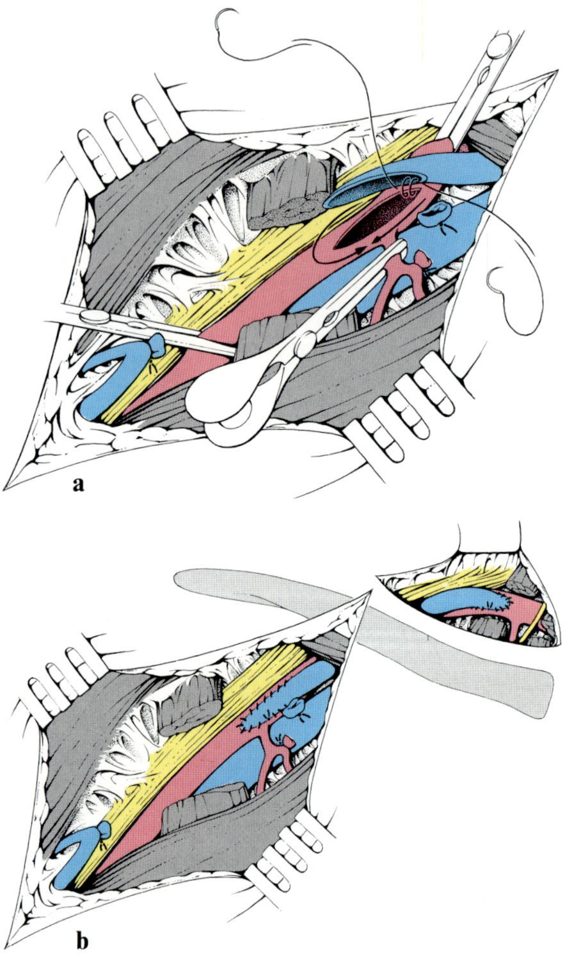

Fig. 19.6a, b. Subclavian-axillary bypass – distal anastomosis. **a** End-to-side anastomosis with loose stitches. **b** Completed anastomosis

1. Vein Bypass

Following exposure of the subclavian and axillary arteries, an incision is made anterior to the ipsilateral medial malleolus for harvesting a sufficiently long segment of the greater saphenous vein. After harvesting the graft, it is turned end for end (vein valves!) and marked with a clamp. The distal end of the vein graft is anastomosed first, then the proximal end. A longitudinal incision is made in the vein graft corresponding to the 1.5-cm ventral incision in the axillary artery, and the projecting flaps are trimmed off. The anastomosis is performed by continuous suture using 5–0 or 6–0 monofilament suture material. It has been found beneficial to start the continuous suture at the proximal corner of the incision. At first, the continuous suture is kept very loose so that every stitch at the proximal corner of the anastomosis can be carefully inspected (Fig. 19.6a). Then the suture is tightened as the vein is guided gently into position in the proximal corner. The continuous over-and-over suture commences again on the side away from the surgeon and proceeds toward and around the distal end of the anastomosis (Fig. 19.6b). The other end of the suture is used to complete the anastomosis. Then, using a long forceps, the vein is carefully passed behind the clavicle and brought into the proper position, care being taken not to twist it. The vein is tailored under slight tension and anastomosed to a ventral incision in the subclavian artery in the same manner as that just described. Here, too, just prior to completion of the suture, the segment is flushed briefly by releasing the clamps (possible thrombi).

To avoid bypass thrombosis, van Dongen generally recommends resection of the first rib when using a transaxillary approach (p. 559).

2. Prostheses

If the vessel caliber is large enough, prosthetic material may also be used for this segment. Most suitable are prostheses made of PTFE or double velour Dacron. The anastomosis is performed in the same way as when using a vein. However, when inserting double-velour Dacron prostheses, it is important that the proximal anastomosis be performed first so that the prosthesis can be clotted by repeated flushing with blood. Vascular pros-

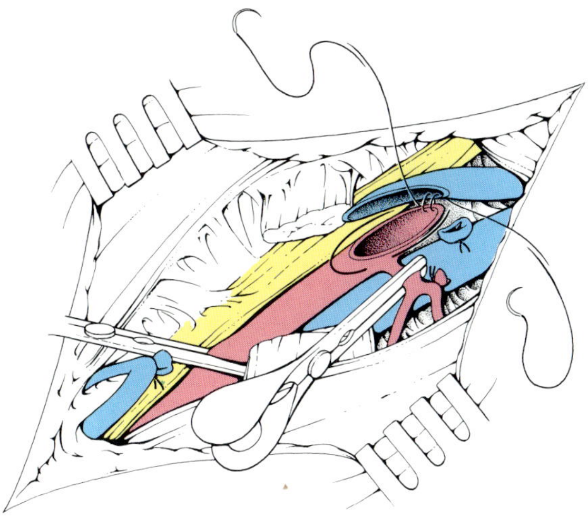

Fig. 19.7. Subclavian-axillary bypass. End-to-end anastomosis and situation following completed anastomosis

theses made of expanded PTFE material (Gore-Tex, Impra) are inserted using the same sequence of steps as with the vein graft. If the costoclavicular space does not allow the graft to be pulled through (risk of compressing the graft), the arterial segment must be resected. Then, at both the proximal and distal ends, a beveled end-to-end anastomosis is constructed, preferably with a longitudinal diameter of 1.5 cm. The loose suture technique, allowing inspection of the corner stitches, is recommended in this instance also (Fig. 19.7).

D. Operative Procedures for Occlusions of the Axillary Artery

I. Positioning and Draping

Axillary artery occlusions require reconstruction extending from the infraclavicular axillary artery to the brachial artery. Therefore, it is necessary to abduct the arm [4, 5]. The patient is placed on the operating table in a supine position with the arm abducted at a right angle and placed on a separate arm table. The supraclavicular fossa, the anterior wall of the thorax, the axillary region, and the whole upper arm are disinfected and draped. The forearm is wrapped to the elbow in a sterile drape. The surgeon stands caudal to the abducted arm. With sterile drapes placed around the operative field, the skin is covered with a transparent incisional drape.

II. Exposure of the Axillary Artery and the Proximal Brachial Artery

With the arm abducted at a right angle, the clavicular head of the pectoralis major muscle almost completely covers the axillary artery. Therefore, it is necessary to make an infraclavicular skin incision parallel to the clavicle (Fig. 19.1), starting medial to the configuration of the deltoid muscle and extending about 8–10 cm. Following division of the skin and the subcutaneous tissue, the pectoralis major muscle is found deep within. It is incised parallel to the clavicle and 1 cm caudal to the insertion, using an electrosurgical knife. Smaller vessels of the muscle are coagulated. Following insertion of a retractor, the axillary artery may be exposed by deep blunt dissection. The axillary vein, usually passing somewhat ventromedially, often has to be retracted medially (Fig. 19.8). Usually this segment of the axillary artery cannot be mobilized sufficiently through this incision. The fibers of the pectoralis minor muscles crossing obliquely are either incised or completely divided to expose the isolated axillary artery over a sufficient length. Special care must be taken that the adjacent fascicles of the brachial plexus are not injured intraoperatively, e.g., by cautery or dissection. The artery is exposed circumferentially and a tape is placed around it.

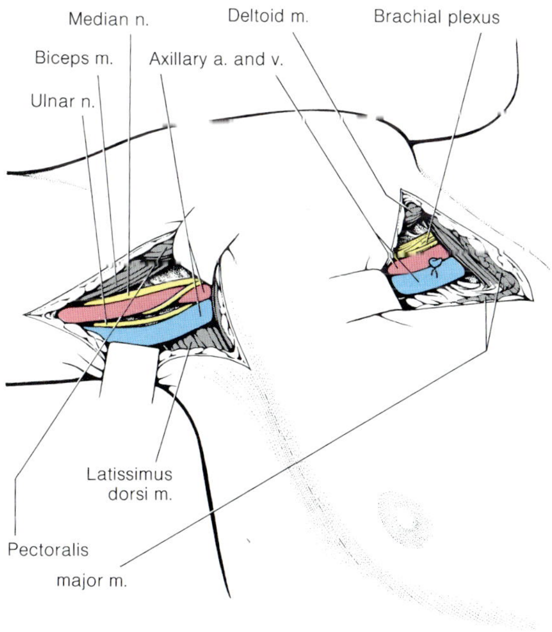

Fig. 19.8. Exposure of the first and third segments of the axillary artery [4, 5, 8]

The proximal segment of the brachial artery is found in the medial bicipital groove of the upper arm (Fig. 19.8), which is easily located by palpation. The skin incision begins at the groove, which is in the proximal third of the upper arm, and continues ventrally in a curve along the contour of the pectoris major muscle (Fig. 19.1). Following division of the skin and the subcutaneous tissue, the brachial fascia is split and dissection carried out in the depths of the medial bicipital groove. The medial cutaneous nerve of the forearm is also located here; it must be preserved at all costs in order to avoid postoperative paresthesia and hyperalgesia. Medially and deep, the brachial vein is found. Laterally and somewhat deeper lies the brachial artery, with the median nerve in close proximity. The nerve must be dissected off the arterial sheath. The brachial artery as well as the profunda brachii artery are isolated circumferentially, and tapes are placed around them. When dissecting, it is often necessary to retract the upper edge of the pectoralis major muscle in the direction of the axillary fossa with a hook. If the operative field is insufficient for exposure of the brachial artery, it may become necessary to incise the pectoralis major muscle at this site. This provides access to a long segment of the brachial artery.

III. Thromboendarterectomy of the Axillary Artery

Usually, angiography does not reveal whether an occlusion of the axillary artery is due to arteriosclerosis, arteriitis, or to trauma. Therefore, one usually decides intraoperatively which type of reconstruction is to be used. Thromboendarterectomy has the advantage that it can be performed quickly by means of two incisions. A disadvantage, however, is that proper evaluation of the results of disobliteration requires painstaking examination of the lumen. Following exposure of the axillary and brachial artery, and following central and peripheral cross-clamping of the artery as well as of the tributaries, a longitudinal incision is made in the infraclavicular segment of the axillary artery as well as in the brachial artery at the level of the origin of the profunda brachii artery, whenever possible (Fig. 19.9a, b). The distal incision must be made in such a way that the thrombus can be loosened from the arterial wall with a spatula and then completely dissected free by means of a ring stripper. The spiraling movement of the ring stripper should not be forced or jerky; otherwise, one risks perforation of the arterial wall. After the thrombus has been dissected as far as the proximal incision, it is cut free from the normal intima, leaving a smooth transition zone.

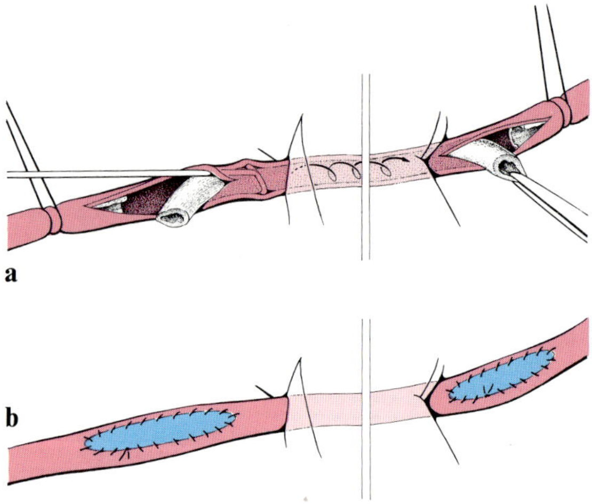

Fig. 19.9a, b. Endarterectomy of the axillary artery. **a** Semiclosed endarterectomy of the axillary artery with a ring stripper, then closure of the arterotomy using a vein patch (**b**)

We have found it very useful to check the operative result by intraoperative vascular endoscopy and to remove any remaining intimal flaps, as these may be the source of recurrent stenoses [9]. After the lumen has been checked, the arteriotomies are closed using venous patch grafts. The graft material can be harvested either from the basilic vein, using the same incision, or from the greater saphenous vein, for which purpose an incision must be made anterior to the ipsilateral medial malleolus. The suturing is begun using the loose stitch technique, which insures precise suture placement and thereby guards against the possible formation of stenoses at the corners of the anastomosis; 5–0 or 6–0 monofilament suture material should be used. Before completion of the suture line, the clamps are released briefly in order to flush out any clots thay may have formed. Following a careful check for hemostasis, Redon drains are put in place, the separated portions of the pectoris major muscle are approximated, and the wound is closed layer by layer.

IV. Vein Bypass or Graft Interposition

The exposure of the axillary and brachial arteries is performed in the same way (Fig. 19.8). Following exposure of the arterial segments to be anastomosed, an appropriate segment of the greater saphenous vein of sufficient caliber is harvested from the lower leg. If the vein cannot be used because of postthrombotic or varicose lesions, the central segment of the greater saphenous vein at the thigh may have to be used. The harvested vein graft is kept for the time being in Ringer's solution, with the proximal and distal ends clearly marked. Following cross-clamping, the brachial and axillary arteries are incised on their ventral aspect in a region that is definitely free of stenoses. The vein is turned end for end, incised to match the length of the anastomosis, and the excess edges are trimmed. Simultaneously, the arteriotomy is tailored to a slightly elliptical shape to avoid overcorrection and pseudodilation (Fig. 19.10a). Using a loose suture technique, the base of the vein is sutured to the proximal corner of the arteriotomy of the brachial artery by a 5–0 or 6–0 monofilament suture. The anastomosis is then completed, beginning on the side away from the surgeon, using a continuous over-and-over suture. At the distal end of the anastomosis one must be careful not to catch too much wall when suturing as the resultant plications may lead to stenoses. After the distal corner has been sutured, the anastomosis is completed on the side nearer the surgeon, using the other half of the suture and proceeding distally. Finally, both sutures are tied together. Afterwards, the vein graft is cross-clamped at the base of the anastomosis and blood is allowed to enter the old vascular bed. It is advisable in this phase of the operation to fill the vein with heparinized saline solution and to occlude the central end with a bulldog clamp. A tunnel is formed digitally from the axillary artery along the vessel as a guideline and behind the pectoralis minor and major muscles down to the brachial artery. Holding the bulldog clamp (marker) with a forceps, one pulls the vein graft through to the proximal arterial incision. The vein must not lie too loosely in place, and above all, it must not be twisted, as this might result in a stenosis. Once the vein has been pulled through, it is tailored to the proper length, special attention being given to the dorsoventral edge. The distal end of the vein is then anastomosed to the axillary arteriotomy in the manner already discussed, using 5–0 or 6–0 monofilament suture and stitching loosely at first, then later tightening the suture (adaptation of vein and artery). In this case, too, the anastomosis is begun on the side away from the surgeon using a continuous suture and passing the proximal edge of the anastomosis. Us-

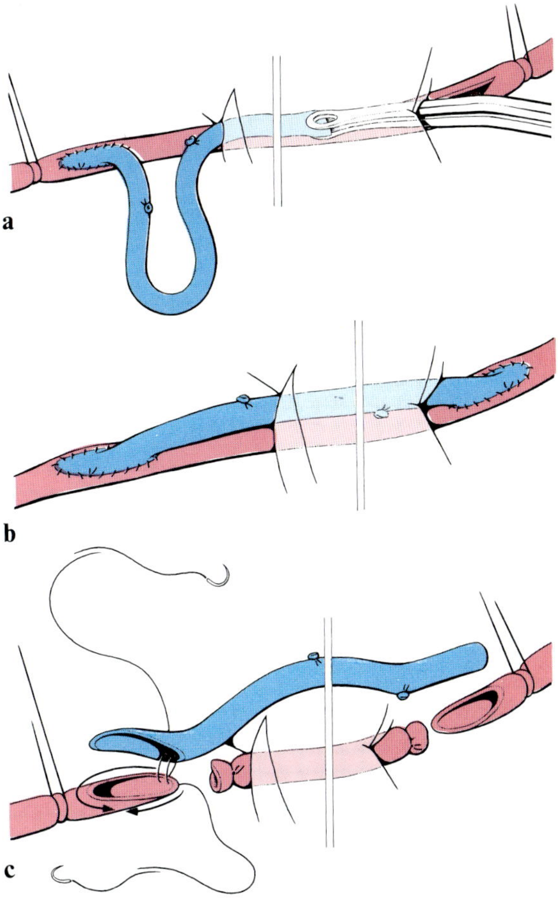

Fig. 19.10a–c. Axillobrachial bypass. **a** End-to-side anastomosis of a vein graft. **b** Situation following completion of the anastomosis. **c** End-to-end anastomosis with exclusion of the axillary artery

ing the other half of the suture, the anastomosis is completed, from the distal to the proximal end. Before completion of the suture the flow is checked by brief flushing. After the suture has been tied, the clamps are removed (Fig. 19.10b). Following a bypass procedure an intraoperative check should be performed to ensure that there are no technical errors making early reocclusion likely. In this vascular region, intraoperative angiography is rather difficult to perform. It may sometimes be possible with a C-arch and the camera fixed to the ceiling. Intraoperative flow measurement has proven useful as an alternative. Here, what is important is the increase in flow following release of the clamps as compared with the flow prior to reconstruction.

Usually, this end-to-side technique is preferred over an end-to-end technique because it is easier to perform. Occasionally, however, if the arterial wall is extremely fibrous or if it has been destroyed in an attempted endarterectomy, it may be necessary to exclude the axillary artery. Extensive dissection and resection of the entire axillary artery is time consuming and does not provide any advantage over simple ligation. In this case, too, the reconstruction starts at the distal anastomosis. Care must be taken to bevel the artery and vein over a long enough distance – about 1.5 cm – as a safeguard against suture-related stenosis (Fig. 19.10c). The ventral aspect of the artery is incised to the appropriate length, and a corresponding incision is made in the caudal end of the vein. Edges are rounded to avoid pseudodilatation of the anastomosis. The end of the artery is sutured to the anastomotic base of the vein using a 5–0 or 6–0 monofilament suture. Both vessels are approximated by tightening the suture. Then, the suture lying on the side away from the surgeon is used to sew the lateral edge of the anastomosis. Care must be taken to avoid the plication effect that results when the sutures are placed too far apart. In particular, one must guard against a stenosis at the distal corner. Therefore, when suturing the end of the anastomosis, the sutures should be placed as close together as possible. When the suture line has been brought around the distal end, the remaining portion of suture is used to complete the anastomosis, and the two suture ends are tied together. Following completion of the anastomosis, the vein is filled with Ringer's solution in the same way as with the end-to-side anastomosis, and the ventral and dorsal edges are marked with a bulldog clamp. A tunnel is created digitally. Then, the vein is pulled through the tunnel with a long forceps to the site of the proximal anastomosis. Following determination of the appropriate length, the vein is shortened and tailored. The proximal anastomosis is performed using the same technique as for the distal anastomosis. Concerning intraoperative control, the same principles apply as earlier described.

E. Operative Procedures for Brachial Artery Occlusions

I. Positioning and Draping

Occlusive disease of the brachial artery usually involves a long segment. This may extend from the origin of the profunda brachii artery to a point just proximal to the cubital joint. This is usually the distal limit of brachial artery occlusions, owing to the numerous collaterals of the rete cubiti. Therefore, the arm is placed on an arm table, providing free movement (Fig. 19.1a). The entire arm from the axilla down to the wrist is disinfected and draped. The hand and the forearm are wrapped in a sterile drape. After wiping off the disinfected skin, a transparent incisional drape is placed in position. To provide full exposure of the cubital region, a folded sheet is introduced under the cubital joint to serve as a fulcrum.

II. Exposure of the Final Segment of the Brachial Artery

For reconstruction, an incision is made over the initial segment of the brachial artery (approach to the proximal brachial artery as described on p. 528). However, the skin incision does not have to be extended along the border of the pectoralis muscle. Access to the distal brachial artery is provided by curvilinear incision following the course of the artery in the cubital fossa (Fig. 19.11). In principle, a straight incision over the cubital fossa could be performed; however, straight incisions tend to cause contractions owing to shrinkage of the scar. Therefore, a slightly curvilinear or S-shaped incision is preferred. Following division of the skin and the subcutaneous tissue, the soft fatty tissue is dissected bluntly. The incision will reveal the basilic and medial cubital veins, which can vary considerably; they should be preserved. Following splitting of the brachial fascia, the aponeurosis of the biceps brachii muscle is divided. The branches of the medial cutaneous nerve of the forearm pass in close proximity and should be preserved whenever possible. Following division of the aponeurosis, the final segment of the brachial artery is found somewhat deeper. This segment is isolated circumferentially, and a tape is placed around it. In order to expose the entire length, collaterals of the concomitant vein of the crossing brachial artery have to be divided between ligatures. While dissecting, special care must be taken of the median nerve passing medial to the artery to avoid concomitant injuries. Following determination of the proximal and distal sites of anastomosis an appropriate segment of the greater saphenous vein can be harvested from the lower leg. It is turned end for end, and both ends are marked. The vein is then placed in Ringer's solution until the anastomosis

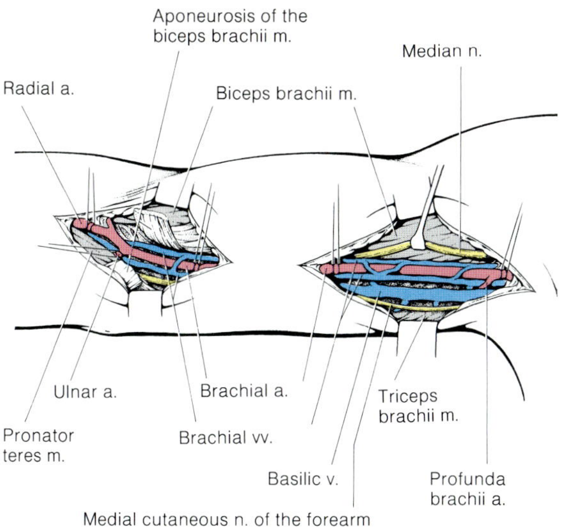

Fig. 19.11. Exposure of the proximal brachial artery [4, 5, 8] and of the distal segment of the brachial artery in the cubital fossa [4, 5, 8]

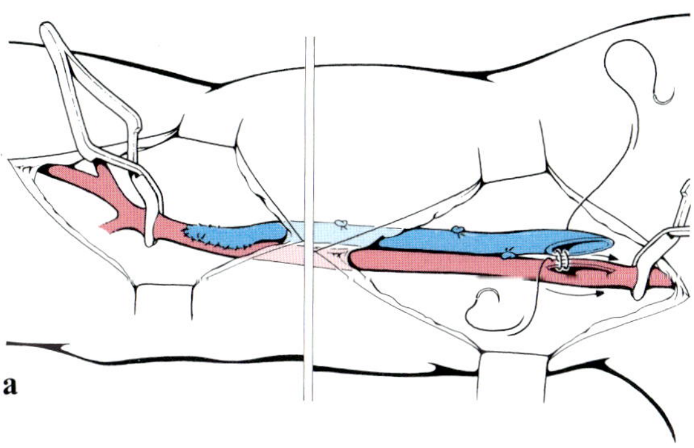

a

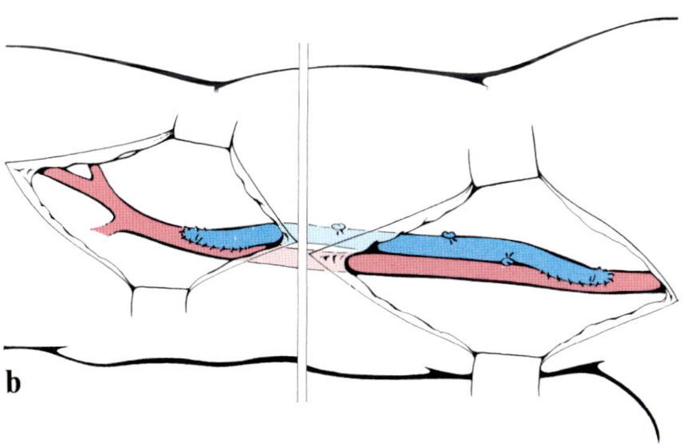

b

Fig. 19.12 a, b. Brachiobrachial vein bypass. **a** Distal anastomosis end-to-side technique; completed distal anastomosis, the vein being passed underneath the fascia to the proximal anastomosis. **b** Proximal anastomosis end-to-side technique; completed proximal anastomosis

is performed. Following proximal and distal cross-clamping, a ventral arteriotomy of the brachial artery is performed (Fig. 19.12a, b). Heparinized saline solution (1:100) is injected into the periphery. If there is an arterial spasm, it is advisable to insert a Fogarty balloon catheter into the distal segment of the artery and to retract the catheter with the balloon inflated (mechanical dilation). The harvested vein is sutured distally to the arteriotomy, which should be about 1.5 cm long (the caudal end of the vein has been incised and tailored beforehand). The basal edge of the vein end is sutured to the proximal corner of the arteriotomy, and, following tightening of the suture, the anastomosis is completed using a continuous over-and-over technique (at the distal corner, especially, the stitches should be placed as close together as possible to avoid a plication effect). With the remaining portion of suture the final stitches are placed in the side nearer the surgeon, and the two ends are tied together. Next, a tunnel is created under the fascia of the medial bicipital groove, using a long forceps. Then the vein is filled with heparinized saline solution and pulled through the tunnel proximally with the forceps (checking carefully for length and guarding against twisting). The vein is tailored and anastomosed end-to-side to the proximal arteriotomy using 5–0 or 6–0 monofilament suture material (Fig. 19.12). Before completion of the anastomosis, possible clots are flushed out by brief declamping. After completion of the suture, intraoperative angiography is performed, the needle being inserted in the region of the central anastomosis and the contrast medium injected in the anterograde direction. To avoid extensive bleeding, the site of puncture is closed by a single suture. Following careful hemostasis, the procedure is completed by the insertion of Redon drains and suture of the subcutaneous tissue and the skin. Reinsertion of the aponeurosis of the biceps muscle or the brachial fascia is not necessary. Occlusions in the region of the brachial artery are mostly limited to the region proximal to the elbow for the reasons already mentioned. If, as happens in rare cases, the terminal segment of the brachial artery is also involved, the vein bypass may be extended beyond the cubital fossa to the radial or ulnar artery. However, there is the risk of graft occlusion provoked by extreme kinking, as in all grafts crossing joints. Therefore, indications for such long reconstructions in the region of the forearm should be judged following exact evaluation of the clinical symptoms and necessity.

REFERENCES

1. Bollinger A (1979) Funktionelle Angiologie. Lehrbuch und Atlas. Thieme, Stuttgart New York
2. Denck H (1976) Chirurgie der peripheren Aneurysmen. In: Vollmar JF (ed) Arteriovenöse Fisteln – dilatierende Arteriopathien. Thieme, Stuttgart New York
3. Gross WS, Flanigan P, Kraft RO, Stanley JC (1978) Chronic upper extremity arterial insufficiency. Arch Surg 113:419–423
4. Haimovici H (1976) The upper extremity. In: Haimovici H (ed) Vascular surgery. McGraw-Hill, New York
5. Leitz KH (1981) Zugangswege in der Gefäßchirurgie. Springer, Berlin Heidelberg New York
6. Loeprecht H (1982) Gefäßverletzungen an der Schulter. In: Burri C (ed) Verletzungen des Schultergürtels, Hefte zur Unfallheilkunde 160. Springer, Berlin Heidelberg New York
7. Pirker E, Stampfel G (1977) Röntgendiagnostik bei arterieller Durchblutungsstörung der oberen Extremität. VASA 6:289–291
8. Platzer W (1982) Atlas der topographischen Anatomie. Thieme, Stuttgart New York
9. Vollmar JF (1982) Rekonstruktive Chirurgie der Arterien, 3rd revised edn. Thieme, Stuttgart New York

20 Extra-anatomic Bypasses in Chronic Arterial Occlusive Disease (Infections, Patients at Risk)

H. MÜLLER-WIEFEL

CONTENTS

A. Indications

Atypical, or so-called "extra-anatomic," bypasses are employed whenever a special local situation (e.g., infection, multiple operations, radiation, stoma) or an unfavorable general condition precludes direct arterial reconstruction or orthotopic placement of the bypass, or when a minimum stress operation must be performed, without opening of a large body cavity.

Whether or not an extra-anatomic bypass procedure is indicated will depend on its value for the specific vascular region involved, as established by comparing the mortality, patency rate, and functional results with those of the classical procedure.

B. Supra-aortic Region

In the supra-aortic region there is a significant *trend toward extrathoracic reconstruction*. This is especially true for bridging a central occlusion of the left subclavian artery by means of a carotid subclavian bypass.

This technique, as well as the other extra-anatomic bypasses in the supra-aortic region, are described in Chap. 15.1 (supra-aortic branches) on p. 508 ff.

C. Axillo(bi)femoral Bypass

The bypass from the major upper extremity arteries to those of the lower part of the body through a partially subcutaneous, partially subfascial tunnel of the lateral thoracic and abdominal wall is usually performed using an 8-mm Dacron velour or PTFE prosthesis. Depending on the individual case, ring-reinforced or helical coil-wrapped grafts are also used as protection against external compression.

General anesthesia is recommended, although one may also consider local anesthesia in extreme cases.

The ipsilateral subclavian artery is most suitable to serve as the *donor artery* for limb revascularization. Additional stenoses of other supra-aortic vessels must also be taken into account so that in individual cases an axillomonofemoral crossover bypass may also be considered when an axillobifemoral bypass is not indicated. The axillobifemoral bypass is usually performed on the right shoulder because the right subclavian artery is significantly less often occluded than the left.

If it is not necessary to shorten the operative time by using a separate team at each of the two anastomotic sites, the procedure is begun by exposing the proximal axillary artery using an oblique or slightly curvilinear infraclavicular approach caudal to the lateral half of the clavicle. The upper arm is abducted almost 90° (Fig. 20.1). Following division of the subcutaneous tissue and the fascia, the pectoralis major muscle is split bluntly, parallel to the direction of the muscle fibers, with the pulsating axillary artery serving as a guide. If necessary, fibers of the pectoralis

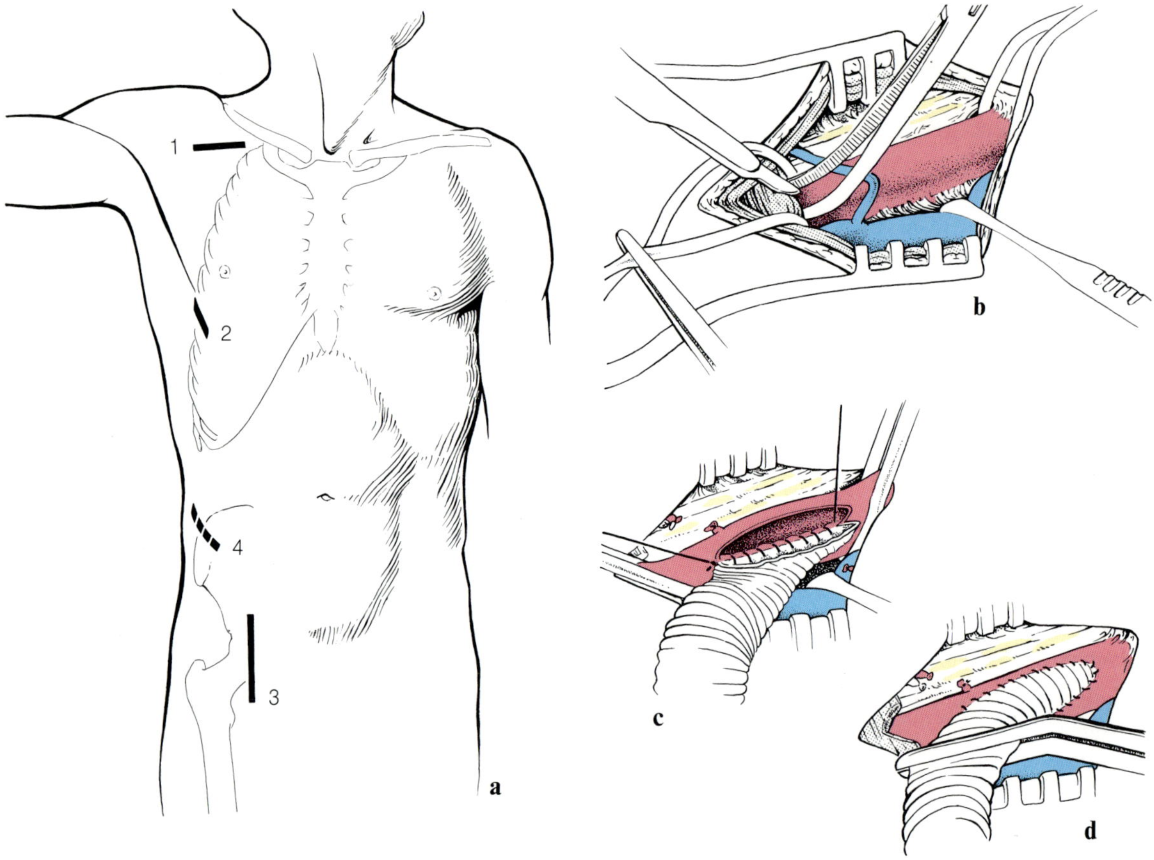

Fig. 20.1. **a** Location of incisions for an axillofemoral bypass. The procedure begins with an infraclavicular incision (*1*). From there a subcutaneous tunnel leads to infrapectoral incision (*2*) and then to the inguinal site of anastomosis (*3*). For an axillobifemoral bypass an additional incision somewhat above the iliac crest (*4*) is provided. **b** The axillary artery, exposed below the clavicle, is dissected as far proximally as possible, and two vessel loops are placed around it. The pectoralis minor muscle may have to be incised to provide more space. **c** Ligation and division of the thoracoacromial artery help to mobilize the axillary artery. At the site of the proximal anastomosis, longitudinal arteriotomy and wall excision to achieve an oval orifice. **d** The proximal anastomosis should be constructed at an angle that is hemodynamically favorable

minor muscle, located in the lateral third of the wound, may be incised additionally. Then, the axillary artery and vein are exposed in the subpectoral fatty tissue. The vein, passing ventrally, is exposed first.

The artery is exposed as far proximally as possible, i.e., up to where it emerges from beneath the clavicle. A tape is placed around it. Usually, ligation and division of the branching thoracoacromial trunk is required in order to mobilize the vessel sufficiently. While dissecting, care must be taken to preserve the branches of the brachial plexus, passing in the cranial and lateral part of the operative field.

After a tape has been placed around the distal segment of the exposed artery, the proximal and distal clamps are placed, and an incision is made over a distance of about 2–2.5 cm on the ventrocaudal aspect of the first one third of the artery, i.e., lateral to the point where it emerges from beneath the clavicle.

This provides a hemodynamically favorable anastomotic angle. Kinking or distortion between artery and graft when moving the shoulder or the arm may thus be avoided.

A Dacron prosthesis may now be clotted using the patient's blood. Afterwards, the vascular bed of the arm is heparinized.

Following extension of the arteriotomy by tailoring an oval orifice, the anastomosis is completed by a continuous over-and-over suture using 5–0 suture material. It should be pointed out that because the wall of the axillary artery is much more vulnerable than other vessel walls, there is always the danger of tearing at the suture line.

Where the operative field is narrow, it is advantageous to use a monofilament synthetic suture such as Prolene, allowing one to place several loops loosely and to tie them later (parachute technique).

Following completion of the suture, the graft is cross-clamped close to the anastomosis and the arterial flow to the arm is released again. If necessary, the graft may be flushed again by brief declamping to achieve further clotting.

The site of the distal anastomosis is prepared by exposure of the femoral bifurcation through a longitudinal incision, using the standard technique (see p. 392). The incision of the skin and the subcutaneous tissue should extend about 3 cm above the inguinal ligament. The distal limit is determined by the extent of the arterial occlusive disease (Fig. 20.2).

Graft placement starts with a transverse incision about 5 cm long between the anterior and middle axillary line and approximately at the level of the sixth interspace. From this incision a tunnel is created to the cranial wound by blunt dissection, using the finger or a curved clamp. The index finger of the other hand simultaneously dissects downward between the pectoralis major and minor muscle to the counterincision – or between the pectoralis major muscle and the outer thoracic wall if the pectoralis minor muscle has previously been incised.

When pulling the graft through the tunnel care must be taken to avoid twisting it, and above all, the graft must be placed so that the proximal anastomosis or the axillary artery is not subjected to excessive tension. Otherwise, there will be the danger later on that vigorous movement of the arm or shoulder might cause tearing at the suture

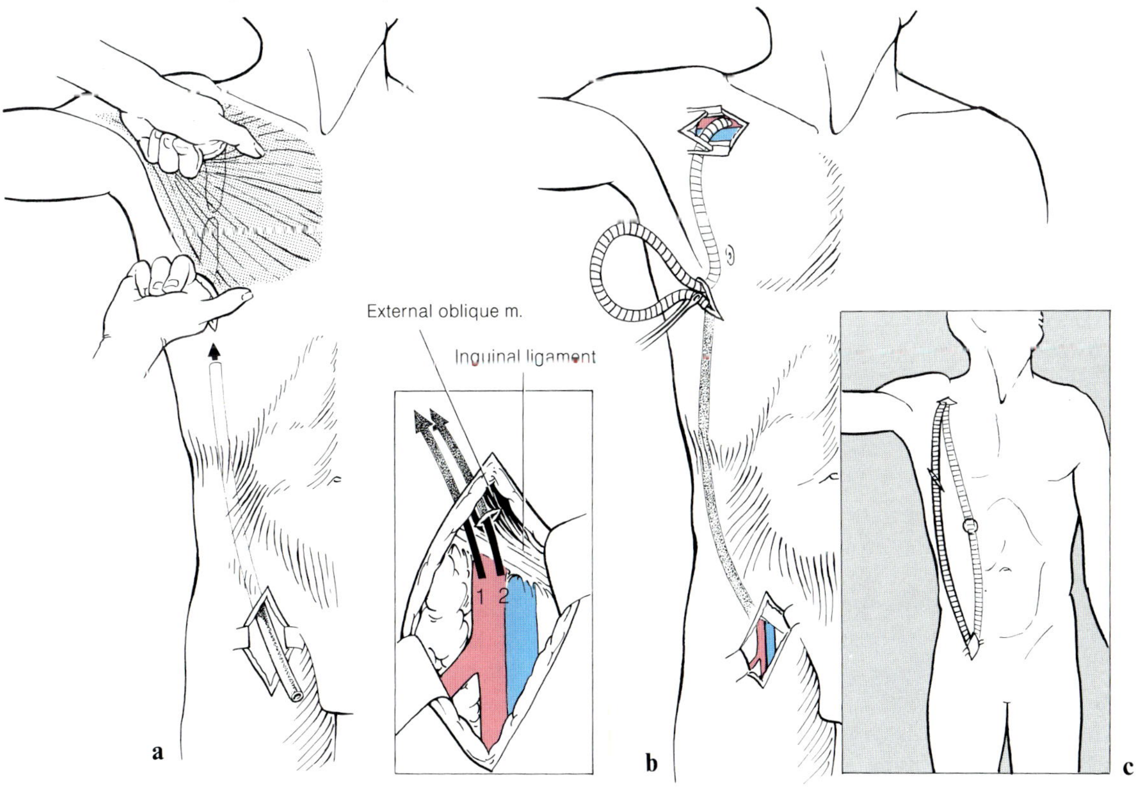

Fig. 20.2. a Following completion of the central anastomosis, a tunnel is created by blunt dissection of the soft tissue between the infraclavicular incision and the counterincision at the lower border of the pectoralis muscle, using both index fingers. Then, using a tunneler, a graft bed is created from the groin to the subpectoral incision. *Inset:* Caudally the prosthesis may be passed either subcutaneously or in the region of the lateral muscles. The tunneler is then inserted ventral to the inguinal ligament or into the muscles following incision of the external oblique muscle. **b** The graft is pulled through the prepared tunnel with a curved forceps. **c** Optimal course of the axillofemoral bypass: anastomosis to the axillary artery as far ventrally as possible and then located in the region of the thorax and the flank within the midaxillary line. A graft passing too far ventrally is more likely to kink where it crosses the costal margin

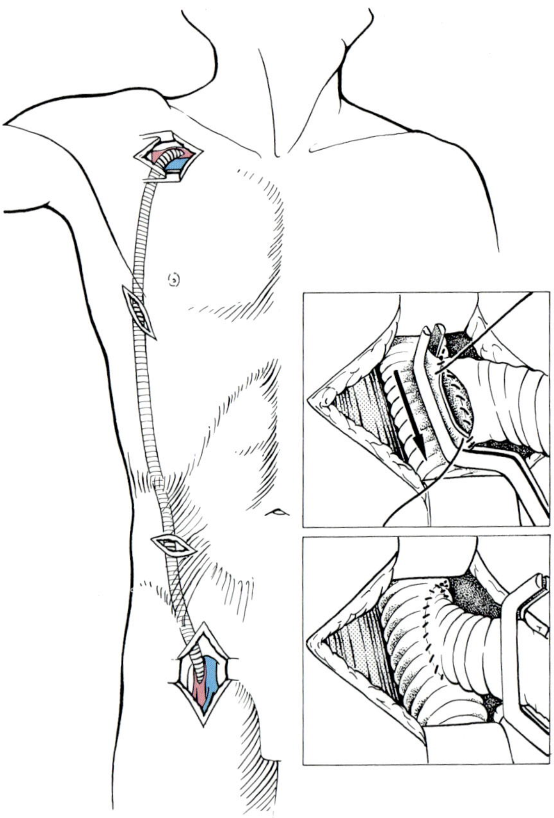

Fig. 20.3. Extending an axillofemoral bypass to form an axillobifemoral bypass. The already functioning unilateral segment of the graft is exposed through an additional incision above the iliac crest (*1*) and an end-to-side anastomosis is performed using a crossover graft of the same caliber

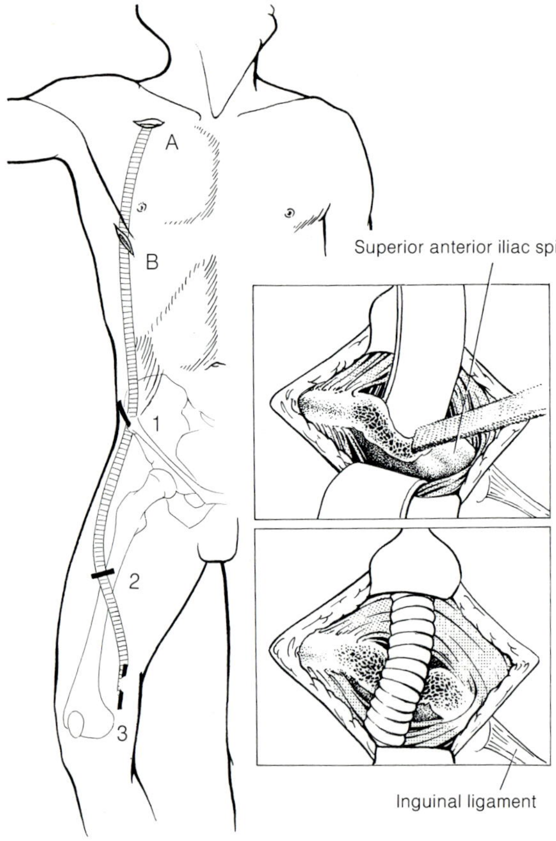

Fig. 20.4. Extension to the femoropopliteal junction: following the classical incision (*A, B*) a counterincision is required somewhat above the iliac crest close to the anterior iliac spine (*1*). There, the iliac crest must be incised to protect the graft and to avoid kinking. From there, with the help of an additional incision (*2*), the graft can be passed down to the site of the distal anastomosis (*3*) along the extensor side of the thigh

line with resultant hemorrhage or formation of a false aneurysm.

A graft which is too long may kink during adduction of the arm and cause thromboembolic complications.

Whether the graft originating from the axillary artery will be passed ventral or dorsal to the axillary vein to avoid venous compression depends upon the situs.

To pass the graft to the site of the peripheral anastomosis in the groin, a tunneler is preferred, but a long, curved forceps may also be used if another short counterincision is made between the groin and the costal margin.

The course of the graft from the costal arch to the groin may be through a subcutaneous tunnel, as preferred by us, or beneath or within the external oblique muscle. In the latter case, the inguinal ligament is slightly incised, the aponeurosis of the external oblique muscle slit open, and a tunneler inserted cranially.

Special care has to be taken to place the bypass sufficiently far dorsally at the flank to avoid kinking where the costal margin is crossed. And, as already mentioned, the length of the graft must be correctly determined as well. If the operating table has been flexed and the head portion elevated to facilitate the operation in the proximal infraclavicular region, it is advisable to place the patient in a completely supine position to determine the final length of the graft.

Before the final placement of the graft within the tunnel, it may be flushed with blood by brief declamping close to the central anastomosis. Afterwards, the graft is filled with heparinized saline solution.

The form and technique of the peripheral anastomosis in the groin or the proximal thigh must be adapted to the situation at the femoral bifurcation; usually, the anastomosis with the common and deep femoral arteries will be end-to-side. For further details see p. 441.

If there is no possibility of anastomosing an axillofemoral bypass in the groin, e.g., because of infection, then the previously mentioned procedure may be *changed* by extending the graft beyond the hip on the lateral side of the extremity. About one third of the way down the outer thigh, the graft is passed from the lateral side of the thigh to the inner side (Fig. 20.4).

In this case an additional incision is necessary along the midaxillary line over the iliac crest. From there, a tunnel is created to the cranial incision at the lower border of the pectoralis muscle. A rounded notch is made in the pelvic bone to protect the prosthesis from kinking as it passes down to the lateral part of the thigh.

One or two additional small skin incisions in the middle of the extensor side of the thigh facilitate passage of the bypass subcutaneously to the distal anastomotic site at the level of the subsartorial canal or the initial segment of the popliteal artery (see p. 394).

When the contralateral lower extremity has to be revascularized in the same operation, an axillo-bifemoral bypass is indicated. The procedure described before is continued, exposing the pulsating graft by a separate incision somewhat above the superior anterior iliac spine, following declamping of the axillofemoral bypass. Then tapes are placed around it cranially and caudally (Fig. 20.3).

For anastomosis of the crossover branch, a Satinsky clamp is placed on the main graft, which is already perfused; the clamped portion is incised over a distance of 1.5–2 cm, and the incision is widened, forming an oval orifice. The crossover graft, which must be of the same caliber and beveled at the end, is anastomosed end-to-side.

The Satinsky clamp is removed and placed on the crossover bypass, close to the anastomosis. Next, the contralateral inguinal region is exposed, and a tunnel is created across the lower abdomen in an oblique direction using bidigital dissection,

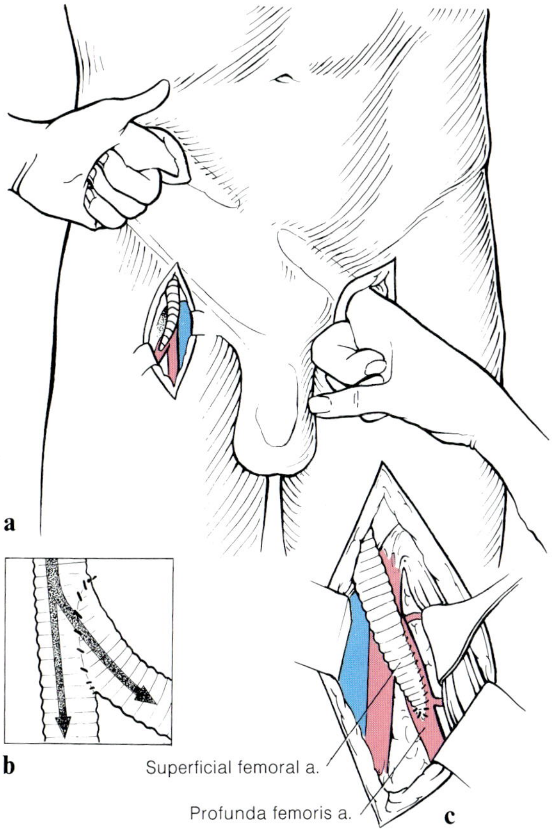

Fig. 20.5. a Creating a subcutaneous tunnel for an axillo-bifemoral bypass by digital dissection from the groin and the suprainguinal incision. **b** The branch of the bypass, crossing obliquely to the contralateral side, should be attached at an acute angle, as this is hemodynamically favorable. **c** If required, the crossover bypass can be anastomosed to the profunda femoris artery, thereby providing the effect of a profundaplasty

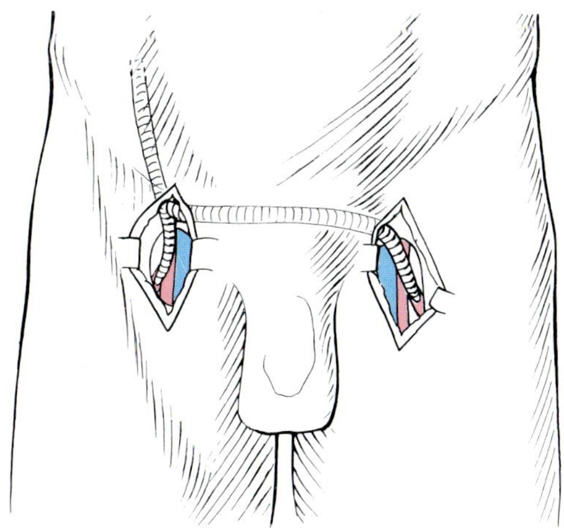

Fig. 20.6. If the suprasymphyseal crossover graft is not ▷ to have a suprainguinal takeoff, the crossover can also be anastomosed end-to-side in the region of the inguinal incision; in this case, of course, the anastomosis will be more or less rectangular

or possibly aided by a curved forceps. Here, too, a subcutaneous course is most suitable, although a preperitoneal course may also be used. If the latter approach is chosen, special care must be taken not to open the peritoneum or to cause bleeding by injuring muscle vessels during the blind tunneling (Fig. 20.5).

An alternative to the hemodynamically favorable acute-angled takeoff of the crossover bypass is the more or less rectangular end-to-side anastomosis of the crossover bypass (Fig. 20.6).

D. Iliofemoral Crossover Bypass

This form of extra-anatomic bypass allows circumvention of a diseased segment of the iliac artery, provided there is sufficient arterial blood flow on the donor side.

The procedure begins with exposure of the external iliac artery through an oblique or slightly curved incision 8–10 cm long, several fingerbreadths above the inguinal ligament. Following division of the abdominal wall muscles parallel to the muscle fibers, the peritoneal sac is retracted medially and cranially. A tape is placed around the external iliac artery proximally and distally, preserving the concomitant vein. Then the artery is occluded with two clamps.

The artery is incised over a distance of 2–3 cm and the beveled end of an 8-mm vascular prosthesis anastomosed end-to-side using a continuous over-and-over suture (Fig. 20.7).

The graft is then passed somewhat ventrally and caudally. If a Dacron graft is used, it must be preclotted with the patient's blood. A tunnel is created by digital dissection as described for the axillobifemoral bypass. The graft is passed through the tunnel to the arterial segment exposed in the contralateral groin for the distal anatomosis.

For an iliofemoral crossover bypass, a subcutaneous course is again recommended. In this case, the prosthesis is passed across to the recipient side in front of the external oblique muscle and the inguinal ligament and terminates in the operative field of the groin.

A more dorsal course may also be used, i.e., through the muscles of the lower abdominal wall or immediately in front of the peritoneum. In this case, the graft reaches the distal site of the anastomosis behind the inguinal ligament, as in an aortofemoral bifurcation bypass.

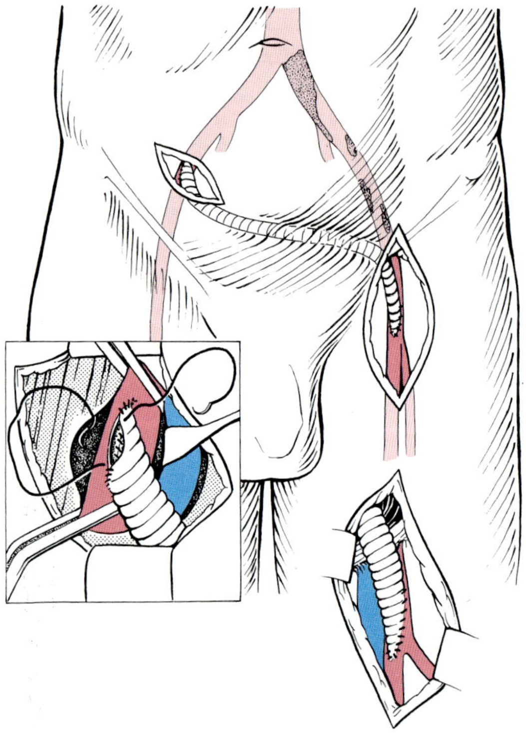

Fig. 20.7. Suprasymphyseal iliofemoral crossover bypass in an S-configuration. The external iliac artery is exposed through a suprainguinal extraperitoneal incision. The graft is anastomosed end-to-side at a hemodynamically favorable acute angle and is passed to the contralateral side through the soft tissue of the anterior abdominal wall, for the most part within a subcutaneous tunnel

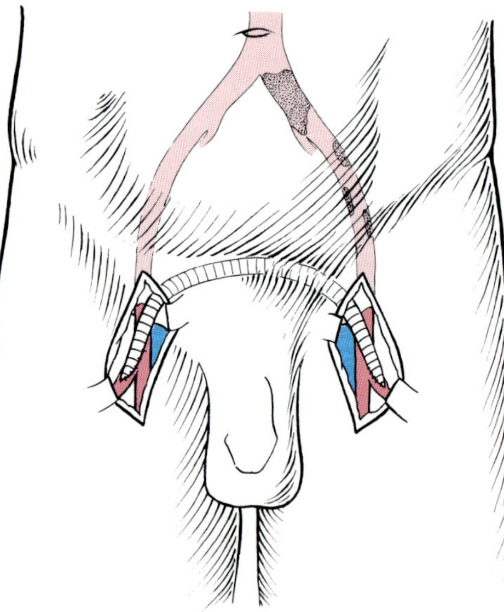

Fig. 20.8. Besides the S-configuration of the suprapubic crossover bypass, a C-configuration from one femoral bifurcation to the other may be considered. This approach is suitable for simultaneous correction of bilateral lesions of the femoral bifurcation

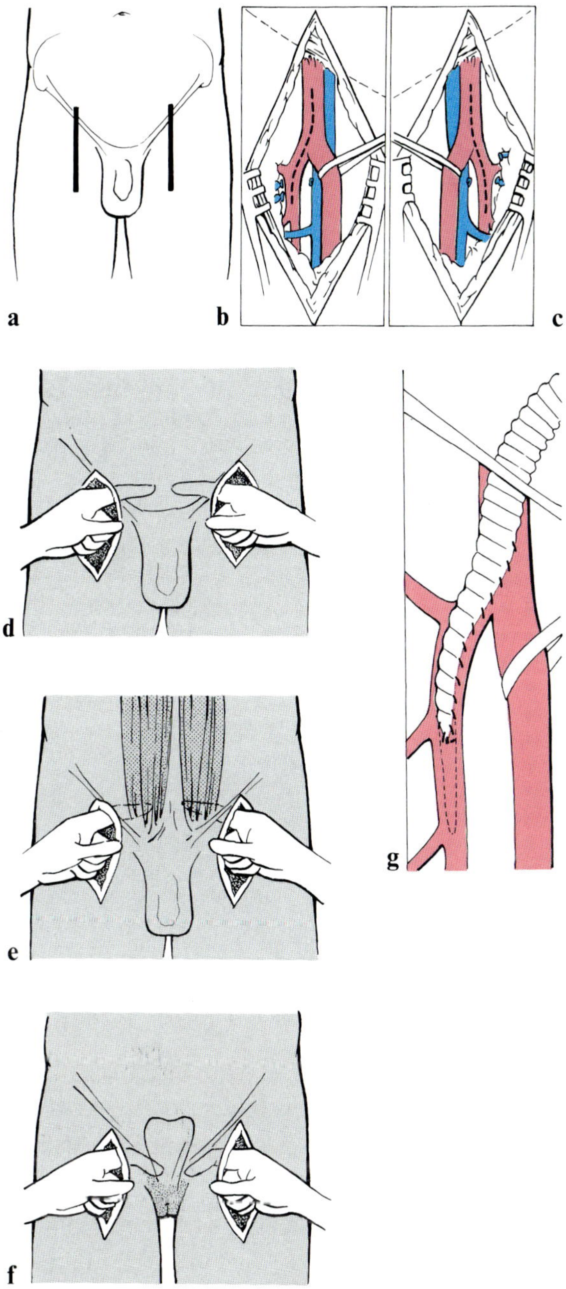

Fig. 20.9 a–g. Steps in the placement of a C-shaped femoral bypass in bilateral stenoses of the femoral bifurcation: skin incisions (**a**), location of the vessels in the groin (**b**, **c**). The course of the graft may be within a subcutaneous tunnel (**d**) or between the peritoneum and the rectus abdominis muscle (**e**). Alternatively, one may consider a perineal approach (**f**). Anastomosis of the bypass to the major trunk of the profunda femoris artery (**g**)

E. Femorofemoral Crossover Bypass

For the so-called suprasymphyseal crossover bypass, an iliofemoral route in an S-configuration is usually preferred for hemodynamic reasons. For a femorofemoral bypass, a C-configuration is used when there are lesions of the femoral bifurcation or the profunda femoris trunk on the donor side that have to be reconstructed as well (Figs. 20.8, 20.9).

Following exposure of both inguinal regions, reconstruction on the donor side is performed. The procedure depends on the local findings; e.g., endarterectomy of the femoral bifurcation or long arteriotomy of the trunk of the profunda femoris artery, leading to a profundaplasty. For the end-to-side anastomosis, the end of an 8-mm vascular prosthesis (occasionally 6 mm) is trimmed to create a long flap that serves as a patch graft for the profunda femoris artery. The tunnel for the graft is made in each inguinal wound with the index finger, just above symphysis. Its course may be either subcutaneous or dorsal to the rectus abdominis muscle through the cavum Retzii.

On the recipient side, the graft is anastomosed to the common femoral artery or to the profunda femoris artery, depending on local and angiographic findings. As a rule, the anastomosis is end-to-side, less often end-to-end.

If a suprapubic course for the graft is impossible owing to the local situation, a subcutaneous course through a perineal tunnel caudal to the insertion of the scrotum and penis may be used.

F. Obturator Bypass

This form is used mainly for the aseptic bypass of an infected groin area. Thanks to the flexibility of the bypass principle, the basic technique can be modified to fit highly variable local situations. The basic principle is that of a bypass from the aorta or an iliac artery, which does not pass in front of the anterior pubic ramus, but through the obturator foramen and finally downward to an artery of the thigh.

For the proximal approach (for details see p. 378), the iliac vessels are exposed transperitoneally or retroperitoneally, and a tape is placed, for example, around the common iliac artery. The distal approach is through a longitudinal incision on the inside of the middle third of the thigh, there-

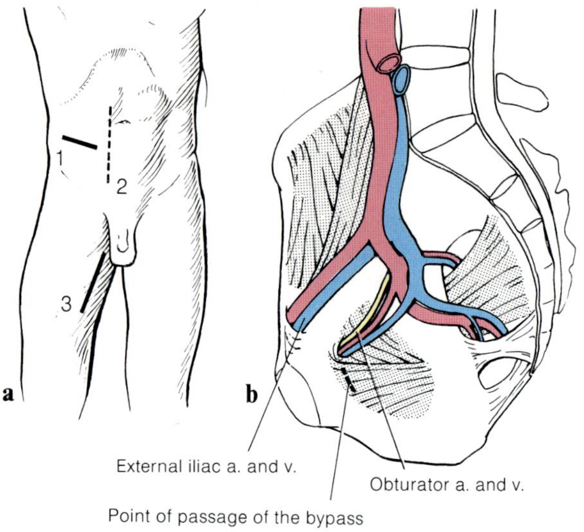

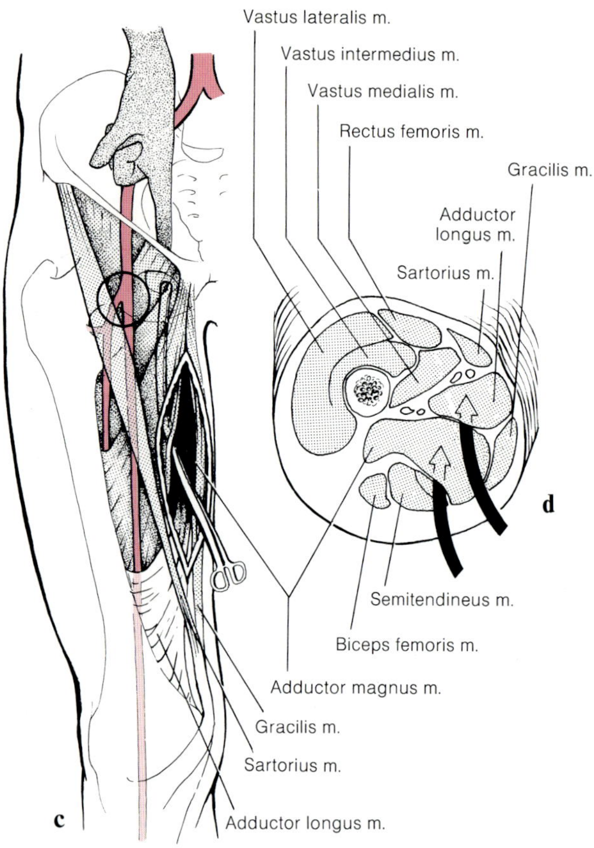

Fig. 20.10. a Location of skin incisions for an obturator bypass. The central anastomosis to the iliac arteries is made through an oblique or curved (*1*) or a longitudinal (*2*) incision. The peripheral anastomosis to the superficial femoral artery is performed on the medial aspect of the proximal or middle thigh (*3*). **b** Topography of the iliac vessels, the obturator vessels, and the point of passage of the bypass through the obturator membrane. **c** Following completion of the central anastomosis, the graft tunnel is created by blunt dissection. With the fingers of the left hand on the pelvic side of the obturator foramen, a long, curved forceps is passed upward from below, perforating the membrane. **d** The tunnel made by the forceps can have two different courses: either between the adductor magnus muscle and the adductor longus muscle or dorsal to the adductor magnus muscle. The latter approach is used when the distal anastomosis must be made to the popliteal artery

by exposing the superficial femoral artery, around which a tape is placed (Fig. 20.10).

After completion of the proximal anastomosis of the iliac artery to the graft (caliber 6–8 mm, depending on the distal anastomosis that is planned) a tunnel is created in the usual manner, either from the suprainguinal operative field or from the incision at the thigh.

Coming from the cranial incision, one can use the superior pubic ramus, which crosses obliquely, for orientation. On its caudal rim, the obturator membrane and the muscles lying on top of it can be palpated. The palpable obturator artery branching off from the iliac artery can serve as a guideline. The point of passage of the bypass should be medial to the obturator vessels so as not to cause lesions which might result in bleeding that is difficult to control.

When the index finger of the surgeon reaches the membrane at the location selected for perforat-

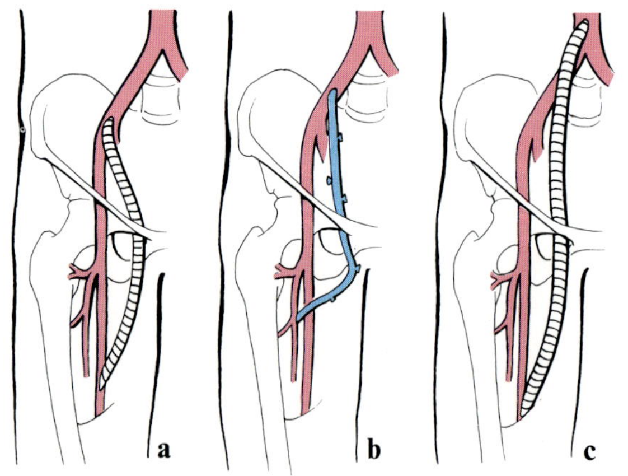

Fig. 20.11. a Completion of the extra-anatomic bypass through the obturator foramen, bypassing the femoral bifurcation in the groin. **b** Obturator bypass to the profunda femoris artery, bypassing the inguinal region. **c** For central anastomosis of the obturator bypass, the common iliac artery or the abdominal aorta may also be considered

ing the foramen, a slightly curved forceps is inserted through the medial incision in the thigh and passed toward the finger so as to create a tunnel by blunt dissection. Slight flexion and external rotation of the leg at the hip joint facilitate this procedure.

The tunneler is passed upward between the adductor longus and magnus muscles if the graft is to be anastomosed to the distal superficial femoral artery. If there is more extensive infection or if the superficial femoral artery is not suitable for distal anastomosis, it is advisable to pass the tunneler dorsal to the adductor magnus muscle so that the prosthesis passes directly down to the initial segment of the popliteal artery, bypassing the subsartorial canal. Care should always be taken not to let the tip of the tunneler deviate too much ventrally as this might result in the accidental opening of the infected inguinal area.

When the tip of the tunneler reaches the obturator membrane, the membrane is perforated bluntly from the pelvic side with the help of the finger. It is seldom necessary to use scissors.

The distal end of the prosthesis is grasped by the forceps and pulled through the hole in the membrane, avoiding twisting and tension. The graft is passed through the soft tissue of the thigh down to the distal wound. There, an end-to-side anastomosis to the superficial femoral artery is performed in the standard fashion.

However, if the distal anastomosis is to be made to the profunda femoris artery, the middle segment of the artery is exposed through an incision on the anterolateral aspect of the thigh (see p. 449). The graft is passed subcutaneously on a curvilinear course across the anterior side of the thigh, using the prepared anastomotic site on the ventromedial side. The best graft material in such a situation is autogenous greater saphenous vein. Alternatively, a ring-reinforced PTFE prosthesis (e.g., Gore-Tex) may be used.

As regards the proximal anastomosis of the bypass, variations are possible in individual cases. For instance, if the iliac artery is not suitable, the prosthesis may be sutured to the distal aorta, exposed by a transperitoneal or retroperitoneal approach (Fig. 20.11).

When an infection of an aortobifemoral graft is definitely limited to the inguinal anastomotic region, the graft segment close to the bifurcation may be exposed transperitoneally, divided, and anastomosed end-to-end to the new extra-anatomic graft through the obturator foramen (Fig. 20.12).

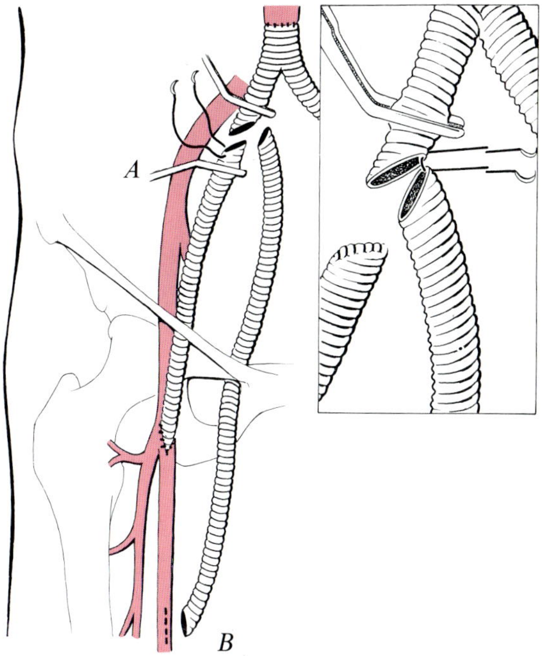

Fig. 20.12. Extra-anatomic bypass through the obturator foramen when infection of an aortobifemoral graft is limited to the groin. The old prosthesis is divided obliquely, close to the bifurcation (*A*). The distal anastomosis of the obturator bypass is marked *B*

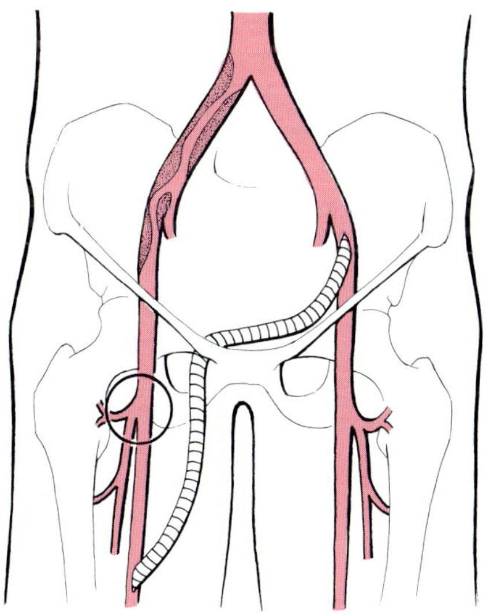

Fig. 20.13. Obturator bypass from the contralateral iliac artery in the case of severe stenosis of the ipsilateral iliac vessels

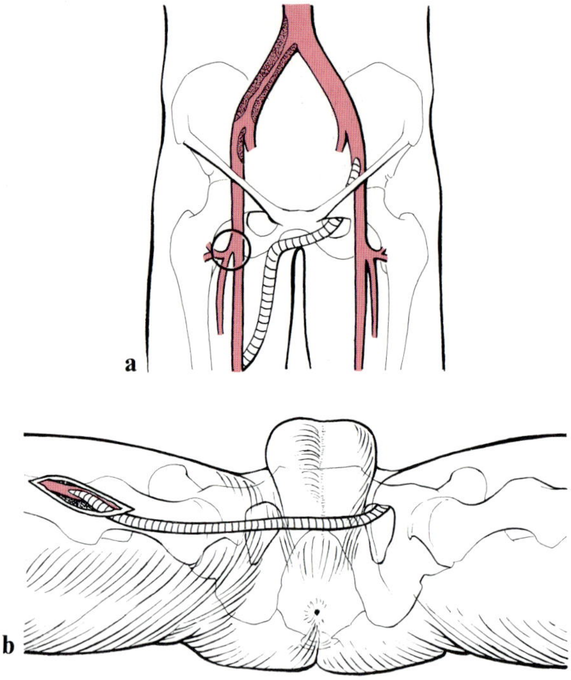

Fig. 20.14. **a** If a crossover obturator bypass cannot be passed through the ipsilateral obturator foramen, it can be passed through the foramen of the donor side. **b** The graft passes perineally and subscrotally to the contralateral femoral artery

Also, it may occasionally be necessary to perform the central anastomosis of an obturator bypass on the contralateral side, e.g., to the external iliac artery. This procedure initially corresponds to that of the iliofemoral crossover bypass (see p. 544; Fig. 20.13).

Finally, there is a variation of the crossover bypass in which the graft is passed through the obturator foramen on the side of the proximal anastomosis. The graft then leaves the pelvis and passes through the perineum to the anteromedial side of the thigh being revascularized. The anastomosis is then made to the superficial femoral artery (Fig. 20.14).

G. Lateral Aortofemoral or Iliofemoral Bypass

If extra-anatomic bypasses through the obturator foramen, including their various anastomotic sites and courses, are not suitable and if there is no possibility of an axillofemoral bypass, a graft from the terminal aorta or the common iliac artery to the vessels of the thigh may be used (Fig. 20.15).

Following retro- or transperitoneal exposure of the proximal anastomotic site on the abdominal aorta or iliac artery, an end-to-side anastomosis of the graft is performed in the usual fashion. This anastomosis is best located on the anterolateral aspect of the artery.

Following curvilinear placement through the retroperitoneum and through a tunnel created by blunt dissection through the muscle layers of the lateral abdominal wall, the bypass enters the subcutaneous tissue of a counterincision at the level of the iliac crest, somewhere in the region of the midaxillary line.

Through this incision the iliac crest is incised as already described for the extended axillofemoral bypass. The further course of the bypass to the profunda femoris or the superficial femoral artery is subcutaneous, from the iliac crest downward (see p. 542).

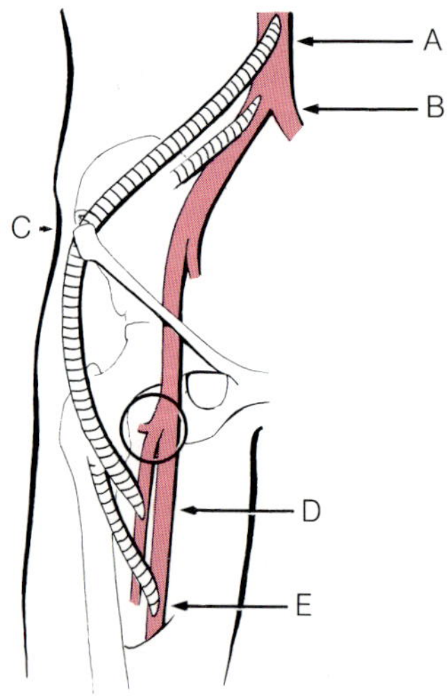

Fig. 20.15. Lateral aortofemoral bypass. *A* and *B* represent the possible sites for proximal anastomosis to the abdominal aorta or the iliac vessels. For the lateral course, an incision of the iliac crest is recommended (*C*). The distal anastomosis of the bypass may be with either the middle profunda femoris artery (*D*) or the middle superficial femoral artery (*E*)

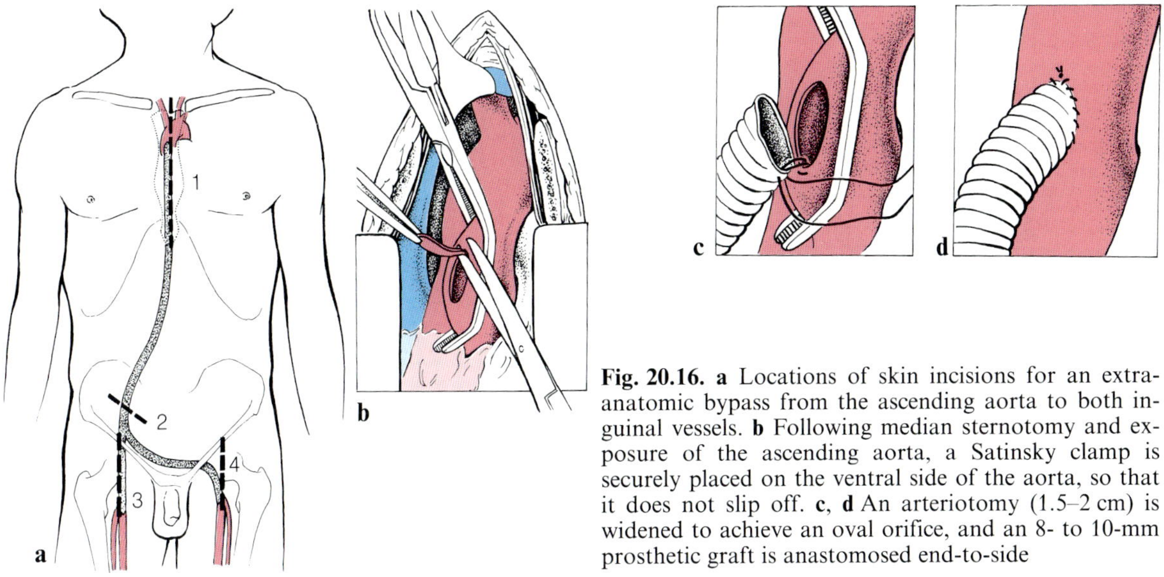

Fig. 20.16. **a** Locations of skin incisions for an extra-anatomic bypass from the ascending aorta to both inguinal vessels. **b** Following median sternotomy and exposure of the ascending aorta, a Satinsky clamp is securely placed on the ventral side of the aorta, so that it does not slip off. **c**, **d** An arteriotomy (1.5–2 cm) is widened to achieve an oval orifice, and an 8- to 10-mm prosthetic graft is anastomosed end-to-side

H. Aortoascendobifemoral Bypass

When there is no possibility of an axillobifemoral bypass because it is necessary to bypass the abdomen extra-anatomically and because of simultaneous supra-aortic lesions, a bypass originating directly on the ascending aorta may be considered as an alternative.

A median sternotomy is performed over the entire length. Following hemostasis and insertion of a thoracic retractor, the ascending aorta in the upper mediastinum is dissected so that a Satinsky clamp can be placed securely on the ventral side. The arteriotomy (1.5–2 cm) is widened by an oval excision of aortic wall. Then, the end-to-side anastomosis with the 8-mm (up to 10-mm) graft is performed using a continuous suture technique (suture size: 3–0; Fig. 20.16). This part of the procedure is the most critical. One must take the greatest care that the Satinsky clamp does not slip off while anastomosing and that the edges of the arteriotomy do not slip back under the clamp. In order to reduce unwelcome leverage effects resulting from transmission of heart movements to the clamp, it is advisable to have the handle of the clamp gently held by an assistant. If the clamp should slip off or the wall of the aorta tear, one should first control the massive bleeding by digital pressure and then try to place a larger clamp with bigger jaws. In such a situation one should also consider inserting and inflating a Fogarty catheter to close the aortic opening (Fig. 20.17).

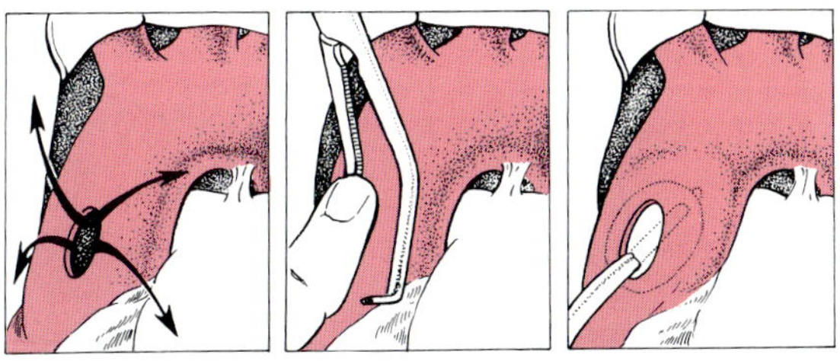

Fig. 20.17. Procedure in case of bleeding while anastomosing the ascending aorta. Control of bleeding by compression with the finger, by placing another, larger Satinsky clamp or by provisional transluminal occlusion using an inflatable balloon catheter

I. Subhepatic Aortofemoral Bypass

Extensive abdominal adhesions and a central anastomotic infection following a classical aortobifemoral bypass are two indications for this type of extra-anatomic bypass.

Through a median or dorsal curvilinear laparotomy, the subphrenic aorta, which is the proximal site of anastomosis, is exposed, and the lesser sac of the omentum is opened over a sufficient length. The esophagus can be retracted somewhat laterally, and the aorta can then be isolated sufficiently to allow a tape to be passed around it and a Satinsky clamp to be placed tangentially on it in a caudocranial direction. A sufficiently long trunk of the bifurcation graft is then anastomosed

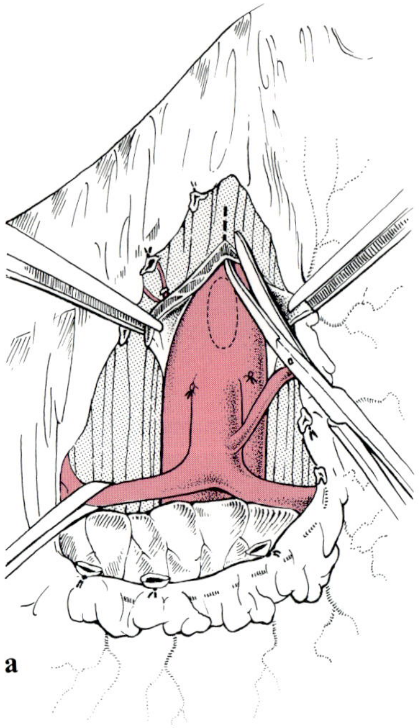

a

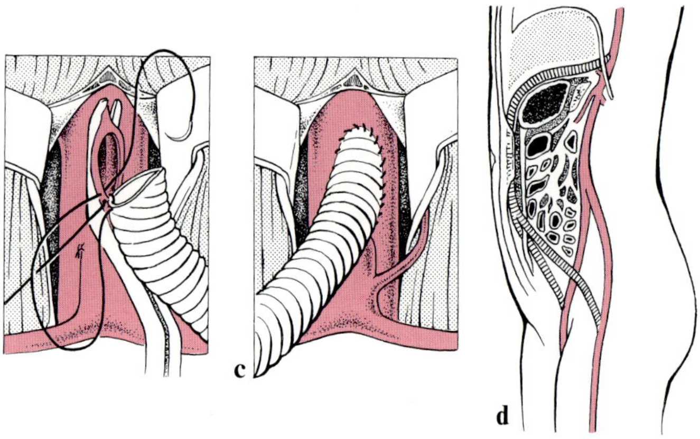

b c d

Fig. 20.18. a Exposure of the subphrenic aorta for a subhepatic bypass. After opening the lesser sac of the omentum, the celiac trunk is exposed and both crura of the diaphragm are divided. Marking the arteriotomy, which is to be widened to form an oval orifice. **b, c** End-to-side anastomosis of an 8-mm prosthetic graft to the supraceliac aorta. **d** Bifurcation graft with distal anastomosis in both groins

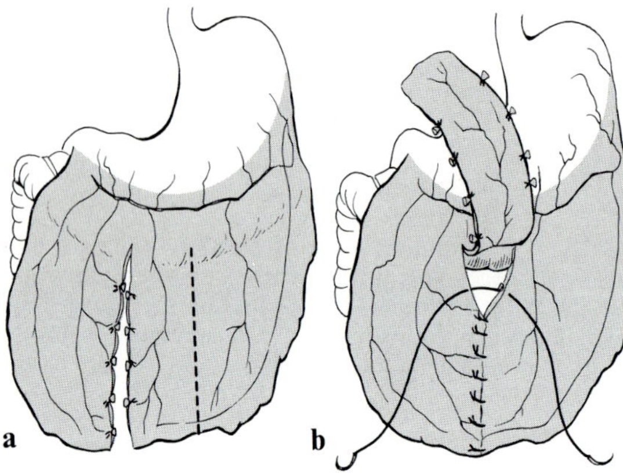

a b

Fig. 20.19 a, b. Creating an omental graft to cover the subhepatic bypass segment. **a** The division lines of the greater omentum are marked. Stepwise division of the omentum between appropriate ligatures. **b** A sufficiently broad patch of the greater omentum is isolated and drawn up. The edges of the omentum are approximated again. The omental patch serves to cover the graft and to separate it biologically from the abdominal viscera

end-to-side in typical fashion to the oval orifice on the anterior aspect of the aorta (Fig. 20.18).

If necessary, the graft may be extended by an additional segment of the same diameter.

The graft is then passed subhepatically through the free abdominal cavity to the anterior abdominal wall. There, a sufficiently large incision of the peritoneum is made on the abdominal side and on the dorsal sheet of the rectus sheath. The graft is located in this sheath. For tunneling, the anterior part of the rectal sheath is opened by a skin incision about where it crosses the right mamillary line and the interspinal line. The muscle is perforated bluntly with a curved forceps. The end of the forceps is passed to the cranial opening from the abdominal side.

Now both limbs of the graft are grasped by the forceps and pulled through the incision in the lower abdomen and passed down to both groins. This procedure is equivalent to that described for an axillobifemoral bypass.

The subhepatic segment of the graft, which is free within the abdominal cavity, is finally covered with a patch of greater omentum and is thus separated from the viscera by vital tissue (Fig. 20.19).

K. Lateral Femorocrural Anterior Bypass

Sometimes, an orthotopic bypass through the popliteal fossa to the terminal segment of the popliteal artery or to one of the crural arteries has to be abandoned as a way of revascularizing the lower leg. In such cases, a bypass to the anterior tibial artery is possible. The prosthesis or the autogenous vein should be passed subcutaneously on the lateral side of the knee joint between the edge of the patella and the outer femoral condyle (Fig. 20.20).

After the distal anastomosis to the anterior tibial artery on the lateral side of the lower leg has been performed, a curved forceps is used for blunt dissection of a subcutaneous tunnel through a counterincision on the anterolateral side of the distal thigh, about one handbreath above the patella. The graft is passed through the tunnel upward without kinking and twisting.

The graft passes on subcutaneously to the groin. The tunnel has been made previously by a forceps or a tunneling instrument. The inguinal anastomosis between the graft and the femoral bifurcation is done in the standard fashion (see p. 398).

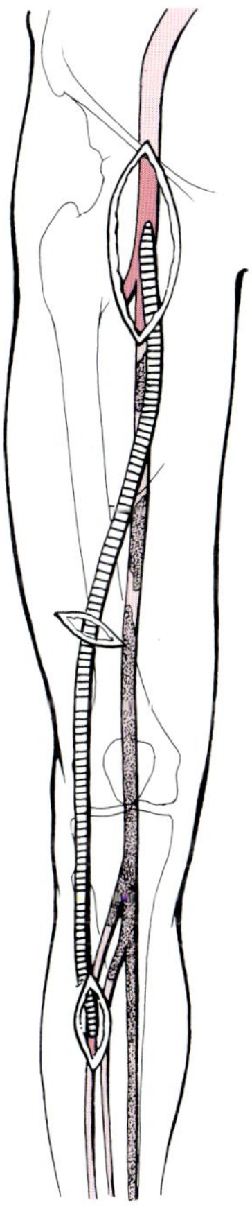

Fig. 20.20. Course of the lateral anterior bypass for femorocrural reconstruction. Following completion of the distal anastomosis, the graft is passed through a subcutaneous tunnel between the lateral femoral condyle and the outer edge of the patella to a counterincision one handbreadth above the knee joint on the anterolateral side of the thigh. The graft is then passed subcutaneously to the femoral bifurcation

REFERENCES

1. Bergan JJ, Conn J (1971) Alternative methods in arterial reconstruction. Surg Clin N Amer 51:85
2. Bergan JJ, Yao JST (eds) (1980) Operative techniques in vascular surgery. Grune & Stratton, New York
3. Blaisdell FW, Hall AD, Lim RC, Moore WC (1970) Aortoiliac arterial substitution utilizing subcutaneous grafts. Ann Surg 172:775
4. Haimovici H (ed) (1976) Vascular surgery – principles and techniques. McGraw-Hill, New York
5. Hershey FB, Calman CH (1973) Atlas of vascular surgery. Mosby, St Louis
6. Linton RR (1973) Atlas of vascular surgery. Saunders, Philadelphia
7. LoGerfo FW, Johnson WC, Corson JD (1977) A comparison of the late patency rates of axillobilateral femoral and axillo unilateral femoral grafts. Surgery 81:33
8. Müller-Wiefel (1974) Iliaco-femoroprofundaler Obturator-Bypass mittels Vena saphena magna. Acta Chir 9:15
9. Müller-Wiefel H (1978) Eingriffe an den Arterien. In: Gschnitzer F, Breitner B, Kern E, Schweiberer L (eds) Chirurgische Operationslehre, vol IV/1. Urban & Schwarzenberg, München
10. Rutherford RB (ed) Vascular surgery. Saunders, Philadelphia
11. Vollmar JF (1982) Rekonstruktive Chirurgie der Arterien, 3rd edn. Thieme, Stuttgart New York
12. Wylie EJ, Stoney RJ, Ehrenfeld WK (1980) Manual of vascular surgery, vol I. Springer, New York Heidelberg Berlin

21 Compression Syndromes

21.1 Neurovascular Compression Syndromes of the Upper Thoracic Outlet and Their Vascular Complications

M.G.M.H. Barwegen and R.J.A.M. van Dongen

CONTENTS

A. Anatomic and Functional Conditions

The neurovascular compression syndrome of the upper thoracic outlet includes all syndromes caused by neurogenic, arterial, or venous compression in the costoclavicular region. The anatomic and functional conditions in this region may be the cause of neurovascular compression at several sites [1]. Depending on the level of the cause and the compression mechanism, the following syndromes are usually distinguished:

1. Cervical rib syndrome
2. Anterior scalene syndrome
3. Scalenus minimus syndrome
4. Costoclavicular compression syndrome
5. Pectoralis minor syndrome or hyperabduction syndrome

I. Cervical Rib Syndrome

In the case of a cervical rib syndrome the subclavian artery and the brachial plexus, but not the subclavian vein, may be compressed (Fig. 21.1.1.). There are several types of cervical ribs:

a) A long C7 process (probably not of significance for the pathogenesis of this syndrome)
b) A rudimentary cervical rib, but with the lateral end not extending beyond the dorsal tubercle

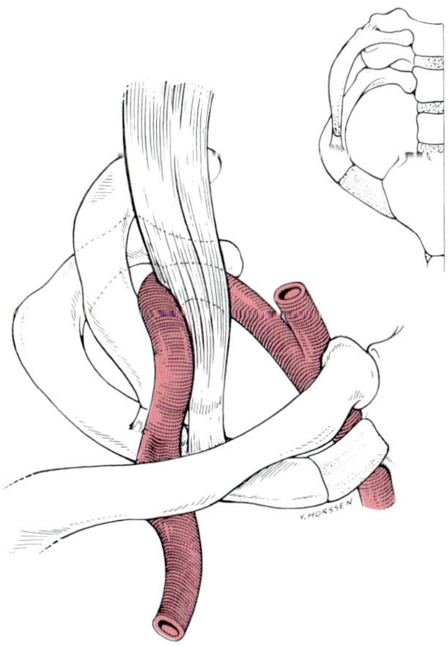

Fig. 21.1.1. The most important variation of a cervical rib. Compression of the cervical artery is possible at the site where the artery crosses over the cervical rib or is compressed against the rib by the anterior scalene muscle

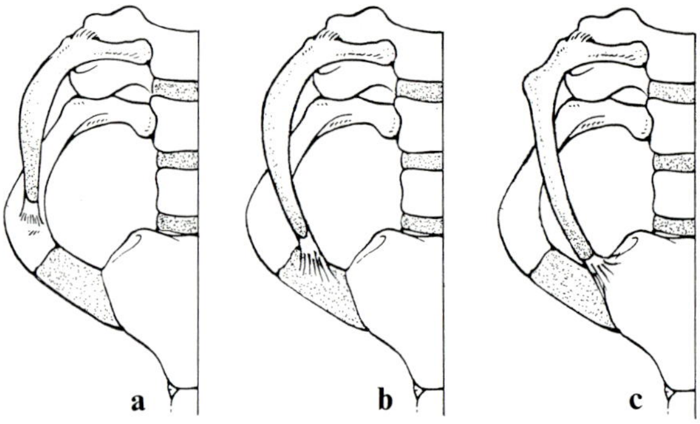

Fig. 21.1.2a–c. The three most common types of cervical rib. **a** A cervical rib attached to the osseous segment of the first rib by a fibrous band. **b** An incomplete cervical rib attached to the first rib by cartilage. **c** The complete cervical rib extending to the manubrium sterni

c) A cervical rib ending free, or attached to the osseous segment of the first rib by a fibrous band (Fig. 21.1.2a)
d) An incomplete cervical rib, attached to the first rib by cartilage (Fig. 21.1.2b)
e) A complete cervical rib, extending to the manubrium sterni (Fig. 21.1.2c)

In most complete cervical ribs, the anterior scalene tubercle is severely protruded. The artery rides just behind this tubercle on the cervical rib, causing kinking and compression. Furthermore, the cervical rib draws the artery through the scalene space upward and anteriorly, compressing the artery against the tendon of the anterior scalene muscle. The brachial plexus is also pushed upward and anteriorly, causing kinking and compression.

II. Anterior Scalene Syndrome

The anterior scalene syndrome is thought to be caused by compression of the artery and the plexus between the anterior and the medial scalene muscles. The scalene triangle is too narrow and becomes even narrower by contraction of the scalene muscles. However, the question remains whether contraction of these muscles alone can cause compression of the artery. It has been suggested that the first rib is drawn upward by the contraction of the scalene muscles, thus narrowing the costoclavicular space and consequently causing costoclavicular compression (Fig. 21.1.3).

III. Scalenus Minimus Syndrome

The scalenus minimus syndrome (Fig. 21.1.4) is caused by the scalenus minimus muscle passing from the transverse process of the sixth and seventh cervical vertebrae to the first rib, where its insertion is located between the anterior and medial scalene muscle. This muscle is very variable. Sometimes, there is only a fibrous band, the cos-

Fig. 21.1.3. Anatomy of the upper thoracic outlet showing the neurovascular bundle leaving the outlet through the scalene triangle

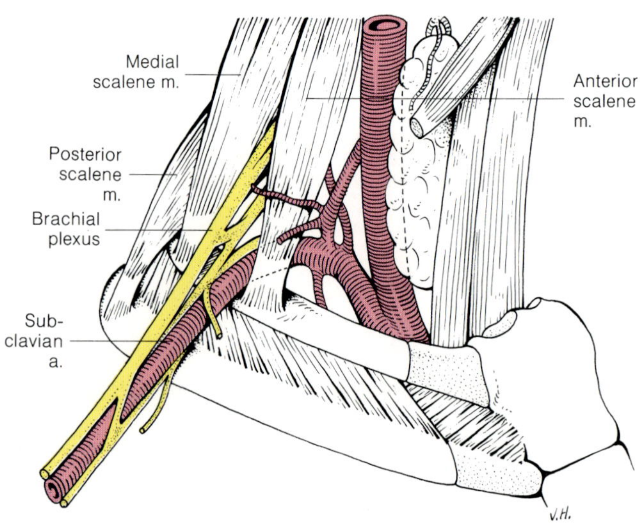

Fig. 21.1.4. Compression of the subclavian artery crossing transversely through the scalenus minimus muscle

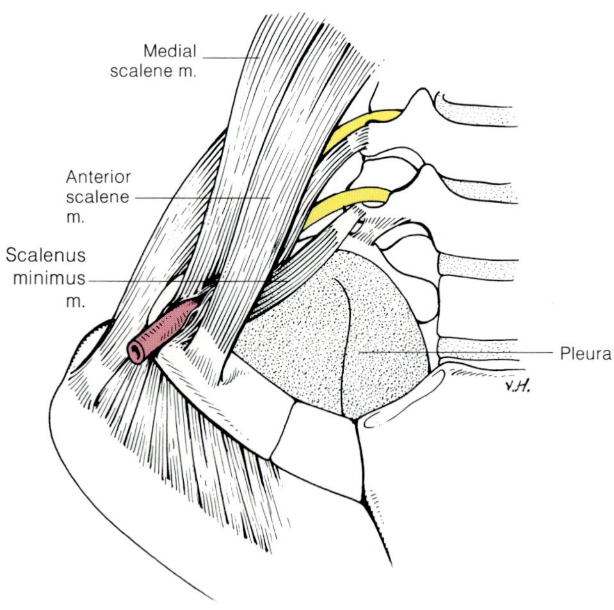

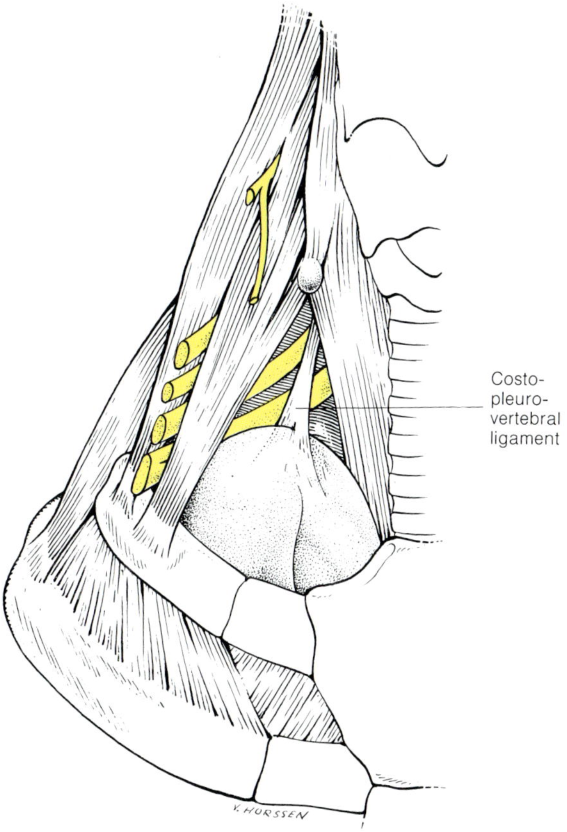

Fig. 21.1.5. The costopleurovertebral ligament, which fixes the apex of the lung, can vary considerably and may cause compression of the neurovascular structures

topleurovertebral ligament (Fig. 21.1.5). The scalene space, which is already small, is narrowed even further because the scalenus minimus muscle passes between the artery and the plexus within the scalene triangle. Sometimes the artery crosses transversely through the muscle, compressing the artery during contraction.

IV. Costoclavicular Compression Syndrome

The costoclavicular syndrome is characterized by compression of the neurovascular bundle between the first rib and the clavicle (Fig. 21.1.6). The clavicle and the first rib, including its fixation to the manubrium sterni create a scissorlike configuration. When the arm is abducted, the clavicle rotates a distance of 2.5 cm dorsally over the first rib, thereby narrowing even further the already narrow costoclavicular space. Usually, the tonus of the shoulder muscles will lift the clavicle from the neurovascular structures. Symptoms result only when this is no longer the case, for instance when the muscles are hypotonic, or as a result of an increase in the weight of the arm. The etiology is very complex and usually not based on a single cause.

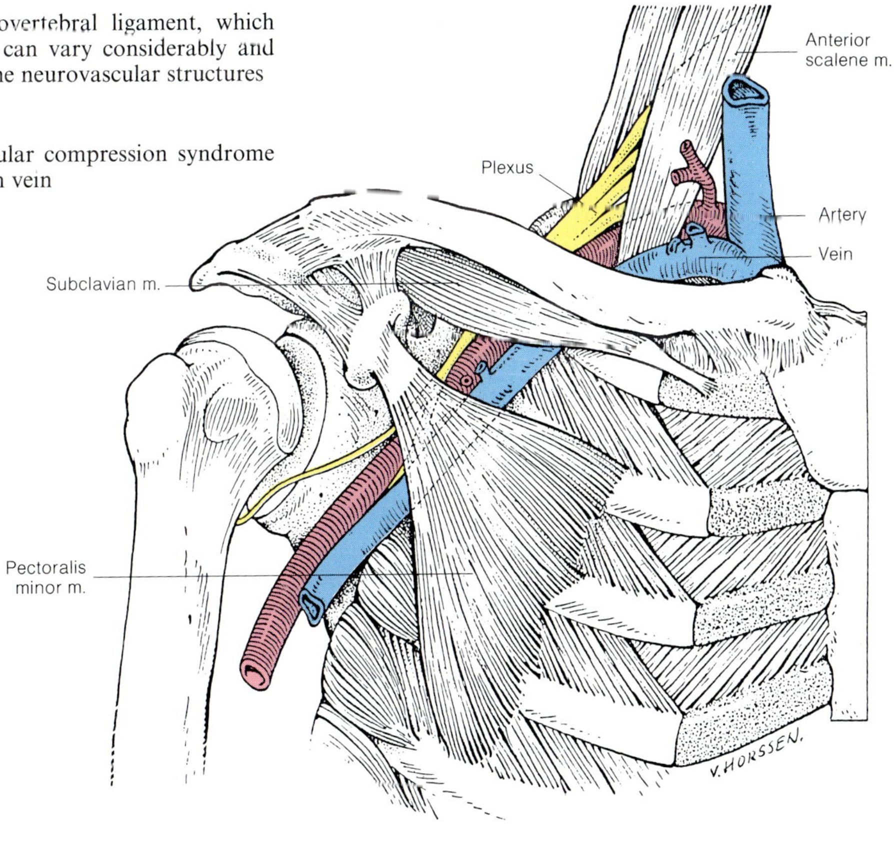

Fig. 21.1.6. The costoclavicular compression syndrome involving also the subclavian vein

V. Pectoralis Minor Syndrome or Hyperabduction Syndrome

On elevation of the arm the neurovascular bundle is forced by the tendon of the pectoralis muscle and its insertion on the coracoid process to assume an angle of nearly 90°. The result may be compression of the subclavian artery (Fig. 21.1.7). As already mentioned, abduction of the arm causes simultaneous narrowing of the costoclavicular space. Consequently costoclavicular compression may be a contributing factor.

Finally, compression of the neurovascular structures in the region of the shoulder may also be caused by a poorly healed fracture of the first rib or of the clavicle, by an exostosis of the first rib, by fusion of the first with the second rib, or by other congenital or aquired anomalies (Fig. 21.1.8).

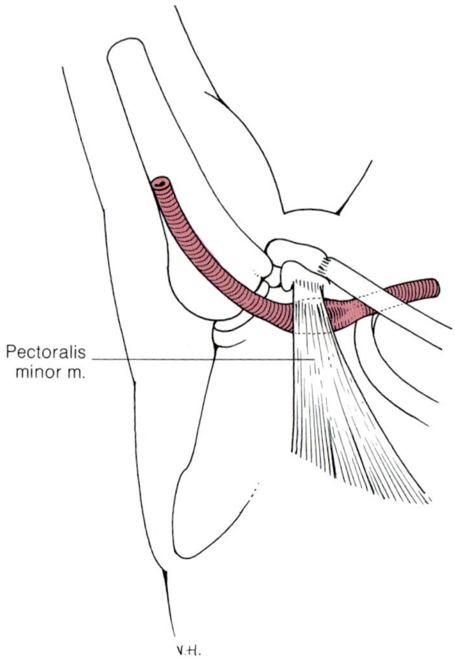

B. Vascular Complications in Neurovascular Compression Syndromes

The three most important *arterial complications* are [2, 3]:

1. Formation of mural thrombi due to local vascular lesions
2. Development of poststenotic aneurysms
3. Thrombotic occlusion of the diseased or aneurysmatic vessel

I. Formation of Mural Thrombi Due to Local Vascular Lesions

Repeated compression of an artery can lead to ulcerative lesions of the intima and the related formation of thrombi which may dislodge and cause peripheral embolic occlusions. An arterial lesion resulting from compression within the costoclavicular space is usually first recognized by the occurrence of peripheral embolisms in the finger arteries and is often misdiagnosed as Raynaud's disease.

II. Development of Poststenotic Aneurysms

Poststenotic aneurysm of the subclavian artery is the result of turbulence in the blood flow following narrowing or kinking of the vessel in the region of a cervical rib or in the costoclavicular space (Fig. 21.1.8). Within these aneurysms, usually

◁ **Fig. 21.1.7.** Distal compression of the subclavian artery by the tendon of the pectoralis minor muscle

Fig. 21.1.8. Compression of the artery between the clavicle and an exostosis of the first rib with development of poststenotic aneurysm

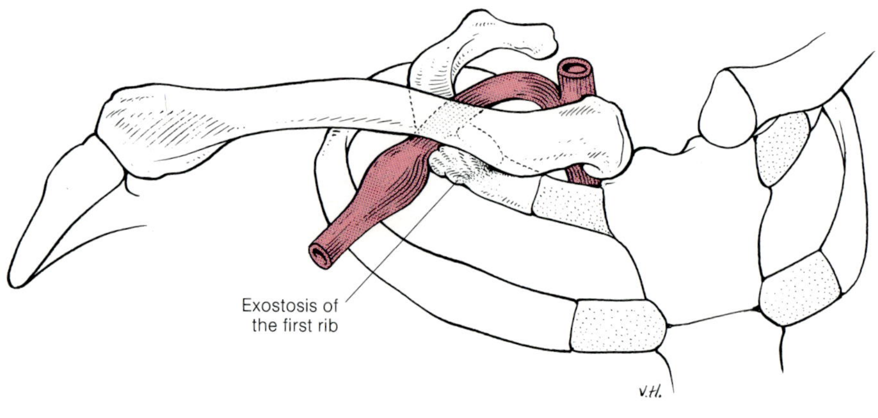

larger thrombi form, which may become detached, causing embolic occlusions of upper- and forearm arteries. The subclavian aneurysm itself usually remains asymptomatic. In the majority of cases, the first symptom is an acute occlusion of an upper extremity artery.

III. Thrombotic Occlusions of the Diseased or Aneurysmatic Subclavian Artery

The third severe complication is acute subclavian artery occlusion, which is caused by mural lesions and the related formation of thrombi or by thrombosis of the poststenotic aneurysm. In such cases, there is the risk of extension of the localized occlusion by additional thrombosis distally or proximally, or even in both directions (see p. 527 ff.).

Distal progression may cause ischemia of the fingers or the hand. Extension in a proximal direction endangers the vertebral artery and, in the case of an occlusion of the right subclavian artery, even the carotid artery.

Venous Complications. Repeated compression of the neurovascular structures may also injure the subclavian vein, resulting in an acute axillary vein thrombosis, i.e., the Paget-von-Schrötter or thoracic inlet syndrome; Fig. 21.1.9). This thrombosis may also extend proximally and distally. Pulmonary embolism is relatively rare. Phlegmasia coerulea dolens with gangrene of the upper extremity is extremely rare.

Fig. 21.1.9. In the case of a costoclavicular compression syndrome not only the artery and the plexus, but also the subclavian vein are compressed

C. Indications for Operative Treatment

The treatment of neurovascular compression syndromes may be conservative or operative [1, 4, 6]. Conservative treatment may be tried in cases with mild or moderately severe symptoms. The patient is advised to avoid certain movements and positions and is put on an exercise program to strengthen cervical and shoulder muscles and to improve posture. However, this conservative therapy does not prevent the development of arterial or venous complications. In patients without symptoms or signs of such complications, surgery is usually not indicated.

Operative correction of compression is indicated when severe symptoms are not improved by conservative therapy. When there are signs of vascular complications, operative treatment is always indicated. Cervical ribs and osseous anomalies of the upper thoracic outlet, e.g., an abnormal first rib and exostosis of the first rib, fusion of the first with the second rib, or exaggerated callus formation following fracture of the clavicle, represent a significantly greater risk of vascular complications. In such cases operative intervention is urgently indicated, even if there has been no evidence of vascular complications.

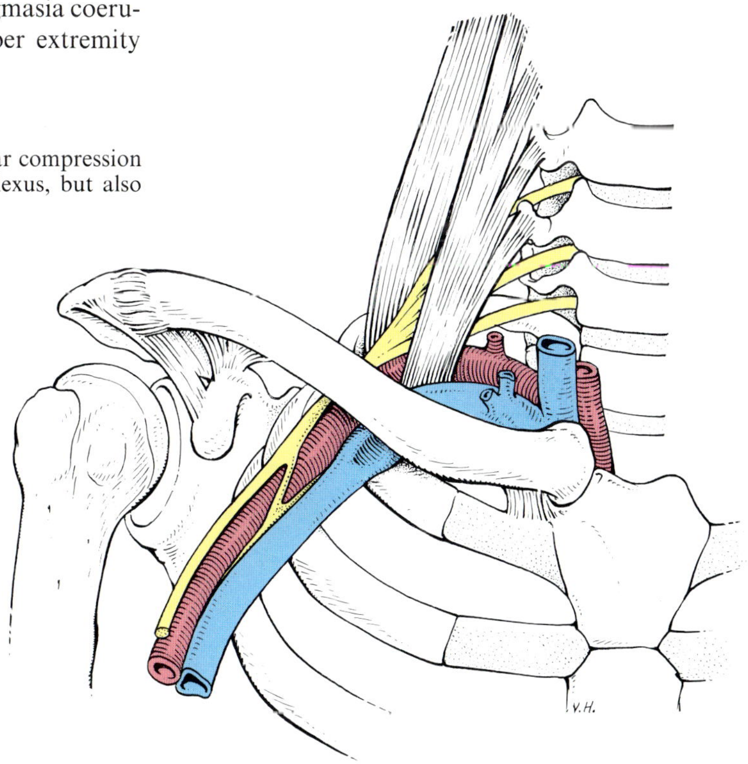

Compression of the subclavian vein in the upper thoracic outlet is an indication for surgery if symptoms are severe and phlebographic findings are significant. Thrombotic occlusion of the subclavian vein may be treated operatively or conservatively. There are several possibilities for treatment of axillary vein thrombosis. Besides conservative or thrombolytic therapy, venous thrombectomy is possible in some cases. It is our opinion that, following successful venous thrombectomy, the first rib must be resected to eliminate the cause of the thrombosis and to prevent early recurrent thrombosis. For the same reason, the first rib should also be resected following successful lysis. Opinions are divided as to whether the rib should be resected following conservative treatment of an axillary vein thrombosis. However, we think that in this case resection is necessary to increase the possibility for undisturbed recanalization of the subclavian vein and for the undisturbed development of sufficient collateral circulation in the costoclavicular space.

D. Operative Approach

There are several possible approaches to the upper thoracic outlet. Using the supraclavicular approach, access can be gained only to the anterior segment of the first rib. The rib cannot be resected far enough dorsally. The infraclavicular approach has the same disadvantage. A combination of supra- and infraclavicular incisions provides good access to the subclavian artery and the anterior segment of the first rib if the clavicle is divided or partially resected. Access to the posterior segment of the first rib, however, is impossible except at great risk to the brachial plexus. In cases of compression syndrome of the upper thoracic outlet, where it is essential that the brachial plexus be decompressed, the posterior segment of the first rib must be resected. Under these circumstances the only possibility of gaining adequate access to the dorsal portion of the rib is the transaxillary approach [1, 4, 6]. This approach has several advantages. First, it is relatively simple. No muscles,

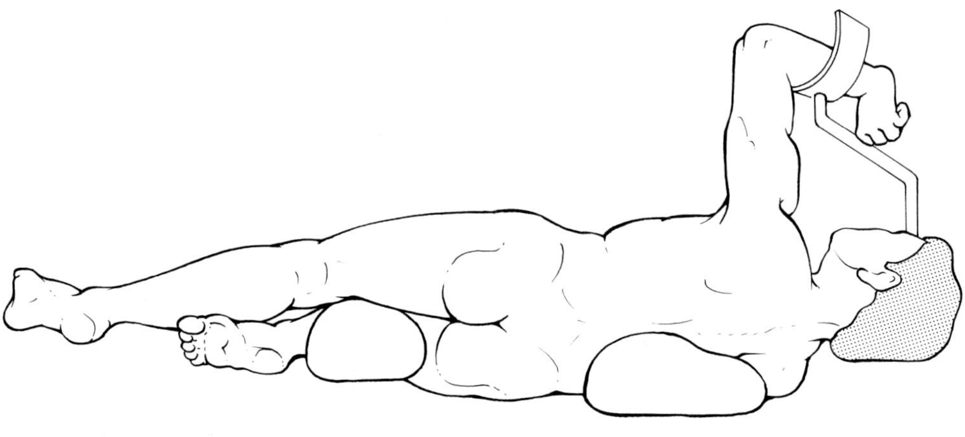

Fig. 21.1.10. Positioning and location of the arm for left side transaxillary rib resection. The arm should not be drawn up nor abducted more than 90°

Fig. 21.1.11. The arm is padded with cotton, suspended ▷ without traction, and abducted 90°

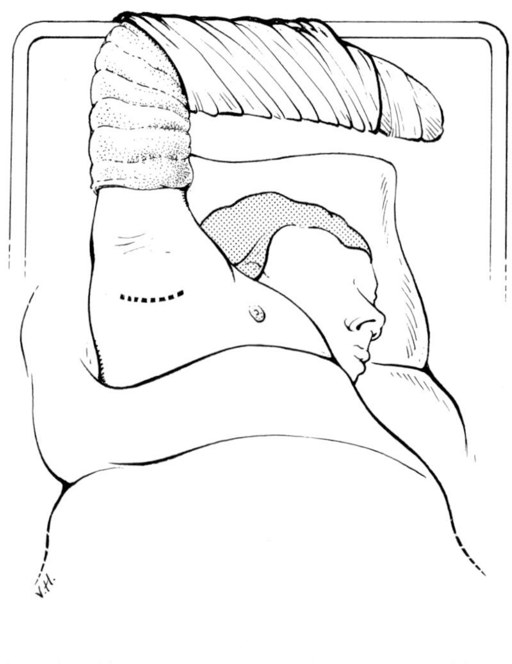

osseous or other vital structures have to be divided, only the skin and subcutaneous tissue. The neurovascular structures are easily exposed and identified. Moreover, wound healing is good and the cosmetic result is excellent. The most important advantage, however, is that the entire neurovascular structure is exposed by a transaxillary incision following resection of the first rib or the cervical and the first rib. Also, if arterial reconstruction is necessary, it presents no problem. An additional thoracic sympathectomy may also be performed without difficulty.

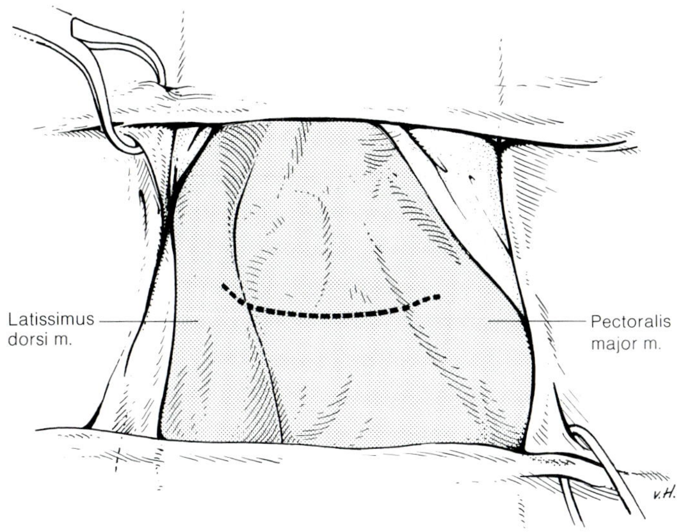

Fig. 21.1.12. The skin incision is made at the level of the third rib

E. Positioning

For transaxillary resection of the first rib and the cervical rib, the patient is placed in a lateral position, with the contralateral lower limb flexed (Fig. 21.1.10). A cushion is placed between the knees. The pelvis and the back are supported. The lower arm is somewhat anteverted and externally rotated and may be used for measurement of blood pressure and for infusion. The arm on the diseased side is abducted and fixed on a holder (Fig. 21.1.11). Care should be taken not to hyperabduct the arm (not more than 90°–100°) and not to elevate it too much; otherwise, the plexus may become overstretched. It is not necessary to have the arm wrapped in sterile drapes and held by an assistant. When the arm is drawn up, the wound becomes deeper and less clearly visible. And, as mentioned above, drawing the arm up too far may cause overstretching of the plexus.

F. Transaxillary Resection of a Rib

The curvilinear incision is located in the region of the axillary hair border at the level of the third rib (Fig. 21.1.12). If the incision is too high, lymph vessels and lymph nodes in the axilla may be injured, resulting in disturbances of wound healing. The lateral thoracic artery and the thoracoepigastric vein pass within subcutaneous tissue in the midaxillary line. They must be sacrificed. The sub-

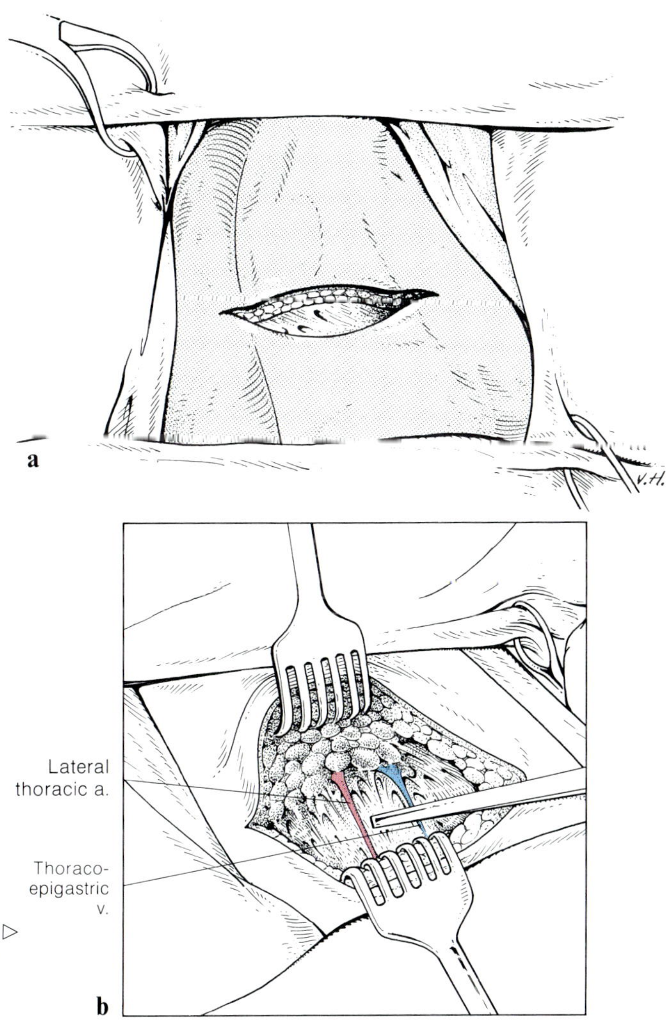

Fig. 21.1.13. a The thoracic wall is reached by division ▷ of the skin and subcutaneous fatty tissue. **b** The lateral thoracic artery and the thoracoepigastric vein are sacrificed

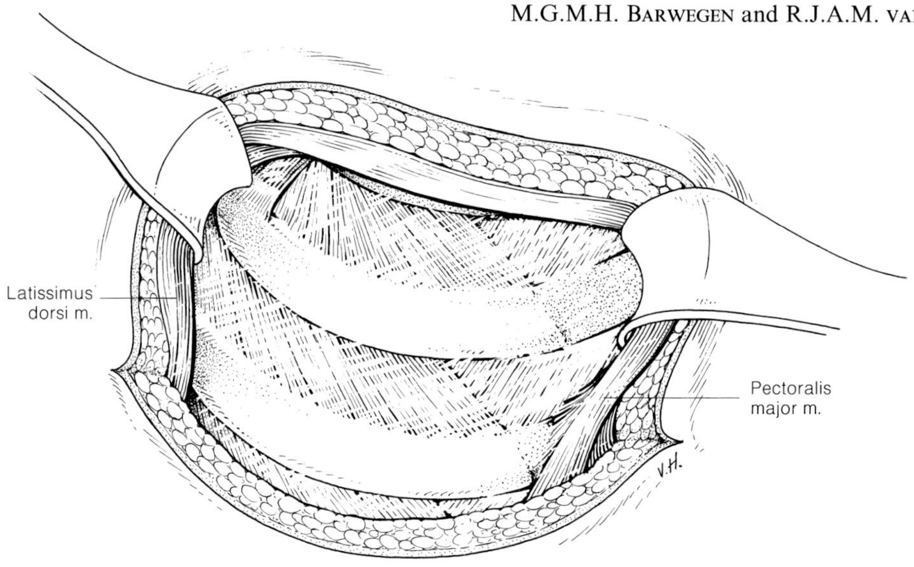

Fig. 21.1.14. On reaching the thoracic wall, the dissection continues cranially through the soft fatty tissue of the axilla, which is liftet off the thoracic wall, together with the lymph nodes

cutaneous fatty tissue is divided in a direct approach to the thoracic wall (Fig. 21.1.13a, b). The anterior border of the latissimus dorsi muscle and the posterior border of the pectoralis major muscle are dissected (Fig. 21.1.14). Exposing the border of the latissimus dorsi muscle, one must be careful not to injure the long thoracic nerve and the thoracodorsal nerve, which pass under the margin of the muscle. Once the thoracic wall has been reached, the soft fatty tissue of the axilla, together with the lymph nodes, are retracted proximally and dissected from the thoracic wall. Dissection is continued cranially over the thoracic wall, in the direction of the first rib. The intercostobrachial nerve, passing from the second interspace to the axilla, is preserved whenever possible (Fig. 21.1.15). Division of this nerve results in anesthesia of the axilla and the dorsal side of the upper arm. The superior intercostal vessels perforating the intercostal muscle of the first interspace are ligated and divided. The axilla and the first rib are now clearly exposed. The subclavian vein is identified ventrally as well as the subclavian artery and the plexus in the middle. As soon as the plexus is identified, it is important to check the tension. If the tension is too great, then the arm has been lifted too high and must be loosened somewhat. Now, in anteroposterior order, the following structures are visible (Fig. 21.1.16):

- The costoclavicular ligament.
- The tendon of the subclavian muscle.
- The subclavian vein.
- The anterior scalene muscle.
- The subclavian artery.
- The brachial plexus.
- The medial scalene muscle attached to the inner wall of the first rib dorsal to the scalene tubercle. The posterior scalene muscle passes dorsal to the second rib. In these circumstances one can determine whether a scalenus minimus muscle exists.

All these muscle insertions are much better visualized and better exposed when the surgeon's left hand presses the second rib firmly inward.

First, the posterior scalene muscle is dissected off the second rib and the medial scalene muscle off the first rib, providing better exposure of the posterior segment of the first rib and of the plexus. Anteriorly, the tendon of the subclavian muscle is divided very ventrally down to the manubrium sterni; for this purpose, the subclavian vein is separated from the tendon of the subclavian muscle by means of a small cotton applicator and retracted (Fig. 21.1.17). Division of the anterior scalene muscle is the next step. The subclavian vein is located on its ventral side, the subclavian artery and the brachial plexus on its dorsal border. If these two structures are carefully retracted using a cotton applicator, a right-angled clamp may be passed underneath the head of the anterior scalene muscle. Only when one is absolutely sure that the artery and the vein will not be injured is the muscle divided 1 cm above the scalene tubercle (Fig. 21.1.18). All the remaining muscle fibers and

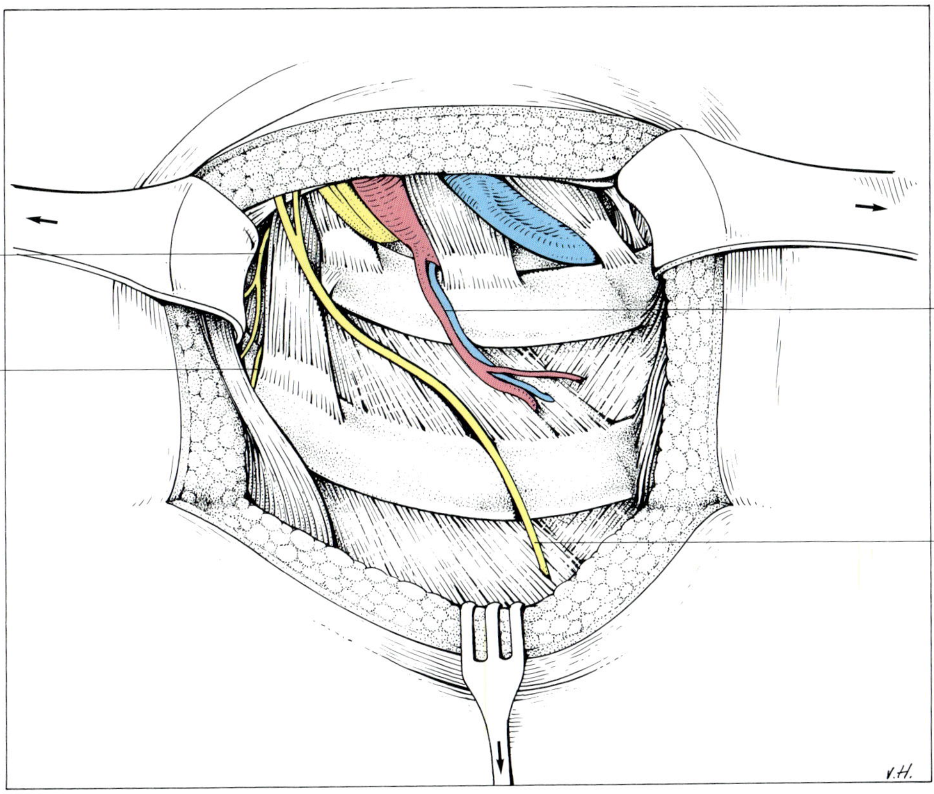

Fig. 21.1.15. The superior intercostal vessels are ligated and divided. The intercostobrachial nerve is preserved whenever possible

Fig. 21.1.16. In anteroposterior order, the following structures are visible: costoclavicular ligament, tendon of the subclavian muscle, subclavian vein, anterior scalene muscle, subclavian artery, brachial plexus, medial scalene muscle, posterior scalene muscle, thoracodorsal nerve, and long thoracic nerve
▽

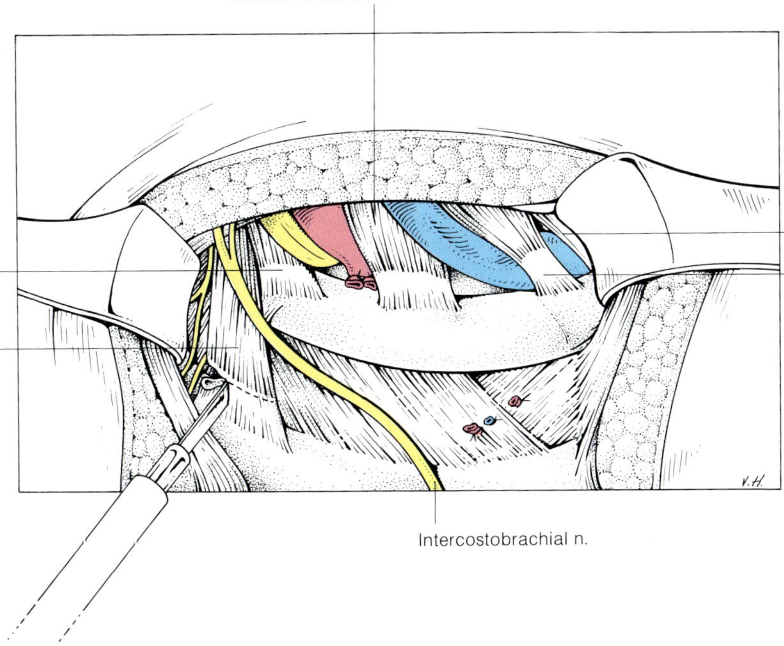

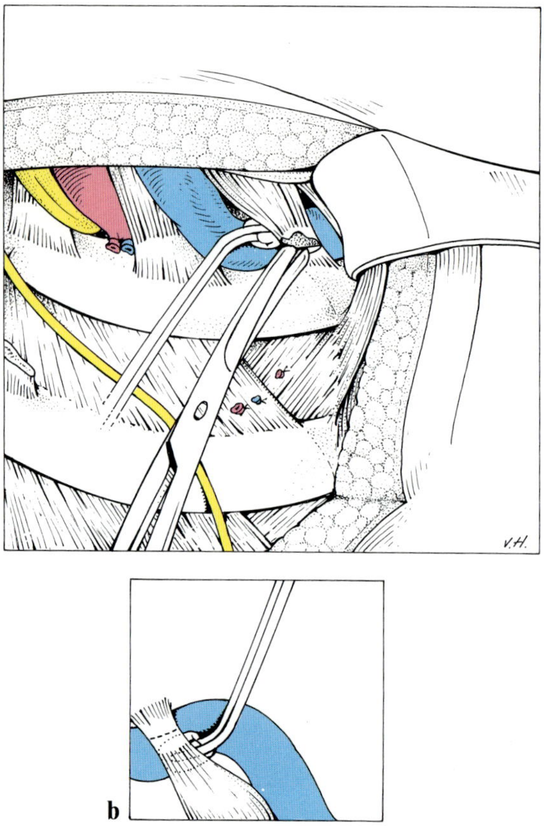

Fig. 21.1.17 a, b. When dividing the tendon of the subclavian muscle, the subclavian vein and the plexus are retracted by a cotton applicator

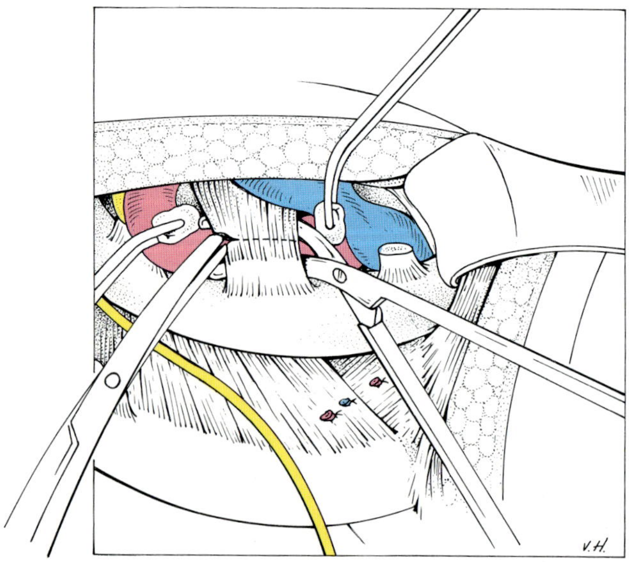

Fig. 21.1.18. A right-angled clamp is passed underneath the anterior scalene muscle and only then is the muscle divided 1 cm above the scalene tubercle

fibrotic structures still attached to the first rib are removed with a right-angled raspatory, carefully preserving the periosteum of the first rib (Fig. 21.1.19).

Within the first interspace the muscles are initially divided by thermocautery and then with scissors until the pleura is reached (Fig. 21.1.20 a). On the ventral side, the incision extends to the sternum, on the dorsal side to the transverse process. The pleura is bluntly dissected off the inner side of the first rib, using the finger (Fig. 21.1.20 b).

Next, all muscles and remaining soft tissue are removed from the first rib with an angled raspatory, sparing the periosteum. In particular, the anterior and posterior segments of the first rib are cleaned. The first rib is now completely isolated and may be resected. Curved (45°) rib scissors of the type developed by Beaujean are best used for the resection. When dividing the rib at the anterior end, the scissors must be placed so that, first of all, the rib is divided directly at the manubrium sterni, and, secondly, the rib is divided completely by a single cut. The scissors are placed somewhat obliquely for definite removal of the entire inner rim of the first rib (Fig. 21.1.21 a). When dividing the rib at the posterior end, care must be taken not to catch the first thoracic root as well. With the nerve retracted dorsally by means of a spatula, the first rib can be divided as far dorsally as possible without danger (Fig. 21.1.21 b). Following resection of the first rib one has to look for sharp or acute borders. If found, they must also be resected to prevent damage of the neurovascular bundle by postoperative arm movements. Second, the artery and vein are carefully examined and remaining fibrotic bands are resected. One should examine the artery carefully for dilatations and wall thickenings.

If the pleura has been injured accidentally, one should not try to close the opening. It can even be extended to allow blood and other fluids to drain from the pleural cavity. It is important that there be no wound hematoma. A hematoma, on becoming organized, causes a fibrotic encapsulation of the neurovascular bundle, resulting in new compression symptoms. Additionally, a Redon drain is placed in position. The suspended arm is loosened somewhat, whereby the wound is almost completely closed. Only the skin and subcutaneous tissue are closed by interrupted sutures. Postoperatively, the arm is abducted 90° to avoid adduction contraction. Mobilization starts on the 1st postoperative day.

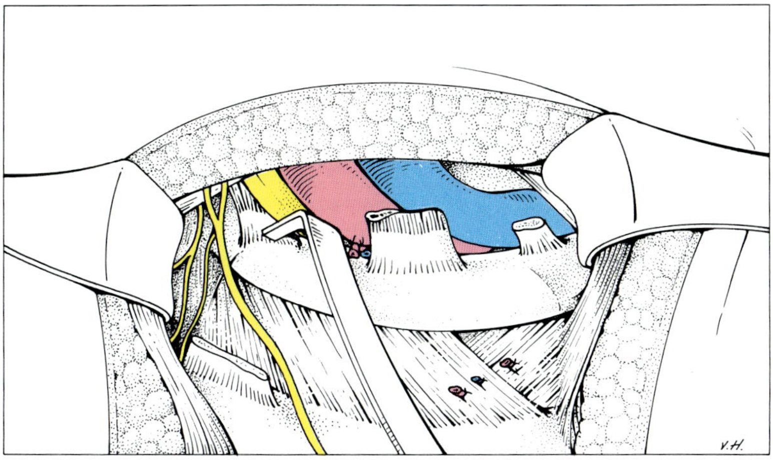

Fig. 21.1.19. Remaining muscle fibers and fibrotic tissue are removed from the first rib with a right-angled raspatory, leaving the periosteum intact

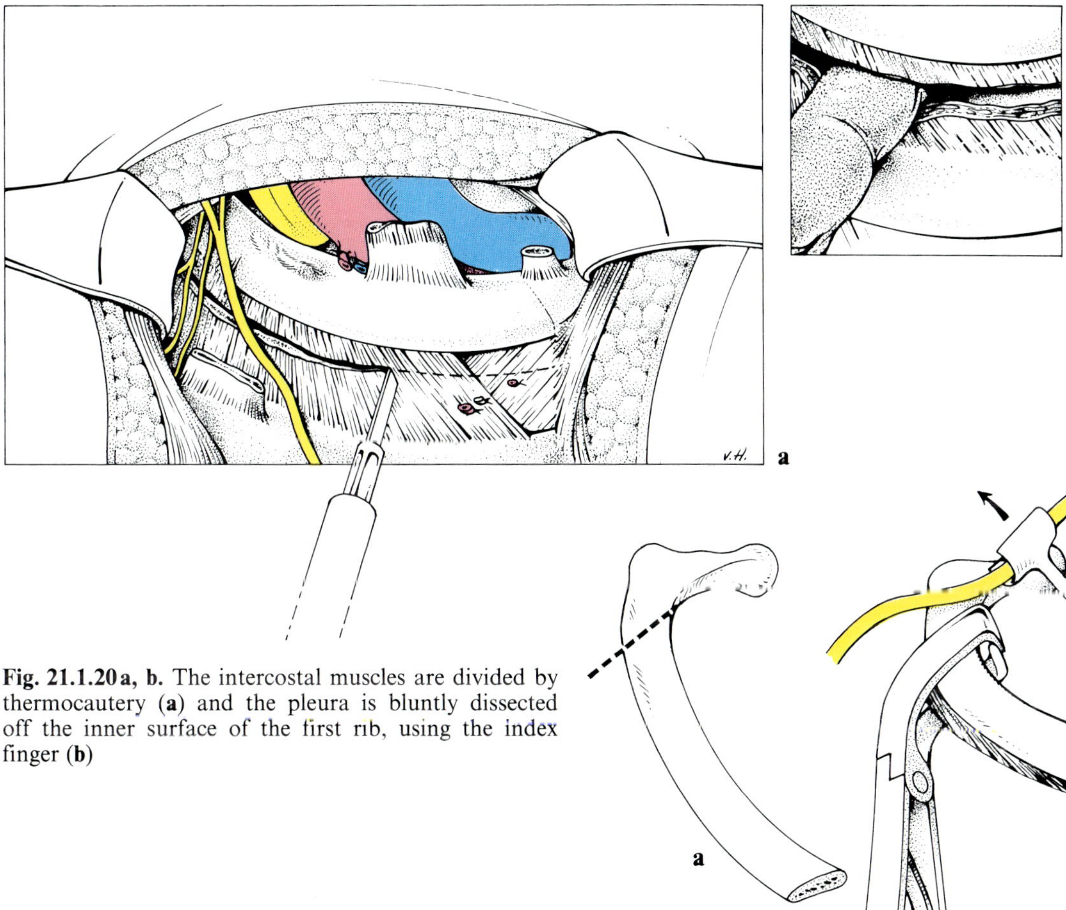

Fig. 21.1.20 a, b. The intercostal muscles are divided by thermocautery (**a**) and the pleura is bluntly dissected off the inner surface of the first rib, using the index finger (**b**)

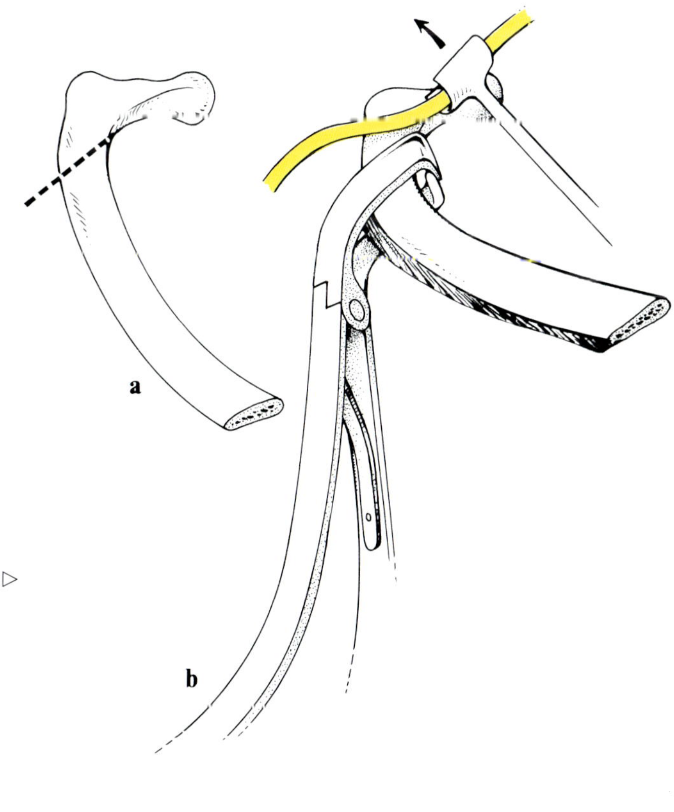

Fig. 21.1.21. **a** The rib scissors are placed somewhat ▷ obliquely on both ends of the rib so that the entire inner border of the first rib can be removed. **b** The first thoracic root of the brachial plexus is retracted dorsally with a nerve spatula while dividing the rib

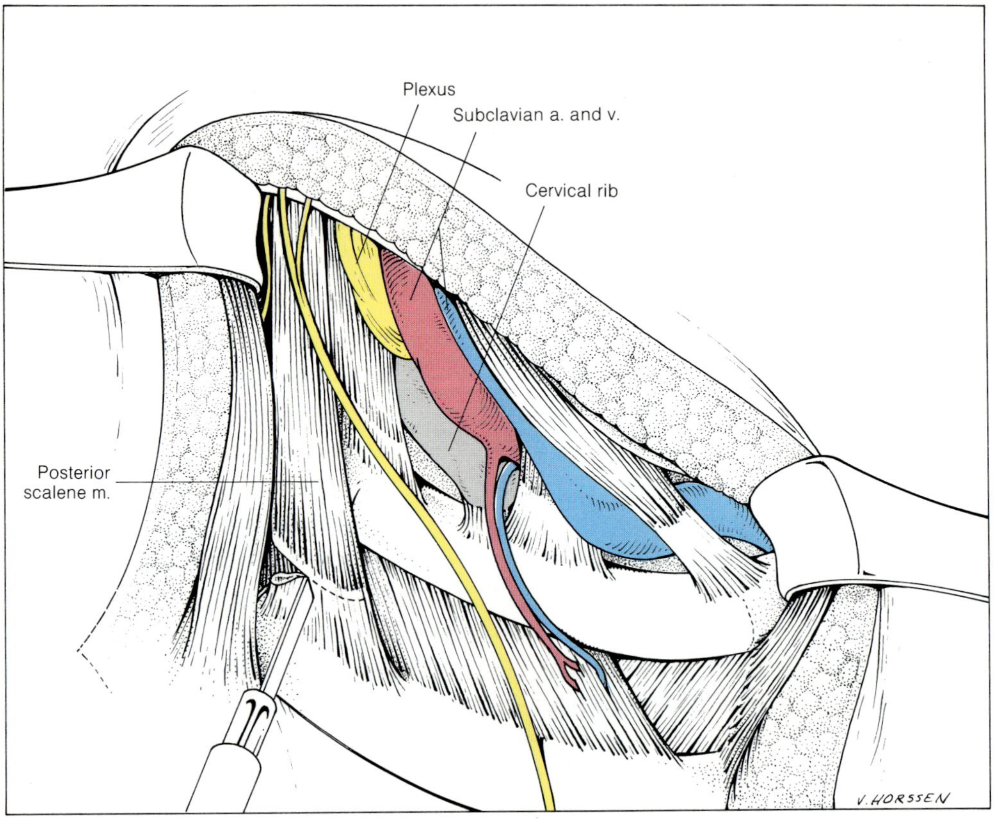
Plexus
Subclavian a. and v.
Cervical rib
Posterior scalene m.
V. HORSSEN

21.1.22

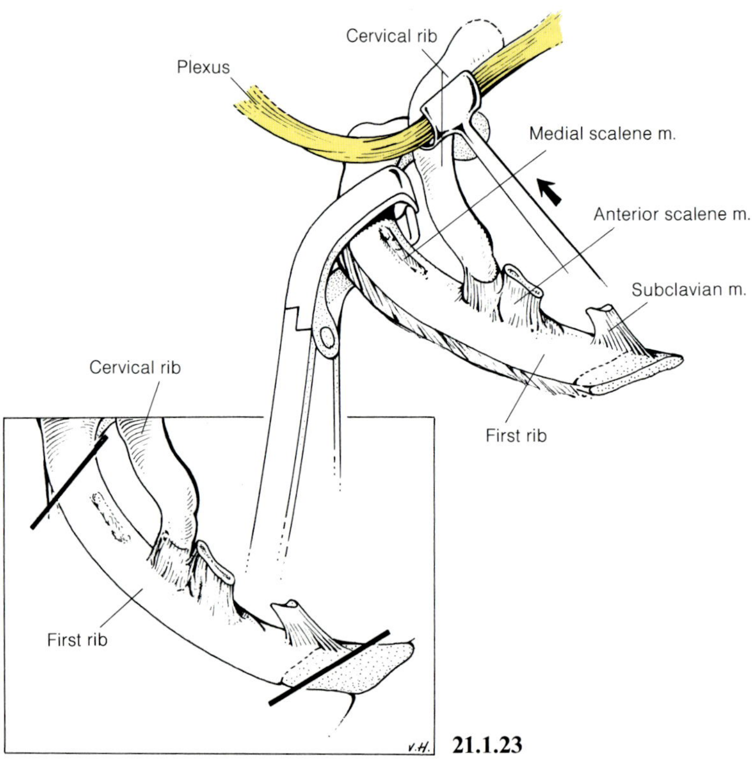
Cervical rib
Plexus
Medial scalene m.
Anterior scalene m.
Subclavian m.
First rib
Cervical rib
First rib
V.H.

21.1.23

G. Transaxillary Resection of a Cervical Rib

Positioning and operative approach are the same as for the transaxillary resection of the first rib (Fig. 21.1.22). The division of the posterior scalene muscle, the subclavian muscle, the scalene muscle, and the intercostal muscles, as well as dissection of the first rib, is performed in the manner described for the resection of the first rib. The anterior scalene muscle is also divided. When a cervical rib is present, the anterior scalene muscle is always hypoplastic and sometimes even rudimentary.

Behind the protruded tubercle of the anterior scalene muscle, the anterior part of the cervical rib and its insertion on the first rib is visualized. The subclavian artery and the plexus are retracted ventrally by a small cotton applicator, allowing visualization of the dorsocranial course of the cervical rib. Sometimes, the cervical rib and the posterior part of the first rib are so close together that it is difficult to feel the gap between them.

Before dissecting the cervical rib, the first rib should be divided ventrally and dorsally (Fig. 21.1.23). A fixation forceps is placed on the first rib. Pulling it toward the surgeon gives better access to the cervical rib. The cervical rib may be dissected up to the C7 transverse process by a small raspatory. When dissecting the cervical rib, again, care must be taken not to damage the lower root of the brachial plexus riding over the cervical rib. It is important always to retract the plexus ventrally with a small cotton applicator when dissecting the cervical rib, so as not to injure it with the raspatory. When dissection is complete, the cervical rib is divided within the joint cavity to the seventh cervical vertebra. Fine, sharply pointed, and either straight or slightly curved bone scissors are most suitable. The specimen – the first rib together with the cervical rib – is then removed. The wound is closed in the manner described on p. 562) (Fig. 21.1.23).

Fig. 21.1.22. For transaxillary resection of the cervical rib the axilla is exposed in the same manner as for the resection of the first rib

Fig. 21.1.23. Initially, the first rib is divided at its dorsal and ventral ends. It is pulled outwards, providing better access to the cervical rib. While dissecting the cervical rib, the plexus is retracted from it

H. Transaxillary Reconstruction of the Subclavian Artery

To date, the transaxillary exposure of the subclavian artery has hardly ever been mentioned in the literature. There are numerous approaches for the reconstruction of the subclavian artery: supra- and infraclavicular approaches or the combination of both with or without division or resection of the clavicle. These procedures are not necessary for the approach to the subclavian segment that extends from the origin of the vertebral artery to the brachial artery. The transaxillary approach provides good exposure, lower risk, less blood loss, a significantly lower postoperative morbidity, and a much better cosmetic result.

It is also important to consider that, with other approaches, it is very difficult, if not impossible, to resect a cervical rib or the first rib when they are causing pathologic changes in this segment of the subclavian artery.

When the pathologic findings are limited to that segment of the subclavian artery distal to the origin of the vertebral artery, positioning and approach are the same as for resection of the first rib. Also, a saphenous vein graft can be harvested from the groin in this position if necessary; however, it is preferable to harvest the vein beforehand with the patient in a supine position. The operation starts with resection of the first (and cervical) rib, as already mentioned. Following removal of both ribs, the subclavian artery is identified and dissected. Double vessel loops are placed around the arterial branches that are to be preserved. Crossing tributaries of the subclavian vein are double-ligated and divided. The subclavian artery can always be exposed up to the origin of the vertebral artery or the internal thoracic artery using this approach. It may even be possible to dissect the subclavian artery proximal to these two branches. However, on the right side, care must be taken of the recurrent nerve.

The artery may be dissected far into the distal axilla. If necessary, the brachial artery can be exposed through a second incision in the medial bicipital groove of the upper arm, between the median and ulnar nerves. Usually, the proximal transection of the subclavian artery is performed just distal to the origin of the vertebral artery. The subclavian artery then has to be cross-clamped just proximal to the origin of the vertebral artery. With the axillary approach, this can be done without difficulty; likewise cross-clamping of the vertebral artery and the internal thoracic artery poses no problem. The same holds for the anastomosis to the proximal subclavian segment. Saphenous vein harvested from the groin is the prefered graft material. Only when the subclavian artery is very wide, or when there is no suitable vein available, a prosthetic graft should be used. Following reconstruction, a Redon drain is placed in position, and the wound is closed.

Postoperatively, the extremity is immobilized and abducted 90° on a pillow in bed. On the 6th postoperative day, mobilization is started. The arm is kept in a sling for another 5 days. Exercises for the shoulder, which are performed under the supervision of a physiotherapist, should not require the arm to be abducted more than 90° for the first few weeks.

REFERENCES

1. Roos DB (1971) Experience with first rib resection for thoracic outlet syndrome. Am Surg 173:429
2. Barwegen MGMH, van Dongen RJAM, Schwilden ED (1980) Arterial complications of the thoracic outlet syndrome. Angio 2:103
3. Dorazio RA, Ezzet F (1979) Arterial complications of the thoracic outlet syndrome. Am J Surg 138:246
4. Roos DB (1966) Transaxillary approach for first rib resection to relieve thoracic outlet syndrome. Am Surg 163:354
5. van Dongen RJAM, Barwegen MGMH, Koning J (1980) Rekonstruktive Chirurgie der Arteria subklavia, transaxillärer Zugang. Angio 2:93
6. van Dongen RJAM (1984) Klinische Diagnostik und operative Erfahrung mit dem transaxillären Zugang beim TOS. In: Hase U, Reulen H-J (eds) Läsionen des Plexus brachialis. de Gruyter, Berlin New York, p 177

21.2 Median Arcuate Ligament Syndrome

E.-D. SCHWILDEN

CONTENTS

A. Definition

Patients presenting with the so-called celiac artery compression syndrome suffer from abdominal symptoms resulting from external compression of the celiac axis or its surrounding structures by the medial arcuate ligament of the diaphragm. The underlying cause is an anatomic disproportion between the aortic hiatus and the origin of the celiac axis [2, 3, 6, 8]. The mechanism of compression is shown in Fig. 21.2.1.

The effects of this compression are sometimes interpreted as disturbances in hemodynamics [1, 2, 4, 10], sometimes as irritation of the celiac plexus [5, 6, 7]. Both versions lack a sound pathophysiologic basis, and this explains that doubts are sometimes expressed concerning the existence of the syndrome [9, 12]. Therefore, it makes sense not to use the term "celiac artery compression syndrome," which suggests an exclusively vascular ischemic etiology, but rather terms like "neurovascular compression syndrome of the aortic hiatus" or "median arcuate ligament syndrome" [11].

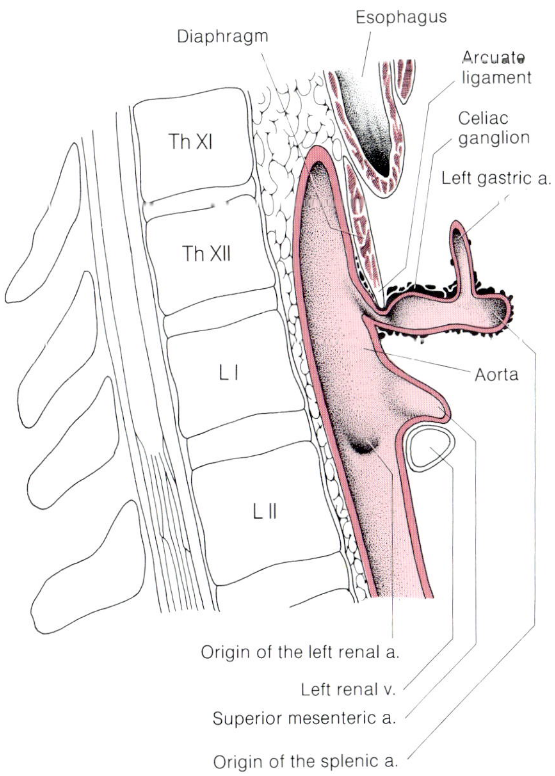

Fig. 21.2.1. Sagittal section of the vertebral column and the aorta at the level of the origin of the celiac axis and the superior mesenteric artery, with eccentric compression of the celiac axis and its surrounding structures by the median arcuate ligament of the diaphragm

B. Anatomy (Fig. 21.2.2)

In 80% of cases, the origin of the celiac axis on the anterior wall of the aorta is located between the lower third of the twelfth thoracic vertebra and approximately the middle of the first lumbar vertebra. A higher origin, at or above the level of the twelfth thoracic vertebra, has been found in 20% of autopsies. The length of the celiac axis may vary between 4 mm and about 4 cm. Usually, it branches into the common hepatic and the splenic artery. In 90% of cases, it shows a third branch, the left gastric artery, which usually branches off alone from the proximal trunk. A common origin of the left gastric, common hepatic, and splenic arteries, forming a tripus, is found in only 25%. The left gastric artery originates directly from the aorta or from one of the branches of the celiac trunk (common hepatic or splenic artery) only rarely, in about 10% of cases. The phrenic arteries originate either directly from the aorta, at the level of the celiac trunk, or, with equal frequency, from the proximal segment of the latter.

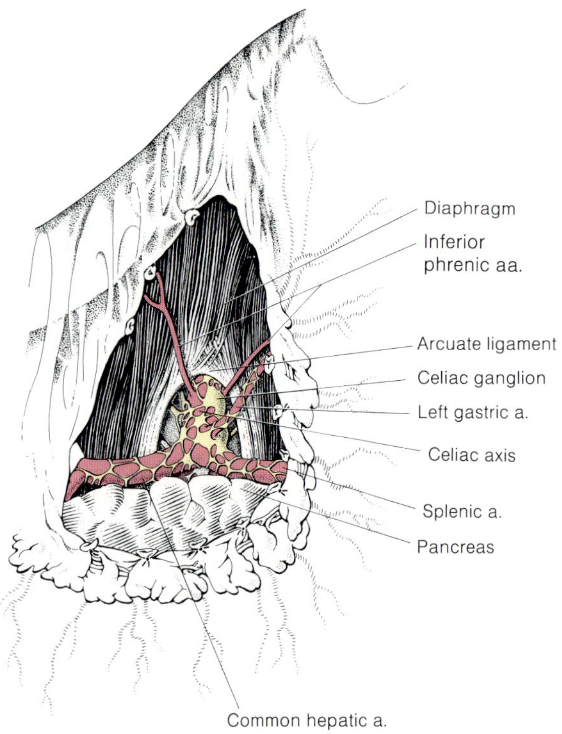

Fig. 21.2.2. Anatomy of the celiac axis with its proximal branches and side branches, the aortic hiatus, and the celiac nerve plexus, as seen through the lesser omentum

The initial segment of the abdominal aorta and the origin of the celiac trunk are confined laterally by the medial diaphragmatic crura, which arise from the first to the third lumbar vertebrae, leaving the aortic hiatus in between. The so-called median arcuate band stretches between both crura in front of the aorta, creating a tendinous arch. The celiac plexus is located on the anterior wall of the aorta, largely comprising the origin of the celiac axis and the initial segments of its branches. The major splanchnic nerves join this largest sympathetic ganglion. These nerves originate from the fifth to the ninth thoracic ganglia, pass over the lateral and anterior aspects of the lower vertebra, and, after passing through the diaphragm, terminate in the celiac ganglion. Parasympathetic fibers of the vagus nerve terminate here as well.

The ganglia of the plexus, which are mostly semilunar in shape, are often merged at the left side of the aorta. On the right side, by contrast, several smaller ganglia may be identified. The ganglia themselves are connected to each other by numerous fibers comprising the origin of the celiac axis and its branches. The nervous networks originating from the plexus itself pass along the arteries to the appropriate organs.

C. Indication for Operation

Given no clear pathophysiologic explanation for the syndrome, and therefore no sound therapeutic concept, the diagnosis of a median arcuate ligament syndrome and the decision to operate should not be forthcoming until all other possible causes of the symptoms – e.g., the more frequent abdominal diseases – have been ruled out.

Mechanical irritation of the celiac plexus seems the most likely cause of the syndrome if the patient's complaints are completely atypical as compared with a true intestinal angina of vascular origin and if there are no angiographic findings, such as collaterals, indicating a hemodynamically effective compression [11]. Besides splitting the arcuate ligament, it is usually beneficial to resect most of the diseased plexus and simultaneously the periarterial sympathetic nerves of the proximal celiac trunk branches. Vascular reconstruction may not be necessary, even if a pressure gradient persists following splitting of the ligament. Also reconstruction is probably not defensible as the only operative measure undertaken.

When the patient's symptoms are typical of intestinal angina, perhaps combined with morphological secondary changes of an abdominal organ of vascular origin, vascular insufficiency of the celiac axis and its branches has to be considered [11]. In this case, reestablishment of normal blood flow is indicated. If this cannot be achieved by simple cutting of the median arcuate ligament, for instance because the stenosis fails to become dilated or is already occluded, a reconstruction of the celiac trunk is required. Simultaneous resection of the plexus should be performed to exclude an additional neurogenic component of the symptoms.

D. Positioning and Location of Incisions

For the operative therapy of the celiac artery compression syndrome, the procedure should be limited to a transabdominal approach whenever possible. More or less the same approaches are used as described for reconstruction of visceral arteries (see p. 592).

Median laparotomy is most suitable. Possible alternatives are a right-side paramedian incision or a transverse incision of the upper abdomen. The left side thoracoabdominal approach, opening two cavities, should be restricted to extreme situations, e.g., when a graft is to be anastomosed to the proximal aorta and this cannot be done using the abdominal approach alone. For all other approaches, patients are placed in a supine position. It is important in positioning and draping of the operative field that access to the saphenous vein also be provided in case a graft is needed for reconstruction of the celiac axis (see p. 592).

E. Exposure of the Celiac Axis

Following laparotomy and careful exploration to exclude other intra-abdominal diseases, the celiac axis is exposed either through the hepatogastric ligament or the gastrocolic ligament (Fig. 21.2.3).

When using the approach through the lesser omentum (Fig. 21.2.3a), the left triangular ligament of the liver is first divided, and the mobilized left lobe of the liver carefully turned down and retracted to the right with a broad speculum. Then, the hepatogastric ligament is split in an avascular region, if possible. Crossing vessels are

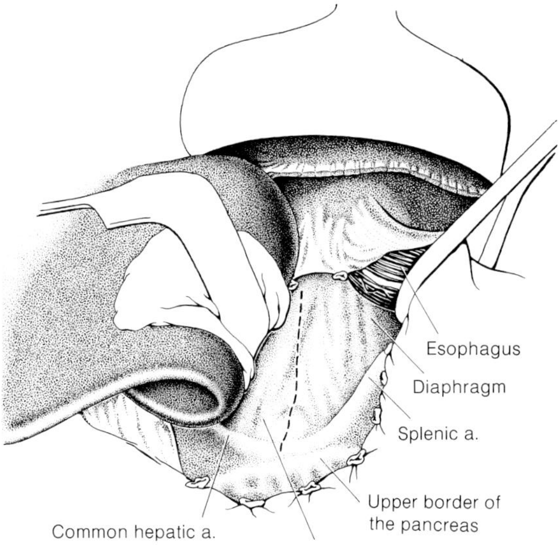

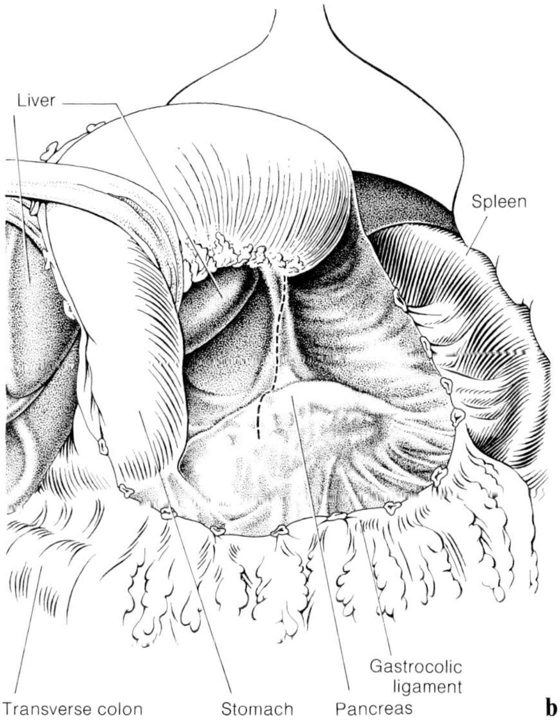

Fig. 21.2.3a, b. Approaches to the celiac axis through the lesser omentum (**a**) and through the gastrocolic ligament (**b**)

double-ligated. The esophagus and stomach confining the operative field on the left lateral side are retracted to the left and downward. This procedure may be facilitated by placing a strong, smooth rubber tube around the esophagus. This procedure exposes the retroperitoneum with the underlying structures: the upper border of the pancreas, the posterior segment of the diaphragm, and the celiac axis with its branches and surrounding nerve plexus.

The approach through the gastrocolic ligament (Fig. 21.2.3 b) begins with dissection of the greater curvature approximately in the middle of the stomach. Reaching up the cardia, the short gastric vessels are divided between ligatures and the fundus of the stomach is dissected off the diaphragm. Reflecting the stomach to the right (facilitated by placing a rubber band around it and pulling the colon downward) exposes the retroperitoneum in the region of the aortic hiatus, with the structures of the celiac axis region below it.

F. Intraoperative Diagnostics

Prior to the completed exposure of the celiac axis and the decision regarding further operative measures, the stenosis of the celiac axis is tested for hemodynamic effectiveness. Besides the subjective assessment of pulsations of the celiac axis branches and the diagnosis of a possible bruit over the stenosis, objective quantitative measurement of the disturbed hemodynamics is performed by comparing intravasal blood pressure in the aorta and in a poststenotic branch of the celiac axis (common hepatic or splenic artery). If collateral circulation via the pancreatic arcades and the gastroduodenal artery is verified angiographically, this artery must be cross-clamped prior to determination of the pressure gradient. The control measurement following division of the celiac band, together with the clinical symptoms, and the angiographic morphology, decide whether vascular reconstruction will be necessary. Electromagnetic flow measurements before and after splitting of the ligament provides quantitative data on the increase of blood flow due to the therapeutic measures. In order to exclude vascular spasm by local manipulations, intra-arterial application of a vasodilator is advisable. If a reconstruction is required, the final measurements of pressure and flow following reconstruction document the hemodynamic properties of the anastomosis.

G. Operative Measures

I. Division of the Ligament and Resection of the Plexus (Fig. 21.2.4)

Following longitudinal incision of the retroperitoneum, the dissection of the celiac axis and its surrounding structures is carried out, first exposing and placing a tape around those branches that are easily exposed, namely, the common hepatic artery and the splenic artery at the upper border of the pancreas (Fig. 21.2.4a). Being in close contact with the vascular wall, the arteries are dissected in the direction of the celiac axis and freed from the surrounding structures of the celiac plexus. The first 1–1.5 cm of the left gastric artery are dissected and denervated as well. One must be careful to note the possible anomaly of a vessel originating from the celiac axis and passing posteriorly, the so-called "anastomosis of Bühler." Following exposure and proximal denervation of the three major celiac branches, dissection is continued on the anterior aspect of the celiac axis. The nerve plexus covering the axis is resected (Fig. 21.2.4b). Care must be taken of any phrenic arteries branching off; if accidentally divided, they may slip back into the retroperitoneal tissue and cause serious bleeding.

Often, nerve fibers and structures of the ganglion may not be clearly identified during the dissection. The entire celiac axis may be covered by a fibrotic mass, significantly impairing the dissection. When exposing a poststenotic dilatation of the celiac axis, special care must be taken not to injure the anterior wall of the artery, which is thin and highly vulnerable.

Dissecting further in the direction of the aorta, the median arcuate ligament is finally exposed. In most cases it is stretched over the celiac axis like a tight band. A dissecting clamp is carefully inserted beneath the band, and it is divided sharply with a scalpel between the jaws of the clamp for a considerable distance proximally (Fig. 21.2.4c). Following division of the ligament, a distinct groove can usually be seen on the artery, indicating where compression was being exerted. Following division of the ligament, the anterior and lateral walls of the aorta at the origin of the celiac axis are also dissected and the surrounding nervous tissue removed. Finally, the celiac plexus is resected between the origin of the celiac axis and the superior mesenteric artery while the upper

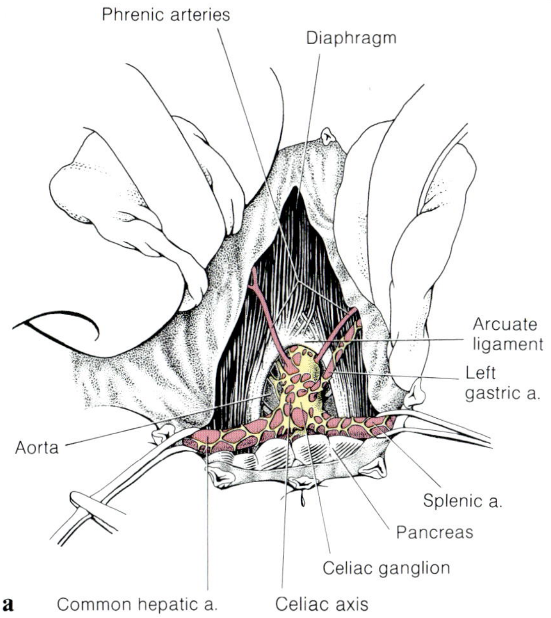

a

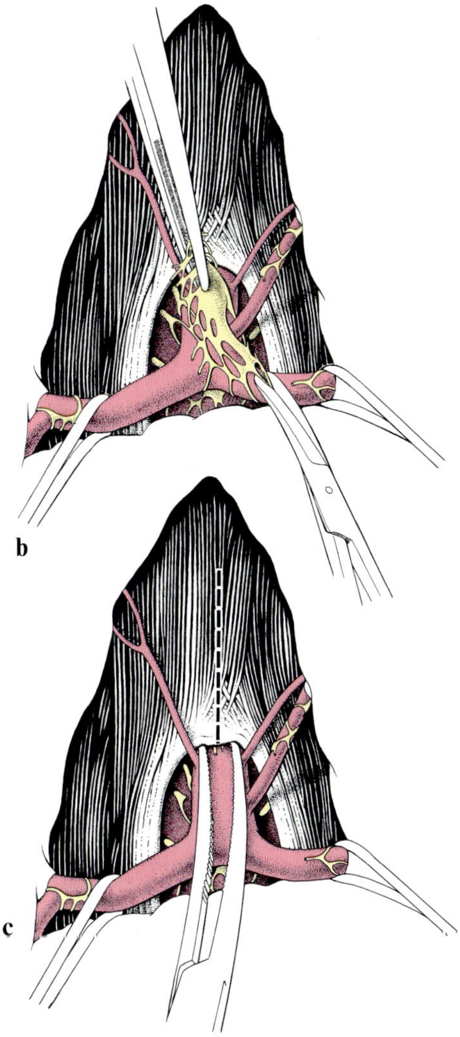

b

c

Fig. 21.2.4a–d. Technique for division of the ligament and resection of the plexus. **a** Following incision of the retroperitoneum, the dissection of the the celiac axis and its surrounding structures starts with the placing of tapes around the common hepatic and splenic artery at the upper border of the pancreas. **b** Dissection and periarterial sympathectomy of the proximal branches of the celiac axis, and resection of the plexus at the anterior wall of the axis. **c** Division of the median arcuate ligament and longitudinal incision of the posterior crura of the diaphragm. **d** Removal of the celiac plexus between the origin of the celiac axis and the superior mesenteric artery

border of the pancreas is mobilized and the celiac axis is retracted with a tape (Fig. 21.2.4d).

Pressure and flow measurements will decide whether any further procedure is called for. If a furrow persists at the upper border of the celiac axis, one may attempt to dilate the stenosis carefully from the inside, using heparinized saline solution while the segment is cross-clamped by two bulldog clamps.

II. Vascular Reconstructions

When reconstruction or revascularization of the celiac axis is required, the following methods may be used, depending on the approach, on local factors such as a narrow costal arch, obesity, etc., and on the anatomic situation at the origin of the celiac axis:

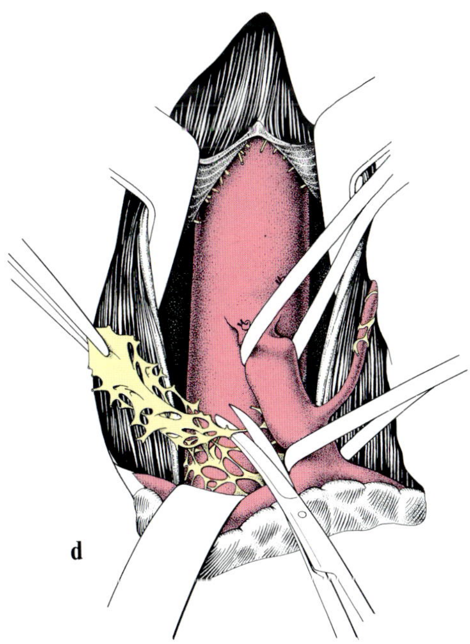

d

1. Resection of the Stenosis and Graft Interposition (Fig. 21.2.5)

For this procedure, exposure of a sufficiently long aortic segment above the origin of the celiac axis is necessary; this is achieved by a large incision of the muscular posterior crura of the diaphragm. In cases of obesity or a narrow costal arch, this dissection of the aorta may cause considerable technical difficulties and may be possible only by a thoracoabdominal approach. The stress caused by opening two body cavities, however, is justified only if local anatomic situations, previous operations, or extensive arteriosclerotic lesions of the distal aorta do not allow other reconstructions. Care should be taken of phrenic arteries originating from the aorta and intercostal arteries branching off dorsally.

Cross-clamping of the aortic segment for anastomosing the graft may be complete or tangential. Tangential cross-clamping guarantees perfusion of the lower part of the body, especially of the kidneys, but it may often be very difficult and is not without risk as the clamp may slip off. Complete cross-clamping of the aortic segment is safer and, provided the anastomosis is not too time consuming, does not entail an excessively long interruption of blood flow to the kidneys (Fig. 21.2.5a). An oval incision is made in the anterior aortic wall for the proximal anastomosis with the graft, which is preferably a segment of great saphenous vein. When the graft has been anastomosed to the aortotomy, it is cross-clamped close to the anastomosis and the aorta is unclamped. The celiac axis is then divided, the proximal stump sutured, and the distal end anastomosed end-to-end to the graft, which has been tailored to the appropriate length (Fig. 21.2.5b).

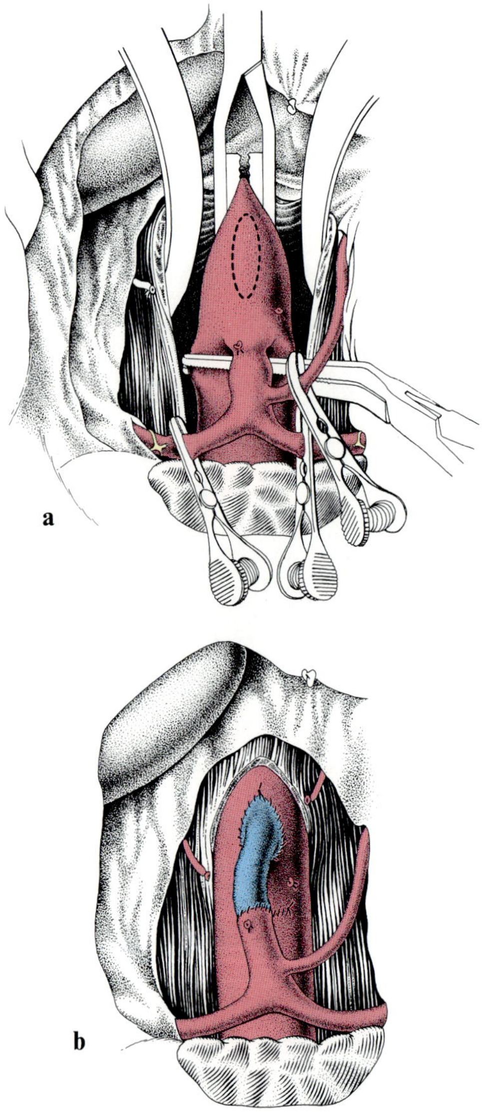

Fig. 21.2.5a, b. Technique for resection of the stenosis and graft interposition. **a** Following complete cross-clamping of the branches of the axis and of the isolated thoracic aortic segment, the anterior wall of the aorta is opened by an elliptical excision. **b** Situation following suture of the proximal celiac axis stump and graft interposition with proximal end-to-side anastomosis to the aorta and distal end-to-end anastomosis to the divided celiac axis

2. Bypass from the Proximal Aorta

Approach, exposure of the aortic segment, and proximal anastomosis are identical to the procedure for graft interposition. The distal anastomosis of the bypass is performed after an appropriate segment has been isolated by cross-clamping. It is either anastomosed end-to-side to the celiac axis itself or to one of its branches, the common hepatic or the splenic artery.

3. Resection of the Stenosis and Reinsertion (Fig. 21.2.6)

Resection of the stenosis and reinsertion of the celiac axis into the aorta at a higher level is usually impossible because the distance is too great; therefore, graft interposition is usually required (see above). The possibility of direct reimplantation of a celiac axis in the aorta below its natural origin depends on the length of the aortic segment between the celiac axis and the origin of the superior

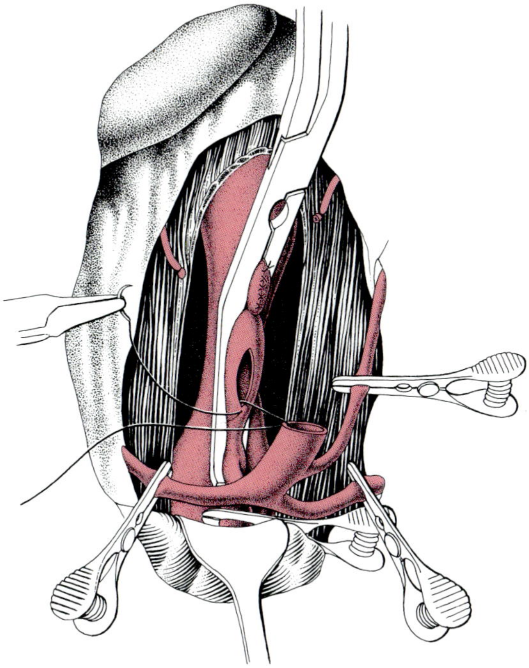

Fig. 21.2.6. Technique for resection of stenosis and reimplantation of the celiac axis. After tangential placement of a Satinsky clamp on the aorta and oval excision of the anterior wall of the aorta between the origin of the celiac axis and the superior mesenteric artery, reimplantation of the divided celiac axis into the aorta is performed by an end-to-side anastomosis

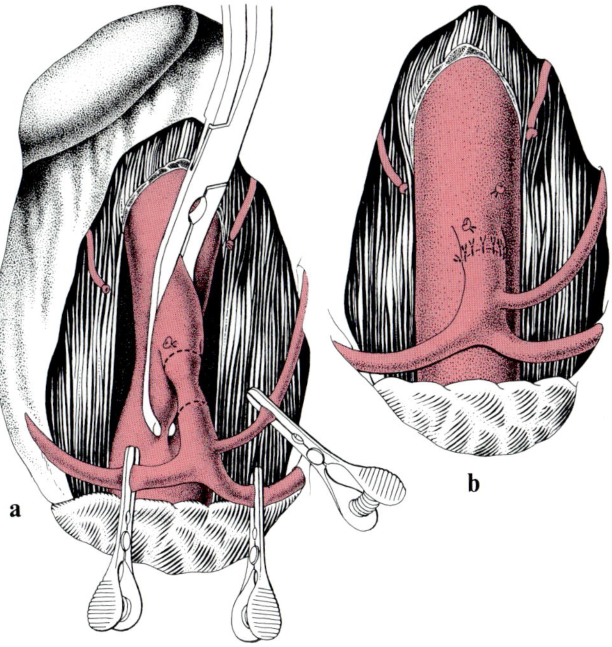

Fig. 21.2.7 a, b. Technique for resection of the stenosis and end-to-end anastomosis. **a** Following placement of a Satinsky clamp on the aorta or complete cross-clamping of the aortic segment at the origin of the celiac axis and cross-clamping of the celiac axis branches, the diseased segment of the celiac axis is resected. **b** The stumps of the celiac axis are anastomosed end-to-end using interrupted sutures

mesenteric artery, which varies between a few millimeters and 2 cm. If the arterial segment is sufficiently long to create a new orifice in the aorta, a new elliptical orifice is excised at the anterior wall of the aorta, between the origin of the celiac axis and the superior mesenteric artery, following complete or tangential cross-clamping of the appropriate segment. The celiac axis itself is divided and the proximal end closed by suture ligation or over-and-over suture. The stenosis is resected at the distal end and the poststenotic segment reimplanted into the aorta.

4. Resection of the Stenosis and End-to-End Anastomosis (Fig. 21.2.7)

This method of reconstruction may be performed when there is a sufficiently long segment of the celiac axis of normal caliber proximal to the site of compression, providing the possibility of reanastomosing the distal celiac axis following resection of the stenosis. Simple proximal cross-clamping of the celiac axis does not provide adequate exposure for resection of the stenotic segment and rejoining of the two stumps of the celiac axis. As with the reimplantation procedure, an area including the entire origin of the celiac axis, together with a segment of the aorta, must be clamped off (Fig. 21.2.7a). The stenosis is then resected and an end-to-end anastomosis of the celiac axis stumps is performed (Fig. 21.2.7b). Luminal discrepancies can be overcome by beveling the end of the smaller vessel.

5. Bypass from the Distal Aorta

A vein bypass from the infrarenal aorta to one of the branches of the celiac axis is the easiest and safest procedure for reconstruction of a celiac axis stenosis. When there is clear indication for operation preoperatively (for instance, celiac axis occlusion), dissection in the region of the celiac axis may be abandoned and the graft anastomosed to the common hepatic artery or the splenic artery. The technique is identical to that for arteriosclerotic occlusions of the celiac axis (see p. 601).

6. In Situ Bypass

Patients suffering from celiac artery compression syndrome are usually not at the age at which patients present with arteriosclerosis. Therefore, in most of these patients, the splenic artery is intact. An aortosplenic in situ bypass may also be considered since stenotic lesions do not usually occur in the region where the celiac artery divides to form the common hepatic and splenic arteries. The disadvantage of this reconstruction consists in the very time-consuming dissection of an appropriate segment of the splenic artery at the upper border of the pancreas. The technique is the same as with the in situ bypass for arteriosclerotic occlusions of the celiac axis (see p. 600).

7. Endarterectomies

A direct open or transaortic endarterectomy of the celiac axis is not usually considered in cases of celiac artery compression syndrome because the stenosis is mostly caused by thickened fibrotic intima, which usually precludes dissection and appropriate endarterectomy.

REFERENCES

1. Carey JP, Stemmer EA, Connolly JE (1969) Median arcuate ligament syndrome. Arch Surg 99:441
2. Cleator I, Macpherson A, Fraser G (1971) Celiac artery compression. Int Roy Coll 16:96
3. Curl JH, Thompson NW, Stanley JC (1971) Median arcuate ligament compression of the celiac and superior mesenteric arteries. Ann Surg 173:314
4. Drapanas T, Bron KM (1966) Stenosis of the celiac artery. Ann Surg 164:1085
5. Dunbar JD, Molnar W, Beman F, Marable SA (1965) Compression of the celiac trunk and abdominal angina. Am J Roentgen 95:731
6. Harjola PT (1963) A rare obstruction of the celiac artery. Ann Chir Gynec Fenn 2:547
7. Klink DD (1973) Celiac axis compression syndrome. Wis Med J 69:133
8. Marable SA, Molnar W, Beman FM (1966) Abdominal pain secondary to celiac axis compression. Am J Surg 111:493
9. Plate G, Eklöf B, Vang J (1981) The celiac compression syndrome: myth or reality. Arch Chir Scand 147:201
10. Schmidt H, Schimanski K (1967) Die Stenose der Arteria coeliaca – ihre Diagnose und klinische Bedeutung. Fortschr Röntgenstr 106:1
11. Schwilden ED (1980) Zur Problematik des Zöliakakompressionssyndroms. Angio 2:251
12. Szilagyi DE, Rian RL, Elliott JP, Smith RF (1972) The celiac artery compression syndrome: does it exist? Surgery 72:849

21.3 Popliteal Artery Entrapment Syndrome

R.G.M. BIEMANS

CONTENTS

A. Anatomy

The superficial femoral artery leaves the subsartorial canal, entering the popliteal fossa proximal and medial to the sciatic nerve to become the popliteal artery (Fig. 21.3.1). The artery passes centrally through the intercondylar notch. Together with the vein and the tibial nerve, the artery passes to the lower border of the popliteal muscle and branches into the tibial artery and the tibiofibular trunk. In the popliteal fossa, the artery gives off a variable number of branches (sural arteries) as well as some important arterial collaterals, namely, the lateral and medial inferior and superior genicular arteries, supplying the arterial network of the knee. At the level of the joint fissure, the medial genicular artery branches off from the anterior aspect of the popliteal artery on its way to the knee joint.

At the distal end of the popliteal fossa, the tibial veins form the popliteal vein. Often, two popliteal veins are found. Between the heads of the gastrocnemius muscles, the short saphenous vein is located in a duplication of the crural fascia. This vein perforates the fascia at varying levels to enter the deeper located popliteal vein (see p. 705). Also, the genicular veins, accompanying the lateral and

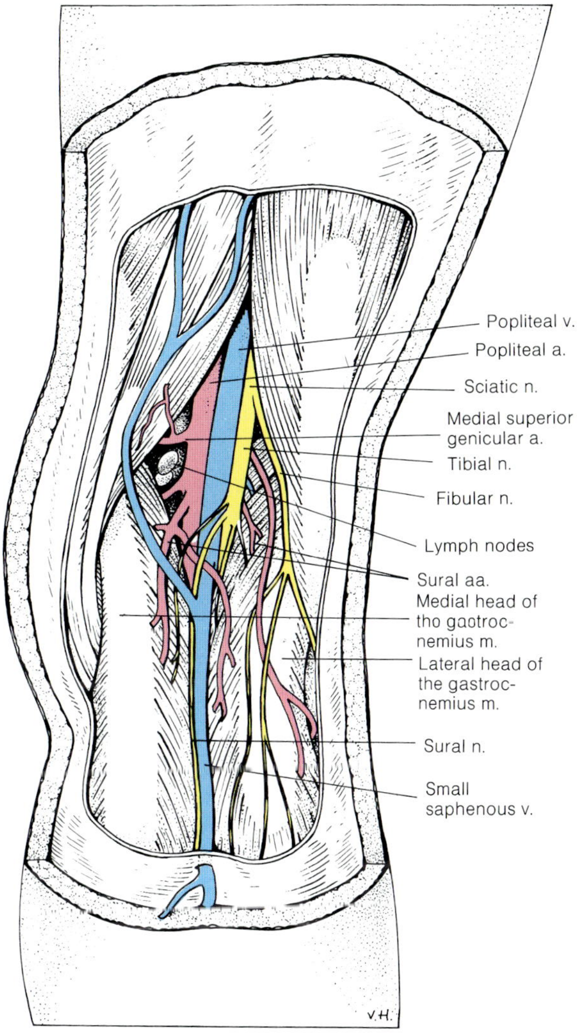

Fig. 21.3.1. The anatomy of the popliteal fossa

medial superior and inferior genicular arteries, join the popliteal vein.

At the upper end of the popliteal fossa, the artery is located medial and the tibia nerve lateral to the popliteal vein. On its course through the popliteal fossa, the artery gradually assumes a more anterior position with respect to the vein, which is covered on its dorsal side by the tibial nerve. Artery and veins are comprised of common connective tissue sheaths and are easily identified, especially at the caudal end of the popliteal fossa.

B. Classification of Entrapment Syndromes

I. According to Insua

Sometimes, owing to anomalous anatomic relations between the popliteal artery – and possibly also the popliteal vein – on the one hand, and the muscles within the popliteal fossa on the other, the artery may be compressed by contraction of the muscle. In such cases the artery is compressed during each plantar flexion, thereby temporarily reducing the blood flow to the lower leg and possibly leading to secondary lesions of the vascular wall and intermittent claudication.

The various relations between the artery and the muscles were divided into four groups by INSUA, YOUNG, and HUMPHRIES [12] in 1970 (Fig. 21.3.2). In the first two groups, the popliteal artery deviates medially. In the other two groups, the artery is located in its normal position, but is compressed by structures crossing the popliteal fossa. All congenital anatomic malformations can be subsumed under these four headings.

The Insua classification of the popliteal entrapment syndrome is as follows:

Type 1: The popliteal artery passes medially over the dorsal surface of the medial head of the gastrocnemius muscle. Further distally, it is located in its normal position ventral to the muscle. In other cases, the artery passes through the medial head [13]. In rare cases, the vein participates in the anomalous course. The muscles do not show any pecularities.

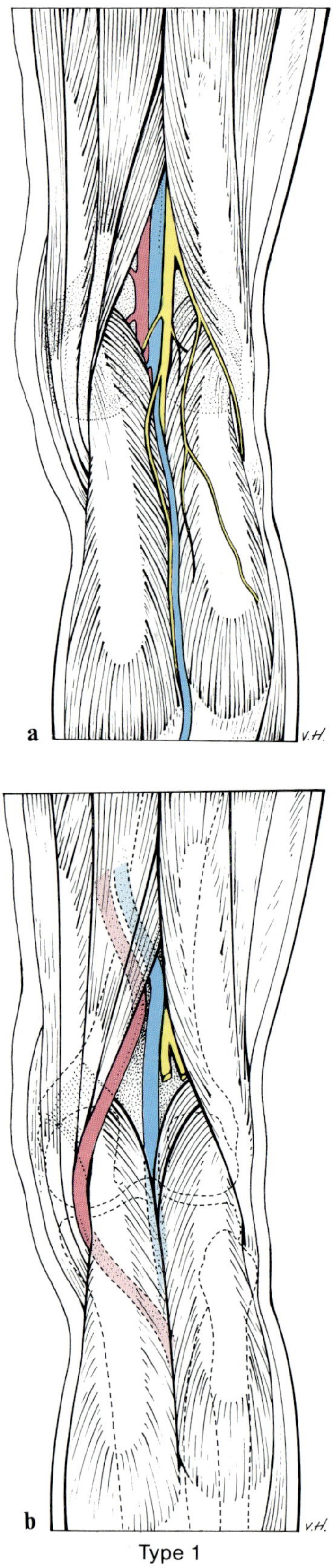

Fig. 21.3.2a–e. Possible anatomic variants of the popliteal fossa. **a** Normal position of the popliteal artery and vein and the surrounding muscles (see Fig. 21.3.1). **b** Type 1. **c** Type 1 a. **d** Type 2. **e** Type 2a ▷

Type 1a: The medial head of the gastrocnemius muscle is displaced in a craniolateral direction. The artery passes in the same way as in type 1, but with less deviation. In this case, also, the vein may accompany the artery [14].

According to Insua, most compression mechanisms belong to types 1a and 1b.

Type 2: The medial head of the gastrocnemius muscle has an accessory head arising more laterally; or, the plantar muscle has an anomalous course. In both cases muscle tissue may compress the artery, even though it may not deviate from its normal course.

Type 2a: Muscle fibers arising from the lateral femoral condyle insert at the medial head of the gastrocnemius muscle instead of centrally at the lateral head. Here, too, a normally coursing popliteal artery may be compressed by anomalous bands of muscle.

II. Other Types of Entrapment

HOHMANN [11] describes a patient in whom the popliteal artery was compressed by an anomalous motoric branch of the tibial nerve to the medial head of the gastrocnemius muscle. The compression caused thrombosis of the artery.

DOWNS [8] and also BAKER [1] described an acquired type of compression. In each case an infragenicular bypass was constructed medial to the gastrocnemius muscle, resulting in compression of the graft. Following transection of the medial head, the graft assumed the normal position. Afterwards the patients were free of symptoms.

An excessive hypertrophy of the gastrocnemius muscle may cause intermittent claudication. The hypertrophic heads of the muscle compress the popliteal artery during contraction. Simultaneously, there may be compression of the popliteal vein as well [2, 3, 18].

The popliteal vein may show an anomalous course, usually together with a displaced popliteal artery [10, 17]. Only once has compression been reported due to an anomalous course of the popliteal vein where the artery was in its normal position [6].

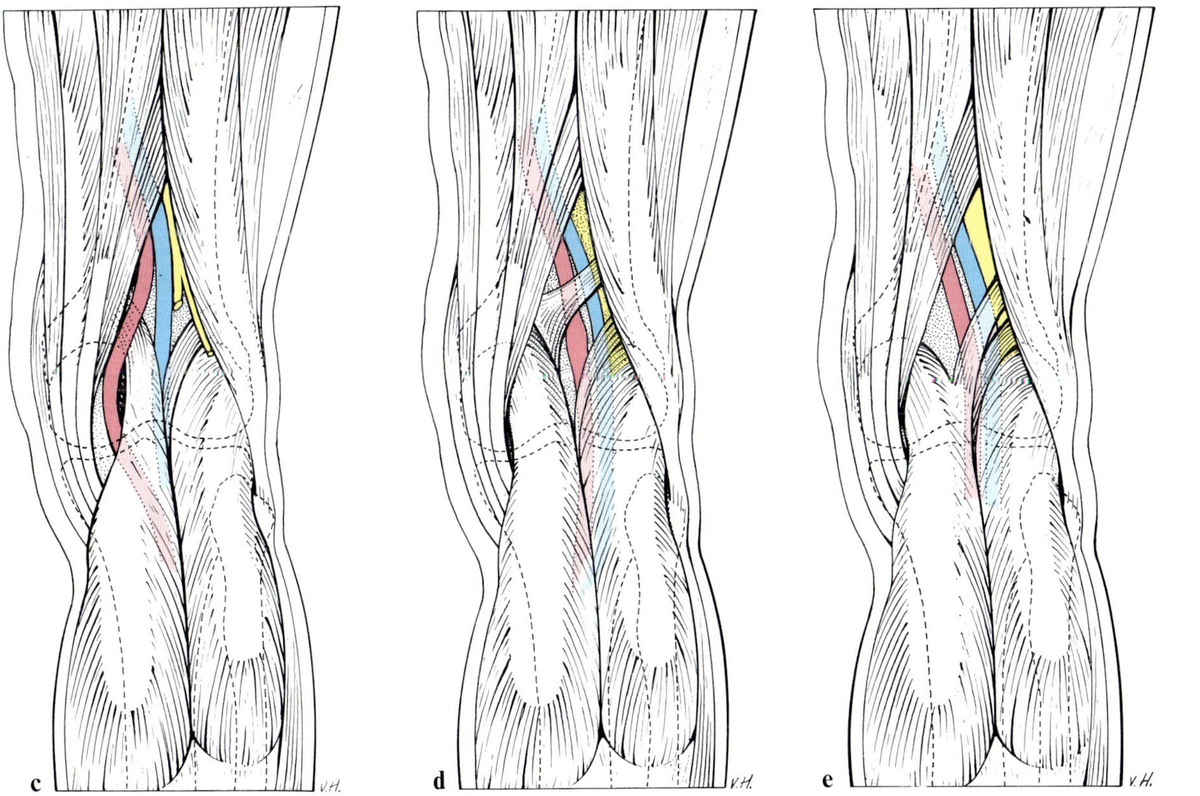

c Type 1a

d Type 2

e Type 2a

C. Indication for Surgery

Treatment of this entrapment syndrome is always surgical. The morphological changes of the vessel wall are initially limited to intimal and medial proliferation. The stenosis is initially reversible, but becomes irreversible. Ulcerative intimal lesions with adherent thrombi may develop, resulting in a complete occlusion. Thrombus growth by apposition may cause complete occlusion of the peripheral vascular bed.

Also, compression of the artery may cause a poststenotic aneurysm with mural thrombi. The thrombi on the aneurysm wall as well as on the ulcerative intimal lesions may cause embolism with peripheral occlusions.

Treatment must begin as early as possible because the complications mentioned are almost always encountered. It is best if treatment can come at a time when only correction of the compression mechanism is necessary. If a reconstruction is required, it is usually much easier to perform in young patients because of the good condition of afferent and efferent vessels. If a compression mechanism is diagnosed on both sides, the asymptomatic limb must also be operated on.

D. Positioning and Operative Approach

Operative procedures on the popliteal artery as well as on the anatomic structures causing compression may be performed using a dorsal or medial approach. When the procedure is limited to the correction of the compression mechanism – perhaps accompanied by local vascular lesions – the dorsal approach is preferred. The patient is placed in a prone position on the operating table with the feet free, in order to provide passive dorsal flexion of the foot during the procedure (Fig. 21.3.3).

The dorsal approach provides good exposure of the anomalous conditions. Not only gross anomalies, such as displaced medial head of the gastrocnemius muscle, but also smaller accessory muscle bundles or anomalous bands may be recognized more easily from the dorsal aspect. These compression mechanisms are much more difficult to recognize by the medial approach.

Also, complications such as local vascular lesions and poststenotic aneurysms that have not yet resulted in complete occlusion may be treated effectively using a dorsal approach. Operating in a prone position allows simultaneous treatment of the contralateral limb [15].

Since 1959, when HAMMING [9] performed the first successful operation for the entrapment syndrome using an S-shaped curve, this method has found general acceptance. The incision starts at the site where the popliteal artery emerges from the subsartorial canal. Localization of this point is facilitated by slight flexion of the knee, allowing the pulse in the popliteal artery to be palpated (Fig. 21.3.4). The incision continues vertically down to the level of the joint fissure. Then, it turns laterally for a few centimeters. Finally, it continues downward again, reaching the level of the junction of both heads of the gastrocnemius muscles (Fig. 21.3.5). The fascia is opened through a longitudinal incision placed centrally between the condyles (Fig. 21.3.6). Care must be taken of the tibial nerve and its branches passing to the medial and lateral heads of the gastrocnemius muscles; they are sometimes located just beneath the fascia. Additionally, there is an important sensory branch, the medial cutaneous nerve of the calf.

In case of complete occlusion, reconstruction over long segments (e.g., a bypass) may be performed in a supine position, as usual. In reconstructions over long segments, the medial approach also has the advantage that a sufficiently long graft of greater saphenous vein may be harvested without changing the patient's position.

Fig. 21.3.3. Position of the patient for the dorsal approach to the popliteal artery. The knee joints are extended. Passive dorsal flexion of the foot is not impaired

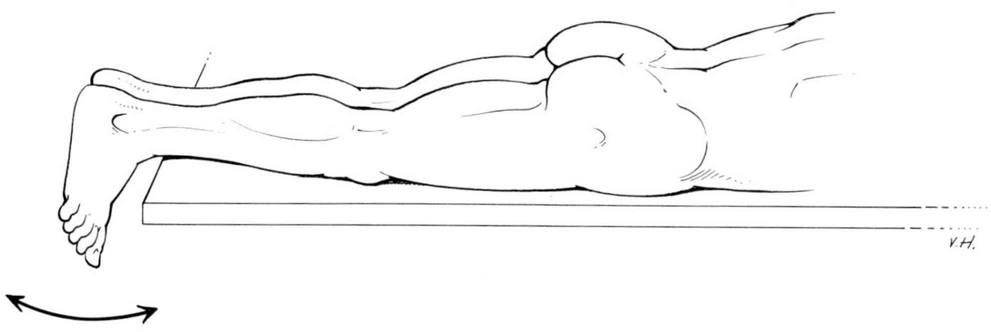

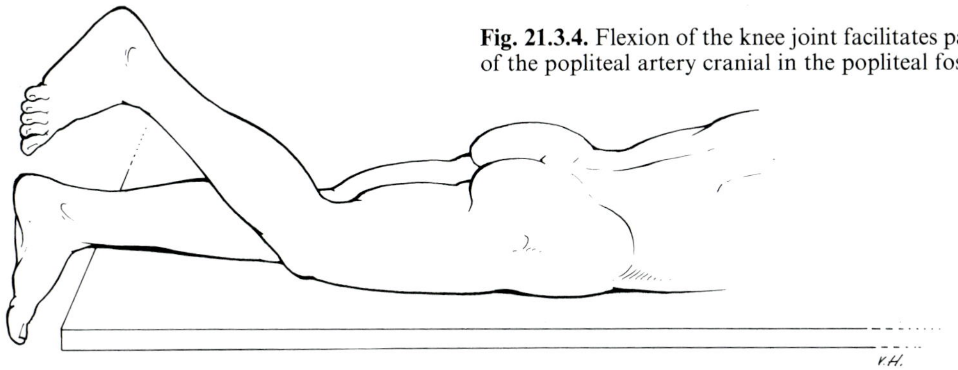

Fig. 21.3.4. Flexion of the knee joint facilitates palpation of the popliteal artery cranial in the popliteal fossa

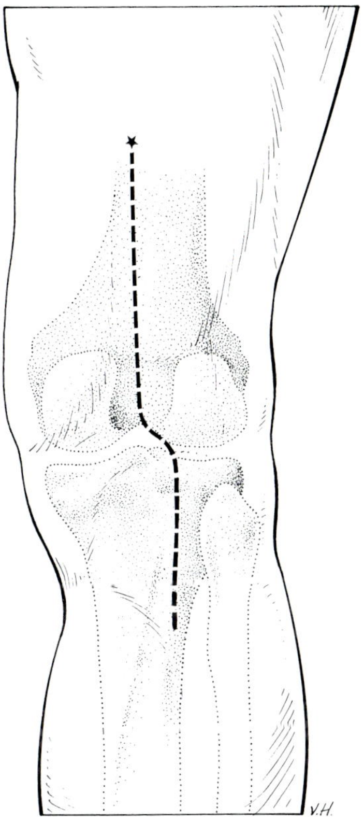

Fig. 21.3.5. Location of skin and subcutaneous incision

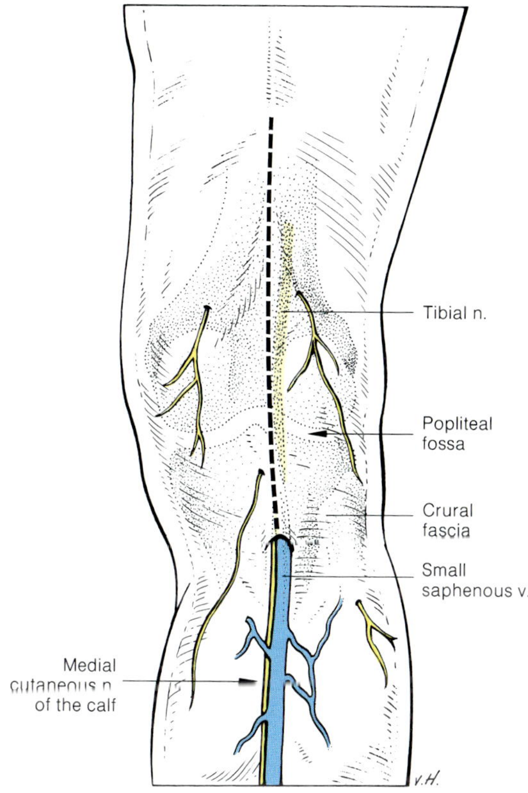

Fig. 21.3.6. Location of popliteal fascia incision

E. Technique of Exposure

For the further steps in the procedure only general guidelines can be given which have to be adapted to the local anatomic situation. The fatty tissue and the connective tissue of the popliteal fossa must be divided along the course of the neurovascular bundle. Exploration in the medial or lateral direction, if required, must be carried out over the bottom of the popliteal fossa so that the popliteal lymph nodes and the accompanying lymph vessels can be preserved. Dissection is carried out between the popliteal artery, which is palpable cranially, and the small saphenous vein distally. The small saphenous vein enters the operative field at the junction of the medial and lateral head of the gastrocnemius muscle and perforates the fascia at a variable level. It serves as a guideline for the exposure of the popliteal vein. The small saphenous vein is located under the fascia, usually very superficially. It is accompanied over its entire length by the medial cutaneous nerve of the calf, which must be carefully preserved. Dissection is often most difficult distal to the popliteal fossa because the nerves and vessels in this region have so many branches, often crossing one another. The tibial nerve with its various branches is visualized superficially, partially covering the popliteal vein. Behind the popliteal vein and somewhat more medially lies the artery. More cranially, the artery is located medial to the vein, while the sciatic or the tibial nerve passes lateral to the vein. When deeper structures, e.g., the popliteal muscle, have to be dissected, it is advisable to mobilize the neurovascular bundle first and then to dissect along the popliteal artery.

F. Intraoperative Diagnostics

The condition of the vascular wall may be judged by palpation. Intraoperative arteriography may give indications of the extent of the stenosis after decompression. However, it should be noted that the initial presence of a stenosis does not imply that it will persist. It is known that a peripheral pulse may become normalized, even some time after correction of the entrapment syndrome. However, a reconstruction will be necessary if the vascular wall is greatly altered or if an aneurysm or occlusion is found.

Careful examination of the location of the arteries and the veins in relation to the other structures of the popliteal fossa is also included in the intraoperative diagnostic measures. One should take careful note of any anomalies in the position of the medial head of the gastrocnemius muscle or any part of it; and one should likewise note accessory muscle fibers passing between both heads of the gastrocnemius muscles, the position of the plantaris muscle and the popliteal muscle in relation to the vessel, and finally the existence of fibrotic bands deep in the popliteal fossa. Darling [7] has drawn attention to the possibility of proving a compression mechanism during the operation by passive dorsal flexion of the foot. A compression caused by hypertrophy of the gastrocnemius muscles may be diagnosed in the same way [18].

G. Operative Techniques

I. Decompression

The preferred treatment of the popliteal entrapment syndrome consists of correction of the compression mechanism. Usually, simple myotomy is sufficient. The blood vessel (usually the artery, sometimes the vein) is dissected by separation of the overlying muscles – almost always the medial head of the gastrocnemius muscle. In case of other anomalies, accessory muscle bundles or crossing fibrotic bands are divided. Then, the blood vessels are placed in their normal position, and the divided muscles repositioned or, if necessary, fixated. The head of the gastrocnemius muscles may remain unsutured without causing loss of function. Anomalous muscle bundles or fibrotic bands are dissected as far as possible. When true muscle hypertrophy is the cause of the compression mechanism, those portions of the heads of the gastrocnemius muscles which lie opposite each other are partially resected. Also in the case of localized lesions of the vessel wall, such as thickening, or in case of a moderate remaining stenosis, simple myotomy is sufficient. However, it may take some months before the peripheral pulse is palpable or becomes completely normal. Occasionally peripheral pulses never become palpable, though the patient is free of symptoms [4, 5, 18].

II. Reconstruction

In cases of extensive vascular lesions over a longer segment, the medial approach is preferred and the popliteal artery is bridged by an infragenicular graft (for technique see p. 397ff.).

For treatment of local stenotic vascular lesions, endarterectomy in combination with a venous patch graft may be performed by a dorsal approach and the use of segment of the small saphenous vein is preferred. The results with this method, however, leave something to be desired. Therefore, it has recently become practice to resect the pathologic vascular segment and to replace it with a venous graft in the normal position between the structures of the popliteal fossa. It is usually necessary to use a segment of the great saphenous vein, but a segment of the small saphenous vein can also be used.

A popliteal artery aneurysm must be completely isolated and continuity restored by means of a vein graft or a bypass (see p. 281).

An additional lumbar sympathectomy should be considered whenever peripheral pulses are absent postoperatively. However, if ischemia is only slight, this procedure is not necessary since gradual improvement in the circulation may be expected without sympathectomy.

REFERENCES

1. Baker WH, Stoney RJ (1972) Acquired popliteal entrapment syndrome. Arch Surg 105:780–781
2. Biemans RGM, Bockel JH van (1977) Popliteal artery entrapment syndrome. Surg Gynecol Obstet 144:604–609
3. Bouhoutsos J (1980) Popliteal artery entrapment syndrome. Vasc Surg 14:365–374
4. Brightmore TGJ, Smellie WAB (1971) Popliteal artery entrapment. Br J Surg 58:481–484
5. Carter AE, Eban R (1964) A case of bilateral developmental abnormality of the popliteal arteries and gastrocnemius muscles. Br J Surg 51:518–522
6. Connell J (1978) Popliteal vein entrapment. Br J Surg 65:351
7. Darling RC, Buckley CJ, Abbott WM, Raines JK (1974) Intermittent claudication in young athletes. J Trauma 14:543–552
8. Downs AR, see discussion Insua JA and M, Ref 12
9. Hamming JJ (1959) Intermittent claudication at an early age, due to an anomalous course of the popliteal artery. Angiology 10:369–371
10. Hamming JJ, Vink M (1965) Obstruction of the popliteal artery at an early age. J Cardiovas Surg 6:516–524
11. Hohmann FR (1974) Chirurgie van de arteria poplitea. Thesis Leiden. Steens, Schiedam
12. Insua JA, Young JR, Humphries AW (1970) Popliteal artery entrapment syndrome. Arch Surg 101:771–775
13. Laubach K, Trede M, Perera R, Saggau W (1973) Das Kompressionssyndrom der A poplitea. Chirurg 44:74–77
14. Rich NM, Hughes CW (1967) Popliteal artery and vein entrapment. Am J Surg 113:696–698
15. Rich NM (1982) Popliteal entrapment and adventitial cystic disease. Surg Clin North Am 62:449–465
16. Servello M (1962) Clinical syndrome of anomalous position of the popliteal artery. Circulation 26:885–890
17. Turner Edmondson H, Crowe JA (1972) Popliteal arterial and venous entrapment. Am Surg 38:657–659
18. Van Bockel JH, Biemans RGM (1976) Popliteal artery entrapment; claudication during youth. Arch Chir Neerl 28:251–260

21.4 Entrapment Syndrome by the Tendinous Arch of the Soleus Muscle ("Soleus Syndrome")

O. Thetter

CONTENTS

Popliteal artery entrapment is mostly found in young healthy males who begin to present increasingly severe symptoms of claudication in the lower leg [4]. Often, these symptoms occur following overexertion or long periods of physical activity. In the last few years, this syndrome has often been diagnosed in joggers and part-time sports participants [6]. These symptoms are believed to be caused by compression of the popliteal artery, which is in turn due to an anomalous anatomic relation between the artery and the muscles in the popliteal fossa [2, 3, 5]. In the vast majority of cases, the course of the popliteal artery is displaced by an anomaly at the origin of the medial head of the gastrocnemius [1]. The deviation of the vessel causes kinking and, especially, a constant mechanical alteration of the arterial wall, which is increased by sports activity.

This chronic trauma leads to intimal lesions and consequently to the formation of thrombi; the final result is an occlusion.

By way of a supplement to the chapter on the popliteal artery entrapment syndrome, this chapter describes another compression mechanism within the popliteal fossa causing not only compression of the artery, but of the entire neurovascular bundle.

A. The Soleus Syndrome

In sports that make special demands on the calf muscles, swelling and hypertrophy of the soleus muscle may cause its tendinous arch (arcus tendineus musculi solei) to compress the popliteal artery and vein as well as the tibial nerve where they enter the popliteal canal. This causes chronic mechanical damage not only to the artery, as in the other compression mechanisms, but also to the vein and the nerve. This finally results in arterial and venous occlusion as well as damage to the tibial nerve.

B. Topography of the Popliteal Fossa Outlet

The popliteal artery and vein, as well as the tibial nerve, are deeply embedded in the fatty tissue of the popliteal fossa and pass distally, following a line defined by the long diagonal of the rhomboid popliteal space. They cross the planum popliteum femoris. They are then located on the posterior wall of the knee joint capsula and finally directly on the popliteal muscle. At the lower border of the popliteal muscle, the neurovascular bundle enters the popliteal canal, passing underneath the tendinous arch of the soleus muscle, fixed to the narrow entrance of the popliteal canal by short fibers of connective tissue [8, 9].

The soleus muscle arises from the posterior surface of the head and proximal third of the fibula, as well as from the popliteal line of the tibia. Both osseus origins are connected by the tendinous arch of the soleus muscle. This tendinous arch also serves as the muscle origin and, together with the lower border of the popliteal muscle, creates a hiatus, the popliteal canal. The popliteal vessels and the tibial nerve pass through this canal. This narrow opening can become even narrower due to swelling or hypertrophy of the soleus muscle; when this happens, the neurovascular bundle is

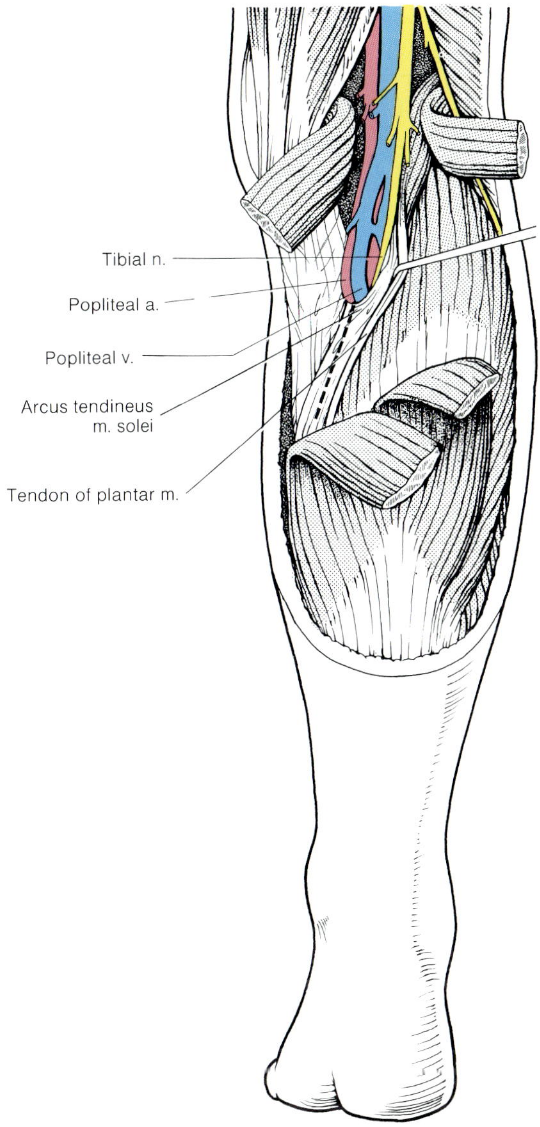

Fig. 21.4.1. Popliteal region with soleus syndrome. The broken line shows the operative approach, dividing the arch of the soleus muscle and dissecting the insertion of the soleus muscle off the posterior edge of the tibia

constricted. Artery, vein, and nerve are stretched over the tendinous arcade of the soleus muscle like a string over the bridge of a violin (Fig. 21.4.1).

C. Symptoms and Diagnosis

The symptoms of this special type of popliteal artery entrapment syndrome are mainly characterized by intermittent claudication or acute ischemia. Additionally, disturbances of the venous flow, as well as paresthesia and a sensation of weakness in the lower leg are described.

In most cases, such patients are first seen when an acute lower leg ischemia has already occurred. The patient describes increasing symptoms of claudication within the last few weeks, especially associated with sports activity.

When the patient is examined upon being admitted, the foot is white and cold, and pulses are absent. Clinical examination, Doppler ultrasonography, and angiography disclose occlusion of the popliteal artery somewhat distal to the knee joint cavity.

If an arterial occlusion has not yet developed, the compression mechanism can be demonstrated by means of provocation tests. A significant sign of the entrapment syndrome is the disappearance of foot pulses upon extension of the knee, extensive plantar flexion of the foot, and a fall in blood pressure, as measured by a Doppler probe.

In case of an acute angiographically proven occlusion of the popliteal artery in a young patient, one tries increasingly to recanalize the thrombotic occlusion by catheter lysis. This is successful in a relatively short time. On withdrawing the catheter, however, one gets the impression of an elastic constriction in this region. Angiography through the catheter placed in the femoral artery reveals compression of the popliteal artery during extension of the knee and plantar flexion of the foot. Following lysis, however, in the majority of cases, segmental thrombosis of the popliteal artery and ischemia of the lower leg recur.

The neurologic examination of the patients should include electromyography or measurement of the velocity of nerve conduction. With these methods, significant indications of compression of the tibial nerve may be revealed even if the symptoms are still tolerable.

Compression of the contralateral neurovascular bundle should be excluded as well, even in the absence of symptoms, because the entrapment may exist on both sides.

D. Therapy

Surgery is always indicated when an entrapment syndrome is diagnosed. Only an operation can provide the needed therapy, which consists of decompressing the artery or, in the case of the soleus syndrome, the artery together with the vein and the nerves.

In a young patient suffering from claudication, one should always regard an entrapment syndrome as indicative of possible ischemic damage. If a thrombotic occlusion has already occurred, the popliteal region must be exposed as quickly as possible. In the early stages of the occlusion, it may still be possible to restore vessel patency. However, if the vessel is already irreversibly damaged or if a thromboendarterectomy is no longer possible, then it is necessary to resect this vascular segment and replace it with a vein graft.

It is seldom possible to diagnose the exact compression mechanism preoperatively.

In the case of the soleus syndrome, the popliteal artery is exposed by a medial approach (see p. 281). The patient is placed in a supine position, with the leg flexed at the hip and rotated externally. The knee is flexed and supported by sterile cushions so that it may be moved intraoperatively. The medial approach always provides exposure of the entire popliteal artery and, if needed, of the superficial femoral artery as well as the branches to the lower leg. For exposure of the third popliteal segment and the trifurcation, a skin incision 1 cm dorsal to the medial edge of the tibia is sufficient. Following division of the fascia, the medial gastrocnemius muscle is retracted dorsally. Deep within the incision, the neurovascular bundle, located on the popliteal muscle, is dissected, a tape is placed around it, and the vessels are inspected. In the case of the soleus syndrome, an extremely hypertrophic soleus muscle will be found. Its tendinous arch presses the neurovascular structures to the inferior border of the popliteal muscle and to the complex of connective tissue within the tibiofibular interosseous space.

The thrombosed vessel is expanded in a bulb-like manner by the thrombus, which becomes conical toward the periphery. The tibial nerve may show a clearly visible furrow.

For correction of the compression mechanism in the case of the soleus syndrome, the popliteal canal must be dilated. This may be accomplished by division of the origin of the soleus muscle at the posterior surface of the tibia.

Additionally, the tendinous arch of the soleus muscle is divided. This procedure eliminates the constriction and provides exposure of the trifurcation. When there is no possibility of performing thromboendarterectomy of the occluded vessel, or when there are severe degenerative lesions [7], the only possible procedures are resection of the occluded segment and interposition of an autogenous saphenous vein graft.

REFERENCES

1. Delaney TA, Gonzales LL (1971) Occlusion of popliteal artery due to muscular entrapment. Surgery 69:97–101
2. Ezzet F, Yettra M (1971) Bilateral popliteal artery entrapment. J Cardiovasc Surg 12:71
3. Haimovici H, Sprayregen S, Johnson F (1972) Popliteal artery entrapment by fibrous band. Surgery 72:789–792
4. Ikeda M, Iwase T, Ashida K, Tankawa H (1981) Popliteal artery entrapment syndrome. Am J Surg 141:726–730
5. Lowe JW, Whelan TJ (1965) Popliteal artery entrapment syndrome. Am J Surg 109:620–624
6. Madigan RR, Mc Campbell BR (1982) Thrombosis of the popliteal artery in a jogger. J Bone Joint Surg [Am] 64:1490–1492
7. Palma EC (1978) The soleus syndrome. J Cardiovasc Surg 19:615–622
8. Sieglbauer F (1927) In: Lehrbuch der normalen Anatomie des Menschen. Urban and Schwarzenberg, Berlin Wien
9. Toldt C, Hochstetter F (1928) In: Anatomischer Atlas, vols 1 and 2, 14th edn. Urban und Schwarzenberg, Berlin Wien

21.5 Brachial Artery Entrapment Syndrome

R.G.M. BIEMANS

CONTENTS

A. Anatomy

At the level of the elbow joint, three muscle groups are located within a rigid space created by the skeleton and the brachial fascia (Fig. 21.5.1). When the elbow joint is flexed, the biceps brachii and brachial muscle glide, as it were, between the two muscle groups located laterally and medially to the cubital fossa and consisting of the bellies of the extensor and flexor muscles of the hand and the forearm (Figs. 21.5.2 and 21.5.5). As more muscles contract, the volume of the muscle bellies increases in direct proportion. The bicipital aponeurosis, a continuation of the tendon of the biceps, also stretches the ulnar portion of the fascia covering the pronator teres muscle. In case of muscular hypertrophy, the brachial artery may then become compressed between the pronator teres muscle and the bicipital aponeurosis. There is no development of collaterals because the most important potential collaterals pass on the volar side

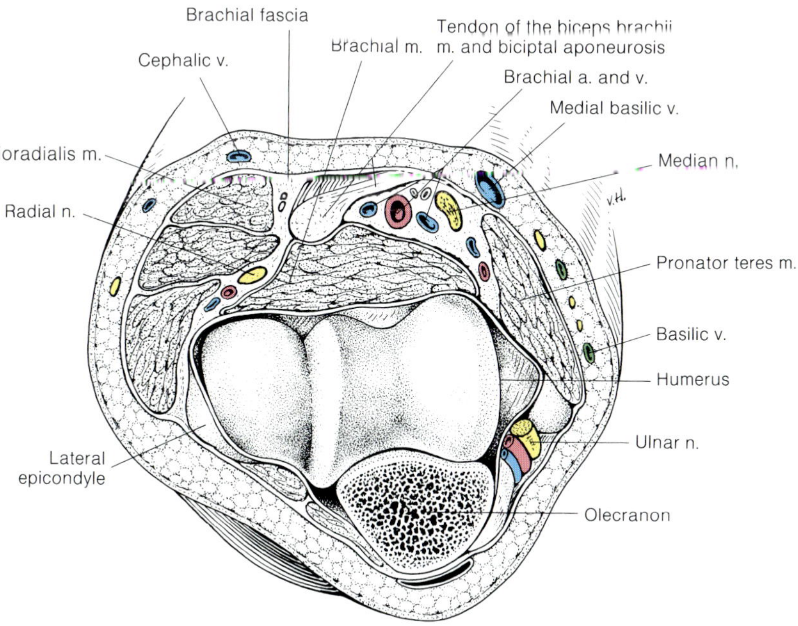

Fig. 21.5.1. Cross section at the level of the elbow joint. The brachial artery surrounded by muscle groups is located within a rigid space created by the skeleton and the brachial fascia

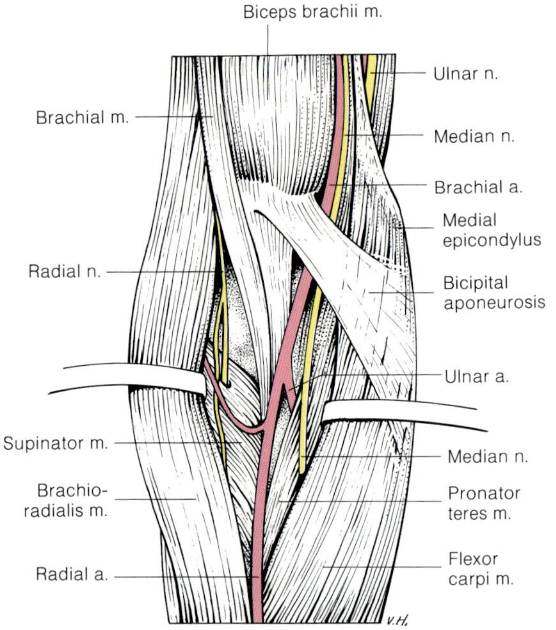

Fig. 21.5.2. The radial and ulnar muscle bellies with the biceps brachii and brachial muscle located in between. The brachial artery lies within the loose tissue of the cubital fossa

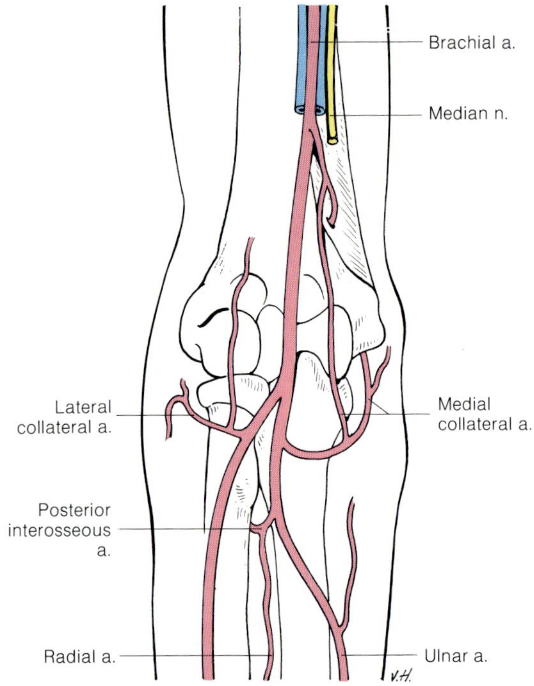

Fig. 21.5.3. The arterial circulation passes mainly volar of the arm bones and within the brachial fascia

Fig. 21.5.4. Division of the bicipital aponeurosis, relationship with the surrounding structures

▽

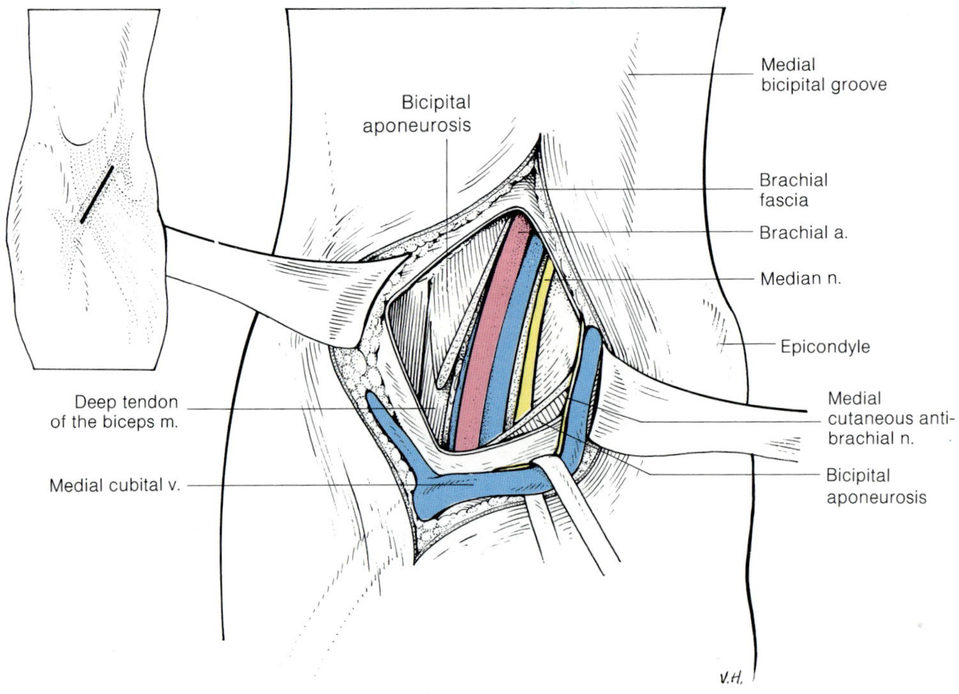

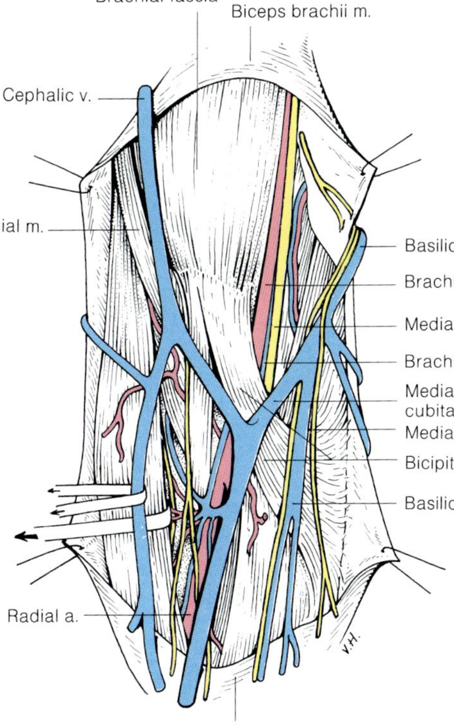

Fig. 21.5.5. As in Fig. 21.5.2, but showing the location of the surrounding structures to be preserved

and are therefore affected by the same mechanism (Fig. 21.5.3). Venous obstruction does not occur because unimpeded venous flow is possible outside the fascia.

B. Indications for Operation

Brachial artery entrapment is found in unusually muscular men who have done heavy work with their arms for many years. Division of the bicipital aponeurosis is indicated when there are symptoms such as early fatigue of the muscles of the hand and the arm, sometimes accompanied by irritation or excessive sensations of cold in the hand. The pulse of the brachial artery disappears just peripheral to the bicipital aponeurosis when the muscles of the hand and forearm are strongly contracted and the elbow is strongly flexed (simulation of the movements required in the work situation). This provocation test may also be performed during angiography.

C. Operative Treatment

The treatment is simple and consists of decompression of the brachial artery by division of the bicipital aponeurosis. The procedure may be performed under local anesthesia at the site where the brachial artery crosses the bicipital aponeurosis, which is palpable if stretched (Fig. 21.5.4). The cubital median vein and the branches of the medial cutaneous nerve of the forearm pass subcutaneously and are carefully preserved. Following exposure of the bicipital aponeurosis over its entire width, it is carefully divided over the brachial artery. Care is taken not to injure the artery and the median nerve.

REFERENCES

1. Biemans RGM (1977) Brachial artery entrapment syndrome. J Cardiovas Surg 18:367–371
2. Biemans RGM (1984) The Popeye syndrome – brachial artery entrapment as a result of muscular hypertrophy. Neth J Surg 36:103–106
3. Lanz T von, Wachsmuth W (1959) Praktische Anatomie, vol I, part 3, 2nd edn. Springer, Berlin Göttingen Heidelberg

22 Revascularization of the Visceral Arteries

R.J.A.M. van Dongen and E.-D. Schwilden

CONTENTS

A. Anatomy

Four arteries contribute to the blood supply of the gastrointestinal tract: the celiac axis, the superior mesenteric artery, the inferior mesenteric artery, and finally the internal iliac artery, which is the only artery not exclusively supplying the intestine (Fig. 22.1).

The *celiac axis*, supplying the organs in the upper abdomen, branches off from the anterior wall of the aorta at the level of the twelfth thoracic or first lumbar vertebra. Its length varies, usually between 0.5 and 4 cm. However, it may measure up to 6 cm. A true tripus, i.e., simultaneous branching into three arteries (common hepatic artery, splenic artery, left gastric artery) is found only in 25%. Bifurcation is more common, consisting of the splenic artery and the common hepatic artery while the left gastric artery arises more proximally as a solitary branch. The inferior phrenic arteries are variable branches of the celiac axis.

The *splenic artery*, which is the largest branch, always – or nearly always – arises from the celiac axis, to the right of the middle of the aorta. The splenic artery crosses the aorta and passes to the left, cranial to the splenic vein and in close contact with the pancreas. The course along the pancreas varies. In 90% of cases, the artery is located at the upper border of the pancreas, in 8% behind the pancreas, and in 2% in front of the pancreas. A striking feature of the splenic artery is its more or less pronounced coiling, allowing one to stretch the vessel to about three times its length. This is encountered in more than 85% of cases. The branches of the splenic artery show many variations in origin, caliber, vascular bed, and topography. To the extent that one may speak of a normal anatomy, the following arteries branch off the splenic artery proceeding from proximal to distal:

1. Dorsal pancreatic artery
2. Greater pancreatic artery
3. Rami pancreatici
4. Left gastroepiploic artery
5. Short gastric arteries
6. Superior and inferior terminal arteries

Variable branches are an upper or lower pole artery, an accessory left gastric artery, and an inferior phrenic artery.

The *hepatic artery* is the second important branch of the celiac axis with respect to revascularization. In its course to the right the gastroduodenal artery branches off at the level of the pylorus. It then continues as the proper hepatic artery, with the right gastric artery branching off. Finally, it branches into a right, left, and sometimes a middle hepatic artery within the hilus of the liver. A right

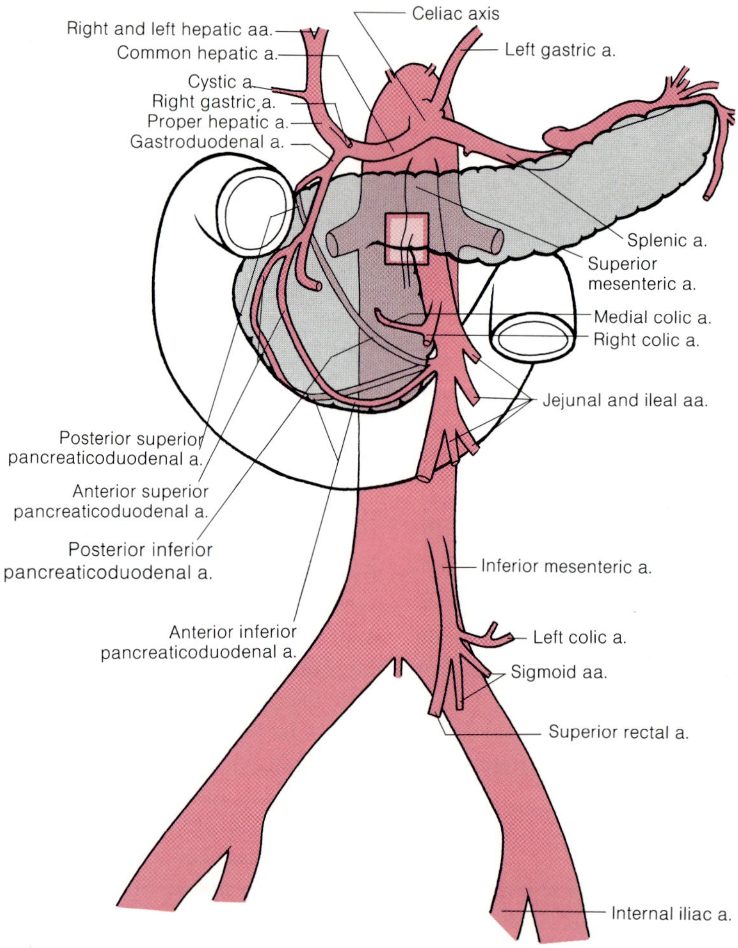

Fig. 22.1. Anatomy of the intestinal arteries. The upper intestinal arteries show many variations, but these are not of great significance for reconstructive procedures. As depicted here, the branches of the mesenteric artery show an anatomic variation that is very frequently encountered. In most cases the inferior pancreaticoduodenal artery branches off the superior mesenteric artery as the first branch before the medial colic artery, as described in the text and depicted in the inset

hepatic artery, originating from the superior mesenteric artery (about 15%) or from an accessory right hepatic artery, is of no significance for revascularization.

The *superior mesenteric artery* takes off from the anterior wall of the aorta between the twelfth thoracic and the second lumbar vertebra. First, it passes behind the pancreas, then crosses the third part of the duodenum as well as the uncinate process of the pancreas, and finally enters the mesenteric root. The first constant branch is the inferior pancreaticoduodenal artery. It either consists of a common trunk, branching later into an anterior and posterior artery, or originates directly as two branches from the superior mesenteric artery. Before entering the mesenteric root (just below the origin of the inferior pancreaticoduodenal artery), the superior mesenteric artery gives off its next branch, the medial colic artery, passing to the right. In about 45% of cases, the vessel is solitary. Otherwise, it shows a common trunk together with the right colic artery. The further course shows a convexity to the left, passing down to the right lower abdominal quadrant. Along its course, further branches to the right are the right colic and the ileocolic artery and to the left the jejunal and ileal arteries.

The *inferior mesenteric artery* originates from the left anterior wall of the aorta, approximately at the level of the third lumbar vertebra, 3–5 cm above the aortic bifurcation. The arterial trunk passes downward over a distance of 2–4 cm, parallel to the aorta. Then, the first branch, the left colic artery, arises from it to pass upward. In its further course, in an oblique direction to the left and downward, several branches to the sigmoid colon take off. Its final segment represents the superior rectal artery, connected to the medial rectal artery by the perirectal anastomoses. The medial rectal artery is either a direct branch of the *internal iliac artery* or a subsidiary branch of internal iliac artery branches supplying the pelvic organs.

B. Indications for Reconstruction

I. Of the Celiac Axis and the Superior Mesenteric Artery

A clear *therapeutic indication for operation* is given in all patients suffering from clinical symptoms of intestinal angina as a result of a proven occlusion or stenosis of the superior mesenteric artery and/or the celiac axis [4, 13, 14, 28]. The operation is indicated, first, to relieve the patient's symptoms and, second, to prevent mesenteric infarction. There is no general indication for prophylactic reconstruction since objective investigations have never demonstrated that, as a rule, an asymptomatic occlusion of a visceral artery leads to an infarction [2, 6, 7, 12, 17, 22, 24]. However, a *prophylactic reconstruction* should be performed in the following cases, provided the criteria for general operability are optimally fulfilled:

1. When there are double occlusions or double stenoses. In such cases, the entire intestine is usually supplied by just one artery, and an additional diminution of this irreplaceable source of collaterals may have deleterious effects. This may happen, for instance, through progression of the underlying disease or as a result of hypotension of various origin (cardiac, operative).

2. When there are simultaneous intra abdominal occlusive diseases to be corrected. This is on the understanding that should a visceral arterial reconstruction later be indicated, access to the operative field would be much more difficult, and the operative risk therefore much higher, as a result of the previous operation.

3. When operations are indicated that require ligation of an artery serving as a collateral. Usually, the artery involved is the inferior mesenteric artery. Ligation of this artery – for example when an aortic aneurysm is resected and there is simultaneous occlusion of the superior mesenteric artery – may have disastrous consequences for the intestinal blood supply.

4. When a renal artery reconstruction for renovascular hypertension is performed. In this case, the collateral circulation may owe its functional effectiveness to hypertension and may therefore suffer serious impairment when blood pressure is normalized.

II. Of the Inferior Mesenteric and Internal Iliac Arteries

Reconstructions of the inferior mesenteric artery and/or the internal iliac artery are practically never undertaken for therapeutic purposes because a single occlusion in these regions has so far not been known to cause intestinal angina. If combined with occlusive disease of the celiac axis and/or the superior mesenteric artery, reconstruction of these latter arteries has absolute priority. Under certain circumstances it may be possible, as a supplementary procedure, to correct a stenosis at the origin of the inferior mesenteric artery by simple, open thromboendarterectomy and patch graft angioplasty. As for prophylactic procedures the intention to preserve an artery that serves as a collateral has priority over reconstruction of a stenosed vessel. This holds above all for reconstructive surgery in cases of aortic aneurysms or aortoiliac occlusive disease. Where there is simultaneous occlusion of the superior mesenteric artery, the inferior mesenteric artery serves as an important collateral and should not be ligated.

And the same holds true if during resection of an aortic aneurysm both internal iliac arteries are ligated simultaneously with the inferior mesenteric artery: the blood supply to the left colon is endangered.

III. Multiple Reconstructions

Enough experience has been gained to indicate that, in cases of multiple occlusions, reconstruction of a single artery is sufficient to relieve the symptoms. Usually, priority is given to the superior mesenteric artery, although it has not yet been demonstrated conclusively that this must be so. On the contrary, it has been said that reocclusion of a single reconstruction usually causes new symptoms, even infarction. However, following double reconstructions, most patients remain asymptomatic, and there is no risk of infarction, even if a thrombosis occurs in one of the reconstructed arteries. Therefore, perhaps one should prefer double reconstruction:

a) When a major operation can be tolerated by the patient
b) When the procedure is technically not too difficult
c) When the venous material for reconstruction is optimal
d) When collateral circulation is poor

C. Positioning

For visceral arterial reconstruction the patient is placed in a supine position if the approach is to be exclusively transabdominal.

For harvesting the great saphenous vein, access should be provided to an area extending from both inguinal regions to the middle of the thigh. External rotation of the thigh and flexion of the knee is advantageous. It is important that both groins be draped in case the greater saphenous vein on one side is not suitable. If only patch grafts are required, the vein segment should not be harvested from the groin, thereby sacrificing the entire vein, but rather from the ankle region. Appropriate draping for this procedure is required.

With a thoracoabdominal approach, it has been shown that it is beneficial to turn the patient slightly to the right and to lift the left half of the thorax by placing a cushion underneath it and simultaneously to elevate the left arm (Fig. 22.2). In relatively obese patients, the approach to the great saphenous vein in the groin may be impaired in this position. In these cases the vein should be harvested before the patient is positioned for the thoracoabdominal incision.

D. Operative Approach

Several incisions may be used to approach the visceral arteries (Fig. 22.3):

1. Median supraumbilical longitudinal incision
2. Right-sided paramedian incision
3. Right-sided pararectal incision
4. Left-sided subcostal incision
5. Transverse supraumbilical incision
6. Left-sided thoracoabdominal incision

The median, paramedian, and pararectal supraumbilical incisions and the transverse supraumbilical incision are suitable for reimplantations, venous

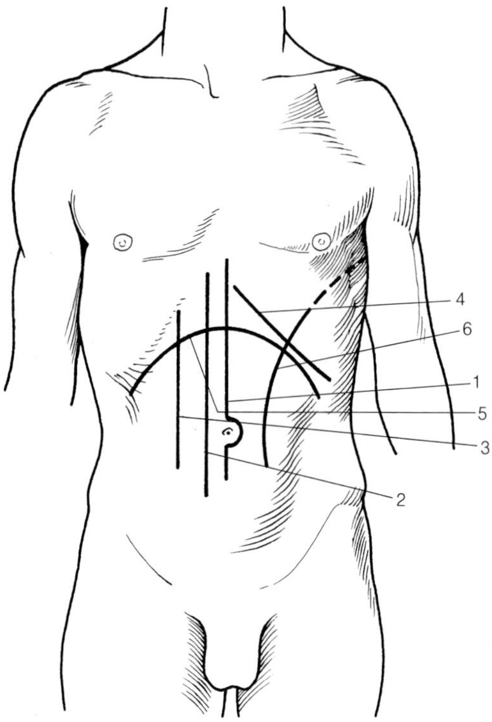

Fig. 22.3. Approaches to the visceral arteries. Skin incisions. *1*, Median longitudinal incision; *2*, right-sided paramedian longitudinal incision; *3*, right-sided pararectal longitudinal incision; *4*, left-sided subcostal incision; *5*, transverse supraumbilical incision; *6*, left-sided thoracoabdominal incision

Fig. 22.2. Positioning for a left-sided thoracoabdominal approach. The left half of the thorax and pelvis are elevated by cushions

▽

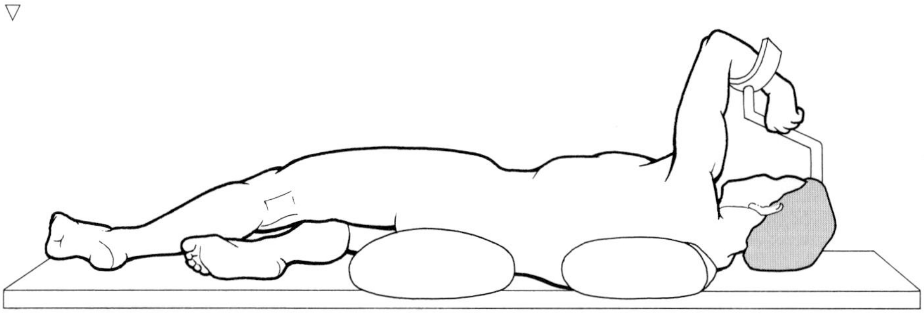

bypasses, or bridge grafts. When simultaneous reconstructions in the aortoiliac region are planned, longitudinal incisions should be preferred. In cases of simultaneous reconstruction of renal arteries, a transverse incision seems to be more suitable.

For the in situ bypass of the splenic artery, a large left subcostal incision may be sufficient when the epigastric angle is wide and the patient is not too obese. If difficulties arise, the incision can simply be extended to the right. More favorable for the in situ bypass of the splenic artery is a small thoracoabdominal incision at the eighth intercostal space, especially in obese patients. The diaphragm is incised over a short distance to provide better access.

Open thromboendarterectomy, with or without patch graft angioplasty at the origins of the visceral arteries, as well as bypasses from the thoracic aorta require a left-sided thoracoabdominal approach, dividing the diaphragm to the hiatus. The exposure should always be performed transabdominally, but not exclusively extraperitoneally, because careful examination of the entire abdomen is always mandatory.

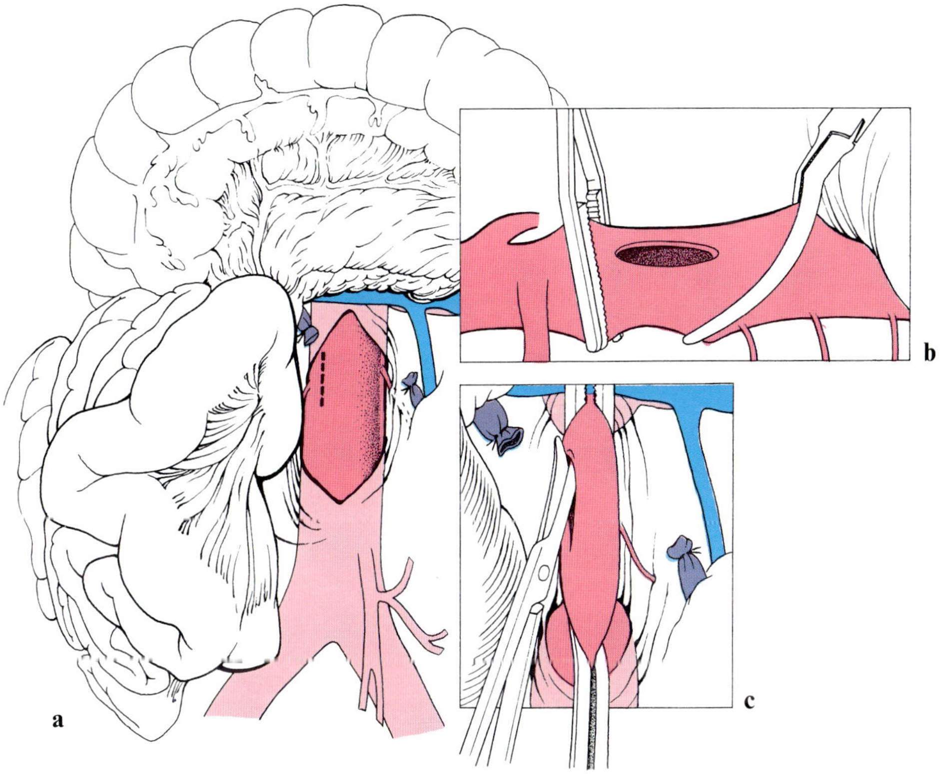

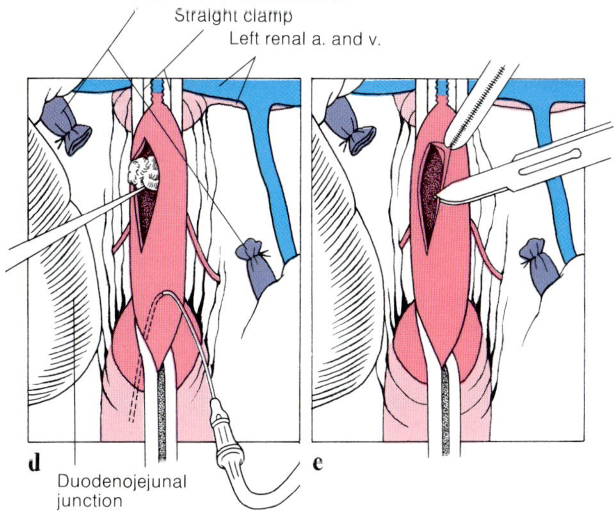

Fig. 22.4a–e. Infracolic exposure and opening of the aorta. **a** The transverse colon is drawn up, the entire intestine is retracted to the right, and the duodenojejunal flexure is mobilized; then the peritoneum is incised over the infrarenal aorta, thereby dividing the inferior mesenteric vein. **b** Clamping of the infrarenal aortic segment from the surgeon's viewpoint. The proximal straight clamp is placed perpendicularly on the aorta below the renal arteries. The distal spoon-shaped or curved clamp is placed obliquely, so as to simultaneously cross-clamp the lumbar arteries. **c** Longitudinal incision in the right anterior wall of the aorta. Extension of the aortotomy using scissors. **d** Inspection of the aortic lumen and removal of thrombi and plaques. Local distal heparinization by continuous heparin infusion. **e** Excision of the edges of the aortotomy and smoothing with Pott's scalpel

E. Technique for Exposure of the Visceral Arteries

I. Aorta

Exposure of the infrarenal aorta is by either an infracolic or a supracolic approach.

With the infracolic exposure (Fig. 22.4a), the transverse colon is drawn up and the entire intestine retracted to the right. Following mobilization of the duodenojejunal flexure, the retroperitoneum is incised over the anterior surface of the aorta, between the origin of the renal arteries and the inferior mesenteric artery. The crossing inferior mesenteric vein can be divided without hesitation.

The supracolic exposure is performed either from the left or from the right (see p. 615).

Dissection of the anterior circumference of the aorta over a distance of about 4–5 cm is sufficient for cross-clamping and anastomosis. Mobilization of the entire circumference of the aorta, including the segmental lumbar arteries, is not required.

There are two ways to clamp the aorta – partial and total occlusion. Partial clamping (e.g., with a Satinsky clamp) is usually not sufficient for an optimal anastomosis with the superior mesenteric artery or a vein transplant because the aortic orifice is not well exposed, and exact placement of the sutures is impaired.

The anastomosis is better performed following complete occlusion provided by two clamps placed perpendicularly. If there is still reflux from a lumbar artery, a spoon-shaped or curved clamp can be placed distally to occlude those arteries as well (Fig. 22.4b). Intraoperative systemic or local heparinization of the distal aorta is required to avoid distal thrombosis (Fig. 22.4d).

Following cross-clamping, the aorta is incised at the site selected for the anastomosis, either transversely, longitudinally, or obliquely, depending on the type of reconstruction (Fig. 22.4c). In most cases, excision of a wall segment measuring about 3 × 8 mm is more favorable than simple incision. The lumen of the aorta is examined and, if necessary, cleaned of plaques (Fig. 22.4d). The same procedure must be carried out at the edges of the orifice, which may have to be smoothed with a small Pott's scalpel (Fig. 22.4e). When exposure and cross-clamping of the aorta have to be performed at the thoracic level or at the origin of the celiac axis and the superior mesenteric artery, only tangential placement of a clamp can be considered, owing to the risk of neurologic or renal complications [1].

II. Origins of the Celiac Axis and Superior Mesenteric Artery

Following a left-sided thoracoabdominal incision (Fig. 22.5a), the colon, spleen, and pancreas are mobilized and, together with the stomach, retracted medially. Using the kidney and the left renal vein at the base of the operative field as a guideline, the dissection is carried out in the direction of the aorta (Fig. 22.5b). The origins of the celiac axis and the superior mesenteric artery are isolated and vessel loops are placed around them (Fig. 22.5c). The distal dissection of both branches

Fig. 22.5a–c. Left-sided thoracoabdominal approach to the origin of the celiac trunk and the superior mesenteric artery. **a** Positioning of the patient, with cushions under the left half of the thorax and the pelvis. Upper pararectal incision on the left side, extending into the seventh intercostal space. **b** Following incision of the diaphragm and incision of the peritoneum lateral to the descending colon, the left half of the colon, together with the spleen and the pancreas, are dissected off toward the right, the left renal vein at the base of the operative field serving as a guideline. Dissection is continued until the aorta and the origin of the celiac axis and the superior mesenteric artery are sufficiently exposed. **c** The celiac axis and the superior mesenteric artery are isolated and vessel loops are placed around them (surgeon's view). Tangential placement of a clamp on the aorta at the level of the origin of the two upper intestinal arteries

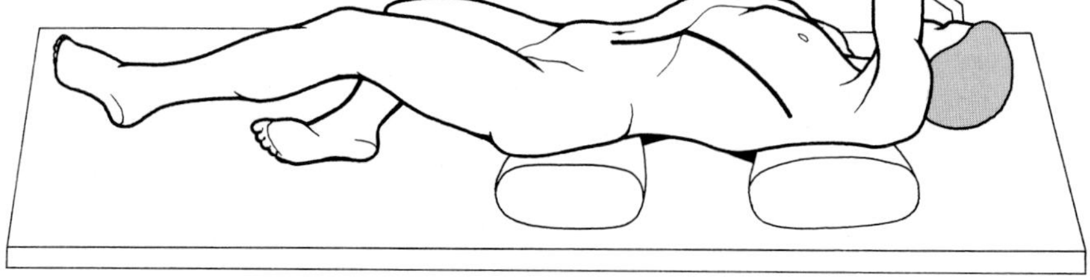

a

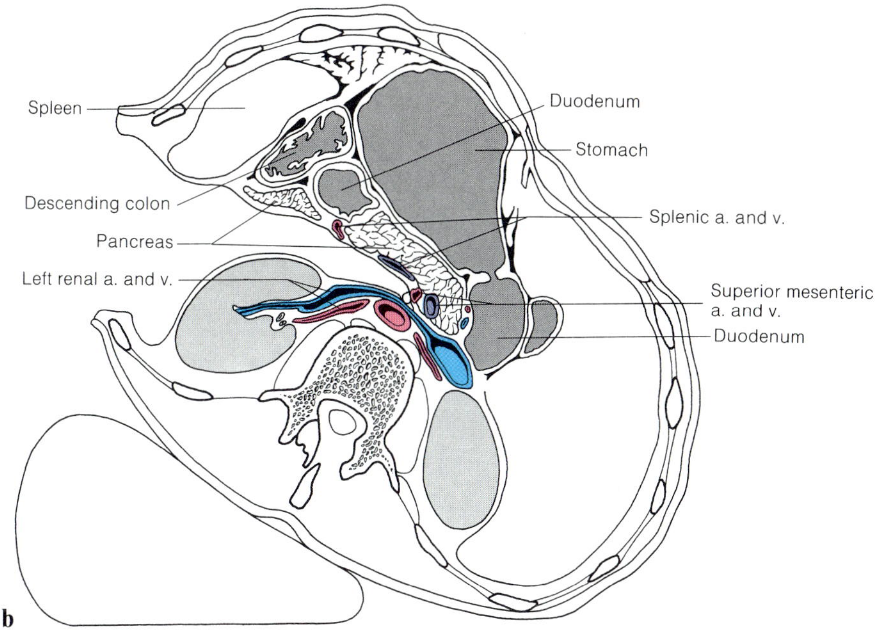
Spleen
Duodenum
Stomach
Descending colon
Splenic a. and v.
Pancreas
Left renal a. and v.
Superior mesenteric a. and v.
Duodenum

b

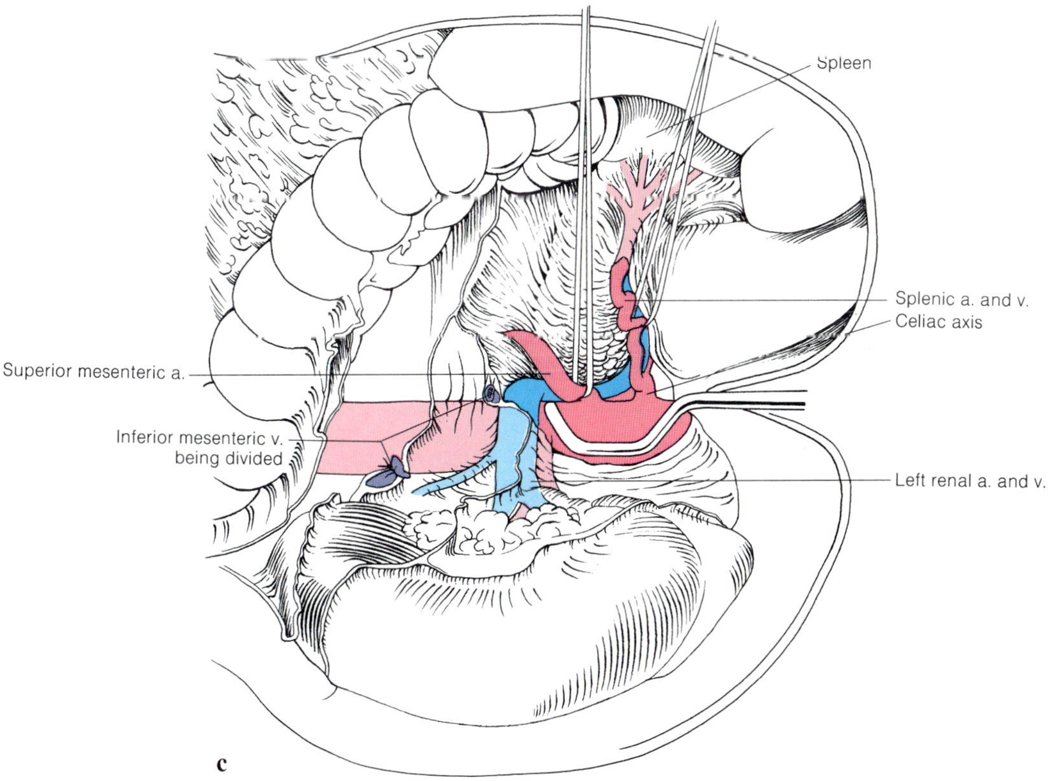
Spleen
Splenic a. and v.
Celiac axis
Superior mesenteric a.
Inferior mesenteric v. being divided
Left renal a. and v.

c

is continued sufficiently far into the disease-free segment. The aorta itself is exposed only to the extent necessary for tangential placement of a clamp (encompassing the origins of the celiac axis and the superior mesenteric artery) without impairing renal circulation (Fig. 22.5c). At the same time, it should be possible to make a sufficiently long incision in each visceral artery; each of these incisions should extend into the aortic wall.

III. Hepatic and Splenic Artery

The dissection of the hepatic artery is carried out through the lesser omentum (Fig. 22.6). The serosa is divided in the region of the hepatoduodenal ligament, and the artery, which is usually located cranial to the bile duct and ventral to the portal vein, is dissected. Vessel loops are placed around the gastroduodenal and right gastric arteries. Prior to the arteriotomy, careful dilation of the arterial segment that will be clamped for the anastomosis is beneficial. The lumen of the artery can sometimes be dilated to a diameter twice as large as the original one. This greatly facilitates the anastomosis.

The dissection of the splenic artery is performed using a supracolic approach through the lesser omentum, with temporary division of the gastrocolic ligament (Fig. 22.7). The splenic artery is usually found at the upper border of the pancreas, or from below, when the artery's course is retropancreatic. Mobilization of the segment required for the anastomosis is carried out by dividing the pancreatic branches, the ends of which are carefully closed by small suture ligatures. Mobilization of the pancreatic tail may facilitate dissection of the artery.

IV. Trunk of the Superior Mesenteric Artery

For exposure of the trunk of the superior mesenteric artery, two approaches may be considered in addition to the left-sided thoracoabdominal one: the infracolic and the right-sided retrocolic or supracolic [16] approach.

Fig. 22.6. Exposure of the hepatic artery through the lesser omentum. Dissection and placement of vessel loops around the gastroduodenal and right gastric arteries. Following cross-clamping of theses two arteries, the proximal common hepatic and the proper hepatic artery, careful dilation of the arterial segment for the anastomosis, with heparinized saline solution. While the solution is being injected, clotting in the isolated vascular segments can be avoided by releasing the clamps one after the other

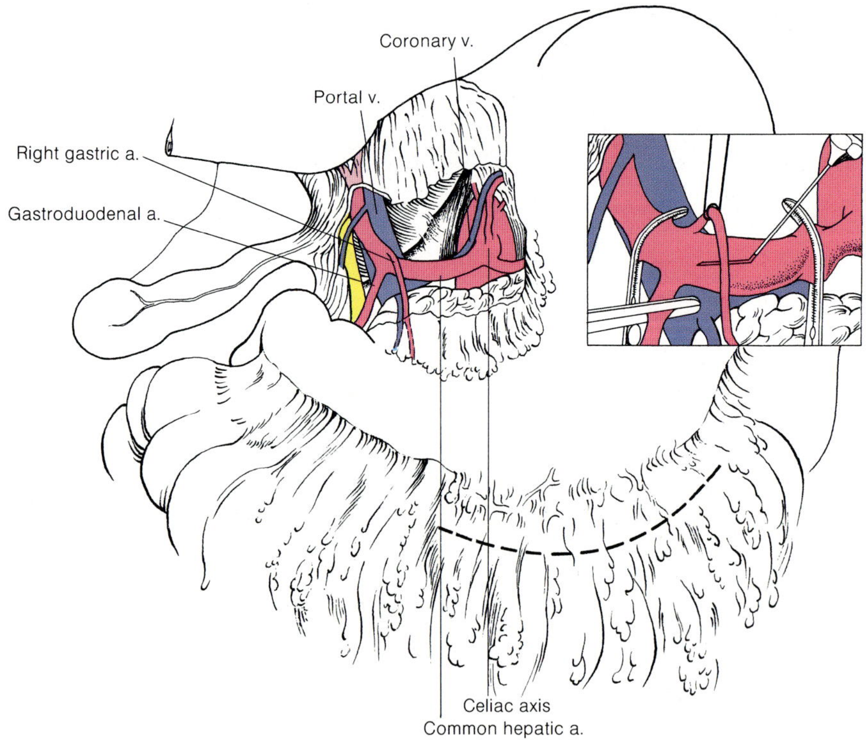

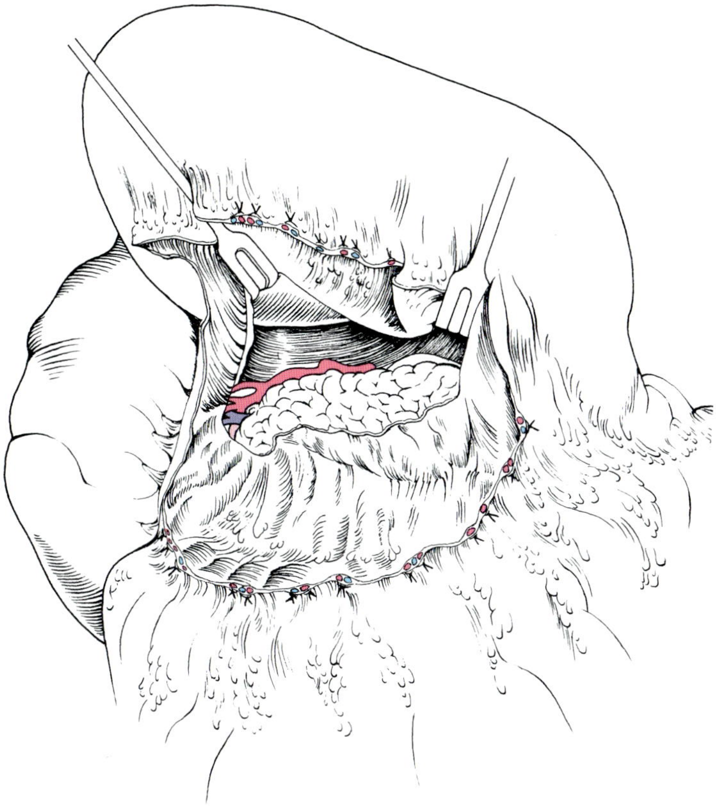

Fig. 22.7. Supracolic exposure of the splenic artery through the lesser omentum following division of the gastrocolic ligament

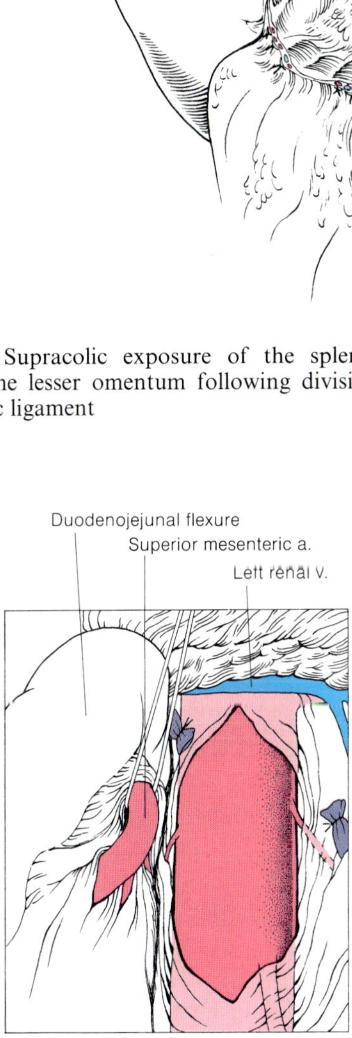

Fig. 22.8. Infracolic exposure of the superior mesenteric artery. The transverse colon is drawn up and the entire intestine retracted; the superior mesenteric artery is then dissected at the root of the mesentery

For infracolic exposure (Fig. 22.8), the colon is drawn up and the entire intestine retracted to the right. While searching for the superior mesenteric artery, palpation of the vessel at the level of the inferior part of the duodenum is beneficial. If one does not succeed in identifying the artery by palpation, the peritoneum is opened at the crossing of the mesenteric vascular bundle and the inferior part of the duodenum. The artery is exposed by careful dissection of the tissue. Side branches may serve as guidelines. Accidental injury to the concomitant veins can be avoided if one bears in mind that the venous mesenteric trunk lies to the right of the artery. Careful dilation of the superior mesenteric artery prior to arteriotomy and anastomosis may be beneficial.

For the right-sided retrocolic or supracolic exposure of the trunk of the superior mesenteric artery (Fig. 22.9a, b), the peritoneum is incised along the lateral duplication of the ascending colon. The duodenum is mobilized according to KOCHER. The colon and duodenum are turned medially. The anterior surface of the vena cava is dissected and the right spermatic or ovarian vein is divided between ligatures near the origin. After the horizontal part of the duodenum is dissected away from

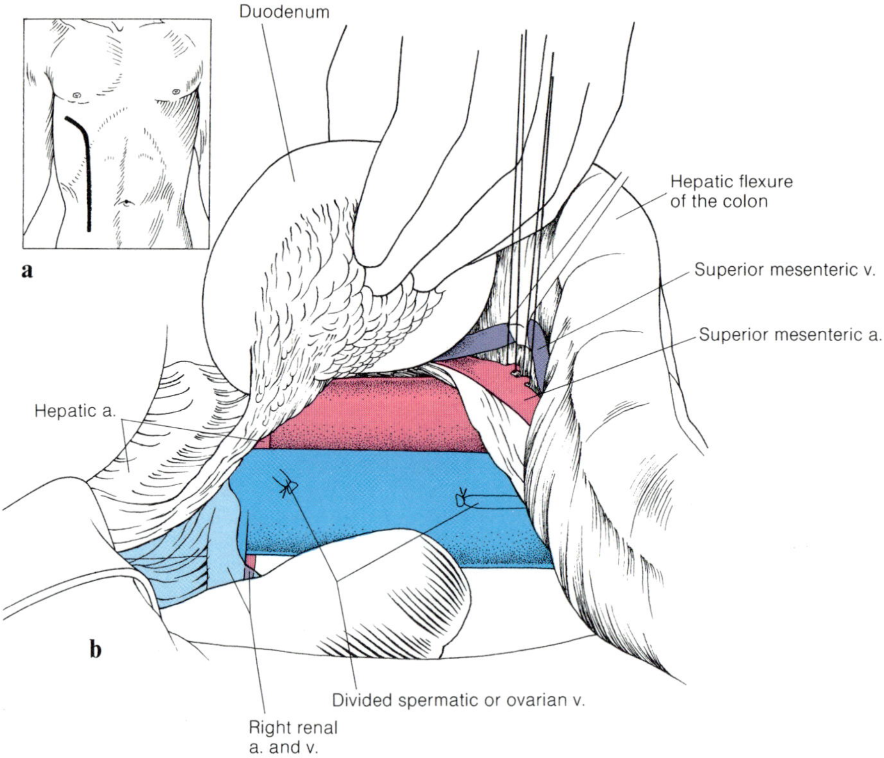

Fig. 22.9 a, b. Right-sided retrocolic or supracolic exposure of the superior mesenteric artery and the infrarenal aorta. **a** Right-sided pararectal incision with short extension beyond the costal arch into the seventh intercostal space. **b** Exposure of the superior mesenteric artery, as seen by the surgeon. The ascending colon, together with the hepatic flexure and the duodenum with the head of the pancreas are mobilized and drawn up, exposing the vena cava. Division of the spermatic or right ovarian vein. Identification and dissection of the superior mesenteric artery at the posterior aspect of the mesentery. Dissection of the infrarenal aorta at the bottom of the operative field to the left of the inferior vena cava

the surroundings, the superior mesenteric artery can be identified at the posterior aspect of the mesentery by bidigital palpation. It is dissected as proximally as possible, and a vessel loop is placed around it. Tourniquets are placed around all jejunal tributaries passing to the left.

At the bottom of the operative field, left of the vena cava, the infrarenal segment of the aorta is exposed without difficulty [5].

F. Intraoperative Diagnosis

By palpation one can assess the occlusion and the degree of stenosis and gain some idea as to the condition of the arterial wall distal to the occlusive disease. Then, the pressure in the aorta, in the postocclusive segment of the artery, and in the patent intestinal arteries is measured. Finally, blood flow in the various intestinal arteries and in the large collaterals (gastroduodenal artery, Riolan arch) is measured.

G. Techniques of Reconstruction

[9, 10, 11, 15, 18, 19, 20, 25, 26]

I. Open Thromboendarterectomy

Historically, this was the first method employed. In principle, it is quite suitable for short stenoses or occlusions where the end point of the atherosclerotic lesion is abruptly separated from the normal fixed intima.

The safest approach and the best exposure are provided by a left-sided thoracoabdominal incision. However, this has the disadvantage of being a two-cavity operation, and it poses problems for the simultaneous correction of extended aortoiliac occlusive disease [3].

The exclusively transabdominal exposure of the celiac axis (through the lesser omentum) and of the origin of the superior mesenteric artery (infracolic or through the lesser sac of the omentum) avoids opening the thorax, but is not recommended. The dissection of the vessel itself does not cause too much difficulty. However, adequate exposure of the appropriate aortic segments requires a relatively large dissection. Additionally, cross-clamping of the aorta at the site of origin of the visceral branches carries some risk. The risky and insecure clamping of the aorta usually does not allow one to suture the patch far enough into the aortic wall to provide for adequate dilation.

Therefore, open thromboendarterectomy with patch graft angioplasty is suitable only for reconstruction of a stenosis at the origin of the inferior mesenteric artery and the rare distal stenosis of the superior mesenteric artery.

II. Transection and Reimplantation into the Aorta

Another method, not requiring difficult dissection of the origins of the celiac axis and the superior mesenteric artery, is the division of the vessels distal to the occlusion followed by reimplantation into the aorta. Reimplantation of the celiac axis may be possible only at a higher level, i.e., the thoracic aorta. A disadvantage is the large abdomino-thoracic incision. Therefore, this type of reconstruction is limited almost exclusively to the superior mesenteric and inferior mesenteric arteries [21].

In the case of the superior mesenteric artery, the peripheral stump is anastomosed end-to-side to the infrarenal aorta following division. For this procedure, the infracolic approach (Figs. 22.8 and 22.10a–d) as well as the left- and right-sided retrocolic approaches for exposure of the superior mesenteric artery and the infrarenal aorta (Figs. 22.5, 22.9, and 22.13) are suitable.

When direct reimplantation of the superior mesenteric artery is impossible without undue ten-

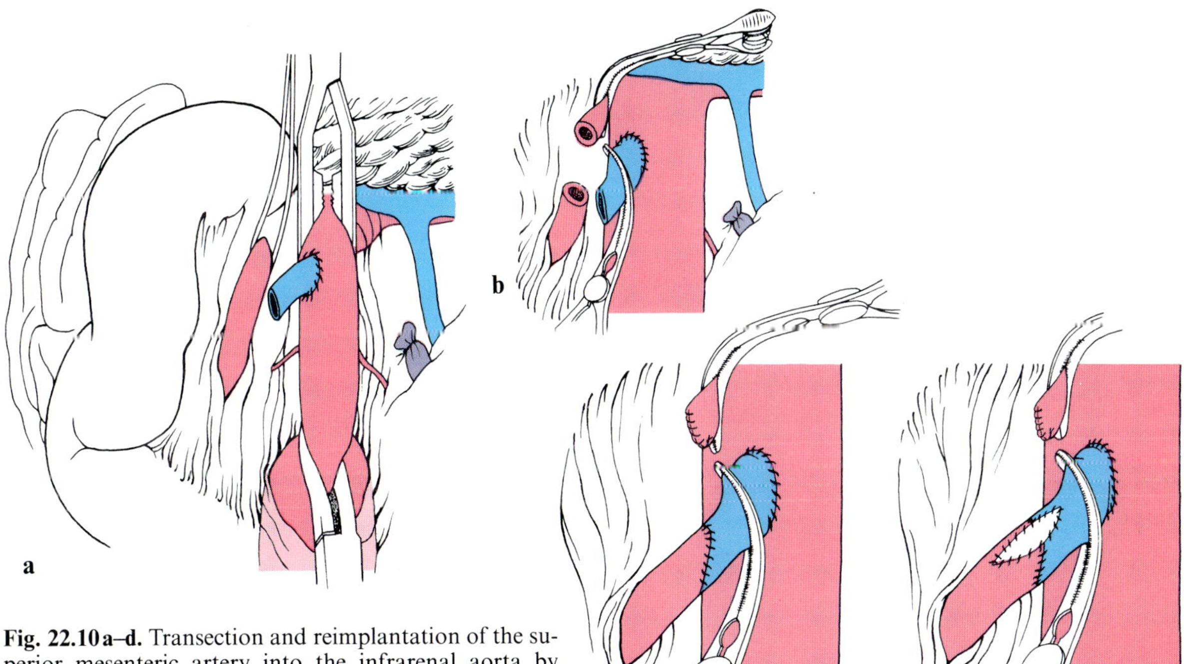

Fig. 22.10a–d. Transection and reimplantation of the superior mesenteric artery into the infrarenal aorta by means of a vein graft. The drawings show the various steps in the procedure following infracolic exposure of the aorta and the superior mesenteric artery. **a** Following dissection of the trunk of the superior mesenteric artery and clamping of the infrarenal aortic segment, the vein graft, with its end tailored to achieve a greater orifice, is anastomosed to an opening in the right anterior wall of the aorta. **b** Cross-clamping of the vein graft close to the anastomosis and declamping of the aorta; division of the superior mesenteric artery distal to the occlusion. **c** Anastomosis of the distal stump of the superior mesenteric artery to the vein graft. Over-and-over suture of the proximal stump of the mesenteric artery. **d** Suture of a venous patch into the distal anastomosis

sion on the anastomosis, a graft can be interposed (Fig. 22.10a–d). For this purpose the great saphenous vein is preferred as a source of material. Its ends can be dilated by several techniques (Fig. 22.17). Instead of venous segments, autogenous arterial grafts, taken from the splenic or the external iliac artery and then replaced by a prosthesis, may be interposed. Segments of internal iliac artery should not be used as this would mean the interruption of an important collateral donor vessel. A precondition for any of these reimplantation techniques is that the wall of the infrarenal aorta is in relatively good condition.

First, the graft is anastomosed end-to-side to the infrarenal aorta (Fig. 22.10a). Following cross-clamping of the graft close to the anastomosis, the blood flow to the distal aorta is released (Fig. 22.10b). Then, the superior mesenteric artery is divided distal to the occlusion, and the proximal stump is closed by atraumatic over-and-over suture (Fig. 22.10c). The end-to-end anastomosis of the graft, tailored exactly to match the length, to the stump of the superior mesenteric artery is performed either obliquely, S-shaped, or semicircumferentially, using a vein patch (Fig. 22.10d).

Reimplantation is the method of choice for maintaining an inferior mesenteric artery that functions as a collateral (Fig. 22.11a, b). That it does in fact function as a significant collateral must be established before it is divided. In such a case, for instance in aortic aneurysm, it should not be divided at its takeoff from the aorta, but should be excised with a Carrel patch. This will facilitate anastomosis to the bifurcated prosthesis, which must be clamped tangentially.

III. In Situ Bypass

Owing to its length, the splenic artery is well suited to serve as an in situ bypass for revascularization not only of the celiac axis, but of the superior mesenteric artery as well. The splenic artery must have a large caliber and must be free of arteriosclerotic lesions. This may be documented by a good preoperative angiogram and intraoperative

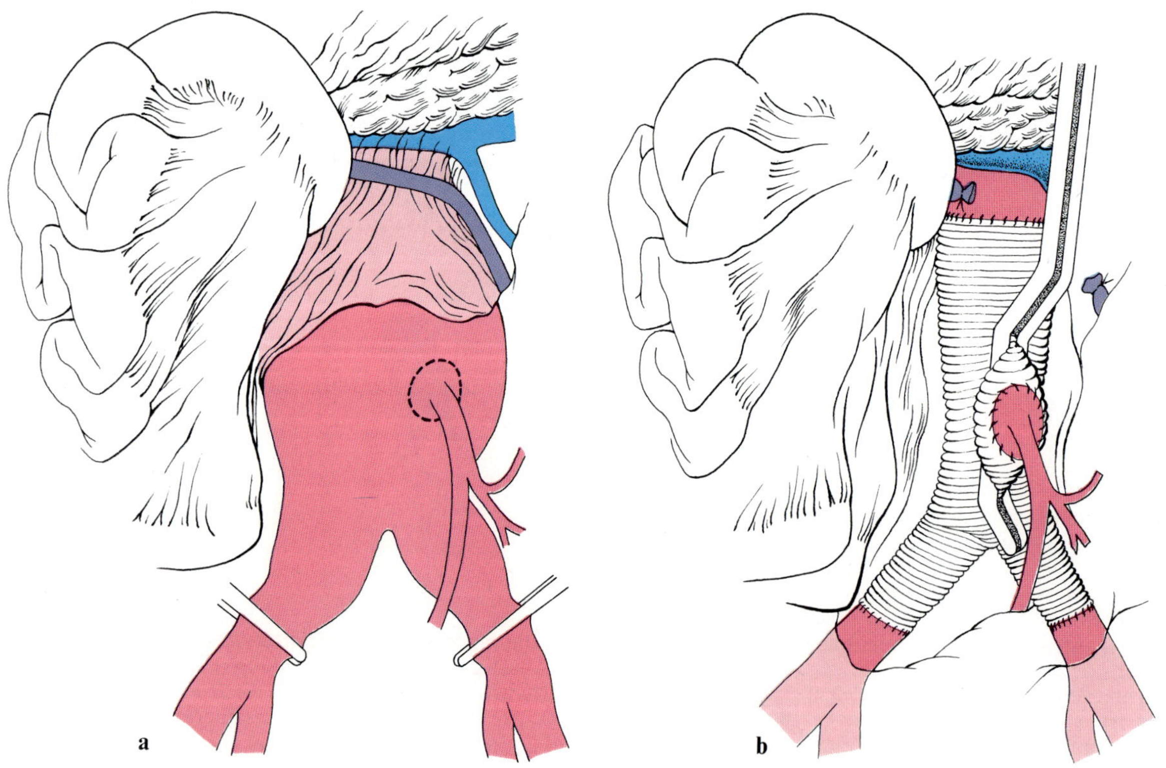

Fig. 22.11 a, b. Reimplantation of the inferior mesenteric artery into a bifurcation prosthesis following resection of an aortic aneurysm. **a** Excision of the origin of the inferior mesenteric artery with a Carrel patch from the aortic wall. **b** Connection of the inferior mesenteric artery to the left anterior wall of the bifurcation graft, which is clamped tangentially

measurement of pressure and flow. Time-consuming and unsuccessful dissection of the artery can thus be avoided.

For the bypass, the splenic artery is dissected free from its origin at the celiac axis to the splenic hilus (Fig. 22.12). At this hilus, it is divided in its branches in such a way that the incised branching can be used for the anastomosis. Usually, splenectomy is not required. The isolated artery should be filled proximally with heparinized solution to avoid thrombosis and then cross-clamped atraumatically. The mobilized splenic artery is passed in front of or behind the pancreas to the infracolic region through a tunnel in the root of the mesentery. Kinking and twisting must be avoided. In the case of an occluded celiac axis, the splenic artery is anastomosed end-to-side to the infrarenal aorta (splenoaortic in situ bypass) after the branched end of the splenic artery has been tailored to create a funnel-shaped orifice. A precondition for this bypass, however, is that the flow of blood is not impaired from the splenic artery past the occlusion in the celiac axis to the hepatic artery.

If the superior mesenteric artery is occluded, the splenic artery may be used for revascularization by anastomosing the funnel-shaped end of the splenic artery end-to-side to the superior mesenteric artery distal to the occlusion (splenomesenteric in situ bypass; Fig. 22.12). Here, the precondition is adequate patency of the celiac axis and the splenic artery.

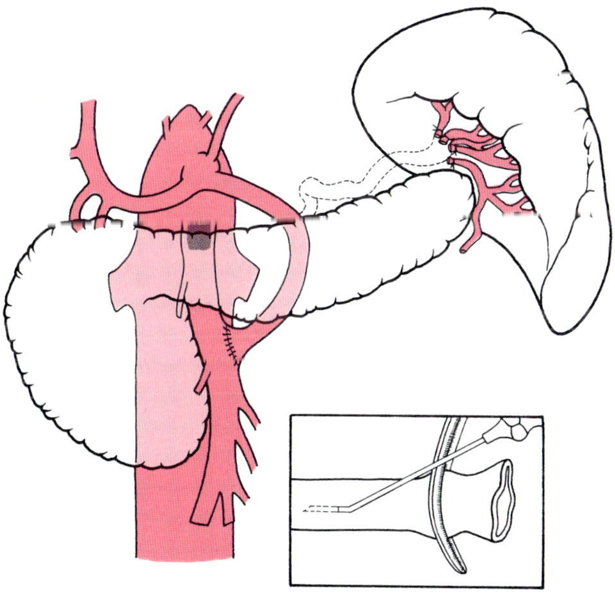

Fig. 22.12. Splenomesenteric in situ bypass for revascularization of the superior mesenteric artery. Dissection of the splenic artery over its entire length and division of the branches in the splenic hilus. Filling with heparinized solution. Passage of the dissected artery in front or behind the pancreas and anastomosis to the superior mesenteric artery, which is dissected infracolically

IV. Bypass Procedures

The bypass procedure is the quickest and technically the simplest procedure for reconstruction of a proximal occlusion of the superior mesenteric artery or of the celiac axis.

In cases of superior mesenteric artery occlusion, the bypass runs from the right anterior wall of the infrarenal aorta to the posterior aspect of the superior mesenteric artery, both being exposed by a retrocolic approach (Fig. 22.13a–c). First, the connection to the infrarenal aorta is performed in the usual fashion. The orifice of the vein graft should be enlarged using one of the techniques shown in Fig. 22.17. For the exact placement of the end-to-side anastomosis to the posterior wall of the mesenteric artery (usually proximal or at the level of the origin of the medial colic artery), the artery may be rotated by vascular clamps prior to the arteriotomy. The bypass must be extremely short as both arteries are parallel and close to each other. Too long a bypass tends to cause kinking when the intestine is brought back into the abdominal cavity. The technique of implanting a long bypass and then shortening it by resecting the middle segment is sometimes advocated as a way of avoiding this complication. In our opinion, however, neither this technique nor that of proximal connection of the graft to the iliac artery can be justified as a routine procedure.

For celiac axis revascularization, the graft may originate from either the thoracic or the infrarenal aorta. The advantages of a thoracic origin are:

1. Favorable hemodynamics with outflow at an obtuse angle to the aorta
2. Hardly any lesions of the wall of the thoracic aorta
3. No risk of intestinal arrosion by the bypass

A disadvantage is the large abdominothoracic incision. Therefore, we prefer the abdominal approach. The only exceptions are where the infrarenal aorta is absolutely unsuitable for anastomosis or where there has been a previous operation in this region. In the latter case, the time-consuming and difficult task of dissecting within the scar

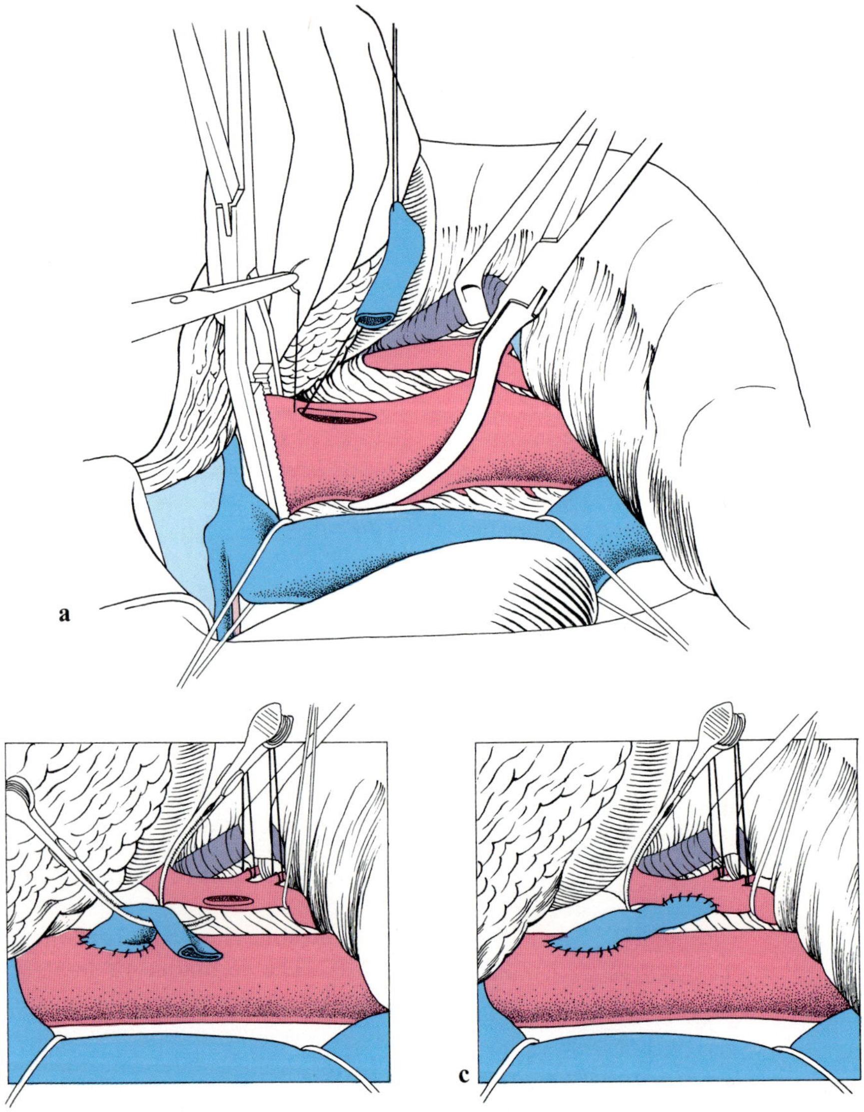

a b c

Fig. 22.13a–c. Aorto-superior mesenteric bypass using a vein graft, following right-sided retrocolic exposure of the superior mesenteric artery and the infrarenal aorta. **a** Following cross-clamping of the infrarenal aortic segment and elliptical excision of the right anterior wall of the aorta, the anastomosis is performed with a vein graft, the end being tailored to achieve a greater orifice. **b** Cross-clamping of the vein graft close to the anastomosis and release of the blood flow in the aorta. Longitudinal incision in the posterior wall of the superior mesenteric artery, rotated by vascular clamps. **c** Distal end-to-side anastomosis of the graft to the superior mesenteric artery

tissue poses an additional, significant risk which can be avoided using a thoracic bypass. In such cases, the iliac vessels, with all their hemodynamic disadvantages, can possibly serve as an alternative donor artery.

With an exclusively abdominal approach, the proximal anastomosis of the vein graft is performed end-to-side to the infrarenal aorta, which is exposed infracolically (Fig. 22.14a, b) or right-retrocolically (Fig. 22.14g, h). Prior to the anastomosis, the end of the vein graft is tailored to achieve a larger orifice (Fig. 22.17). Following cross-clamping of the vein graft, blood flow in the aorta is released. The branches of the celiac axis are more suitable for the distal anastomosis than the trunk itself because their exposure is significantly easier. The bypass is placed in a curvilinear

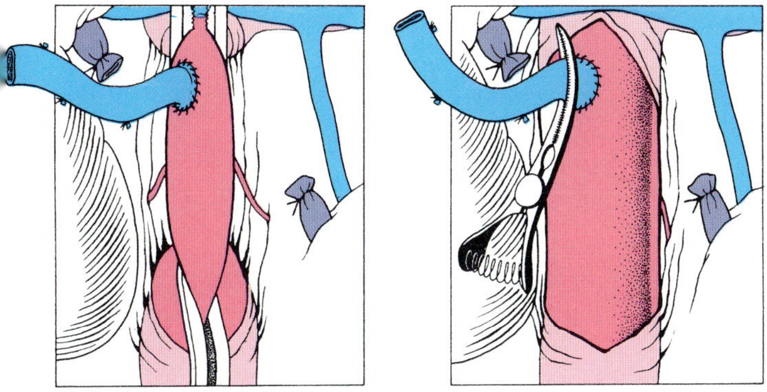

a b

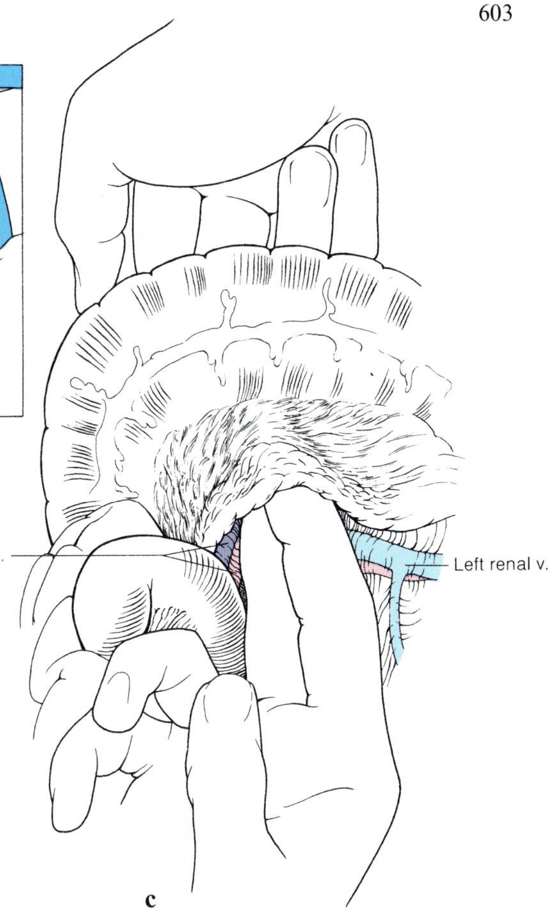

c

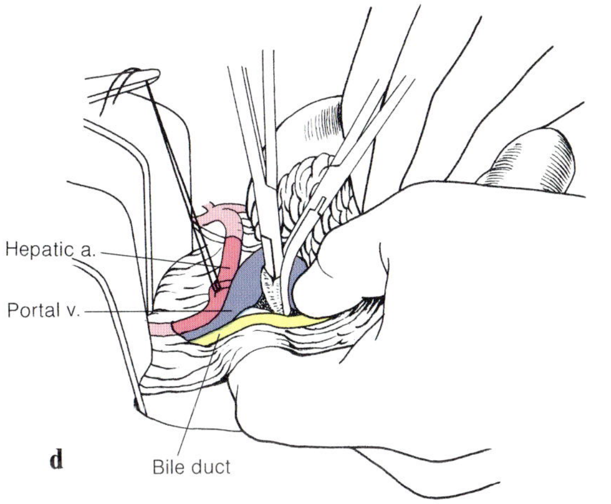

d

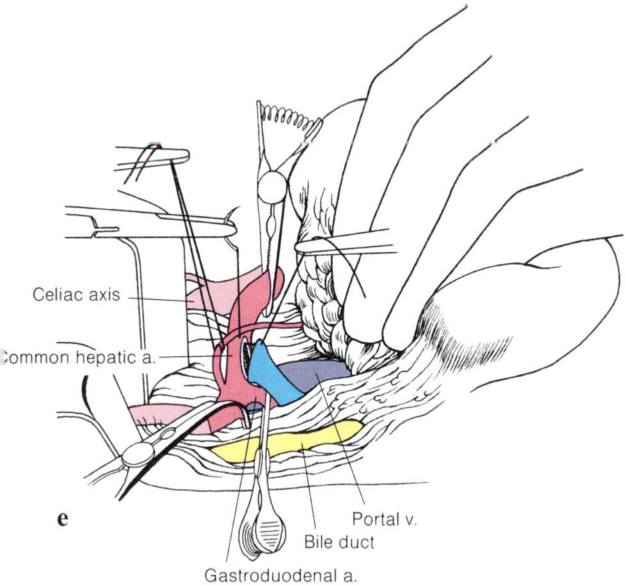

e

Fig. 22.14a–h. Aortohepatic bypass using a vein graft. The figures show the various steps of the procedure following infracolic and right-sided retrocolic exposure of the infrarenal aorta. **a**, **b** Following infracolic exposure and infrarenal cross-clamping of the aorta, the vein graft, tailored at its end to achieve a larger orifice, is anastomosed to an elliptical opening in the right anterior wall of the infrarenal aorta. After completion of the anastomosis, the vein graft is cross-clamped close to the anastomosis and the blood flow in the aorta released. **c** Creation of a tunnel, using both hands, between the infracolic site and the lesser sac of the omentum, behind the pancreatic isthmus along the initial segment of the superior mesenteric artery. **d** The hepatoduodenal ligament, as viewed by the surgeon. The tunnel terminates between the bile duct and the portal vein. There, the space for the vein graft is created by careful dissection. **e** Anastomosis of the vein graft to the distal common hepatic artery directly proximal to the origin of the gastroduodenal artery. **f** Operative view within the hepatoduodenal ligament following completion of the anastomosis of the vein graft to the common hepatic artery. **g** Anastomosis of the vein graft to the infrarenal aortic segment following right-sided retrocolic exposure of the aorta, as seen by the surgeon. **h** The graft is passed from the retrocolic operative field to the common hepatic artery. A tunnel between the bile duct and the portal vein inside the hepatoduodenal ligament is created by careful dissection

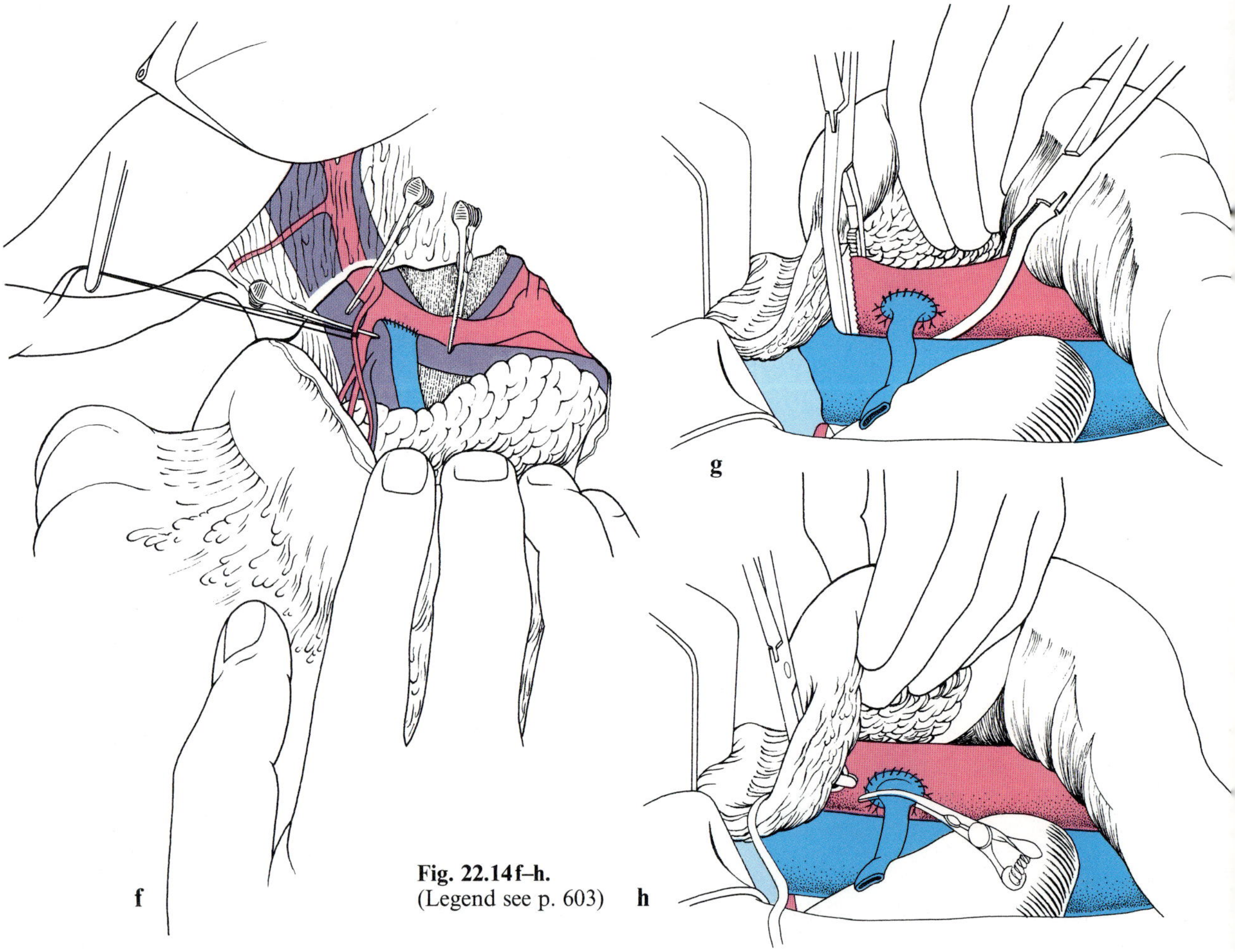

Fig. 22.14f–h. (Legend see p. 603)

course behind the pancreas to the hepatic artery or to the splenic artery. When the aorta is exposed by an infracolic approach, the tunnel to the hepatic artery is created by bidigital blunt dissection of the tissue between the aorta and the pancreas at the level of the superior mesenteric artery (Fig. 22.14c). Creating the tunnel to the common hepatic artery requires dissection between the portal vein and the bile duct (Fig. 22.14b). While pulling the bypass through the tunnel, twisting or kinking must be meticulously avoided. The distal connection is performed end-to-side to the splenic or the common hepatic artery (Fig. 22.14e, f). The preconditions for an anastomosis to the splenic artery are:

1. The vessel must not show arteriosclerotic lesions.
2. The stenosing lesions at the celiac axis must not extend into the bifurcation, thereby impairing the circulation from the splenic artery to the vascular bed of the liver.

When there are doubts as to whether the splenic artery is hemodynamically intact, anastomosis to the common hepatic artery should be preferred in every case [27].

V. Reconstruction of Multiple Occlusions

For reconstruction of double stenoses or occlusions of the superior mesenteric artery and the celiac axis, all of the methods previously described can be used in combination. In our hospital, we are most satisfied with the so-called venous bridge bypass graft (Fig. 22.15).

Following exposure of the anastomotic sites of the visceral arteries, the infrarenal aortic segment is dissected and cross-clamped. The superior mes-

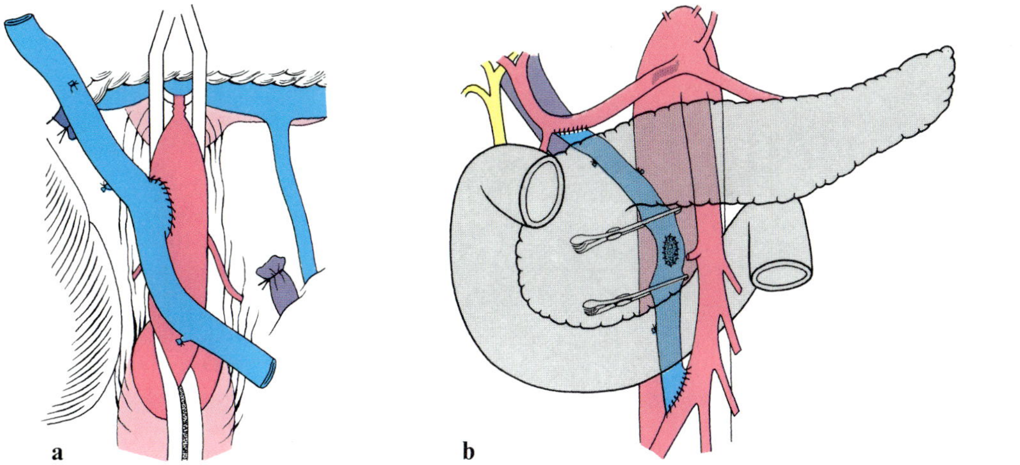

Fig. 22.15 a, b. Venous bridge graft for the treatment of double stenoses or occlusions of the superior mesenteric artery and the celiac axis following infracolic exposure of the infrarenal aorta. **a** The venous graft, with its valves already resected (Fig. 22.16), is first anastomosed side-to-side to an oblique elliptical orifice in the right wall of the infrarenal aorta. **b** Both ends of the graft are cross-clamped separately, close to the aorta, and the blood flow in the aorta is released. The upper end of the graft is passed behind the pancreas to the common hepatic artery and the lower end to the superior mesenteric artery. Both distal anastomoses are performed obliquely end-to-side

enteric artery may be better exposed infracolically or retrocolically from the right side. An oblique elliptical orifice is excised out of the right wall of the infrarenal aorta, the edges being cleaned of arteriosclerotic lesions. The vein graft is incised eccentrically and longitudinally because of the different lengths of the graft ends (Fig. 22.15a) and anastomosed side-to-side to the aorta. After completion of the anastomosis, the inflow lumen of each segment is checked by inserting olives from both directions. Both ends of the graft are then cross-clamped close to the aorta and the blood flow to the aorta released. Finally, both ends of the graft are passed to the appropriate segments of the superior mesenteric artery and the celiac axis (hepatic artery, splenic artery) and anastomosed end-to-side (Fig. 22.15b).

Graft Material. Usually, the visceral arteries are relatively fine and are thin walled, not suitable for anastomosis to the relatively thick walled alloplastic vascular grafts. Other disadvantages are the significant differences in caliber and the secondary loss of graft lumen. For these reasons and also because of the higher biologic value, autoplastic vascular grafts should be used for the reconstruction of visceral arteries whenever possible. The graft of choice is the great saphenous vein. When no vein is available, arterial segments of the splenic artery or the external iliac artery may be used (the latter being replaced by a prosthesis). The internal iliac artery should be saved as a collateral donor artery whenever possible.

Preparation of the Graft. The harvested vein segment is kept in heparinized patient's blood. The graft is everted over a bulb-headed probe and the vein valves are resected under direct vision in order to anastomose the wide proximal end of the great saphenous vein segment anterograde to the aorta (Fig. 22.16). After the vein is reinverted, it is

Fig. 22.16. Preparation of the vein graft to serve as a bridge bypass. The vein is everted using a bulb-headed probe. The valves are resected with fine scissors

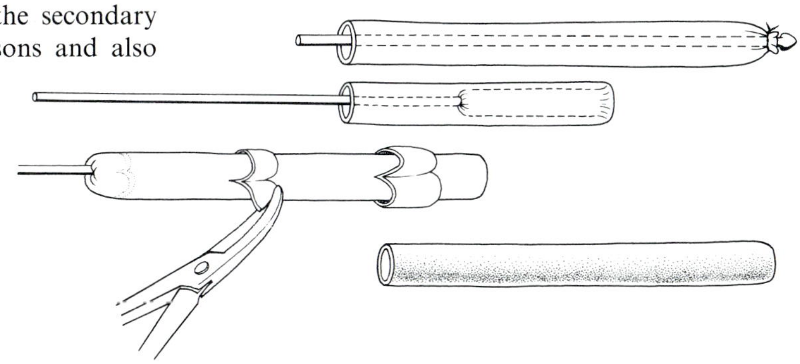

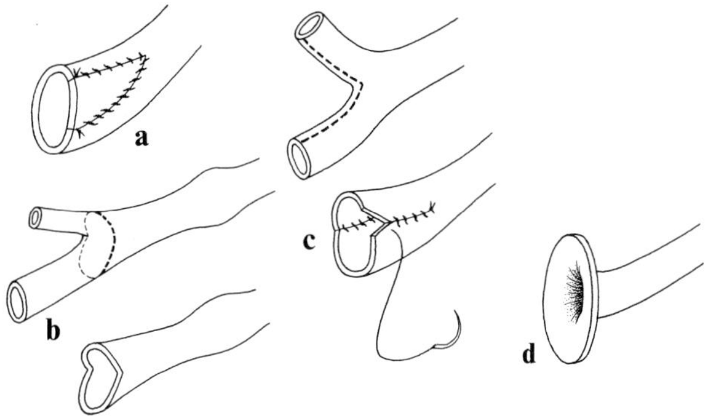

Fig. 22.17 a–d. Several techniques for enlarging the end of the vein graft to be anastomosed to the aorta. **a** Tulip-shaped enlargement of the graft end by means of a wedge-shaped vein patch. **b** Trumpet-shaped graft end achieved by obliquely tailoring the major branch and one branch. **c** Funnel-shaped enlargement of the graft end using a vein dichotomy. **d** Vein graft with Carrel patch. Resection of valves is required in all these cases

checked for any remaining valves and for leaks by filling it in each direction with heparinized blood.

The same graft preparation is required for the bridge graft.

Other possibilities of enlarging the graft end to be anastomosed to the aorta are shown in Fig. 22.17.

H. Postoperative Complications

Postoperative complications following reconstructions of intestinal arteries do not differ from those following other arterial reconstructions. In the event of bleeding, immediate reintervention is indicated. The same is true for an early occlusion. However, except for signs of intestinal infarction, it may not be easy to diagnose such a reocclusion early enough.

I. Reoperation of Intestinal Arteries

An early occlusion following visceral artery reconstruction should always be reoperated immediately [8, 23]. The earlier the operation is performed, the fewer adhesions and scars will be found in the operative field and the easier the access to the region of reconstruction will be.

In the majority of cases, the cause of early reocclusion is found in the region of the distal anastomosis. Therefore, this anastomosis should be opened first, evaluated, and corrected. Thrombectomy, if required, is performed from this side, using a Fogarty catheter.

Rarely, an early reocclusion is accompanied by clinical signs of intestinal ischemia. In such cases, the procedure should be the same as for primary acute occlusion of a visceral artery. Depending on the severity of ischemia, a reconstruction can be done, possibly in combination with bowel resection or bowel resection alone. A second-look operation eventually must be discussed.

In late reoperations necessitated by recurrent stenosis or occlusion, one may attempt to correct the reconstruction. The exposure of the previous operative region and the corrective procedure itself (suturing a patch graft, endarterectomy, or graft replacement) usually present considerable difficulties and also carry the risk of injury to the concomitant structures.

Under such circumstances, exposure of the appropriate visceral artery distal to the previous site of anastomosis is preferred. It goes without saying that there may still be significant difficulties.

Independent of the first operation, only bypass procedures are considered for the reintervention. Autogenous material, if still available, should be used for the bypass in any case. Often, the site of the proximal anastomosis of the graft can only be determined intraoperatively, following evaluation of the local anatomic conditions and the type of previous operation. When there is still good access to the aorta distal to the previous bypass anastomosis or to the distal aorta, the new graft should be anastomosed there. Under certain circumstances, the common iliac artery or the lower thoracic aorta may be used for the graft connection.

When the splenic artery is suitable, an in situ bypass using this artery may be considered as a second operation. Here, the splenic artery is mobilized and divided at the hilus of the spleen, and anastomosed to the infrarenal aorta or the superior mesenteric artery distal to the previous anastomosis.

REFERENCES

1. Adeshek K, Wittenstein G (1979) Mesenteric revascularization: an operative approach. Am J Surg 137:821
2. Buchardt-Hansen HJ, Engell HC, Ring-Larsen H, Randek L (1977) Splanchnic blood flow in patients with abdominal angina before and after arterial reconstruction. Ann Surg 186:216
3. Crawford ES, Morris GC Jr, Myhre HO, Roehm JOF Jr (1977) Celiac axis, superior mesenteric artery and inferior mesenteric artery occlusion; surgical considerations. Surgery 82:856
4. Dick AP, Gregg DMcC (1972) Chronic occlusions of the visceral arterial. Clin Gastroenterol 1:689
5. Dongen RJAM van (1970) Atlas of reconstructive arterial surgery. HE Stenfert Kroese, Leiden
6. Dongen RJAM van (1976) Abdominal angina; diagnosis and surgical treatment. Minerva Chir 31:415
7. Dongen RJAM van, Schwilden ED (1976) Die chronischen intestinalen Durchblutungsstörungen. Operationsindikationen, Wiederherstellungsmethoden, Ergebnisse. Chirurg 47:366
8. Dongen RJAM van, Schwilden E-D (1980) Reinterventionen an den Visceral- und Nierenarterien. Chirurg 51:7
9. Eidemiller LR, Nelson JC, Porter JM (1979) Surgical treatment of chronic visceral ischemia. Am J Surg 138:264
10. Eklof B, Hoevels J, Ihse I (1978) The surgical treatment of chronic intestinal ischemia. Ann Surg 187:318
11. Giessler R, Hoffmann K, Heberer G (1973) Akute und chronische Verschlüsse der Viszeralarterien. Dtsch Med Wochenschr 98:1112
12. Hansen HJB (1976) Abdominal angina. Results of arterial reconstruction in 12 patients. Acta Chir Scand 142:319
13. Heberer G, Dostal G, Hoffmann K (1972) Zur Erkennung und Behandlung der chronischen Mesenterialarterieninsuffizienz. Dtsch Med Wochenschr 97.750
14. Hertzer NR, Beven EG, Humphries AW (1977) Chronic intestinal ischemia. Surg Gynecol Obstet 145:321
15. Hollier LH, Bernatz PE, Pairolero PC, Payne WS, Osmundson PJ (1981) Surgical management of chronic intestinal ischaemia: a reappraisel. Surgery 90:940
16. Jaumin P, Fastrez J, Goenen M, Kestens-Servaye Y, Schoevaerdts J, Dautrebande J (1975) Revascularization of the superior mesenteric artery. J Cardiovasc Surg 16:548
17. Nunn DB (1972) Chronic intestinal angina: a report of two patients treated succesfully by operation. Ann Surg 175:523
18. Pokrowsky AV, Kasantchjan PO, Spiridonov AA (1980) A new method of one-stage revascularization of the visceral arteries. Experience with 25 operations. J Cardiovasc Surg 21:659
19. Robb HJ, Ketonen P, Ketonen L, Luosto R, Matilla S (1978) Clinical experience with surgical treatment of chronic intestinal ischemia. Ann Chir Gynaecol 67:70
20. Robicsek F, Daugherty HK, Cook JW, Owen BJ (1977) A new method to revascularize the celiac axis. Vascular Surgery 11:34
21. Santavirta S, Nieminen J, Kauste A, Ahonen J (1978) Revascularization in mesenteric infarction by reimplantation of the superior mesenteric artery. Acta Chir Scand 144:185
22. Schwilden E-D, Dongen RJAM van (1978) Angina intestinalis. Fortschr Med 96:839
23. Semb BKH, Halvorsen JF, Fossdal JE, Eide J (1977) Visceral ischaemia following coeliac- and superior mesenteric artery occlusion. Acta Chir Scand 143:185
24. Solheim K, Rosseland A, Lund B-L (1977) Intestinal angina. Report of two operated cases. Scan J Thorac Cardiovasc Surg 11:1141
25. Stoney RJ, Olcott C (1979) Visceral artery syndromes and reconstructions. Surg Clin North Am 59:637
26. Stoney RJ, Ehrenfeld WK, Wylie EJ (1977) Revascularization methods in chronic visceral ischaemia caused by atherosclerosis. Ann Surg 186:468
27. Wichterman KA, Stansch HC Jr (1979) Simplified splanchnic artery revascularization using extra-anatomic bypass grafts: a report of ten cases. Arch Surg 114:1052
28. Zelenock GB, Graham LM, Whitehouse WM Jr, Erlandson EE, Kraft RO, Lindenauer SM, Stanley JC (1981) Splanchnic arteriosclerotic disease and intestinal angina. Arch Surg 115:497

23 Renal Artery Occlusive Disease

F.W. Eigler and H.D. Jakubowski

CONTENTS

A. Anatomy

The renal vessels may show variations in their number and branches. If there is only one major renal artery on each side, both originate from the aorta at the level of the intervertebral disk between the first and second lumbar vertebra. The origin is often asymmetrical: the right renal artery usually takes off somewhat deeper. Close to the hilus, the renal artery gives off several branches. The majority of these enter the parenchyma in front of the renal pelvis. The suprarenal artery and the testicular or ovarian artery originate along the course of the renal artery from the aorta to the hilus of the kidney (see p. 19).

In about 25% of humans, the kidney is supplied by two or more arteries, directly originating from the aorta. These variant vessels can cause compression effects in the region of the renal pelvis and the ureters, with consequent impairment of urinary flow as well as the risk of accidental ligation. Renal hypertension may develop, depending on which region of parenchyma is no longer supplied.

Additional arteries may enter the kidney at the hilus itself, but also somewhat outward. They may be expected above as well as below the hilus. The origin of the right renal artery is covered by the venous crossing, which is formed where the two renal veins join the inferior vena cava; extensive dissection of this crossing is necessary for adequate exposure of the renal artery.

The Collateral System of the Kidney. The renal arteries are usually considered to be terminal arteries since in cases of acute occlusion, the existing collaterals are not sufficient for maintaining an adequate blood flow. However, when the renal arteries gradually narrow, owing to an occlusive disease, preexisting collaterals may develop so that at least basic metabolism is maintained. Collateral circulation may be developed by arteries to the adrenals via the junction to the superior suprarenal arteries, by the arteries of the capsule via the lumbar arteries, and by the ureter vessels. The ureter vessels are supplied by the renal artery in the upper region, by the ovarian or spermatic artery in the middle region, and by the common iliac artery in the lower region [12]. When serving as collaterals, the ureteral vessels show this very clearly on the intravenous pyelogram; these images serve as a sure diagnostic sign of a functionally significant stenosis of the renal artery.

B. Renovascular Hypertension, Indications for Operation

Renovascular hypertension is the most common reason for operations on the renal arteries. Therefore, procedures for the treatment of this condition will be discussed before those that are used in acute occlusion, in trauma, or following renal transplantation.

I. Definition, Incidence

Renovascular hypertension is a syndrome in which normalization of the blood pressure may be achieved by reconstruction of the appropriate renal artery lesions outside of the parenchyma [17]. Lesions of intraparenchymatous arteries and arterioles, on the other hand, are not included. However, the term "renovascular hypertension" is not used uniformly in the literature. Among all types of hypertension, renovascular hypertension may account for less than 1% [6].

II. Etiology

The most common cause of renal artery stenosis is *arteriosclerosis* [9] close to the aorta, in the first third of the renal artery. The stenosis is more or less concentric with a poststenotic dilatation. It is impossible to say whether the renal artery arteriosclerosis is caused by essential hypertension or vice versa.

The second most frequent disease is *fibrodysplasia*, occurring in four different forms [13]:

1. The rare, so-called fibromuscular dysplasia with a circumferential stenosis caused by thickening of the artery muscles
2. Intimal fibroplasia, causes also constricting lesions with poststenotic dilation
3. Medial fibrodysplasia, characterized by a series of stenoses alternating with aneurysmal dilatations, resembling haustration
4. Subadventitial (perimedial) dysplasia

The lesions, typically located in the periphery, are often bilateral and combined with a so-called mobile kidney.

These lesions may also appear in other vascular regions, but are then not as widespread as in arteriosclerosis.

It is controversial to what extent the classification of the various forms, as already diagnosed by the angiogram may have therapeutic consequences. The forms of revascularization that are necessary may differ greatly from those required for arteriosclerosis [22].

III. Pathophysiology

A common feature in all lesions is the impairment of renal blood flow, resulting in characteristic changes in the affected kidney, as compared with the contralateral one, which is exposed to a higher systemic blood pressure [3]. Reduction of blood flow causes an increase in the concentration of the initial urine and a decreased sodium concentration of the final urine as a result of reduced filtration. Previously, the indication for operation was based on tests of the functional differences on both sides [14], but because these tests were too complicated and caused too much stress on the patient, they have been abandoned.

Moreover, decreased blood flow, resulting in an increase of blood pressure via the renin–angiotensin system, is probably perpetuated via the aldosterone system by changes in the sodium metabolism. Administration of the converting enzyme inhibitor captopril may reveal the significance of the renin–angiotensin system by decreasing the blood pressure [20]. Care must be taken in the case of a single kidney because of the possibility of acute renal failure. Only in exceptional cases should the decision to operate be based on the results of this test.

IV. Diagnosis

History and clinical examination will not reveal peculiarities in patients with renovascular hypertension. The only basis for a clear suspicion is a reliable report of the sudden onset of hypertension. An abdominal bruit may be of similar significance, but is open to several interpretations, especially in patients with arteriosclerosis.

The intravenous pyelogram, so often used in the diagnosis of hypertension, is very useful as a screening test. A unilateral small kidney of smooth configuration with delayed, but concentrated excretion and with visible indentations of the renal pelvis and the ureter as a result of collateral circulation may suggest unilateral or unilaterally pronounced renal artery stenosis [14]. In the future, digital subtraction angiography may be used as a screening test [15], while all other procedures, including isotope renography, show nonspecific effects. Precise angiography is an indispensable prerequisite in deciding whether surgery is indicated. When percutaneous angioplasty [16] is indicated, the Seldinger procedure should be used (see p. 121).

Angiography usually reveals the underlying etiology of the stenosis. For all practical purposes, a distinct poststenotic dilatation proves that the stenosis is hemodynamically significant.

V. Operative Indications

The indication for surgical treatment of renovascular hypertension primarily depends on local and general factors. When considering the local situation, the indication for renal artery revascularization is always given if there are clear signs of a functionally effective stenosis (poststenotic dilatation, collateral circulation, and possibly a unilateral increase of renin concentration in the renal venous blood), and if percutaneous transfemoral angioplasty has failed or is not suitable. Absolute indications for an operative procedure are complete renal artery occlusion, an unfavorable course of the vessel, extreme poststenotic dilatation with risk of perforation, or suspicion of a primary aneurysm. It should be mentioned here that when a kidney transplant is performed, any existing stenosis of the renal artery should be corrected in the primary operation as there can in this case be no development of collateral circulation.

Where there is danger that kidney function will be lost, surgery is contraindicated only by life-threatening diseases. But, with regard to the correction of hypertension, the indication for surgery as well as for angioplasty will be subject to certain limitations imposed by the general condition of the patient. When considering whether angioplasty is indicated, one should always bear in mind that in a small percentage of cases this procedure eventuates in an emergency operation. Therefore, the general contraindications for an operation also apply to angioplasty (see p. 121).

In patients under 40 years of age with hypertension an operation is practically always indicated. With increasing age and in generalized arteriosclerosis, one should hesitate because the operative mortality beyond 50 years of age increases significantly and the long-term results do not measure up to expectations. Coronary artery disease, diabetes, and cerebral vascular disease must also be included among the risk factors.

Due to very effective medical antihypertensive therapy, the problem of patient selection has become more the problem of maintaining the function of the diseased kidney, especially in older patients. This is especially true for patients with one kidney or only one functional kidney.

C. General Surgical Aspects

I. Tolerable Ischemic Time

The ischemic time tolerated by the kidney must be considered under three headings, namely:

1. Normal preoperative renal blood flow on both sides and unilateral operation, i.e., temporary acute renal failure on one side without consequences
2. Necessity of interrupting blood flow on both sides in cases of preoperative normal blood flow or of a single kidney, i.e., absolute necessity of avoiding acute renal failure
3. Operation on a renal artery because of gradual impairment of renal blood flow or complete occlusion, where collateral circulation has already developed

1. When a unilateral operation is undertaken and it has been demonstrated that the contralateral side is functioning adequately, the ischemic time may be extended beyond 45 min because postoperative acute renal failure on the side of the operation and its sequelae for the whole organism should be compensated by the "healthy" kidney. Under these circumstances, interruption of blood flow up to 1.5 h seems to be possible. Operations on renal arteries requiring this much time are almost unknown; only in the case of a difficult aneurysm would an operation of this length be necessary.

2. When attempting immediate restoration of kidney function following the vascular procedure, the interruption of the blood flow at body temperature should not exceed 45 min. Such a long clamping time is only safe if circulatory parameters before and after interruption of blood flow are normal. The induction of diuresis by furosemide or osmotically by 20% mannitol prior to the ischemia is recommended [1].

When the interruption of the blood flow is projected to last longer than 1 h, the sequelae of ischemia can be ameliorated by decreasing the temperature in the organ by means of hypothermic perfusion. However, continuous cooling requires additional drainage of the renal vein. Superficial cooling using special bags requires complete mobilization of the kidney with the sacrifice of possible collaterals. Therefore, this procedure is not recommended.

3. The major indication for renal artery surgery is chronic occlusive disease due to lesions of the major renal arteries. Practically speaking, there are no time limits, provided there is no peripheral thrombosis, because under such conditions, the collateral circulation has sufficiently developed to supply the basic metabolism, and sometimes even part of the stress metabolism. Peripheral thrombosis may be avoided by local heparinization and periodic checks of retrograde flow.

II. Preoperative Management

Hypertension is usually present and should be carefully controlled. In contrast to earlier views, perioperative management at normal blood pressure is now preferred. Electrolyte disturbances should be corrected; this is especially necessary in the case of hypokalemia, which is often caused by the use of diuretics. Digitalis should be administered in accordance with the cardiac situation. When there is severe impairment of renal function, the situation should be normalized as far as possible by carefully monitoring the fluid balance.

The general statement that obesity is a risk factor for major procedures is particularly true in cases of renal reconstruction. Since there is usually no great urgency involved in scheduling the operation, obese patients should be put on a consistent weight reduction program. This is also recommended when "only" a percutaneous angioplasty is contemplated; for, in the event of a complication – admittedly rare with this procedure – obesity poses an especially high risk. And finally, weight reduction not only facilitates anatomic dissection, but may also help to alleviate hypertension.

III. Intraoperative Management

Intraoperative circulatory fluctuations, especially in patients with arteriosclerotic stenoses, should be avoided since there are, or are likely to be, similar lesions in other vascular regions. We recommend cross-clamping the origin of the renal artery, and not complete occlusion of the aorta, whenever possible. However, current techniques of intra-arterial measurement of blood pressure and the Swan-Ganz catheter provide immediate correction of significant alterations of the blood pressure by intravenous administration of antihypertensive drugs in cases of hypertension, or administration of fluid in cases of a fall in blood pressure (see p. 197).

In any case, prior to cross-clamping the renal artery intraoperatively, diuresis using 20% mannitol or, if there is a risk of cardiac overloading, furosemide should be ensured in order to keep the renal ischemic sequelae to a minimum [1].

When there is a stenosis close to the ostium, care is taken to identify other causative lesions close to the origin of the renal arteries. If these renal artery stenoses are of arteriosclerotic origin, a tendinous band is often found directly adjacent to the aorta, consisting of a deep portion of the diaphragm. The renal artery may lie across it, and the continuing pulsations against the band can result in arteriosclerosis at this site. We recommend division of this tendinous band under vision, at least in cases where no bypass is considered. Moderate bleeding can easily be stopped by electrocoagulation.

Following extensive exposure of the renal artery origin and prior to any further measures, there is a final opportunity to verify the hemodynamic effectiveness of the stenosis. Flow measurement by means of an electromagnetic probe, in combination with the determination of blood pressure by direct puncture of the aorta and poststenotic dilatation, is ideal. A pressure gradient exceeding 15 mmHg is considered to be significant where there is proven flow through the artery. If flow has almost ceased, one has to remember that the pressure behind the stenosis is equal to the pressure in the aorta, independent of the degree of stenosis.

IV. Postoperative Management

Following operations on the renal arteries, generally intensive monitoring has to be assured. Fluctuations in blood pressure are not rare and require immediate correction. Especially in patients with hypertension of arteriosclerotic origin, significant deviations from a systolic pressure of 150 mmHg and a diastolic pressure of 90 mmHg should be corrected either by antihypertensive drugs or, in case of hypotension, by fluid therapy. Simultaneously, urine output has to be recorded continuously. A urine output of 100 ml/h should be achieved. With enforced diuresis there is the risk of hypokalemia and in cases of oliguria the risk of hyperkalemia. Also, a slight increase of serum sodium may result in higher blood pressure. Therefore, several measurements of electrolytes should be made within the first 24 h.

An abrupt decrease in urine output with a simultaneous increase of blood pressure is indicative of renal artery reocclusion. In cases of acute renal failure, the intravenous urogram and scintigram may fail; if so, angiography (digital subtraction angiography, whenever possible) should be performed without delay to corroborate the diagnosis. If the findings are positive (hematoma, arterial thrombosis), immediate reoperation is indicated.

D. Operative Approach

For the operation, the patient is placed in a supine position. The ventral approach to the renal arteries through the abdomen is performed either by a midline incision, extending upward as high as possible, or a transverse, supraumbilical abdominal incision (Fig. 23.1). While a longitudinal incision is of greater advantage where the epigastric angle is acute, the transverse supraumbilical abdominal incision is better in case of a very wide angle. However, one should consider that the renal arteries originate relatively high up on the aorta, at the level of the intervertebral disk between the first

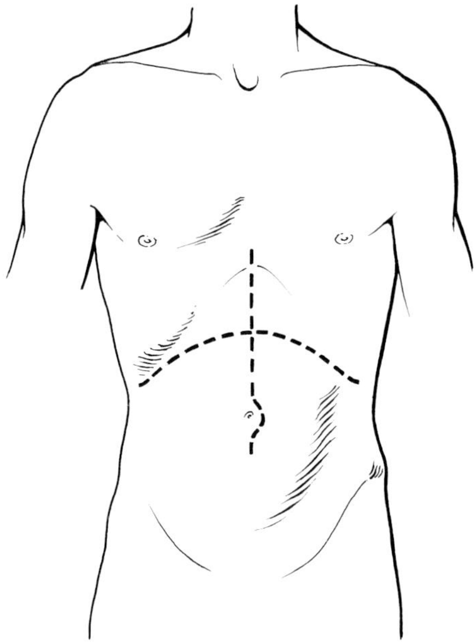

Fig. 23.1. Location of skin incision for renal artery exposure. Generally, the approach to the renal arteries is possible by medial longitudinal abdominal incision or transverse supraumbilical abdominal incision. When placing the incision, the relatively high origin of the renal arteries from the aorta have to be considered

and second lumbar vertebra. For exposure of the renal artery itself, there is the choice of an infracolic approach through the mesocolon or a supracolic approach following dissection of the left or the right flexure of the colon, depending on the diseased renal artery. The procedure depends on whether there are lesions close to the aorta and whether the patient is obese. If the lesions are located close to the aorta and there is an intra-abdominal mass of fat, the direct infracolic approach is preferred.

I. Infracolic Approach (Fig. 23.2a, b)

For the infracolic approach, the transverse colon, together with the greater omentum is drawn upward, the small bowel is retracted to the right, and the peritoneum is excised over the aorta by dissecting the duodenojejunal flexure. One first encounters the left renal vein, which crosses the aorta. A tape is placed around it. If the left renal artery originates somewhat above the vein, the suprarenal vein is divided between ligatures just before it joins the renal vein. Suture ligation is recommended, at least at the junction of the veins, as a safeguard against the bleeding that would re-

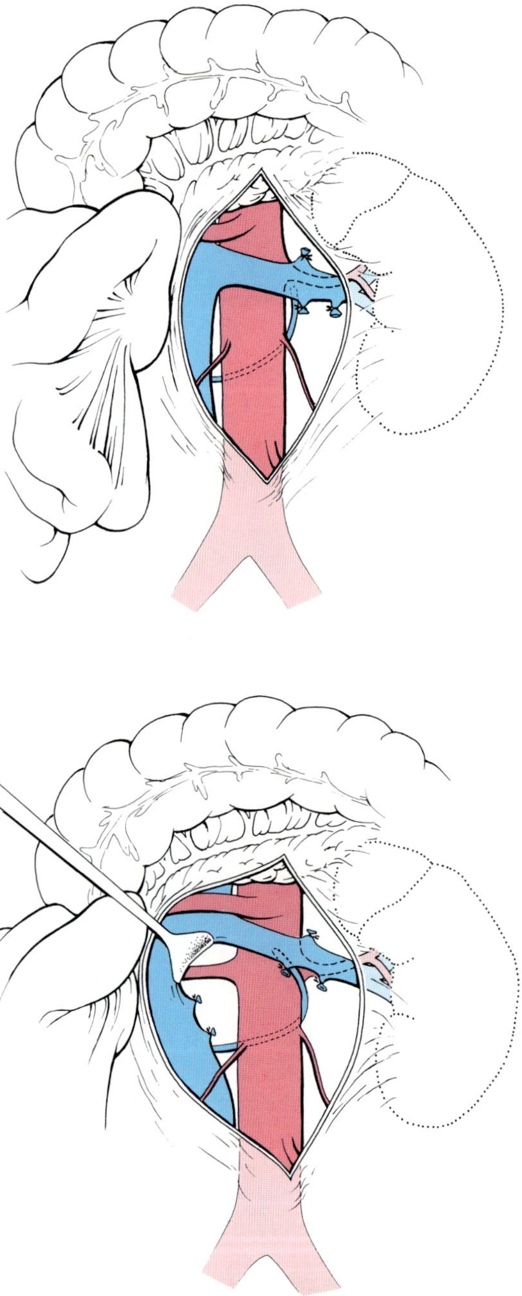
a

b

Fig. 23.2a, b. Infracolic approach to the renal arteries. a Exposure of the left renal artery. Following dissection of the duodenojejunal flexure and the mesentery, longitudinal incision of the retroperitoneum over the aorta and dissection of the left renal vein away from the fatty tissue. Tributary veins, such as the suprarenal, ovarian, or spermatic vein, are ligated and divided to achieve better mobilization. Usually, the origin of the renal artery is exposed directly at the crossing of the left renal vein and the border of the aorta. b For exposure of the origin of the right renal artery, the venous intersection (vena cava and both renal veins) must be dissected and retracted to the right

sult if a ligature would slip off during dissection. When the artery is located more distal to the renal vein, the ovarian or spermatic vein is divided following ligation to facilitate retraction of the renal vein (Fig. 23.2a). When there is doubt as to the location of the renal artery, the vein is initially retracted upward using a vein hook and the dissection is carried on stepwise toward the arterial wall. The palpating finger can then easily detect the renal artery at the lateral origin by its pulsations. If the artery is occluded, it can at least be palpated as a band. Very often in cases of arteriosclerotic renal artery lesions, many adhesions to lymph vessels and lymph nodes are found. Sometimes, one may get the impression that the renal artery is compressed by this tissue. When this suspicion exists, blood pressure in the aorta and in the peripheral renal artery should be measured as soon as possible in order to confirm a pressure gradient. Only when a proven pressure gradient disappears following dissection of the vessel it is justifiable to assume a stenosis by exogenous compression and not to open the renal artery itself. In cases of adhesions, the dissection must be carried out by small steps as the adventitia of the aorta and the renal artery are otherwise easily injured. It may be helpful to begin by passing a tape around the aorta.

When both origins of the renal arteries, or predominantly the right one, have to be dissected, the procedure is performed as described. Then, the junction of the renal vein with the inferior vena cava is dissected to expose at least the left side of the vena cava. Although the origin of the right renal artery is located directly below the junction of the left renal vein with the inferior vena cava, one should be careful when dissecting and placing tapes around the vena cava. If peripheral segments of the right renal artery must also be exposed, the right renal vein will have to be dissected. Sufficient mobilization can be achieved by dissecting along the vena cava, dividing the lumbar veins if necessary. Adequate visualization of the origin of the right renal artery is obtained by placing a vein hook in the angle of junction of the left renal vein (Fig. 23.2b). If the lesions extend into the periphery, the right side of the vena cava must be retracted to the left in order to carry on the dissection. While performing this maneuver, care is taken of renal vein tributaries joining the vena cava relatively centrally. Tearing may cause troublesome bleeding. Stopping the bleeding may be difficult when these veins join the renal vein at

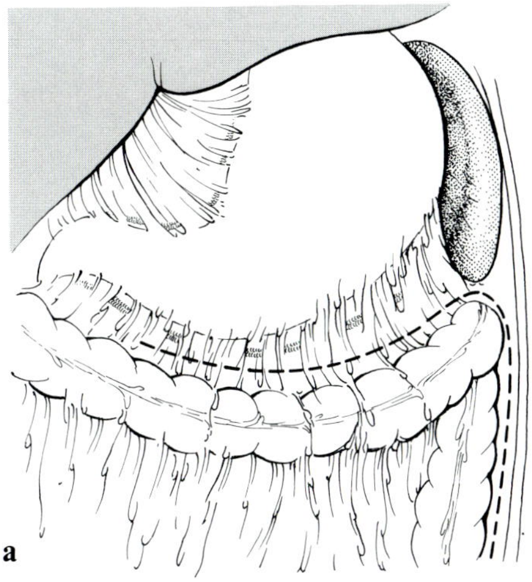
a

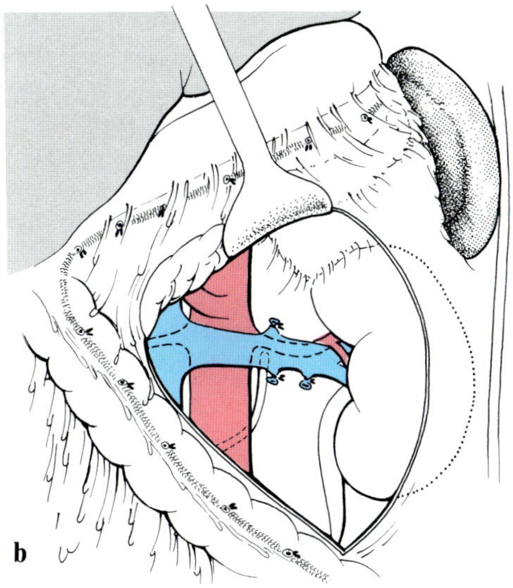
b

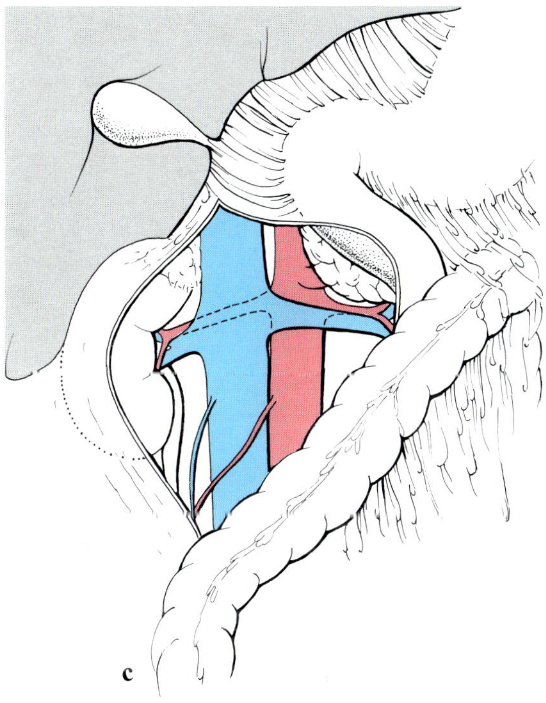
c

Fig. 23.3a–c. Supracolic approach to the renal arteries. **a, b** Exposure of the left renal artery. After the gastrocolic ligament is divided and the left colon flexure is dissected free of adhesions to the posterior abdominal wall, the flexure, together with its mesocolon, is retracted medially and the renal vein dissected free; the left renal artery can then be found beneath the vein. **c** Exposure of the right renal artery. Following incision of the retroperitoneum around the duodenum and the right colon flexure, both bowel segments are dissected off the perirenal fatty tissue and the capsule, and retracted medially. The origin of the right renal artery is located directly under the point where the inferior vena cava and both renal veins cross

the posterior circumference. However, hemostasis may be achieved by careful exposure of the posterior wall and suture ligation with atraumatic 5–0 or 6–0 sutures.

II. Supracolic Approach (Fig. 23.3)

When the lesions extend very far peripherally or can only be located there, the supracolic approach must be chosen either additionally or primarily.

On the left side (Fig. 23.3a), the adhesions of the left colon flexure to the spleen have to be divided and the flexure mobilized to the right until the left renal vein is exposed (Fig. 23.3b). Depending on the situation, the ovarian or spermatic vein and the suprarenal vein, which always joins the renal vein, is divided following ligation. By retracting the renal vein with an appropriate hook (see p. 616), exposure of the renal artery origin at the aorta is achieved without difficulty.

On the right side (Fig. 23.3c) the hepatic colon flexure, together with the duodenum, are mobilized according to Kocher and dissected away from the renal capsule and the perirenal fatty tissue. Identification of the renal vein is relatively easy. Because of its large diameter, it is readily distinguished from other veins, especially mesenteric veins. If the right suprarenal vein joins the renal vein, it is advisable to divide it between ligatures in order to create enough space to retract the renal vein for renal artery exposure.

Generally, it should be emphasized that good exposure of the renal artery beyond the diseased segment is essential for secure cross-clamping and later revision. With the infracolic approach, the retroperitoneum should be closed by interrupted sutures or continuous suture following completion of the operation on the renal arteries. Fixation of the colon flexures is usually not required; it is sufficient to return the bowel to its normal position. Drainage is rarely necessary.

E. Operative Procedures

Special instruments. For renal artery operations, the standard vascular instruments are usually sufficient. However, long instruments should be available because of the depth of the operative field. For retracting the veins and the vena cava, we use a special vein hook. In cases of peripheral dysplasia, coronary surgery instruments may also be used. For dilation of renal artery branches, thin plastic dilators are especially suitable.

The suture material for the aorta is a 5–0 monofilament, nonabsorbable, atraumatic suture. For the renal artery, a 6–0 or 7–0 suture is used, depending on the caliber (close to the aorta or very peripherally).

I. Endarterectomy

It is essential for direct endarterectomy [11] to cross-clamp a sufficiently large aortic segment at the ostium of the renal artery because the lesions usually extend farther into the aorta than suggested from outside or by angiogram (Fig. 23.4).

By means of a curved clamp (Cooley clamp, or sometimes a Satinsky clamp), this may be achieved quite well. Depending on the degree of stenosis, the vessel is incised longitudinally over the stenosed segment. A clamp is also placed peripherally because of the massive retrograde flow that is to be expected. The plaque is then dissected in the normal way (Fig. 23.4a). Usually, its end point will leave a smooth transition zone not requiring fixation of the intima. The situation in the aorta may cause more problems due to significant arteriosclerotic lesions of the aortic wall. This segment of the aortic wall has to be examined to avoid residual stenoses or even postoperative thrombosis. If it is reasonably clear that the original arterial

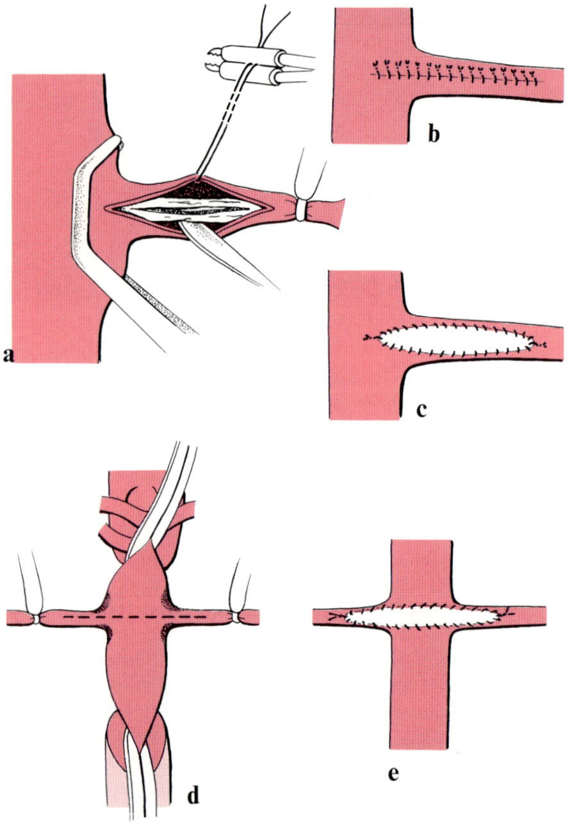

Fig. 23.4a–e. Endarterectomy of an arteriosclerotic renal artery stenosis close to the aorta. **a–c** Direct endarterectomy of a unilateral stenosis. Longitudinal arteriotomy of the renal artery following cross-clamping at its origin on the aorta and dissection of the constricting intimal lesion (**a**). Usually, the plaque separates, leaving a smooth distal transition zone. Otherwise, the intima must be fixed from inside. The arteriotomy is then closed with a vein patch using a continuous 6–0 suture (**c**). If the lumen of the segment following endarterectomy is greater than normal, a direct continuous suture may be feasible (**b**). In the region of the aortic wall, 5–0 interrupted sutures are used. The renal artery may be closed by a 6–0 continuous suture. However, it must be ensured that there are no stenotic strands located posteriorly. If there are any, they will have to be divided. **d, e** Transaortic direct endarterectomy of the ostia of both renal arteries through a transverse aortotomy. Following proximal and distal cross-clamping of the aorta, the incision is made transversely over the ostia of both renal arteries. The procedure is especially recommended where the major lesions are limited to the origin. Following endarterectomy, it is advisable to suture a venous or prosthetic patch into the arteriotomy

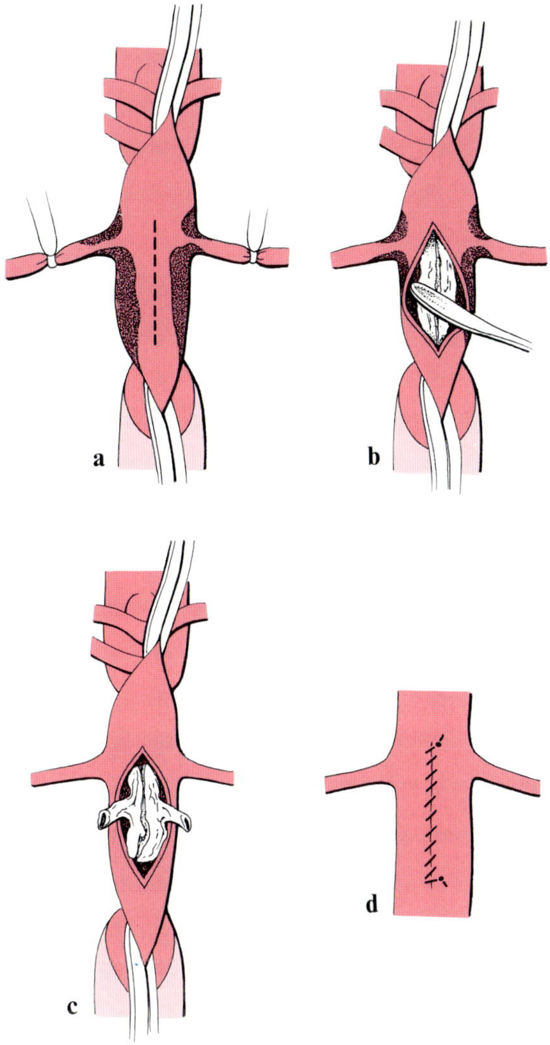

Fig. 23.5a–d. Indirect transaortic endarterectomy of both renal arteries following longitudinal incision. After proximal and distal cross-clamping, the aorta is incised longitudinally on the anterior wall (**a**) and the plaque dissected off the intima (**b**). Ideally, one may succeed in removing the specimen as a complete cylinder (**c**). The intima must be torn off at the proximal and distal clamps. After ensuring that a smooth transition zone is left at the distal intima, the aorta is then closed by a continuous 5–0 suture (**d**)

lumen can be preserved after plaque removal and closure, we prefer to close the artery by direct suture rather than with a venous patch graft (Fig. 23.4b). This way, it is possible to achieve a result that is indistinguishable from a normal renal artery. For the arteriotomy, we use 5–0 interrupted sutures in the region of the junction with the aorta. The renal artery itself is closed by a continuous suture using 6–0 nonabsorbable monofilament synthetic material. This procedure cannot succeed, of course, unless the arterial wall is sufficiently strong to ensure a secure suture following endarterectomy.

Otherwise, patch graft angioplasty, using autogenous venous material, is the safer technique (Fig. 23.4c). Here, the critical point is the juncture of the renal artery with the aorta. The initial sutures should be placed opposite one another on both sides of the juncture in order to prevent distortion. Flushing is especially important before release of the blood flow. Especially in cases of bilateral stenosis, it is advisable to incise the aorta transversely (Fig. 23.4d) or longitudinally (Fig. 23.5a–d) in the osteal region and to perform an endarterectomy of the ostium coming from inside. The advantage of this procedure is the possibility of rapid closure following completion of the endarterectomy [24]. A significant disadvantage of the longitudinal incision is that the peripheral end, which can be of essential importance for the success of the procedure, may not be visualized. With the transverse aortotomy (Fig. 23.4d, e), however, the incision can be extended into the renal arteries and later closed with a venous or Dacron patch.

II. Resection and Renorenal End-to-End Anastomosis (Fig. 23.6a–d)

In short stenoses of fibrodysplastic origin – especially of the rare constricting fibromuscular type – resection of the diseased segment may be considered (Fig. 23.6a). The corresponding vessel ends should be beveled to achieve the widest possible anastomosis (Fig. 23.6b). Depending on the diameter of the vessel, the anastomosis is performed either partially or completely using a continuous suture (Fig. 23.6c). If there is doubt, a patch graft should be considered (Fig. 23.6d). For a lesion of the arterial segment extending over a longer distance, an end-to-end anastomosis may be achieved if there is a mobile kidney, which is often the case in fibrodysplastic disease. By ap-

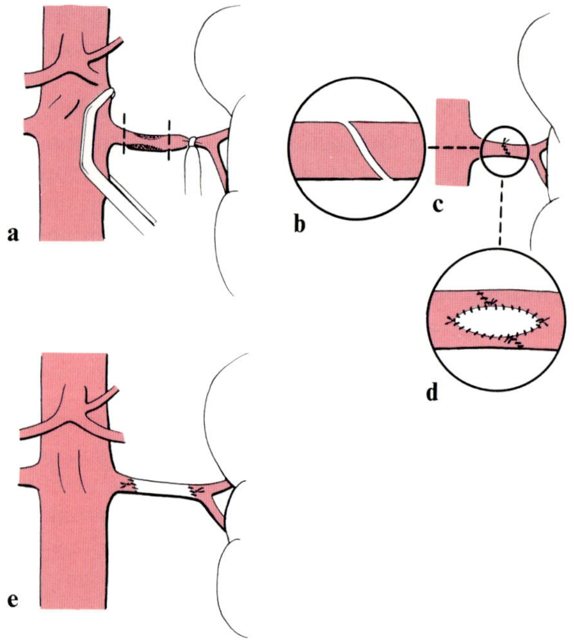

Fig. 23.6a–e. Resection of the stenosis and renorenal end-to-end anastomosis. When the stenosis is located in the middle of the renal artery, resection of a diseased segment following cross-clamping may be the simplest procedure (**a**). Great care should be taken to bevel the ends to be anastomosed (**b**, **c**). If the artery is of very small caliber, interrupted sutures are preferred, or a vein patch is used to enlarge the anastomosis (**d**). **e** Resection of the stenosis and renorenal graft interposition. Following resection of the stenosis, a vein graft is sutured between the proximal stump at the aorta and the peripheral renal artery. This approach has the advantage of maintaining the original renal artery ostium at the aorta. However, it has the disadvantage that both anastomoses are performed while the renal artery is cross-clamped. Usually, the aortorenal vein graft is preferred

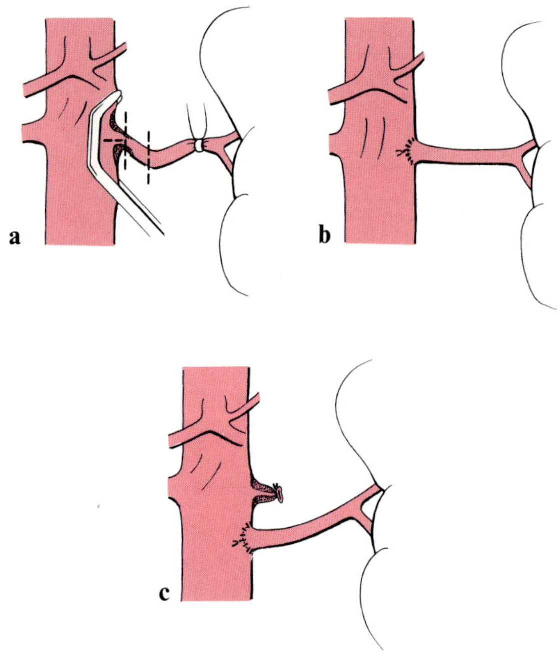

Fig. 23.7. a, b Division of the renal artery close to the aorta, endarterectomy of the ostium of the renal artery, and reimplantation of the vessel at its aortic origin. This procedure may be used when coiling of the artery has occurred in the region of the stenosis (**a**). Following division of the renal artery relatively close to the aorta and endarterectomy of the renal artery, a careful endarterectomy is performed at the ostium. The incision on the anterior wall of the renal artery is extended to the aorta (**a**). Following endarterectomy, the renal artery is sutured again to its origin at the aorta, using a continuous suture (**b**). By incising the posterior wall of the renal artery and matching it to the incised origin, a wide anastomosis is achieved. **c** Aortic reimplantation of the renal artery. When the condition of the ostial renal artery is too unfavorable, and if there is only a very short stenosis, the renal artery may be directly reimplanted into the aorta. Care is taken to create a sufficiently wide new ostium and to perform a sufficient endarterectomy of the aortic wall in the appropriate region. Continuous sutures with two interruptions as well as interrupted sutures are possible

proximation of the kidney, the two renal artery stumps can be brought together and anastomosed without tension.

III. Resection and Renorenal Graft Interposition (Fig. 23.6e)

In long resections, prosthesis or vein graft interposition should be performed, based on the assumption that surgical restoration of normal renal artery ostia is possible only in exceptional cases. The disadvantage of such a procedure is the prolonged ischemic time, as two anastomoses have to be sutured while the renal artery is cross-clamped. Therefore, this procedure has largely been replaced by aortorenal graft interposition.

IV. Resection and Renorenal End-to-End Anastomosis at the Ostium of the Renal Artery (Fig. 23.7a, b)

When there are renal artery lesions of arteriosclerotic origin, elongation of the vessel and kinking in the region of the stenosis are often encountered (Fig. 23.7a). It may be of advantage to divide the renal artery approximately 1 cm beyond its origin at the aorta. An endarterectomy of the renal artery and the renal artery ostium is performed, and the renal stumps are reconnected (Fig. 23.7b). The posterior wall may be sutured continuously; however, the anterior wall should be closed by interrupted sutures. The ends to be anastomosed should be beveled as much as possible to achieve a wide anastomosis. In cases of arteriosclerosis of the aorta, this procedure is preferable to reimplantation because the original conditions of the renal artery ostium may be reconstructed or maintained.

V. Reimplantation of the Renal Artery into the Aorta (Fig. 23.7c)

For lesions close to the aorta, an especially unfavorable location, the simplest procedure is to ligate and divide the renal artery at its origin and reimplant it at a selected site on the aorta [23]. Care must be taken to ensure that a sufficiently large ostium is excised at the new takeoff site and that the aorta is properly endarterectomized in this region. When the aorta is only partially cross-clamped, one must be sure that the true lumen has been opened; for in cases of intimal thickening, the intima may be pushed inside, thus simulating a lumen. As a result of endarterectomy, the aortic wall may be thinner at the origin of the renal artery; this ameliorates the disadvantage of anastomosing a relatively thick wall (aorta) to the often very thin wall of the poststenotically dilated renal artery.

VI. Aortorenal Graft Interposition (Fig. 23.8a–c)

Graft interposition from the aorta to the peripheral arterial end following resection of short or long stenoses may be used [10] in practically all situations. The aorta is completely or partially cross-clamped distal to the origin of the renal artery at a readily accessible site. At the lateral aortic wall, an orifice is created matching the caliber of the renal artery. The prepared vein graft is sutured in place. VAN DONGEN advises making the anastomosis as wide as possible, either by means of a bifurcated segment of great saphenous vein whose branches are slit longitudinally, thus allowing the edges to be sewn together to form a large single orifice, or by means of a patch at the orifice of the vein graft (Fig. 23.8c). During this maneuver, blood flow in the kidney is normally maintained. Following completion of the anastomosis and test-

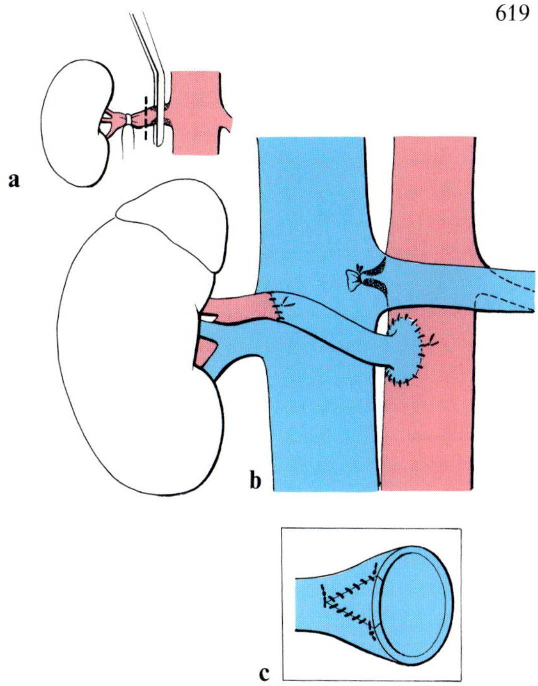

Fig. 23.8a–c. Aortorenal graft interposition. It is presumed that venous grafting material can be harvested from the patient. In principle, prosthetic material can also be used; however, in the case of the renal arteries it has the disadvantage of low elasticity. VAN DONGEN recommends that one achieves an especially wide anastomosis at the aorta, either tailoring the vein at a bifurcation or using an additional vein patch to achieve a greater circumference (**c**). In this way, one should be able to avoid vein dilatations, which have been variously described and which can be interpreted as poststenotic dilatation. For anastomosis with the peripheral renal artery the graft is passed in front of the vena cava; this facilitates the anastomosis, which should be beveled for greater longitudinal diameter

ing it for tightness, the renal artery is divided, following proximal ligation. Then the anastomosis of the vein is performed end-to-end to the healthy or poststenotic segment. The end-to-side anastomosis in the periphery is no longer performed, for hemodynamic reasons.

VII. Aortobirenal Graft (Double End Bypass) (Fig. 23.9)

In cases of bilateral renal artery lesions, the vein graft is anastomosed to the aortic wall side-to-side. Then, each vein end is again anastomosed end-to-end to the appropriate peripheral end of the renal artery. Essentials to this procedure, suggested by VAN DONGEN [7] are a good primary anastomosis of the aorta to the graft and resection of the vein valves.

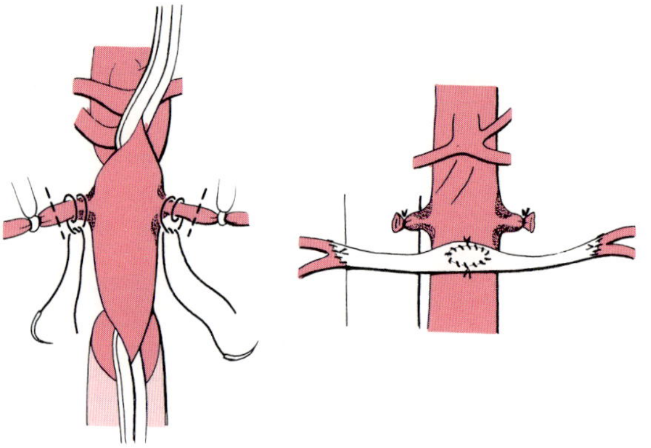

Fig. 23.9. Aortobirenal graft interposition. In cases of bilateral renal artery stenoses, a double-end bypass graft may also be used. A sufficiently long vein graft is anastomosed to the anterior wall of the aorta side-to-side. Then the renal arteries were anastomosed one after the other to the ends of the bypass graft

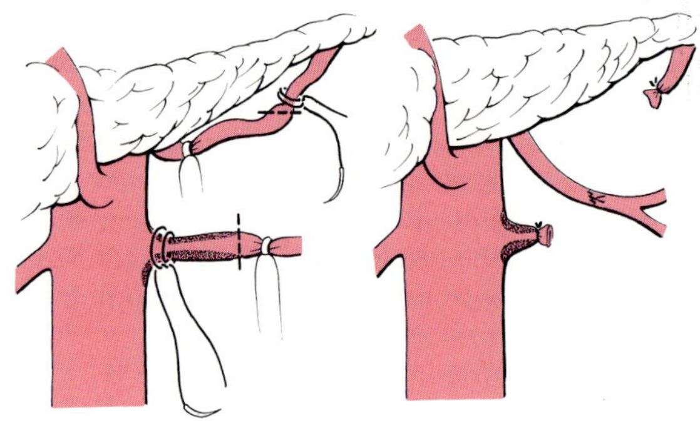

Fig. 23.10. Splenorenal end-to-end anastomosis to the left renal artery. The advantage of this procedure is that it requires only one peripheral anastomosis. However, there is the disadvantage that the splenic artery is affected very early by arteriosclerotic lesions

VIII. Extra-anatomic Reconstructions

Under special circumstances, other bypass procedures may be used. For a time, the most common procedure consisted of dissecting the splenic artery, dividing it peripherally, and then anastomosing it end-to-side or end-to-end to the poststenotic dilatation of the renal artery [4] (Fig. 23.10). Objections are based on the fact that the splenic artery is usually the first abdominal vessel affected by arteriosclerosis, a circumstance which rather seriously limits its long-term potential as a vascular graft. An interposition graft between the superior mesenteric, the hepatic [18], or the gastroduodenal artery and one of the renal arteries is, practically speaking, no longer indicated (Fig. 23.11a, b). In contrast, iliacorenal interposition may be an alternative under special circumstances (Fig. 23.11c). The procedure is the same as for aortorenal vein graft interposition; however, one should be aware that the region of the iliac vessels is a prime location for arteriosclerotic lesions, even when there are no lesions in the distal aorta.

IX. Autotransplantation (Fig. 23.12a–c)

Under certain circumstances, when vascular lesions are located very peripherally, renal autotransplantation, analogous to renal homotransplantation, has been suggested as a way of facilitating the treatment. This procedure is not indicated when the lesions are of arteriosclerotic origin, i.e., close to the aorta, because it requires down-

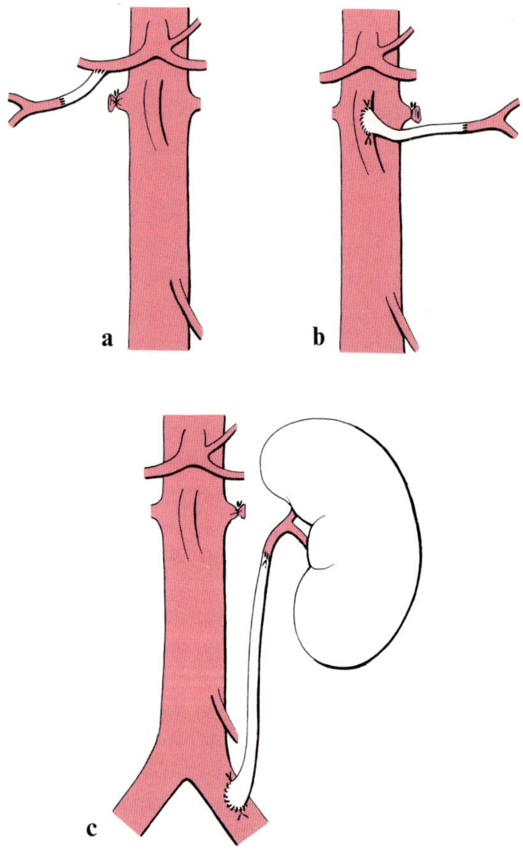

Fig. 23.11a–c. Special types of extra-anatomic reconstructions. In rare cases, especially for reoperations, it may be necessary to interpose a vein graft from the hepatic artery to the right renal artery (a), from the superior mesenteric artery to the left renal artery (b), or from the common iliac artery to the peripheral renal artery (c). In normal practice, however, these procedures are of little or no significance

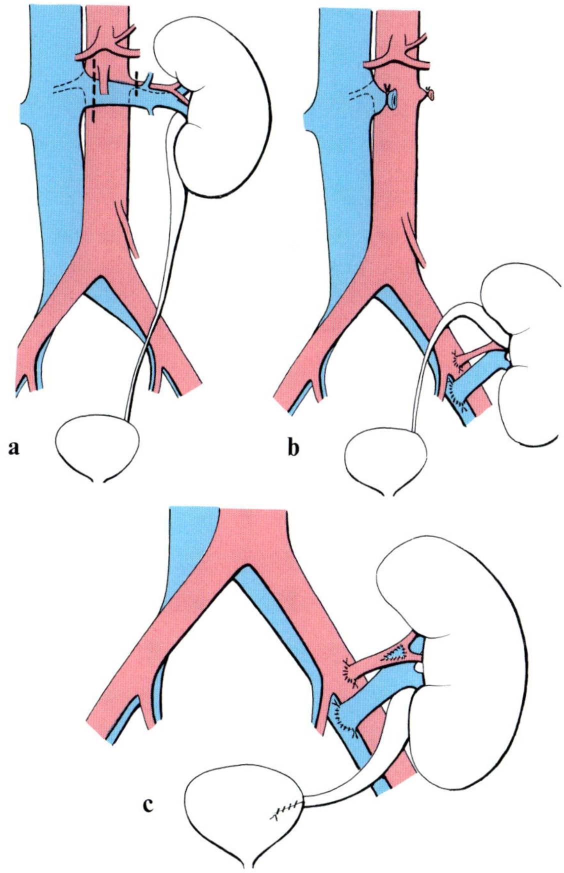

Fig. 23.12 a–c. Autotransplantation of the kidney. The continuity of the ureter may be maintained by moving the upper pole of the kidney downward (**b**) or total autotransplantation may be necessary following complete removal and hypothermic perfusion of the kidney and ex situ reconstruction of stenotic branches, e.g., with a V-shaped patch of greater saphenous vein (**c**)

ward displacement of the kidney into the minor pelvis and anastomosis of the renal vessels to the iliac vessels, in which extensive arteriosclerotic lesions may also be present. Moreover, all renal collaterals will be destroyed. In cases of very peripheral lesions, however, one should consider a complete autotransplantation, involving ex situ "workbench" surgery [2]. Simple autotransplantation, however, is more often used in cases of long ureteral defects to locate the kidney as close to the bladder as possible. The details of simple autotransplantation are the same as for organ harvesting from a living donor (Fig. 23.12c). In the meantime a perfusion with a hypothermic solution is recommended (see PICHLMAYR, Organtransplantation, vol. III, Allg. u. spez. Operationslehre).

X. Ex Situ "Workbench" Surgery, Total Autotransplantation [2]

In this procedure, the kidney is completely removed, as in homotransplantation. Special care must be taken of the vascular supply to the ureter within the surrounding fatty tissue. Following hypothermic pulsatile perfusion, peripheral vessels can be reconstructed under the microscope. After its connection to the iliac vessels in the minor pelvis (preferably by end-to-side anastomosis), the ureter is implanted into the bladder, as in homotransplantation (Fig. 23.12c).

F. Special Situations in Children

Even in infants, renal artery lesions may cause hypertension [21]. When correcting these lesions, one has to consider that the organism is still growing and that continuous sutures must therefore be avoided. Often, one may use 7–0 suture material for the very small vessels. Usually, the diseased or changed segment is resected, and either an end-to-end anastomosis or a reimplantation of the artery is performed. Of course, other reconstructive procedures may be considered, but prosthetic material should not be used.

G. Arterial Occlusion Based on a Preexisting Renal Artery Constriction

Often, primary medical treatment of renovascular hypertension may result in progression of the stenosis and finally in complete occlusion, especially with lesions of arteriosclerotic origin. Similar problems are present in cases of renal artery occlusion following percutaneous transluminal angioplasty. This special situation, as compared with an acute arterial occlusion, is usually characterized by well-developed collaterals [12, 25]. Therefore, even urine output, or in any case sufficient blood flow for the basic metabolism, can be maintained. Typically, the kidney behind such an occlusion is small and shows a smooth outline. An operation is indicated for maintenance of renal function if the patient is otherwise in good general condition. Nephrectomy should be performed only in cases of proven atrophy of pyelonephritic origin. Of course, the indication is urgent in cases of a single kidney or of bilateral occlusion. Owing to the special pathophysiology, the time of operation depends on the urgency of the situation. The operative approach corresponds to that for arteriosclerotic lesions of the renal artery. The prognosis is always favorable if a good retrograde flow is achieved.

A rare indication may also be given in patients already presenting with chronic renal insufficiency, where hypertension is hard to control and renal function worsens because of a renal artery stenosis. In rare cases, the time of first dialysis may be significantly delayed through revascularization [25].

H. Renovascular Hypertension Following Renal Transplantation

Following renal transplantation, hypertension may also be caused by a renal artery stenosis [5]. The data in the literature report up to 10%. Three reasons are given:

1. Unfavorable location of the anastomosis or secondary shrinking of the anastomosis
2. Intimal lesion of the renal artery resulting from cannulation for hypothermic perfusion
3. Immunologic phenomena of the intima relating to graft rejection

In such cases, it is difficult to determine whether the patient's own remaining kidney could be the cause of the hypertension or the transplanted functioning kidney. When the hypertension is difficult to control and renal function worsens, angiography should be performed to verify the diagnosis.

For reconstruction several especially important points must be considered:

A transperitoneal approach should be used. For the usual end-to-side or end-to-end anastomosis of the renal artery to the iliac artery, exposure of these vessels is much easier by this approach than by the extraperitoneal one, where the artery is reached by dissecting through the graft bed. Proceeding from the proximal anastomotic region, one can achieve good exposure of the anastomosis itself as well as distal vascular segment. While dissecting, one should bear in mind that the renal graft does not show any collaterals, in contrast to the case where there is gradual development of a stenosis in the patient's own kidney in its normal position. Accordingly, one must assume that the ischemic time that can be tolerated without acute renal failure is much shorter. The fastest procedure must therefore be chosen if one wishes to avoid conservation by perfusion. If the stenosis is located at the anastomosis, the site can usually be incised and a vein patch employed to achieve widening. In certain cases, and especially for end-to-end anastomoses, resection of the anastomosis followed by reanastomosis may be of greater advantage. If these principles are observed, the loss of the graft should be avoidable. On the basis of our own experience, we believe that surgical correction is preferable to percutaneous transluminal angioplasty (see p. 120). In the event of a complication, especially arterial thrombosis during angioplasty, quick action is the only way to save the kidney, since collateral circulation is lacking.

I. Acute Occlusion of an Originally Normal Renal Artery [19]

Acute occlusions of a renal artery which did not previously show any changes are caused either by embolism, trauma, or, in exceptional cases, by a spontaneous thrombosis. The acute occlusion of a vessel which was not previously stenosed should always be considered as an emergency because the sequelae of ischemia are bound to be more severe after 1 h due to the lack of collateral circulation. Therefore, in order to avoid permanent dialysis, the operation should always be performed as quickly as possible, especially when there is only a single kidney or when bilateral lesions are present. It is not possible to say with certainty how long an occlusion may persist and still allow partial function of the kidney since the degree to which collateral circulation has developed will obviously vary greatly from case to case. In cases where the time of ischemia is relatively long, there is the risk of massive postoperative urinary bleeding, due to tissue necrosis. This may eventually lead to secondary nephrectomy. While in cases of trauma the symptoms may be more or less clear, embolism can be accompanied by an acute pain attack. In any event, the presence of nearly complete anuria strongly suggests total occlusion of the renal artery, and appropriate diagnostic measures are urgently indicated. In these situations, digital subtraction angiography may well be the diagnostic procedure of choice [15]. Indirect methods, e.g., isotope nephrogram or intravenous pyelogram, may fail. When in doubt, angiography

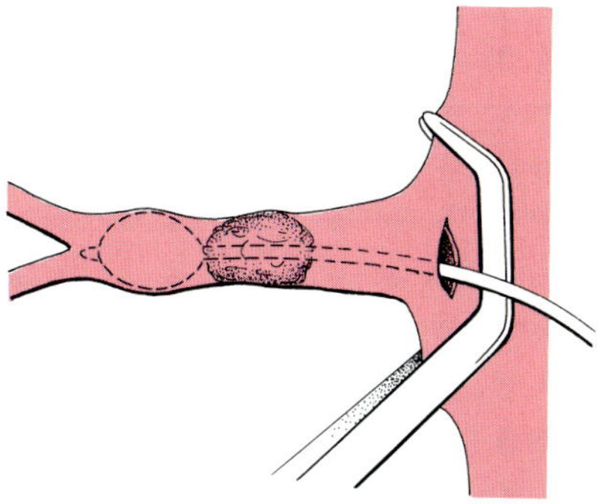

Fig. 23.13. Renal artery embolism. The embolus is removed with a Fogarty catheter inserted through a longitudinal arteriotomy on the aorta. Afterward, the arteriotomy is closed with a short continuous suture. Alternatively, the procedure shown in Fig. 23.14 may be used

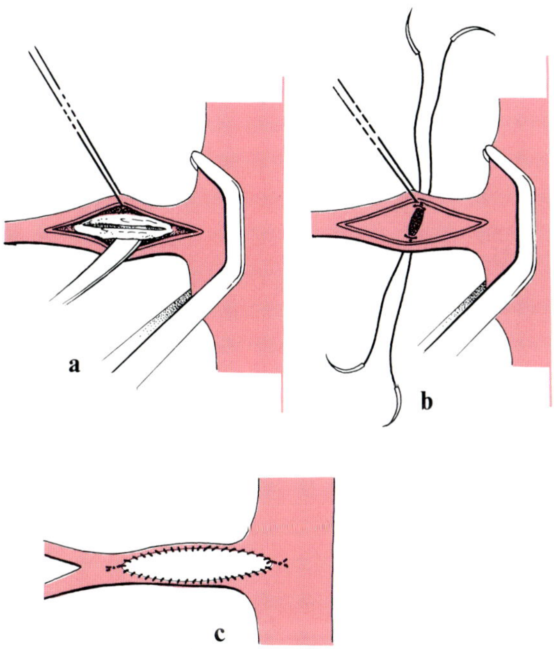

Fig. 23.14a–c. Renal artery trauma with intimal dissection and subsequent thrombotic renal artery occlusion. Thrombectomy is performed through a longitudinal arteriotomy (**a**). Intimal defects are fixed by transluminal sutures (**b**). Since the lumen of the renal artery is of normal width in this situation, the arteriotomy should be closed with a vein patch (**c**)

should be used. If the diagnosis is certain and there are no contraindications, one should operate immediately. Following dissection and placement of tapes around the diseased artery, transverse incision of the vessel approximately 1 cm distal to the ostium is convenient, given an otherwise normal vascular situation. When there is a risk of stenosis, an incision may be made in the partially clamped aortic wall at the takeoff of the renal artery (Fig. 23.13). If an embolus is found here, it is easily removed following incision of the artery. The prepared clamp is immediately placed on the aorta and residuals of embolic or secondary thrombi are removed from the periphery by means of a Fogarty catheter. In every case, retrograde flow should be achieved. Following flushing with heparinized Ringer's solution, the arteriotomy is closed with 6–0 interrupted sutures. If there is suspicion of simultaneous arteriosclerotic lesions, a longitudinal incision of the artery with subsequent enlargement using a vein patch as described for chronic lesions is more favorable. When the acute occlusion has been caused by trauma, involvement of the intima must almost always be assumed (Fig. 23.14a). Even if the artery exhibits only minor changes externally, a longitudinal incision is necessary, both for good exposure of the traumatized area and for fixation of the peripheral end of the intima (Fig. 23.14b). The incision is then closed using a vein patch (Fig. 23.14c).

K. Additional Procedures in Renovascular Hypertension

Fibrodysplastic renal artery lesions are often associated with a floating kidney. If the kidney is clearly hypermobile, nephropexy should be performed in addition to shortening the renal artery. This may be achieved by means of sutures passing around the lowest rib and crossing the upper pole of the kidney. If the renal artery branches are not to be revascularized, resection of the appropriate renal parenchyma should be considered. To define the border of the appropriate parenchyma it is advisable to inject indigocarmine into the renal segment. Following resection of the diseased parenchymatous segment, the remaining parenchyma is closed by continuous suture of the capsule.

L. Complications and Reoperations of the Renal Arteries [8]

Reoperations may become necessary for postoperative complications such as bleeding or early reocclusion, or later for restenosis, gradual occlusion, or development of an aneurysm. In the event of abrupt changes in blood pressure or renal function, postoperative rebleeding or rethrombosis have to be excluded. If the changes are serious, this should be done by angiography as soon as possible. If reintervention becomes necessary, one should quickly gain access to the appropriate renal vessels, as in the first operation. It is urgently recommended that the vessels are reexposed and that loops are placed around them again.

In case of *rebleeding* from incisions or anastomoses, brief cross-clamping cannot be avoided. If there is a *rethrombosis*, it is absolutely essential that the reconstruction has to be checked for possible technical errors as these are usually the principal reasons for rethrombosis. A vein patch may have to be sutured into an occluded segment, or it may even be necessary to implant a venous interposition graft.

Late reoperations due to *restenosing* or *development of aneurysms* at the suture line or graft may be difficult, especially the dissection. The region not previously exposed should now be exposed first; dissection is then continued in the direction of the diseased artery, which usually lies amid dense adhesions. If the lesions are too serious, vein interposition may offer the best means of bypassing the diseased area. However, as long as one can detect renal parenchyma capable of recovery, nephrectomy should be avoided in favor of revascularization.

REFERENCES

1. Abbott WM, Austen WG (1974) The reversal of renal cortical ischemia during aortic occlusion by mannitol. J Surg Res 16:482
2. Belzer FO, Raczkowski A (1982) Ex vivo renal artery reconstruction with autotransplantation. Surgery 92:642
3. Breslin DJ (1982) Pathophysiology of renovascular hypertension: An overview. In: Breslin DJ, Swinton NW, Libertino JA, Zinman L (eds) Renovascular hypertension. Williams & Wilkins, Baltimore London, p 36
4. Brewster DC, Darling RC (1979) Splenorenal arterial anastomosis for renovascular hypertension. Ann Surg 189:353
5. Brölsch Ch, Meiners G, Ringe B, Rippel W, Mellmann J, Tidow G, Lauchart W, Bunzendahl H, Pichlmayr R (1984) Causes and treatment of renal allograft stenosis. In: Eigler FW, Jakubowski HD (eds) Surgery in chronic renal failure. Thieme, Stuttgart New York, p 230
6. Danielson M, Dammström BG (1981) The prevalence of secondary and curable hypertension. Acta Med Scand 209:451
7. Dongen RJAM van (1972) Renovaskuläre Hypertonie – chirurgische Behandlung und Ergebnisse. Thoraxchir 20:361
8. Dongen RJAM van, Schwilden E-D (1980) Reinterventionen an den Visceral- und Nierenarterien. Chirurg 51:7
9. Eigler FW, Dostal G, Bock K-D, Löhr E (1984) Die Nierenarterienstenose arteriosklerotischer Genese. Dtsch Ärztebl 81:271
10. Ernst CB, Stanley JC, Marshall FF, Fry WJ (1972) Autogenous saphenous vein aortorenal grafts. Arch Surg 105:855
11. Freeman NE, Leeds FH, Elliott WH, Roland SI (1954) Thromboendarterectomy for hypertension due to renal artery occlusion. JAMA 156:1077
12. Hallwachs O, Vollmar J (1971) Totalverschluß der Nierenarterie: Nephrektomie oder Ravaskularisation? Dtsch Med Wochenschr 96:53
13. Harrison EG, McCormack LJ (1971) Pathologic classification of renal arterial disease in renovascular hypertension. Mayo Clin Proc 46:161
14. Heberer G, Eigler FW, Albrecht KF (1963) Diagnostische und chirurgische Möglichkeiten bei Hochdruckkranken mit Nierenarterienstenosen. Langenbecks Arch Klin Chir 302:159
15. Hillman BJ (1983) Digital subtraction angiography in the evaluation of hypertension. In: Schilfgaarde R van, Stanley JC, Brummelen P van, Overbosch EH (eds) Clinical aspects of renovascular hypertension. Martinus Nijhoff, Dordrecht, p 46
16. Madias NE, Millan VG (1982) Percutaneous transluminal renal angioplasty in the treatment of renovascular hypertension. In: Breslin DJ, Swinton NW, Libertino JA, Zinman L (eds) Renovascular hypertension. Williams & Wilkins, Baltimore London, p 148
17. Maxwell MH, Bleifer KH, Franklin SS, Varady PD (1972) Cooperative study of renovascular hypertension. Demographic analysis of the study. JAMA 220:1195
18. Novick AC, Palleschi J, Stratton RA (1979) Experimental and clinical hepatorenal bypass as a means of revascularization of the right renal artery. Surg Gynecol Obstet 148:557
19. Sarkissian J, Dubernard J-M, Devonex M, Pugeat G (1980) Chirurgie conservative dans les ruptures traumatiques fermées du tronc de l'artère rénale. J Traumatol 1:55
20. Staessen J, Bulpitt Chr, Fagard R, Lijnen P, Amery A (1983) Long-term converting-enzyme inhibition as a guide to surgical curability of hypertension associated with renovascular disease. Am J Cardiol 51:1317
21. Stanley JC, Fry WJ (1981) Pediatric renal artery occlusive disease and renovascular hypertension: etiol-

ogy, diagnosis and operative treatment. Arch Surg 116:669
22. Stanley JC, Whitehouse WM, Graham LM, Cronenwett JL, Zelenock GB, Lindenauer SM (1982) Operative therapy of renovascular hypertension. Br J Surg 69:63
23. Stansel HC (1964) Complicated renal artery stenosis. N Engl J Med 270:770
24. Trippel OH, Bergan JJ, Simon NM, O'Connor VJ (1964) Bilateral simultaneous renal endarterectomy. Arch Surg 88:818
25. Whitehouse WM, Kazmers A, Zedenock GB, Erlandson EE, Cronenwett JL, Lindenauer SM, Stanley JC (1981) Chronic total renal artery occlusion: effects of treatment on secondary hypertension and renal function. Surgery 89:753
26. Woodruff MFA, Doig A, Donal KW, Nolan B (1966) Renal autotransplantation. Lancet I:433

24 Supplementary and Palliative Procedures of the Extremities

24.1 Sympathectomy

L. Sunder-Plassmann

CONTENTS

Sympathectomy is performed for permanent sympathetic denervation of the lower, and less often the upper extremity; it serves as an indirect means of increasing blood flow or as a supplement to vascular reconstruction.

Fig. 24.1.1 a–c. Thoracic sympathectomy. **a** Skin incision. **b** Exposure of the sympathetic chain. **c** Resection

A. Thoracic Sympathectomy

I. Indications

Indications are Raynaud's disease, Raynaud's phenomenon, peripheral embolism, or thrombosis, thromboangitis (rarely), and finally, excessive hyperhidrosis of the hands. Usually the therapeutic effect on the sudomotor fibers is definitive; however, 1–2 years after the operation an increasing regeneration of vasoconstrictive fibers may occur. Therefore, it is indispensable to obtain appropriate informed consent of the patient.

II. Operative Technique

The patient is in the lateral position. The approach is through a small axillary thoracotomy at the upper edge of the third rib. A curvilinear skin incision is made along the course of the third rib, between the dorsal edge of the pectoralis muscle and the anterior edge of the latissimus dorsi muscle

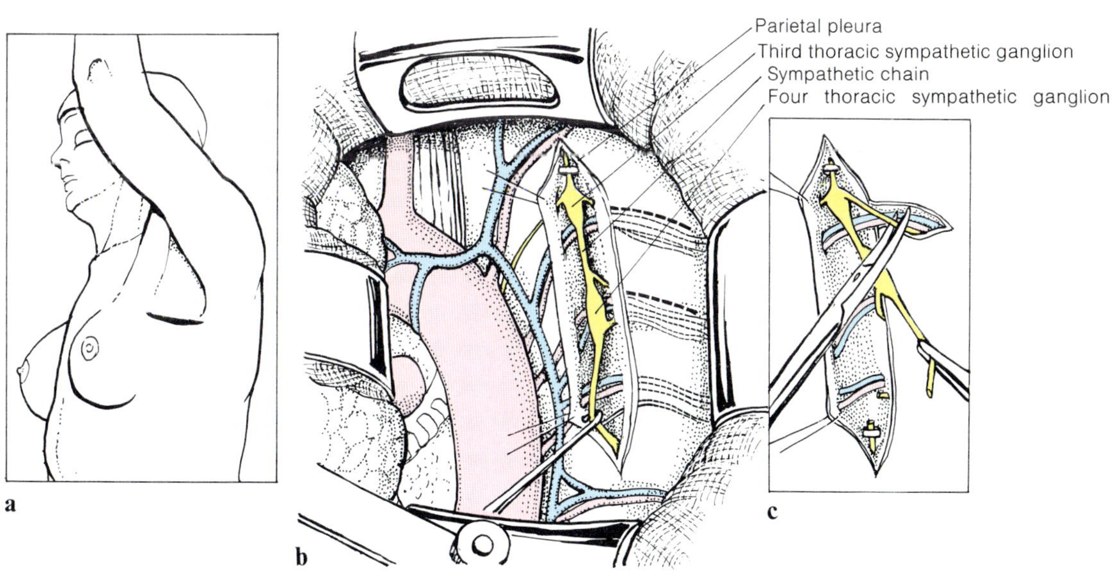

(Fig. 24.1.1a). The serratus muscle is split in the direction of its fibers, and the thorax is opened at the upper edge of the third rib. The upper lobe is retracted laterally and caudally. The thoracic sympathetic chain, located paravertebrally is visible through the parietal pleura which is divided longitudinally (Fig. 24.1.1b). The stellate ganglion is identified. The sympathetic chain between the third and fourth thoracic ganglia is drawn up with a clamp or a nerve hook. The chain is divided and resected as far as the caudal portion of the stellate ganglion (Fig. 24.1.1b). Injury to the ganglion must be avoided at all costs as a Horner syndrome will otherwise result. The thorax is closed with three or four pericostal interrupted sutures. Placement of a chest tube may be abandoned if the continuous suture of the serratus muscle is pulled tight when the lung is inflated. Complete lung extension, however, must be confirmed by X-ray prior to extubation. It is safer to drain the region for 24 h, using a small-caliber chest tube (16–20 Charrière) attached to a water-seal drainage system.

B. Lumbar Sympathectomy

I. Indications

The indication for lumbar sympathectomy alone is still controversial. However, lumbar sympathectomy as a supplementary procedure to increase the blood supply to the crural region is performed more often [1, 2, 3, 4, 6, 7]. Removal of the ganglia L2 to L4 results in an interruption of the vasoconstrictive fibers to all peripheral lower extremity vessels of the skin as well as of the muscles. This causes an increase in blood flow to the cutaneous vessels and also to most of the arteriovenous shunts of the extremities, which serve as temperature regulators. Recently, there have been clinical as well as experimental results showing an increase in muscle blood supply, at least for a short time [2, 6]. If lumbar sympathectomy alone is planned, without vascular reconstruction, there must be a certain minimal perfusion pressure of the arteries in the region of the ankle (about 50 mmHg), as lumbar sympathectomy usually causes an additional decrease in the peripheral pressure. Unmeasurable peripheral pressures are a contraindication for lumbar sympathectomy in all cases. In a given case, the effect of lumbar sympathectomy on the nutritive cutaneous perfusion as well as on the thermoregulatory arteriovenous shunts may be accurately estimated preoperatively by peridural anesthesia and determination of transcutaneous oxygen pressure at the wrist, as well as by skin temperature measurement using a thermocamera [6]. This method permits preoperative identification of paradoxical ischemia following sympathectomy.

II. Operative Technique

For lumbar sympathectomy, the approach is retroperitoneal. The skin incision may be either pararectal or in the flank area (Fig. 24.1.2a). We prefer a relatively cranial, almost transverse incision in the direction of the fibers of the transversus muscle, the latter being split over its whole length. The transversalis fascia is carefully retracted laterally or the peritoneum bluntly pushed medially, using the hand, until the lateroventral edge of the iliopsoas muscle is palpated. From there, the plane is developed medially to the vertebral column (Fig. 24.1.2b). The muscles and the peritoneum are retracted with two broad hooks. The sympathetic chain between the vertebral column and the medial edge of the iliopsoas muscle can now be identified; a clamp is passed underneath it, and it is divided (Fig. 24.1.2c). Dissection of both segments is continued caudally (L3/L4) and cranially as far as possible, in order to be able to remove ganglion L2 for denervation of the thigh as well, if desired. Afterwards, the operative field is briefly compressed with two hot sponges, and bleeding from lumbar veins is controlled. Placement of a drain is usually not required. The wound is closed by continuous suture of the transversus muscle and interrupted sutures of the fascia.

The sympathetic chain segment being resected should always be identified histologically, as in thoracic sympathectomy.

REFERENCES

1. Heberer G, Rau G, Löhr HH (1966) Aorta and große Arterien. Springer, Berlin Heidelberg New York, p 398
2. Heyden B, Vollmar J (1980) Die Bedeutung der Profundaplastik in der rekonstruktiven Gefäßchirurgie der unteren Extremität. In: Müller-Wiefel H (ed) Mikrozirkulation und Blutrheologie. Therapie der peripheren arteriellen Verschlußkrankheit. Witzstrock, Baden-Baden, p 182
3. Lynn RB, Barcroft H (1950) Circulatory changes in

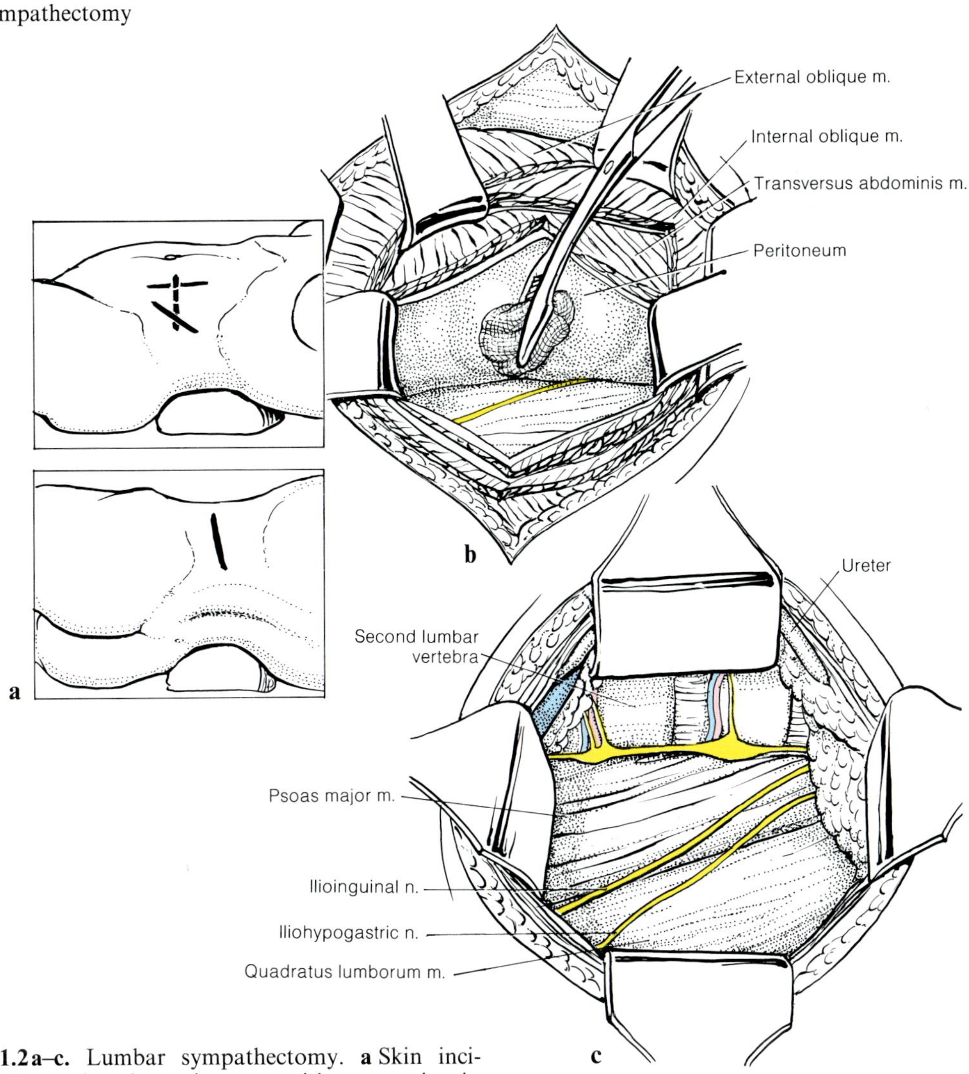

Fig. 24.1.2 a–c. Lumbar sympathectomy. **a** Skin incisions. **b** Retracting the peritoneum without opening it. **c** Exposure of the sympathetic chain, identification of the ureter

the foot after lumbar sympathectomy. Lancet 17:1105
4. Simeone FA (1979) The anatomy of the lumbar sympathetic trunk in man. J Cardiovasc Surg 20:283
5. Strandness DE (1966) Long term value of lumbar sympathectomy. Geriatrics 21:144
6. Sunder-Plassmann L (1981) Verbesserung der Mikrozirkulation und Kollateralstrombahn bei arterieller Verschlußkrankheit: Experimentelle und klinische Befunde. Habilitationsschrift, München
7. Sunder-Plassmann P (1953) Sympathicus-Chirurgie. Thieme, Stuttgart

24.2. Amputations

R.G.H. BAUMEISTER

CONTENTS

Except for emergencies, the goal of lower extremity amputation is to restore the patient to ambulatory status, even though this usually entails a certain impairment of physical capability. In any individual case, the vascular situation is of decisive importance. One should no longer accept the long-held opinion that lower extremity ischemia of vascular origin is best treated by an above-knee amputation. In elderly patients who are to receive a prosthesis, more distal levels of amputation have considerable practical advantages over above-knee amputation and should therefore be selected whenever feasible [1].

A. Indications for Operation

The pathophysiologic indication for operation is given when the perfusion of a limb or limb segment falls below the minimum required to maintain metabolism and correction by operative or conservative measures is not possible.

Characteristically, the clinical symptoms are intractable pain and progressive infection. Local mummification per se is no indication for amputation.

The general condition of the patient and the risk factors must be evaluated prior to any amputation. Metabolic deviations as well as cardiac, pulmonary, and renal disturbances must be treated [6]. Prior to the amputation one should also ascertain by angiography whether reconstructive vascular procedures may still be possible, if this has not already been done prior to a previous vascular procedure.

Exceptions are emergency amputations of a nonvital extremity in acute life-threatening situations.

Preexisting active infections endanger the result of amputation. Therefore, infection should be controlled prior to amputation whenever possible. This may be achieved, for example, by local drainage procedures such as removal or fenestration of necrotic skin areas with subsequent local antiseptic therapy. This is especially successful in the foot. When the infection cannot be controlled by these procedures, open amputation should usually be performed [11].

The parameter ultimately determining the level of amputation is perfusion, which must be evaluated intraoperatively by direct observation of the blood flow remaining at the selected level. Another parameter is the capability of the muscles to contract following transverse incision during the amputation.

B. Selection of Amputation Levels

I. Limited Amputation

Clear demarcation may often be detected in diabetic peripheral angiopathy, where macroangiopathy is missing or not important, and also following successful arterial reconstruction. In both cases, one is able to achieve the most peripheral amputation level possible, removing only the necrotic segments of the member and preserving the defense mechanisms in the region of demarcation. Limited amputations are most often performed on the toe. However, they may also be performed in cases of segmental extension of necrosis to the forefoot.

II. Forefoot

Necroses involving the entire forefoot are usually not considered suitable for a limited amputation. In most cases, transmetatarsal amputation must be performed. The level of the metatarsal joint is generally considered to be the most proximal site for amputations of the forefoot. Parts of the base of the second metatarsal protruding proximally are preserved in order to achieve a uniform amputation level. Disarticulations at Chopart's joint, without additional complicated stabilizations, are not beneficial. Over longer periods of time, they will result in deformities of the equinovarus type, owing to a lack of symmetric muscle insertions; they therefore require either in the primary or in a second operation complex corrections that cannot be recommended in ischemic extremities. Most necroses are so extensive and the circulation so limited that only ankle disarticulation, i.e., the next higher level, is considered.

Local pressure necrosis of the heel is a special case. Excision of the necrotic tissue, together with partial or complete amputation of the calcaneus, may be performed. Thus, primary wound closure is possible. Careful tailoring following partial amputation of the calcaneus serves as prophylaxis against subsequent pressure damage [1].

III. Ankle

In the frequent femoral and popliteal artery occlusions, amputation between the metatarsals and the lower leg is indicated only very seldom. In these rare cases Syme's amputation may be considered as a simple procedure to achieve an end-weight-bearing stump. Two sessions may be necessary in cases of impaired circulation, especially when infections are present. During the primary session, only disarticulation is performed. Later, osteotomy of the ankle has to be carried out through small incisions. Usually, a patent third popliteal segment (trifurcation) is required for this amputation level. In cases with sufficient collaterals of the profunda femoris artery, the superficial femoral artery may also be occluded.

IV. Below Knee

From the point of view of rehabilitation, below-knee amputation is preferred whenever there is macroangiopathy due to more proximal occlusions, and knee function is preserved. Usually, a well-perfused profunda femoris artery is necessary for this amputation level. Below-knee prostheses bear the weight on both femoral condyles or on the tibial head. Besides making it easier to put on and take off the prosthesis, this amputation level provides relatively safe, unimpaired ambulation. However, for this type of prosthesis, the stump of the tibia has to measure at least 6 cm. Tibial tuberosity must be preserved.

V. Knee

For a long time, amputation at the knee was looked upon with disfavor because of the difficulties it posed for prosthetic management. However, with the recent development of prostheses equipped with mechanical knee joints, this attitude is no longer justifiable [2, 7]. Knee disarticulation usually requires patent iliac arteries and a sufficiently perfused profunda femoris artery.

Following knee disarticulation the stump ultimately bears the weight, in contrast to the above-knee amputation. This facilitates ambulation with the prosthesis, especially in patients of reduced physical capability. The amputation does not impose great stress on the patient as there is only very minor soft tissue trauma, owing to the lack of muscles.

VI. Thigh and Hip

If tissue perfusion in the region of the knee is insufficient, above-knee amputation must be performed. The adductor muscles in particular show reduced perfusion, so that often a relatively high amputation level is indicated. The trochanter major, however, must be preserved completely, because its amputation would mean that muscular guidance of the stump could no longer be guaranteed. If perfusion is not sufficient at this level, amputation at the hip is preferable. It may be possible to preserve the head of the femur and parts of the femoral neck.

VII. Upper Extremities

Upper extremity amputations due to vascular disease are rare and are therefore discussed only in general terms. For the most part, these procedures are necessitated either by distal end necroses of an extremity in cases of thromboangitis obliterans or by a peripheral embolism. In such cases, one should try to keep the amputation level as peripheral as possible by vascular reconstructions or by simultaneous medical angiologic therapy. The extremity should be preserved as long as possible, especially the fingers, which are most often affected. However, this should not be done at the price of closing a wound under tension, because perfusion will never be sufficient to supply the skin flap. Flaps are likewise unsuitable for closure of the stump in this situation, although they are widely used elsewhere.

C. Operative Technique

I. General Approach

Amputations are performed in tissues of greatly reduced vitality. Therefore, the operative technique must be as atraumatic as possible. Compression trauma, careless handling with hooks, and tensile stress on the suture line may quickly result in tissue necrosis. The use of electric coagulation should be completely avoided.

Placement of a tourniquet is out of the question in patients undergoing amputation. Skin flaps with an unfavorable length–breadth ratio often result in distal end necrosis. Additional trauma during osteotomy must also be avoided. Therefore, clean-cut edges should be achieved. When using electrical saws, the bone must be cooled by water.

Approximating antagonistic muscle groups of the stump (myoplasty) or suturing them to the bone (myodesis) gives the best functional results [5]. However, as a rule, this procedure cannot be used in patients suffering from vascular diseases as muscle perfusion is often limited.

II. Toe Amputation (Fig. 24.2.1)

In the region of the toes, as well as in cases of partial forefoot demarcation, limited amputation is possible. The tissue is divided transversely just distal to the demarcation zone. The stump should always be left completely open; it will be closed by wound contraction and epithelial growth from the margins. For the complete and final amputation of a toe, disarticulation at the metatarsophalangeal joint, with preservation of the head of the metatarsal, should be the objective. The bradytrophic tendons are resected at a higher level whenever possible.

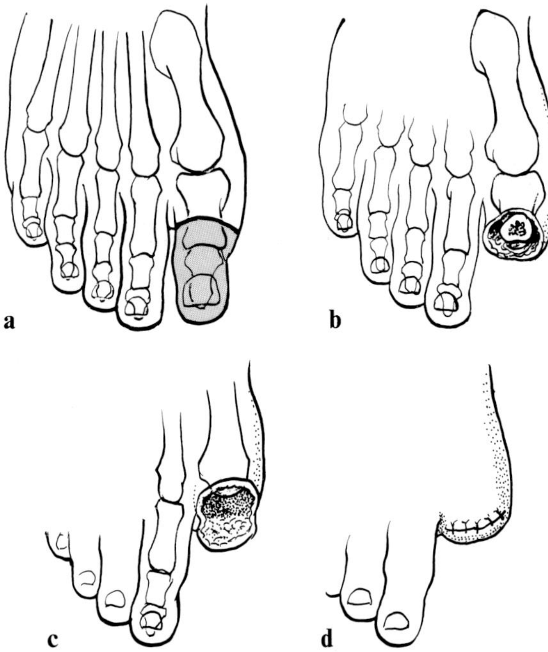

Fig. 24.2.1 a–d. Toe amputation. **a** Partial necrosis of the first toe. **b** In cases of clear demarcation the toe is divided just distal to the demarcation. Closure of the wound is not required. **c** When there is no clear demarcation, a metatarsophalangeal disarticulation is performed, preserving the head of the first metatarsal. **d** Following disarticulation, the wound is closed by a plantar soft-tissue flap

III. Forefoot Amputation (Fig. 24.2.2)

In cases of clear demarcation not involving the entire forefoot, limited amputation may also be performed. In extensive necrosis, transmetatarsal amputation at the level of the proximal third of the metatarsal is indicated. A soft tissue flap is created on the plantar side and turned dorsally. The small foot muscles may be severed first to achieve better trimming of the skin flap for wound closure. The metatarsals are divided in the spongy proximal region at such an angle as to achieve a "sled runner" effect as a safeguard against pressure sites. Disarticulation at the metatarsotarsal joint should not be performed in an undulating plane; one should take care to achieve a level amputation plane. This may be accomplished by preserving part of the second metatarsal head.

IV. Ankle Disarticulation (Fig. 24.2.3)

Ankle disarticulation according to Syme, with primary or secondary osteotomy at the outer and inner ankle, provides an end-weight-bearing stump. The patient walks on the skin of the heel, which is preserved. The skin is incised transversely on the anterior surface of the ankle. The incision extends distally at a right angle in front of the ankle. In this way, the skin of the entire heel is preserved. The extensor muscles are divided and the joint is opened. The talus and calcaneus are resected, together with the metatarsals and forefoot. Care has to be taken that the skin flap around the ankle is not too thin. A transverse osteotomy of the fibula and the tibia is made primarily, or better, secondarily, in the ankle region, especially if an infection is present. Two large Re-

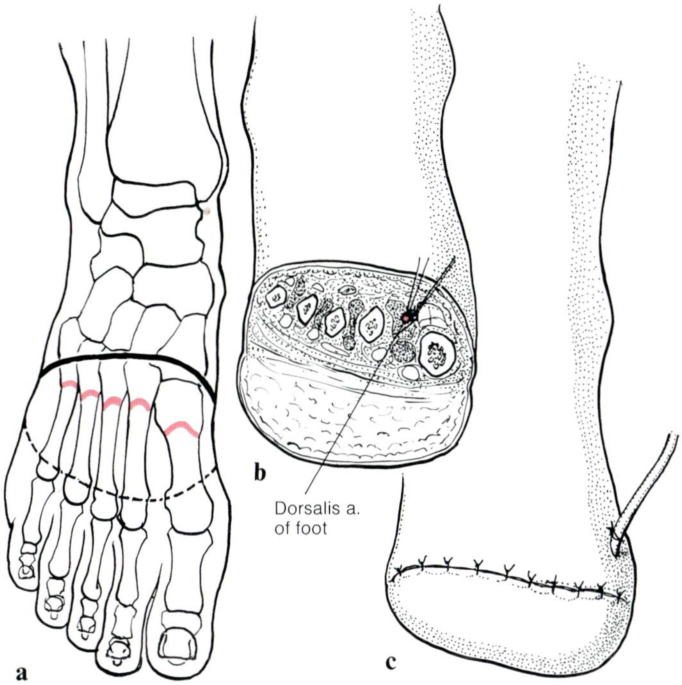

Fig. 24.2.2a–c. Forefoot amputation. **a** The forefoot is incised approximately at the level of the proximal third of the metatarsals, and a long plantar flap is created. The metatarsals are tailored to achieve a curvilinear sled-runner shape as a safeguard against pressure damage. **b** The flexor tendons and the small flexors of the toe are amputated for better approximation of the plantar flap. The dorsalis pedis artery and vein are ligated separately. **c** For wound closure, the plantar flap is turned dorsally. The walking surface is free of scar tissue

Fig. 24.2.3a–c. Ankle disarticulation according to SYME. **a** The curved incision before the ankle joint is extended downward perpendicularly, preserving the skin of the heel. In cases of infection, an osteotomy in the region of the malleoli should not be performed primarily. **b** Disarticulation is performed at the ankle joint. **c** The preserved skin flap of the heel is turned to the volar surface, achieving a good end-weight-bearing stump

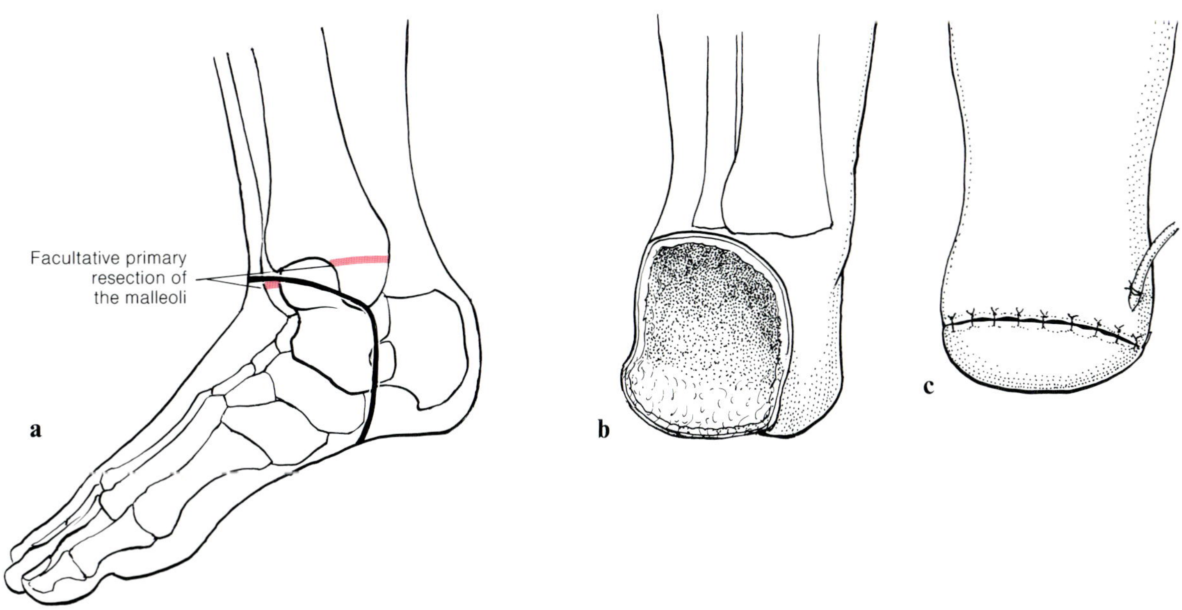

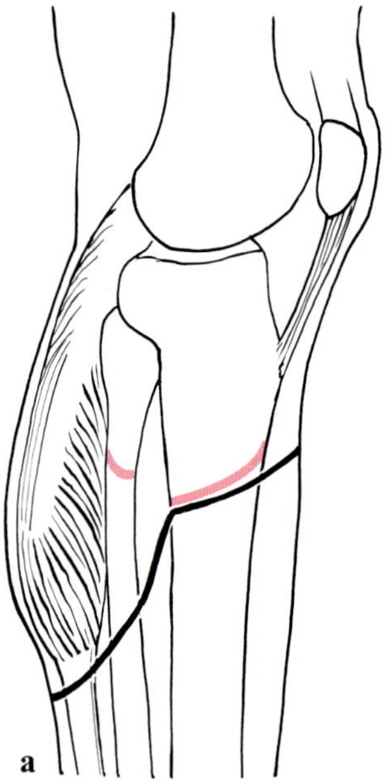

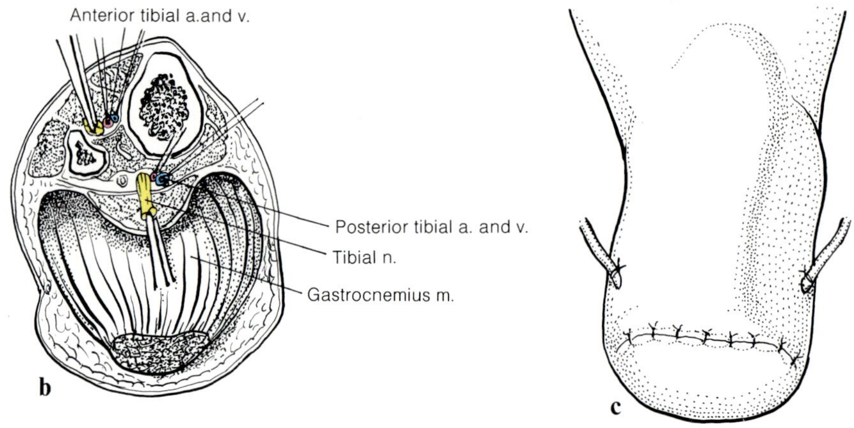

Fig. 24.2.4a–c. Below-knee amputation. **a** A circular incision is placed so as to provide a flap approximately 13–15 cm long. The tibia has to be divided distal to the tubercle of the tibia. The bone is beveled on its ventral surface to avoid pressure damage. The fibula is divided approximately 1 cm above this. **b** The soleus muscle is resected to achieve a better stump shape. The vessels are ligated at the amputation level, the nerves being divided approximately 3 cm proximally. **c** Following placement of drains, the stump is closed using the dorsal flap

don drains are placed. The skin flap is turned ventrally, and the wound is closed.

V. Below-Knee Amputation (Fig. 24.2.4)

In most below-knee amputations for vascular occlusions, a dorsal flap according to BURGESS is suitable [3, 4]. Also, two lateral flaps according to PERSSON [10] are recommended for lower leg ischemia. The dorsal flap must be relatively long (13–15 cm). The soleus muscle may be resected to achieve a slim stump. Resection of the muscles at the junction to the subcutaneous tissue should be avoided as it may result in disturbed perfusion of the flap. Prior to the osteotomy of the tibia, the periost can be incised and pulled up beyond the suggested site of the osteotomy. Following osteotomy, the periost is then be pulled back over the site of resection and sutured. Thus, the physiologically increased pressure within the bone cavity is preserved. The osteotomy of the tibia must always be performed distal to the tibial tuberosity, because otherwise the stump cannot be guided following resection of the tendon of the quadriceps femoris muscle.

As a rule, the stump of the tibia should measure at least 6 cm. The optimal length of the tibia is about 12 cm. The end of the tibia should be carefully filed smooth to avoid later pressure sites by the prosthesis. Furthermore, the ventral crest should be beveled. Removal of the bone marrow should be avoided, because ring-shaped sequestra may result.

The fibula is divided approximately 0.5–1 cm proximal to the tibia. A very small fibular end should be resected completely. The vessels are ligated separately at the amputation level whenever possible. The nerves should be divided approximately 3 cm higher up, so that the developing neuroma does not lie within the soft tissue covering the stump.

VI. Knee Disarticulation (Fig. 24.2.5)

For knee disarticulation also, the patient can be placed in a supine position. The skin incision begins below the tibial tuberosity and continues as two bilateral curved incisions down to the popliteal fossa, forming two lateral flaps. Thus, the suture line will lie between the condyles outside the pressure zones. The patellar ligament is divided just above the tibial tuberosity. Later, it can be fixed to those portions of the cruciate ligaments that are left over. Traction by the retinacula, however, will keep the patella in place, so that this additional fixation may be abandoned. In fact, the shape of the stump is even more suitable for a prosthesis if the patella is slightly retracted cranially. The knee joint ligaments are divided cranially and the menisci resected. Following division of the posterior capsule, the vessels are exposed and may be isolated and ligated. In this case, too, the nerves must be divided approximately 3–5 cm proximal to the amputation level. The heads of the gastrocnemius muscles are resected as well. Following placement of a large caliber drain, simple wound closure is sufficient.

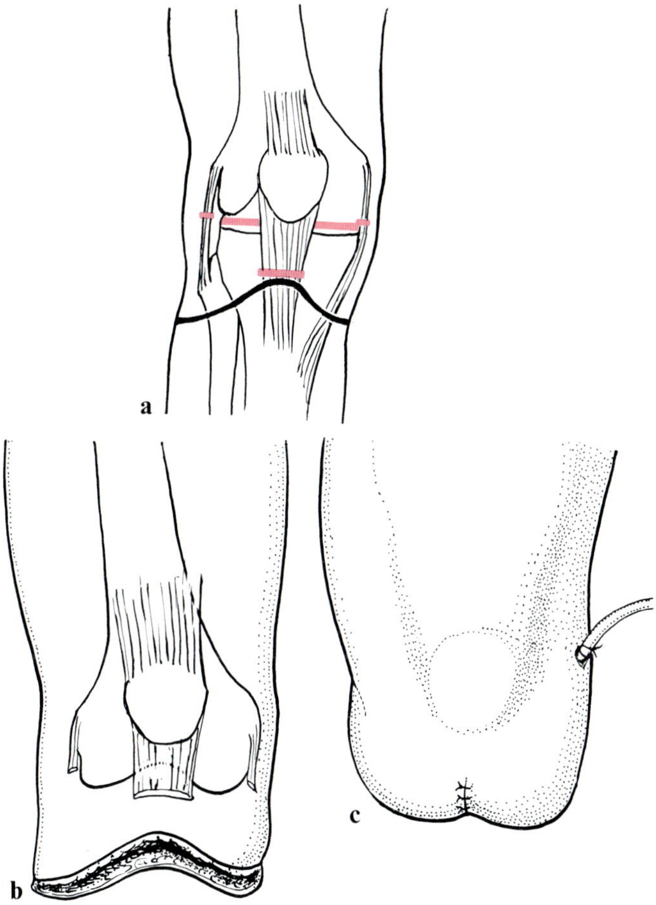

Fig. 24.2.5 a–c. Knee disarticulation. **a** Below the knee joint, two lateral flaps are formed. The patellar ligament is divided at the tibial tuberosity, and all structures within the knee joint are resected, except the insertions of the cruciate ligaments. **b** Following division of the dorsal capsule, the structures within the popliteal fossa may be ligated even when the patient is in a supine position. **c** Because of the two lateral flaps, the sutures are located within the intercondylar space, outside the weight-bearing area

Fig. 24.2.6 a–c. Above-knee amputation. **a** The skin incision with a fishmouth configuration provides a longer dorsal flap. **b** Following osteotomy and smoothing of the bony edges, the vessels are ligated at the amputation level, the nerves 3 cm above it. The muscles are sutured together loosely, combining agonists and antagonists. **c** Following placement of large caliber drains, a shorter volar flap is sutured to the longer dorsal flap
▽

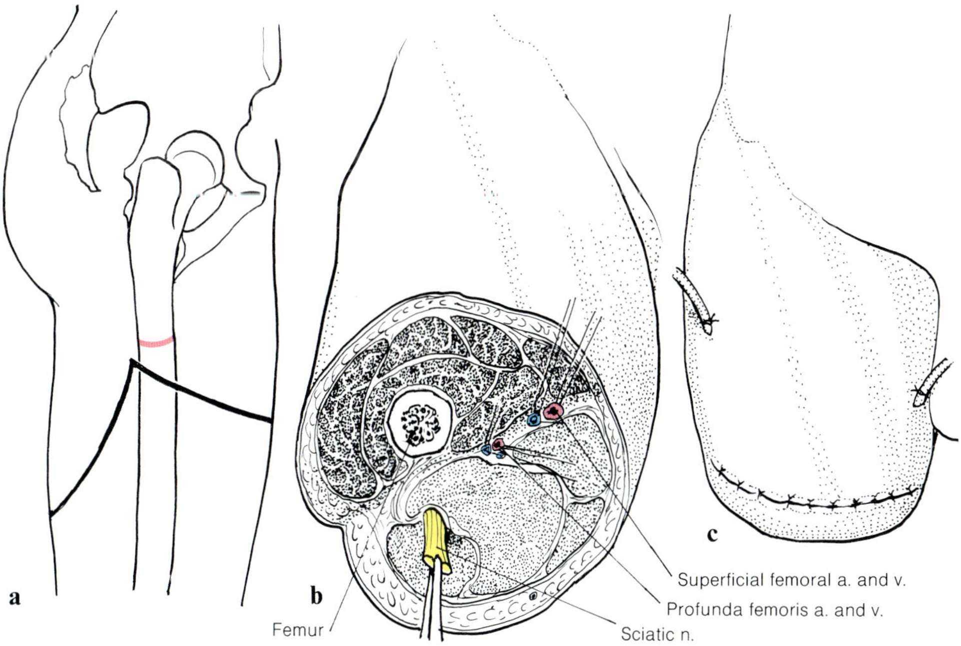

VII. Above-Knee Amputation (Fig. 24.2.6)

At the thigh, an anterior and posterior flap are usually provided. In most cases, a larger dorsal flap is recommended because of better blood supply to the flexor muscles. The femur may be divided just below the greater trochanter. The opposing muscles are sutured loosely in front of the bone, which is filed smooth. The vessels are ligated at the amputation level, the nerves approximately 3 cm proximally. Large drains are placed to achieve sufficient drainage of the secretions.

VIII. Hip Disarticulation (Fig. 24.2.7)

A dorsal flap is normally used to cover the wound. The ventral muscles are divided below the inguinal ligament. It is not always necessary to remove the femur within the hip joint; often, resection of the neck of the femur is sufficient. The dorsal skin flap remains attached to the gluteus maximus muscle.

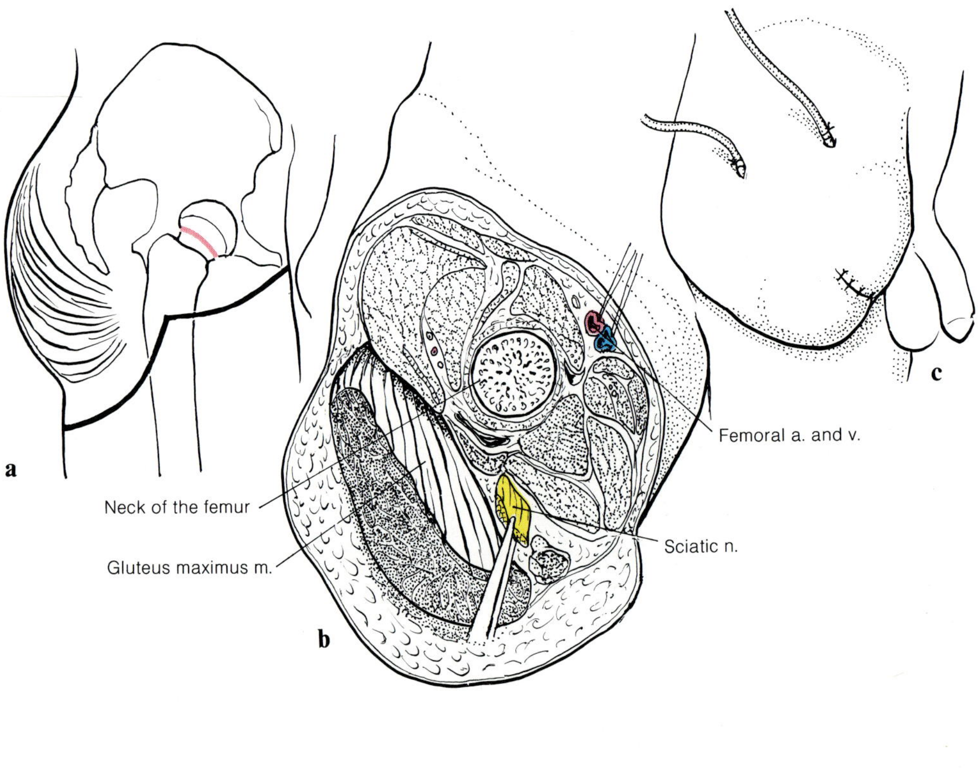

Fig. 24.2.7 a–c. Modified hip disarticulation. **a** Following division of the soft tissues below the inguinal ligament, a dorsal skin-muscle flap is provided. The osteotomy is made at the neck of the femur. **b** The vessels are ligated at the inguinal ligament and the nerves divided above it. **c** Following placement of large caliber drains, the wound is closed by turning the dorsal flap ventrally

IX. Upper Extremity Amputations

Fingers are amputated depending on the extent of the necrosis. Whenever possible, a longer palmar flap should be provided to avoid a scar in the region of the gripping surface. In thromboangitis obliterans, a finger often has to be resected completely or only a short segment of the proximal phalanx remains. Suturing the tendons of the extensor muscles to those of the flexor muscles must be avoided because the gliding of adjacent tendons would be impaired. In the case of higher amputations, the stump should be as long as the local blood supply will allow, since the longer the stump, the less complex the problems of prosthetic management. In disarticulations of the wrist or elbow, the condyles should be preserved as this is more favorable for a self-bearing prosthesis. Again, one must take care to ligate the vessels at the amputation level and to divide the nerves more proximally [8].

D. Fundamentals of Postoperative Management

It is necessary to distinguish between immediate and early postoperative fitting of the prosthesis. In the former case, a temporary cast is applied while the patient is still on the operating table. In the latter case, the stump is first wrapped with an elastic bandage, which is never circular and constrictive, and wound healing is checked at short intervals. When healing is complete, usually within about 14 days, an initial prosthesis is applied. In our experience, early postoperative fitting is usually called for in patients suffering from vascular disease because detection of impaired wound healing has priority. However, good results have also been reported in patients who underwent immediate fitting [5, 9].

Postoperatively, flexion, perhaps from cushions under the joints, must be carefully prevented. Abduction of a femoral stump and placement of cushions under the lumbar vertebrae should be avoided as well. Also, prolonged sitting may result in joint contractures.

Physiotherapy should prevent contractures and achieve full motility, as well as increasing muscle function of the stump. In addition, the patient has to be prepared for the stress of ambulation training. In elderly patients, special attention must be paid to strengthening the muscles of the arm, e.g., by use of a chest expander, in order to facilitate walking on crutches. However, it should also be noted that many patients over 75 years of age find it impossible to get about either with a prosthesis or on crutches. We believe it is best to accustom these patients as soon as possible to the use of a more feasible aid, such as a wheelchair.

REFERENCES

1. Baumgartner R (1979) Amputationen bei gefäßbedingten Nekrosen. Med Welt 30:556
2. Baumgartner R (1983) Exartikulation im Kniegelenk und prothetische Versorgung. Therapiewoche 33:2402
3. Burgess EM, Romano RL, Zettl JH, Schroek RD jun (1971) Amputations of the leg for peripheral vascular insufficiency. J Bone Joint Surg 53:874
4. Burgess EM (1983) Amputations. Surg Clin North Am 83:749
5. Dederich R (1970) Amputation der unteren Extremität. Thieme, Stuttgart
6. Kretschmer G, Piza F (1973) Die Rolle der Amputation im Behandlungsplan der chronisch arteriellen Verschlußkrankheit der unteren Extremität. Wien Med Wochenschr 9/10/11:150
7. Mäder M (1979) Otto-Bock-Modular-Prothesen für die unteren Extremitäten: Ein neues Knieexartikulationsgelenk. Orthopädie-Technik 8:132
8. Marquardt E, Martin AU (1979) Gesichtspunkte der Amputationschirurgie der oberen Extremitäten. Z Orthop 117:622
9. Neff G (1980) Postoperative Behandlung von Amputationsstümpfen einschließlich Sofort-, Früh- und Übungsprothesenversorgung. Orthopädie-Technik 12:181
10. Persson BM (1974) Sagittal incision for below-knee amputation in ischaemic gangreen. J Bone Joint Surg [Br] 56:111
11. Vollmar J, Marquardt E, Schaffelder G (1971) Amputationen bei arteriellen Durchblutungsstörungen. Chir Praxis 15:1983

24.3 Fasciotomy

L. Sunder-Plassmann

CONTENTS

A. Introduction

Some of the muscle compartments of the upper and lower extremities are completely separated by fasciae. The intracompartmental pressure is usually only a few mmHg. For various reasons, an increase in pressure may occur in such a compartment which can only be treated by complete division of the fascia. If an increased pressure above the capillary perfusion pressure (approximately 30 mmHg) persists over several hours, irreversible muscle necrosis, with subsequent scarred contracture, will result. Although the final etiology and pathogenetic mechanism of the increased compartment pressure, up to 90 mmHg, has not yet been clearly established [3, 4], it is generally accepted that there is only one therapeutic possibility: immediate longitudinal division of the fascia.

B. Causes and Indications

The most frequent cause of increased pressure is massive arterial bleeding within a compartment following direct vascuclar injury. The bleeding will sometimes stop by self-tamponade, but not until intracompartmental pressure approaches the arterial blood pressure. The second major cause is interstitial postischemic muscle edema resulting from increased permeability of the capillary walls following hypoxia. This type of edema occurs especially following reperfusion after distal circulation has been interrupted for several hours, or following late embolectomy, or when a tourniquet for hemostasis has been applied too long. Particularly extreme situations are encountered when both causes are present: direct arterial bleeding from a vascular injury and subsequent tissue hypoxia from a tourniquet applied for several hours to achieve temporary hemostasis. If the vascular bed is reperfused after 2–4 h in such a situation, a compartment syndrome will result in 100% of cases, with consequent neuroparalysis and muscle necrosis, unless fasciotomy is performed.

The relation between increased intracompartmental pressure and subsequent muscle necrosis or irreversible impairment of nerve conduction is characterized by hypoxia of ischemic origin; owing to the high hydrostatic pressure within the interstitial tissue, the postcapillary venules are first compressed, and later the capillaries and precapillary arterioles as well [1, 2, 5]. The initial capillary outflow block results not only in capillary stasis with subsequent tissue hypoxia, but also in an increase of the transcapillary filtration pressure and increased transcapillary filtration, with tissue edema.

Hypoxia causes an increased permeability of the capillary endothelium, resulting in a further increase of the edema, despite a sometimes enormously increased interstitial pressure.

Owing to interrupted capillary perfusion, tissue oxygen pressure also decreases to almost 0 mmHg within a short time. Anaerobic glycolysis produces lactate, resulting in severe local acidosis [6].

The compartment syndrome is therefore characterized by tissue edema, necrosis, and irreversible hypoxic nerve damage [2, 5]. Following decompression, hemodynamic changes such as those associated with tourniquet shock may result from reperfusion: metabolic acidosis, fall in blood pressure, hyperkalemia, and renal failure due to myoglobin deposits. As in all hypoxic states, only time will tell whether hypoxic damage of myoneural structures will be irreversible or not. The only therapeutic approach, therefore, is decompression as early as possible by dividing the investing fascia over its entire length.

C. Operative Technique

In cases of a localized compartment syndrome involving only one isolated compartment, e.g., the anterior tibial compartment, decompression is usually achieved by simple fasciotomy and closure of the skin incision. However, when all compartments of the extensor and flexor muscles are involved, complete decompression can be achieved only by a simultaneous extensive skin incision, which is not closed at first.

Fig. 24.3.1 a–d. Lower leg fasciotomy. **a, b** Isolated opening of the anterior tibial compartment. Direction and extent of the fasciotomy and division are indicated by the *broken line*. **c** Transverse section of the lower leg. The *arrows* mark the sites of fasciotomy: *1*, anterior tibial compartment; *2*, peroneal compartment; *3*, dorsal compartment. **d** Location of skin incisions for severe compartment syndrome with additional division of skin and subcutaneous tissue

I. Limited Fasciotomy

Limited fasciotomy means decompression of the anterior tibial compartment. The fact that this compartment is most frequently involved can be explained on anatomic grounds. It is a completely enclosed space, bounded medially by the tibia, dorsally by the interosseous membrane, ventrally by the deep fascia of the tibialis anterior muscle, and laterally by the intermuscular septum. It contains four muscles, the tibialis anterior muscle, the extensor digitorum longus muscle, the extensor hallucis longus muscle, and the peroneus tertius muscle (Fig. 24.3.1 a). The motor innervation of all four muscles is provided by the anterior tibial nerve, passing obliquely through the compartment. Damage to the anterior tibial nerve and muscle necrosis are especially common because the compartment is closed absolutely tight. The surface of the fascia is exposed by one or two small lateral longitudinal skin incisions, and is incised longitudinally over several centimeters. Then the fascia is split downward as far as the lateral malleolus using long blunt scissors opened only a few millimeters (Fig. 24.3.1 b). Division of the fascia is extended cranially to the knee joint, special care being taken to preserve the anterior tibial nerve at the level of the head of the fibula.

Injury to the nerves, vessels, and muscle fibers can be avoided if the scissors, which are opened only a few millimeters, are simply pushed forward,

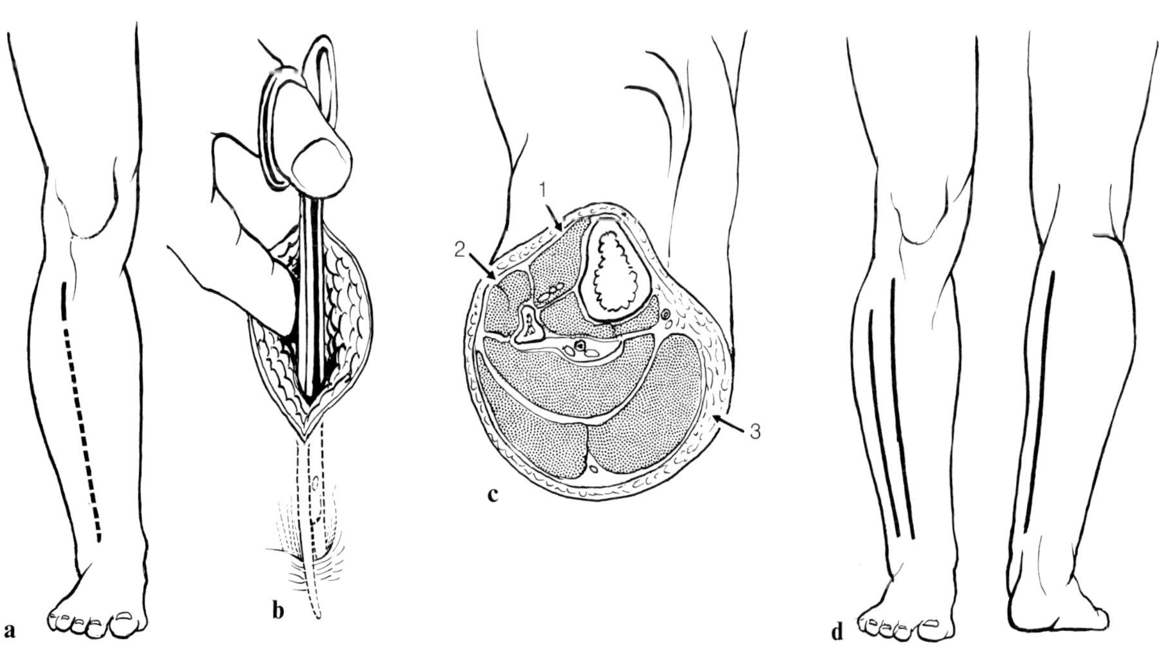

with no snipping action. When the edematous muscle fibers protrude over the skin level, the incision is left open for 5–7 days and is secondarily approximated by interrupted sutures or strips.

II. Extensive Fasciotomy

The limited skin incision and fasciotomy of the anterior tibial compartment are not usually sufficient in cases of hard edema of the entire lower leg, e.g., following injury of the popliteal artery, following delayed embolectomy and complete ischemic syndrome, or following application of a tourniquet for several hours. In such cases, the lateral longitudinal skin incision starts just distal to the head of the fibula and terminates a few centimeters proximal and ventral to the lateral malleolus (Fig. 24.3.1c, d). A second skin incision is made on the flexor side, somewhat lateral to the midline, and the compartments of the gastrocnemius and the soleus muscle are opened by extensive fasciotomy. After the gastrocnemius and soleus muscles are retracted laterally, the flexor digitorum muscles, the flexor hallucis longus muscles, and the posterior tibial muscle lying underneath are exposed and inspected. Wet sterile dressings are placed on the skin incisions for 5–7 days. The skin will be closed later by means of dressings that effect an approximation of the edges. The extremity is placed on a splint elevated by about 20° to reduce the transcapillary pressure and to accelerate absorption of the edema. Of course, constricting circular dressings are contraindicated. Detumescence may be accelerated by administering drugs such as diuretics, with simultaneous administration of heparin as a safeguard against thrombosis.

D. Upper Extremity Fasciotomy

Vascular injuries, tourniquet, and postischemic syndromes following embolectomy of the upper extremity are rare. Fasciotomy must be considered, especially following injury of the axillary or the brachial artery, where perfusion is restored only after several hours. Fasciotomy should also be considered when peripheral nerve damage occurs which is not a result of injury to the plexus or when an initially palpable pulse disappears owing to increasing swelling of the extremity. The postischemic syndrome following replantation of an extremity almost always requires fasciotomy in the upper and lower arm. In the lower arm, incisions may be required on the volar as well as the dorsal side, originating proximal to the wrist and terminating distal to the elbow. The fasciae are opened selectively and the muscle compartments carefully retracted. In this case also, the skin is usually left open before approximation is achieved by dressings after 5–7 days.

REFERENCES

1. Ashton H (1975) The effect of increased tissue pressure on blood flow. Chir Orthop Relat Res 113:15
2. Echtermeyer V, Oestern HJ (1983) Kompartment – Syndrom – Ätiologie – Pathophysiologie – Lokalisation – Diagnostische Therapie. Hefte Unfallheilkd 162:75
3. Mubarak SJ, Owen CA, Hargens AR, Goretto LP, Aheson WH (1978) Acute compartment syndromes: diagnosis and treatment with the aid of wick catheter. J Bone Joint Surg [Am] 60:1091
4. Whitesides TE Jr, Honey TC, Morimoto K, Hivada H (1975) Tissue pressure measurements as a determinant for the need of fasciotomy. Clin Orthop 113:43
5. Wissing H, Schmidt-Neuerburg KP (1982) Diagnose und Differentialdiagnose des Kompartment-Syndroms. Unfallheilkunde 85:133
6. Zweifach SS, Hargens AR, Evans KJ, Gonsalves MR, Smith RK, Mubarak SJ, Aheson WM (1980) Skeletal muscle necrosis in pressurized compartments associated with hemorrhagic hypotension. J Trauma 20:941

25 Vascular Access for Hemodialysis

D. RÜHLAND and F. HUSEMANN

CONTENTS

A. General Remarks and Differential Indications

I. Preoperative Requirements

Even today, extracorporeal hemodialysis still represents the only chance of survival for many patients suffering from renal insufficiency. For this therapy, which is sometimes lifelong, the individual must be connected to an "artificial kidney" one to three times per week. An appropriate angioaccess is absolutely necessary for hemodialysis. In patients undergoing long-term hemodialysis an arteriovenous fistula must be established. In the Federal Republic of Germany today, about 18000 patients undergo hemodialysis. Each year there will be approximately 3500 new patients. These figures indicate the significance of circulatory access for hemodialysis.

The creation of arteriovenous fistulas is therefore an important and significant field for the vascular surgeon. Shunt surgery represents a peculiarity because it is not performed for the sake of the blood vessel itself, but in order to change the original anatomic situation so that an appropriate vascular segment may withstand repeated punctures. Careful preparation and examination of the patient is a precondition for the successful creation of fistulas. Usually no invasive measures such as angiograms are required. It is necessary to preserve the superficial veins of the arms prior to hemodialysis as these veins will be so important for the shunt. It is also necessary to search carefully for alternatives to the venous outflow by manual examination prior to the operation. Only where problems arise, e.g., in reoperations, is it normally justified to perform invasive preoperative diagnostics to evaluate the operative indication for the appropriate fistula.

II. Possible Angioaccesses and Their Assessment

In order to perform maintenance hemodialysis, the shunt vessels must be easily accessed, and there must be sufficient blood flow, i.e., about 150–250 ml/min laminar flow. The dialysis may be venovenous, arteriovenous, or arterioarterial.

1. Arteriovenous Dialysis

For arteriovenous dialysis, a direct connection between the arterial high pressure system and the venous low pressure system is constructed. This short circuit utilizes the physiologic pressure gradient. The appropriate flow rate (150–250 ml/min) is practically always provided and may be exceeded significantly in many cases. The pump of the dialysis machine supports the flow during treatment. Four types of arteriovenous shunts may be constructed to perform arteriovenous hemodialysis:

a) Puncture of an Artery and a Vein. An easily accessible artery (e.g., the superficial femoral artery) is punctured percutaneously with a metal cannula. The blood is returned to the venous system following passage through the dialyzer.

b) External Shunt. In this procedure, Teflon cannulas are inserted into the vessels, and a short circuit is established by means of two silastic limbs.

c) Subcutaneous Arteriovenous Fistula. An artery and a vein are connected together directly or by graft interposition. All parts of the fistula are underneath the skin. For each treatment, 1–2 punctures are performed with large caliber cannulas that are connected to the dialyzer by plastic tubing.

d) Biocarbone Valve. This is a new shunt connecting an artery and a vein by a prosthetic graft. A biocarbone valve arises from the graft (through the skin) which is connected to the dialyzer by tubing.

2. Venovenous Dialysis

With this technique, the blood is taken from a large caliber vein by percutaneous cannulation. Following passage through the machine, it is returned to the same or another suitable vein. A blood pump is always required to achieve sufficient flow.

3. Arterioarterial Dialysis

Another possibility for hemodialysis is the arterioarterial technique. This requires arterioarterial cannulation, which of course takes a lot of effort. However, it is feasible to displace an artery subcutaneously (e.g., the superficial femoral artery), and then to cannulate it. Furthermore, it is possible to implant an arterioarterial bypass subcutaneously and then to cannulate it.

4. Assessment of the Various Shunts, Differential Indications

When the internist recommends hemodialysis, the surgeon has to decide which type of shunt will offer the patient the most favorable angioaccess for hemodialysis.

Here, one has to distinguish between urgent angioaccess for hemodialysis (e.g., acute renal failure, intoxication) and routine maintenance.

Acute hemodialysis requires immediate angioaccess, e.g., direct major vein cannulation performed by the nephrologist. However, when larger shunt volumes are required (e.g., in intoxication) a surgeon may consider an external fistula (e.g., a Quinton-Scribner shunt) for acute hemodialysis. Today, the indication for an external Quinton-Scribner shunt is limited largely to acute angioaccess. The relatively short life of this fistula, together with the fact that there is simultaneous destruction of an important vascular region, has lead to great reservations regarding the indication. However, when the shunt is necessary, it should be placed in the lower leg whenever possible, thus preserving the arm for a subcutaneous fistula that may eventually become necessary. If acute renal failure turns into chronic renal failure and a Quinton-Scribner fistula is present in the arm, the external fistula should be converted into a subcutaneous arteriovenous fistula.

In all types of chronic renal failure, early construction of a subcutaneous arteriovenous fistula is recommended, especially to provide time for the veins to become sufficiently dilated and arterialized. As all subcutaneous fistulas wear out from frequent cannulations, it is essential that a peripheral fistula be established first, and preferably a Brescia-Cimino fistula [4] between the cephalic vein of the forearm and the radial artery proximal to the wrist, consideration being given to which hand is the dominant one. When there are problems, one has to search further proximally. It depends on the local situation whether the operation is performed on the ipsilateral arm or whether the peripheral vessels of the contralateral lower arm are used.

Today, subcutaneous fistulas of the elbow are also of special significance. Although in this case the segment formed for cannulation is shorter, it is nevertheless adequate for dialysis if the "single needle" technique is used.

In view of the availability of prosthetic material for fistula construction, it is doubtful whether repositioning of the major subcutaneous veins (e.g., basilic, saphenous vein) is still necessary, especially when one considers that the subcutaneous venous retrograde flow will be disturbed significantly and suitable sites for connection of prosthetic grafts may be lost.

Subcutaneous fistulas utilizing prosthetic grafts should also be viewed with suspicion because of the risk of infection (when implanting and cannulating). It should be noted that cannulation of this fistula should be started 3 weeks postoperatively at the earliest, in order to allow the large wound to heal and the graft to settle, thus avoiding the riks of early complications, hematomas from the cannulation, and infections.

With every subcutaneous fistula, all possibilities for reintervention should be fully exhausted in order to make the most effective possible use of the superficial veins, which are of such limited availability.

B. Construction of External Fistulas (Quinton-Scribner Shunt) [16]

Permanent external shunts were first described by QUINTON, DILLARD, and SCRIBNER in 1960. This technique began a new chapter in the treatment of patients requiring maintenance hemodialysis. Here, only the most important types of external shunts are described since nowadays other fistulas have largely replaced this procedure.

I. Placement of a Shunt in the Lower Leg Between the Posterior Tibial Artery and the Greater Saphenous Vein

1. Anatomy

The sensibility of the medial side of the lower leg is provided by the rami cutanei cruris mediales of the saphenous nerve. The skin veins represent a large network which is the source of the great saphenous vein on the medial side and of the small saphenous vein on the lateral side. The great saphenous vein passes upward in a slight curve in front of the inner malleolus, receiving several tributaries in this segment. It continues on rather straight and in a proximal direction to the posterior aspect of the medial femoral condyle. The vein is accompanied by the saphenous nerve. In the distal two thirds of the lower leg, the nerve, being a sensory subcutaneous end branch of the femoral nerve, usually passes in front of the vein. In the proximal third, it passes behind the vein. The posterior tibial artery and its veins as well as the tibial nerve represent the medial neurovascular bundle of the lower leg. This bundle descends from the popliteal fossa down into the deep compartment of the flexor muscles, remaining underneath the tendinous arch of the soleus muscle; hence, together with the posterior tibial muscle, which can serve as a guideline, it continues its descent, remaining underneath the lamina profunda fasciae cruris. Along the way, the posterior tibial vessels course closer and closer to the medial side. Finally, they emerge from beneath the soleus muscle at the junction of the middle and distal third of the lower leg (behind the flexor digitorum longus muscle). Here, the neurovascular bundle is located directly underneath the fascia; it finally passes through the third tendon compartment of the flexor retinaculum down to the foot. In the operative field, the tibial nerve is located behind the vessels. Sometimes, it divides here into its two end branches, the medial and lateral plantar nerve, the latter crossing underneath the posterior tibial artery and its concomitant veins. The dorsal artery of the foot and the anterior tibial nerve reach the foot below the inferior extensor retinaculum. They can be exposed lateral to the tendon of the extensor hallucis longus muscle, which usually protrudes significantly.

2. Positioning

Because the posterior tibial artery must be ligated, one must be certain prior to the operation that the anterior tibial artery is functioning properly. When the shunt is to be constructed in the lower leg, the patient is placed in the supine position. Slight flexion, abduction and external rotation at the hip is advantageous as well as a 45° flexion of the knee.

3. Operative Approach (Fig. 25.1.a)

The approach is through two separate longitudinal skin incisions about 5 cm long. Care must be taken to ensure that the ankle joint and the shunt do not impair each other in their respective functions. The skin incision over the great saphenous vein should be performed at a proximal level to achieve sufficient soft tissue to cover the prosthetic material above the inner malleolus. The incision over the posterior tibial artery, however, should be placed further distally, over the site where the vessel emerges from beneath the deeper layers of fasciae and muscle; an incision here will facilitate dissection of the artery. If both vessels are rather close to each other, a single longitudinal incision between the posterior tibial artery and the great saphenous vein is possible.

Fig. 25.1 a–k. External fistula according to QUINTON and SCRIBNER [16] in the lower leg. **a** Operative approach to the great saphenous vein and the posterior tibial artery through two separate skin incisions, each about 5 cm long. **b** The great saphenous vein is exposed, ligated distally and a suture is placed around it proximally. T-shaped incision of the vein. **c** Creating a subcutaneous pocket for the silastic tubing. **d** Insertion of the tip of the Teflon cannula ("vessel tip") into the saphenous vein, the tip being connected to the silastic tubing. **e**, **f** The vein is fixed to the vessel tip and secured by tying the ligatures over the Silastic tubing and the vein. **g** The silastic tubing is pulled through the skin through a separate incision. **h** Exposure of the posterior tibial artery and insertion of the vessel tip into the artery. **i** External fistula in the lower leg according to QUINTON and SCRIBNER [16]. The two silastic limbs are short-circuited by means of a Teflon connector. **j** Modified external shunt ("winged-in-line shunt") according to RAMIREZ [17] (in the lower leg). Two stabilizing wings are connected to the limbs to achieve better fixation. **k** Instead of a simple connector, a T-shaped Teflon connector may be used, allowing flushing of the fistula with heparinized solution through the side arm

4. Surgical Technique

First, the saphenous vein is exposed and dissected free of the subcutaneous tissue over a length of at least 2 cm; two sutures are placed around it. The vein is then ligated, using the distal stay suture. Once tied, the suture should not be cut since it will be used later for fixation of the silastic tubing (Fig. 25.1 b). The vessel is incised transversely, using a scalpel or scissors, so that half of the circumference is open. The venotomy may also be T-shaped to facilitate subsequent cannulation. Immediately afterward, the lumen is flushed and filled with heparinized saline solution, using a bulb-headed cannula to avoid intraoperative formation of thrombi and at the same time to verify venous outflow. If necessary, the vein may also be gently dilated by the flushing. Dilation of the vein with probes or a Fogarty catheter is not recommended, owing to the likelihood of intimal injury.

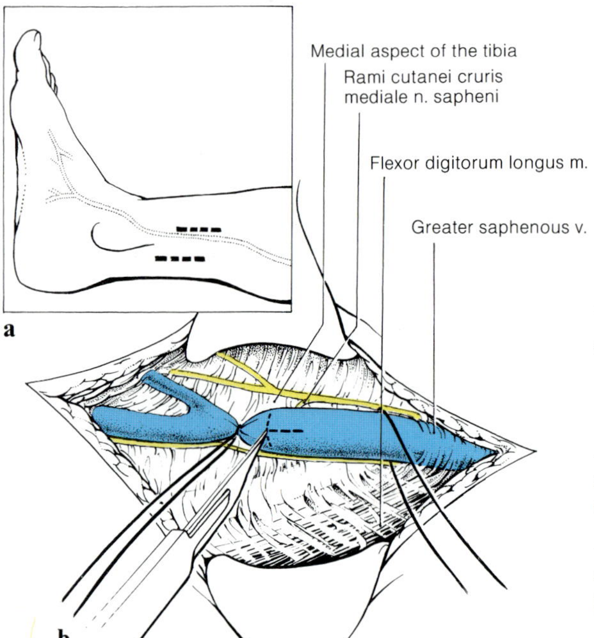

a

b

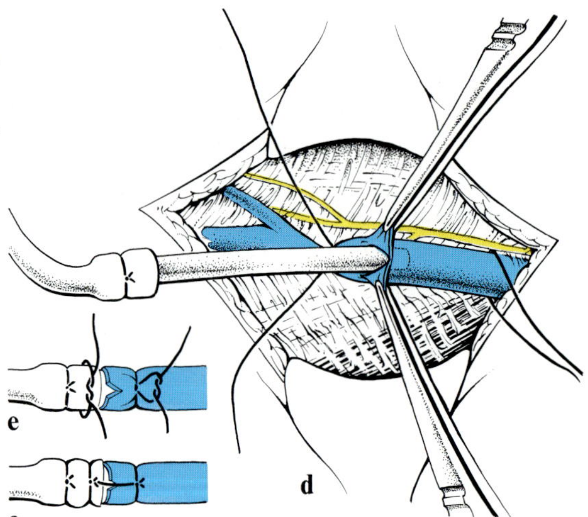

e

f

d

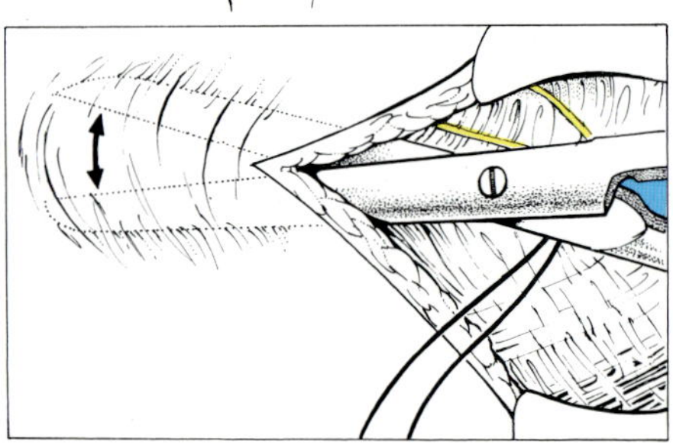

c

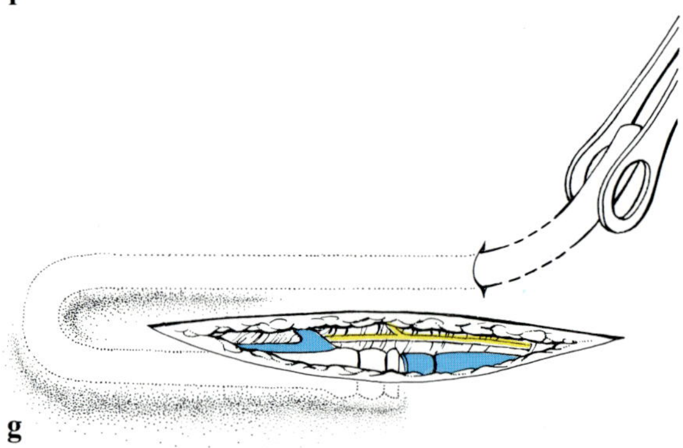

g

Prior to cannulation, a tunnel is formed to accomodate the subcutaneous portion of the Silastic tubing (Fig. 25.1c).

The graft segment lying underneath the skin serves to fix the system. The dimensions and course of the subcutaneous pocket must therefore correspond precisely to those of the tubing. The tubing is to be inserted under the skin without kinking or twisting, and once in place, it must be completely immobile, so that kinks cannot subsequently develop. The already assembled venous limb of the shunt, consisting of the Teflon tip and the Silastic tube, can be used as a guide for creation of the pocket and also, once the hooks have been removed, for marking the site where the tube will pass through the skin (cf. Fig. 25.1g).

To cannulate the blood vessels, the Silastic tubing is mounted on the tip of the Teflon cannula. The connection may be reinforced by a suture tied around the tube (Fig. 25.1.d). Choosing the right Teflon cannula is of great importance for the function of the shunt. The diameter of the tip should approximately match the inner diameter of the vessel. When the caliber of the cannula is too large, atraumatic insertion and fixation within the vein is impossible. The rigid vessel tip scrapes along the vessel wall, inevitably injuring the endothelium, and thereby creating a predisposition to thrombosis. If the cannula is too small, it will not be adequately fixed within the vascular lumen, and its movement will likewise cause intimal lesions. Moreover, the difference in caliber causes turbulence in the blood flow and stagnation of the blood between the vessel wall and the cannula, thereby adding to the risk of thrombosis.

The Teflon tip of the venous limb is now filled with heparinized saline solution and then inserted carefully into the vascular lumen (Fig. 25.1.a). The vessel tip is then tied to the vein to achieve fixation and is also tied to the stay suture on the saphenous vein (Fig. 25.1.e, f). Prior to the final placement of the Silastic tubing, it is necessary to create an opening for the passage to the surface. The wound hooks are removed, and the skin is brought back to its original position. The incision must be placed so that a tight connection with the tubing is achieved without narrowing the tubing significantly. The Silastic tubing is then pulled out through the skin using a small clamp after the curved limb of the shunt has been placed within the subcutaneous tissue (Fig. 25.1g).

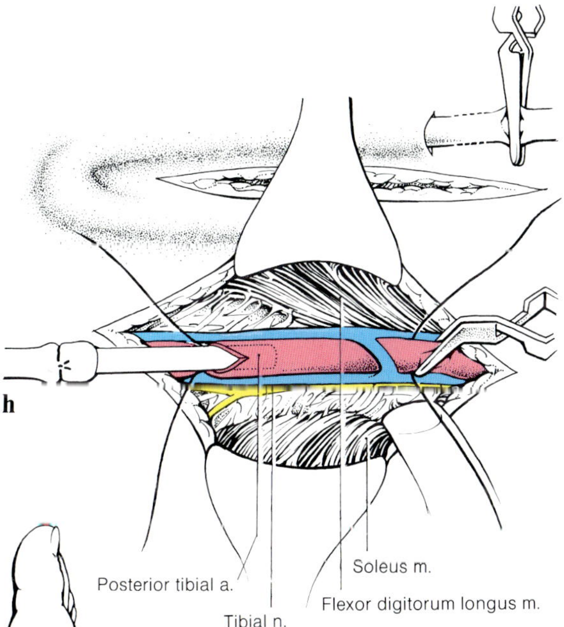

h

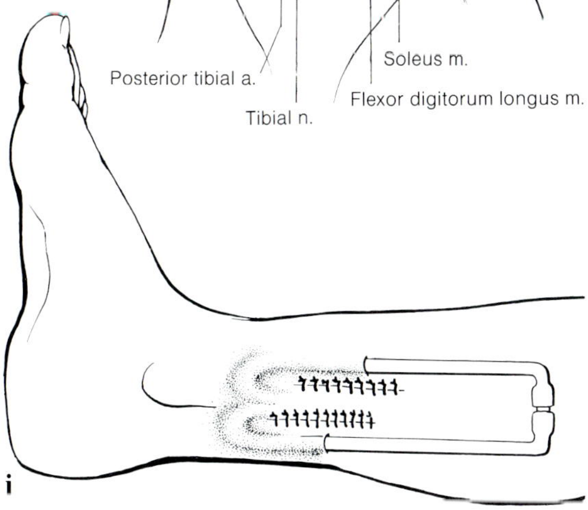

i

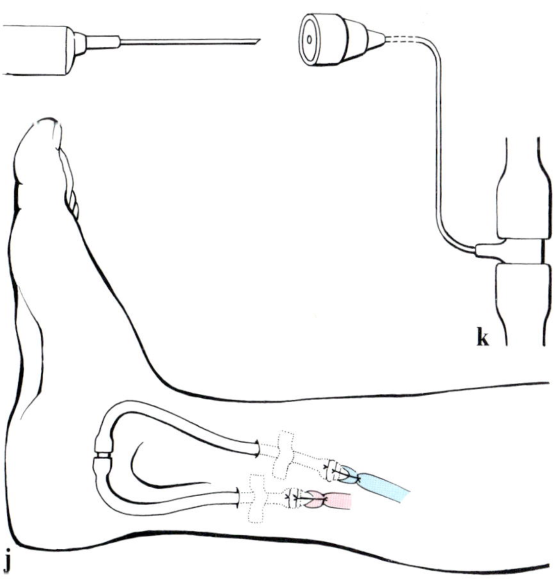

k

j

The arterial limb of the shunt is fixed in place using essentially the same procedure. A second longitudinal incision is made somewhat distally (Fig. 25.1a). Afterwards the fascia cruris is split and the posterior tibial artery exposed underneath the soleus muscle. Two tapes are placed around it and the exposure is extended, matching the length of the cannula (Fig. 25.1h). A much more extensive proximal exposure of the artery, as compared with the vein, is required so that the Teflon tip can be inserted without interference from the clamp that is to be used later for temporary interruption of the blood flow. The artery is ligated distally using the stay suture. Care should be taken to fill the occluded vessel with heparinized saline solution and to dilate it carefully. Fixation of the vessel tip is accomplished in the same manner as with the venous limb.

The arterial Silastic tubing is then passed through the skin. Both limbs of the shunt are connected together by a small tube. Prior to the connection the air is removed from the Silastic tubing (Fig. 25.1i). Instead of a simple straight Teflon connector, a T-shaped connector with a side arm may be used, allowing continuous administration of heparin (Fig. 25.1k).

Among the numerous types of external shunts reported in the literature only one modification the so-called winged-in-line shunt according to RAMIREZ [16] is mentioned here (Fig. 25.1j). In this type the 180° Silastic tubing segments are omitted. The fixation is provided by two wings connected to the Silastic tubing in the subcutaneous tissue, providing better fixation of the whole system. The operative approach is largely identical to that of the Silastic Teflon Quinton-Scribner shunts.

II. Placement of a Shunt in the Lower Arm

A Quinton-Scribner shunt can be placed in the lower arm, utilizing the radial artery or the ulnar artery as the arterial limb and the cephalic or basilic vein as the venous limb. It should be emphasized once again that an external shunt in the lower arm traumatizes a vascular region that is important for maintenance hemodialysis and may eventually render it unusable. Therefore, this procedure should be used only in exceptional cases.

For details of anatomy, positioning, and operative approach see pp. 647–649.

1. Surgical Technique

Because of the close proximity of the radial artery to the cephalic vein of the forearm, only one incision about 4–5 cm long is required. Following dissection, the vein is ligated distally again, incised transversely or "T-like," flushed with heparin, and filled with saline solution. A subcutaneous tunnel is created. Again, one must match the extent of the subcutaneous pocket to the length and position of the tubing. Insertion of the vessel tips and of the Silastic tubing is performed in the same way as described for the foot (Fig. 25.2a). In the arm, the so-called Ramirez winged-in-line shunt may be used as an alternative [17].

III. Postoperative Complications

With external fistulas the risk of infection is high because the prosthetic graft passes through the skin. Therefore, a daily sterile change of wound dressings is important. In cases of infection in the operative field, the prosthetic material has to be removed and the vessels ligated.

The major complication of this fistula, however, is thrombosis of the vein or the artery at the junction of the vessel tip and the intima; this explains the relatively short life of these fistulas. Today, early local fibrinolysis is a means of thrombus removal and recanalization. Reinterventions using a small balloon catheter may also be successful. Especially after the fistula has been functioning for a long time, chronic vessel damage by intimal hyperplasia has to be expected. Here, one may try to reinsert the tubing system proximal to the old site of implantation. In many cases, however, the Quinton-Scribner fistula has to be reconstructed, with the renewed risk of definitive injury to other vascular regions which are important for maintenance hemodialysis. Therefore, subcutaneous fistulas are preferred because they remain functional for a longer period of time and offer a good possibility for successful reintervention.

C. Subcutaneous Arteriovenous Fistulas

I. Fistulas Utilizing Autogenous Vessels

In subcutaneous fistulas created using autogenous vessels, the blood, following the path of least resistance, is short-circuited directly from the artery into the vein, bypassing the capillaries. This produces changes in the wall structure of the arterialized vein. The thin-walled vein is usually dilated by the high intraluminal pressure and may often become visible along the entire course of the appropriate outflow. In addition to this dilatation, however, after a few days or weeks there is a pronounced hypertrophy of the media with augmentation of the smooth muscle; as a result, the vessel wall becomes significantly thicker and more resistant. The most important subcutaneous arteriovenous fistulas utilizing autogenous vessels are listed below. The sequence does not reflect a judgement, but is merely according to anatomic position. The most important anastomotic techniques are described in more detail in the section on the classical Brescia-Cimino fistula.

1. The Arteriovenous Fistula Distal to the Wrist [10]

For anatomy and positioning see below.

a) Operative Approach. To construct an arteriovenous fistula distal to the wrist, a longitudinal incision about 3 cm long is made in the tabatière, i.e., between the tendon of the extensor pollicis longus muscle and the extensor pollicis brevis muscle.

b) Surgical Technique. First, the cephalic vein of the forearm is exposed entirely over a length of 2–3 cm, avoiding injury to the superficial branch of the radial nerve. Following division of the fascia manus, the radial artery is dissected over the same length. The gap in the fascia should not compress the vessel. For the anastomotic technique see the following section.

2. Arteriovenous Fistula Proximal to the Wrist Between the Radial Artery and the Cephalic Vein (Brescia-Cimino Fistula) [4]

a) Anatomy. The skin of the forearm is elastic and mobile. On the extensor side, the skin is stronger than on the flexor and radial side. Sensory function is provided by the musculocutaneous nerve on the flexor and radial side, by the anterior branch and the ulnar branch of the musculocutaneous nerve on the flexor and ulnar side. The superficial branch of the radial nerve perforates the fascia in the distal third of the lower arm and provides the sensory function of the radial dorsum of the hand and the extensor side of the proximal phalanx of the thumb, the index finger, and part of the middle finger.

The coarse-mesh venous network of the back of the hand is the source of both great skin veins of the lower arm, the cephalic and the basilic veins. Both pass over to the extensor side in a screwlike fashion, usually in the distal third of the forearm. On the flexor side they pass upward to the elbow, being connected to each other by several tributaries. The cephalic vein exhibits an oblique course and is relatively straight when looked upon from the radial side. A few centimeters proximal to the processus styloideus radii (in the operative field) one often finds a pronounced bifurcation where it is joined by a separate dorsal vein of the hand or a tributary connecting with the basilic vein on the extensor side.

After branching off from the brachial artery in the middle of the bend of the elbow, the radial artery passes straight to the processus styloideus radii (mostly distal to the joint cavity). The vessel, together with both its concomitant veins and the superficial branch of the radial nerve, is located superficially along its entire length in the forearm and may be exposed in the proximal third between the pronator teres muscle and the brachioradialis muscle (serving as a guideline) and the distal two thirds between the brachioradialis muscle and the flexor carpi radialis muscle (Fig. 25.2c). In the region of the wrist, a superficial palmar branch, usually thin, leaves the radial artery and passes to the superficial palmar arch. The radial artery then passes under the extensor retinaculum to the tabatière, crossing the tendons of the abductor pollicis longus muscle and the extensor pollicis brevis muscle. Finally, it crosses under the extensor pollicis longus muscle and, after perforating the interosseus muscle I, it forms the deep palmar arch.

The ulnar artery first passes downward on the deep flexors of the forearm, crossing under the median nerve. Only in the distal third is it located more superficially, together with the ulnar nerve and its concomitant veins, between the flexor digitorum superficialis muscle and the flexor carpi ulnaris muscle.

Both arteries of the lower arm are connected through several anastomoses in the region of the hand, so that one vessel is usually sufficient to provide adequate blood supply to the hand. Prior to the operation, however, it must be demonstrated that both arteries are functioning (Allen test).

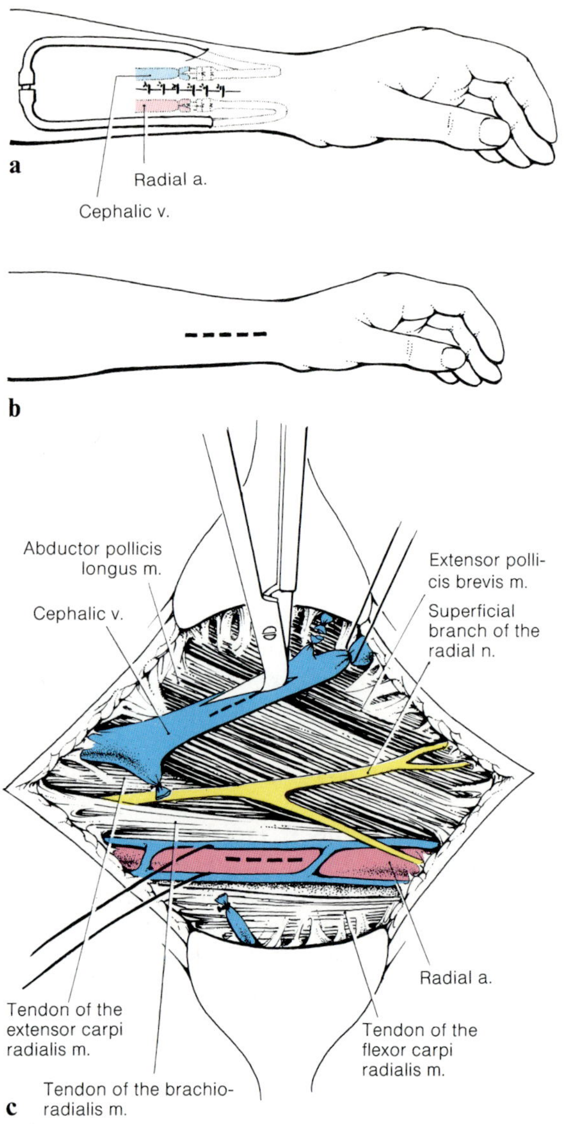

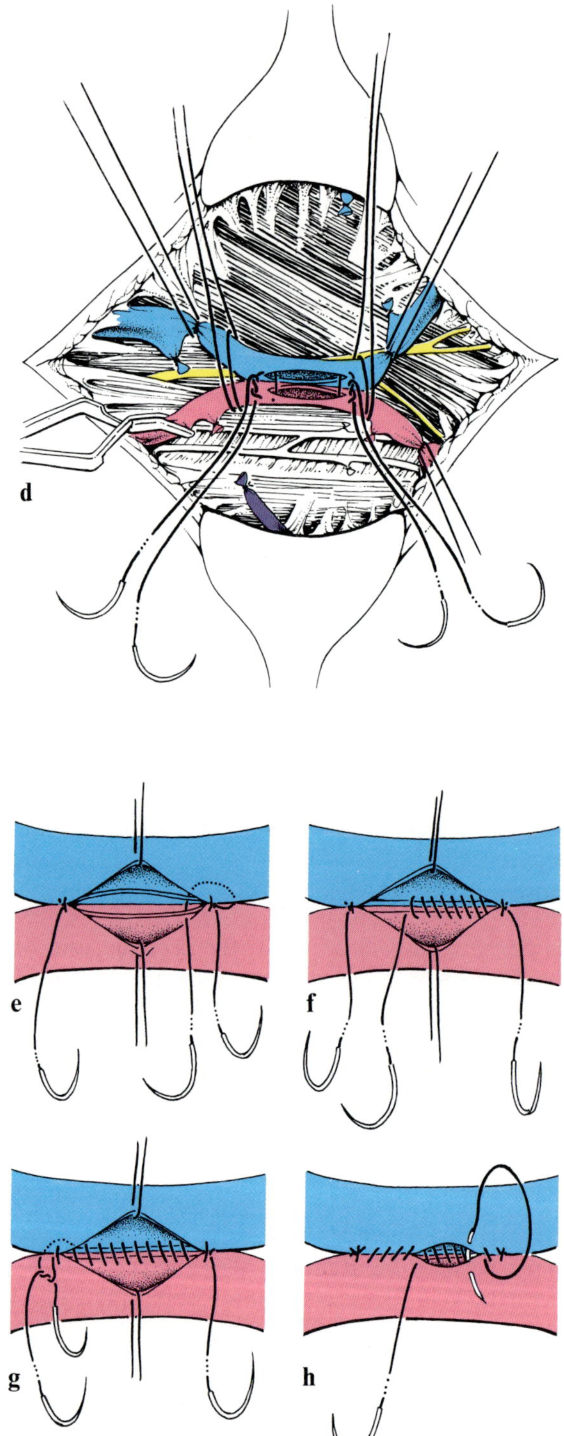

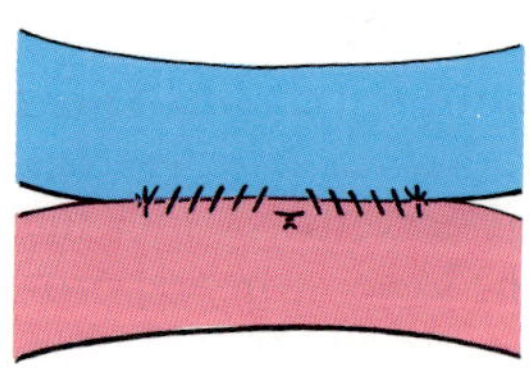

Fig. 25.2 a–i. External fistula in the lower arm, between the radial artery and the cephalic vein according to QUINTON and SCRIBNER [16]. **a** Defined situs. **b** Operative approach for construction of a subcutaneous Brescia-Cimino fistula in the lower arm, between the radial artery and the cephalic vein. **c** Brescia-Cimino fistula in the lower arm, between the cephalic vein and the radial artery. The fascia of the forearm has been divided. **d** Beginning the side-to-side anastomosis with two double corner sutures. The vein is occluded by two suture tourniquets, the radial artery by fine clamps. **e** Insertion of the needle into the distal posterior wall of the artery. **f** Continuous suture of the posterior wall of the vein and the artery from inside. **g** Passing the suture out of the vein from within, and tying the proximal corner suture. **h**, **i** The anterior wall may be sutured continuously, from both ends, so that the knot is placed in the middle of the anastomosis

b) Positioning. Placement of an arteriovenous fistula in an upper extremity is always done with the patient in a supine position and the arm abducted 90° and extended. The hand is in an intermediate position between pronation and supination. For operative procedures on the ulnar artery, it may be necessary to change the position of the arm.

c) Operative Approach. The approach is through a longitudinal incision 4–5 cm long, proximal to the processus styloideus radii, between the radial artery and the cephalic vein (Fig. 25.2b). To construct the curvilinear fistulas two incisions may be made adjacent to each other or over both vessels (see below; Fig. 25.4).

d) Surgical Technique

α) Side-to-Side Anastomosis. One should always expose the cephalic vein first and check the condition of its wall intraoperatively. Often the vein will have been damaged to some extent or may show hitherto undetected strictures, as this region also represents one of the most important sites of puncture.

The vein is dissected over a length of 4–6 cm, according to the distance between the vein and artery. Tapes are placed around it. The course of the superficial branch of the radial nerve must be carefully noted. Tributaries are ligated and divided, thereby making it possible to achieve an anastomosis free of tension and a concentrated retrograde flow through just one vein.

Following division of the lower arm fascia, the radial artery is exposed between the tendons of the brachioradial muscle and of the flexor carpi radialis muscle (Fig. 25.2c). The vascular compartment should be dissected free upward and downward as far as possible to avoid later kinking or constriction in this region. The artery is dissected free of the surrounding tissue and its concomitant veins over a length of about 4 cm. Smaller side branches are ligated and divided. These ligatures must be performed. They must not become the cause of postoperative bleeding or later stenoses due to a hematoma of the arterial wall. The cephalic vein is closed distally, using a suture tourniquet or a small bulldog clamp. The incision is made with a scalpel and extended, using fine scissors, to achieve a maximal opening of 1 cm (Fig. 25.2c). The vein is then flushed with heparinized saline solution through a bulb-headed cannula. The vein may also be carefully dilated by this flushing, and sufficient patency should be ascertained. Dilation of the veins with a balloon catheter or bougienage should be avoided whenever possible (intimal lesions).

The radial artery is carefully occluded proximally and distally using fine vascular clamps. An incision is made in the artery, corresponding to the position and length of the venotomy. Heparinized saline solution is injected into the artery as well. Dilation of the vessel using probes or catheters is not recommended.

The radial artery and cephalic vein are placed side to side so that the incisions match exactly. There should be no tension or kinking (Fig. 25.2d).

The anastomosis is performed with a continuous suture of 6-0 or 7-0 absorbable or nonabsorbable suture material (Fig. 25.2e–i). Two double corner sutures are passed through the vein and artery from inside and tied. It is recommended that the posterior wall be sutured continuously from inside, proceeding as follows: the distal corner suture is first inserted into the posterior wall of the artery or the vein, depending on the situation of the vessels at that end of the anastomosis (25.2e). Upon completion of the continuous suture of the posterior wall, the suture must be passed from the inside outward before being tied to the suture already in place at the proximal corner (Fig. 25.2f, g). The anterior anastomotic wall is then completed, either starting at the proximal end and proceeding to the distal end or starting from both ends and completing the suture in the center (Fig. 25.2h, i). When the vessels are small, it is best to place 3–5 interrupted sutures at the proximal corner in order to avoid stenoses (periarterial tissue).

This procedure was described by Brescia and Cimino [4] in 1966. It may be changed into a functional end-to-side anastomosis by ligation of the cephalic vein distal to the fistula or into a functional end-to-end anastomosis by distal ligation of both vessels, to drain the entire arterial blood volume into the central vein.

β) End-to-Side Anastomosis. Following exposure of the blood vessels, the mobilized cephalic vein is ligated distally. Prior to the ligation, the end is beveled, matching the incision of the artery. The radial artery is again incised up to 1 cm on the side facing the vein (Fig. 25.3a). The beveled vein end may now be incised longitudinally at the prox-

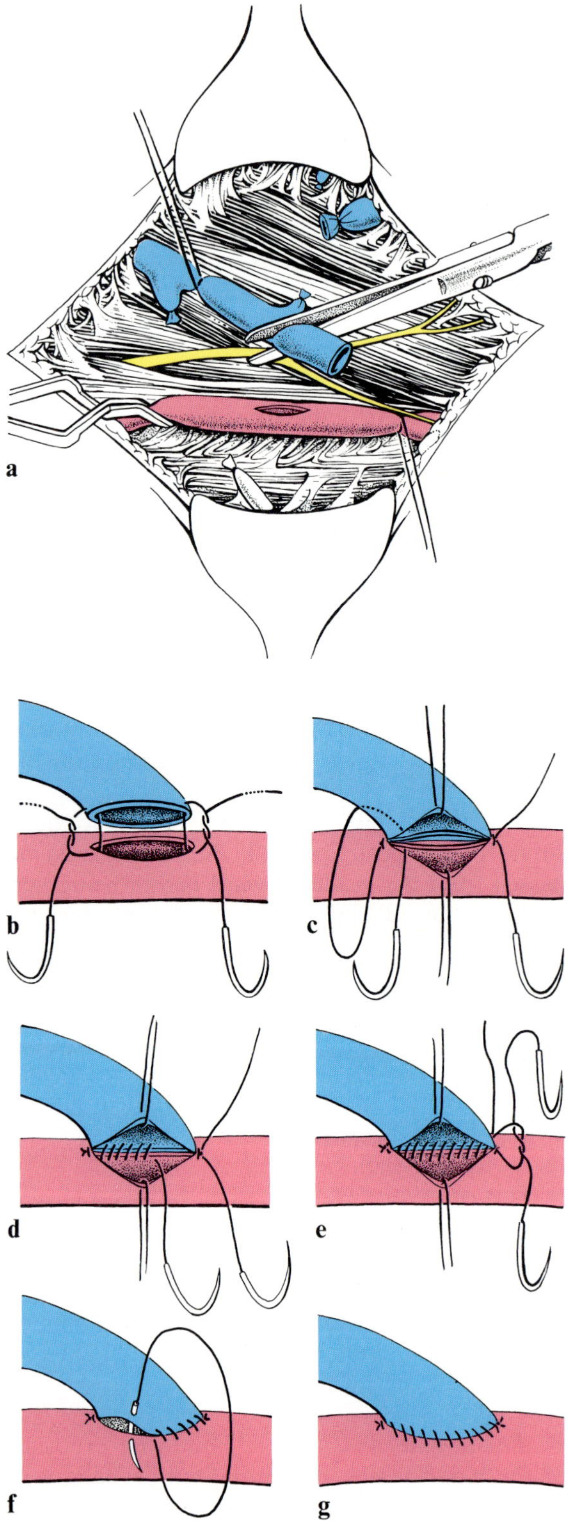

◁ **Fig. 25.3 a–g.** End-to-side anastomosis of the cephalic vein to the radial artery, the vein entering at an acute angle. **a–g** Following dissection, one first divides the vein transversely. Then, a longitudinal incision is made in the artery on the side facing the vein. Completion of the end-to-side anastomosis by continuous suture of the posterior wall from inside, the anterior wall being retracted carefully by two stay sutures. After completion of the posterior suture, the anterior wall is sutured continuously, as in the side-to-side anastomosis

imal corner to match the length of the anastomosis with the arteriotomy. The beveled end enters at an acute angle, avoiding kinking as far as possible. Approximation of the vessels is provided by a continuous suture, as with the side-to-side anastomosis (Fig. 25.3 b–g, f). Also in this case, interrupted sutures may be placed in the proximal corner of the anastomosis to avoid a stenosis.

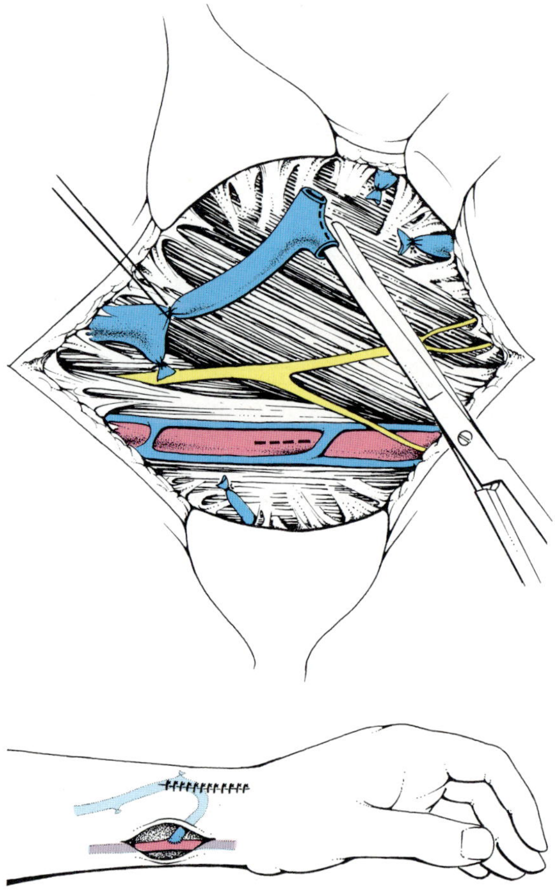

Fig. 25.4. Curved end-to-side anastomosis of the cephalic vein to the radial artery in the distal lower arm. The operative approach is through two staggered longitudinal incisions made alongside (or over) each vessel. These incisions make it possible to mobilize a vein segment that is long enough to form a curve; they also allow for an anastomosis free of tension and twisting

Fig. 25.5a–d. End-to-side anastomosis of the cephalic ▷ vein to the radial artery utilizing a vein branch (natural patch graft angioplasty). The cephalic vein often has large bifurcations. They are ligated approximately 5 cm distal to the dichotomy, (**a**) divided transversely and tailored like a patch (**b**). Afterward the vein thus prepared is anastomosed end-to-side to the radial artery as described before (**c**, **d**)

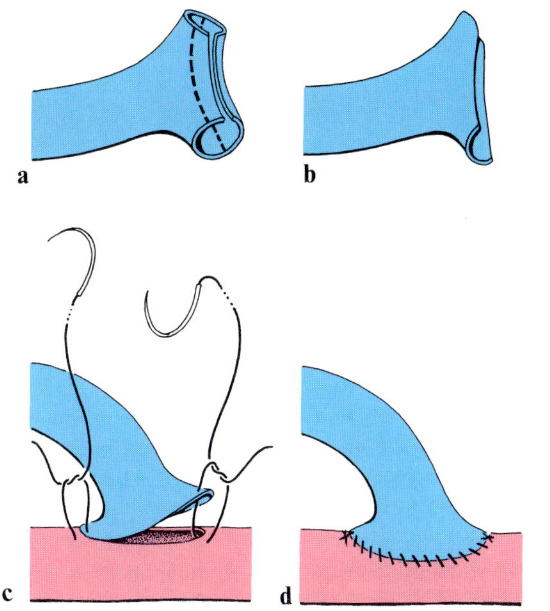

Another technique for maintaining laminar blood flow in the fistula is the so-called smooth loop anastomosis. Here, the vein forms an arch which provides for nearly turbulence-free blood flow. A drawback, however, is the increased risk of kinking (Fig. 25.4). If the cephalic vein is bifurcated at the anastomotic site, it can be incised and tailored in such a way as to increase the diameter of the anastomosis (Fig. 25.5a–d).

γ) *End-to-End Anastomosis.* Here, as with the side-to-end anastomosis, there are essentially two possibilities. The "tennis racket" fistula, distinguished by its acute angle (Fig. 25.6), will be discussed first. Following dissection, both vessel ends are beveled and brought together, creating a V-shaped connection. A continuous suture can be used, as with a side-to-side or side-to-end anastomosis. At the corners, interrupted sutures may help to avoid stenosis. With sufficient dissection, it is possible to suture the posterior wall from outside. In constructing this type of anastomosis, however, it is more convenient to connect the vein to the artery end-to-side and then to ligate the artery distally, thereby creating a functional end-to-end anastomosis.

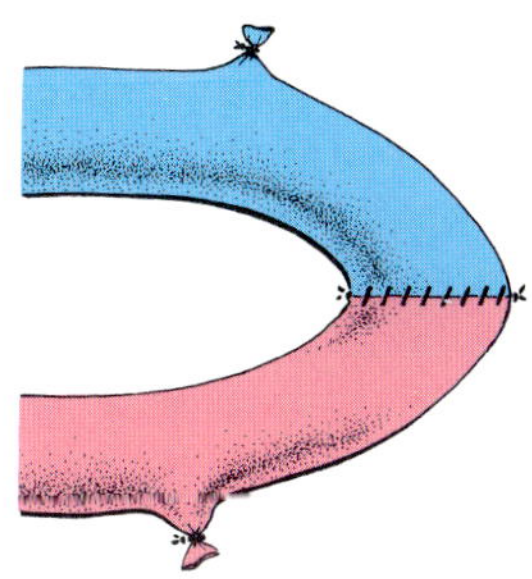

Fig. 25.6. "Tennis racket" fistula. End-to-end anastomosis of the radial artery to the cephalic vein in the distal forearm, the radial artery entering at an acute angle. Following dissection, both vessels are divided transversely and the ends beveled. The anastomosis is performed by the usual technique

Another possibility for an end-to-end anastomosis is the so-called loop of the radial artery as shown in Fig. 25.7. As a rule, the vein may be used for the arch as well. In 1975, while investigating the various procedures, GERLACH and LYMBEROPOULOS pointed out that the U-shaped end-to-end anastomosis is the only one that provides an almost laminar flow. Furthermore, the regions of stagnation and turbulence are smallest when the end-to-end anastomosis to the arterial arch is constructed in a straight line. Other authors [12] place the anastomosis exactly at the apex of the loop. Concerning the anastomotic technique, one should always use interrupted sutures for an end-to-end anastomosis. With vessels of especially small caliber, the anastomosis may be facilitated by previous contralateral longitudinal incisions of the

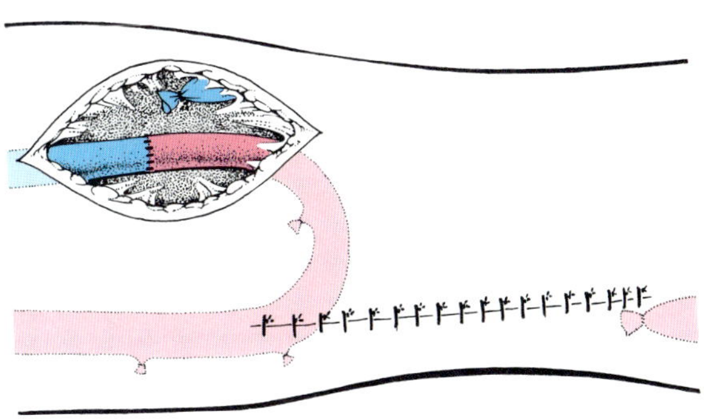

Fig. 25.7. Completed end-to-end anastomosis, producing an arterial vascular arch. In this case, too, the approach is made through two displaced longitudinal incisions

vascular ends. However, it should be pointed out that the end-to-end anastomosis described may kink much more easily, especially after a long period of time, when the fistula has become dilated and stretched by the shunt.

3. Arteriovenous Fistula Proximal to the Wrist Between the Ulnar Artery and the Basilic Vein (Ulnar Shunt)

For details of anatomy and positioning see pp. 647, 649.

a) Operative Approach. The operative approach is through a longitudinal incision about 3–5 cm long, between the ulnar artery and the basilic vein, 2 cm proximal to the ulnar head. When using the curved type of fistula as described above, it may be helpful to have two separate incisions.

b) Surgical Technique. Following exposure and mobilization of the basilic vein of the forearm, which is often less straight and passes further from the appropriate artery than the cephalic vein, the fascia is divided and the ulnar artery exposed between the tendons of the flexor carpi ulnaris muscle and the flexor digitorum superficialis muscle. Concerning the anastomotic technique see Sect. C.I.2. (p. 647).

4. Basilic Vein Repositioning in the Forearm

For details of anatomy and positioning see pp. 647, 652, 653.

a) Operative Approach. With this procedure the basilic vein is exposed through several skin incisions. In the region of the elbow, a transverse incision is made according to the anatomic situation (Fig. 25.13a).

b) Surgical Technique. Following dissection of the basilic vein, the tributaries joining the vein are ligated and divided. The vessel is then ligated at the level of the wrist, and the end is beveled. Also in this case the occluded vessel is filled with heparinized saline solution during venous stasis. The further steps in the procedure are shown in Fig. 25.13b–d. Using an appropriate tunneling instrument, a subcutaneous tunnel is formed, leading to the radial artery. The vein is pulled through the tunnel to the artery, care being taken not to twist the vein. Care must also be taken to ensure that the vein lies just beneath the skin in order to facilitate cannulation.

The anastomotic technique is the same as that described on pp. 649–650.

5. Arteriovenous Fistula in the Elbow

Given the ever-increasing number of patients on maintenance dialysis, there are correspondingly more cases in which arteriovenous fistulas in the periphery of the arm have led to complications. As a result, the elbow has begun to assume greater importance as an alternative site for fistula construction [7]. All too often, a prosthetic graft is used for management of such complications. But because it is possible nowadays, using the single needle technique, to get by with only a relatively short shunt, a functional fistula at the elbow, utilizing the cephalic or the basilic vein, will normally be sufficient for effective hemodialysis [15].

a) Anatomy. The sensory innervation of the thin elastic skin of the anterior and medial side of the upper arm and elbow is provided by the medial cutaneous nerve of the arm (Fig. 25.8). The medial cutaneous nerve of the forearm, which lies on the brachial artery in the medial bicipital groove, reaches the subcutaneous tissue approximately in the middle of the upper arm, usually together with the basilic vein, through a gap in the fascia having the same name. Often, it has already divided to form its two major branches (anterior ramus, ramus ulnaris nervi cutanei antebrachii medialis) (Fig. 25.8).

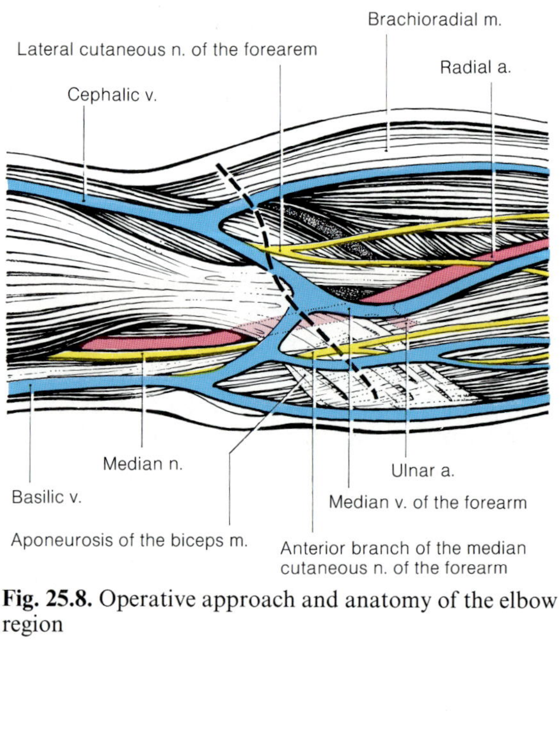

Fig. 25.8. Operative approach and anatomy of the elbow region

They pass through the elbow in a manner similar to that in which the lateral cutaneous nerve of the forearm perforates the fascia in the distal one third of the upper arm. The sensory innervation of the lower arm, except for the extensor side, is provided by all three nerves together.

The skin veins in the region of the elbow (and of the forearm) are extremely variable. Essentially two patterns can be distinguished:

- The cephalic vein and the basilic vein are connected by a median cubital vein passing from radial-distal to ulnar-proximal. In this case, the median vein of the forearm is often underdeveloped or absent.
- There may be a third large skin vein of the forearm, the median vein of the forearm, branching V-shaped into the median basilic and the median cephalic vein in the elbow. After a short distance, these veins join the major cutaneous veins of the arm having the same names (Fig. 25.8).

The superficial veins of the elbow are almost always connected to the deep veins by a perforating branch. The cephalic vein continues through the flat lateral bicipital groove, often almost ventrally across the biceps muscle, to the shoulder, and then through the sulcus deltoideopectoralis to Mohrenheim's fossa.

The larger basilic vein usually passes in the medial bicipital groove above the fascia. Somewhat distal to the middle of the arm, it passes through the basilic hiatus into the deep region and soon joins the brachial vein; indeed, it might be seen as the continuation of the latter (Fig. 25.14a).

The brachial artery has a large branch, the profunda brachii artery, originating in the proximal third of the upper arm, passing over to the extensor side together with the radial nerve between the long and the medial head of the triceps muscle. In the middle of the upper arm, the neurovascular bundle still consists of the brachial artery with its two or three concomitant nerves, the ulner nerve accompanying it medially, the median nerve running lateral and ventral to it, and the medial cutaneous nerve of the forearm. The ulnar nerve soon perforates the septum intermusculare brachii medialis and passes medially to the extensor side (Fig. 25.14b, c). In contrast, the brachial artery and the median nerve approach the elbow. There, the median nerve lies on the ulnar side of the artery (Fig. 25.8). Both pass underneath the aponeurosis of the biceps muscle within connective and fatty tissue. The brachial artery then branches off into its two end arteries: the radial and ulnar artery (usually somewhat distal to the joint cavity). The radial artery crosses the tendon of the biceps muscle and the pronator teres muscle and may be easily approached throughout its entire length. The ulnar artery, together with the median nerve, disappears under the flexor antebrachii superficiales muscles and passes later to the ulnar flexor side of the wrist, accompanied by the ulnar nerve.

b) Operative Approach. For all fistulas a transverse, perhaps also S-shaped incision about 4 cm long is made just below the elbow (Fig. 25.8). The length and the position of the incision may be changed according to the individual vascular situation and the suggested type of anastomosis. However, the remaining scar should neither shorten the segment for cannulation, nor impair the mobility of the arm at the elbow.

c) Surgical Technique. The following points must be considered when constructing a fistula in the elbow:

1. The fistula should be constructed as a "proximal" forearm fistula, distal to the joint cavity whenever possible in order to avoid compression and kinking of the fistula when the joint is flexed. This also has the advantage of a longer segment of shunt vein for cannulation.

2. Whenever possible, the proximal radial artery should be utilized for anastomosis because that way only the radial artery is endangered in the event of complications or reintervention. However, the ulnar artery will still guarantee blood flow to the forearm.

3. In the region of the elbow, only side-to-side or end-to-side anastomoses of the vein to the artery are recommended because end-to-end anastomoses may endanger the blood flow to the hand.

4. In most arteriovenous fistulas in the region of the wrist, it is only flow in the proximal direction that is intended and of significance for cannulation. However, fistulas in the elbow may develop a flow in proximal or distal directions, independent of the type of anastomosis.

α) Side-to-Side Anastomosis. In the elbow region, for purely topographic reasons, the chosen subcutaneous vein is dissected first. The next step is to divide the fascia and, if necessary, part of the aponeurosis of the biceps muscle as well. The radial artery is then exposed over the long tendon of the biceps muscle, between the ulnar flexors and

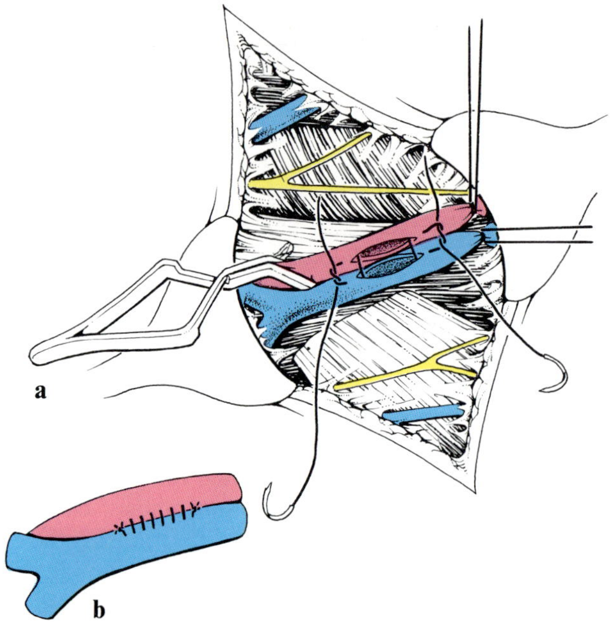

Fig. 25.9 a, b. Anastomosis of the vessels in the elbow. **a** Following division of the fascia and the aponeurosis of the biceps muscle, the radial artery is brought up and cross-clamped just distal to its origin at the brachial artery. The artery and vein must lie next to each other without tension. Following corresponding longitudinal incisions, the vessels are approximated by means of two corner sutures and by continuous suture of the posterior and the anterior wall. **b** Completed side-to-side anastomosis distal to the elbow fold (proximal forearm fistula)

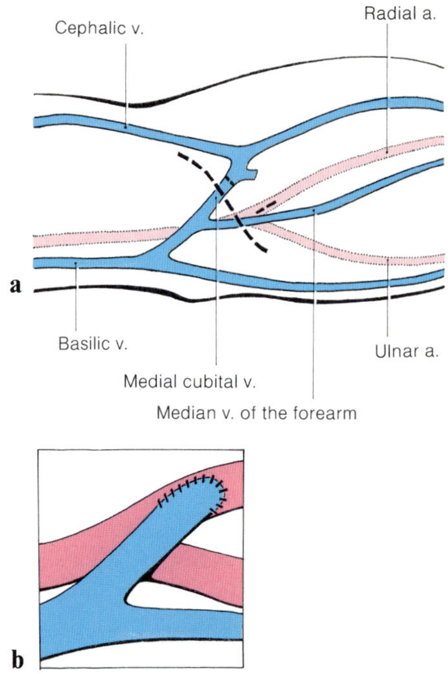

Fig. 25.10. a Schematic drawing of the veins showing a strongly developed median cubital vein. **b** Completed end-to-side anastomosis of the median cubital vein to the radial artery

the brachioradial muscle, and a tape is placed around it. It may also be necessary to expose the brachial artery and the ulnar artery and to place tapes around them in order to achieve a better view. Because the distance between the two vessels is greater in the region of the elbow, one must be especially careful not to create tension at the anastomosis. The anastomotic technique is the same as for the side-to-side anastomosis in the case of the Brescia-Cimino fistula (Fig. 25.9 a, b; see also pp. 648–649). An example of a side-to-side anastomosis of the cephalic vein to the brachial artery is shown in Fig. 25.11. Other side-to-side fistulas not shown may be performed between any suitable adjacent vein and either the brachial or the radial artery.

β) End-to-Side Anastomosis. An end-to-side anastomosis to the radial artery or brachial artery may be required when vessel branching is suitable or when the vessels are occluded peripherally, as shown in Figs. 25.10 a, b and 25.12.

The anatomic variety of veins in the elbow offers numerous possibilities for the construction

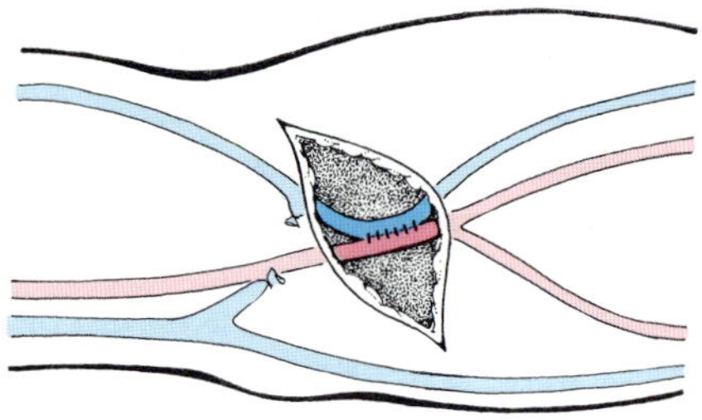

Fig. 25.11. Side-to-side fistula of the brachial artery to the cephalic vein

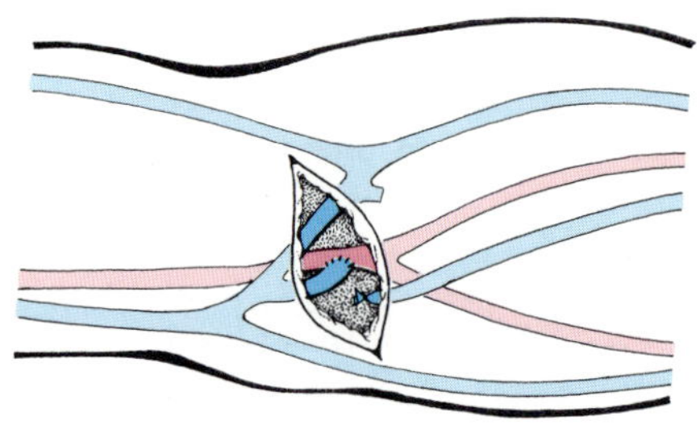

Fig. 25.12. End-to-side fistula of the median vein of the forearm to the brachial artery

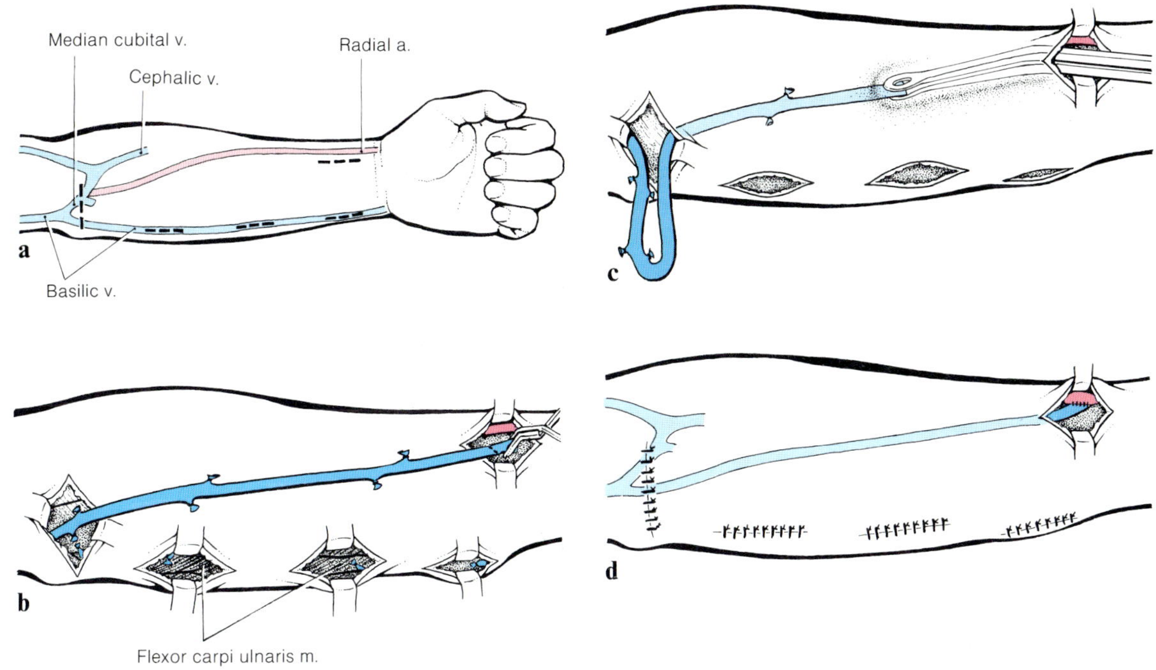

Fig. 25.13a–d. Basilic vein repositioning in the forearm. **a** Operative approach and schematic drawing of the subcutaneous veins. **b** Dissected basilic vein showing its length. **c** The basilic vein is pulled through a preformed subcutaneous tunnel to the radial artery. **d** End-to-side anastomosis of the basilic vein to the radial artery

of fistulas. The basic principles of shunt surgery, i.e., to construct as long an angioaccess as possible without destroying many vessels, is of special importance in this area.

6. Basilic Vein Repositioning in the Upper Arm

Special anatomy see pp. 652–653.

a) Positioning. For basilic vein repositioning, the patient is placed in a supine position with the arm abducted 90°, extended, and supinated.

b) Operative Approach. The approach is either through a skin incision, about 12–15 cm long, somewhat curved distally and extending from the axillary fossa to the elbow, or through two or three separate incisions over the vein.

c) Surgical Technique. The basilic vein is exposed and dissected from the basilic hiatus down to the elbow, preserving the medial cutaneous nerve of the forearm and its branches. Sufficient mobilization must be ensured distally to achieve a sufficient length of vein for subsequent lateroconvex repositioning.

The brachial fascia is divided longitudinally from the hiatus to the axillary fossa, to achieve further exposure of the vessels. The basilic vein joins a deep concomitant vein, usually a few centimeters proximal to the point where it perforates the fascia. Proximal to this site, the brachial vein is displaced (see Fig. 25.14a–c).

One must be careful of the three large nerves of the arm, which course here in very close proximity to one another.

Furthermore, one has to consider that the wall of the basilic vein becomes thinner proximally and may be injured more easily. Secure ligation of all tributaries plays an especially important role in this procedure, as insecure ligatures may cause significant bleeding.

Short broad stumps of the vein may be better closed using a continuous suture. Following dissection of the vein, the fascia is closed again underneath, providing a sufficiently large gap. A subcutaneous tunnel is created by means of a forceps, and the vein is passed through in a lateroconvex arch. As a result of this procedure, it will be possible later to avoid the scar tissue when cannulating the vein. Finally, the vein is anastomosed end-to-side to the brachial artery.

Considering the possibilities offered by synthetic grafts, the technique of repositioning the brachial vein in order to create a shunt should be

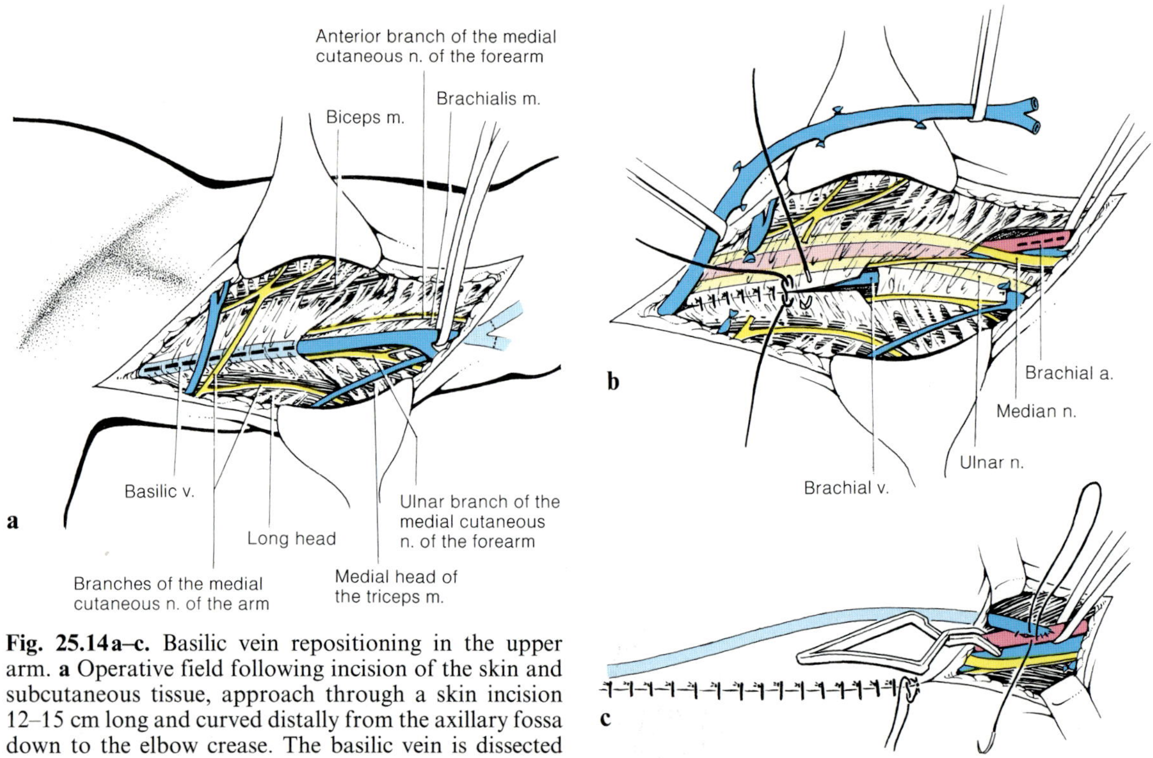

Fig. 25.14a–c. Basilic vein repositioning in the upper arm. **a** Operative field following incision of the skin and subcutaneous tissue, approach through a skin incision 12–15 cm long and curved distally from the axillary fossa down to the elbow crease. The basilic vein is dissected up to the basilic hiatus, and a tape is placed around it. The brachial fascia is divided to bring up the vein, marked by the *broken lines*. **b** Suture of the brachial fascia following complete mobilization and distal division of the basilic vein. **c** The basilic vein, repositioned closer to the surface of the skin, is anastomosed to the brachial artery

viewed with reserve; for, if the repositioned brachial vein ever becomes occluded, no further shunts can be constructed in that entire arm.

7. Repositioning of the Greater Saphenous Vein in the Thigh

For details of anatomy and positioning see below.

a) Operative Approach. Local repositioning of the great saphenous vein in the thigh is done by bringing the vessel up and keeping it straight for anastomosis with the first segment of the popliteal artery. It is also possible, using three curved counterincisions on the lateral thigh, to place the vein directly under the skin for anastomosis to the superficial femoral artery (Fig. 25.20c).

One must be careful not to twist or kink the vein. Furthermore, the vessel must be placed just beneath the skin. For the operative mobilization technique and the possible anastomotic procedures see pp. 650, 658.

8. Saphenous Vein Transplantation to the Forearm

For details of the technique of vein harvesting see p. 397.

Saphenous vein transplantation to the forearm is similar to the use of synthetic grafts for arteriovenous fistulas in this region (see pp. 659, 661). Care must be taken to place the vein segment so that the blood flow is anterograde, i.e., not counter to the action of the valves. Furthermore, kinking and twisting must be avoided.

One should be cautious about utilizing the saphenous vein as a shunt because of its importance as a potential source of autogenous graft material for coronary surgery and bypass surgery of the peripheral arteries. Furthermore, it should be borne in mind that using the saphenous vein for graft material also means that it will no longer be available as a venous connection for the construction of arteriovenous fistulas in the thigh.

9. Superficialization of the Superficial Femoral Artery

a) Anatomy. The ventral thigh has firm skin as compared with other extremity regions. It also has the strongest muscles, as well as large caliber pe-

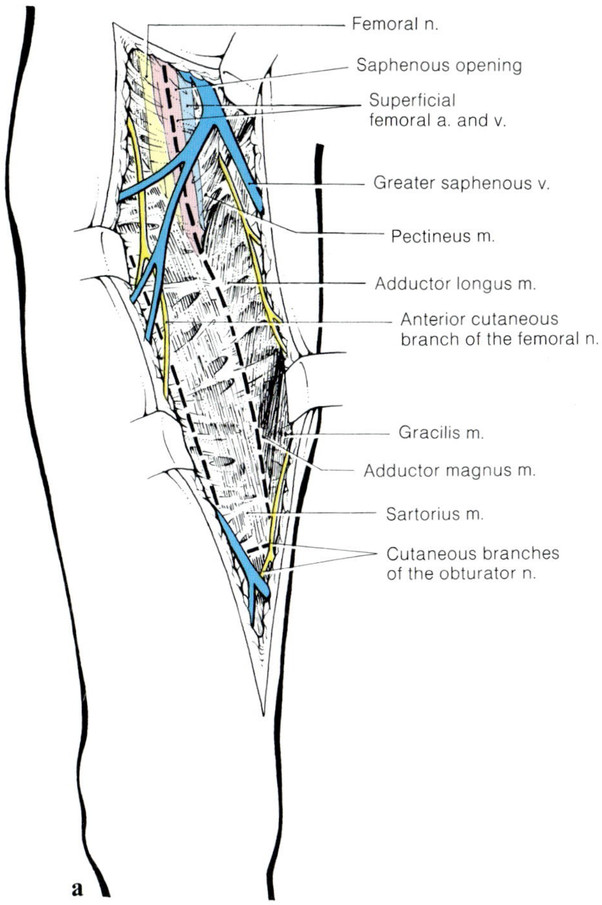

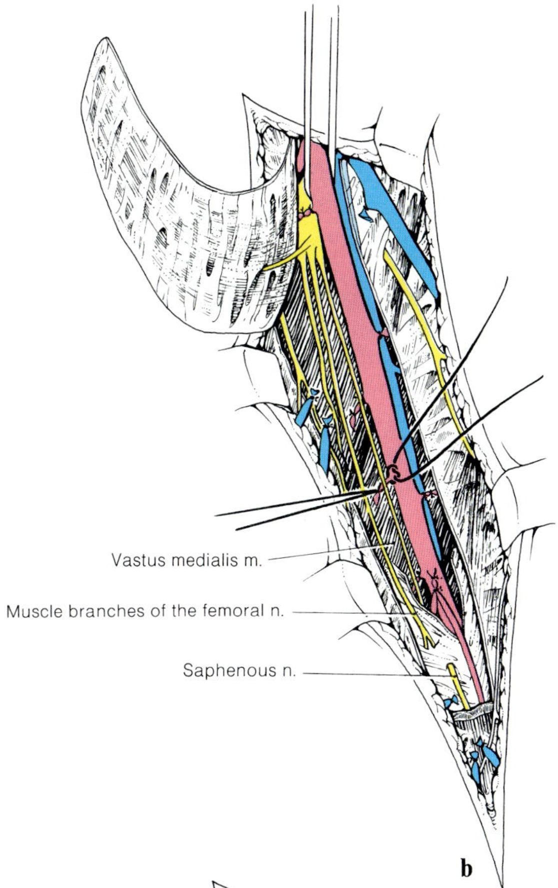

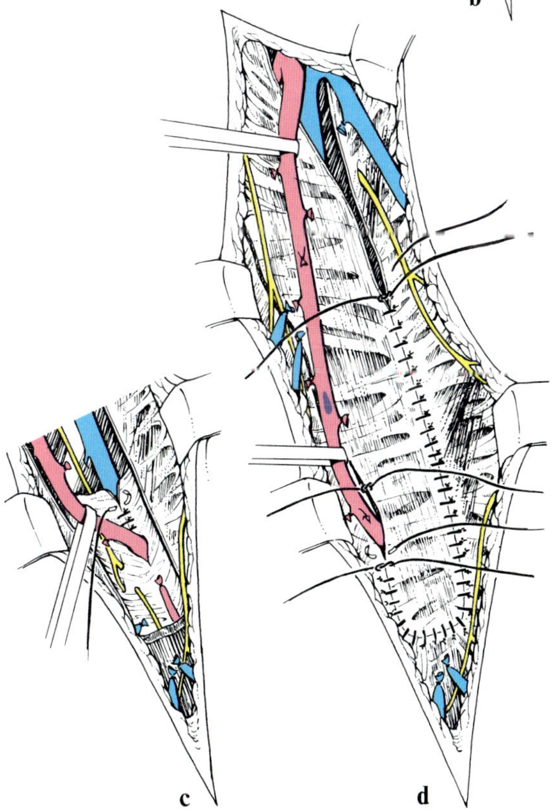

Fig. 25.15a–d. Antepositioning of the superficial femoral artery. **a** Operative field following division of the skin and subcutaneous tissue. Approach through a slightly curved longitudinal incision on the anteromedial side of the thigh. Splitting of the fascia lata and division of the sartorius muscle as marked in the figure. **b** Splitting of the fascia, medial and lateral to the sartorius muscle, the sartorius muscle divided transversely and drawn up. Dissection of the superficial femoral artery from the groin down to the hiatus tendineus, with opening of the subsartorial canal. **c** Reconstruction of the subsartorial canal by suturing the lamina vastoadductoria, leaving a gap in the fascia for the artery. **d** The sartorius muscle is drawn back to its original position and reanastomosed. The fascia lata is closed underneath the repositioned superficial femoral artery

ripheral nerves and veins. The sensory innervation of the skin is mainly provided by the anterior cutaneous rami of the femoral nerves (by the femoral branch of the genitofemoral nerve in the region of the saphenous hiatus). Further medially the innervation is provided through cutaneous branches of the obturator nerve (Fig. 25.15a), while the lateral side is innervated by the lateral cutaneous nerve of the thigh.

Coming from the lower leg, the major vein of the limb, the great saphenous vein reaches this region behind the medial condyle of the femur and passes on the ventral and medial side of the thigh to the saphenous hiatus, receiving several branches. There, other major veins of the groin and the abdominal wall often join the greater saphenous vein (superficial epigastric vein, superficial circumflex iliac vein, external pudendal veins) to form the venous junction. The great saphenous vein joins the femoral vein after perforating the lamina cribrosa fasciae latae (see p. 701).

While the femoral artery and vein pass through the lacuna vasorum, located medial to the trigonum femorale, the femoral nerve, together with the iliopsoas muscle, descends lateral to the iliopectineal arch. The cutaneous branches to the anterior femoral region arise a few centimeters below the inguinal ligament. Then it branches into several muscle rami (to the quadriceps femoris, the sartorius, and the pectineus muscles). Its final branch, the saphenous nerve, accompanies the great vessels (Fig. 25.15b).

The femoral artery follows a straight course over the entire length of the thigh. The proximal one third of the artery lies superficially, directly underneath the strong fascia lata (here it is also called the common femoral artery). Approximately 3–5 cm distal to the inguinal ligament, the profunda femoris artery, which is of almost the same size, branches off. Usually, the medial circumflex artery and the lateral circumflex artery originate from the profunda femoris artery (see p. 22). At the junction of the proximal and middle third of the thigh, the femoral artery then disappears under the sartorius muscle in its own fascia. It then passes medial to the strong quadriceps femoris muscle into the subsartorial canal after giving off several branches to the muscles (Fig. 25.15b). The subsartorial canal is bounded by the vastus medialis muscle, the adductor longus muscle, and the lamina vastoadductoria connecting these two muscles. The vessels pass in this canal from the ventral side of the thigh down to the popliteal fossa. There the descending genicular artery, the last branch of the femoral artery, has its origin. The saphenous branch of the genicular artery perforates the lamina vastoadductoria and accompanies the saphenous nerve.

In the groin, the femoral vein is located farthest medially. The farther peripherally, the more nearly it lies behind the artery; beyond the hiatus tendineus it becomes the popliteal vein and courses lateral to the artery.

b) Positioning. The patient is placed in a supine position with the limb extended, abducted, and rotated externally.

c) Operative Approach. A slightly curved longitudinal incision is made along the entire length of the thigh, originating about 5 cm below the middle of the inguinal ligament and extending downward to the medial condyle of the femur (Fig. 25.15a).

d) Surgical Technique. Since the superficial femoral artery, over its entire length, is to be repositioned in front of the fascia lata, it must first be dissected off the neurovascular bundle and freed of all tissue surrounding the sartorius muscle. Then, the fascia lata is split from the saphenous hiatus down nearly to the other end of the skin incision, medial to the sartorius muscle, and the sartorius muscle is divided above its insertion (pes anserinus). This division should not be performed too far distally, but should be distal to the subsartorial canal. The muscle is now dissected, mobilized up to the groin, and drawn upward (Fig. 25.15b).

Next, the superficial femoral artery is dissected off the vascular sheath, and its branches are ligated and divided. It is also necessary to open the subsartorial canal by splitting the lamina vastoadductoria down to the hiatus tendineus.

Finally, the anatomic situation is restored insofar as possible. First, the lamina vastoadductoria is sutured again. Then, the sartorius muscle is passed underneath the femoral artery and reattached to its insertion. One must be careful to achieve a large enough gap in the fascia to allow passage of the femoral artery (Fig. 25.15c, d).

The artery is placed in the subcutaneous tissue, lateral to the resulting scar, so that subsequent cannulation will be easy and safe. It is carefully fixed in this position by several subcutaneous sutures.

This procedure is not without importance today, but is used only in rare cases, after all other arteriovenous fistulas have been tried, or in the event of problems with the synthetic graft material.

II. Subcutaneous Arteriovenous Fistulas Utilizing a Prosthetic Graft

In numerous instances, there are no autogenous vessels available for use in constructing a fistula, either because they simply do not exist or because the superficial vein system of the arm has been injured by multiple cannulations or intravenous infusions. Furthermore, the superficial veins are often so damaged by previous operations that they, too, are useless for creation of a fistula. In such cases, synthetic grafts can be used to construct a shunt for maintenance dialysis. The requirements for an ideal vascular graft serving as a shunt are:

- Ease of cannulation
- Easy to obtain and always available
- Easy technical utilization
- Immunologically inert
- A wall structure as nearly natural as possible
- Resistant to infections
- Low cost

According to our present knowledge, the following materials may be considered for use as vascular grafts for maintenance hemodialysis:

a) Autogenous material: great saphenous vein
b) Homologous material: denatured umbilical vein, denatured great saphenous vein
c) Heterologous material: denatured calf or bovine carotid artery
d) Alloplastic material: polytetrafluoroethylene (PTFE) prosthesis

All grafts show certain advantages and disadvantages. The reader is referred to the appropriate chapters of this book (see p. 175ff.).

Today, the heated microporous polytetrafluoroethylene (PTFE) prostheses and the denatured homologous umbilical vein have the greatest significance in shunt surgery. Heterologous material, such as calf or bovine carotid arteries, are less often used because of the risk of aneurysm formation [9, 11, 14, 18].

An implanted prosthetic graft may be straight, U-shaped, or loop-shaped. When choosing the appropriate procedure, it is useful to consider the anatomic possibilities and always to select the procedure which least impairs the blood flow of the extremity and would interfere least with further shunt operations that might be needed.

1. Interposition Prosthetic Graft Fistulae in the Forearm

Sometimes, it can only be decided intraoperatively on the basis of the anatomic situation – especially the matter of venous outflow – which vessels can be connected to the graft; often, the patients have been previously operated on. Whenever superficial veins cannot be palpated or inspected, phlebography is useful for demonstrating deep venous flow in veins which could be utilized for the shunt.

The anastomosis of a graft to the radial artery and the median vein of the forearm is described here as being representative of the numerous possibilities for creating dialysis fistulas using synthetic grafts. It may be performed in a loop or in a straight line (Figs. 25.16a–d, 25.17, 25.18, and 25.19).

a) Detailed Anatomy and Positioning (see pp. 647, 649).

b) Operative Approach. For this procedure, too, a transverse incision is made just below the elbow to expose the vessels. The incision may be modified to become somewhat S-shaped. Furthermore, two other counterincisions are made in the forearm to facilitate the implantation of the graft in a curve (Fig. 25.16). With a straight graft interposition, an incision is made over the appropriate vessel in the forearm. Dissection of the vessels to be connected in the elbow and in the region of the peripheral radial artery is performed as described on pp. 647, 653–654.

c) Surgical Technique

α) Curved Course of the Graft (Fig. 25.16a–d). When the graft is implanted in a curve, one should take care that it lies without tension in a subcutaneous tunnel created by a forceps or a tunneling instrument and that the graft does not show any direct contact with the skin incisions (risk of infection). The suture technique for the anastomosis is not significantly different from the techniques described earlier. However, one must use only nonabsorbable suture material, e.g., 6-0, when working with prosthetic material.

β) Straight Graft. This type of fistula should be considered when a radial artery is significantly dilated by preexisting fistulas. Thus, there will be no great difference in caliber between the usual 6 mm graft and the artery. For the implantation technique, see Figs. 25.17 and 25.18. The ulnar ar-

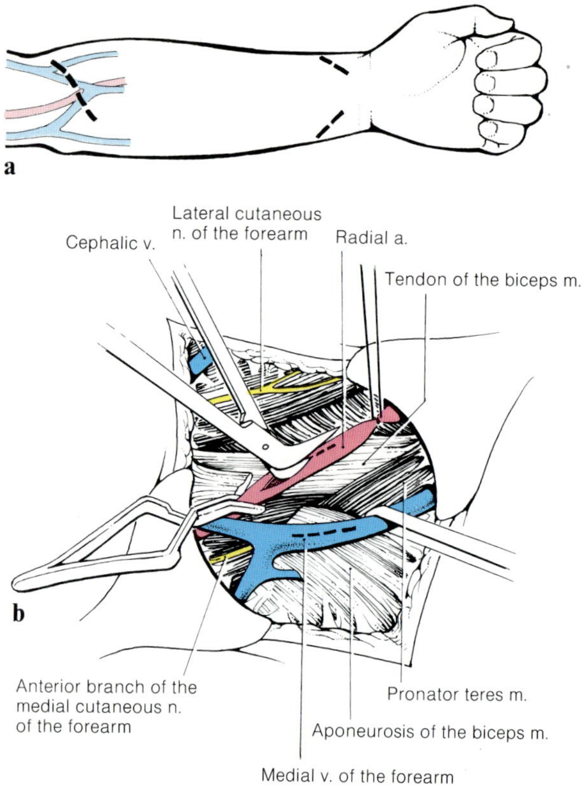

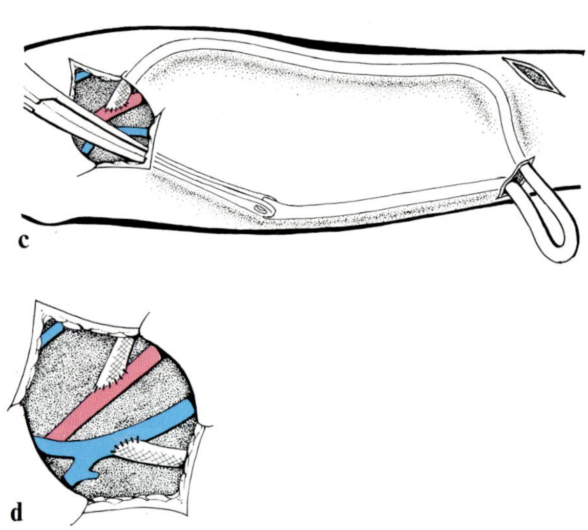

Fig. 25.16a–d. Implanting a curved vascular graft in the forearm from the radial artery to the median vein. **a** Transverse incision of the skin below the elbow fold with two counterincisions in the region of the medial (to distal) forearm to create a tunnel for the graft. **b** Exposure of the fully dissected vein and artery in the region of the elbow. The site of incision is marked on the vessel. **c** Anastomosis of the graft to the radial artery and subcutaneous pull-through in a curve in the preformed tunnel. **d** Situation in the elbow after completion of the arterial and venous anastomosis

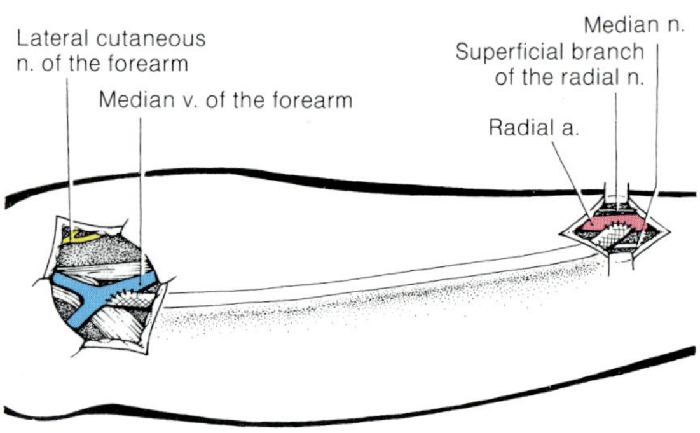

Fig. 25.17. Implantation of a vascular graft in a straight position from the distal radial artery to the median vein of the forearm

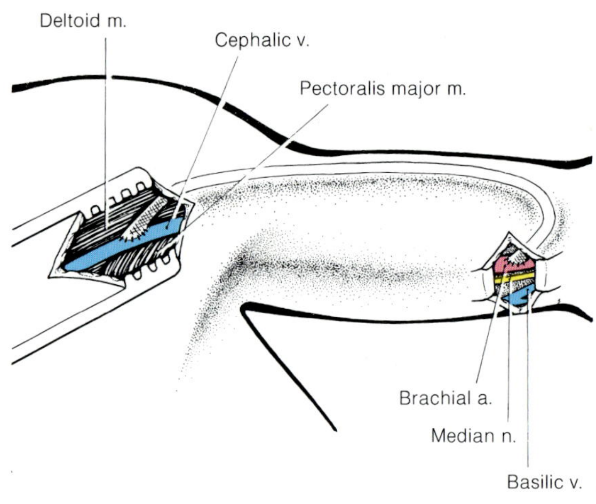

Fig. 25.19. Graft implantation in the upper arm from the distal and brachial artery to the cephalic vein, and end-to-side anastomosis of the graft to the brachial artery, which is curved to achieve good flow

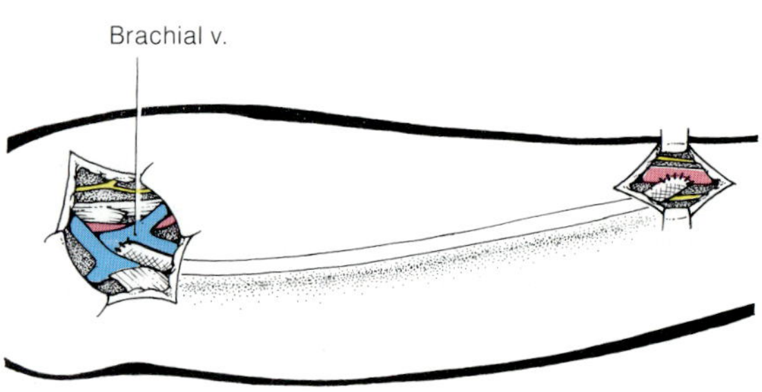

◁ **Fig. 25.18.** In cases where the superficial veins are insufficient, the brachial vein, which is usually well developed, may be used for the anastomosis

tery must be functioning well if one is utilizing the radial artery (Allen test). In the event of a difference in caliber, interrupted suturing of the anastomosis is beneficial.

2. Interposition Graft Fistulas in the Upper Arm

For details of anatomy and positioning see pp. 652, 653.

a) Operative Approach. The approach is through two incisions about 3–4 cm long over both vessels, placed in the region of the suggested anastomosis (Fig. 25.19). It may be necessary to make an additional incision in the lateral portion of the middle upper arm in order to pull the graft through the tunnel and to achieve an advantageous curvilinear course for it in the subcutaneous tissue.

b) Surgical Technique. Following division of the fascia, first the brachial artery is exposed over a short distance of about 2–3 cm. Then, the cephalic vein is exposed as well, but preferably not too far proximally (shoulder joint). It is advisable to implant the graft in the upper arm so that it is C-shaped to achieve favorable flow conditions (Fig. 25.19).

3. Further Possible Arteriovenous Fistulas Utilizing Prosthetic Grafts

Besides the standard procedures described, there are other possibilities for constructing arteriovenous fistulas utilizing synthetic grafts. Included here in particular is the bridging of autogenous veins and arteries with prosthetic grafts for the ultimate purpose of using the autogenous vein for cannulation. Furthermore, there is the possibility of interposing synthetic grafts in old shunt veins so that these valuable vessels are still available for cannulation proximal and distal to the synthetic graft. If required, prosthetic grafts may also be used for crossing the elbow joint. In such regions, which carry the risk of kinking, reinforced prostheses (ring or spiral type) are suitable. However, the segment to be cannulated should not be reinforced.

4. Interposition Graft Fistula in the Thigh

Here, a graft is interposed from the superficial artery to – whenever possible – the great saphenous vein. Only in special cases should the femoral vein be used. The graft may be curved or straight.

a) Detailed Anatomy (see pp. 656–658)

b) Positioning. The patient is placed in a supine position with the arm extended and abducted. For an anastomosis within the subsartorial canal, additional slight external rotation is recommended.

c) Operative Approach. A skin incision about 6–8 cm long is made to expose the two vessels that are to be connected by a curved graft. The incision starts below the inguinal region at the level of the saphenous hiatus and extends downward, parallel to the neurovascular bundle (Fig. 25.20a).

Three other incisions are necessary to place the graft as shown in Fig. 25.20b, c.

When placing the graft in a straight position in the thigh, a small incision is made over the great saphenous vein at the site where it joins the femoral vein. Another incision is made medially and above the knee joint at the end of the subsartorial canal to allow dissection of the superficial femoral artery (Fig. 25.21).

d) Surgical Technique

α) Curved Graft. First the great saphenous vein is exposed in the proximal thigh and a tape is placed around it. Following division of the fascia and starting from the saphenous hiatus, the superficial femoral artery is exposed a short distance beyond where it branches off from the common femoral artery. It is advisable to suture the beveled end of the graft end-to-side to the superficial femoral artery. One should fill the clamped vascular ends with heparinized saline solution. The graft is then passed through a preformed loop-shaped tunnel in the subcutaneous tissue so that its free end can be anastomosed end-to-side with the saphenous vein where the latter joins the femoral vein (Fig. 25.20a–c). Care must be taken not to kink the graft. Furthermore, the graft should not be in direct contact with the incisions. The saphenous vein should not be ligated distal to the anastomosis.

β) Straight Graft. In this procedure, the graft is sutured to the superficial femoral artery in the region of the subsartorial canal. It is passed subcutaneously to the saphenous vein, to which its beveled end is then anastomosed end-to-side (Fig. 25.21). The anastomotic technique is similar to the procedures described earlier.

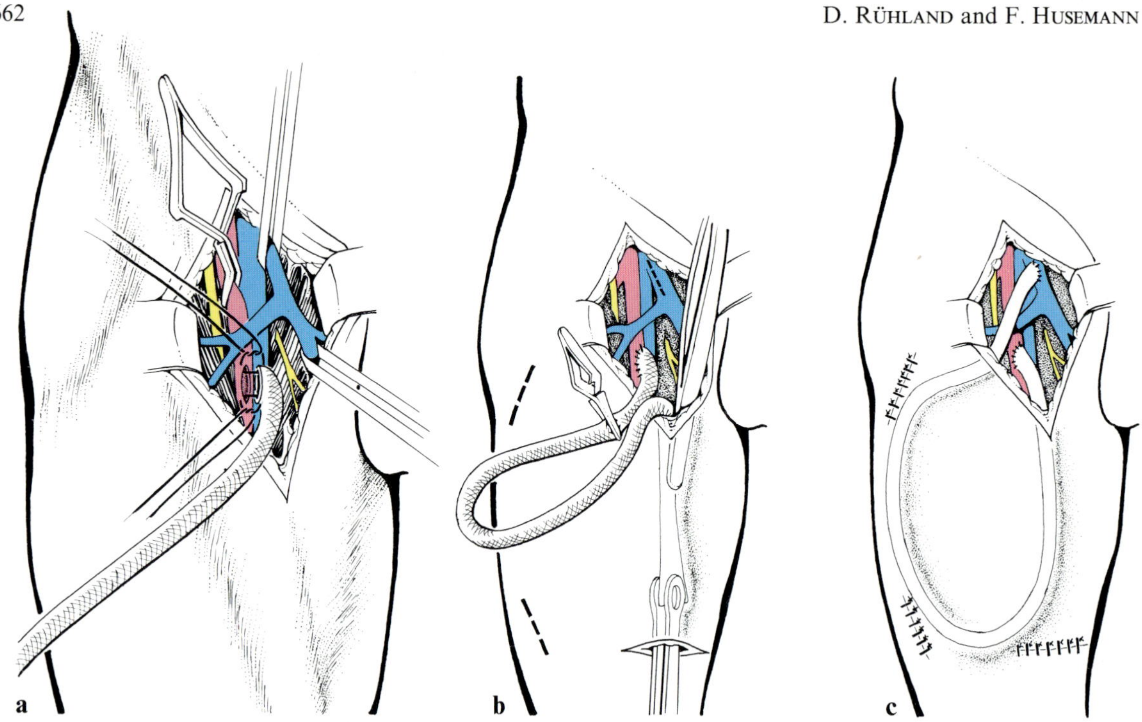

Fig. 25.20 a–c. Curved placement of a vascular graft from the proximal superficial femoral artery to the great saphenous vein. **a** End-to-side anastomosis of the graft to the superficial femoral artery. **b** The graft is pulled through a preformed subcutaneous tunnel, first distally and then laterally. Finally, it is pulled proximally in the direction of the junction of the great saphenous vein with the femoral vein. **c** Completed arteriovenous fistula between the femoral artery and the saphenous vein utilizing a graft

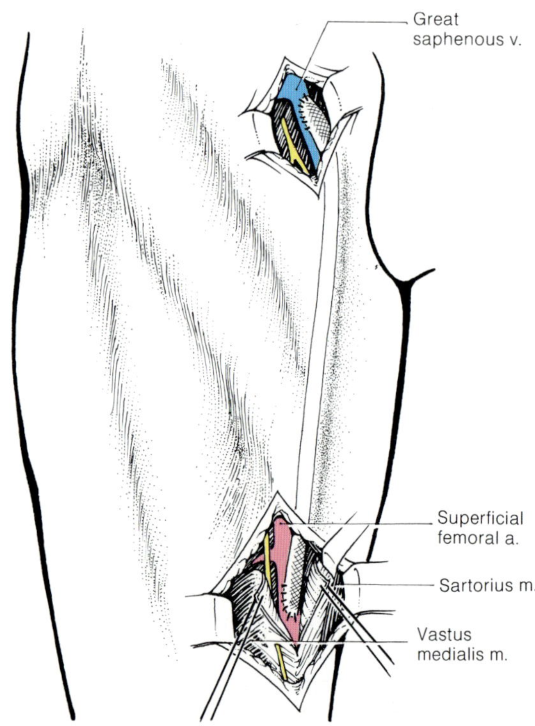

Fig. 25.21. Straight graft from the distal superficial femoral artery to the great saphenous vein

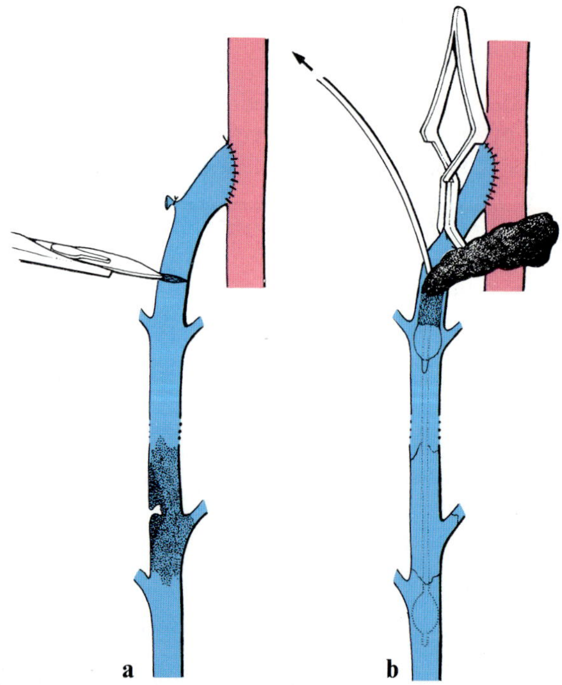

Fig. 25.22 a, b. Thrombotic occlusion of the venous limb of a shunt at the site of the puncture. **a** Transverse incision of the vein. **b** Removal of the thrombus by means of a Fogarty catheter

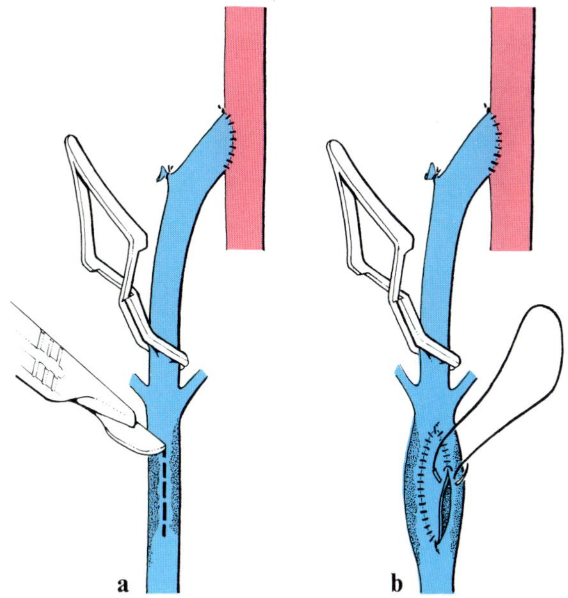

Fig. 25.23a, b. Stenosis due to a scar at the site of puncture of the shunt vein. **a** Incision of the stenosis. **b** Suturing the patch graft (venous patch) to reconstruct the vessel

III. Complications of Subcutaneous Arteriovenous Fistulas and Their Treatment

When treating complications of subcutaneous arteriovenous fistulas, one's first concern should be to preserve or to restore the function of the old shunt so that the patient can be put back on routine maintenance dialysis as soon as possible.

Fig. 25.24. Occlusion of an old PTFE prosthesis by intimal hyperplasia and consequent thrombosis of the anastomosis. First, the thrombus is removed using a Fogarty catheter

Fig. 25.25. If a sufficient lumen cannot be achieved in the anastomosis following thrombectomy, a patch graft is required. Fixation of the tailored patch by interrupted sutures. Continuous suture of the patch graft to the vessel wall. Completed patch graft angioplasties at the arterial and venous anastomoses of the graft

Fig. 25.26. If the occluded anastomosis cannot be reconstructed (as is often the case with the venous anastomosis), the venous limb of the graft can be extended proximally to reconstruct the old prosthetic shunt

▽

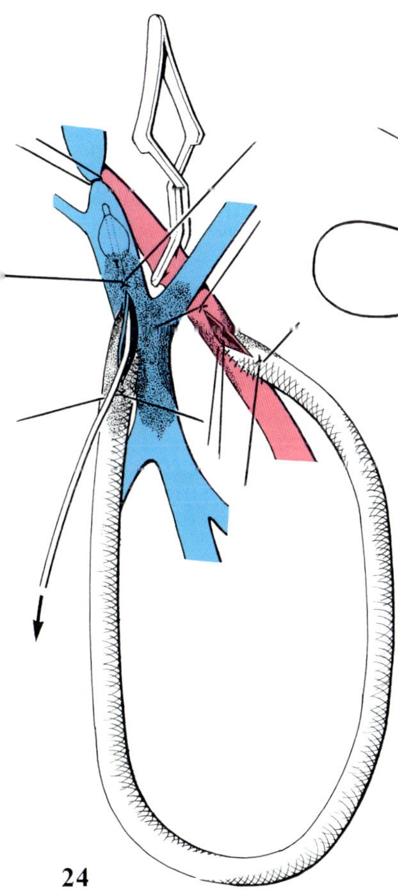

24

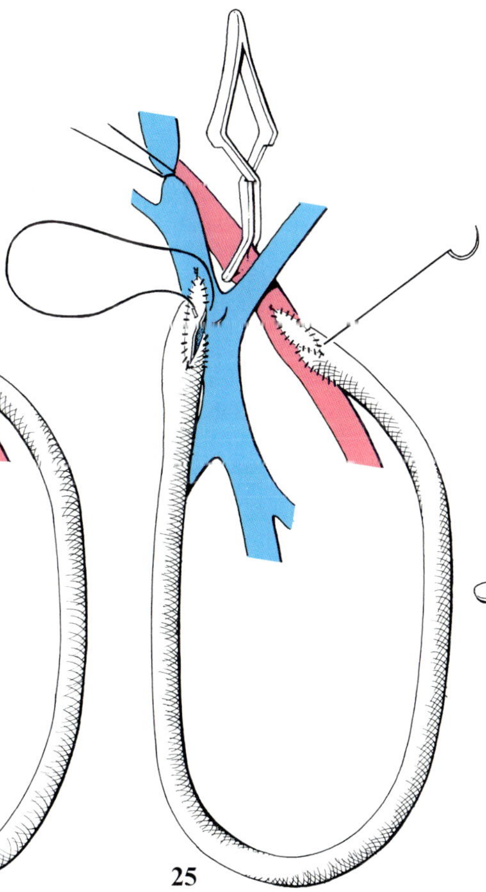

25

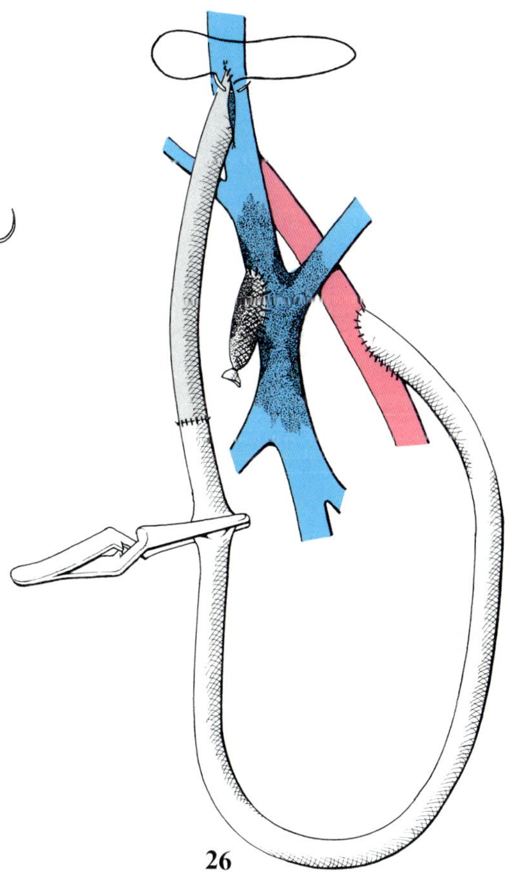

26

1. Stenoses and Occlusions

With fistulas constructed of autogenous material, stenoses and occlusions are observed in the region of the anastomosis and at the cannulation sites [13]. When a stenosis or occlusion occurs, it is advisable to reconnect to the – usually dilated – arteries and veins at a new site above the old anastomosis, thereby avoiding an operation in scar tissue. At the same time, this removes the cause of the stenosis or occlusion. If a new anastomosis above the complication is not possible, thrombectomy may be tried (Fig. 25.22a, b). When there are constricting stenoses due to scars in the region of the cannulation sites, restoration of improved flow may be achieved by patch graft angioplasty (Fig. 25.23a, b).

Especially where prosthetic implants are used for fistula construction, hyperplasia of the intima and, consequently, stenoses at the site of the anastomosis are observed. In such cases the prosthetic graft was implanted after multiple failures with autogenous material; the restoration of function is therefore especially urgent. Thromboendarterectomy of the stenosed or occluded anastomosis and widening it by means of patch graft angioplasty may restore flow. In many cases, however, extensive patch graft angioplasty following endarterectomy is required [3]. As a safety precaution to prevent tearing of the vessels during thromboendarterectomy, stay sutures are placed at the corners of the incisions in the graft, the shunt artery, and the vein (see Fig. 25.24). Furthermore, it is beneficial to widen the arterial or venous anastomoses using a patch graft (see Fig. 25.25). If the restoration of the venous anastomosis fails, extension of the shunt and anastomosis to the vein further proximally is often possible (Fig. 25.26).

2. Aneurysms

Aneurysms are another relatively frequent complication of all arteriovenous fistulas. They develop in the anastomosis as well as at the site of cannulation [13].

When anastomotic aneurysms develop, they should be removed because they can be expected to grow, and they are often symptomatic. With this complication it is also advisable to resect the aneurysm and to create a new arteriovenous fistula proximally, utilizing the same vessels in order to preserve the old cannulation sites.

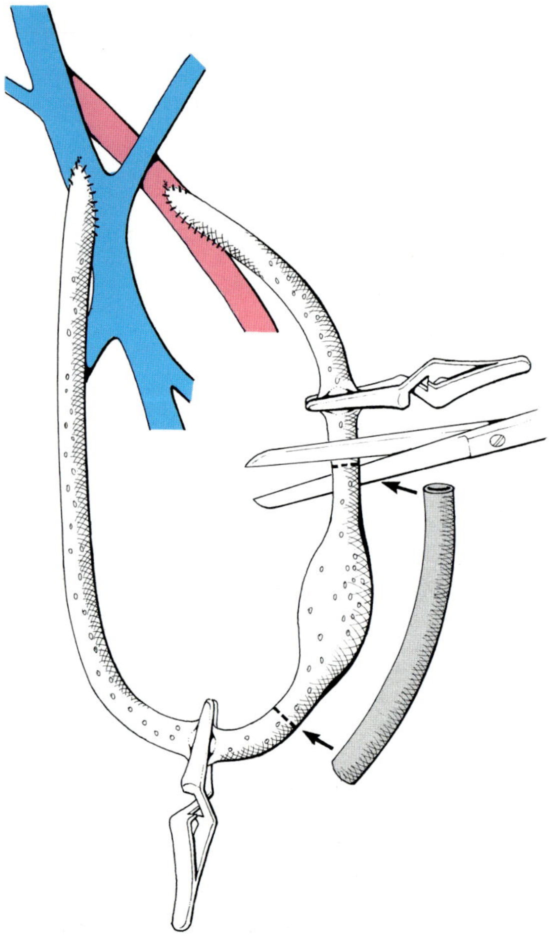

Fig. 25.27. Large aneurysms of a vascular graft may be restored by graft interposition

Aneurysms of subcutaneous arteriovenous fistulas involving autogenous veins, where the lesion is a result of multiple cannulations, constitute a special case. It is recommended that one wait, especially if there are other possible cannulation sites. However, it this is not the case, the aneurysm can be resected and the fistula preserved by interposing a vascular graft.

Aneurysms are observed especially often in fistulas utilizing synthetic grafts. In this case also, it is beneficial to resect the aneurysm and to interpose a new graft in order to preserve the old shunt (Fig. 25.27).

3. Infections

Infections of fistulas are often life threatening and should be treated immediately as the short circuit between the artery and the vein may bring the bacteria directly into the vascular bed of the lungs, causing sepsis.

a) Early Infections. When infections occur postoperatively in a subcutaneous arteriovenous fistula utilizing autogenous vessels (e.g., infected hematoma), one may in exceptional cases try to preserve the fistula if there are no symptoms of sepsis. When there are early postoperative infections following implantation of a prosthetic graft, the graft should be removed immediately and the old vascular bed restored [1, 2, 5].

b) Late Infections. Whether the fistula in question was constructed using autogenous vessels or prosthetic material, late infections are for the most part infections of suture canals. For fistulas that utilize autogenous vessels, it is recommended that one ligate the infected area and perform another anastomosis above the infection. However, it is also possible to resect the infected area and to perform an end-to-end anastomosis of the shunt vein. Afterwards, thorough drainage of the operative field is necessary.

It also makes sense to try to preserve infected fistulas constructed of synthetic material, especially if other methods of shunt creation present difficulties. However, an essential prerequisite is that only an isolated area is infected. The infected segment of the graft is then resected and the remaining graft ligated. When the operative field has healed, it is possible, after thrombectomy of the old prosthesis, to interpose a new prosthetic segment – or, if necessary, to bypass the area of infection. However, this procedure is recommended only when the conditions for a new shunt are extremely unfavorable (Fig. 25.28a, b).

4. Rare Complications

Rare complications are the so-called steal phenomenon, following construction of an arteriovenous fistula in the forearm [6] and cardiac overload with enlargement of the heart due to an excessively large shunt volume. In both complications, it is possible to narrow the fistula by means of incomplete ligation in order to reduce the shunt volume. In the case of a steal phenomenon with ischemic symptoms of the hand, it is also possible to interrupt the steal mechanism of peripheral fistulas by ligating the appropriate artery (usually the radial artery). Before this is attempted, though, it must be demonstrated that the other artery is functional.

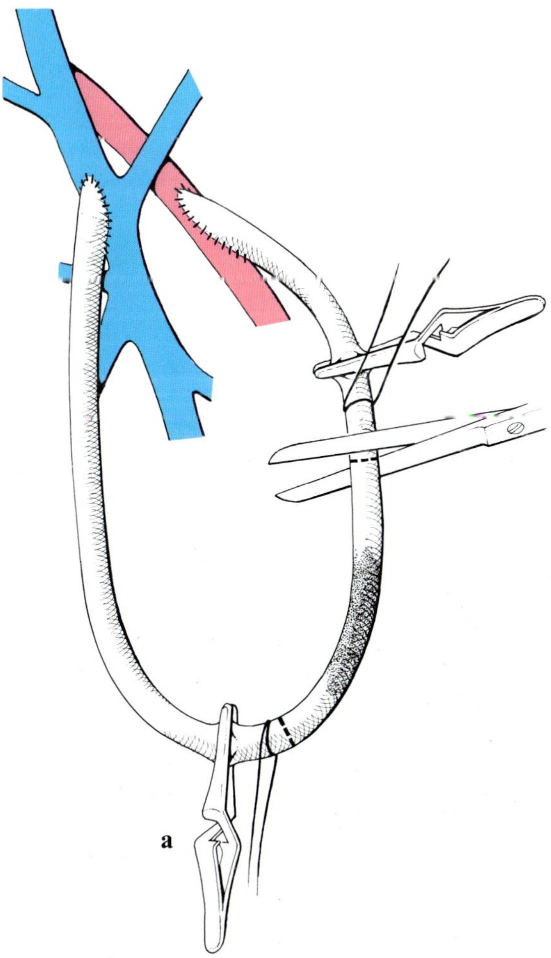

a

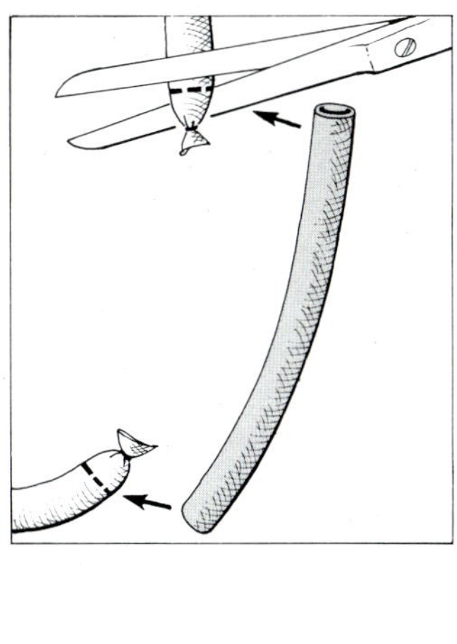

b

Fig. 25.28a, b. Old vascular graft with local infection (due to cannulation). **a** Excision of the infected graft segment. **b** Interposition of a new graft following healing of the infection, or bypassing the infected area, if necessary

REFERENCES

1. Appel GB (1978) Vascular access infections with long term haemodialysis. Arch Intern Med 138:1610
2. Bhat DJ, Tellis VA, Kohberg WI, Driscoll B, Veith FJ (1980) Management of sepsis involving expanded polytetrafluoroethylene grafts for haemodialysis access. Surgery 87:445
3. Bone GE, Pomajzl MJ (1980) Prospective comparison of polytetrafluorethylene and bovine grafts for hemodialysis. J Surg Res 29:223
4. Brescia MJ, Cimino JE, Appel K, Hurwich BJ (1966) Chronic hemodialysis using venepuncture and a surgically created arteriovenous fistula. N Engl J Med 275:1089
5. Buckels JAC, Ezzibdeh MY, Barnes AD (1983) The management of infected vascular access grafts. In: Kootstra G, Jörning PJG (eds) Access surgery. MTP Press, Lancaster Boston The Hague, pp 217–222
6. Bussel JA, Abbot JA, Lim RC (1971) A radial steal syndrome with arterio-venous fistula for hemodialysis. Ann Intern Med 75:387
7. Dagher FJ, Gelber RL, Ramos EJ, Sadler JH (1976) The use of basilic vein and brachial artery as an AV-fistula for long term hemodialysis. J Surg Res 20:373
8. Gerlach D, Lymberopoulos S (1975) Erfahrungen mit AV-Fisteln zur Langzeitdialyse unter besonderer Berücksichtigung der Ellenbeugenfisteln. Zit. in Horntrich J, Müller D (1980) Z Urol Nephrol 73:337
9. Haimov M, Burrous L, Baez A, Neff M, Slivkin R (1974) Alternatives for vascular access. Experience with autogenous vein autografts and bovine heterografts. Surgery 75:447
10. Harder F, Tondelli P, Haenel P (1977) Hämodialyse – die arteriovenöse Fistel distal des Handgelenks. Chirurg 48:719
11. Hollinger A, Largiadèr F (1973) Das freie Venentransplantat für die Langzeithämodialyse. Chirurg 44:274
12. Kalkowski H, Rinke W (1977) Die Anlage einer AV-Fistel zur Vorbereitung der Dialyse. Zentralbl Chir 102:24–31
13. Kemhes BM, Borchard F (1983) Complications and surgical treatment after angio access. In: Kootstra G, Jörning PJG (eds) Access surgery. MTP Press, Lancaster Boston The Hague, pp 203–210
14. May J, Tiller D, Johnson J, Stewart J, Sheil AGR (1969) Saphenous vein arteriovenous fistula in regular dialysis treatment. N Engl J Med 280:770
15. Moris C, Kinnaert P (1983) Arteriovenous fistula at the elbow for maintenance hemodialysis. In: Kootstra G, Jörning PJG (eds) Access surgery. MTP Press, Lancaster Boston The Hague, pp 25–29
16. Quinton WE, Dillard DH, Scribner BH (1960) Cannulation of blood vessels for prolonged hemodialysis. Trans Am Soc Artif Intern Organs 6:104
17. Ramirez O, Swartz C, Onesti G, Mailoux L, Brest AM (1966) The winged-in-line-shunt. Trans Am Soc Artif Intern Organs 12:220, 227
18. Zehle A, Schulz V, Hottmann J, Schmitt N, Pichlmaier H (1979) Arteriovenöse Gefäßverbindungen für die Langzeitdialyse. Chirurg 50:345

26 Further Arterial Procedures

26.1 Regional Chemotherapy

K. SCHWEMMLE and K. AIGNER

CONTENTS

A. Introduction

In advanced stages of cancer the operative procedure may remove the primary lesion, but may not significantly influence the further course of the disease. In such cases, additional chemotherapy is becoming increasingly important. Systemic therapy, however, has two restrictions: an unfavorable relation between the dose and the side effects and limited effectiveness against solid tumor masses. However, the therapeutic synergism of surgery for removal, or at least reduction of the tumor and systemic chemotherapy for certain types of tumors, e.g., osteosarcoma, has improved the therapeutic results.

Intra-arterial administration of cytostatic drugs for inoperable primary tumors or for localized metastases seems to be a rational procedure since the effectiveness of cytotoxic drugs also depends on their concentration at the site of reaction. In 1950, KLOPP reported for the first time on favorable results following infusion of nitrogen mustard into the artery supplying the tumor. With this method significantly higher local concentrations are achieved than with systemic treatment. Therefore, a greater toxic effect on the tumor (growth inhibition, tumor reduction, in some cases local tumor destruction) can be achieved without aggravation of the side effects.

B. Intra-arterial Infusion

I. Infusion Utilizing an Angiography Catheter

As a rule, the vascular supply of each body region can be reached by a catheter used for selective angiography. Once the catheter has been positioned under X-ray supervision, arterial infusion of the diseased organ with cytostatic drugs can begin. If the catheter is to be left in situ for several days, prophylactic measures are required in order to avoid thrombosis (heparin prophylaxis) and dislocation of the catheter tip (bed rest).

1. Approach from the Femoral Artery

Puncture of the femoral artery is performed with the patient in a supine position, under local anesthesia. The palpable artery is punctured below the inguinal ligament, the arteriography catheter is inserted using the Seldinger technique, and the tip of the catheter is placed as superselectively as possible into the artery supplying the tumor. It is advisable to push the catheter 2–3 cm forward into the appropriate artery in order to avoid later dislocation. If the major artery is short, one may be obliged to place the catheter in a segmental artery to avoid dislocation. The catheter should be fixed to the skin with a suture to prevent it slipping off.

Prophylaxis against thrombosis is urgently required (low dose prophylaxis with 5000 I.U. heparin t.i.d.). Furthermore, following each infusion of cytostatic drugs the catheter in the femoral artery is flushed with heparinized solution (1 ml heparin dissolved in 9 ml physiologic saline solution) before being closed. During a series of treatments, which may last 2–6 days, depending on the type of tumor, the patient must stay in bed to prevent dislocation of the catheter.

Local infection with the risk of septic thrombosis and bacteremia represents a severe complication, requiring removal of the catheter. However, because such difficulties are very rare, prophylaxis using antibiotics is, in our opinion, unnecessary. Of course, it is recommended in cases where, due to technical difficulties, the introduction of the catheter takes a long time, thereby increasing the risk of infection.

a) Hepatic Artery Infusion. The main indication for the infusion of cytostatic drugs into liver arteries are liver metastases of colorectal carcinoma, embryonic tumors, sarcomas, and also primary liver-cell carcinomas in cases where resection is impossible or must be supplemented by cytostatic treatment. Anatomic variants of the vascular supply occasionally impair selective regional chemotherapy. A relatively common anomaly is the gastroduodenal artery arising from the right hepatic artery (in 10%–15%). In such cases, only one lobe of the liver may be perfused by placing the tip of the catheter far into the left or right liver artery.

If the catheter were placed in the proper hepatic artery in such a situation, the gastroduodenal artery would also be perfused, resulting in general (nausea, vomiting) and local side effects (duodenal ulcers).

When angiography shows that the right liver lobe is supplied by the superior mesenteric artery, only one half of the liver can be perfused. In this case, either a second catheter must be inserted via the contralateral femoral artery or the treatment of the other liver lobe is postponed until a second session.

b) Stomach. The indication for intra-arterial infusion of the stomach is very rare and limited exclusively to cases of inoperable stomach cancer where it can be used in an attempt to inhibit tumor growth. In rare cases, reduction of the tumor can be achieved by regional chemotherapy, allowing later resection [15]. Because the gastric arteries are not end arteries suitable for isolated perfusion, the dose of the drug must be lower than for the liver. The tip of the catheter is placed selectively into the celiac axis [13], superselectively into the left gastric artery or into the gastroduodenal artery.

c) Extremities. Intra-arterial infusion is indicated mainly for melanomas and soft tissue sarcomas, either as adjuvant chemotherapy following prophylactic resection against recurrence or as palliative treatment for relief of severe symptoms caused by tumor invasion of vessels and nerves.

Technical approach: in the leg, puncture is always performed in the contralateral groin. The catheter is pushed beyond the aortic bifurcation into the diseased extremity. For treatment of upper extremity neoplasia, the catheter is introduced selectively into the axillary or brachial artery via the femoral artery or, even better, it is pushed into the artery predominantly supplying the tumor.

d) Internal Iliac Artery. For tumors in the small pelvis, especially invasive gynecologic tumors [9, 11], or for tumors originating from the rectosigmoid colon, a catheter is again inserted in the contralateral femoral artery and pushed beyond the aortic bifurcation into the internal iliac artery. The most important indication for this procedure is pain that is resistant to other therapies [5, 9].

e) Other Tumors. In cases of breast cancer, the indication for regional chemotherapy is given in advanced stage III with invasion of the thoracic wall and/or the skin. The catheter is either pushed through the brachial and the internal thoracic artery or through the superior epigastric artery [14, 15].

In the ENT region, access to tumors may be achieved by means of a catheter inserted directly into the external carotid artery or transfemorally. In many cases, however, it is advisable to expose the vessel surgically and cannulate it under vision [8].

2. Approach Through the Brachial Artery

The brachial artery can also be used for virtually all of the indications mentioned earlier, in particular for infusion of the liver artery [10]. The puncture is made on the inner side of the upper arm. While the approach to the selected organ artery may be shorter, it also has more curves, so that it may be difficult to push the catheter forward and to place it correctly. Moreover, with this approach complications occur more frequently – occasionally even cerebral embolism. In our own practice, we use the brachial artery only if we fail to position the catheter via the femoral route.

II. Operative Implantation of a Catheter

This is indicated when the intra-arterial infusion is expected to be repeated several times or to be performed over a longer period. The advantages of surgical placement under vision are the diminished risk of catheter dislocation and the possibility of mobilizing the patient very quickly. In cases of repeated therapeutic cycles, the treatment can sometimes be performed as an outpatient procedure. In principle, a catheter may be inserted operatively into any major artery. The most common sites of application are the liver arteries via the gastroduodenal arteries and the major peripheral arteries (iliac artery, femoral artery, axillary artery).

1. Approach Through the Gastroduodenal Artery

Following a median supraumbilical longitudinal laparotomy, extending from the xiphoid to the umbilicus, the liver artery is dissected within the hepatoduodenal ligament, usually located above the bile duct and well palpable. One must ascertain by palpation whether there is a separate right hepatic artery supplying the right lobe of the liver; in most cases, it originates from the superior mesenteric artery. The common hepatic artery is dissected free in the vicinity of the duodenum and the upper border of the head of pancreas; this also involves ligation and division of the smaller arteries and veins supplying the stomach and the duodenum. The gastroduodenal artery, which passes downward and to the left in the direction of the duodenum, is exposed, then ligated as close as possible to the duodenum, and finally closed at its takeoff from the hepatic artery by means of a crocodile clamp.

Close to the ligature, approximately 6–10 mm away from the liver artery, the gastroduodenal artery is incised transversely, and an Implantofix catheter (Braun, Melsungen) is inserted and pushed forward so that the tip of the catheter barely projects into the hepatic artery. The catheter is fixed in place by means of two ligatures of nonabsorbable suture material just behind the fixation ring (Fig. 26.1.1). The catheter should not be pushed too far into the liver artery, so as not to provoke thrombosis. However, it should not be placed too far peripherally either, owing to the risk of thrombosis in the stump of the gastroduodenal artery and a resulting loss of catheter function. The Implantofix catheter we use is equipped

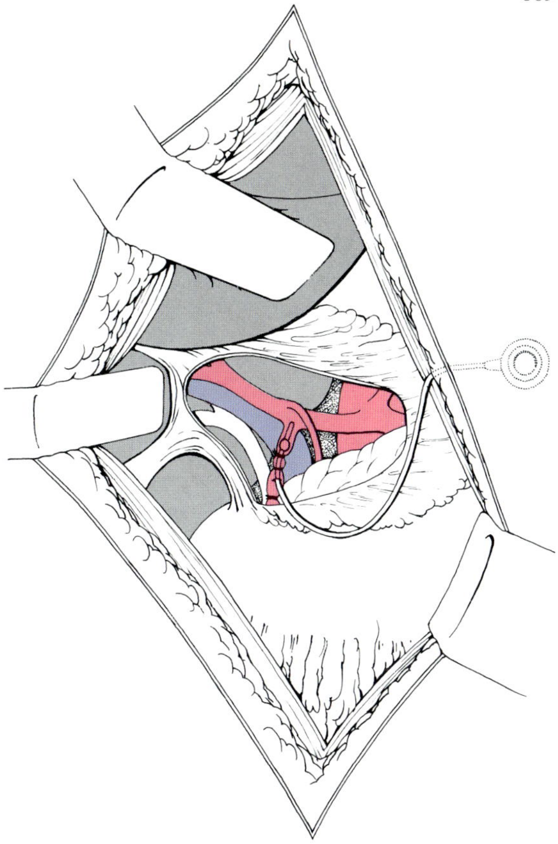

Fig. 26.1.1. Hepatic artery Implantofix catheter in situ. The gastroduodenal artery is ligated at the duodenum. The tip of the catheter projects 1–2 mm into the hepatic artery and is fixed with two ligatures of nonabsorbable suture material. The reservoir of the catheter is placed into a subcutaneous pocket beside the wound and may be fixed to the fascia by sutures

with a valve mechanism at the tip which prevents retrograde blood flow into the catheter and thereby acts as a safeguard against thrombosis. Catheters with an open end have to be flushed once a week with heparinized saline solution (5000 I.U. heparin in 9 ml saline solution) for prophylaxis against thrombosis. The injection device at the end of the catheter (a small reservoir equipped with a puncturable membrane) is placed in a subcutaneous pocket [4].

The same technical approach is recommended for implantation of an infusion pump (Infusaid, Fresenius, Bad Homburg). The catheter is not inserted directly into the hepatic artery, but through a branch, preferably the gastroduodenal artery. The pump itself may be placed in a subcutaneous pocket of sufficient size. In cachectic patients it may also be placed underneath the aponeurosis of the external abdominal muscle or in the rectus sheath.

2. Approach Through Peripheral Arteries

Implantation of an arterial catheter in peripheral arteries using the same technique may be considered when repeated cycles of local intra-arterial therapy are planned. Major indications are metastasizing malignant melanomas, soft tissue sarcomas, and osteosarcomas.

a) Femoral Artery. The femoral artery is exposed by a longitudinal incision perpendicular to the inguinal ligament. Vision may be improved by partial incision of the inguinal ligament. Approximately at the level where the femoral artery crosses under the inguinal ligament a branch of the artery is located, mobilized, and ligated peripherally. The tip of the Implantofix catheter is inserted into the vascular stump, as described for the gastroduodenal artery, and fixed by ligatures. The reservoir is placed either in the proximal and lateral region of the thigh or above the inguinal ligament in the subcutaneous tissue of the lateral lower abdomen.

b) Axillary Artery. The neurovascular bundle within the axilla is exposed through an incision along the anterior fold of the axilla or via a transverse incision below the axilla. The axillary artery is identified and sparingly mobilized. The subscapular artery is then dissected and ligated approximately 1 cm peripheral to the origin of the axillary artery and the Implantofix catheter is inserted through a transverse incision so that its tip just projects into the axillary artery. The catheter is fixed with two ligatures of nonabsorbable suture material and passed around the border of the pectoralis muscle. The injection device is placed infraclavicularly in a subcutaneous pocket in the sulcus deltoideopectoralis.

3. Regional Perfusion

The principle of regional or isolated perfusion consists of in situ isolation of a body region from the circulation by cannulation of afferent and efferent vessels and their connection to an extracorporeal circulation consisting of oxygenator, heat exchanger, and blood pump. Within this system, it is possible not only to adjust the temperature of the blood, and therefore also of the tissue, but also to administer cytostatic drugs. The dose depends on the maximal tissue tolerance without systemic side effects. A better toxic effect on the tumor may be expected as a result of the very high local temperature and the additional hyperthermia. Perfusion of the extremities was first described by CREECH and KREMENTZ in 1957 [7] and is most often used for the treatment of melanoma. Isolated perfusion of the liver is indicated in metastases of colorectal tumors, including carcinoid tumors, as well as in hepatocellular carcinoma, provided that there are no distant metastases.

a) Lower Extremity. The limb can be perfused either by an iliac, femoral, or a popliteal approach. We prefer an approach as high as possible in the iliac or the upper femoral region not only for primary perfusion, but also for repeated perfusions, in order to keep the perfused region as large as possible.

Iliac Perfusion. A pararectal incision is made starting approximately two fingerbreadths medial and cranial to the superior anterior iliac spine and extending over the femoral artery which is palpable below the inguinal ligament. Following division of the aponeurosis of the external oblique and the internal oblique muscles, of the fascia of the transversus abdominis muscle, and after medial retraction of the peritoneal sac, the external iliac vessels are exposed at the level of the origin of the internal iliac artery and vein. The fatty tissue containing the parailiac lymph nodes is resected for histologic staging, as is the lymphatic chain on the lateral wall of the pelvis, extending to the obturator foramen. Care must be taken not to injure the obturator nerve, which passes through the foramen. The obturator vein, passing below and somewhat lateral to the nerve, is closed with a clip to avoid later leakage between extracorporeal and body circulation. For the same reason, arterial and venous collateral vessels must be ligated and divided above the inguinal ligament. Vision is significantly improved by dividing the inguinal ligament.

After heparinization the usual surgical technique is as follows: first, the external iliac artery is cannulated through a transverse incision. Care must be taken to place the tip of the arterial catheter above the origin of the profunda femoris artery; otherwise, the vascular bed supplied by this artery will not be perfused. The external iliac vein is cannulated through a longitudinal incision. If vein valves impede the forward movement of the tube, this resistance can be overcome rather easily by using rotating movements. Prior to the initiation of extracorporeal circulation, the blood vessels within the soft tissue must be compressed by

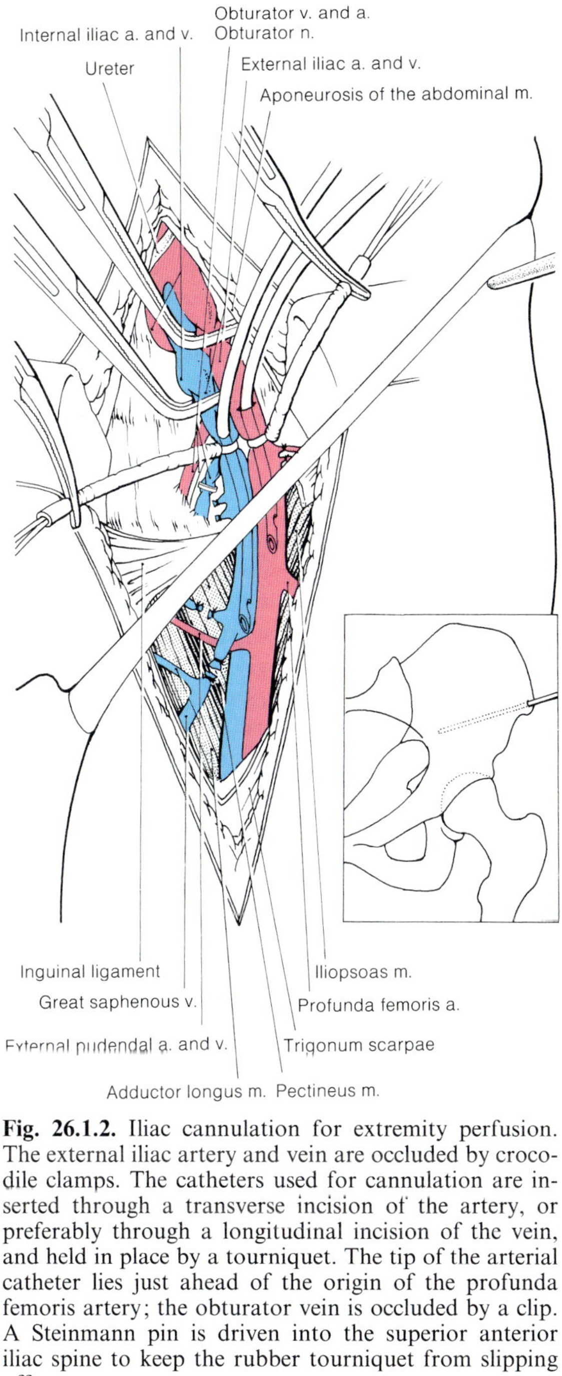

Fig. 26.1.2. Iliac cannulation for extremity perfusion. The external iliac artery and vein are occluded by crocodile clamps. The catheters used for cannulation are inserted through a transverse incision of the artery, or preferably through a longitudinal incision of the vein, and held in place by a tourniquet. The tip of the arterial catheter lies just ahead of the origin of the profunda femoris artery; the obturator vein is occluded by a clip. A Steinmann pin is driven into the superior anterior iliac spine to keep the rubber tourniquet from slipping off

a rubber band tourniquet held securely in place by means of a Steinmann pin driven into the iliac crest (Fig. 26.1.2). Heat loss is reduced by wrapping the extremity in metal foil or by placing it on a mattress perfused with warm water.

After the air is removed from the catheters, they are connected to the heart-lung machine and the perfusion begins, first at a blood temperature of 38° C, which is quickly increased to 41.5°–42° C, measured within the perfusion circulation. A tissue temperature of 40° C can be expected. This is continuously recorded by four needle probes in the thigh and lower leg. The probes are placed as follows:

1. In the proximal vastus lateralis muscle
2. In the lower portion of the vastus intermedius muscle, close to the knee joint and as close to the bone as possible
3. In the upper portion of the tibialis anterior muscle
4. Subcutaneously in the distal lower leg, as close to the tumor as possible if the primary tumor or the metastases are located in the lower third of the lower leg

Only when the desired tissue temperature is achieved are cytotoxic drugs added. The flow rates during limb perfusion are between 300 and 600 ml/min. The cytostatic drug most often used to date is melphalan (Alkeran). Currently, we are using a combination of melphalan and cisplatin (Platinex, Cis-Platin Medac) for malignant melanoma.

Following perfusion for 60 min the fluid is removed from the leg by disconnecting the venous catheter at the machine; the volume is replaced by 1 l Ringer's solution through the arterial side of the heart-lung machine. Afterwards, the arterial side of the limb is filled using packed erythrocytes and 250 ml plasma protein solution until the veins on the wrist seem to be well filled. Only then can the vein be decannulated and the vessel closed by continuous suture. Following the release of the physiologic venous blood flow the rest of the oxygenator blood may be added. Following decannulation, the artery is also closed using a continuous suture, and the operative wound is sutured layer by layer. In advanced tumor stages, the trigonum scarpae is dissected free. Prior to perfusion, dissection in the groin should be avoided at all costs; otherwise, an unnecessary blood loss from the operative field during perfusion can be expected (heparinization!).

Femoral Perfusion. For a second perfusion a femoral approach is recommended, as secondary iliac perfusion requires a significantly more difficult dissection with the risk of complications such as bleeding. The approach below the inguinal ligament, however, often allows only selective perfusion of the superficial femoral or the profunda femoris artery. Therefore, we recommend separate

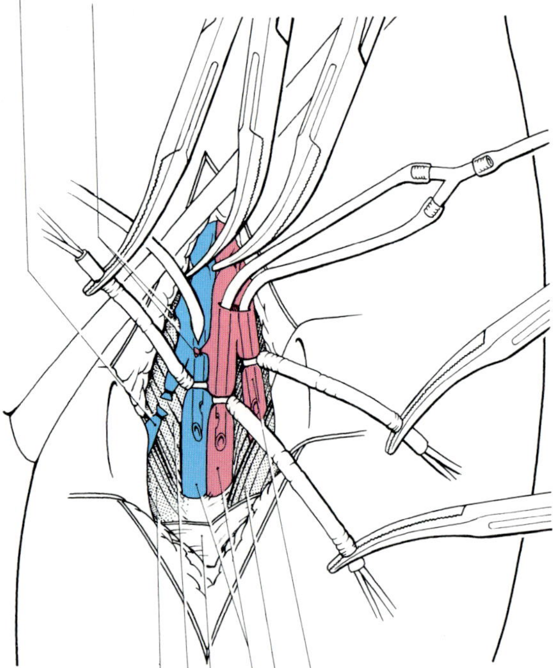

Fig. 26.1.3. Arterial double cannulation for multiple perfusions. Just proximal to the origin of the profunda femoris artery, both catheters are inserted through a transverse incision and fixed by tourniquets. The cannulation of the vein is performed at the level of the former junction with the great saphenous vein

cannulation (Fig. 26.1.3) of both arteries of the thigh [3].

This allows perfusion of the thigh and the lower leg. The skin incision originates 1–2 cm above the groin and extends distally 7–8 cm, excising the scar of the previous incision. The easily palpated femoral artery and the initial segment of the profunda femoris artery are exposed; the femoral vein, which passes medially, is also exposed. Rubber bands are placed around the femoral and the profunda femoris arteries below the bifurcation. Next, the femoral artery is occluded with a vascular clamp and incised transversely, approximately 1–1.5 cm proximal of the origin of the profunda femoris artery; through this arteriotomy a catheter is inserted into the profunda femoris artery and another into the superficial femoral artery. The tourniquet is then pulled tight. A fixation ring behind the tips of the catheters prevents the catheters from slipping off (Braun, Melsungen). Both catheters are connected to the oxygenator by a Y-adaptor. Afterward, the venous catheter is also inserted. Following heating of the leg to the desired temperature, perfusion with cytostatic drugs can begin.

b) Upper Extremity Perfusion. The patient is placed in a supine position with the arm abducted. The approach to the axilla is through a curved incision, starting at the border of the pectoralis muscle and continuing along the anterior fold of the axilla to the proximal upper arm. The procedure for perfusion of the arm contrasts with that used for the lower extremity. The fatty tissue, including the lymph nodes, is dissected as far as the axillary vein; the subscapular artery and vein are preserved. The nerves supplying the serratus anterior and the latissimus dorsi muscles must be exposed and preserved. Following careful separation of the fibers of the plexus, the axillary artery and the axillary vein are exposed and tapes are placed around them. The subscapular artery and vein are temporarily occluded by a suture loop. Cannulation of both axillary vessels may be performed following longitudinal division and separation of the fibers of the pectoralis major muscle, or as shown in Fig. 26.1.4, after the border of the muscle has been firmly drawn up with a hook. Sometimes, it may be difficult to push the venous catheter forward, owing to the numerous venous valves. However, one usually succeeds in overcoming such resistance by rotating the catheter while pushing it back and forth. Here, as in the case of the lower extremity, a Steinmann pin serves as support for a strong rubber tourniquet that interrupts blood flow to the vessels of the skin and muscles. The pin is driven into the head of the humerus from lateral to medial through the deltoid muscle, the tendon of the long head to the biceps muscle being under digital control during this step. Following connection to the heart-lung machine and after the desired tissue temperature of about 39.5°–40° C is achieved, perfusion with cytostatic drugs is carried out for 1 h, at a flow rate of 150–250 ml/min. Decannulation from the heart-lung machine is performed as described for leg perfusion: division of the venous catheters, flushing of the arm with 1 l physiologic saline solution, refilling with packed erythrocytesin solution, decannulation, and suture, first of the vein and then of the artery.

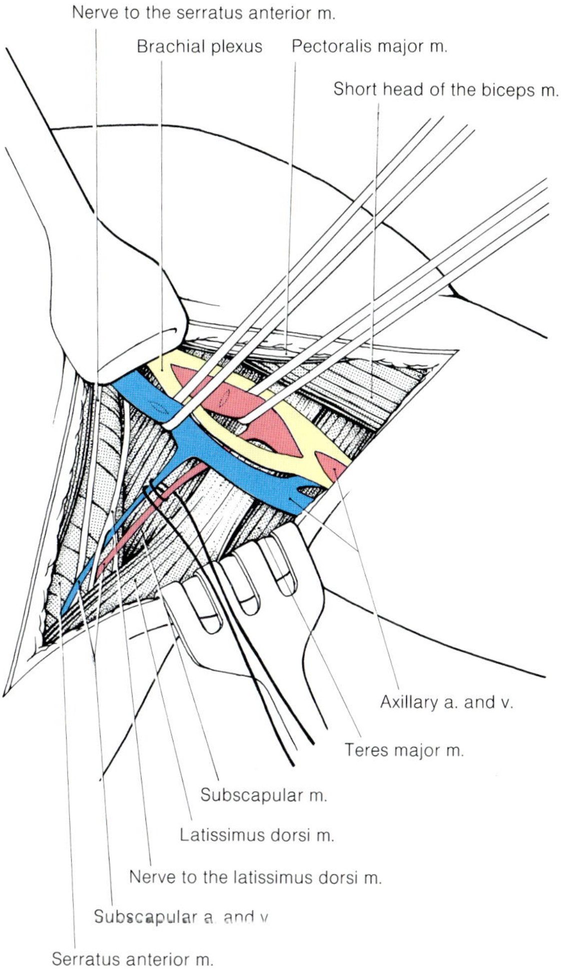

Fig. 26.1.4. Isolated perfusion of the upper extremity. The axilla is dissected. The subscapular artery and vein are temporarily ligated, and tapes are placed around the axillary artery and vein; the artery is exposed by retracting the bundles of the arm plexus

c) Isolated Regional Liver Perfusion. The liver is the first filter against the hematogenous spread of gastrointestinal carcinomas. The tumor cells infiltrate through the portal vein, but soon come into contact with the arterial system as they continue to grow [6]. Later, the metastases are supplied mainly by the artery. The application of cytotoxic drugs via the hepatic artery is therefore logical. Only at the margins of the tumor are there anastomoses between the arterial and the portal vein systems.

Regional liver perfusion is indicated for primary inoperable liver tumors and also for metastases where the primary tumor has been resected radically and no other metastases have been found. These latter conditions are limited almost entirely to colorectal cancer. In these cases, as with perfusion of the extremities, high concentrations of cytostatic drugs are combined with hyperthermia up to 40° C [1, 2, 12, 16].

Removing the venous blood from the liver is naturally more difficult than in the case of extremity perfusion. It is performed by means of a special catheter (Perfufix II, Braun, Melsungen) inserted into the inferior vena cava. The arterialized blood passes through the hepatic artery and the portal vein to the liver, two separate roller pumps being used to achieve approximately physiologic pressures (mean arterial pressure 110 mmHg, portal pressure 20 mmHg). The flow rate in the hepatic

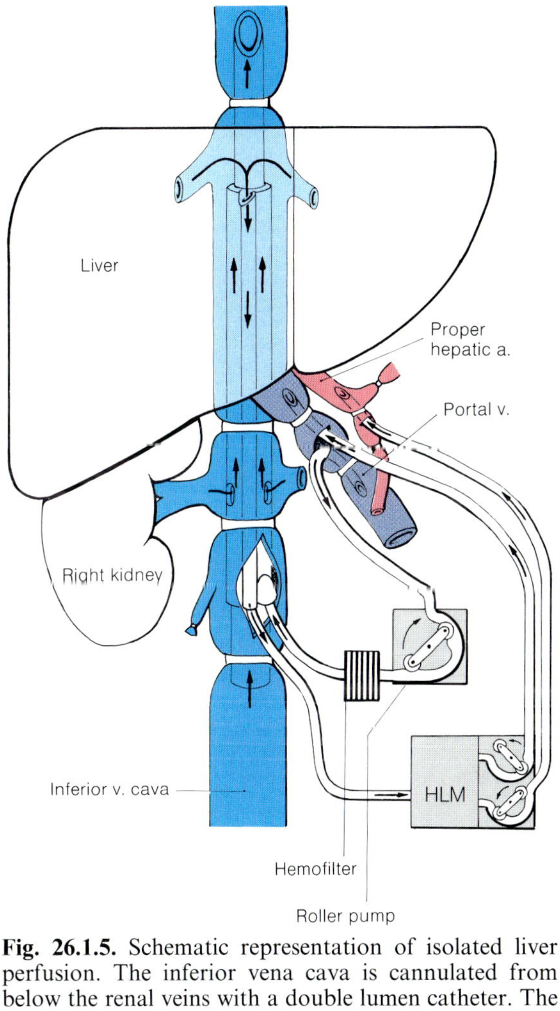

Fig. 26.1.5. Schematic representation of isolated liver perfusion. The inferior vena cava is cannulated from below the renal veins with a double lumen catheter. The venous blood of the liver is selectively removed and oxygenated by the heart-lung machine (*HLM*) and, after heating (42° C), is reperfused into the hepatic artery and the portal vein. Ammonia is removed through a hemofilter interposed in the portocaval shunt, and the blood is returned to the double lumen perfusion catheter

artery is about 300 ml/min, in the portal vein about 150 ml/min. During perfusion, i.e., during that phase of the operation when the liver is isolated from the body circulation, the portal vein blood coming from the gastrointestinal tract is bypassed through a portocaval shunt (Fig. 26.1.5). A hemofilter interposed in this circulation (Plastik für die Medizin, Sürth/Köln) reduces the ammonia concentration of the blood to normal values and probably also eliminates other toxic metabolic products. However, filtration may be omitted.

Dissection Within the Hepatoduodenal Ligament. For the operative approach, we prefer a median supra- and infraumbilical longitudinal laparatomy. An umbilical tape is placed around the hepatoduodenal ligament. The gastroduodenal artery is located superficially and exposed in the direction of the duodenum, and a tape is placed around it. Proceeding from the origin of the gastroduodenal artery, dissection continues along the common hepatic artery in the direction of the aorta and along the proper hepatic artery in the direction of the liver. A tape is placed around the common hepatic artery. On drawing it upward by the tape and retracting the bile duct caudally, access to the portal vein is achieved. The portal vein is exposed preferably over a length of 20 mm, but no less than 15 mm, between the duodenum and the hilus of the liver, and two tapes are placed around it (Fig. 26.1.6). Tributaries are ligated and divided.

Dissection of the Inferior Vena Cava. Following division of the falciform ligament, the liver is retracted caudally and the pars affixa sharply dissected off the diaphragm until the anterior circumference of the vena cava is exposed. Some 2 cm lateral to the vena cava a transverse incision about 5 cm long is made in the centrum tendineum of the diaphragm and in the adjacent pericardium.

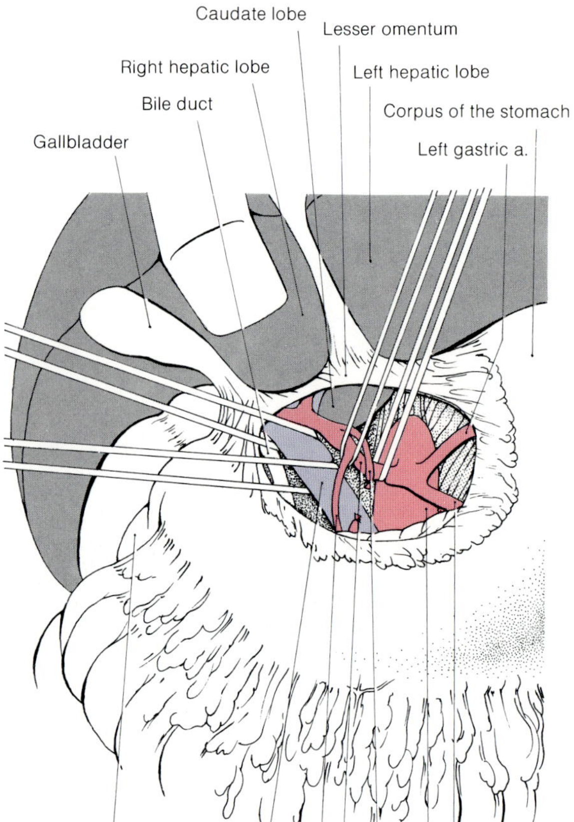

Fig. 26.1.6. Vessels at the hilus of the liver with tapes placed around them. The right gastric artery is divided and tapes are placed around the hepatic and gastroduodenal arteries. Double tapes are placed around the portal vein

Fig. 26.1.7. Placement of a tape around the inferior vena ▷ cava within the pericardium. The liver is mobilized at the pars affixa, and the diaphragm as well as the pericardium are incised transversely, just above the point of passage of the inferior vena cava. A tourniquet is placed around the vena cava intrapericardially

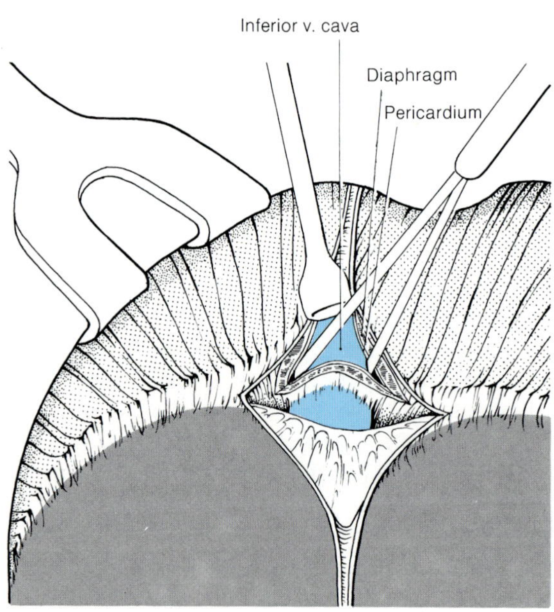

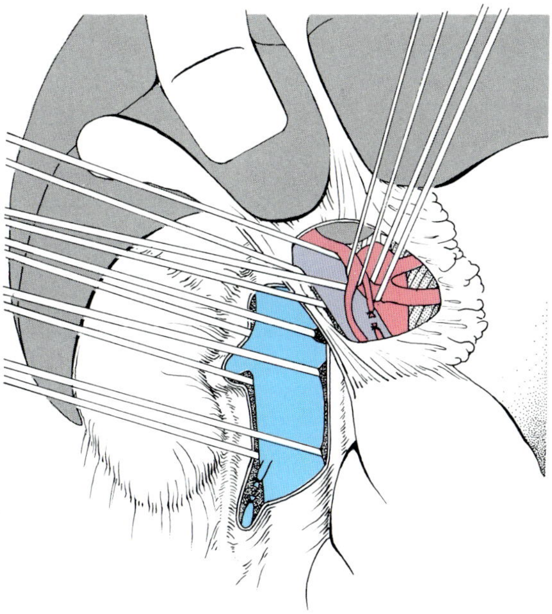

Fig. 26.1.8. Placement of tapes around the inferior vena cava. The spermatic or the ovarian vein is divided and ligated. One tape is placed around the inferior vena cava above the renal veins, and two tapes below

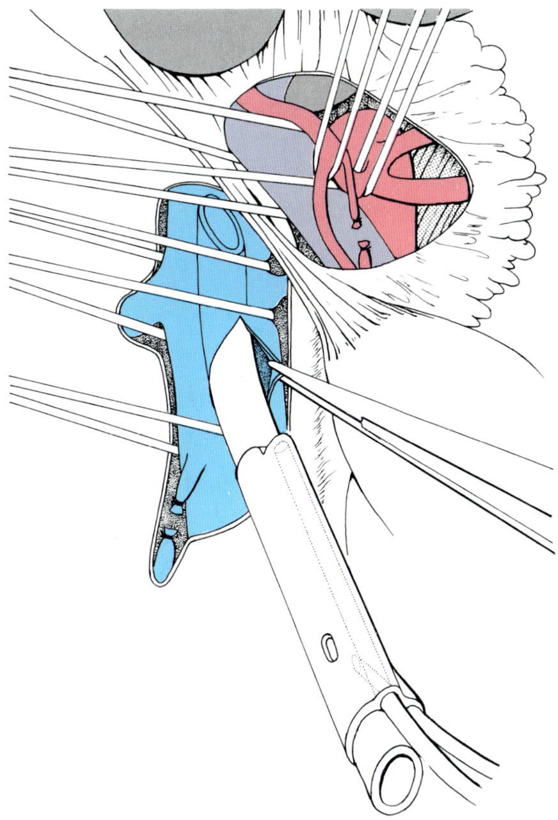

Fig. 26.1.9. Insertion of the perfusion catheter into the ▷ inferior vena cava. The inferior vena cava is incised longitudinally between the two lower tourniquets. The tip of the perfusion catheter lies above the renal veins. Lumbar veins must never be left open. One must be able to inspect this segment of the vena cava in its entire circumference

Within the pericardium, a strong clamp is carefully passed around the inferior vena cava just distal to where it joins the right atrium, and an umbilical tape is placed around it (Fig. 26.1.7). Slight, sometimes pulsating bleeding at the incision of the diaphragm must be stopped carefully.

Access to the infrahepatic segment of the inferior vena cava is achieved through extensive mobilization of the duodenum according to KOCHER. The vena cava is dissected free over a length of 8–10 cm, including the junction of the renal veins; during this step several lumbar veins must be ligated and divided. The right spermatic or ovarian vein is also divided at the respective junction below the right renal vein. Three tourniquets are then placed around the mobilized inferior vena cava, one above and two below the junction with the renal veins (Fig. 26.1.8).

Cannulation of the Inferior Vena Cava. Following systemic heparinization (200 I.U. heparin per kilogram body weight) the inferior vena cava is incised longitudinally. The incision begins 1 cm distal to the right renal vein and extends over 3 cm. The perfusion catheter, closed by an internal rubber trocar, is inserted through this incision (Fig. 26.1.9). Once the two lateral openings receiving renal venous blood are situated cranial to the middle tourniquet, this tourniquet is fixed, the trocar is pulled out of the catheter, and the end of the catheter immediately clamped. The end is then completely immersed in the inferior vena cava. Before the lowest of the three tourniquets – positioned below the venotomy – is tightened, the catheter is pushed downward somewhat. When both of the two lower tourniquets have been properly tightened, the clamp can be removed, thereby releasing the blood flow through the catheter. The two catheters leading off toward the side, one of them to be connected to the heart-lung machine and the other to the portocaval shunt, remain closed at this time. The next step is to tighten the upper infrahepatic tourniquet so that the renal venous blood will pass through the lateral openings of the perfusion catheter to reach the right atrium.

Arterial Cannulation and Connection to the Extracorporeal Circulation. First, the portal vein is incised transversely between two crocodile clamps. A catheter is inserted toward the liver (arterial line) and another in the opposite direction (for the portocaval shunt); both are then fixed in place by tightening previously positioned rubber bands. The portocaval shunt becomes functional when the portal vein catheter, remote from the liver, is connected via the hemofilter to the appropriate side tube of the perfusion catheter. A roller pump provides sufficient flow (600 ml/min). The filtered fluid is replaced completely with Ringer's solution.

Next, the central portovenous catheter and the venous retrograde flow tube from the perfusion catheter are connected to the heart-lung machine. By tightening the intrapericardial tourniquet, the normal retrograde flow of venous blood from the liver is interrupted. Simultaneously, the hepatic artery is occluded with a bulldog clamp. The liver can then be perfused, at first only through the portal vein as a partial bypass. The gastroduodenal artery is ligated peripherally and incised transversely approximately 1 cm from its origin. Through the arteriotomy, a special catheter (Braun, Melsungen) is inserted and pushed forward into the proper hepatic artery (Fig. 26.1.10). This arterial catheter is also connected to the extracorporeal circulation. The total bypass then begins, with the portal vein and the liver artery being supplied by separate roller pumps so as to achieve physiologic flow rates and pressures (Fig. 26.1.5). After ca. 10 min, when a tissue temperature of 39°–39.5° C has been achieved in the liver, the cytostatic drug is administered through the liver artery catheter. To date, we have used mainly mitomycin C and 5-fluorouracil (Fluoroblastin Farmitalia, 5-FU Roche).

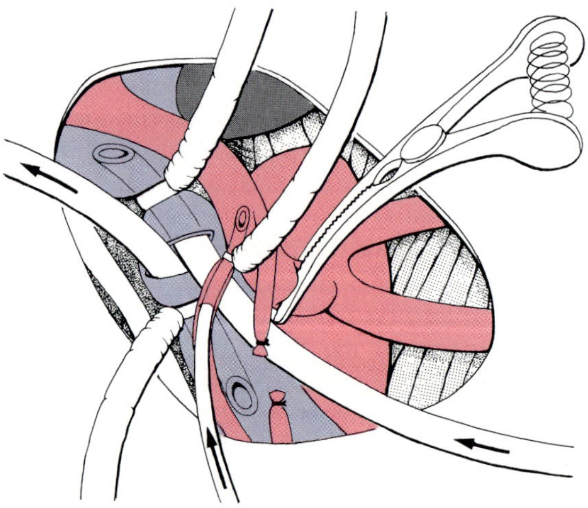

Fig. 26.1.10. Cannulated vessels at the hilus of the liver. The portal vein is incised transversely and cannulated proximally (arterial line) and distally (portocaval shunt), and the tubes are fixed by tourniquets. A bulldog clamp is placed on the common hepatic artery, and the vessel is cannulated through the gastroduodenal artery. The catheter is also fixed by means of a tourniquet. The direction of blood flow within the tubes is indicated by *arrows*

Decannulation. As with isolated perfusion of the extremities, the venous catheter is cut after 1 h of perfusion, the perfusate is then drained and the liver flushed with 1 l Ringer's solution. After the intrapericardial tourniquet has been loosened, the organ is refilled with packed erythrocytes and 250 ml plasma solution. Further decannulation proceeds stepwise as follows:

1. Removal of both tubes from the portal vein and closure of the portal vein using a continuous suture
2. Removal of the hepatic artery catheter from the gastroduodenal artery and temporary occlusion of this vessel with a bulldog clamp
3. Removal of the perfusion catheter from the inferior vena cava and continuous suture of the venotomy

Finally, the Implantofix catheter is inserted into the gastroduodenal artery according to the technique described in Sect. B.II.1. in order to continue intra-arterial infusion. Following placement of soft silicone drains beneath the liver and in the pericardium, the laparotomy is closed layer by layer, leaving the incision of the diaphragm and the pericardium open.

REFERENCES

1. Aigner KR, Walther H, Tonn JC, Krahl M, Wenzl A, Merker G, Schwemmle K (1982) Die isolierte Leberfusion mit 5-Fluorouracil (5-FU) beim Menschen. Chirurg 53:571
2. Aigner KR, Walther H, Tonn JC, Link KH, Schoch P, Schwemmle K (1984) Die isolierte Leberperfusion bei fortgeschrittenen Metastasen kolorektaler Karzinome. Onkologie 7:13
3. Aigner KR, Schwemmle K (1983) Technik der isolierten Extremitätenperfusion. Erfahrungen an 171 Fällen. Langenbecks Arch Chir 359:113
4. Aigner KR, Link KH, Schwemmle K (1984) Die intermittierende arterielle Kurzinfusion zur lokalen Chemotherapie von Tumoren und Metastasen der Leber. Chirurg 55:494

5. Beyer JH, Heyden HW von, Bartsch HH, Klee M, Nagel GA, Schuster R, Romatowski HJ von (1983) Intra-arterial perfusion therapy with 5-fluorouracil in patients with metastatic colorectal carcinoma. In: Schwemmle K, Aigner KR (eds) Vascular perfusion in cancer therapy. Springer, Berlin Heidelberg New York, (Recent results in cancer research, vol 86, p 33)
6. Breedis C, Young G (1953) The blood supply of neoplasms in the liver. Am J Pathol 30:969
7. Creech O, Krementz ET, Ryan RF, Winblad JN (1958) Chemotherapy of cancer: regional perfusion utilizing an extracorporeal circuit. Ann Surg 148:616–632
7a. Klopp CT, Alford TC, Bateman J, Berry GN, Winship T (1950) Fractionated intra-arterial cancer chemotherapy with methyl bis-amine hydrochloride; a preliminary report. Ann Surg 132:811–832
8. Kreidler JF, Petzel JR (1983) Combined treatment of maxillofacial carcinoma by intra-arterial proliferation block and irradiation. In: Schwemmle K, Aigner KR (eds) Vascular perfusion in cancer therapy. Springer, Berlin Heidelberg New York, (Recent results in cancer research, vol 86, p 152)
9. Lathrop JC, Frates RE (1983) The use of nitrogen mustard in the treatment of intractable pelvic pain. In: Schwemmle K, Aigner KR (eds) Vascular perfusion in cancer therapy. Springer, Berlin Heidelberg New York, (Recent results in cancer research, vol 86, p 26)
10. Oberfield RA (1983) Prolonged and continous percutaneous intra-arterial hepatic infusion chemotherapy in advanced metastatic liver adenocarcinoma from colorectal primary. In: Schwemmle K, Aigner KR (eds) Vascular perfusion in cancer therapy. Springer, Berlin Heidelberg New York, (Recent results in cancer research, vol 86, p 49)
11. Oberfield RA (1983) Intra-arterial infusion in tumors of the pelvis. In: Schwemmle K, Aigner KR (eds) Vascular perfusion in cancer therapy. Springer, Berlin Heidelberg New York, (Recent results in cancer research, vol 86, p 15)
12. Schwemmle K, Aigner KR (1984) Die Extremitätenperfusion bei malignen Melanomen und Sarkomen. Med Klin 79:53
13. Stephens FO, Harker GJS, Dickinson RTJ, Roberts BA (1979) Preoperative basal chemotherapy in the management of cancer of the stomach: a preliminary report. Aus NZ J Surg 49:331
14. Stephens FO, Crea P, Harker GJS, Roberts BA, Hambly CK (1980) Intra-arterial chemotherapy as basal treatment in advanced and fungating primary breast cancer. Lancet 2:435
15. Stephens FO (1983) Clinical experience in the use of intra-arterial infusion chemotherapy in the treatment of cancers in the head and neck, the extremities, the breast and the stomach. In: Schwemmle K, Aigner KR (eds) Vascular perfusion in cancer therapy. Springer, Berlin Heidelberg New York, (Recent results in cancer research, vol 86, p 122)
16. Vaupel PW, Otte J, Manz R (1982) Oxygenation of malignant tumors after localized microwave hyperthermia. Radiat Environ Biophys 20:289

26.2 Reconstructive Procedures in Tumor Surgery

H. HAMANN and E.-U. VOSS

CONTENTS

A. Pathomorphology

I. Extravasal Tumors (Benign Tumors, Carcinoma, Sarcoma)

Larger arteries and veins are usually resistant to tumor growth over a long period of time. Even malignant tumors exhibiting rapid expansive and infiltrating growth do not infiltrate the vessel wall in the majority of cases.

It is primarily the veins that are affected by *enveloping* or *invasive tumors*, e.g., the superior vena cava in cases of mediastinal tumors, or the inferior vena cava or its branches in cases of renal or genital tumors (see below).

Even in vessels completely surrounded by a tumor, invasion of the vascular lumen with the risk of life-threatening *bleeding* or *tumor embolism* is relatively rare. More often, adjacent veins are completely compressed by the tumor.

By contrast, an *arterial* wall usually undergoes only a more or less pronounced stenosis, thanks to the higher internal pressure. The stenosis may often be removed by annular dissection of the tumor. Frequently, vascular lesions may be encountered. Radical resection is only seldom achieved [2].

Operative therapy in cases of *carotid body tumor* is of special surgical significance [17, 30, 31].

Embryologically, the normal carotid body, located in the adventitia of the carotid bifurcation, is a chemoreceptor (stimulation by pH, pCO_2, and pO_2), having the form of a 2×3 mm lentiform nodule. *Enlargement* of this nodule up to a diameter of 1 cm is often found in people living at altitudes greater than 4000 m above sea level (Andes, Tibet); the condition is also referred to as *chemodectoma*. A benignly or malignantly growing carotid body contains proven neurotransmitters in up to 10% of cases, but is not *endocrine active* itself. Therefore, the condition is more correctly referred to as a *paraganglioma* of the carotid body, or, to use the clinical term, a carotid body tumor [16, 26, 31]. The vascular supply of the normal carotid body arises from the vasa vasorum in the immediate region of the carotid bifurcation. In cases where the carotid body has undergone tumorous enlargement, branches from the external carotid artery are usually found.

1. Classification

Based on clinical observations, *three types* of tumors are distinguished (Fig. 26.2.1). This classification is especially helpful with respect to the operative approach. Since the tumor is benign in about 90% of cases, the maintenance of continuity following resection is also justified with types II and III. Microscopic examination of tumor tissues reveals the predominant tendency of the tumor to imitate the normal structures of the carotid body, producing both chief cells and sustentacular cells [1]. They may vary from a type that is rich in vessels and similar to an angioma, to an adenoma-like type. According to the predominant feature *three major types* are distinguished: *paraganglion-*

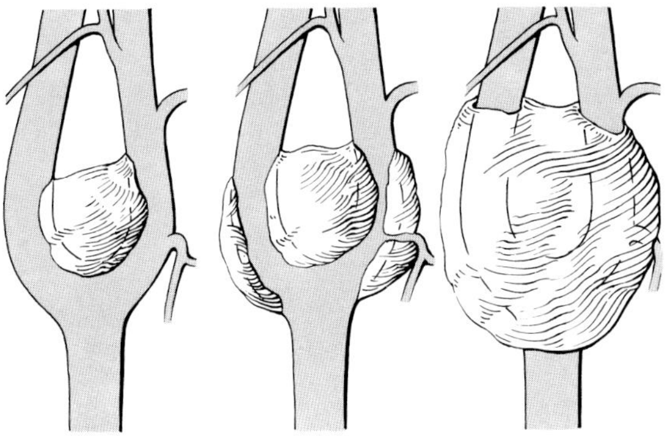

Fig. 26.2.1. Clinical classification of carotid body tumors (according to F. LINDER) [17]

ic, *angiomatous*, and *adenomatous*. This morphological classification, however, is only of minor clinical significance as no conclusions concerning the malignancy may be drawn from it. With respect to *carcinomatosis*, one must distinguish between locally infiltrating growth and the certain proof of actual carcinomatosis with metastases in local lymph nodes or, in rare cases, with distant metastases (in the lung and the bones).

2. Diagnosis

The differential diagnosis of lateral neck tumors deserves special mention, owing to the fact that 80% of carotid body tumors are only partially resected, that is to say, the preoperative diagnosis is correct in only a few cases. Usually the diagnosis is either *lateral cervical cyst* or *lymphoma*.

Carotid body tumors are mostly asymptomatic until the tumor diameter reaches 3 cm. After several years, a hard, indolent mass develops, recognizable by a lateral protrusion on the neck. Larger tumors may cause *symptoms* in *adjacent structures* with lesions of the hypoglossus nerve and also of the vagus or recurrent nerve. Irritations of the adjacent sinus nerve with bradycardia and syncope are also observed.

In case of clinical suspicion (signs of mobility, pulsation, localization; [31]), *arteriography* is indicated, which usually reveals a *typical separation of the carotid body* and also of the tumor itself in the late phase. Computed tomography may be of help in judging the operability of larger tumors [10].

II. Vascular Tumors

Benign or malignant tumors *originating from the vessel wall itself* are extremely rare.

These may include *leiomyomas*, *leiomyosarcomas*, *fibrosarcomas*, *hemangioendotheliomas*, and *hemangiopericytomas* of the vena cava and its branches, the portal vein, the aorta, and also the iliac and leg arteries [3, 4, 7, 8, 14, 15, 18, 19, 22, 24, 25].

Occasionally, in cases of untreated primary tumors, *intra-arterial tumor emboli* may require surgical intervention.

B. Operative Indications

In *malignant* tumors (carcinomas and sarcomas), the indication for an *extended tumor operation* with resection of larger arteries in continuity is relatively *rare*: the tumor already involving adjacent vessels are mostly inoperable for other reasons (distant metastases, invasion of other adjacent structures). Therefore, the indication for vascular resection in tumor surgery is subject to strict criteria [23].

Also for malignant *vascular tumors* (leiomyosarcoma, fibrosarcoma) vascular resection with graft interposition is usually too late.

An *operative indication*, however, is given in cases of:

1. *Benign* and semimalignant tumors – elective, curative surgery
2. *Malignant* tumors in cases of *vascular complications* (bleeding, tumor embolism) – emergency, palliative procedure

C. Techniques of Reconstruction

I. Neck

1. Combined Resection of the Carotid Artery in Neoplastic or Inflammatory Disease

Sometimes, radical surgery for tuberculous lymphomas of the neck and for pharyngeal and laryngeal carcinomas is impossible without a carotid artery resection, with preservation of continuity [5, 20].

Operative Technique. While the external carotid artery may usually be ligated without sequelae, *re-*

construction of the *internal carotid artery* should always be attempted. In many cases the blood supply to the brain can be restored by *vein graft* interposition. It is advisable to use an intraluminal shunt to keep the interruption of the blood flow as brief as possible (see p. 471).

2. Carotid Body Tumor

The *operative treatment* of carotid body tumors requires knowledge of vascular surgery because of the carotid body's close contact with the carotid bifurcation; in one third of cases, reconstructive measures of the internal carotid artery become necessary (direct suture, patch graft angioplasty, transposition).

Operative Technique. The *aim* of surgical therapy is radical removal of the tumor, preserving or restoring the vascular system of the internal carotid artery [28, 29]. With the operative technique described below, i.e., a *dissection method* consisting of three steps, a reconstructive procedure is not necessary in over 60% of cases (Fig. 26.2.2a).

The first step consists of common carotid artery *exposure* (central vascular control).

In the second step, the initial segment of the external carotid artery is exposed. When the artery is completely surrounded by the tumor (type III), the tumor must be divided down to the arterial wall (Fig. 26.2.2b). Ligation and division of the external carotid artery at its origin almost completely interrupts the blood supply to the tumor (Fig. 26.2.2c). In the case of smaller tumors, the external carotid artery may be divided between ligatures distal to the tumor.

The third step consists of *dissecting the tumor* off the carotid bifurcation and sharply dissecting the internal carotid artery within the adventitial layer (Fig. 26.2.2d). There, the tumor is grasped with a clamp in the region of the external carotid artery stump and pulled ventrally. This maneuver provides exposure of the border of the internal carotid artery. If the internal carotid artery is completely encircled by the tumor, the tumor must be divided down to the vascular wall. The tumor, including the interrupted segment of the external carotid artery, is mobilized by this approach in the direction of the base of the skull and dissected free, step by step, preserving the continuity of the internal carotid artery. Only in case of injury to the internal carotid artery is interruption of the blood flow with clamps required. If the leak cannot be closed by *direct suture*, an appropriate reconstruction must be performed by *patch graft*, *graft interposition*, or *transposition* of the internal carotid artery to the stump of the external carotid artery (see p. 268; Fig. 26.2.3).

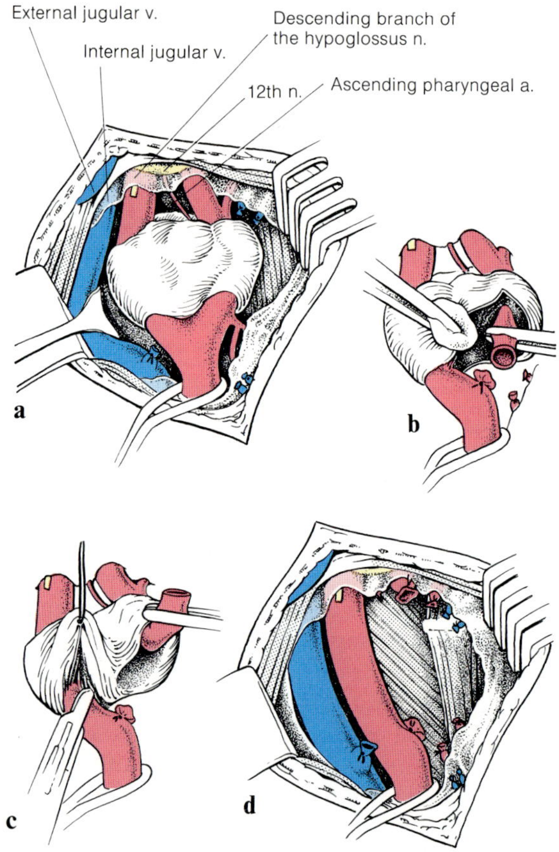

Fig. 26.2.2a–d. Operative technique. **a** Exposure of the common carotid artery. **b** Isolation, ligation, and division of the external carotid artery at its origin. **c** Ventral and cranial mobilization of the tumor to expose the carotid bifurcation and the internal carotid artery, dissection of the tumor in the wall of the internal carotid artery. **d** Complete removal of the tumor, preserving the continuity of the internal carotid artery

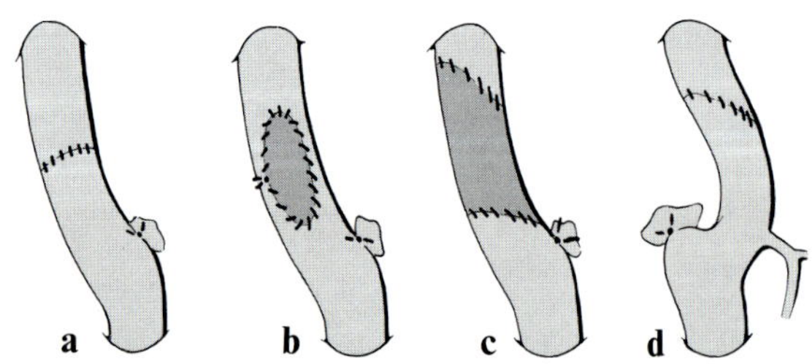

Fig. 26.2.3a–d. Possible reconstructions. **a** Direct suture. **b** Patch graft angioplasty. **c** Interposition. **d** Transposition with end-to-end anastomosis of the internal carotid artery to the external carotid artery

II. Thorax

1. Leiomyoma or Leiomyosarcoma

Leiomyoma or leiomyosarcoma are the most common vascular tumors of the superior vena cava. Congested upper veins, dyspnea, coughing, pain, and hoarseness are the most common clinical symptoms. Venography and computed tomography are absolutely necessary for the planning of the operation.

The *exploration* of the tumor is performed through either a *right-sided posterolateral thoracotomy* or a *median sternotomy*.

The operative method of choice for benign tumors is local *tumor excision* with *tangential suture*.

Malignant tumors are usually *inoperable* (infiltration of the pericardium, pleura, lung, etc.; distant metastases). However, radical tumor excision with *sacrifice* of *the superior vena cava* and subsequent *vascular transplantation* may be possible [7, 9].

Large caliber grafts with reinforced outer walls (e.g., ring-enforced PTFE prostheses) to avoid collapse of the vessel in the venous low pressure system (Fig. 26.2.4) are suitable for replacement of the vein.

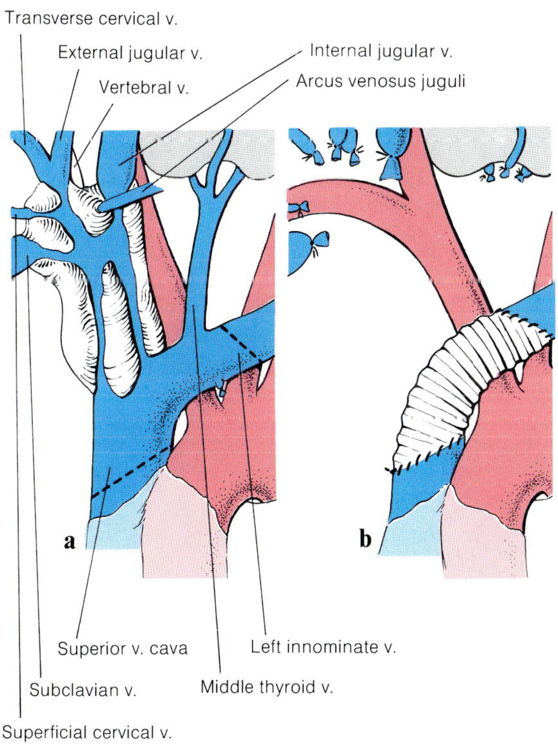

Fig. 26.2.4a, b. Leiomyosarcoma of the superior vena cava. **a** Radical tumor excision, including the superior vena cava. **b** Restoration of continuity by interposition of the ring-reinforced expanded PTFE prosthesis

2. Malignant Vascular Tumors of the Thoracic Aorta

These are extremely rare [14, 24] and are usually inoperable by the time they are diagnosed. *Only cases of polyploid type* of *primary fibrosarcoma* of the aorta have been reported in the world literature as being successfully operated on [14]: The operative excision of the tumor is performed following aortotomy by shelling out the intraluminally growing tumor.

3. Hemangiopericytoma of the Thoracic Aorta

Hemangiopericytoma (facultatively malignant) of the thoracic aorta can usually be dissected off the vascular adventitia and the surrounding tissue without injuring the vessel [3, 8].

III. Abdomen and Retroperitoneum

1. Intestinal Tumors

Intestinal tumors, operable only by resection of larger vessels, have a poor prognosis. This is shown, for instance, by the results of 840 pelvic exenterations, in 55 of which the iliac vessels (artery, vein, or both) had also been resected. The 5-year survival is only 20%. Among those patients who had undergone an extended tumor operation including the major iliac vessels, only four survived for 5 years (11%; [2]).

The 5-year survival rate is only 20%. Among those patients who had undergone an extended tumor operation including the major iliac vessels, only four survived for 5 years (11%) [2].

In the case reported by Moore in 1958, the recurrent tumor of a sigmoid carcinoma was radically excised in two sessions, including the left ureter, the left kidney, and the aortic bifurcation. Some $5^1/_2$ years postoperatively, the patient was still healthy and free of recurrence [21].

In 1968 Yoshida et al. [33] reported on a patient with a *duodenal reticulosarcoma* encircling the *superior mesenteric artery* which was curatively resected by duodenal and small bowel resection, left-sided nephrectomy, and division of the superior mesenteric artery. Restoration of continuity of the superior mesenteric artery was achieved by interposition of a vein graft (greater saphenous vein) from the central stump of the visceral artery to the ipsilateral internal iliac artery.

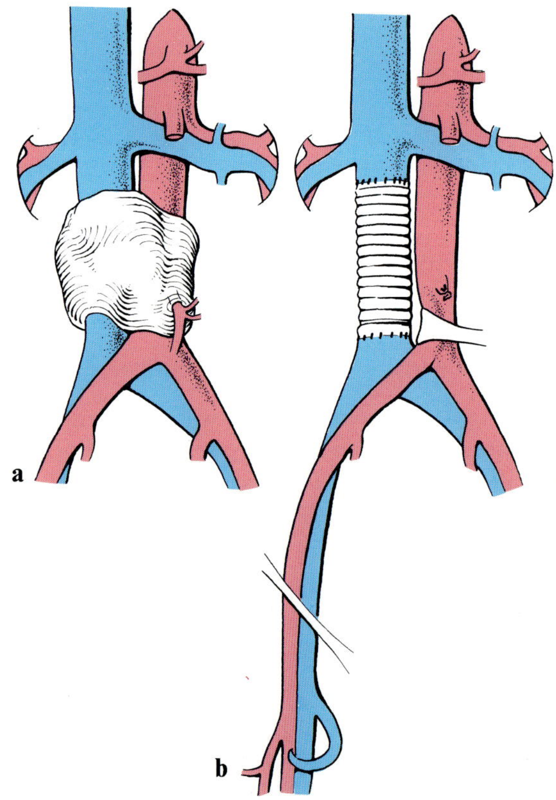

Fig. 26.2.5a, b. Retroperitoneal ganglioneuroma encircling the inferior vena cava and the infrarenal aorta. **a** Exposure of the tumor following medial supra- and infraumbilical laparotomy: dissecting the tumor off the aorta, stepwise mobilization, sacrificing the lumbar arteries and veins branching off dorsally, en bloc resection and resection in continuity of the inferior vena cava. **b** Replacing the vein defect by interposition of a ring-reinforced expanded PTFE prosthesis, construction of an arteriovenous fistula in the groin (see p. 462)

Fig. 26.2.6a–c. Hypernephroma plug in the inferior vena ▷ cava in a case of left-sided hypernephroma. **a** Median supra- and infraumbilical laparotomy, exposure of the inferior vena cava, the right and left renal vein, and the left kidney, central ligation of the renal vein, including the tumor plug. **b** Digital subdiaphragmatic occlusion of the inferior vena cava and inspiratory standstill (PEEP = positive end-expiratory pressure) the patient being placed in an anti-Trendelenburg position, incision of the inferior vena cava at the level of the junction of the left renal vein and resection of the intracaval tumor plug by digitally pushing it caudad. **c** Following closure of the inferior vena cava by continuous suture, tumor nephrectomy is performed in the usual fashion, with resection of the fatty capsule, the adrenal, and the regional lymph nodes

2. Primary Benign Retroperitoneal Tumors

Primary benign retroperitoneal tumors (e.g., *ganglioneuromas*) encircling the vena cava and the aorta are an indication for extended tumor resection. Usually the tumor is dissected off the infrarenal and aortic wall without difficulty; however, *resection of the inferior vena cava* is often unavoidable [12].

Operative Technique (Fig. 26.2.5). Following systemic heparinization and interruption of the blood flow, the inferior vena cava is resected, tributary lumbar veins are ligated, and vascular continuity is restored by interposition of a large graft with a reinforced outer wall (e.g., ring-enforced PTFE prosthesis).

Graft implantation should always be performed under the protection of a *temporary arteriovenous fistula* created in the inguinal region (it can be surgically closed after 3–6 months).

3. Renal Tumors

In cases of hypernephroma, the most common renal tumor in adults, tumor invasion of the inferior vena cava is diagnosed in 4%–6%.

Leaving such tumor plugs during palliative nephrectomy disposes to a generalized metastasis

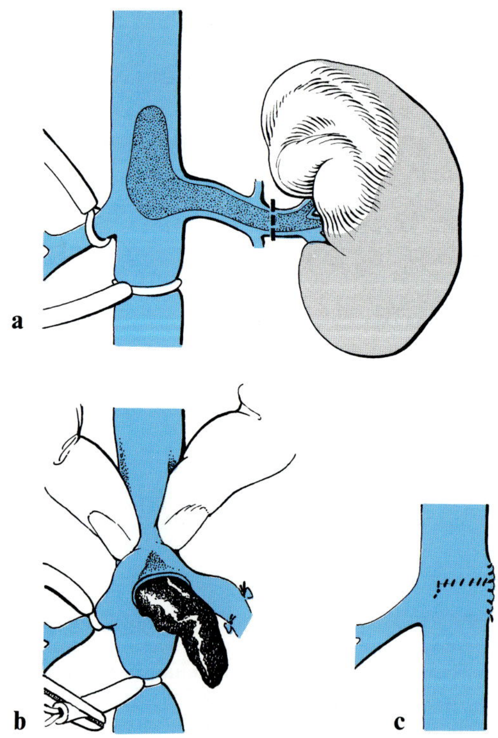

within 1 year. Resection of a *right-sided tumor* invading the inferior vena cava may be possible by resection of the inferior vena cava in continuity and ligation of the left renal vein: collateral circulation through the suprarenal vein, inferior phrenic vein, spermatic vein, ureteric vein, and ascending lumbar vein provides sufficient outflow for the left kidney [32].

For radical *left-sided tumor nephrectomy*, a similar procedure cannot be used because insufficient venous collateral circulation may remain following ligation of the right renal vein.

Operative Technique

1. *Endarterectomy* during inspiratory standstill (Fig. 26.2.6)
2. *Resection of the inferior vena cava in continuity* and *graft interposition* under the protection of an inguinal arteriovenous fistula (Fig. 26.2.7)

If necessary, the contralateral vein can be anastomosed to the graft end-to-side [27].

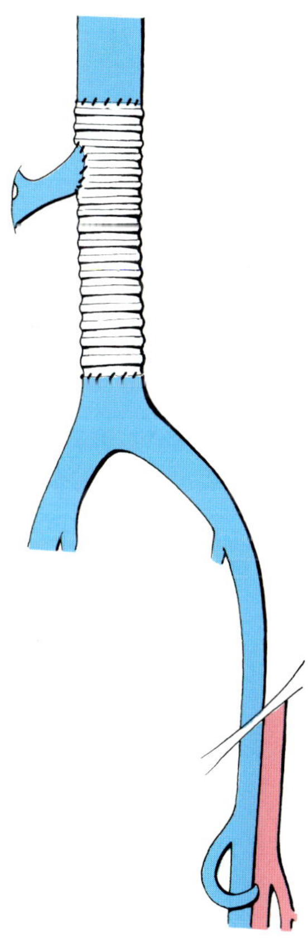

Fig. 26.2.7. Inferior vena cava resection in continuity, interposition of a vascular prosthesis, and reimplantation of the contralateral (right) renal vein into the graft

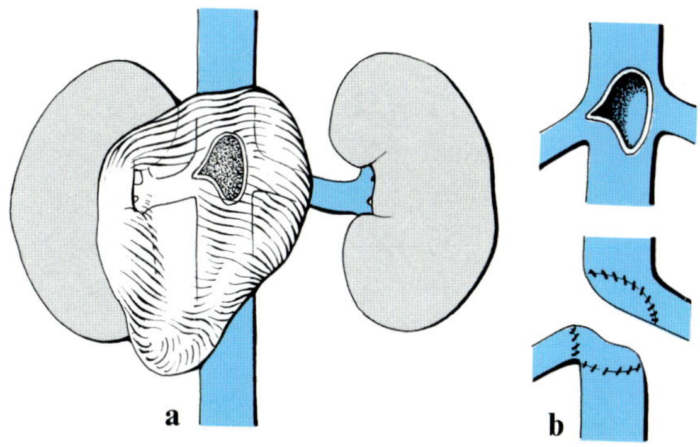

Fig. 26.2.8. a Resection of the tumor including the anterior wall of the inferior vena cava between the junction of (the patent) renal veins. **b** Oblique division of the posterior wall of the inferior vena cava, reconstruction of both caval stumps with a posterior flap

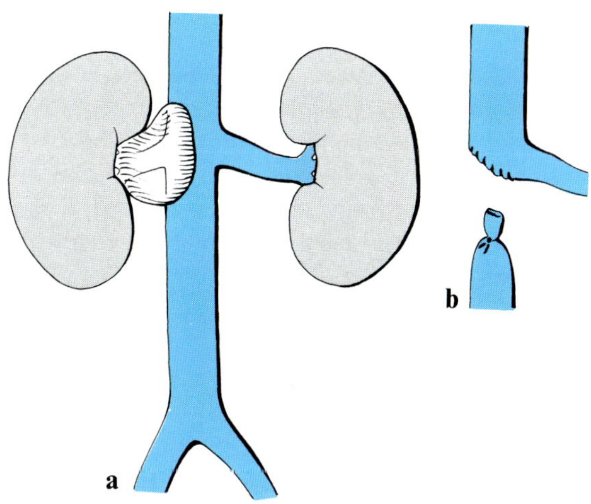

Fig. 26.2.9. a Resection of the tumor, including the right kidney and the renal vein. **b** Maintaining patency at the junction of the left renal vein by reconstruction of the proximal stump of the inferior vena cava

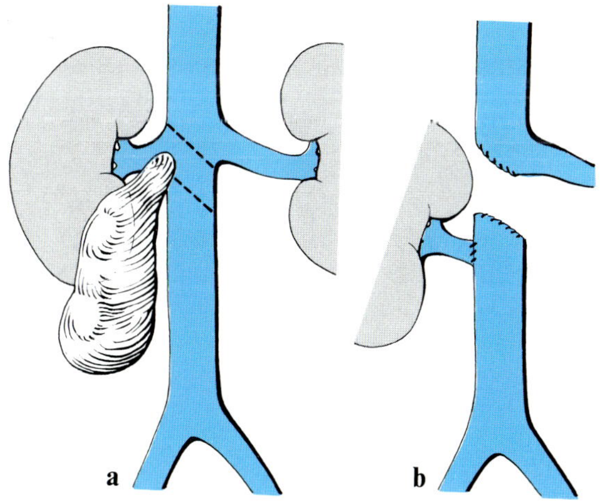

Fig. 26.2.10 a, b. Resection of the tumor, end-to-side anastomosis of the right renal vein to the distal inferior vena cava

4. Vascular Tumors of the Inferior Vena Cava

Vascular tumors of the inferior vena cava are curatively operable when they are:

a) *Benign (leiomyomas)*
b) *Malignant (leiomyosarcomas)* or *facultatively malignant (hemangioendotheliomas),* but limited to the middle and distal third of the inferior vena cava [19]

Tumors of the proximal third of the inferior vena cava involving the liver veins (Budd-Chiari syndrome) are for the most part inoperable [18].

The *operative technique* is the same as in Sect. C. III: vascular resection, graft interposition (eventually reinserting the renal veins), and inguinal temporary arteriovenous fistula [4].

The *procedures* described by COUINAND [6] (Fig. 26.2.8), GUEDON [11] (Fig. 26.2.9), or STUART and BAKER (Fig. 26.2.10) may be used, depending on the extent of the tumor.

In case of less extensive tumors, especially tumors of the anterior wall, local excision and tangential suture of the inferior vena cava may be successful [25].

IV. Extremities

1. In the extremities vascular reconstructions are considered for *en bloc resection* of *soft tissue* and *bone sarcomas* [13], the resected artery being replaced by autogenous vein (greater saphenous vein) or a fabric prosthesis.

In the rarer benign and semimalignant *vascular tumors (leiomyomas, hemangiopericytomas), excision* of the tumor, together with the involved artery, followed by reconstruction using a vein graft is the operative method of choice.

2. Another indication for arterial reconstruction is the presence of deep *ulcers* at the base of which major arteries may be exposed and therefore susceptible to arrosion. In the majority of cases it is an *ulcus radiologicum*, much more rarely a carcinomatous or sarcomatous crater.

The preferred localization is the groin. Erosion of the femoral artery may cause life-threatening bleeding. Ligation of the artery in the infected tumor is seldom successful (frequently, the ligatures cut through the arterial tissue and cause bleeding). Simple ligation usually causes a more or less severe ischemia of the limb.

Ligation of the afferent and efferent arteries (external iliac artery, superficial femoral artery, and profunda femoris artery) within healthy tissue, i.e., outside the tumor, and restoration of the vascular system by means of a *graft* is the *operative method* of choice. For bypassing the groin, the so-called *obturator bypass* from the external iliac artery to the superficial femoral artery is primarily used (see p. 545). Here, the same principles of reconstruction apply as in postoperative infection in the groin.

REFERENCES

1. Acker H, Pietnuchka F (1977) Meaning of the type I cell for chemoreceptive process. In: Acker H (ed) Chemoreception in the carotid body. Springer, Berlin Heidelberg New York, p 92
2. Barber HRK, Brunschwig A (1967) Excision of major blood vessels at the periphery of the pelvis in patients receiving pelvic exenteration: common and/or iliac arteries and veins 1947 to 1964. Surgery 62:426
3. Blenkinsopp WK, Hobb JT (1966) Pedunculated hämangiopericytoma attached to the thoracic aorta. Thorax 21:193
4. Brewster DC, Athanasoulis CA, Darling R (1976) Leiomyosarcoma of the inferior vena cava. Diagnosis and surgical management. Arch Surg 111:1081
5. Conley J (1975) Carotid artery surgery in the treatment of tumors of the neck. Arch Otolaryngol 65:437
6. Couinaud C (1973) Tumeurs de la veine cava inférieure. J Chir (Paris) 105:411
7. Davis GL, Bergmann M, O'Kane MB (1976) Leiomyosarcoma of the superior vena cava. A first case with resection. J Thorac Cardiovasc Surg 72:408
8. Feldman F, Seaman W (1964) Primary thoracic hemangiopericytoma. Radiology 82:998
9. Gomes MN, Hufnagel CA (1975) Superior vena cava obstruction: A review of the literature and report of two cases due to benign intrathoracic tumors. Ann Thorac Surg 20:344
10. Gretchen A, Gooding W (1979) Gray scale ultrasound detection of carotid body tumors. Radiology 132:409
11. Guédon J, Mesnard J, Poisson J, Kuss R (1970) Hypertension réno-vasculaire par léiomyosarcome de la veine cave inférieure. Guérison de l'hypertension et survie de 2 ans après intervention chirurgicale. Ann Méd Intern (Paris) 121:905
12. Hamann H, Vollmar J (1979) Expanded PTFE-Gefäßprothesen – ein neuer Weg des Arterien- und Venenersatzes? Chirurg 50:249
13. Imparato AM, Roses DF, Francis KC, Lewis MM (1978) Major vascular reconstruction for limb salvage in patients with soft tissue and skeletal sarcomas of the extremities. Surg Gynecol Obstet 147:891

14. Kattus AA, Longmire WP, Cannon JA, Webb R, Johnston C (1960) Primary intraluminal tumor of the aorta producing malignant hypertension successful surgical removal. N Engl J Med 262:694
15. Kremer K, Palomba PP, Sandmann W (1976) Leiomyom der Vena portae. Bericht über eine erfolgreiche chirurgische Behandlung. Chirurg 47:214
16. Lack EE, Cubilla AL, Woodruff JM, Farr HW (1977) Paraganglioma of the head and neck region. Cancer 39:397
17. Linder F (1953) Tumoren der Karotisdrüse. Langenbecks Arch Chir 276:165
18. Lintner F, Faust U, Nowotny CH (1978) Ein maligne entartetes primäres Leiomyom der Vena cava inferior (Leiomyosarkom) unter dem klinischen Bild des Chiari-Budd'schen Syndroms. Wien Klin Wochenschr 90:485
19. Markov J, Dontschev T (1967) Hämangio-Endotheliom an der Bifurkation der unteren Hohlvene. Zentralbl Chir 92:38
20. Mehmke S (1965) Gefäßchirurgische Möglichkeiten im HNO-Bereich. Mschr Ohrenheilk 99:321
21. Moore SW (1958) A report on a patient five years following resection of the abdominal aorta for recurrent carcinoma. Surg Gynecol Obstet 107:709
22. Nickels J, Kalima TV (1979) Leiomyosarcoma of the inferior vena cava. VASA 8:333
23. Rob CG, Vollmar JF (1959) Die Chirurgie der Bauchaorta. Ergebn Chir Orthop 42:569
24. Salm R (1972) Primary fibrosarcoma of the aorta. Cancer 29:73
25. Schildberg FW, Kuntz RM (1977) Leiomyosarcomas of the inferior vena cava. Report of a case and review of the literature. Thoraxchirurgie 25:28
25a. Stuart FP, Baker WH (1973) Palliative surgery for leiomyosarcoma of the inferior vena cava. Ann Surg 177:237
26. Thevent A (1976) Tumeurs du corpuscule carotidien. Dans: Encyclopédie médico-chirurgicale, Ed. by Editions Techniques, Paris (4-4-09), 1–4, 43205
27. Vollmar J, Loeprecht H, Nadjafi AS (1973) Die akute Vena cava inferior-Unterbrechung: Ligatur oder Rekonstruktion? Münch Med Wochenschr 115:978
28. Vollmar J (1975) Rekonstruktive Chirurgie der Arterien, 2nd edn. Thieme, Stuttgart, p 409
29. Vollmar J (1978) Chirurgie der Gefäße. Arch Otorhinolaryngol 219:197
30. Vollmar JF, Voss EU, Mohr W (1980) Carotid body tumors – diagnostic and surgical aspects. Angéoiologie 32:253
31. Voss EU, Vollmar J, Meister H (1977) Tumoren des Glomus caroticum. Diagnostische und therapeutische Aspekte. Thoraxchirurgie 25:1
32. Walz PH, Schlag P, Altwein JE (1980) Radikale Exstirpation eines linksseitigen Hypernephroms mit Tumorzapfen in der Vena cava inferior. Urologe 19:60
33. Yoshida Y, Matsuda S, Yamane M, Yamaguchi T (1968) Reconstructive vascular surgery for radical resection of malignant duodenal tumor. Am J Surg 116:917

27 Surgery of Veins

27.1 Injury of the Large Veins

K.H. GÄNGER † and A. SENN

CONTENTS

A. Anatomy

The system of large veins of the trunk extends from the upper aperture of the thorax to the lacunae vasorum in both groins (see p. 247). It consists of four separate drainage systems (Fig. 27.1.1):

1. Superior vena cava,
2. Pulmonary veins,
3. Inferior vena cava,
4. Portal vein.

I. Superior Vena Cava

The superior vena cava measures 4–5 cm in length and – separated from the thoracic wall – extends from the costomediastinal angle and the right first intercostal space to the sternal end of the third rib. At this point, it enters the pericardial sac obliquely. It is formed by the juncture of the two brachiocephalic veins. Because the junction of these veins is located behind the right margin of the sternum, the left brachiocephalic vein is longer than the right. As it descends obliquely downward and to the right behind the manubrium, the left brachiocephalic vein crosses the left subclavian artery, the left common carotid artery, and the brachiocephalic artery.

II. Pulmonary Veins

The pulmonary veins collect the blood from the pulmonary capillaries; in addition, the blood from the small bronchial veins empties into these vessels. Like the branches of the pulmonary artery, they follow the course of the bronchial tree and form in general two upper and two lower venous trunks in the pulmonary hilus. The superior pulmonary vein lies anterior to the hilus and the inferior pulmonary veins caudad to the respective bronchus. The part which lies within the pericardial sac is characterized by a perivascular cuff of heart muscle which keeps the vessel open and prevents kinking during systole [8].

III. Inferior Vena Cava

The inferior vena cava is formed by the junction of the two common iliac veins at the level of the fourth lumbar vertebra. This junction is situated caudal and to the right of the aortic bifurcation by which it is partially covered. At the level of the second lumbar vertebra, it runs to the right

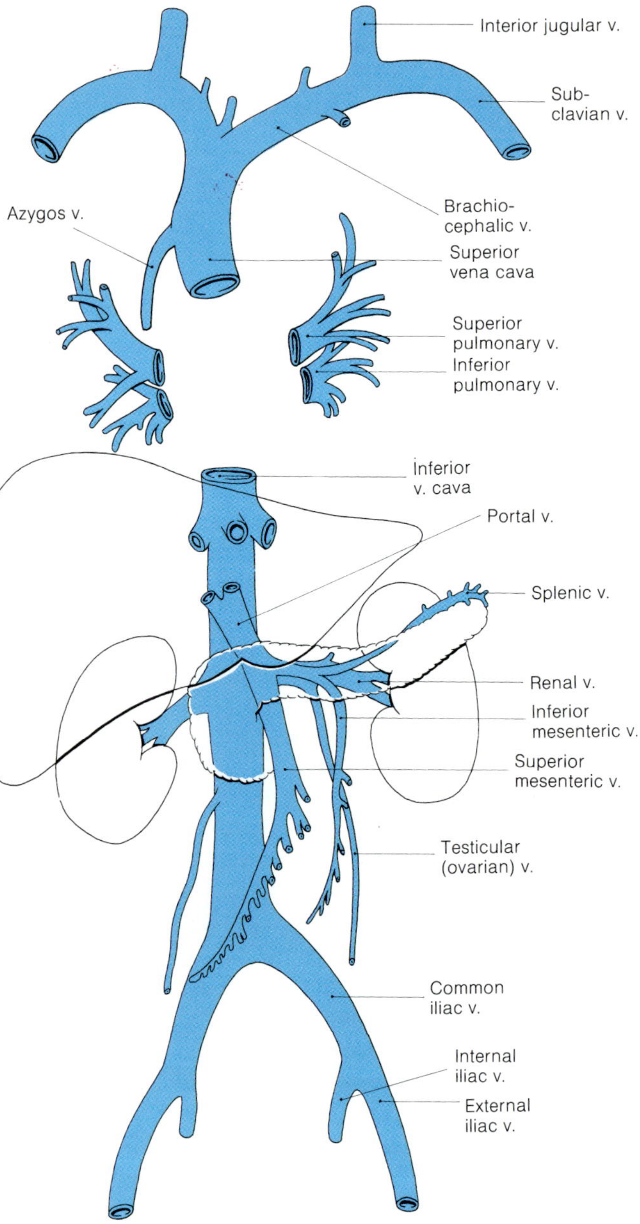

Fig. 27.1.1. Anatomy of large veins

of the aorta and anterior to the vertebral column. It passes under the root of the mesentery at the level of the third lumbar vertebra. Cephalad, it separates from the aorta and passes close to the upper pole of the right kidney, through the sulcus behind the liver, and finally via the opening named after it through the diaphragm. Without accepting any more branches, it passes through the thorax and empties into the right atrium. The vena cava transports approximately two thirds of the venous return. Its major tributaries are the iliac veins, the renal veins, the three hepatic veins, the lumbar veins (usually four), the testicular or ovarian veins, the suprarenal veins, and the phrenic veins [8].

IV. Portal Vein

The portal vein is formed by the confluence of the superior mesenteric and the splenic vein. A short distance distal to this junction, the inferior mesenteric vein drains into the splenic vein. The junction is situated behind the head of the pancreas; from there the portal vein continues cephalad for 5 cm behind the first part of the duodenum and reaches the hilus of the liver as part of the hepatoduodenal ligament [8]. Between 65% and 80% of the perfusion of the liver is derived from the portal vein. The liver is usually drained by three veins which enter the inferior vena cava beneath the diaphragm and contribute approximately 50% of the entire blood volume that passes through the inferior vena cava.

B. Causes of Venous Injuries

Venous injuries can be caused by trauma, or they can be iatrogenic.

I. Traumatic Venous Injuries

Traumatic venous injuries are caused by blunt or penetrating trauma of the thorax or the abdomen. Isolated injuries to the veins are rare because of their protected position deep within the cavities of the body. Usually, other structures, such as arteries, parenchymatous organs, or the gastrointestinal tract, are injured simultaneously.

II. Iatrogenic Venous Injuries

With advances in medicine and the increasing use of invasive diagnostic and therapeutic manipulations, the incidence of iatrogenic venous injuries has increased rapidly. They make up approximately 10% of all vascular injuries, but this is probably an underestimate [14, 27, 31]. One distinguishes intraoperative iatrogenic injuries and lesions caused by catheters.

1. Intraoperative Iatrogenic Injuries

Even though all forms of venous injury during surgery are possible, they can usually be avoided by exact knowledge of the anatomy and careful surgical technique. However, inflammatory changes, scars, and invasive tumor growth will lead to incidental venous injuries, even though all precautions are taken. The most common iatrogenic injuries in the thorax are the laceration of the left brachiocephalic vein during sternotomy [11] and the incidental biopsy of the vena azygos during mediastinoscopy. In the abdomen, injuries of the inferior vena cava and the common iliac veins are common during operative procedures on the spine [23]. Lacerations of the vena cava are common during right lumbar sympathectomy, resection of abdominal aortic aneurysms and other operations of the abdominal aorta, right lumbar sympathectomy, and right radical nephrectomy. Injuries to the iliac veins most commonly occur during iliac endarterectomy, operations in the region of the hip, and gynecologic procedures.

2. Catheter Injuries

If central venous catheters remain in place for a long period they can lead to an erosion of the venous wall with resultant hemorrhage. This is especially the case with subclavian hemodialysis catheters, which are made of Teflon. Small polyethylene catheters usually have a low complication rate. While jugular catheters are regarded as safe, central venous catheters advanced from the arm have a high complication rate. Moving the arm can advance the catheter as much as 10 cm with the risk of perforating the superior vena cava and the right atrium [13, 14]. Intraluminal cava filters developed by MOBIN-UDDIN or KIM-RAY-GREENFIELD can also lead to a perforation of the inferior vena cava [20]. As a rule, catheter or puncture injuries do not require surgical intervention.

C. Indications for Operative Intervention

I. Principles

Surgery is an integral part of resuscitation in patients with hypovolemic shock. The diagnosis of a venous injury can usually be made only intraoperatively. The indications for surgery are therefore the magnitude of the injury and the condition of the patient. When a large vein is injured, one always observes hemorrhagic shock. This clinical picture in connection with suspected injuries of other organs such as spleen, liver, pancreas, or bowel is an indication for emergency surgery [1, 6, 15].

II. Indications for the Exploration of Retroperitoneal Hematoma

The following findings are indications for exploration:

- Expanding retroperitoneal hematoma,
- Pulsating retroperitoneal hematoma,
- Suspected injury of other retroperitoneal organs (duodenum, pancreas, colon),
- Already opened retroperitoneum,
- Hemodynamic instability during the observation.

If the retroperitoneal hematoma is not pulsating one has time for a thorough inspection of the entire abdominal cavity, the repair of other injuries, procurement of enough blood for transfusion, and, depending on the circumstances, proximal and distal control of the large vessels. After hemodynamic stabilization, and, if necessary, enlargement of the incision, the retroperitoneal exploration can proceed without haste according to the criteria given. Retroperitoneal hematomas following fractures of the pelvis or the vertebrae should as a rule not be explored [21, 22, 25, 29].

D. Positioning

Because injuries to the large veins are usually diagnosed only intraoperatively, the position of the patient is determined by the associated injuries.

I. Thorax

After thoracic trauma, the patient is usually positioned in the standard thoracotomy position, the uninjured side down. A supine position is used if a transsternal approach is planned.

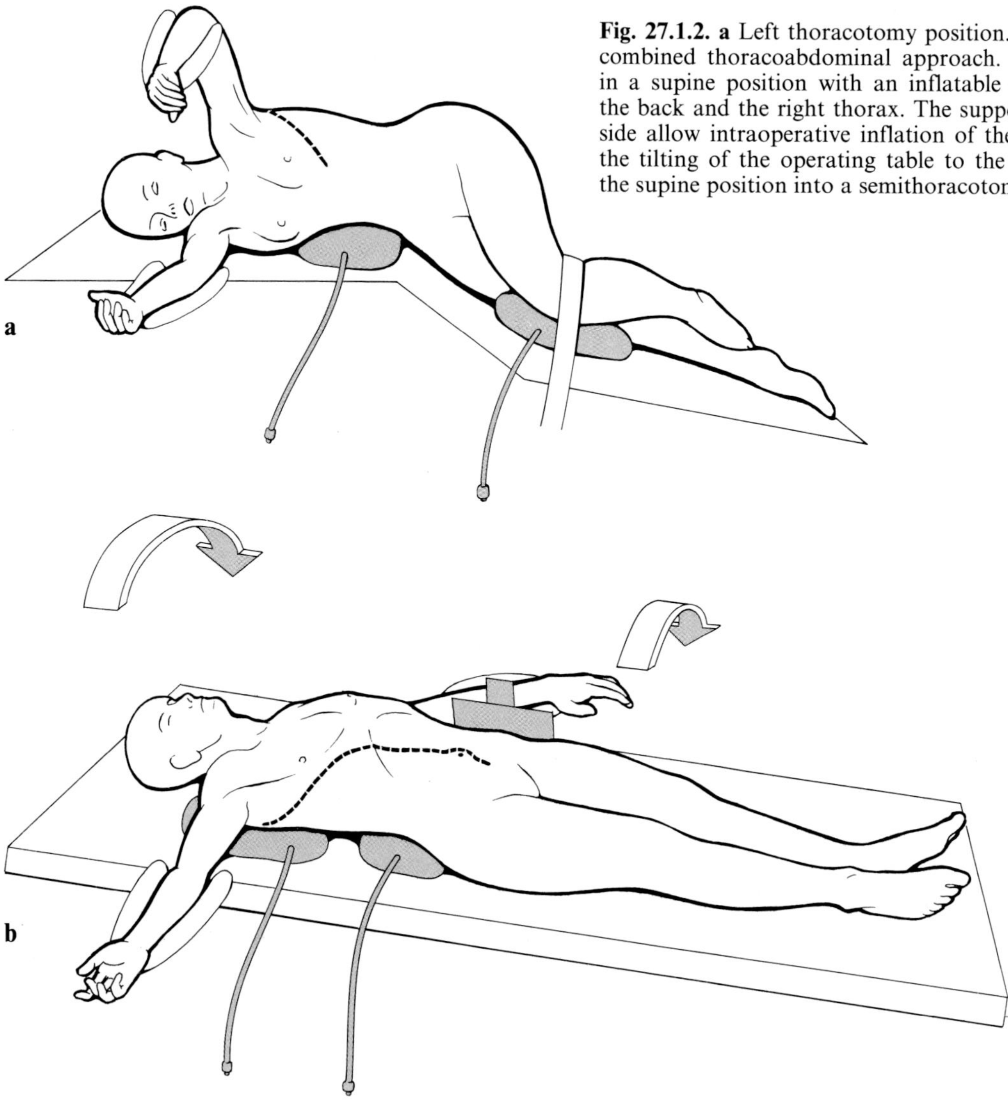

Fig. 27.1.2. **a** Left thoracotomy position. **b** Position for combined thoracoabdominal approach. The patient is in a supine position with an inflatable cushion under the back and the right thorax. The supports on the left side allow intraoperative inflation of the cushions and the tilting of the operating table to the left to change the supine position into a semithoracotomy position

II. Abdomen

After abdominal trauma, the supine position is best for exploration of the veins. An inflatable cushion is positioned under the lumbar spine to facilitate the surgical procedure. Side supports on the left side and an inflatable cushion under the right hemithorax allow for intraoperative repositioning of the patient in a right hemithoracotomy position to facilitate a thoracic extension of the incision for a better approach to the suprarenal vena cava inferior (Fig. 27.1.2a, b). Side supports on the contralateral side of the operating table facilitate the exposure of pelvic veins.

E. Approaches (Fig. 27.1.3)

I. Superior Vena Cava

The superior vena cava can be approached through an anterolateral thoracotomy in the fourth intercostal space on the right with the patient in the thoracotomy position, or through a median sternotomy in the supine position. The decision which approach to use depends on the suspected concomitant injuries. If a massive hemothorax on the right is the main preoperative finding, one should choose a right thoracotomy. If, however, an enlarged mediastinum raises the suspicion of additional injuries of the heart or the aorta, a transsternal approach is preferable. If a right thoracotomy is used, the parietal pleura over

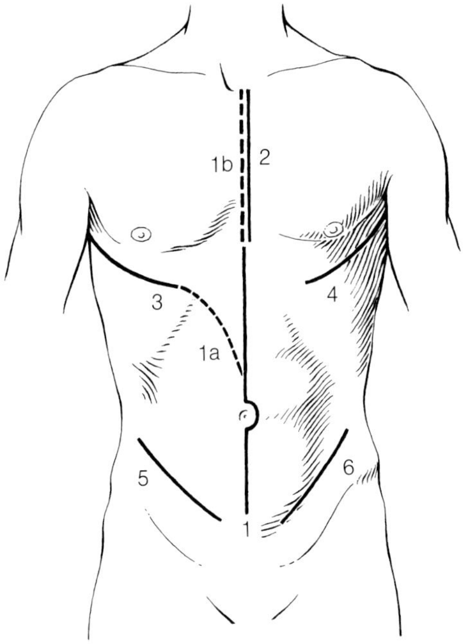

Fig. 27.1.3. Skin incisions. (*1*) Median laparotomy, (*1a*) anterolateral thoracotomy extension (*5*) and (*6*), (*1b*) sternal extension, (*2*) median sternotomy, (*3*) and (*4*) flank incision for the retroperitoneal approach to the iliac veins

the superior vena cava is incised, care being taken not to injure the right phrenic nerve, which is found lateral to the vein. The pericardium is opened longitudinally, and the superior vena cava can be encircled without difficulty, just cephalad of its junction with the right atrium. After median sternotomy, the right pleural reflection must be retracted toward the hilus of the lung, and a large thymus may have to be removed. Exposure of the superior vena cava is then possible without difficulty. During dissection, it is best to use the easily identifiable brachiocephalic vein as a guide. When incising the pericardial sac, one must again be careful not to injure the phrenic nerve [12, 24].

II. Pulmonary Veins

Intrapericardial injuries of the pulmonary veins present with the clinical picture of cardiac tamponade and are usually approached through a median sternotomy because of the suspected cardiac injury. Intrapleural injuries of the pulmonary veins lead to an ipsilateral hematothorax which, because of the suspected lung injury, is usually treated using an anterolateral thoracotomy in the lateral thoracotomy position [4].

III. Inferior Vena Cava (Fig. 27.1.4a, b)

In an injured patient, the approach to the inferior vena cava should always be transperitoneally, through a median laparotomy. The best exposure of the entire inferior vena cava is obtained when the vessel is approached from the right side. If the injury is located in the infrarenal part, an incision of the retroperitoneum around the cecum and along the base of the mesentery up to the ligament of Treitz and mobilization of the colon is sufficient. If one wants to explore the junction of the renal veins with the vena cava, one must also incise the peritoneal reflection along the ascending colon, the phrenocolic ligament as well as the duodenocolic ligament, until the entire right colon is mobilized and can be retracted toward the left side. A special dissection of the testicular/ovarian vessels and the right ureter is not necessary. The duodenum is mobilized with a Kocher maneuver, incising the peritoneum along the second portion of the duodenum after traction has been put on the liver in a cephalad direction. Duodenum and pancreas can now be mobilized bluntly and retracted medially. It is difficult to expose the suprarenal vena cava. Thoracoabdominal incisions or an additional sternotomy and extracorporeal circulation have been recommended in the literature, but the emergency use of these maneuvers is rarely possible; they represent an additional risk for the patient with multiple trauma [2, 15, 17, 18, 21]. The transdiaphragmatic intrapericardial approach from the abdomen, to control the inferior vena cava, as described by Heaney [10] (Fig. 27.1.5), appears to be the quickest and simplest way of controlling massive bleeding from the suprarenal vena cava in a traumatologic emergency. The round ligament and the falciform ligament are transected, and the liver is retracted caudally. The triangular ligament is incised down to the suprahepatic portion of the inferior vena cava. An L-shaped incision in the diaphragm is made, the angle of which is directed posterolaterally toward the vena cava, and the pericardium is opened on the left side of the vena cava. The thin pericardial reflection can now be opened bluntly with a finger, along the posterior wall of the vena cava, and the vessel can be encircled with an appropriate clamp. One should not hesitate to cross-clamp the vein since a reversal of flow has occurred as a result of the massive venous injury distally. If the reconstruction takes a longer time, an intra-abdominal shunt can be advanced from the abdomen into

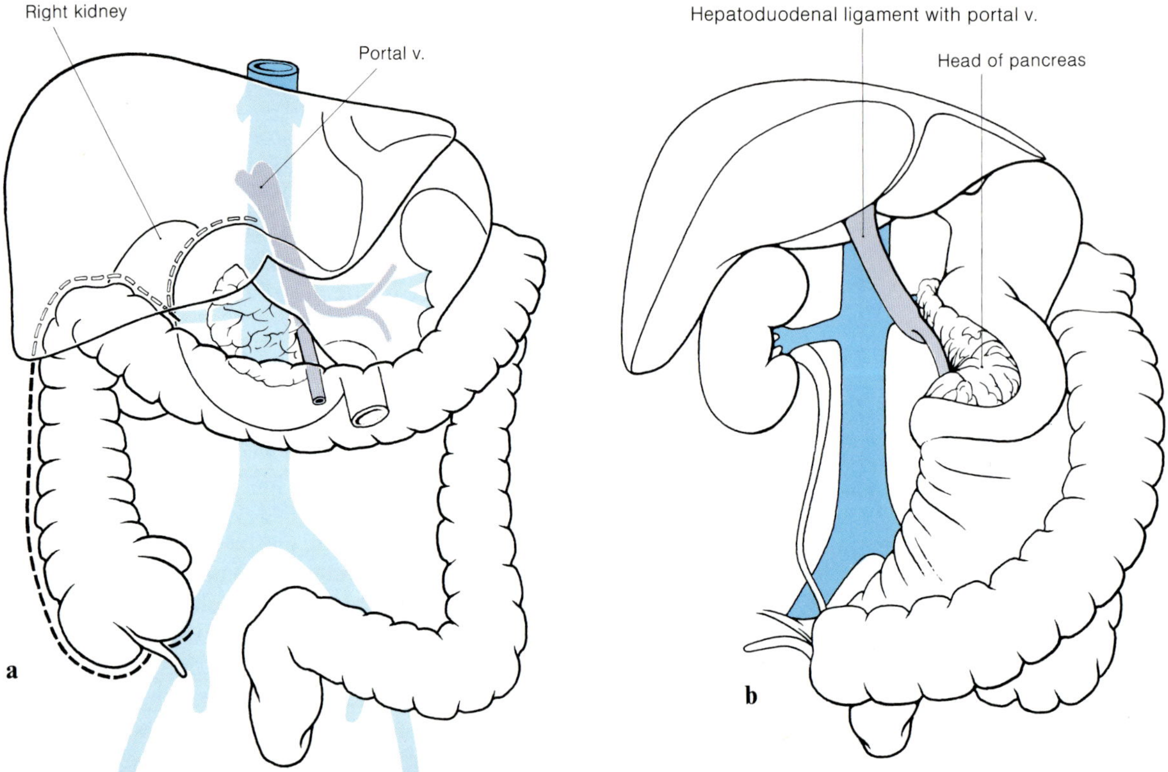

Fig. 27.1.4a, b. Exposure of the entire inferior vena cava, the portal vein, and the renal veins from the right.
a Peritoneal incision of the peritoneum along the right colon, division of the phrenicocolic ligament and the duodenocolic ligament, extension of the incision around the cecum and along the inferior small bowel as far as the ligament of Treitz. **b** Reflection of the right colon toward the left and mobilization of the duodenum using a Kocher maneuver, retraction of the duodenum and the head of the pancreas to the left

Fig. 27.1.5. Transabdominal, transdiaphragmatic intrapericardial exposure of the inferior vena cava as described by HEANEY. Approach from below after transection of the round ligament, the falciform ligament, and the triangular ligament. L-shaped incision in the diaphragm and the pericardium. Intrapericardial encircling of the inferior vena cava, if needed, with an intracaval shunt
▽

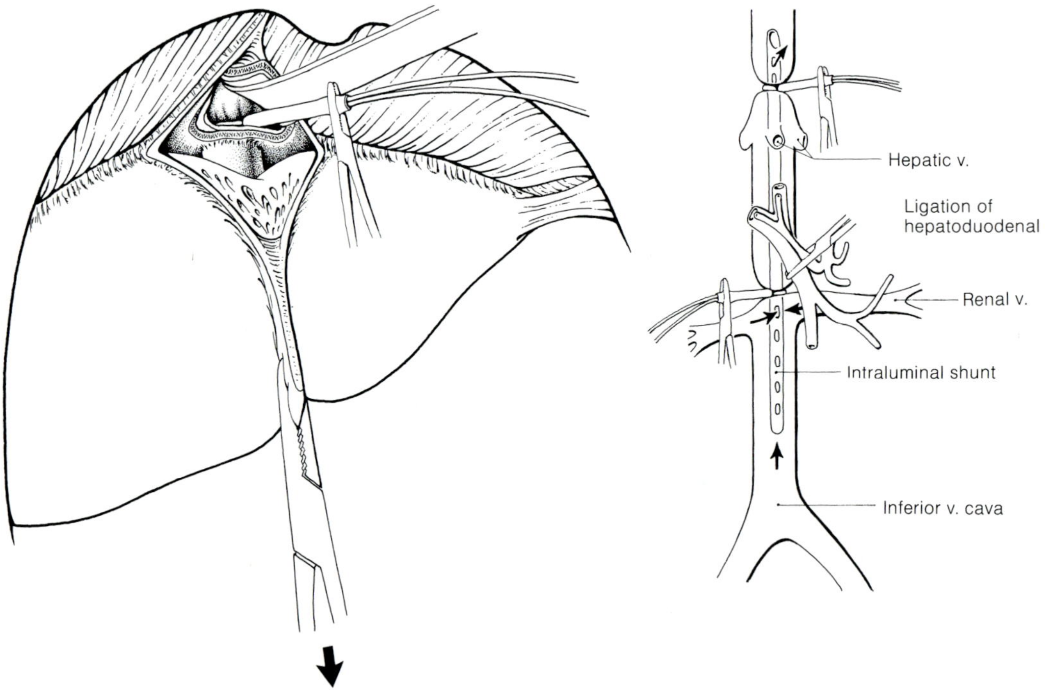

the right atrium and secured by circular bands which are placed below and above the liver. In emergency situations, a thoracostomy tube can be used as a shunt. Complete isolation of the liver from the circulation is achieved by occluding the hepatoduodenal ligament with a clamp (Pringle maneuver). The liver will tolerate normothermic ischemia for 30 min [5].

IV. Portal Vein

The portal vein is approached in the same way as the middle section of the inferior vena cava, i.e., by mobilization of the right colon and the duodenum using the Kocher maneuver. The isolation of the portal vein in the hepatoduodenal ligament requires a longitudinal incision of the peritoneum on the right side of the ligament and retraction of the common duct and the hepatic artery medially. The portal vein should be encircled as close to the liver as possible in order to avoid the branches which enter the vein from a medial direction. The exposure of the retropancreatic portal vein remains problematic. It is not always possible to get sufficient exposure by medial retraction of the duodenum and the head of the pancreas. If necessary, the pancreas can be transected distal to its head. After hemostasis is achieved, the distal pancreas is drained into a Roux Y-loop and the proximal cut end of the pancreas is closed with sutures [2, 7].

F. Surgical Technique

The primary purpose of all operative procedures in cases of venous injury is hemostasis, and secondarily the reconstruction – if possible – of the injured segment of the vessel.

I. Hemostasis

1. Principles

The most reliable instrument for the control of venous bleeding is a compressing finger. Prerequisites for control of bleeding are good exposure through a wide incision, effective suction devices, good light, and adequate assistance.

2. Tamponade

If the source of bleeding cannot be located immediately, unnecessary blood loss is prevented by temporary tamponade with warm compresses. After the patient has been stabilized, the compresses are removed gradually; it should then be possible to locate the source of bleeding and deal with it appropriately. Occasionally the patient can be saved only if the surgeon abandons the search for the bleeding point. In such desperate cases, the patient can be saved from exsanguination only by extensive tamponade. Tamponade in these cases is surely better than exsanguination. Even though tamponade should not be the primary aim during exploration for massive venous hemorrhage, it occasionally presents the only solution, and the surgeon is wise to keep it in mind for extreme situations. It is most easily done with several meters of wide impregnated gauze, the ends of which are passed through the abdominal wall to the outside. After the hemodynamic situation has stabilized for several days, the tampon is removed stepwise.

3. Ligature

While tamponade is usually unsatisfactory, ligature represents a safe method for hemostasis. One should, however, know how ligature of the different venous section is tolerated [28].

a) Tolerance to Ligature. Small veins can be ligated without hesitation. However, the main veins proximal to the elbow joint and the knee joint should be reconstructed as long as there are no life-threatening concomitant injuries which make a reconstruction impossible. Ligature of the brachiocephalic vein, as well as one internal jugular vein is tolerated without sequela. Ligature of the superior vena cava leads to the superior vena cava syndrome but is compatible with life because a collateral circulation over the inferior vena cava develops. Ligature of the pelvic vein does not necessarily lead to post-thrombotic changes if the distal venous bed is unaltered. The same holds true for ligature of the infrarenal vena cava.

Ligature of the suprarenal vena cava, however, is problematic. If the left kidney is functional, usually only a temporary renal insufficiency with the need for dialysis results because the necessary venous drainage from the left kidney occurs over the extensive preformed collaterals. Ligature of branches of the hepatic veins should be followed by resection of the corresponding liver segments. Ligature of the suprahepatic vena cava is not compatible with life. If, for technical reasons, surgical reconstruction in this difficult-to-expose area is not possible, extensive tamponade is preferable to ligature performed out of desperation. Ligature of the inferior mesenteric vein as well as the splenic vein is tolerated without difficulty. Ligature of the superior mesenteric vein is possible if the temporary hypovolemia which results from the pooling of large amounts of blood in the portal drainage area is corrected by volume substitution. Ligature of the portal vein is controversial. An emergency portosystemic shunt with distal ligature of the portal vein within the first 48 h leads to severe encephalopathy in patients without portal hypertension. Recently, successful ligation of the portal vein without a shunt has been described. The main problem here is the sequestration of blood in the portal drainage area during the first 72 h, which can be compensated with massive transfusion guided by the central venous pressure and the pulmonary artery pressure [2, 7, 26].

Even though ligation of any major vein – except the suprahepatic and, in most cases, the suprarenal vena cava – is compatible with life, it should be emphasized again that a reconstruction should always be attempted.

b) Technique. The following technical principles should be observed when ligating large veins:

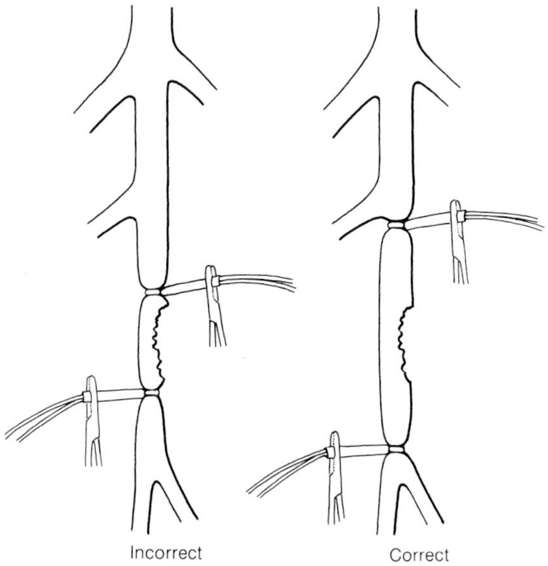

Fig. 27.1.6. Principle of ligation of large veins. To avoid stasis, ligatures are placed proximally and distally as close as possible to the next branch

Proximal and distal thrombectomy should be done prior to ligation to allow for optimal collateralization.

The proximal ligature should be placed as close as possible to the next branch and the distal ligature as close as possible to the last branch, to avoid the danger of stasis, thrombosis, and embolism [28] (Fig. 27.1.6).

II. Reconstruction

Sufficient exposure of the vascular lesion prior to any attempt at reconstruction is essential. The decision on which method to use can, therefore, only be made after temporary hemostasis has been achieved. Three methods are possible: simple suture, patch graft, and reconstruction with a graft.

Absence of tension and free inflow and outflow are essential for successful reconstruction. The absence of tension is assured by choosing the appropriate method, and free inflow and outflow is secured by the use of a balloon catheter prior to completion of the reconstruction.

1. Direct Suture

Most injuries of veins, especially penetrating and intraoperative lesions, can be dealt with by direct suture. Small lacerations can be sutured under finger compression, with 4-0 or 5-0 atraumatic nonabsorbable monofilament suture material. Depending on the extent of the injury, interrupted sutures, U-sutures, or a continuous suture are used. A narrowing of the lumen up to 50% can be tolerated. If it is possible to encircle the injured vein segment from behind with the finger and the finger is lifted slightly, thereby achieving hemostasis, then the suture can be done under vision rather than under finger compression (Fig. 27.1.7b). If control cannot be achieved digitally, a tangential atraumatic vascular clamp can be used (Fig. 27.1.7c). Vascular clamps must be used very sparingly and cautiously in venous surgery, as their uncontrolled use can lead to an enlargement of the laceration. Furthermore, placement of a tangential clamp is dependent on good mobilization of the venous segment. Instead of using clamps, one can achieve hemostasis by compressing the vein proximal and distal to the lesion with a sponge held in place by an assistant. Hemostasis, however, is rarely complete, owing to the rich col-

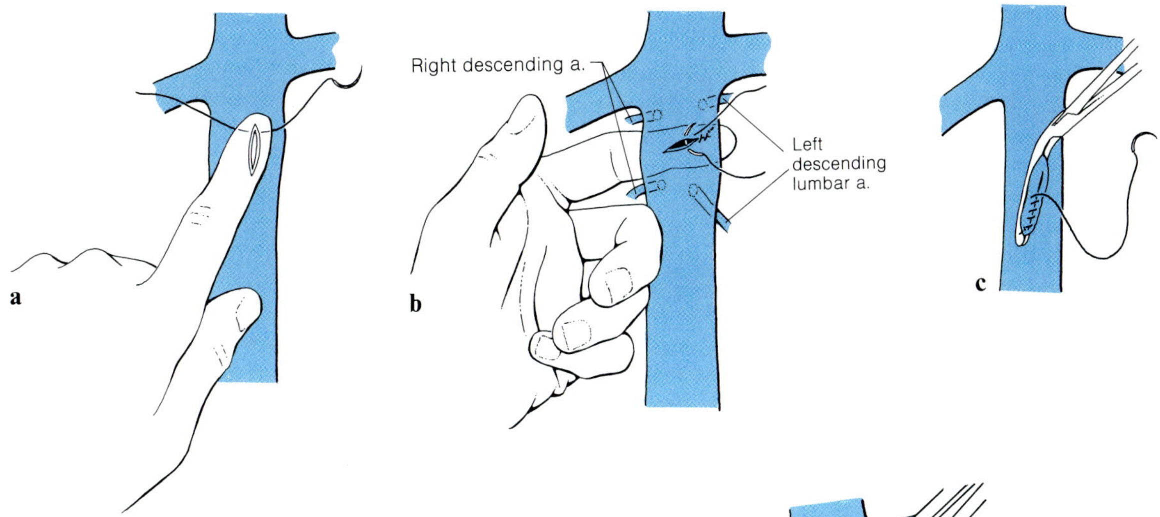

Fig. 27.1.7 a–e. Technique of direct venous suture. **a** Technique of direct suture under finger pressure. **b** Technique of venous sutures with finger pressure from behind. **c** Temporary hemostasis for the tangential placement of a clamp with direct suture. **d** Temporary hemostasis by combination of finger compression and proximal distal compression with sponges. **e** Transcaval suture technique with digital compression and compression with sponges for suture of lacerations of the posterior wall

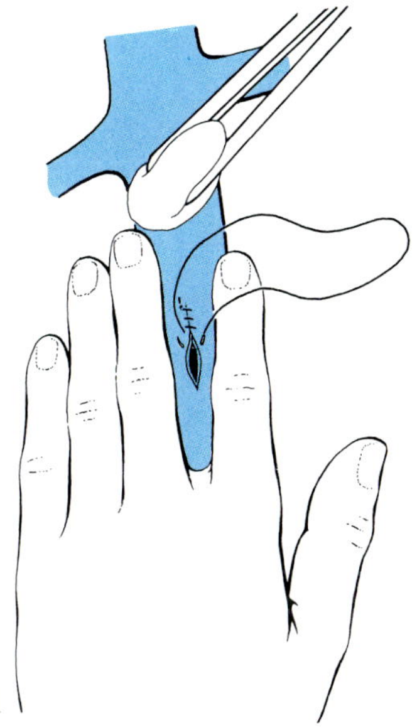

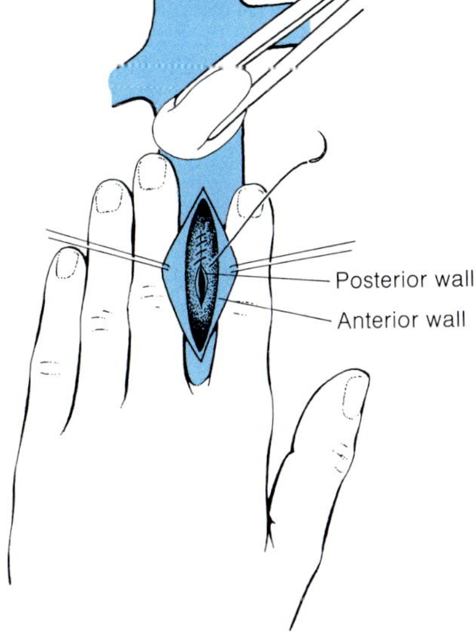

laterals, especially of the vena cava. If, in addition, the index and middle finger are placed on both sides of the vena cava, the lumbar veins, which empty dorsally, can be controlled and the laceration can be sutured under vision (Fig. 27.1.7d). The suture of a defect in the posterior wall is more complicated. The vena cava is fixed in place by a rich net of collaterals and cannot be freed without time- and blood-consuming dissection. Therefore, since the laceration of the posterior wall is usually associated with lesions in the anterior wall, access to the posterior wall can, if necessary, be gained by enlarging the opening in the anterior wall (Fig. 27.1.7e). The combination of proximal and distal control of blood flow by compression with sponges as well as by digital compression achieves the temporary hemostasis necessary to deal with these through-and-through injuries. Long catheters, inserted either directly through the defect or from the periphery, can also effect temporary hemostasis and thereby produce appropriate conditions for reconstruction [16, 24, 28].

2. Patch Graft

Direct suture will lead to a narrowing of the lumen if large lacerations with a tissue defect are present. If, in such cases, the narrowing would be over 50%, a patch graft is indicated. A segment of the saphenous vein, preferably from the distal calf, is the material of choice. As second choice, one may use artificial material, i.e., a PTFE patch. The tailoring and sewing of the patch follows the usual vascular technique.

3. Reconstruction Using a Graft

In contrast to arterial reconstruction, placement of a graft in the low pressure system is considered the least favorable method of reconstruction. Before it is applied, one must weigh the additional surgical effort and the uncertain prognosis against the risk of simple, careful ligature of the vein. Only if ligature of an injured vein is likely to have life-threatening complications, as is the case with the renal and suprahepatic segments of the inferior vena cava or the portal vein, reconstruction with autogenous vein or alloplastic material is justified.

a) Autogenous Vein Grafts. Because no autogenous veins with a wide enough lumen are available, the surgeon has to fashion the graft by combining two segments of saphenous vein (Fig. 27.1.8). An additional incision, in the thigh, involving appropriate preparation and draping, is the disadvantage of this method. Therefore, synthetic material is frequently used in emergency situations, even though the results with autogenous material are superior (Fig. 27.1.9).

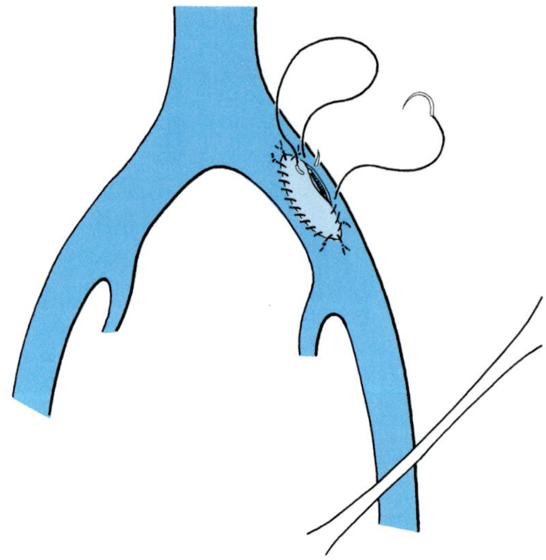

Fig. 27.1.9. Repair of a defect of an iliac vein with autogenous vein or prosthetic material

b) Synthetic Graft. Various materials, such as Dacron, velour, and PTFE, have been used as grafts. Recently, synthetic graft material reinforced by plastic rings has become available, eliminating the risk of a postoperative occlusion due to collapse of the graft. If there is no contamination of the operating field, the use of reinforced PTFE prostheses seems to be justified.

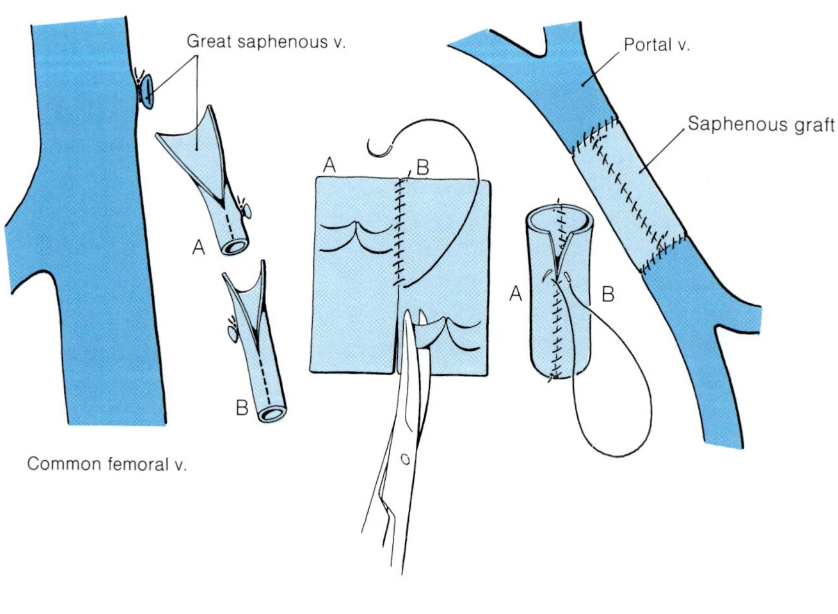

Fig. 27.1.8. Construction of a venous graft with a large lumen. Two segments of saphenous vein are split longitudinally and sutured together after the valves have been excised

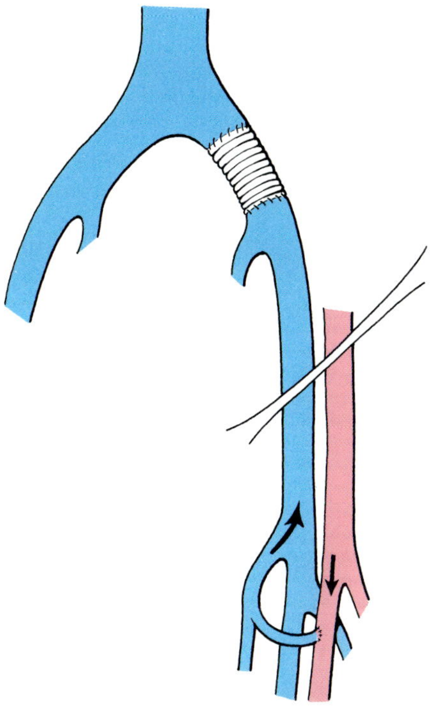

Fig. 27.1.10. Placement of a protective arteriovenous fistula after implantation of a synthetic prosthesis in the common iliac vein. End-to-side anastomosis of a branch of the saphenous vein to the superficial femoral artery

c) Protective Arteriovenous Fistula. After interposition of a graft, especially at the level of the iliac vein, the additional construction of a protective arteriovenous fistula between a branch of the femoral vein and the superficial femoral artery is recommended (Fig. 27.1.10) (see p. 723).

G. Postoperative Complications

The postoperative complications following injuries to the veins are basically the same as after all vascular surgical interventions. After multiple trauma, they are often the consequences of concomitant injuries. Specific vascular surgical complications include bleeding, thrombosis, embolus, and infection. In the case of bleeding and large retroperitoneal hematomas, the patient should be operated on promptly and the hematoma evacuated as soon as the general condition permits. If the hematoma is left in place, complications, e.g., thrombosis as a result of compression and infection, are likely. During the first operation a drain should be placed prophylactically in the retroperitoneal space. Postoperative thrombosis of the reconstructed vein does not in itself represent an indication for reoperation, because in most cases an adequate collateral circulation will have developed. Anticoagulation, however, can prevent the development of a mural thrombus and other thromboembolic complications. Posttraumatic arteriovenous fistulas occur as a result of simultaneous injury to an artery and vein and have been dealt with in Chap. 13 (see p. 251).

H. Prognosis

The success of the surgical treatment of venous injuries depends on a quick and sufficient hemostasis as well as on the magnitude of the concomitant injuries. One must therefore be careful when comparing the results of different authors. It is estimated that approximately half of all traumatized patients who have sustained a penetrating injury of the large veins will exsanguinate before reaching the hospital. The mortality of patients who reach the hospital alive ranges from 40% to 60% [17, 18]. The chance of survival is directly dependent on the time elapsed between injury and treatment. In patients with injuries to the venous system, mortality has remained 50% over the last few decades. Reports involving small numbers of patients sometimes give the false impression of an improvement; but that is because injuries to the mesenteric veins are included, for which the prognosis is much more favorable [26]. The prognosis of iatrogenic injuries, especially intraoperative lacerations, is of course much more favorable since they can be treated without delay and concomitant injuries are not present.

Venous injuries remain a challenge for the skill, experience, and diligence of the surgeon. Not only vascular surgeons, but all surgeons should be familiar with the principles of their treatment.

REFERENCES

1. Agarwal N, Shah PM, Clauss RH, Reynolds BM, Stahl WM (1982) Experience with 115 civilian venous injuries. J Trauma 22:827–832
2. Busuttil RW, Kitahama A, Cerise E, McFadden M, Lo R, Longmire WP Jr (1980) Management of blunt and penetrating injuries to the porta hepatis. Ann Surg 191:641–648
3. Byrne DE, Pass HI, Crawford FA Jr (1980) Traumatic vena cava injuries. Am J Surg 140:600–602

4. DiMarco RF, Layton TR, Manzetti GW, Pellegrini RV (1983) Blunt traumatic rupture of the right atrium and the right superior pulmonary vein. J Trauma 23:353–355
5. Duke JH Jr, Jones RC, Shires GT (1965) Management of injuries to the inferior vena cava. Am J Surg 110:759–763
6. Graham JM, Mattox KL, Beall AC Jr, DeBakey ME (1978) Traumatic injuries of the inferior vena cava. Arch Surg 113:413–418
7. Graham JM, Mattox KL, Beall AC Jr (1978) Portal venous system injuries. J Trauma 18:419–422
8. Hafferl A (1957) Lehrbuch der topographischen Anatomie, 2nd edn. Springer, Berlin Göttingen Heidelberg
9. Hamann H (1983) Iatrogene Gefässverletzungen bei diagnostischen und therapeutischen Eingriffen. Angio 5:153–161
10. Heaney JP, Jacobson A (1975) Simplified control of upper abdominal hemorrhage from the vena cava. Surgery 78:138–141
11. Hines GL (1981) Avulsion of the innominate vein during median sternotomy. J Cardiovasc Surg 22:349–352
12. Leitz KH (1981) Zugangswege in der Gefässchirurgie. Springer, Berlin Heidelberg New York
13. Kappes St, Towne J, Adams M, Kauffman HM, Maierhofer W (1983) Perforation of the superior vena cava. A complication of subclavian dialysis. JAMA 249:2232–2233
14. Krog M, Berggren L, Brodin M, Wickbom G (1982) Pericardial tamponade caused by central venous catheters. World J Surg 6:138–143
15. Mattox KL (1982) Abdominal venous injuries. Surgery 91:497–501
16. May R (1974) Chirurgie der Bein- und Beckenvenen. Thieme, Stuttgart
17. Millikan JS, Moore EE, Cogbill TH, Kashuk JL (1983) Inferior vena cava injuries – a continuing challenge. J Trauma 23:207–212
18. Misra B, Wagner R, Boneval H (1983) Injuries of hepatic veins and retrohepatic vena cava. Am Surg 49:55–60
19. Ochsner JL, Crawford ESt, DeBakey ME (1981) Injuries of the vena cava caused by external trauma. Surgery 49:397–405
20. Phillips MR, Widrich WC, Johnson WC (1980) Perforation of the inferior vena cava by the Kimray-Greenfield filter. Surgery 87:233–235
21. Quast DC, Shirkey AL, Fitzgerald JB, Beall AC Jr, DeBakey ME (1965) Surgical correction of injuries of the vena cava: an analysis of sixty-one cases. J Trauma 5:3–10
22. Rich NM (1982) Principles and indications for primary venous repair. Surgery 91:492–496
23. Schlosser V, Spillner G, Breymann T, Urbanyi B (1982) Vascular injuries in orthopaedic surgery. J Cardiovasc Surg 23:323–327
24. Schwarz H (1977) Verletzungen des Herzens und der großen Gefässe. Huber, Bern
25. Starzl TE, Kaupp HA, Beheler EM, Freeark BJ (1962) The treatment of penetrating wounds of the inferior vena cava. Surgery 51:195–204
26. Stone HH, Fabian TC, Turkleson ML (1982) Wounds of the portal venous system. World J Surg 6:335–341
27. Vollmar J (1968) Iatrogene Gefässverletzungen in der Chirurgie. Langenbecks Arch Chir 322:335–339
28. Vollmar J, Loeprecht H, Nadjafi AS (1973) Die akute V.-cava-inferior-Unterbrechung: Ligatur oder Rekonstruktion? Münch Med Wschr 115:978–985
29. Wright CB, Hiratzka LF, Hobson RW, Collins GJ, Rich NM (1981) Management of vena caval injuries. The Vietnam vascular registry review. J Cardiovasc Surg 22:203–212

27.2 Primary Varicose Veins

R. May †

CONTENTS

A. Anatomy

See Chap. 2 for general anatomy and Sect. A.I. of Chap. 27.3: for anatomy of acute venous occlusion.

B. Indications and Preoperative Work-up

The following pathophysiologic aspects should be kept in mind from the outset: With the patient standing, blood stagnates completely in varices. This has been proven through measurement of flow and venous pressure [4, 11, 12]. During movement, it is pushed forward, i.e., proximally, for short distances, then rushes distally again (blow-down), flowing through the incompetent perforating veins into the deep venous system (blow-in) (Fig. 27.2.1 a, b). In patients with severe and long-standing varicose veins, therefore, the deep venous system is overloaded. Because they are measurably enlarged, one must regard primary varicose veins as a mixed venous disease. The aim of every operative intervention is the complete elimination of the blow-down. Ligation of the incompetent perforating veins is necessary since blow-out will increase once blow-down has been abolished (see Chap. 27.4) (Fig. 27.2.2a, b).

One can distinguish between simple and complicated varicose veins. Patients who have no symptoms, except an occasional feeling of heaviness, have uncomplicated varicose veins which represent a relative indication for surgery:

1. For cosmetic reasons,
2. Because of complaints (feeling of heaviness),
3. For prophylactic reasons to decrease the risk of thromboembolic complications prior to other operations (operations on the hip joint).

An absolute indication for surgery is present in patients whose varices have led to one or more of the following complications:

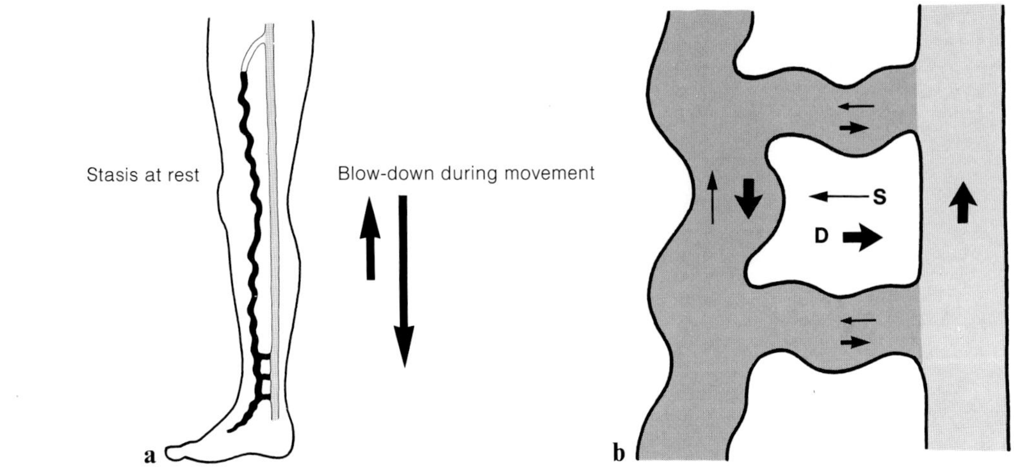

Fig. 27.2.1 a, b. Primary varicose veins. **a** Because of the incompetence of the superficial veins, the blow-down is increased during movement. **b** Because of the increased venous filling, the perforating veins become incompetent. During systole, there is a backflow of venous blood into the superficial system. Nevertheless, the blow-in during diastole is stronger than the blow-out during systole

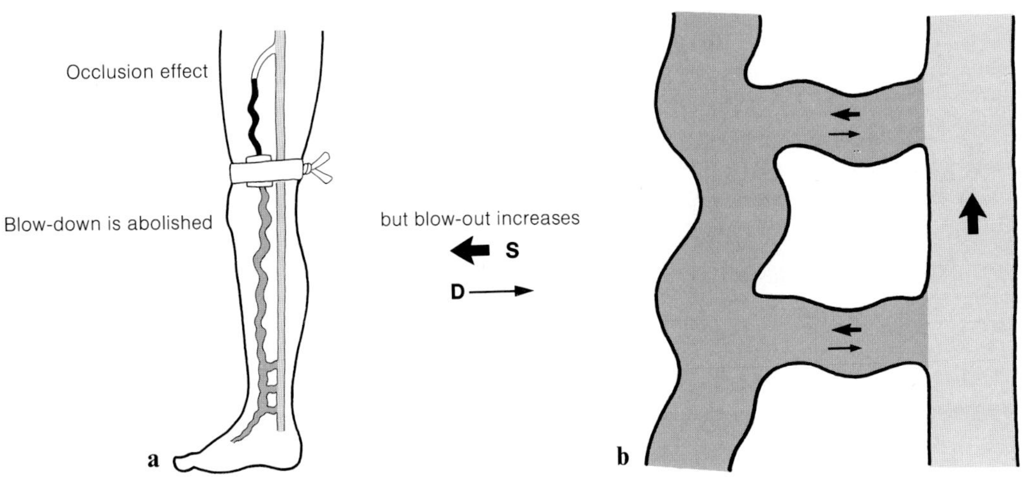

Fig. 27.2.2 a, b. Primary varicose veins postoperatively, simulated by occlusion. **a** The blow-down is eliminated by occlusion. **b** At the junction with the incompetent perforating veins, the flow is reversed. The blow-out is now stronger than the blow-in

1. Bleeding of the varicose veins,
2. Superficial thrombophlebitis (subsided),
3. Eczema,
4. Infiltration, induration, and stasis,
5. Venostasis ulcers.

I. Relative Contraindications

The relative contraindications are:

1. Severe concomitant disease,
2. Patient confined to bed,
3. Recent febrile or purulent disease in the patient's environment,
4. Pregnancy,
5. Combination with other operations, i.e., herniorrhaphies,
6. Obesity (danger of recurrence),
7. Nocturnal "charley horses" (these are never caused by varicose veins).

II. Absolute Contraindications

1. Competent main venous trunks: a prophylactic operation cannot be justified in view of the importance of the veins as a source of graft material.

2. Peripheral arterial disease: in patients with peripheral arterial disease, the complaints are often falsely attributed to incidentally present varicose veins. If a well-collateralized arterial occlusion and venostasis ulcers are present at the same time, the indication for surgery of the varicose veins and ligature of incompetent perforating veins may be forthcoming from an exact evaluation of the arterial tree.

3. Post-thrombotic occlusion of the deep venous system: varices which serve as collaterals following occlusion of the deep venous system should never be removed. It is, therefore, mandatory that a venography be done if there is a history of edema, phlebitis, or pleurisy following trauma, operations, or delivery (see p. 728).

4. Primary and secondary lymphedema (see p. 785): this can be worsened by varicose vein surgery. One should make sure that it is possible to raise a crease in the skin of the toes. Objective evidence can also be obtained by injecting 0.4 ml methylene blue in the interdigital space between the first and second toe. This should normally color the lymph vessels, but results in a deep blue spot if lymphedema is present.

5. Surgery is contraindicated in cases of acute and chronic inflammatory change. Infiltrations, indurations, and venostasis ulcers should be treated with diligent compression for many months to achieve the best possible preoperative situation. A history of erysipelas, often combined with venostasis ulcers, requires antibiotic treatment for 6 weeks postoperatively.

The importance of competent venous segments for aortocoronary bypass operations requires the preservation of all competent segments of the greater and lesser saphenous veins. Veins are also superior to prosthetic grafts in arterial reconstructive surgery of the leg. The long-recommended schematic radical operation of the greater and lesser saphenous vein therefore, can, no longer be justified; the preservation of competent venous segments is essential. A preoperative sketch showing the procedures to be performed – this is shown to the patient – facilitates the localization of competent venous segments for later grafting.

III. Preoperative Investigation

1. Evaluation of arterial circulation using Doppler ultrasound (with foot pulse measurement) [6].

2. Exclusion of lymphedema by history and clinical investigation. If there is the slightest suspicion of lymphedema, a color test should be done (see p. 796).

3. Phlebography of the deep and superficial system is not essential. However, if there is the slightest suspicion that the deep venous system is compromised, the patency must be ascertained radiologically. Patency of the deep veins can also be proven, albeit with less accuracy than with radiologic methods, by Doppler ultrasonography and light reflex rheography. In the superficial system, venography is helpful in preventing a recurrence because it allows the assessment of details which may be overlooked during clinical examination [6, 8, 9].

C. Positioning

Operations on the great saphenous vein and its branches are usually possible with the patient in a supine position; surgery on the lesser saphenous veins requires a prone position. Because of the prone position as well as the necessity for diligent surgical technique, general anesthesia is necessary.

D. Surgical Technique

I. Ligature of the Greater Saphenous Vein in the Groin [2, 5, 10]

1. Surgical Technique

A skin incision is made in the groin or two fingerbreadths above it (Fig. 27.2.3a). This incision was recommended by Brunner [2] to avoid injury to the lymphatic vessels which collect in this area. In our experience, injury to these lymph vessels can be prevented by meticulous surgical technique. To demonstrate the close relationship between lymphatics and the greater saphenous vein, one can inject methylene blue underneath the skin of the first interdigital space. The superficial fascia is divided in the direction of the skin incision with a scalpel. Subcutaneous fat is pushed distally with

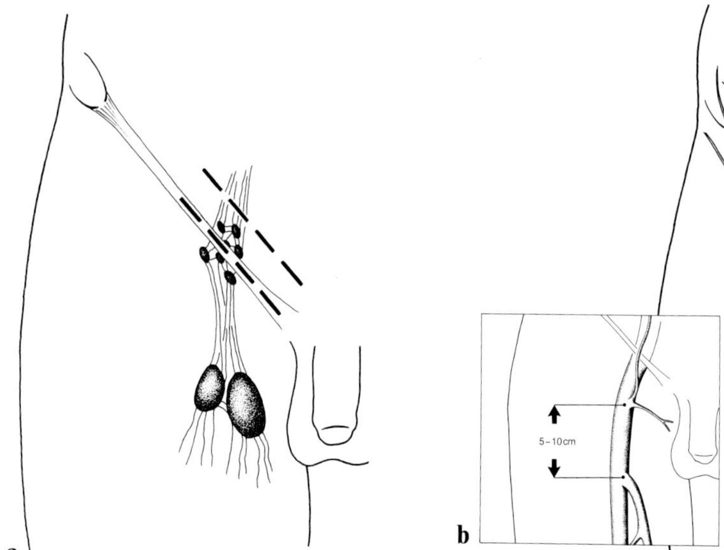

a b

Fig. 27.2.3a–d. Exposure of the venous junction in the groin. **a** Skin incision of the groin or two fingerbreadths above it. **b** The junction of the greater saphenous vein. **c** Variations of the saphenous junction. **d** Suture of the greater saphenous vein without compromising the lumen of the femoral vein

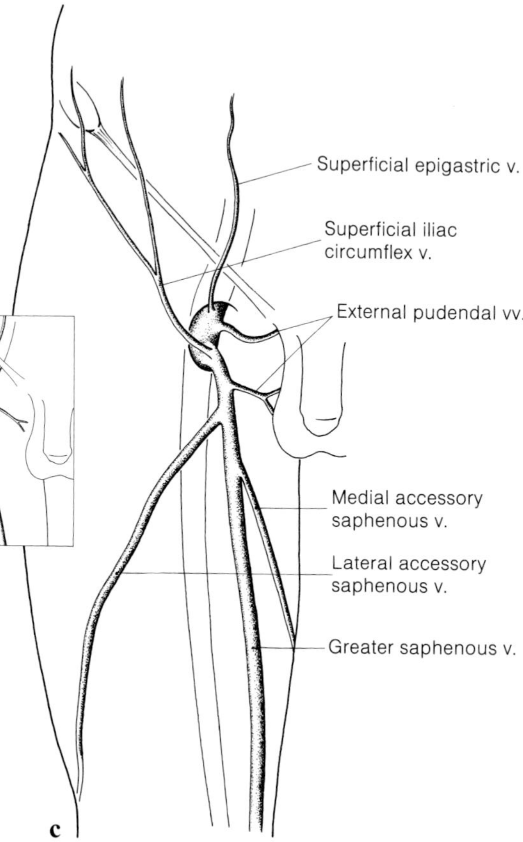

c

a sponge until the first larger vein is encountered. This vein is followed in the direction of its junction with the femoral vein by blunt dissection. Since there are many variations in this junction (Fig. 27.2.3b) and the position of the femoral vein, no larger vein should be ligated or grasped with a forceps before the location of the femoral vein has been ascertained by finger palpation. In addition, the femoral vein should be dissected free ventrally and medially for 1 cm. Complete dissection of the femoral vein should be avoided since it destroys the suspensory ligaments.

Only this approach makes certain that an encountered vein is really the greater saphenous vein. In addition, the direct tributaries of the femoral vein, i.e., the epigastric vein, which approaches proximally, and the pudendal veins, which approach medially and are the main source of recurrences, can be identified and ligated. A variation that is especially dangerous is the deep junction of the femoral and greater saphenous vein, approximately 3–4 fingerbreadths distal to the junction of the smaller veins (Fig. 27.2.3c). For example: the surgeon finds the venous junction, but not the greater saphenous vein, and tries to insert the stripper from the ankle proximally. It can be advanced effortlessly into the deep vein which is then erroneously ligated.

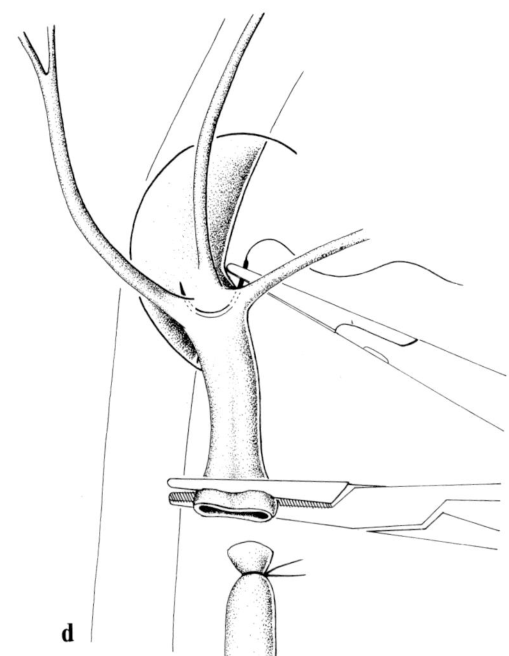

d

After the incision of the fascia, one often finds a large venous aneurysm. This aneurysm should have been diagnosed prior to the operation with the patient standing up, and it must be differentiated from a femoral hernia. This aneurysm usually has a very thin wall and is dissected bluntly along the venous wall. The neck of the aneurysm is usually very short and has to be freed from the ventral and medial part of the femoral vein prior to ligature.

If a femoral hernia is present, it is taken care of prior to ligation of the greater saphenous vein. After the anatomic situation has been clarified completely, the greater saphenous vein is transected between clamps, approximately 2 cm distal to the junction (Fig. 27.2.3d). Leaving the stump long facilitates the next step of the operation. The branches which join the femoral artery directly can be ligated easily. The distal ends of these branches are not ligated if they are not too large in caliber. Usually they can be pulled out for 10–15 cm and evulsed.

Not infrequently, a large lateral branch is encountered. It is followed with a small stripper down to the region lateral to the knee joint and is stripped out through a small stab wound. The constant medial side branch joins the greater saphenous vein approximately 4 cm distal to the saphenous junction. It is followed until its branches can be pulled out. Not infrequently, this vein continues as the so-called femoropopliteal vein or vena Giacomini, curving toward the medial side of the thigh to the lesser saphenous vein in the popliteal fossa. The stripper is advanced down to this vein, and the whole system is stripped.

Ligation of the greater saphenous vein is always done by suture ligature to eliminate the possibility of slipping. Also, a narrowing of the lumen of the deep vein occurs not infrequently if a simple suture is placed around the lesser saphenous vein close to the junction.

2. Complications

a) Lymphatic Fistula, Lymphoceles. If a lymphatic vessel is injured, a lymphatic fistula with a point exit, for example in the groin, may develop. Up to 100 ml lymph may empty every day. Compression treatment is advisable. If this is not successful, the lymph vessel is ligated. If the lymph cannot escape through the skin after injury, it collects and forms a lymphocele with a size of up to 100–200 ml. This lymphocele should be aspirated and afterward compression should be applied. This treatment must be continued over several months but will eventually lead to the disappearance of the lymphocele [2].

b) Small Tear in the Deep Femoral Vein. This can be controlled easily as described by FISCHER [5]. The remnant of the small vessel should be twisted with a clamp; this leads to immediate hemostasis. An atraumatic suture will close the tear.

c) Larger Lacerations of the Femoral Vein. The femoral vein is a large and important vessel which should never, under any circumstances, be narrowed, or even ligated. A large number of tragic incidents are the result of the fact that varices are operated on in small institutions, even on an outpatient basis, and under local anesthesia. If the common femoral vein is injured, the operative field is flooded with dark blood; clamping blindly will injure the venous wall further, or even the artery. When a large laceration is present, the following procedure should be adhered to:

1. Do not use clamps, hemostasis can always be obtained with compression.
2. Assure sufficient help.
3. Put the patient in the Trendelenburg position, with the legs elevated.
4. Enlarge the incision and be sure to use a suction device. After exposure of the defect, the stump of the saphenous vein can be twisted.
5. Dissect the artery and retract it laterally. The lacerated and compressed vein should be ignored for the moment; the artery is dissected free, encircled, and retracted laterally out the danger zone.
6. Expose the deep vein.

While hemostasis is obtained by means of a sponge, the vein can be dissected free proximally and distally. The assistant compresses the vein proximally and distally with the finger, suction will then allow a clear view. If the defect is closed with a running vascular suture, the problem is solved. However, if a complex and severe injury to the femoral vein occurs in a hospital where there are neither vascular instruments nor a surgeon skilled in vascular surgical technique, the following course of action is mandatory. No further surgical procedures should be attempted under inadequate working conditions. In every case, venous bleeding can be stopped by compression, which can be maintained with a bandage around the hip joint and the groin in a crosswise fashion. The patient is transferred, accompanied by the surgeon to a specialized hospital, which has been informed beforehand by phone. The courts have held that an injury to the femoral vein, or even an injury to the femoral artery is inconsequential for the surgeon if arrangements are made for appropriate transport of the patient to the specialized hospital without delay. A surgeon skilled in vascular surgery can then dissect the proximal and distal end of the femoral vein while hemostasis is maintained by digital compression. Up to this point, the use of clamps is contraindicated, because they could destroy the paper-thin venous wall. After the defect has been exposed, Fogarty hydrogrip clamps can be applied. In the most favorable situations, a direct linear vascular suture is sufficient. In most other cases, the defect can be closed with a vein patch. If this is not possible, a graft, fashioned from two pieces of saphenous vein, should be interposed.

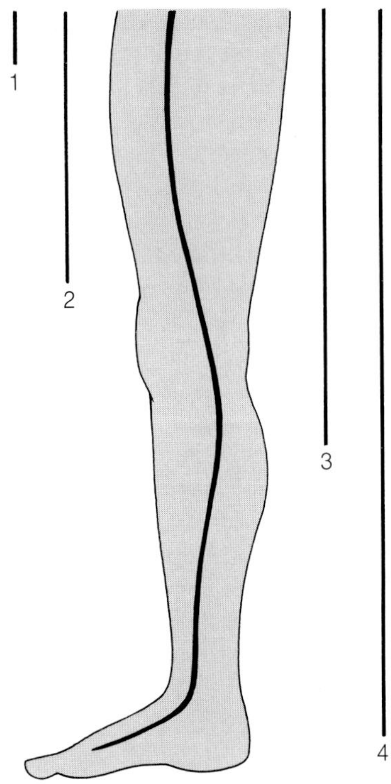

Fig. 27.2.4. Classification of varicose veins in the region of the greater saphenous vein

II. Resection of the Greater Saphenous Vein and Its Branches

1. Preliminary Remarks

Stripping of the main vein and its long branches must be considered the safest method of removing varicose veins. The combination of surgery plus sclerosing, scraping of the intima with special instruments, destruction of the intima by fulguration, multiple percutaneous ligatures, etc. have not stood the test of time. However, one should keep the following points in mind.

Variceal changes of the main trunk of the greater and lesser saphenous vein progress from proximal to distal. One should, therefore, determine in each case whether the distal part of the vein can be saved. This can be done by Doppler ultrasonography, but more precisely by venography. According to the proposal of HACH [6], we grade the varicose changes of the greater saphenous vein in four groups (Fig. 27.2.4). Varicose changes end, depending on their grade, immediately at the juncture with a large side branch or an incompetent vein. HACH has called this "the distal point of insufficiency." If one saves the distal functioning part of the vein, it usually remains functional and does not take part in the general progression of the varicosities.

In rare cases, the greater saphenous vein does not become incompetent at the level of groin, but further distally, immediately distal to the juncture of an incompetent perforating vein (distal insufficiency).

In this case, the starting point of the insufficiency is moved away from the groin distally, but it has been shown that the proximal part of the saphenous system always becomes incompetent later, therefore, it does not make any sense to save it. The competent greater saphenous vein is, therefore, also removed from the groin to the proximal point of insufficiency. The incompetent perforating veins must be ligated under all circumstances; the remaining varicose greater saphenous vein is stripped.

2. Removal of the Varicose Greater Saphenous Vein and Its Branches [4, 10]

The day before surgery, the varicose vein and its branches are marked with a pen, with the patient standing up. The incompetent perforating veins, which can be suspected by bulging and a palpable defect in the fascia, are marked by rings or arrows. When a venography has been done, the markings on the legs of the patient are done according to the radiologic picture. During venography, the most important perforating veins can be exactly localized. We call these "key perforating veins." Usually one encounters two or three key perforating veins the ligating of which is crucial for the success of the procedure.

a) Side Branches. If varicose changes are present, these branches should be removed surgically as radically as possible, to limit later sclerosing therapy to small branches. For this purpose, we use small incisions (up to 15). With an anatomic dissecting clamp, the tip of which has longitudinal and transverse grooves, the convoluted varices can easily be removed by twisting (e.g., Rochester Carmalt, 16 cm, BH 801, Aesculap).

The distal end does not have to be ligated but must be compressed for 10 min.

b) Dissection of the Distal Greater Saphenous Vein. Investigations have shown that the greater saphenous vein should be dissected in the middle of the forefoot, as described by FISCHER [5], rather than through the commonly used incision at the level of the ankle (Fig. 27.2.5). Lymphatic vessels are not disturbed and the cosmetic result is better. At the tip of the arch between the inner and dorsal part of the foot, the vein can easily be marked preoperatively. A longitudinal incision, long enough to accept the tip of the stripper, is performed, and the vein with its branches at this point is dissected free. The distal end is ligated and transected. Proximal to the branch, a venotomy is made, and the stripper is inserted. It is important that the accompanying nerve be carefully dissected away.

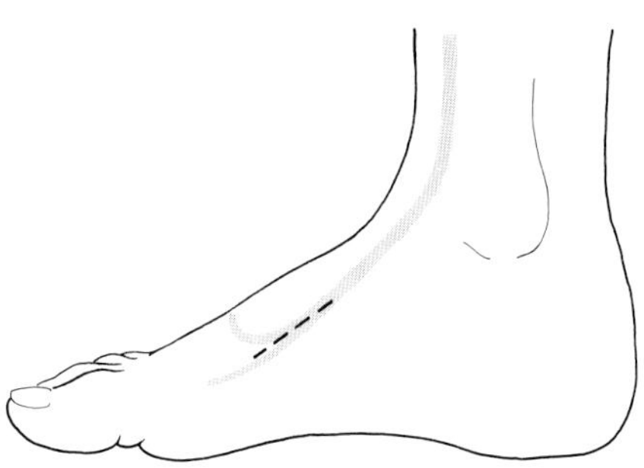

Fig. 27.2.5. Incision for exposure of the distal greater saphenous vein

c) Insertion of the Stripper. The stripper is usually made of plastic material and has an olive at each end. Proximally, a handle for extraction and distally, a tip of the appropriate size, depending on the diameter of the varicose veins, can be attached.

After the venotomy is made, the olive is introduced, and the stripper is advanced through the tortuous vein, guided by palpation through the skin. If the vein is not occluded, it can be advanced up into the groin, where the olive can be palpated. If the greater saphenous vein is only partially open, an elastic resistance prevents further advancement. In this case, the stripping distance has to be diminished and one proceeds stepwise.

d) Dissection of the Proximal Stripping Point. This is done as described for the exposure of the greater saphenous vein in the groin (see p. 701). If the probe is palpated at this point and the venous structures have been identified, a venotomy is made just distal to the junction with the femoral vein, and the stripper is pulled out. The saphenous vein is then transected and the small veins are removed as described earlier (see p. 701).

e) The Stripping Procedure. The stripping is done from distal to proximal. For this reason, the appropriate stripper head is attached distally and the handle for extraction proximally. If the extraction of the veins is done slowly, injuries to the cutaneous nerve are rare. These injuries can be further diminished if a stripper head is chosen that will not remove subcutaneous tissue.

The stripper is pulled out carefully and stepwise. As soon as a side branch is encountered, a small incision is made, and it is pulled out with a long, narrow, curved forceps. The stripping is then continued. The stripped varices are checked for completeness. If some vessels remain, they are removed through small stab wounds afterward.

III. Resection of the Lesser Saphenous Vein

1. Preliminary Remarks

During the last few years, the opinion of French surgeons that the lesser saphenous vein should be removed together with the greater saphenous vein has steadily gained ground. Indeed, the medial branches of the greater saphenous vein nearly always connect with the lesser saphenous vein. If there are only minimal varicose changes, the prob-

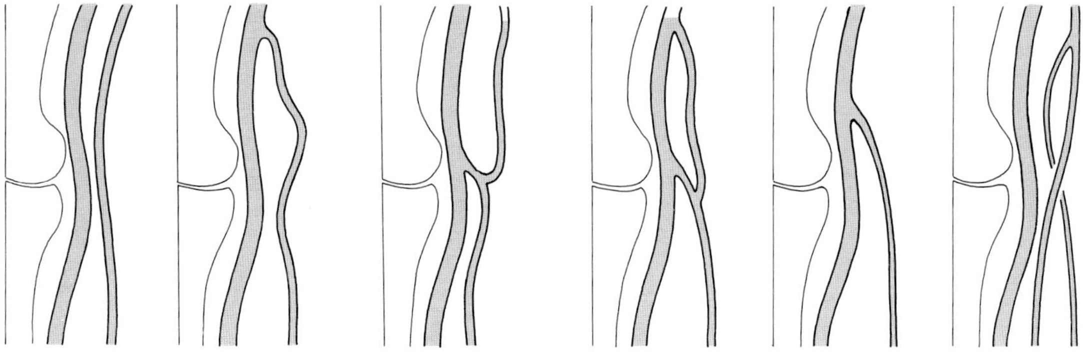

Fig. 27.2.6. Anatomic variations of the junction of the lesser saphenous vein, with frequency in percentages

lem of removal is solved more safely if they are pulled from both sides. Late results of this combined operation are definitely better. Furthermore, we know from experience that patients who present with a varicose greater saphenous vein, but whose lesser saphenous vein is still sufficient at that time, develop varicosity of the latter vein within several years. Nevertheless, today it is no longer permissible to remove a competent vein which might be used as a graft. We inform the patient of this situation in order to explain the necessity of the second operation. Another question is whether the lesser saphenous vein should be partially removed. The lesser saphenous vein is composed of two parts: the lower part runs subcutaneously, the upper part is located beneath the fascia but does not (as always reported and as one would expect) influence the extension of the varicose changes. Often, there are severe varicosities in the upper part down to the incompetent and often multiple perforating veins, which empty into the vv. gastrocnemiae (May's perforating veins). In these cases, it is superfluous to resect the lower competent part. This part can be used for an aortocoronary bypass. Varicose changes of the greater and lesser saphenous vein develop, related to the pressure gradient from proximal to distal. If the upper part of these varicose changes is ligated correctly, i.e., immediately at the junction of a deep vein, and the remaining segments, including the perforating veins which are always the end point of the resection, are removed, the competent distal segments of the greater and lesser saphenous vein remain functional for the rest of the patient's life. It is furthermore very important to know how many variations there can be in the site where the lesser saphenous vein empties into the popliteal vein.

Most anatomy books say that the lesser saphenous vein empties into the popliteal vein at the level of the knee joint. This is not true. On the basis of 1000 venographies, we have described six variations (Fig. 27.2.6). If one ligates the lesser saphenous vein at the level of the knee joint, one leaves a stump which will frequently lead to recurrence.

The reason for this recurrence is that just distal to where the lesser saphenous vein empties into the popliteal vein, it gives off a small branch that is known to physicians as the femoropopliteal vein (Fig. 27.2.7).

If this branch is not ligated, the same sequela occurs as in the case where a small venous branch remains following ligation of the great saphenous vein in the groin. Owing to the pressure from proximal, i.e., the blow-down, an ugly varicose vein will appear in the popliteal fossa. This explains why the follow-up after ligation of the lesser saphenous vein reveals a recurrence rate of 25%.

The name femoropopliteal vein is surely incorrect. This vein never connects the femoral vein with the popliteal vein. If the valve is functioning, it is simply a high side-branch of the lesser saphenous vein that connects via a perforating vein with the deep venous system in the mid-thigh region or below the gluteal fold. The vein can also curve along the inside of the thigh and join the greater saphenous vein. The postmedial branch of the greater saphenous vein then connects directly to the lesser saphenous vein. This vein is called vein of Giacomini [5, 10].

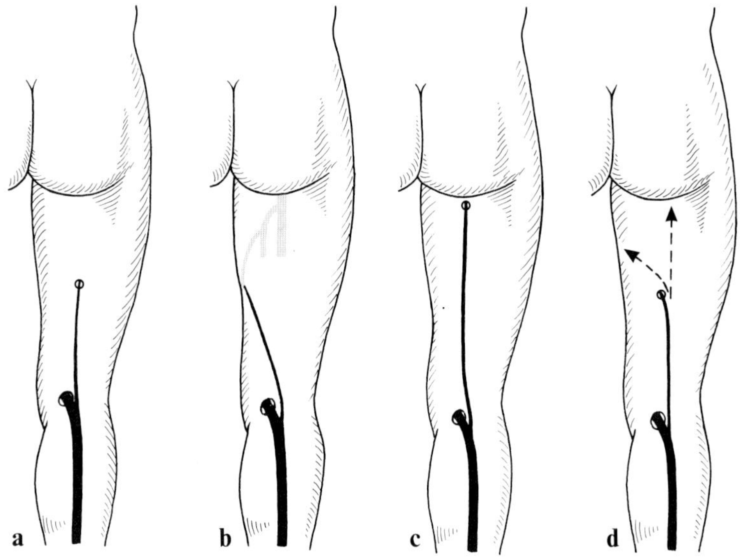

Fig. 27.2.7 a–d. The most common types of femoropopliteal vein

2. Roentgenologic Visualization of the Junction of the Lesser Saphenous Vein

This is a simple procedure which every surgeon must be able to perform. With the patient in the lateral position, any enlarged branch of the saphenous system is punctured. During the injection, the operating table is lowered slightly so that the junction can be visualized under fluoroscopic control and documented. As the injection continues, the foot of the X-ray table is lowered, allowing the distal portion of the lesser saphenous system to be visualized. Because of the different degree of venous filling, the junction should be documented with at least two or three films [3].

3. Summary of Guidelines for Ligation of the Lesser Saphenous Vein

1. Ligation of the lesser saphenous vein is correct only if the junction of the ever-present femoropopliteal vein is also resected.

2. Even if the femoropopliteal vein is not visualized during venography, because of incompetent valves, it nevertheless must be ligated.

3. If the femoropopliteal vein empties into an incompetent perforating vein at the mid-thigh level or below the gluteal fold, this perforating vein must be ligated. If it is small, it can also be evulsed. This junction is seen best when the patient is standing up, because the vein may disappear into the depth of the tissue.

4. If a vein can be probed with a stripper, it should be removed. This is especially true for the vein of Giacomini.

5. If the entire lesser saphenous vein is incompetent, the distal part, between the lateral ankle and the Achilles tendon, is clearly visible and easily marked with the patient standing up.

4. Positioning and Exposure

Prior to the operation, the lesser saphenous vein is located and marked in the popliteal fossa. This is easily done by having the patient stand and then bend the knee slightly. For the operation, we prefer the prone position. We begin with a 2 cm incision at the site previously marked in the popliteal fossa (Fig. 27.2.8). The fascia is opened transversely, the vein is grasped between two clamps, and the proximal end is put under tension and ligated proximal to the junction of the femoropopliteal vein. If the vein empties into the deeper system higher than normal, it is exposed first in the popliteal fossa. From the X-ray picture, the junction has been measured and marked on the skin. Pulling on the proximal stump allows a very small skin incision at the correct level. The proximal stump is pushed up to the second incision and put under tension. Without this second step, the incision will be significantly longer, and therefore cosmetically unfavorable, because the popliteal vein and its junction with the lesser saphenous vein is located deeper in the tissue at this point. The popliteal vein can be clearly visualized only in very slim patients.

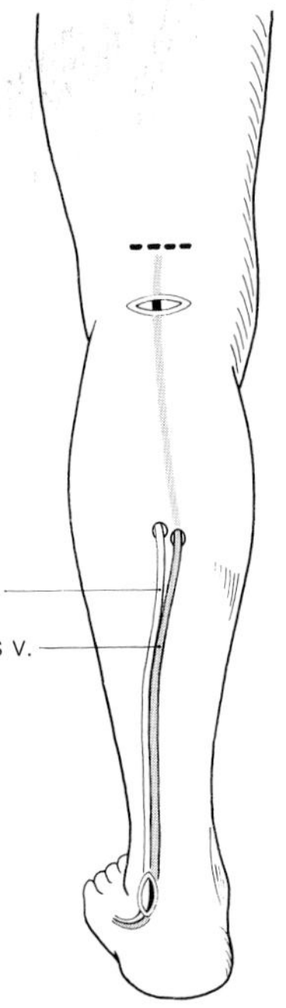

Fig. 27.2.8. Skin incision for the resection of the lesser saphenous vein

Nevertheless, one should be careful not to encroach on its lumen by pulling on the proximal stump of the lesser saphenous vein. The common mistake is to ligate the lesser saphenous vein too far distally.

5. Stripping of the Lesser Saphenous Vein

After the lesser saphenous vein has been ligated, the distal stump of the vein is probed. The stripper is inserted down to the previously marked incompetent perforating vein. At this point a skin incision of only ca. 6 mm is needed to bring the stripper out and to ligate the perforating vein and the distal stump. The fascial defect in the popliteal fossa is closed with a U-stitch.

If the lesser saphenous vein is incompetent over its entire length, the stripper will advance effortlessly down to the ankle region. Here, too, owing to the palpability of the stripper and the presence of a preoperative marking, only a small longitudinal skin incision is required. The sural nerve, lying close beside the vein, must be dissected away with great care. At the level of the distal ligature of the lesser saphenous vein, one frequently encounters a branch extending across the ankle; because this branch can be difficult to sclerose, it should be removed through a small stab wound. If it is difficult to advance the stripper from a distal direction during total stripping of the lesser saphenous vein, one can first expose the distal part of the vein and then advance the stripper proximally. The lesser saphenous vein, however, is always stripped from proximal to distal, to avoid injury to the sural nerve.

IV. Ligature of Incompetent Perforating Veins

The necessity of legating incompetent perforating veins has been repeatedly discussed. If one keeps in mind the principles of venous circulation according to Bjordal [1], which were described at the outset of this chapter, it is just as wrong to ligate all radiologically visible perforating veins as it is to abandon any attempt to ligate these veins. Experience shows that only those incompetent perforating veins should be ligated that are explicitly singled out and are radiologically significant. The ligation should be done subfascially. The defect in the fascia should be closed with a U-suture. The more distal the perforating vein is situated, the more important is its exclusion. In the lower leg, we ligate only those perforating veins which are especially large or which are located at the transition from a competent to an incompetent venous segment. In most cases, the ligature of two or three perforating veins is sufficient [13].

The technique is described in the chapter on post-thrombotic syndrome (see p. 731).

V. Surgery of Varicose Veins of the Inner and Outer Ankle Region

These varicose veins pose a special problem. They are not removed during the usual stripping procedure. Even though they are not very thick, they are difficult to sclerose, and are cosmetically disturbing for many patients. The failure of sclerotherapy is explained by the fact that these varices always have their origin in perforating veins (Fig. 27.2.9a, b).

Direction of flow in these perforating veins is, even under physiologic conditions, completely different from those of the leg. In the foot and also in the region of the inner and outer ankle, blood flows from the deep to the superficial veins during weight bearing. Therefore, the superficial veins of the foot, including the distal ends of the greater and lesser saphenous vein, are under more stress

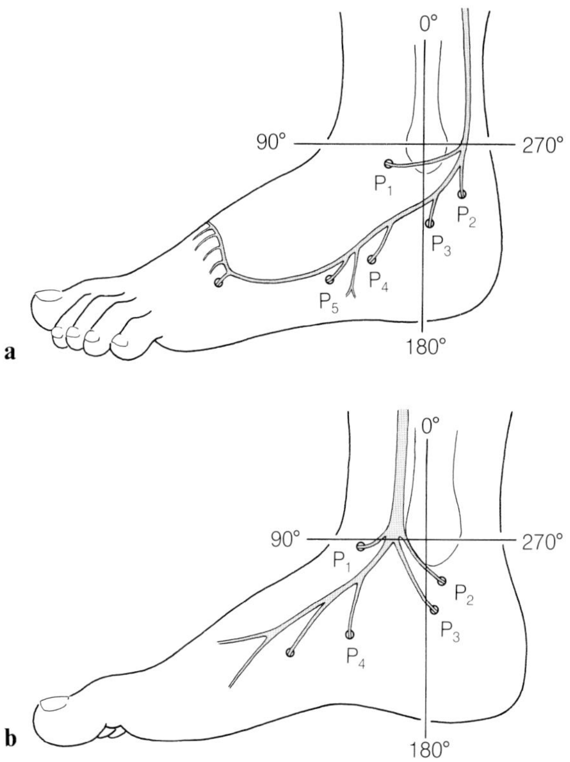

Fig. 27.2.9a, b. Varicose veins in the region of the ankle (perforating veins of Kuster). Localization is facilitated by the use of a system of coordinates with a zero point at the internal medial or lateral malleolus. **a** Lateral malleolus. **b** Medial malleolus

than they would be if they only had to drain blood from the skin and subcutaneous tissue. This becomes obvious if one of the perforating veins is evulsed. The brisk hemorrhage is impressive, even if the perforating vein is obviously competent. These perforating veins are often without a valve, or have only one valve, which directs the blood flow toward the surface. Therefore, the following therapy is necessary.

The perforating veins must be ligated. With the patient standing up, the veins are marked. Venography is not necessary. The anatomy of the perforating veins is for the most part constant. Usually, only from one to three branches exhibit varicosities, which means that at most three perforating veins have to be ligated. In order to keep a complete and precise record, we use the diagram and the grading system proposed by KUSTER, LOFGREN, and HOLLINSHEAD. We have suggested calling these perforating veins the "perforating veins of Kuster". Exposure of these perforating veins is done with the same instruments used for the dissection of lymphatic vessels. We carry out the dissection under magnification.

Resection of Varicose Veins on the Dorsum of the Foot. Varicose veins of the dorsum of the foot are removed only under special circumstances, using very fine instruments. The skin incisions have to be longitudinal in order not to injure the lymphatic vessels. Careful compression with foam rubber prevents hematoma formation.

VI. Recurrent Varices

Because patients with varices have a predisposition to this type of vascular disease, recurrences are common, even if optimal surgical technique is used. Therefore, patients should see a phlebologist every 1–2 years. In most cases, minor sclerosing treatments are sufficient.

Surgical intervention is indicated under the following circumstances: elimination of the blow-down in recurrent varices that originate from the groin, i.e., from the stump of the greater saphenous vein or directly from the femoral vein; elimination of the blow-down in the region of the popliteal vein; elimination of the blow-out, i.e., varicose veins that originate from the bigger incompetent perforating veins.

After these surgical interventions, remaining varicose veins can be easily sclerosed.

1. Operative Approach in Groin Recurrences [10]

Occasionally, recurrence results when the greater saphenous vein has not been ligated precisely at the level of the femoral vein. However, the recur-

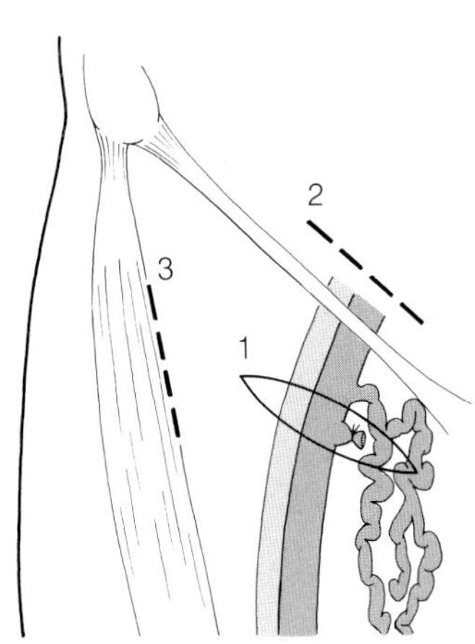

Fig. 27.2.10. Surgical approaches in recurrent varicose veins of the groin

rence usually originates from a superficial epigastric vein that has not been ligated and therefore continues to empty directly into the femoral vein, or even more often from an overlooked external pudendal vein. It is very surprising how large a varicosity can develop out of the unresected small branches through the dynamics of the blow-out. A recurrence in the groin, however, is not always caused by a technical mistake during the first operation. New collateral varicose veins may develop directly through the operation scar as a result of pressure from above (Fig. 27.2.10).

a) Surgical Technique According to LI. This technique consists of a wide excision at the root of the varicosity. We do not recommend this approach. It involves extensive destruction of lymphatic vessels, as demonstrated by the frequent development of postoperative lymphocele. In the scar tissue, which contains many small varices, an injury to the femoral vein is possible.

b) Exposure According to LUKE (Fig. 27.2.11a, b). We recommend this technique in almost every case. The femoral vein is dissected out in a region where no scars are encountered. A large transverse incision 2–3 fingerbreadths above the old scar is easily made. Once the artery has been dissected free, one can approach the femoral vein directly. Since the dissection is carried out from a lateral direction, it is very easily freed bluntly at its medial aspect. The roots of the varices are doubly ligated and transected. We always ignore the old scar. The varices, which are located distal to the old scar, can usually be extracted proximally with a fine curved forceps, or distally, with little effort. After the root has been ligated, bleeding is surprisingly minimal.

Only when the old scar is located in the groin do we use the approach of JUNOD, which is technically easier. Following an incision along the anterior border of the sartorius muscle, the artery is dissected free and retracted; then the femoral vein is exposed.

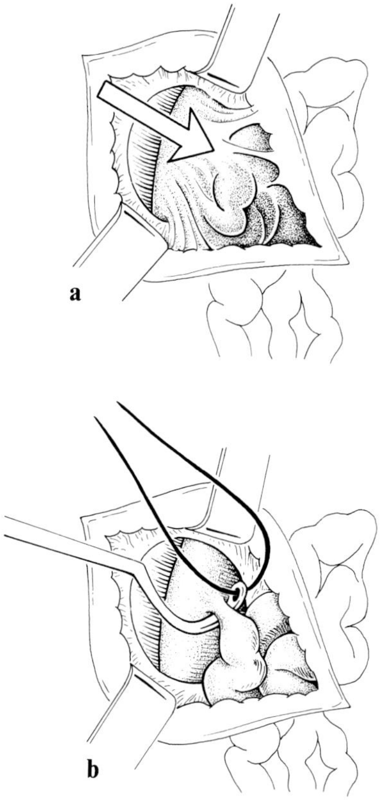

a

b

Fig. 27.2.11a, b. Ligation of the basis of the recurrent varicose veins in the groin. **a** With a lateral approach, the femoral artery and vein are identified. **b** The branch supplying the recurrence is doubly ligated and transected. In this way, one can avoid the more dangerous approach through the agglomeration of varices

2. Recurrence in the Popliteal Fossa

In this case venography is indispensable. The contrast medium injected into a superficial varicose vein shows that the recurrence originates from the stump of the lesser saphenous vein.

Circumstances will decide whether it is necessary to excise the old scar. We nearly always make a new skin incision more proximally. Since the incision has to be of sufficient length, cosmetic considerations are not appropriate here. However, we close the wound with intercutaneous sutures. We have never encountered injuries to the popliteal artery or vein. Only once did we notice an injury to the tibial nerve.

Recurrence in the popliteal fossa can also originate from a vein that empties directly into the popliteal vein independently of the lesser saphenous vein. This variation, which is not really rare, is called "popliteal fossa vein." The X-ray picture obtained by direct injection of the contrast material into the varicose vein, guides the surgical approach.

3. Ligation of Newly Formed or Previously Overlooked Perforating Veins

After radiologic localization, these veins are ligated subfascially through a small transverse incision.

Defects in the fascia and in the skin are closed (see p. 731). Sclerotherapy of remaining varicose veins can then proceed without difficulty.

VII. Surgery of the Venostasis Ulcers

After normal arterial circulation has been assured, one can distinguish between a venostasis ulcer with normal deep veins and a post-thrombotic venostasis ulcer where the deep veins have been damaged by a previous thrombosis. Even though the therapy is identical, the prognosis and postoperative treatment differ. A venostasis ulcer is easily managed, provided the deep veins are normal. The post-thrombotic stasis ulcer, even after optimal surgical therapy, requires lifelong compression treatment, since only the sequelae of the chronically damaged vein have been treated.

Venostasis Ulcer. Optimal treatment is surgical, because it removes the cause. The treatment consists of three surgical measures:

a) Removal of the blow-down: i.e., removal of the radiologically localized varicose veins.
b) Exact exposure and ligation of the incompetent perforating veins.
c) In case of extensive ulcer scars, wide total resection, either simultaneously or in a later procedure. Whether the defect is covered with a split-thickness skin graft, Reverdin grafts, or mesh graft is of secondary importance.

Our Procedure. Every venostasis ulcer will heal under compression treatment, but recurrence must be expected. Only venography will determine the exact cause. The radiologic findings determine the therapy in each case: ligation of the incompetent perforating veins, elimination of the blow-down. These procedures can be done simultaneously with the excision and grafting of the ulcer, if necessary. Frequently, the X-ray pictures will show that the responsible incompetent perforating veins are not to be found beneath the ulcer.

VIII. Surgical Correction of Primary Incompetent Valves

Primary incompetence of vein valves is so frequent and the complaints are so minimal that it is debatable whether surgical correction is really justifiable in such cases. The decision must be made on an individual basis. The objective parameters do not always correspond to the complaints of the patient. If there is a tendency toward swelling and a feeling of heaviness, surgical intervention can be considered. In the beginning we were very skeptical because the venous valves consist of only two layers of endothelium with a very thin layer of connective tissue in between at the base. Injury to the valves leads to shrinkage. Since shrinkage after suturing of a valve has not been observed in animal experiments, a plastic operation on the vein valves in selected cases may have a future. One should observe the classification proposed by SANDMANN [14]:

Type A. Increased length of the valve leaflets through loss of elasticity, as described by KISTNER [7]. If the central venous pressure is elevated, the valves will collapse, and reflux will occur.

Type B. Enlargement of the annulus of the valves secondary to ectasia of the vein. One can also include in this group slight cases of post-thrombotic injury to the femoral vein with destruction of the valves.

The distinction between the two groups is essential for the operative treatment. Only with type A does a valvuloplasty as described by KISTNER [7] make sense. In type B patients, one can take advantage of the fact that, even if there is a post-thrombotic injury of the femoral vein, the strong valve at the proximal end of the femoral vein remains intact.

Preparation for Surgery. If there are varicosities in the distribution of the greater saphenous vein, these must be eliminated if the occlusion test is positive, as must incompetent peripheral perforating veins. Many of the procedures on the deep veins that have now been abandoned showed positive results because they were combined with other proven methods. The incompetence of valves can be demonstrated by Doppler ultrasonography with the Valsalva maneuver. The accuracy of Doppler ultrasonography is surprisingly high; nevertheless, we still perform retrograde pressure venography in all cases. A good X-ray picture provides the most exact intraoperative information about the status of the valves. But in view of the reliability of Doppler ultrasonography, we agree with Sandmann [14], that venography will not be necessary in all cases in the future.

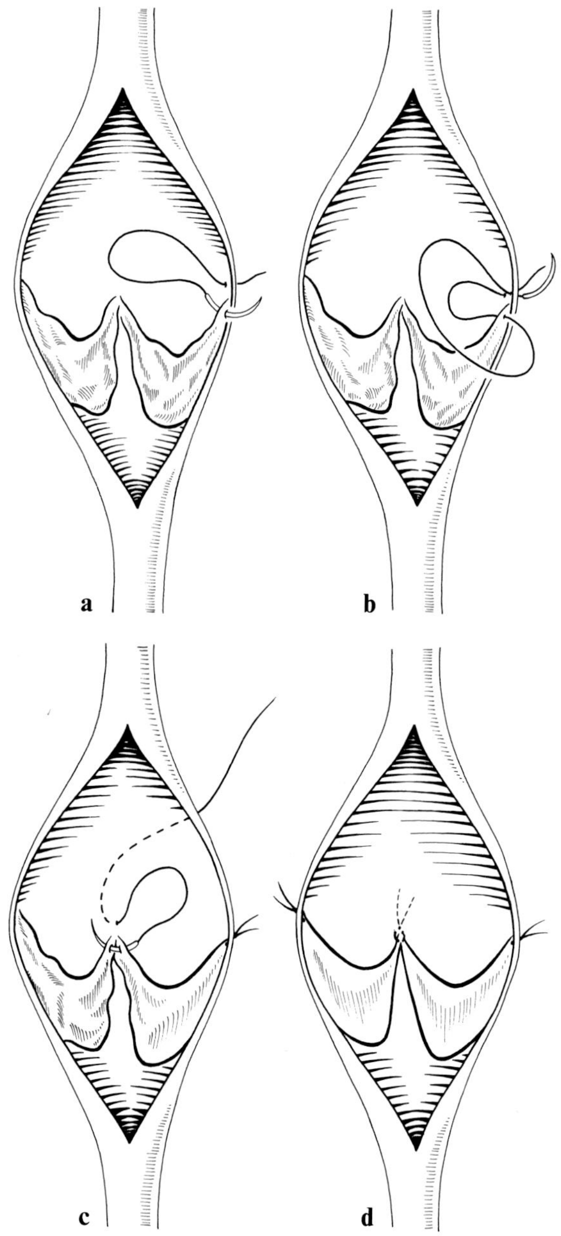

Fig. 27.2.12a–d. Valvuloplasty for incompetent valves. **a, b** With 7-0 monofilament nonabsorbable suture material the medial and lateral suspensions of the valves are shortened; the knot lies on the outside of the vessel. **c, d** In the same manner, the valves are shortened in the commissure

1. Type A: Elongation of the Valve Edges with Reflux During the Valsalva Maneuver: Surgical Technique

The following figures illustrate the Kistner technique (quoting from Sandmann [14]):

"The operation should be done under regional anesthesia to ensure cooperation of the patient for the Valsalva maneuver with Doppler sonography before and after the valve reconstruction. The femoral vein is dissected free over a long distance, including its tributaries, which are occluded with silicone bands. The femoral vein is then opened anteriorly between two stay sutures, and with the aid of magnification the elongated cusps of the valves are fixed at the posterior and anterior commissure with 1 or 2 7-0 monofilament, nonabsorbable sutures. The closure of the venotomy is done with the same suture material" (Fig. 27.2.12a–d).

2. Type B: Incompetence of the Valvular Annulus Resulting from Ectasia of the Vein or Post-thrombotic Damage to the Valves of the Femoral Vein

This procedure can be of importance when the valves are congenitally absent. Even in these cases, the important valve at the proximal end of the femoral vein is intact.

Again, we report the surgical procedure according to Sandmann [14]:

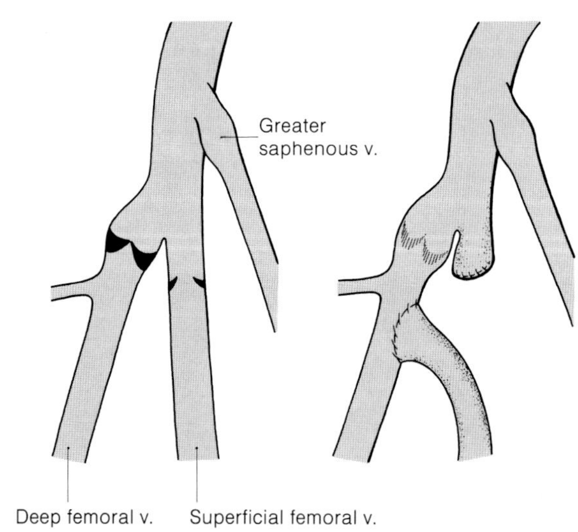

Fig. 27.2.13. Transposition of the superficial femoral vein in the case of an incompetent valve. The functioning valve at the junction of the deep femoral vein stops venous reflux

"The deep femoral vein is dissected free over a long distance, and the valve at its emptying point is localized. It is isolated from the venous circulation by means of a tourniquet band, and a longitudinal venotomy is made distal to the valve. The superficial femoral vein is divided and its distal stump anastomosed to the venotomy with 7-0 interrupted sutures. Its proximal stump is closed with a continuous suture immediately distal to the junction with the deep femoral vein. The procedure is monitored intraoperatively and postoperatively by ultrasonography" (Fig. 27.2.13).

Most authors report favorable late results. Our experience indicates that this surgical procedure may withstand the test of time.

3. Transplantation of Valve-Bearing Segments of the Brachial Vein

We can only mention this procedure; owing to the small number of cases and the lack of late follow-up, no final judgment is possible.

E. Postoperative Treatment

Just before the skin is closed, the leg is elevated and hematomas are expressed. After suture of the skin, a compression dressing is applied, which is supplemented by rubber foam sheets; this dressing remains in place until the sutures are removed. After removal of the sutures, the compression dressing is renewed every 10 days, until all indurations and hematomas have disappeared. This postoperative treatment largely determines the success of the procedure. If necessary, sclerotherapy can be done after approximately 6 weeks.

Until the treatment has been terminated, the legs should always be elevated when the patient is lying down.

The length of the hospital stay and whether the procedure can be done on an outpatient basis depends on the local conditions.

F. Complications

I. Injury to the Nerves (Saphenous Nerve and Sural Nerve)

Because of the close proximity of the nerves to the main venous trunks, minor loss of sensation cannot always be avoided. Most authors report that the direction of the stripping is important: when the stripping is done from proximal to distal, there is less injury to the nerves. It is important to note that the risk of injury to the sensory nerves is less if the subcutaneous fat is thick. If the circumference of the calf is above 29 cm, injury to the nerves is hardly possible. In our experience, it is essential to proceed carefully. If the head of the stripper is so large that one also removes subcutaneous fat, the corresponding nerves can also be injured. We usually strip the greater saphenous vein from proximal to distal. Contrary to the reports of other authors, we did not find that stripping in the opposite direction produced any significant sensory loss. Temporary loss of sensation in the lower leg, up to an area the size of the palm of the hand, cannot always be avoided and is of no consequence. If one strips the lesser saphenous vein, the distal part of the sural nerve is endangered. It is again impossible to avoid some local loss of sensation along the lateral margin of the foot, but the patient will tolerate such a loss. It is important to inform the patient that the circulation is not compromised. However, when we strip the lesser saphenous vein, under no circumstances do we extract it from distal to proximal.

II. Lymphedema and Lymphocele

Persistent swelling after surgery for varicose veins is usually caused by lymphatic problems. It is important to know that the number of lymph vessels and their ability to compensate can vary considerably. BRUNNER [3] emphasizes that one should avoid narrow places where lymph vessels lie close together (Fig. 27.2.14). Some degree of damage to lymph vessels is unavoidable even when the operation is technically flawless. Minimal damage must be the objective. Therefore, in every operation for varicose veins, from the first incision to the last, one should be mindful of the need to spare the lymph vessels, which are, of course, doubly vulnerable because they are invisible. The smallest possi-

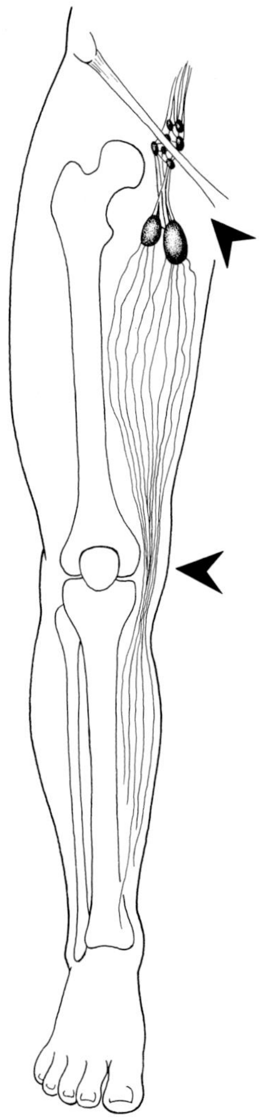

Fig. 27.2.14. Narrowing of the lymphatic vessels according to BRUNNER [13]. Injury in the area marked by *arrows*, including large incisions, can lead to secondary lymphedema

ble incisions should be the rule. One must never "dig" into the subcutaneous fat. If a swelling is noted postoperatively, a compression dressing should be applied carefully until the swelling has completely subsided, even if this takes months.

1. Lymphoceles in the Groin

We occasionally observe lymphoceles in the groin after operating for recurrences. After the lymphocele has been emptied, it disappears, usually within a few weeks.

2. Lymphoceles of the Lower Leg

These lymphoceles are rare but apparently not completely avoidable. We have seen such lymphoceles as far as 4 cm from the nearest, very small incision. Performing surgery for varicose veins 800 times a year, we see such a lymphocele about every 2 years.

The number has been reduced during the past 5 years, since we ligate the distal greater saphenous vein only at the level of the arch of the foot.

3. Therapy

Therapy consists of aspiration and carefully applied compression dressings. If the lymphocele is not diminished in size after 6 weeks, one cannot expect a spontaneous resolution. Total excision of the lymphocele is often futile. We recommend coloring the lymphatic vessels by means of a subcutaneous injection of methylene blue in the first and second interdigital space. Then 4 h later, the cyst is opened. If the leg is massaged, one can see the leak in the lymphatic vessels by the appearance of the blue dye. A suture ligature resolves the complication.

III. Erysipelas

After surgery for varicose veins, even after 2–3 years, we see this complication not infrequently. It should probably be regarded as one of the late sequelae of an injury to the lymphatic vessels.

IV. Thrombotic Complications

While thrombosis following surgery on the legs can never be completely avoided, thrombotic complications after surgery for varicose veins are astonishingly rare. Persistent swelling as a result of damage to the deep veins occurs, with few exceptions, in patients in whom this damage was already present preoperatively. In the varicose vein operation functionally significant collateral circulation is removed, and, as a result, the preexisting swelling, which was hardly noticeable before, becomes much worse. The steady stream of claims for compensation in such cases points up the importance of preoperative radiologic evaluation of the deep veins in all doubtful cases.

V. Ligation or Stripping of the Femoropopliteal Vein

This complication will not occur if one adheres to the guidelines described here for exposure of the greater and lesser saphenous vein. In addition, the stripper should always be advanced through the greater saphenous vein carefully and under digital control, from distal to proximal. One can probe from proximal to distal only when performing a partial resection of the lesser saphenous vein, and then only if the anatomic situation is certain. If the stripper meets resistance and cannot be advanced further by means of careful rotation, one should make a small incision rather than apply more force to the stripper, as this will only increase the risk of perforation.

Even when the X-ray picture is clear, an injury to the popliteal vein is possible if the stripper is advanced through an incompetent perforating vein into the deep system or if one makes the cross-incision in the popliteal fossa at the wrong level, even though the X-ray picture is clear. The lesser saphenous vein must lie immediately beneath the fascia. Then too, the junction of the lesser saphenous vein might have been incorrectly marked when the patient was in the standing position with the knee bent. If one is not able to find the lesser saphenous vein immediately beneath the fascia, it is wrong to look for the head of the stripper in the deep tissues. One should then make a small incision in the skin more proximally, where one can just feel the stripper head through the skin. If any doubt remains, under no circumstances should one ligate or strip. The rule is: never proceed if in doubt! If there is the slightest suspicion of an injury to the deep veins, one should always assume the worst, terminate the operation, apply compression, and consult a vascular surgeon, or arrange for helicopter transport to an appropriate hospital and accompany the patient during the transport. Because of the severe bleeding and the variability of the deep venous system, a nonvascular surgeon will have difficulty in clarifying the situation. If a partial stripping of the femoral or popliteal vein has occurred, it is impossible to give guidelines. Each case requires individualized measures. Intentionally to terminate the operation by ligating the popliteal vein or the femoral vein can no longer be justified.

VI. Injury to the Femoral Artery

Every surgeon should be able to deal with small injuries to this artery (see p. 247). However, every year there are reports of major injuries, even stripping of the artery from the groin to below the knee. Smaller defects can be managed with vein grafts, following careful removal of clots from the distal stump. Larger defects require longer grafts. In all cases that have come to our attention, the greater saphenous vein on one side was fortunately intact and able to be used as a graft. If the patient complains of severe pain following surgery, the compression dressing must be removed temporarily, allowing the arterial circulation to be checked by Doppler ultrasonography and documented on the chart. In most cases, one is dealing with hypersensitive patients, and more often than not, the problem is simply that the compression dressing is too tight. However, the diagnosis of psychologic instability is no reason for delaying treatment.

VII. Hematomas

Hematomas should always be evacuated through an opening in the skin incision. Evacuation of hematomas in the region of the groin is especially important, because the healing of the wound is here especially endangered. One should keep in mind that it is good practice to compress the area of stripping for 10 min at the end of surgery. However, this does not eliminate the need for suturing large side branches.

VIII. Wound Infections

Wound infections are possible following the ligation of incompetent perforating veins cranial to healed venostasis ulcers, even if meticulously sterile technique is used. If an elevation of temperature occurs, all surgical wounds should be inspected. Only then can one decide whether surgical drainage or antibiotic therapy is indicated.

IX. Septicemia (Mostly Due to Streptococci)

This complication is very rare, but it carries a high mortality. The clinical impression of a severely ill patient should make the diagnosis or at least raise suspicions. Septic temperatures and chills are suspicious signs. However, they can occur late, even if antibiotics have not been used. The results of blood analysis can also be indeterminate in the early phase. The following measures are indicated: all surgical wounds must be inspected by an experienced surgeon and, if necessary, opened. In some cases, a wide incision (without regard to later cosmetic results) should be made. Before bacteriologic results are available, massive antibiotic therapy (for example penicillins, cephalosporins) is indicated (see p. 167).

REFERENCES

1. Bjordal R (1981) In: Venae perforantes. Urban & Schwarzenberg, München
2. Brunner U (1979) Die Leiste. Huber, Bern
3. Brunner U (1975) Die Kniekehle. Huber, Bern
4. Cockett B (1976) In: Dodd H, Cockett FB (eds) The pathology and surgery of the veins of the lower limb. Churchill Livingstone, Edinburgh
5. Fischer R (1976) In: Die chirurgische Behandlung der Varizen. Huber, Bern
6. Hach W (1981) In: Spezielle Diagnostik der primären Varikose. Demeter, Gräfeling
7. Kistner RL, Sparkuhl MD (1979) Surgery in acute and chronic venous disease. Surgery 85:31–43
8. May R, Nißl R (1973) In: Die Phlebographie der unteren Extremität. Thieme, Stuttgart
9. May R, Weber J (1984) In: Funktionelle Phlebographie der Bein- und Beckenvenen. Thieme, Stuttgart
10. May R (1979) In: Surgery of the veins of the leg and pelvis. Thieme, Stuttgart
11. May R, Kriessmann A (1978) In: Periphere Venendruckmessung. Thieme, Stuttgart
12. May R (1984) In: Die Licht-Reflexions-Rheographie – LRR. Perimed, Erlangen
13. May R, Partsch H, Staubesand J (1981) Venae perforantes. Urban & Schwarzenberg, München
14. Sandmann W (1982) Chirurgische Therapie der primären Femoralklappeninsuffizienz. In: Hach W (eds) Die Chirurgie der Venen. Schattauer, Stuttgart

27.3 Acute Venous Thrombosis (Upper and Lower Extremities)

H. STIEGLER and L. SUNDER-PLASSMANN

CONTENTS

A. Lower Extremity

I. Anatomy

Venous blood returns by the veins of the superficial and deep system. While the superficial veins are, as a rule, single vessels, in the deeper system two veins usually accompany an artery; proximal to the knee joint, however, the deep veins are also predominantly single vessels (Fig. 2.1.13, see p. 26), [6].

Superficial venous system: They lie above the crural and femoral fascia in the subcutaneous tissue and are, therefore, not influenced by the muscle pump; they are connected with the deep veins through the perforating and communicating veins. The valves of the perforating and communicating veins are arranged in such a way that the blood flow is directed only from the superficial to the deep system as long as the valves are functioning. In the region of the foot, there are also perforating and communicating veins, but without valves. A reversal of flow is pathologic, causing venostasis ulcer and its sequelae. The superficial venous drainage of the foot follows a medial course into the greater saphenous vein, which passes in front of the medial malleolus, then behind the medial condyle, and finally, 2–3 cm below the inguinal ligament, empties into the femoral vein through the oval fossa. In 3.8%–27.0% of all cases, a doubling of the greater saphenous vein occurs. Even a division into three vessels has been reported. Abnormalities of the junction include a distal junction (emptying into the superficial femoral vein in the middle of the thigh) and a proximal junction (emptying, for example, into the inferior epigastric vein). The lesser saphenous vein arises from the lateral rim of the venous arch on the dorsum of the foot and empties into the popliteal vein.

Deep venous system: This consists of the entirety of the subfascial veins, which carry over 90% of the venous blood of the lower extremity. As a rule, they accompany the corresponding arteries and are known as the anterior and posterior tibial veins and the fibular veins. The perforating and communicating veins receive the blood from the superficial system. In 28% of healthy patients the communications between these veins can be found. The popliteal vein, arising from this system, can be single, double, or triple. Arising from the adductor canal, the superficial femoral vein carries the main burden of the venous return. In 21% of cases it is double, and further division (3%) is known. In the region of the lower leg, valves occur at relatively short intervals of 3–5 cm. The intervals are greater in the region of the thigh, where one can expect only 1–3 (maximally 6) venous valves.

Between the superficial femoral vein and the deep femoral vein a distal connection can occur at the level of the adductors, which can function as important collaterals if a proximal obstruction occurs. Above the inguinal ligament, the iliac vein is located medial to the artery in its distal course.

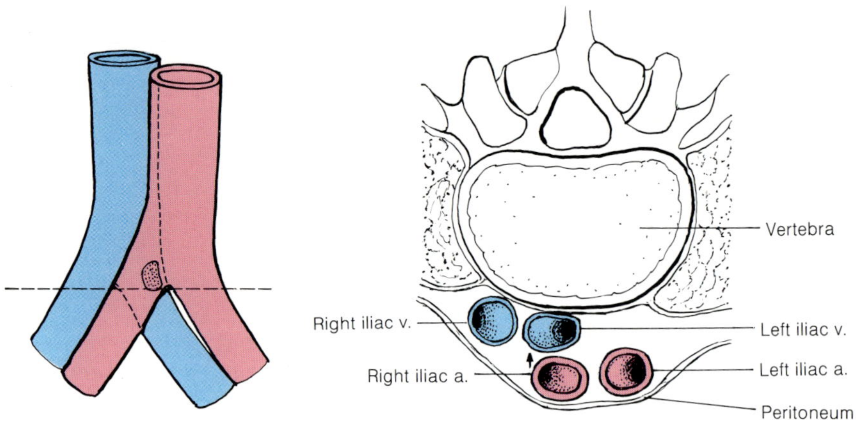

Fig. 27.3.1. Pelvic vein spur. As a result of the pulsation of the right iliac artery against the left iliac vein (which lies on top of the anterior longitudinal ligament and therefore cannot move) intimal lesions develop, which produce the spur in its chronic form (see p. 735)

On the right side, the artery crosses the vein proximally 5 fingerbreadths above the inguinal ligament. This can be seen on venograms. In its course, it accepts the deep iliac circumflex vein and the inferior epigastric vein. After accepting the internal iliac vein, thereby becoming the common iliac vein, it joins the inferior vena cava at the level of the fifth lumbar vertebra. Prior to the venous bifurcation, the iliac vein accepts the ascending lumbar vein, which carries blood from the paravertebral plexus. This vein can assume an essential collateral function, particularly in case of a venous spur. Such a spur is present in 20% of all adults. It occurs on the left side and results from the microtraumatic pulsing action of the right common iliac artery against the left common iliac vein, which, lying behind the artery on the anterior longitudinal ligament, cannot give way (Fig. 27.3.1 and see p. 735) [7, 8, 12]. This spur can become a significant risk factor leading to decompensation in the form of a thrombosis, e.g., in cases where immobilization (cast, operation, etc.) is involved.

This assertion is supported by the fact that two-thirds of all spontaneous deep vein thromboses occur on the left side. The external and common iliac vein and the inferior vena cava have, with very few exceptions, no valves.

II. Indications for Venous Thrombectomy

For the treatment of acute venous thrombosis of the lower extremity, there are three options.

1. Immobilization for at least 8 days and heparin therapy afterward, mobilization under anticoagulant medication (unless contraindicated) and compression therapy
2. Systemic fibrinolysis; rarely, local fibrinolysis [2]
3. Thrombectomy/heparin.

The first option is chosen if there are contraindications to fibrinolysis or surgery.

Contraindications to fibrinolysis (see also p. 106) are:

a) *Absolute:*
   Coagulation defect
   Previous surgery (less than 10 days before)
   Operations on the central nervous system
   Trauma to the central nervous system
   Cerebrovascular accident
   Hypertension
   Peptic ulcer
   Renal calculi
   Acute pancreatitis
   Endocarditis
   Progressive malignancy
   Intramuscular or intra-arterial injections (less than 10 days before)
   Pregnancy
   Phlegmasia cerulea dolens
b) *Relative:*
   Patient's age (about 70 years)
   Diabetes mellitus
   Age of the thrombosis (more than 14 days)

Contraindications to surgery are:

a) *Absolute:*
Progressive malignancy
Isolated venous thrombosis of the lower leg
Intolerance of general anesthesia
Danger of local wound-healing problems (i.e., folliculitis)
b) *Relative:*
Age of the thrombosis (older than 14 days)
Patient's age (older than 70 years)
Clinically significant pulmonary emboli

In cases of uncontrolled malignancy in patients above 70 years of age, treatment with heparin and perhaps warfarin remains the therapy of choice, because the patient will not live long enough to experience the post-thrombotic syndrome. As a rule, therapy should also be limited to heparin if the thrombosis is older than 2 weeks and already in the stage of organization, because by neither operation nor fibrinolysis (except in special cases) can one achieve a complete restoration, saving the function of the venous valves (late lysis, late thrombectomy). If the thrombosis is older than 14 days, one can expect good results with lysis and surgery only if the pelvic level alone is involved. In other words, exceptions to the 14-day rule make sense only for thrombosis at the level of the pelvis. This is especially true if one cannot demonstrate collaterals radiologically, and a significant difference in circumference of the legs is present.

If the thrombosis is 8–14 days old and if only the pelvic veins are involved, the therapy of choice is either surgery or lysis. If the veins of the upper and lower leg are also affected, one will also opt for surgery or fibrinolysis. In these cases, the prognosis with regard to a post-thrombotic syndrome is determined by the residues on the upper and lower leg [3].

If the thrombosis is limited to the deep veins of the upper and lower leg, the chances for its complete removal after the eighth day by means of indirect maneuvers (manual compression, Esmarch bandage compression, see p. 722) are considerably diminished. However, if no local collaterals can be demonstrated radiologically and the symptoms are severe, one will, nevertheless, decide in favor of surgery or thrombolysis.

If the clinical course is characterized by two episodes, the time of the second episode should be used to determine the age of the thrombosis, especially in cases where the symptoms during the second episode are more pronounced than during the first.

One can hardly expect full recovery after heparin therapy alone. Therefore, it should never be the therapy of first choice.

Criteria for and against surgery are:

1. *Phlegmasia cerulea dolens:* If the venous lumen becomes completely occluded, the resulting disturbance in the arterial circulation can easily lead to gangrene. Here, the time factor is decisive for the prognosis; immediate operative intervention is indicated.

2. *Venous thrombosis in patients with contraindications to fibrinolysis:* Immobilization, especially postoperative immobilization, is a frequent cause of venous thrombosis. Because of the danger of bleeding and/or wound complications after the tenth postoperative day, thrombectomy is the method of choice.

3. *Venous thrombosis following unsuccessful fibrinolysis:* If one has not achieved success with fibrinolysis after 6 days, operative intervention should be considered. With fibrinolysis, the degree to which the thrombus adheres to the vascular wall seems to decrease, and the chance of removing it mechanically is enhanced.

4. *Venous thrombosis with recurrent pulmonary embolus:* If, for example, a paraplegia is present, and therefore the risk of immobilization cannot be reduced, a blocking operation should be considered in cases of recurrent pulmonary emboli (caval umbrella, caval clip, ligation of a vein, see p. 745) in order to prevent further emboli. A venous thrombectomy or lysis promises long-term success only if the underlying risk factors can be influenced. If one decides to treat the thrombosis actively, systemic fibrinolysis should be preferred over surgery, because it also reduces the stress on the right heart caused by the pulmonary embolism. Subsequent treatment with warfarin should reduce the risk of recurrent thrombosis and of pulmonary emboli. If recurrent pulmonary embolus occurs in spite of this, interruption of the vena cava is indicated, if the pulmonary embolus is clinically compensated (see p. 744) [15].

5. *Isolated venous thrombosis* in the region of the lower leg. Here, one should not operate, since the

results without surgery (heparin therapy) are just as good. If venography shows a complete occlusion of the lumen and there is significant swelling of the lower leg, lysis therapy is indicated.

6. *In venous thrombosis not older than 14 days* and without contraindications to lysis, both approaches are justified. At the level of the pelvis, an operation – possibly with the additional construction of an arteriovenous fistula – promises greater success; at the level of the upper and lower leg, however, the results with lysis seem to be better. The decision can be made only after a prospective randomized trial. Until then, the method chosen should be that with which one has the greatest experience.

7. One should determine the possibility of *isolated perfusion of an extremity with streptokinase or urokinase* alone, or in combination with venous thrombectomy [13].

III. Positioning

A thrombectomy at the level of the pelvis is done in a supine position with the body elevated 40° (reverse Trendelenburg position) (Fig. 27.3.2). The entire leg is prepared for surgery, as this allows for free manipulation during manual compression or expression with an Esmarch bandage. Furthermore, except for the inguinal region, the entire abdomen and the thorax should be prepared, so that an immediate sternotomy with pulmonary artery embolectomy can be performed in the event of a fulminant pulmonary embolism (see p. 741). If a perforation occurs as a consequence of maneuvering the balloons in the vena cava or in the pelvis, a laparotomy or an extraperitoneal approach to the retroperitoneal area should be possible. Preparation of the contralateral side is not necessary. During a unilateral operation the opposite side can be protected by ipsilateral blocking [1, 6, 8].

IV. Surgical Approach and Exposure of Vessels

The exposure of the venous structures at the level of the groin are done through a slightly curved 8-cm incision, ending cephalad at the level of the inguinal ligament (Fig. 27.3.3). A transverse incision should be avoided so as not to damage the lymphatic vessels. After the subcutaneous tissue is transected and the common femoral artery has been identified by palpation, the femoral vein can be exposed medial to the artery. If this is difficult, especially in obese patients, the greater saphenous vein can be identified and used as a guide for the dissection cephalad and deep. In no case should

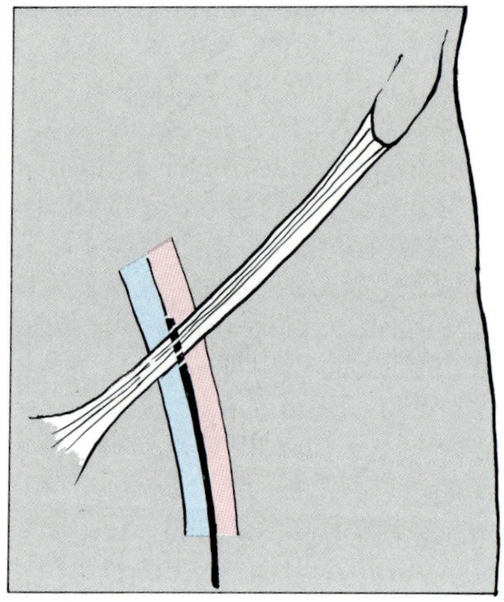

Fig. 27.3.3. Skin incision for thrombectomy. The lateral lymphatic collectors are not touched. The incision can be extended proximally by incising the inguinal ligament

Fig. 27.3.2. Positioning (reverse Trendelenburg)

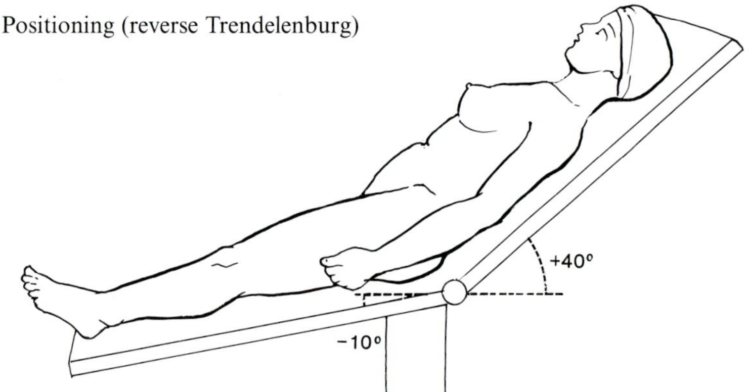

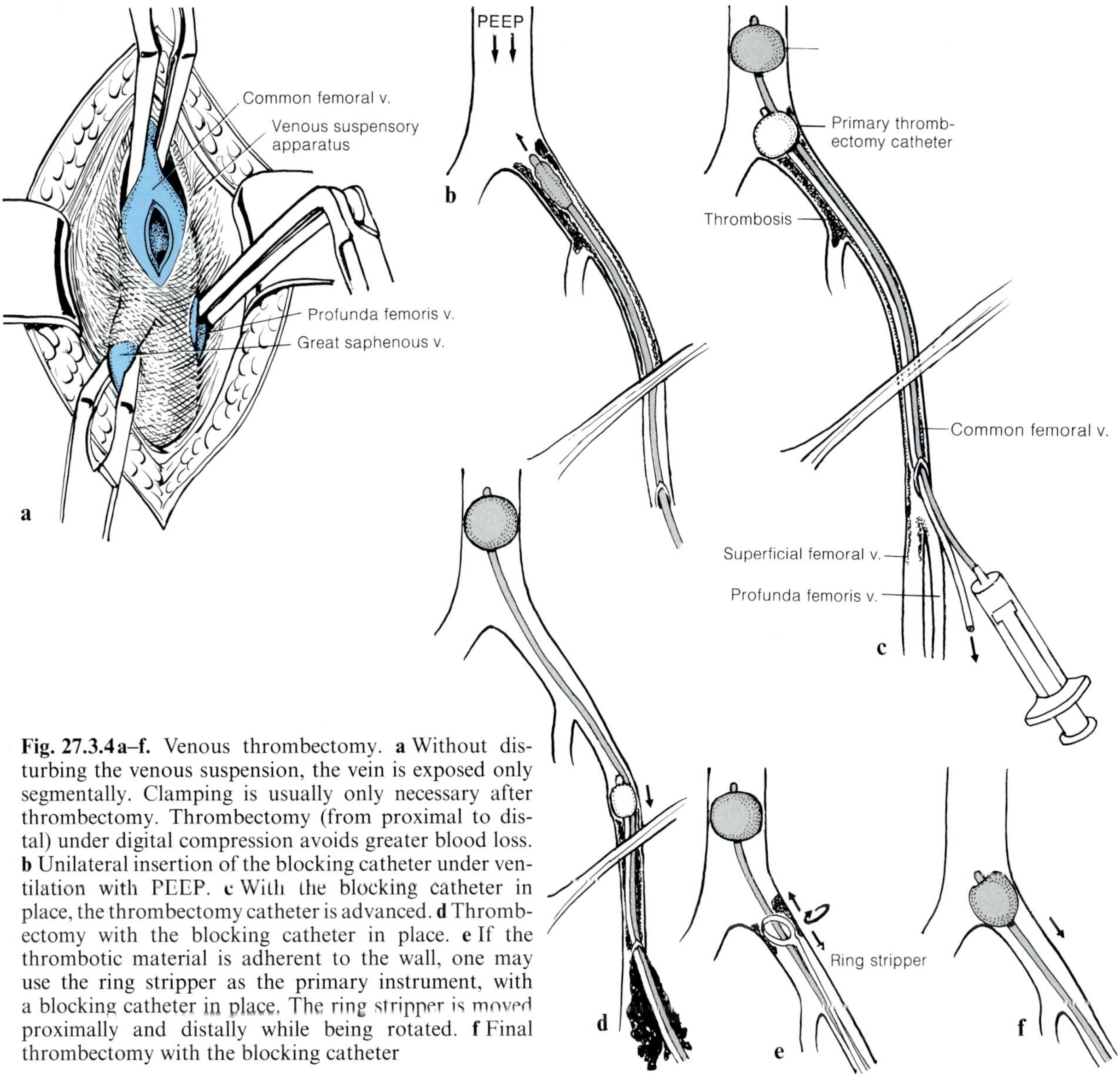

Fig. 27.3.4a–f. Venous thrombectomy. **a** Without disturbing the venous suspension, the vein is exposed only segmentally. Clamping is usually only necessary after thrombectomy. Thrombectomy (from proximal to distal) under digital compression avoids greater blood loss. **b** Unilateral insertion of the blocking catheter under ventilation with PEEP. **c** With the blocking catheter in place, the thrombectomy catheter is advanced. **d** Thrombectomy with the blocking catheter in place. **e** If the thrombotic material is adherent to the wall, one may use the ring stripper as the primary instrument, with a blocking catheter in place. The ring stripper is moved proximally and distally while being rotated. **f** Final thrombectomy with the blocking catheter

the venous junction be destroyed by ligation, as it represents collaterals. In cases of a thrombotic occlusion, the femoral vein is engorged. In contrast to the usual technique of encircling arteries with a tape, dissection of the vein should be limited to the shortest possible segments at the sites where clamps are to be placed. It is not necessary to encircle them. The reason for this limited preparation is that the suspension in the surrounding tissues prevents the collapse of the vein (Fig. 27.3.4a).

It is essential that the deep femoral vein, which comes from a dorsolateral direction, be exposed over a distance of 1–2 cm. Thrombectomy of this vessel assumes an importance similar to that of an embolectomy of the corresponding artery, since the femoral vein can accept collaterals from the popliteal region when the superficial femoral vein is occluded. Exposure of the proximal greater saphenous vein is also necessary to remove thrombotic material.

If the junction of the deep femoral vein is situated rather high, the incision can be extended by partially transecting the inguinal ligament. Depending on the extent of the incision, reconstruction of the inguinal ligament is necessary to prevent the development of a femoral hernia. If, during the operation, an arteriovenous fistula is indicated, the superficial femoral artery is exposed and encircled.

V. Thrombectomy

Systemic heparinization should be started with an intravenous bolus (10000 I.V. heparin iv) after the diagnosis is made or, even better, when a deep venous thrombosis is suspected. Heparinization should be continued by controlled infusion to maintain a partial thromboplastin time (PTT) between 80 and 120 s: This approach makes heparin injection after clamping of the veins unnecessary. Because clamping can provoke a pulmonary embolism, the intubated patient is ventilated with PEEP by hand. The PEEP should be high enough to cause a marked reduction of venous return, resulting in a drop in blood pressure. This kind of ventilation is maintained until the thrombectomy of the proximal segment is completed. This diminishes the venous return from the lower half of the body to the heart, and a thrombus which is only slightly adherent to the endothelium can be passed and extracted. Because a steady, high, positive and extraperitoneal pressure is possible only under general endotracheal anesthesia, thrombectomy should not be performed with local anesthesia. The Valsalva maneuver which the patient is asked to perform does not always assure the reduction of venous return.

After the clamps are applied, the femoral vein is incised longitudinally over a distance of 1–1.5 cm about 1 cm proximal to the junction with the deep femoral vein (Fig. 27.3.4a). Then a brown Fogarty catheter is introduced, without a guide wire, and advanced to the inferior vena cava (Fig. 27.3.4b). There the blockade is formed by filling the catheter with 40 ml of normal saline solution. A second brown or white Fogarty catheter is then introduced at the same level, filled, and pulled back, care being taken not to apply undue force (Fig. 27.3.4c, d). It is important to take into account the difference in diameter between the inferior vena cava and the left common iliac vein. The spur, which is located at this point, can also pose an obstacle to the withdrawal of the catheter and possibly cause perforation of the vein. The maneuver is repeated until no more thrombotic material can be extracted. Then, the blocking catheter is also retracted with slight pressure against the venous wall.

It should be mentioned that, in addition to the ipsilateral blockade, contralateral blockade has also been described [1]. However, this technique does not seem necessary if continuous PEEP is used. Furthermore, venous thrombectomy with a Fogarty catheter has also been done without blockade, apparently without increased risk of pulmonary embolism.

A good proximal reflux, especially under PEEP, is an indication of free passage. If one has the impression that irregularities of the vessel wall remain, one can remove additional thrombotic material by means of a ring stripper and extract it with the blocking catheter (Fig. 27.3.4e, f). If a blockage remains at the level of 20 cm on the left side, it is usually related to the spur. Nevertheless, a

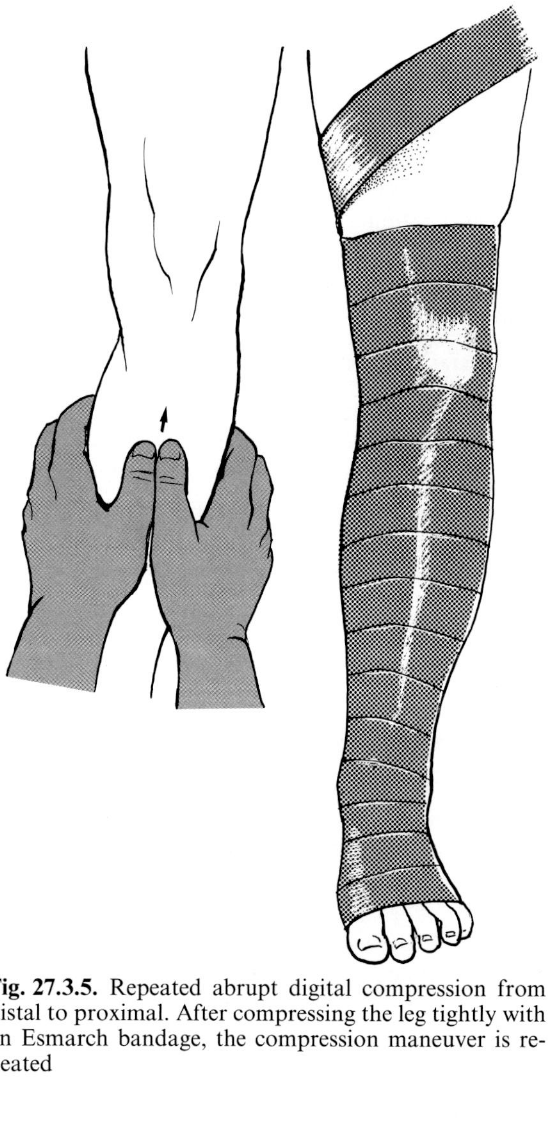

Fig. 27.3.5. Repeated abrupt digital compression from distal to proximal. After compressing the leg tightly with an Esmarch bandage, the compression maneuver is repeated

thrombectomy of all reachable material should be done, since venous blood can drain via the internal iliac vein to the contralateral side and further via the ascending lumbar vein [7]. Next, the thrombectomy of the leg is performed (Fig. 27.3.5). After opening the clamps on the superficial and deep femoral veins, the calf is compressed from distal to proximal with both hands. In most cases, the thrombus can be mobilized by strong blows with the fist. The compression is continued up to the proximal thigh, where thrombotic material protrudes through the venotomy. To avoid large blood loss, digital compression of the venotomy is recommended, the pressure to be released only as the calf or the thigh is compressed. The use of a cellsaver diminishes blood loss. Following the intermittent compression the entire leg, including the foot, is compressed with an Esmarch bandage and the compression maneuver is repeated. If the anterograde venous flow is insufficient, one can insert a brown Fogarty catheter distally, which is usually possible up to 35 cm. The retraction, however, has to be done with very carefully adjusted filling pressure because of the valves. Definite proof that a spur is present should not be taken as an indication for local dissection, since a spur resection and a venous patch angioplasty increase the magnitude of the operation significantly and entail a high risk of rethrombosis. Rather, one should construct an arteriovenous fistula and await spontaneous collateralization; this technique, together with the spontaneous lysis, often makes the Palma procedure unnecessary. The operation of Palma (venous crossover bypass with the greater saphenous vein or ring-reinforced Gore-Tex, see p. 736) should be reserved for secondary interventions. As a primary intervention combined with a thrombectomy, it should be the exception, to be used only when there is an extreme increase in the volume of the upper and lower leg and an occlusion of the pelvic veins [5].

VI. Intraoperative Diagnosis

Intraoperative venographic control of the pelvic veins should always be performed prior to closure of the incision. After closure of the venotomy with a continuous suture of 6–0 Prolene, the common femoral vein is punctured with a butterfly cannula. More elegant is the introduction of a small subclavian catheter into a side branch of the venous junction. Venography provides information about the pelvic veins. If there is a blockage or an irregularity of the wall, one should repeat the thrombectomy maneuver. With the construction of an arteriovenous fistula and the consequent increased pressure from a distal direction, the danger of a thrombosis is diminished and the chances of collateralization improved. By means of intraoperative venoscopy, the pelvic veins can be evaluated three-dimensionally, and especially the region of the spur can be directly visualized [8]. If residues on the venous walls are observed, the use of a ring stripper is recommended. This elaborate diagnostic method has not become intraoperative routine.

VII. Arteriovenous Fistula

Since the development of a thrombosis is dependent on the flow velocity of the venous blood, it can be assumed that the incidence of recurrent thrombosis can be reduced by using an AV fistula to increase the flow velocity. Not only can the rate of recurrence be lowered by an AV fistula, but the changes of recanalization and collateralization are increased as well. The danger of congestive heart failure does not exist if the fistula is unilateral (shunt volume 1000 ml/min) and there is no history of heart disease. Since the flow volume of the fistula increases with time, closure is recommended after 3–6 months.

Fistulas are constructed in the shape of a basket handle or a letter N.

To construct the basket-handle fistula, a long branch of the venous junction or the greater saphenous vein (most likely the first medial branch) is dissected distally, and the end is anastomosed side-to-end with the superficial femoral artery using 6–0 Prolene (Fig. 27.3.6a–c). To make it easier to find the shunt later on, a sterile wire is passed around the base of the loop, and then both ends of the wire are brought through the skin approximately 2 cm distal to the wound, transected, and allowed to retract into the subcutaneous tissue. The length of the wire loop should be determined using a sterile ruler. If the fistula is to be closed, this wire is used as a guide during dissection. Occlusion of the fistula using the wire is not an acceptable substitute for dividing it between ligatures. After the fistula is opened, a definite thrill can be palpated. After closure of the incision, the functioning of the fistula can be checked with a stethoscope (continuous bruit). Spontaneous closure of the basket-handle fistula is likely as a result

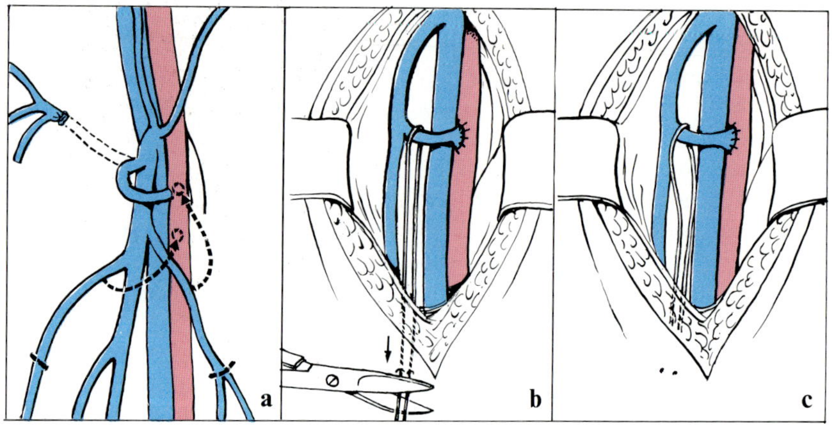

Fig. 27.3.6a–c. Arteriovenous fistula (basket-handle shunt). **a** Depending on the size of the lumen, a branch of the greater saphenous vein (ideally the first medial branch) is moved toward the superficial femoral artery. **b** Longitudinal incision of the superficial femoral artery and construction of the fistula with 6–0 Prolene. Encircling the shunt with the wire, which is then brought through the skin 2 cm distal to the lower wound angle. Before cutting the wire, it is put under minimal tension. **c** After cutting the ends, the wire retracts into the subcutaneous tissue; the wire must not be under tension

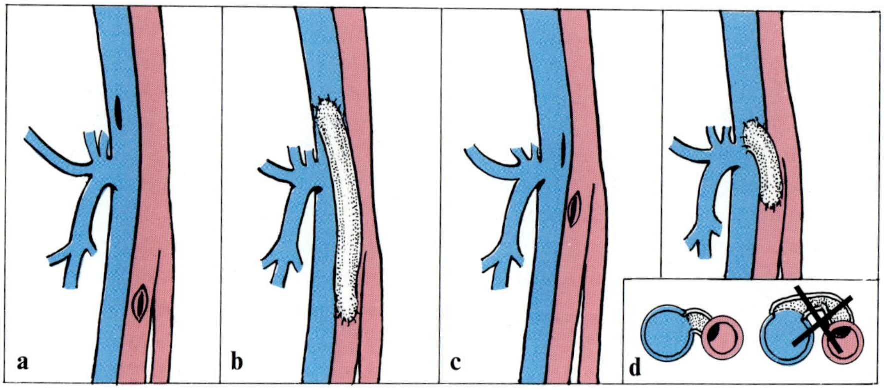

Fig. 27.3.7a–d. Arteriovenous fistula (N-shaped shunt with Gore-Tex). **a**, **b** Venotomy and arteriotomy (with minimal oval-shaped enlargement) if the shunt is longer than 3 cm. **c**, **d** If the shunt is short, the openings in the vessels have to face each other to avoid kinking

of kinking (up to 50%), the N-shaped fistula is a good alternative. A 5-mm Gore-Tex graft is interposed between artery and vein by means of a side-to-end (arterial side) and an end-to-side (venous side) anastomosis. When the anastomosis is done with running 6–0 suture (Fig. 27.3.7a–d), it is advisable to enlarge the arteriotomy by excising an oval-shaped piece of the wall. If the N-shaped shunt is longer than 3 cm, venotomy and arteriotomy can be placed in the middle. If the shunt is shorter, however, venotomy and arteriotomy should face each other to avoid kinking. One should keep this complication in mind during the thrombectomy if the venotomy has been done first.

The closure of the fistula with the wire in place is done as described above. If a marking wire is not used, one should expose the artery distal to the fistula and dissect proximally. During this dissection, the fistula can be located medially. It should be transected between two ligatures, foreign material remaining in the wound.

Indications for an arteriovenous fistula at the level of the groin are:

1. Radiologically proven stenosis of the pelvic veins.
2. Very old thrombotic material from the pelvic veins, suggesting significant trauma to the endothelium.

It should be mentioned that some authors require an arteriovenous fistula whenever the pelvic veins are involved. Fistulas at the level of the adductors are technically more difficult to construct, and fistulas at the level of the medial malleolus suffer from a high spontaneous occlusion rate. On the other hand, they achieve the goal of increasing the flow in only one of the six veins of the lower leg [11].

VIII. Intraoperative and Postoperative Complications

Intraoperative pulmonary embolus and perforation of the vessel, postoperative bleeding, and recurrent thrombosis are the most important complications. An intraoperative pulmonary embolus should be approached surgically if the symptoms dictate this. This complication should already be taken into consideration while the patient is being prepared and draped. In our own experience, we found 3 intraoperative pulmonary emboli in 234 operations. All 3 cases were operated on at the stage of multiple, frequently recurrent pulmonary emboli.

Perforation of a vein is a very rare complication and is manifested by visible blood loss or deterioration of circulatory parameters. After the diagnosis is made by venography or on clinical grounds, a laparotomy or a retroperitoneal approach is indicated (see p. 691).

Postoperative bleeding, usually in the region of the incision, is usually the result of heparin therapy. Diligent hemostasis, local compression and appropriate control of the regulatory parameters (PTT 80–120 s) can control this complication. Large hematomas present in the groin should be evacuated because of the danger of infection.

IX. Postoperative Treatment

The advantage of the operation is immediate postoperative mobilization, with compression (grade II support stocking) and heparinization. During rest, the vein is elevated on the splint.

On the third postoperative day, heparin (by continuous infusion and guided by PTT) is gradually replaced by warfarin. If a PT is doubled, the patient is weaned from heparin over 1–2 days. Discharge from hospital is possible, if the prothrombin time is stable. Prophylaxis with warfarin should be maintained for 6–12 months. The patient should be advised to wear the compression stockings throughout the day. The compression should be discontinued only after the clinical examination, venographic or Doppler ultrasonographic investigation, *and* phlebodynamometry have been normal for 6 months. If compression can be discontinued, long-term follow-up is necessary.

Therapeutic successes should not obscure the fact that an acceptable operative result can be achieved with only 50% of patients. Long-term observations show an even higher risk of post-thrombotic syndrome [3, 10, 14, 16].

Since the risk of thromboembolic complications is difficult to judge and thrombosis is an individual risk, the essential measure is general pharmacologic prophylaxis with 3 × 5000 I.U. heparin subcutaneously, 2 × 5000 I.U. heparin Dihydergotamine mesulate subcutaneously, or intravenous dextrane, if the patient has to be immobilized. Physiotherapy supports this treatment but is not in itself sufficient [4, 9].

B. Upper Extremity

Thromboses in the region of the upper extremity are essentially different from thrombosis of the veins of the leg and the pelvis, because the hydrostatic pressure in the arms presents only an inconsequential stress. Therefore, post-thrombotic syndromes, comparable to those in the lower extremities, are very rare in the arm.

Thromboses of the upper extremity develop under the following circumstances [5]:

1. Tumor compression,
2. Following subclavian/jugular catheterization,
3. In thoracic outlet syndrome.

1. Mediastinal tumors (benign, malignant, inflammatory), goiters and large bronchial metastases (suprainfraclavicular and axillary) can lead to a stenosis, with eventual blockage of the main ve-

nous drainage of the arm, and secondarily to the development of a thrombosis in the periphery. On radiologic examination, one usually sees a marked development of collaterals, especially via the veins in the region of the scapula. Therefore, one should always search for a tumor by clinical and technical means. Further therapy depends on the underlying tumor. A thrombectomy is usually not indicated, because the developed collaterals are sufficient for venous drainage. Frequently the cause of the thromboses cannot be removed, even in cases of palliative treatment of the tumor.

2. The increasing frequency of invasive diagnostic measures as well as the frequent use of central venous catheters, has lead to an increased incidence of thromboses of the subclavian vein and consequently an increased incidence of pulmonary emboli in autopsy statistics.

As a rule, these thromboses cause more symptoms than those caused by tumors, since collaterals are missing. Moreover, they are forced by hyperemia resulting from muscle activity. In these cases, local lysis should be considered. The doses of streptokinase or urokinase by direct injection into the thrombus are so low that the indications for this technique are broader than for systemic fibrinolysis (following the technique of local fibrinolysis for arterial thrombosis, see p. 106ff.). Thrombectomy is not appropriate in this case, since the rate of recurrence is high and since satisfactory results are usually obtained by waiting for the spontaneous development of collaterals.

A thrombectomy should, however, be considered if phlegmasia cerulea is evident and the entire venous lumen is occluded. In this case the proximal brachial vein or the axillary vein is exposed (analogous to the exposure of the artery, see p. 533). The proximal thrombus is extracted with a Fogarty catheter. The distal thrombus can be removed by use of a bandage or manual compression (see p. 722).

3. The veins, arteries, and nerves in the region of the shoulder girdle are especially subject to mechanical stresses, which are explained by both the anatomy and the mobility of the arm. Predominant pathologic anatomic features are:

- Cervical rib,
- Hyperostosis after clavicular fracture or deformity of the clavicula,
- Atypical ventral course of the phrenic nerve.

Furthermore, the subclavian vein can be mechanically impaired by costoclavicular compression, when the shoulder is adducted at a right angle and moved dorsally. This can lead to thrombosis [5]. The involvement of nerves and arteries as described dominates the clinical picture and determines the indication for operative treatment (e.g., resection of the first rib see p. 559).

An isolated intervention on the vein (thrombectomy or even a venous reconstruction with the interposition of a Gore-Tex graft or a patch graft) is not indicated after the cause of the compression has been removed, because the recurrence rate is high and the spontaneous collateralization is sufficient.

However, if exposure of the nervovascular bundle is necessary because of a thoracic outlet syndrome or a nerve compression, a reconstruction of the vein (Gore-Tex interposition or patch graft) can be added, especially if, following thrombectomy or fibrinolysis, the lesion in the venous wall at the site of the costoclavicular compression can be demonstrated venographically. In this case, a thrombectomy is performed through a venotomy in the subclavian vein. The thrombus can be removed proximally with a Fogarty catheter after a PEEP is established. The thrombus is removed from the arm by means of the compression technique used for the leg (hitting with the fist and bandaging). Reconstruction (suture of the vein, patch graft angioplasty, or interposition of ring-reinforced Gore-Tex) follows the rules of atraumatic venous surgery (see p. 732ff.).

REFERENCES

1. Baumann G (1974) Operative Technik bei der akuten Bein- und Beckenvenenthrombose unter Berücksichtigung von Venenverletzungen. Vasa 3(1):34–38
2. Bloom AL, Thomas DP (1981) Haemostasis and thrombosis. Churchill, Livingstone
3. Brunner U, Wirth W (1971) Spätresultate nach Thrombektomie bei Ileofemoralvenenthrombose im klinisch-radiologischen Vergleich. Schweiz Med Wochenschr 101 (37):1327–1334
4. Comerota AJ, Sasahara A, DiSerio FJ, Cranley JJ (1983) Postoperative deep vein thrombosis using Dihydroergotamine-Heparin. Lecture, American College of Surgeons, 69th Annual Clinical Congress, Atlanta
5. Ehringer H, Fischer H, Netzer CO, Schmutzler R, Zeitler E (1979) Venöse Abflußstörungen. Enke, Stuttgart, p 407ff.
6. Hach W, Salzmann G (1982) Die Chirurgie der Venen. Schattauer, Stuttgart

7. Höflinger C, Wirth W (1976) Kollateralwege bei einseitiger Beckenvenenthrombose. Vasa 5(3):185–193
8. Hutschenreiter S, Vollmar J, Loeprecht H, Abendschein A, Rödl W (1979) Rekonstruktive Eingriffe am Venensystem – Spätergebnisse unter kritischer Bewertung funktioneller und gefäßmorphologischer Kriterien. Chirurg 50(9):555–563
9. Kakkar VV (1975) Deep vein thrombosis. Circulation 51:8–19
10. Kriessmann A, Rupp N (1977) Natürlicher Verlauf der venösen Drainagen-Insuffizienz bei Becken- und tiefer Beinvenenthrombose. Vasa 6(2):124–127
11. Loeprecht H, Vollmar J, Heyes H, Paulini K, Spohn B (1976) Beeinflussung des Spontanverlaufs der Phlebothrombose und ihre operativen Behandlungsergebnisse durch Änderung der Haemodynamik. Vasa 5(2):135–141
12. May R (1974) Die Problematik des Beckenvenensporns. Vasa 3(1):28–33
13. Nachbur BB, Beck EA, Senn A (1980) Can the results of treatment of deep venous thrombosis be improved by combining surgical thrombectomy with regional fibrinolysis? J Cardiovasc Surg 21:347–352
14. Partsch H, Weidinger P, Mostbeck A, Olbert F, Denck H (1980) Funktionelle Spätergebnisse nach Thrombektomie, Fibrinolyse und konservativer Therapie von Bein-Beckenvenenthrombosen. Vasa 9(1):53–61
15. Pollak EW, Sparks FC, Barker WF (1974) Inferior vena cava interruption: indications and results with caval ligation, clip and intracaval devices in 110 cases. J Cardiovasc Surg 15:629–635
16. Raithel D, Söhnlein B (1981) Die venöse Thrombektomie – Technik und Ergebnisse. Vasa 10(2):119–124

27.4 Post-thrombotic Syndrome of the Lower Extremity

R. May †

CONTENTS

A. Introduction

In a healthy individual, some 90% of the venous blood is transported through the deep venous system. After a deep venous thrombosis, this venous return is impaired up to 80%–85% as a result of valve destruction and irregular recanalization. The impedance is progressive in character. Many surgical procedures have been tried in the past. However, upon critical examination, only a few can be said to have withstood the test of time.

B. Anatomy

The reader is referred to the chapter (2.2) on the general anatomy of the veins and to the anatomical sections of the chapters on primary varices and acute venous occlusion (see p. 717).

C. Surgical Options

I. Procedures on the Superficial Venous System

1. Resection of Secondary Varices

a) Indication. Following deep venous thrombosis there are, in 80% of cases, residual changes that have a general tendency to progress. One type of such a residual change is secondary varices. They must be distinguished from primary varices by means of venography. Whether anything is to be gained by eliminating secondary varices can be determined by an occlusion test.

Two methods are available:
1. Determination of the peripheral venous pressure [6] (Fig. 27.4.1 a–c),
2. Light-reflex rheography [5].

With the patient standing up, a vein of the dorsum of the foot is punctured, allowing insertion of a catheter that is connected to a properly calibrated manometer or Statham apparatus. One measures the pressure with reference to the equilibrium level, i.e., the level at which the same pressure is present, independent of the position of the body. It is located one handbreadth below the diaphragm. The muscle pump is activated by having the patient repeatedly stand tiptoe (ten times in 15 s, if possible, according to a metronome). Depending on the function, the pressure drops. Figure 27.4.1 a shows such a pressure drop from 90 to 70 mmHg after ten elevations on the toes. Depending on the behaviour of the pressure in the superficial varices upon occlusion (for this it is best to use a compress that has been folded several times), the following conclusions can be drawn (Fig. 27.4.1 b):

1. If the pressure drops markedly after occlusion, removal of the varicose vein is not only permissible but essential to the improvement of venous return.

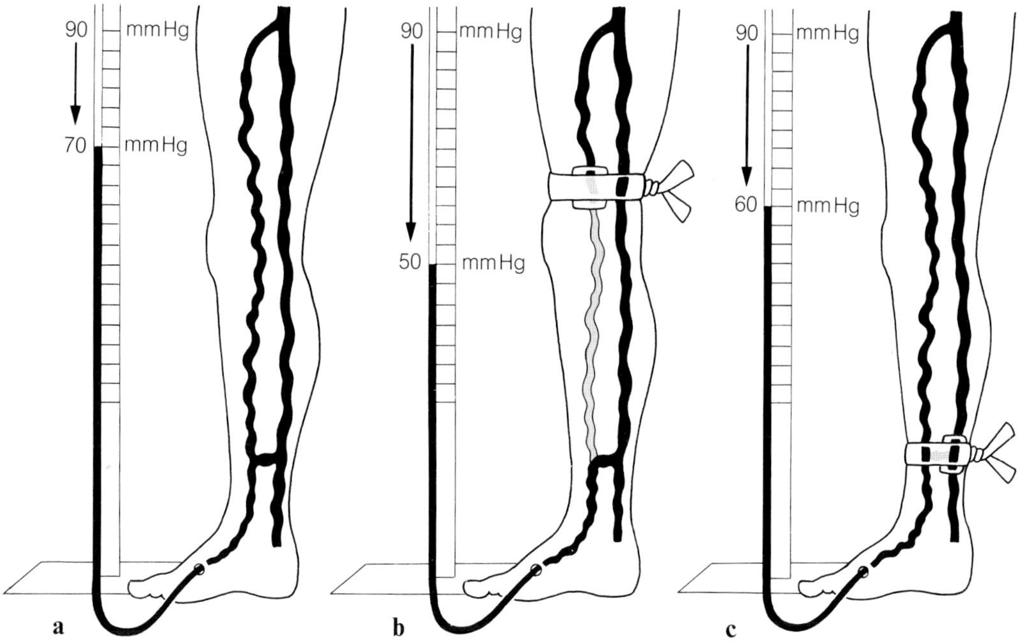

Fig. 27.4.1 a–c. Measurement of peripheral venous pressure according to MAY and KRIESSMANN [6]: **a** After puncture of a vein of the dorsum of the foot, tubing is connected via an amplifier to a pressure gauge. Measurements under resting conditions are taken until a steady state is reached (starting point here: 90 mmHg). The patient stands ten times on tiptoe within 15 s. If the venous outflow is impeded, a pressure drop of 50–60 mmHg occurs. A pressure drop of only 20 mmHg indicates a severe outflow impedance. **b** By occlusion of the superficial veins, the change in pressure is eliminated if it is the sum of several factors. **c** Functional improvement through elimination of the incompetent perforating vein is clarified by the compression test

2. If the pressure does not change after occlusion, the operation is optional and of essentially cosmetic importance.
3. If the pressure rises after occlusion, the varicose vein is essential for the venous return, and operative removal is contraindicated.

As an alternative to invasive pressure measurement one can use light-reflex rheography for an assessment of the cutaneous venous plexus, which, because it connects the superficial and deep venous systems, can provide information about the function of both. The essential parameter is the refilling time after ten dorsal flexions of the foot with the heel supported. This examination can be combined with the occlusion test.

b) Positioning, Exposure, Operative Technique, Complications, and Postoperative Treatment. For details see Chap. 27.2, p. 701).

2. Insufficient Perforating Veins

a) Introduction. The perforating veins communicate between the superficial and deep venous systems. By means of valves they direct blood flow in such a way that during relaxation of the muscles (diastole) there is a blow-in, i.e., a flow from the superficial to the deep veins (Fig. 27.4.2). The blow-out, i.e., flow in the opposite direction during muscle contraction (systole), is pathologic. The pathologic reversal of flow is much stronger in the case of insufficient perforating veins (as a result of a deep vein thrombus) than it is with primary varicose veins. The incompetent perforating veins are ligated during vein stripping, because the blow-out through the incompetent veins increases after the blow-down (reflux to the varices) has been eliminated. The functional improvement through ligation of the perforating veins can be shown by the compression test (Fig. 27.4.1 c).

In post-thrombotic syndrome, the blow-out can be very strong and is sometimes referred to as systolic jet-out. In most cases, it is the direct cause of a post-thrombotic venostasis ulcer (see p. 711).

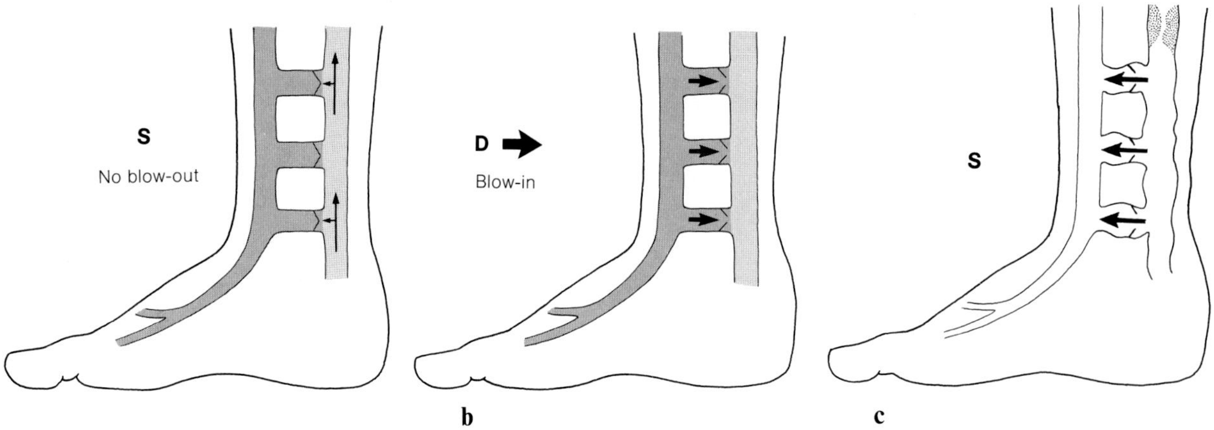

Fig. 27.4.2a–c. Flow conditions between the superficial and the deep venous systems. **a, b** During systole (muscle contraction) the valves of the perforating veins are closed under normal conditions. During diastole, a pressure gradient between the superficial and the deep venous systems is built up, and the valves open. **c** If the perforating valves are incompetent (owing to changes in the valve cusps themselves or because of an overall increase in valve diameter), the valves do not close on systole, and reflux from the deep to the superficial venous system occurs

Fig. 27.4.3a, b. Typical location of incompetent perforating veins. **a** Medial side. **b** Dorsal side
▽

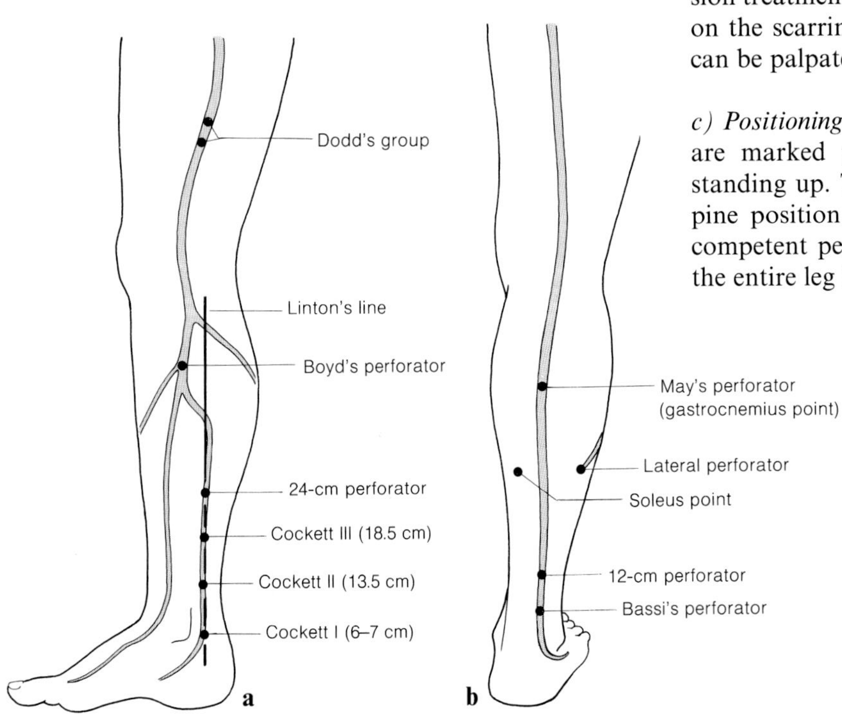

b) Indication

1. Only functional perforating veins should be eliminated. The exact determination is possible by means of the compression test, after they have been located clinically or by venography. If the venous pressure improves, the perforating vein in question is functionally active.

2. Incompetent perforating veins may be functionally unimportant; however, in the classic positions [1, 2] they are usually functional active (Fig. 27.4.3).

3. If a venostasis ulcer is present, this should be treated by compression. At the very least, careful wound cleansing is necessary. Under compression treatment, the edema subsides and, depending on the scarring, the incompetent perforation vein can be palpated as an opening in the fascia.

c) Positioning. The incompetent perforating veins are marked prior to surgery, with the patient standing up. The procedure itself is done in a supine position. In this position, all important incompetent perforating veins can be reached after the entire leg has been prepared.

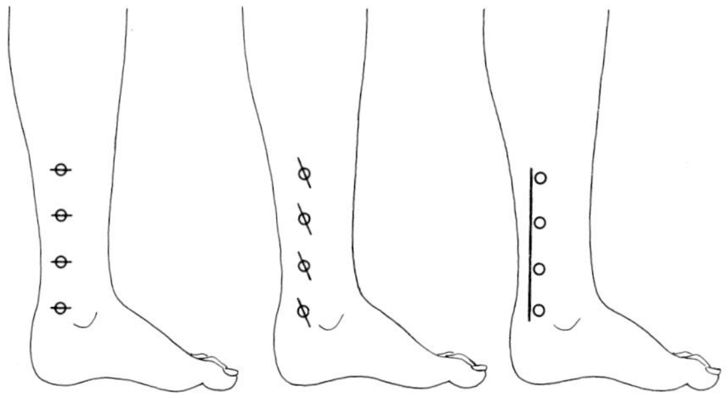

Fig. 27.4.4. Multiple small oblique or transverse incisions are made dorsal to the perforating veins. They are preferable to the long longitudinal incision of Cockett. The more severe the skin changes are, the farther from the incompetent perforating veins the incisions should be made

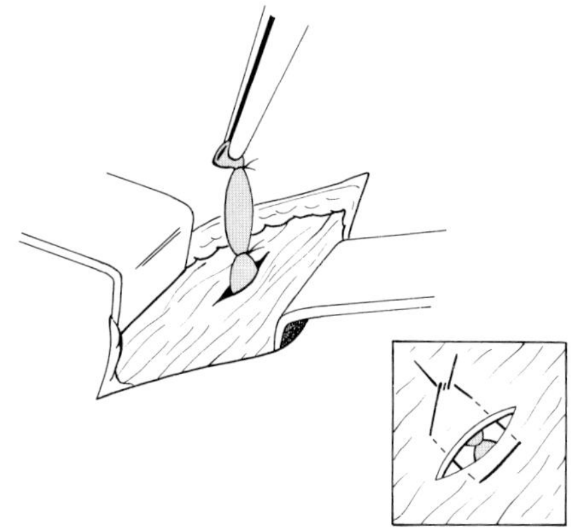

Fig. 27.4.5. Double ligature of the perforating vein, the stump of which retracts beneath the fascia. Closure of the fascia with a U-suture

d) Exposure. Under local anesthesia; if multiple procedures are necessary, then under endotracheal anesthesia; in the latter case, one or more incisions 2–3 cm long are made in the direction of the skin folds (Fig. 27.4.4). Depending on the condition of the skin and the subcutaneous fatty tissue, smaller incisions are possible. These incisions should be cephalad or caudad of the perforating veins in order to avoid significant skin changes. A longitudinal incision, as described by COCKETT [1], is only done in exceptional cases. It is indicated only if severe induration necessitates a dorsal approach through healthy skin. If a venostasis ulcer is excised, the ligation is performed through the site of excision.

e) Surgical Technique. After the skin incision, the subcutaneous tissue is divided down to the fascia. The fascia is opened, usually starting from the entry point of the perforating vein. The vein is ligated in such a way that, after transection, the vessel retracts beneath the fascia. The hole in the fascia is closed with a U-suture. Finally, the subcutaneous tissue is approximated, and the skin incision is closed with interrupted sutures (Fig. 27.4.5). It should be mentioned that incompetent perforating veins can be evulsed, e.g., by the use of sharp retractors inserted through the small incisions. Another method proposes the subfascial division of all perforating veins within reach with scissors. Bleeding must be controlled by prolonged compression (at least 10 min). We, however, prefer the selective approach [8]. A recent development is endoscopic splitting of perforating veins.

3. Venostasis Ulcer (Secondary to Varicose Veins or Deep Venous Thrombosis)

a) Indication. Venostasis ulcer can be caused by a deep venous thrombosis or by varices. The cause in both cases is a hemodynamic alteration brought about by varicosis (primary or secondary and/or incompetent perforating veins). The goal of the procedure is to remove these local causes; however, despite the elimination of the varicosities, the damage to the deep venous system in the post-thrombotic state remains irreparable, and the prognosis is therefore doubtful [1, 2].

Prerequisites for therapy are:

1. Exclusion of arterial insufficiency as the underlying cause. If peripheral arterial disease is present, the healing of the ulcer can be accomplished only by improving perfusion (conservatively or surgically). This takes precedence over venous problems.
2. With local cleansing and antiseptic treatment, as well as local compression, a venostasis ulcer should heal or at least show clean granulations. If extensive scarring is present, complete healing by conservative means usually cannot be achieved.

b) Positioning. The procedure is carried out with the patient in a supine position and under general anesthesia. Local anesthesia is usually contraindicated because of the poor skin condition. The leg is prepared in such a way that all marked places are included in the operative field and can be reached by appropriate manipulation.

c) Exposure and Operative Technique. The procedure and the extent of the operation depend on the degree of damage and its cause. The surgical technique for both kinds of venostasis ulcers is the same, but the prognosis is different.

A venostasis ulcer secondary to varicose veins usually heals under compression; however, recurrences are the rule. Etiologic treatment consists of excision of the varicose vein as well as ligation of the incompetent perforating vein. Both causes should be exactly delineated prior to surgery by radiologic means. The excision of the ulcer is usually not necessary as long as the deep veins are intact. Excision of the scars, either immediately or in a second procedure, is recommended only if there is marked scarring of the skin secondary to the ulcer. The skin defect is covered with a mesh graft or a split-thickness skin graft. Depending on the condition of the wound, the latter can be done either primarily or secondarily.

For a venostasis ulcer secondary to deep vein thrombosis, the surgical procedure is identical to that for ulcers secondary to varicose veins. The damage to the skin is usually more extensive; therefore, a bloc resection of the ulcer and the scar is done more frequently. Incompetent perforating veins are eliminated during the same procedure.

d) Complications. The most serious complication is of course local wound infection that may progress into a phlegmon of the lower leg. Here, the risk depends on the degree of preoperative wound infection. Therefore, meticulous conservative therapy prior to surgery is highly recommended. If the clinical signs of purulent infection are present, incision and drainage are necessary.

e) Postoperative Treatment. After an extensive operative procedure (wide excision of the ulcer with primary skin graft), bed rest for 1 week with the leg elevated, physiotherapy, and pharmacologic prophylaxis against thrombotic complications are indicated. If the only procedure to be performed after healing of the ulcer is ligation of the perforating vein, this can be done under local anesthesia and on an outpatient basis. After discharge from the hospital, compression treatment for several months is recommended. Thereafter, no further therapeutic measures are required provided the venostasis ulcers were the result of varices. When the ulcers are secondary to deep vein thrombosis, however, further therapy with compression stockings is necessary. Indeed, in order to prevent a recurrence, these stockings should be worn throughout the day for life. Recurrence is due either to an overlooked incompetent perforating vein or to insufficient compression treatment.

II. Procedures on the Deeper Veins of the Leg

1. Introduction

The main difference between surgical procedures on the arterial and the venous systems is the higher rate of thrombosis during venous surgery. Damage to the endothelium, which usually heals in arteries because of the high perfusion pressure, leads more frequently to thrombosis in the veins owing to the low intravascular pressure and the low flow velocity. This requires from the surgeon:

a) Atraumatic and careful handling of the endothelium,
b) Proper decision regarding creation of a temporary arteriovenous fistula distal to the anastomosis.

Under heading (a), the four basic rules for careful handling of the endothelium during venous sutures are:

1. The vein itself should not be touched by the hand of the surgeon or with a clamp. It should be grasped on the adventitia or by means of a long ligature (Fig. 27.4.6a).

2. Bleeding from the anastomosis should not be controlled with a sponge, but rather by irrigation with normal saline followed by suction (Fig. 27.4.6b).

3. The anastomosis should be sutured without touching the edge of the vessels with the forceps. Usually, an everting vascular suture gives the best results (Fig. 27.4.6c).

4. Traction will damage the endothelium. However, the intima is not damaged when the vessel is expanded in order to locate leaking collaterals (Fig. 27.4.6d).

5. Connective tissue, which connects with the adventitia of the femoral vein and keeps the vein open, independently of the position of the leg, should remain. Dissection for clamping, therefore, should be done very sparingly, and circular dissection is to be condemned. By contrast with the artery, the vein is only completely filled during the time of strong venous return; most of the time,

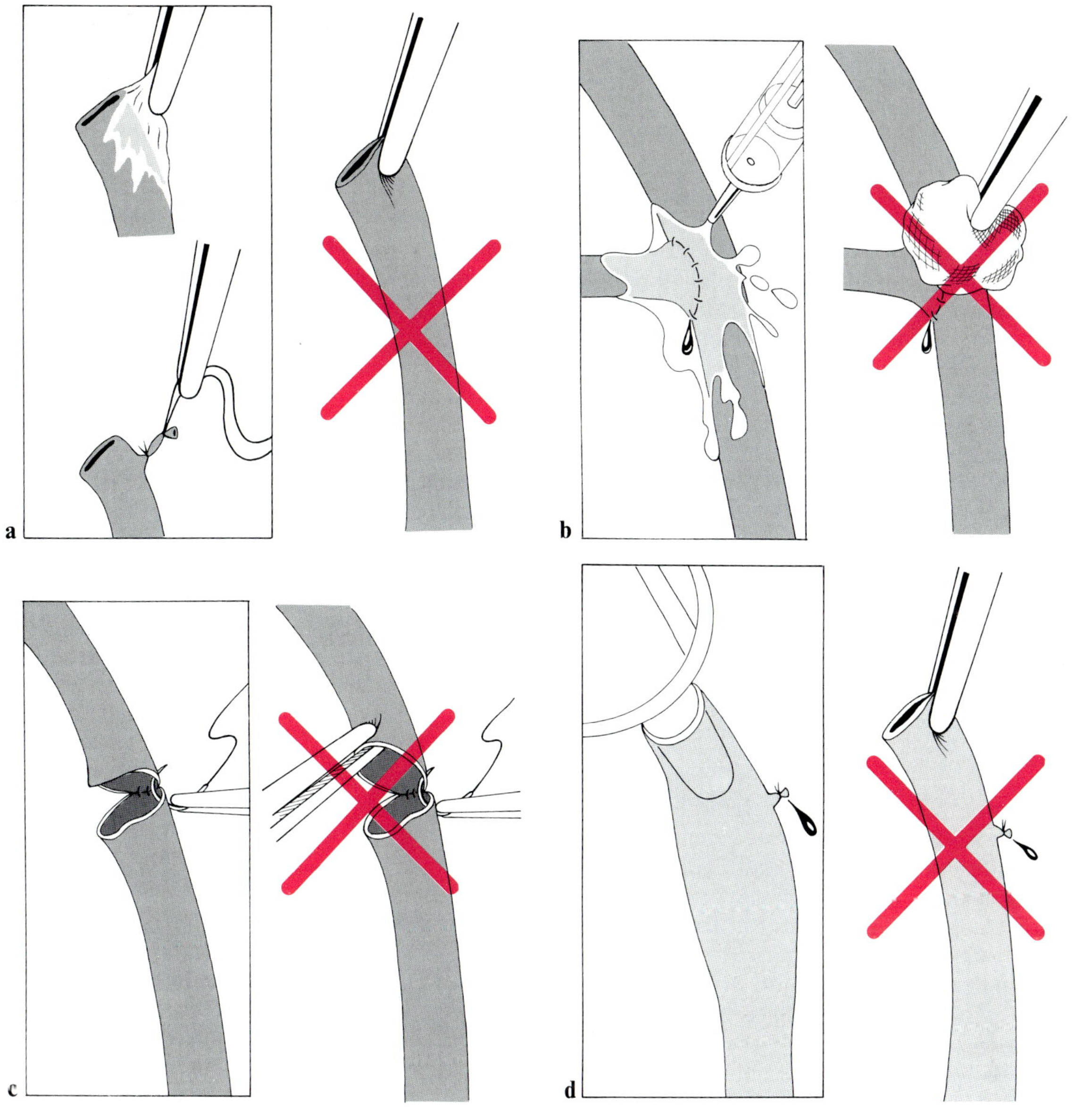

Fig. 27.4.6 a–d. Atraumatic surgical technique. **a** Only indirect handling of the vein with a stay suture or on the adventitia. **b** Local cleaning by irrigation, not with a sponge. **c** Venous suture without use of a forceps. **d** Avoidance of traction on the vein

however, it has an oval-shaped diameter. Circular dissection of the vein at the level of the inguinal ligament would greatly increase its tendency to collapse. This principle led to the technique of suspension within a ring, developed by Kunlin (Fig. 27.4.7). If a vein must be clamped, this should be done with a Fogarty hydrogrip surgical clamp (Edwards laboratories), which keeps the damage to the endothelium at a minimum

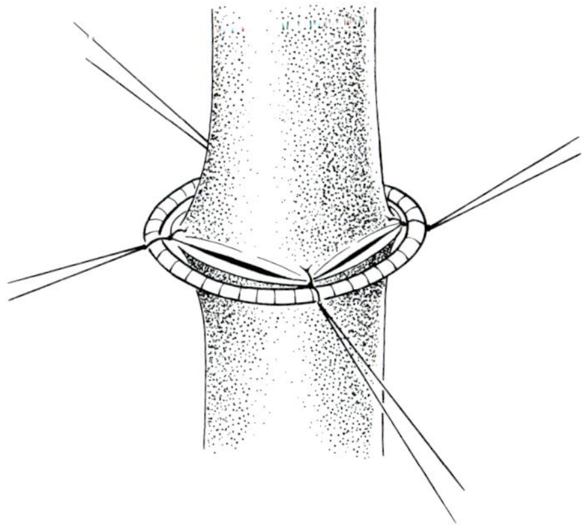

Fig. 27.4.7. Ring suspension as described by Kunlin

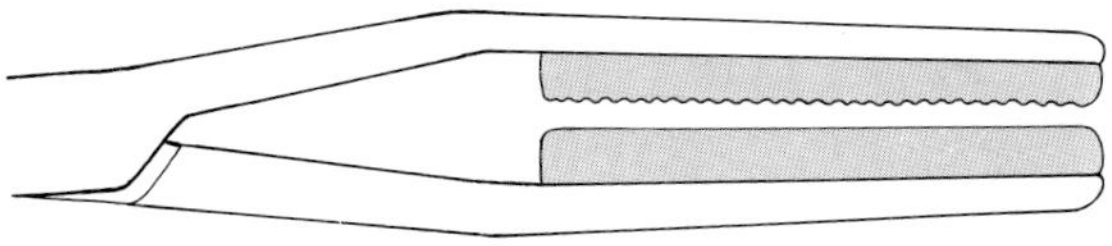

Fig. 27.4.8. Fogarty hydrogrip clamp for avoiding trauma to the endothelium

(Fig. 27.4.8). Its branches are clipped with exchangeable soft rubber cushions. For partial exclusion, a Satinsky clamp is recommended. Its teeth destroy only small islands of endothelium, which are rapidly endothelialized from the edges.

With respect to (b; temporary arteriovenous fistula), the technique is described in the chapter on acute venous occlusion (see p. 723).

Femoral bypass according to MAY and HUSNI [4]. If it is primarily the femoral vein that is damaged as a result of thrombosis, it can obviously be bridged by the saphenous vein, which is in that case implanted into the popliteal vein. Unfortunately, the greater saphenous vein tends to develop varices. The operative result, therefore, is dependent on the function of the valves.

2. Indications

An indication for surgery is a severe obstruction to venous outflow, demonstrated venodynamically, together with the appropriate clinical symptoms. Venography will usually show the obstruction to be located in the superficial femoral vein. An ideal case would be an isolated trauma with appropriate sequelae at the level of the thigh. If there are post-thrombotic changes at the level of the lower leg, the result of the operation can be jeopardized by the progressive nature of the disease. A further prerequisite is an intact greater saphenous vein. However, even if the valves are competent, the tendency to develop varices is great.

3. Positioning

The operation is performed with the patient in a supine position, the entire leg prepared and draped. The distal thigh is supported by two surgical gowns in order to allow external rotation of the leg and flexing of the knee.

4. Exposure and Surgical Technique

A skin incision of approximately 8 cm is made, parallel to the tibia (one fingerbreadth medial to its edge). The incision begins immediately below the medial epicondyle. After the skin has been cut, one encounters the greater saphenous vein (one should try preoperatively to mark it, with the patient standing up); the vein is dissected distally with strict observance of the rules for atraumatic procedure. After incision of the deep fascia and retraction of the gastric muscle, the popliteal vein is located on top of the artery in the loose areolar tissue. It is dissected out and clamped with small atraumatic clamps. After the periphery has been locally heparinized with 10000 I.U. heparin, a venotomy 3–4 cm long is made. The venotomy should be placed as far distally as possible, since this part remains unchanged, even in cases of severe post-thrombotic damage. The greater saphenous vein is then transected as far distally as possible and anastomosed to the popliteal vein, side-to-end and without tension (Fig. 27.4.9a, b). For an accurate measurement of the length of the greater saphenous vein, the patient's knee should be extended.

The fascia is left open, and the wound is closed after a suction drain has been inserted. If in addi-

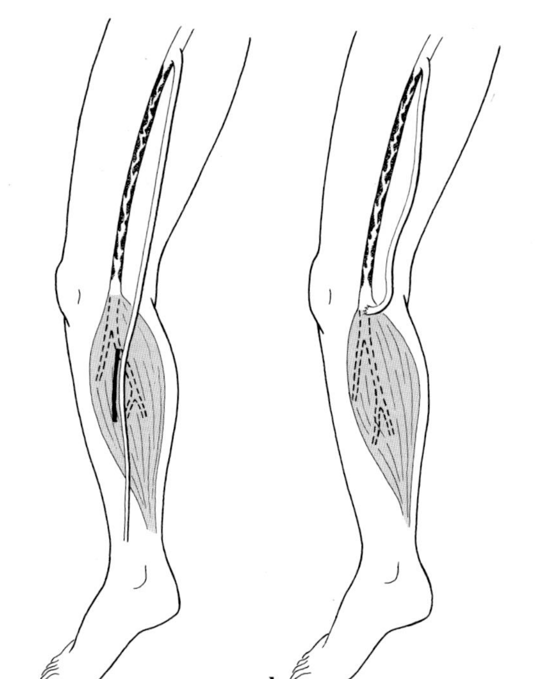

Fig. 27.4.9a, b. Femoral bypass according to MAY and HUSNI. **a** In cases of isolated (rare!) thrombosis of the superficial femoral vein, the healthy greater saphenous vein is transected approximately one handbreadth below the knee joint (skin incision is marked by a full line). **b** The distal end is anastomosed side-to-end to the popliteal vein without torsion or tension

tion incompetent perforating veins are present, they are ligated during the same procedure. Postoperatively, the patient is heparinized by continuous infusion (the PTT should be increased to two or three times the normal value), foot exercises are done, and the leg is elevated for 5 days. An arteriovenous fistula of the ankle may be added.

5. Complications

Because of the anticoagulation with heparin, postoperative bleeding is possible and may lead to a thrombosis by compression of the vein graft. Therefore, meticulous hemostasis is essential. Minor bleeding from the anastomosis usually stops spontaneously. Here, there is great danger that interrupted sutures will lead to stenosis.

6. Postoperative Treatment

Early evaluations show improvement in the venous pressure curve. However, late results after 5–7 years are disappointing. The reason for this is that, as a rule, occlusion of the superficial femoral vein is not isolated; there are usually additional post-thrombotic changes at the level of the lower leg. These are progressive and lead to a worsening of the post-thrombotic syndrome. Therefore, it should be decided very carefully whether this procedure is indicated. After surgery, long-term compression treatment is necessary. Also, warfarin anticoagulation therapy under precise control (doubled prothrombin time) is necessary. Problems that can be treated surgically (e.g., incompetent perforating veins) should be discovered in annual checkups and treated appropriately.

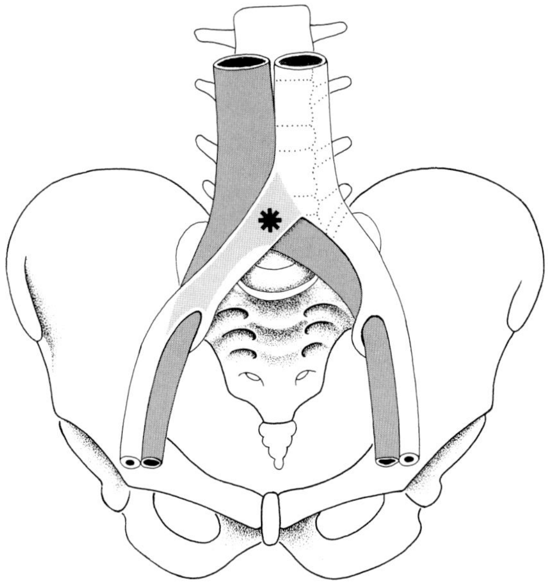

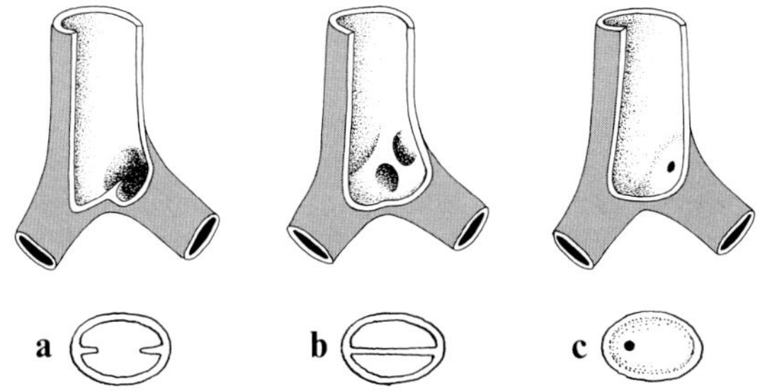

Fig. 27.4.10a–c. Pelvic vein spur. Microtraumas resulting from the pulsating action of the right common iliac artery against the left iliac vein leads to lesions of the intima and development of the spur. These start medially and laterally (**a**) and develop over time into septation (**b**) and to a complete obliteration (**c**) of the vessel

III. Spur of the Pelvic Veins

1. Anatomy

The left common iliac vein lies directly on the vertebral column and cannot yield to the pulsating action of the right common iliac artery, which lies against it in front; as a result, the intima of the vein undergoes changes in varying degree. Such lesions of the intima lead to platelet aggregation, then to a fibrous reaction, and finally to the development of three different forms of vein spur. These spurs must be distinguished from the many anatomic variations of the veins that are observed in this region (Fig. 27.4.10).

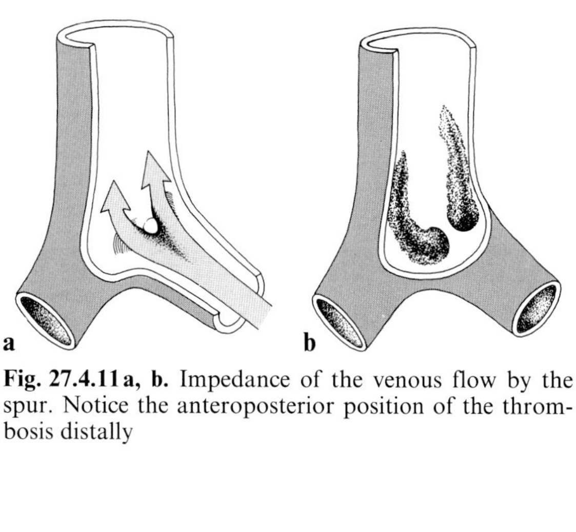

Fig. 27.4.11a, b. Impedance of the venous flow by the spur. Notice the anteroposterior position of the thrombosis distally

The spur occurs in 20% of all adults. However, not every spur impedes the venous return; one must distinguish between functionally unimportant and functionally active spurs. In any event, the spur is responsible for the fact that thromboses of the lower extremities occur twice as often on the left side as on the right. Bilateral thromboses are rare (Fig. 27.4.11) [7, 9].

2. Indications

A functionally active spur does not necessarily cause symptoms. Frequently, however, venous congestion or acute thrombosis of the left leg will point to the presence of a spur. In either case, immediate venographic clarification is necessary.

Thrombosis and spur. If an acute thrombosis is present, it determines the therapeutic approach (see Chap. 27.3, p. 717). If one finds the spur intraoperatively, it is not touched. An arteriovenous fistula is created to promote the development of collaterals. The fistula is ligated after approximately 3 months. Any further intervention should be postponed for 1–2 years following the acute thrombosis, because it is only after that period of time that no further improvement in collateralization can be expected. When the spur is large and the symptoms correspondingly severe, another approach is to correct the spur (Palma operation) immediately following thrombectomy, in the same operative session; this approach is indicated especially in cases where no collateralization can be documented venographically.

Spur. If an isolated spur is present with no evidence of thrombosis, the indications for surgery are as follows:

1. Severe symptoms,
2. The spur can be demonstrated radiologically, if necessary, by venous puncture at the level of the groin. Evaluation of both legs, including the pelvis, is essential,
3. Determination of venous pressure,
4. Only minor post-thrombotic changes in upper and lower leg.

Determination of venous pressure. With the patient lying down, the femoral vein is punctured bilaterally and connected to a properly calibrated pressure gauge (apparatus manufactured by F. Hellige, Freiburg, and W. Wilken, Karlsruhe). First, the resting pressure is registered. Then, the pressure curve is registered while the foot is dorsally flexed 20 times. Under normal conditions, the pressure rises only minimally. However, if a significant flow obstruction is present, the pressure rises markedly. A threefold increase in pressure difference is an indication for surgery.

$$\frac{(\text{P exercise diseased side} - \text{P rest diseased side})}{(\text{P exercise normal side} - \text{P rest normal side})} = \frac{3}{1}$$

Excavation of the vertebral body lying beneath the crossing of the artery and vein has not been successful. Extensive transposition, for example with a vascular prosthesis, is limited to rare special cases. At the present time, there are two procedures to choose from.

a) Resection of the Spur. With the patient in a supine position an oblique incision is made in the flank, and the aortic bifurcation and the left common iliac vein are exposed from the right, using a retroperitoneal approach. The aortic bifurcation is encircled and retracted, and the vein is clamped above the spur. A longitudinal venotomy is made, and the spur is removed. The venotomy is closed with a patch of autogenous vein or alloplastic material. An arteriovenous fistula at the level of the groin is recommended (see p. 723).

Because of its extreme technical difficulty and the high recurrence rate associated with it, this procedure has been replaced to a large extent by the Palma operation.

b) Bypass Procedure. Here, the Palma procedure and the high Palma procedure should be mentioned. These operations are also indicated if a unilateral pelvic vein occlusion is present. They are dealt with in the following section.

IV. Palma Procedure (Fig. 27.4.12a–d) [7, 9]

1. Indications

The indications are:

1. Unilateral occlusion of the pelvic veins or a decompensated spur which has been demonstrated radiographically and functionally (with dynamometry). The contralateral side must be normal.
2. Normal veins in both legs, only minor damage should be tolerated.
3. Severe clinical symptoms, i.e., "venous claudication," meaning that the leg swells up during exercise because of reactive hyperemia and forces the patient to rest.

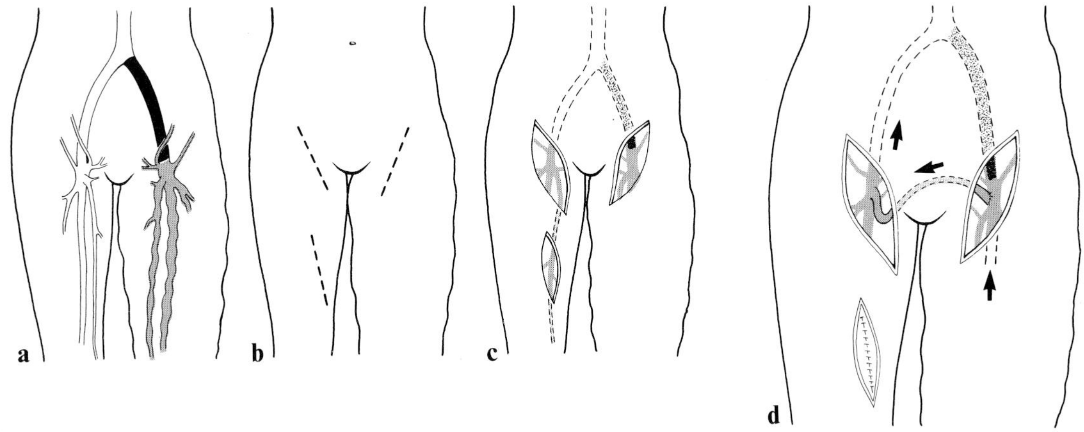

Fig. 27.4.12a–d. Palma operation. **a** Typical venographic appearance of the indication: occlusion of the left pelvic veins. **b** Skin incision. **c** Exposure of the greater saphenous vein on the uninvolved side, distal transection after determining the length with a ruler. **d** The graft is up into the right groin and through a tunnel to the left groin. Here, the anastomosis with the common femoral vein is performed

4. Venous pressure measurement. A threefold increase must be observed (see p. 728).

Completely isolated damage to the pelvic veins is the ideal indication. However, one should never forget that complaints of patients in these cases are frequently so minimal that no operation is necessary. Even a total occlusion at the level of the common iliac vein can be completely compensated by venous dynamometry if the necessary collaterals are present. In these cases, a high initial pressure difference after ten elevations on tiptoe is observed, which normalizes after a short time. The decision to operate is easier if the thrombosis is 1–2 years old and a further improvement of collateralization cannot be expected. In an acute occlusion which can be treated neither surgically nor by fibrinolysis, a primary bypass operation can be recommended.

2. Positioning, Exposure, and Surgical Technique

With the patient in a supine position, both thighs, including both groins, are prepared down to the knee. A 10 cm longitudinal inguinal incision is made on the normal side to expose the deep veins. The greater saphenous vein is exposed medially. If it has a very small diameter, further dissection is abandoned, and one must resort to a reinforced PTFE prosthesis. If the greater saphenous vein can be used, the femoral vein on the diseased side is exposed. It is important to perform the anastomosis in an unaltered segment of the femoral vein. Depending on the circumstances, either the common femoral vein, the superficial femoral, or the deep femoral vein is chosen for anastomosis.

The ideal site of anastomosis is the common femoral vein. At this point, the flow is especially high because the deep femoral vein empties just distally. We do not recommend implantation into the greater saphenous vein on the diseased side. Even though this procedure is technically very easy, the rate of later occlusion is remarkably high. In no case is the femoral vein dissected free about its entire circumference, as this might disturb the suspension of the vein [9]. The greater saphenous vein on the healthy side is then dissected free through two or three 10-cm skin incisions down to a level just above the knee. The appropriate length is measured with a sterile ruler; then, the vein is transected between ligatures, fully extracted through the inguinal incision, and flushed with heparinized saline solution. Prior to the transection of the saphenous vein, 10000 I.U. heparin should be given systematically. By finger dissection a tunnel is then created over the symphysis and secured with a plastic tube. The vein is pulled through this tube to the opposite side, great care being taken not to stretch or twist the vessel. The plastic tube is then removed. It should be carefully ascertained whether there are any varicosities in the region of the symphysis, and any that are found should be removed. Using a Satinsky clamp, the femoral vein on the diseased side is tangentially clamped and incised longitudinally over a distance of 1.5 cm. The end of the greater saphenous vein is tailored so as to fit the venotomy in the femoral vein. Then, beginning at the proximal corner, the end-to-side anastomosis is performed with running sutures of 6–0 Prolene. The anastomosis should be done without forceps, using stay sutures, under magnification. After the removal of the Satinsky clamp, suction drains should be placed in both wounds. Reversal of heparinization is not recommended. Postoperatively, the patient receives 5000 I.U. heparin subcutaneously t.i.d., or continuous heparinization. In the past, this procedure has been done without construction of a distal arteriovenous fistula, but today the construction of this fistula is the rule (see p. 723).

3. Results

The success rate is approximately 85%–90%. Early occlusions are usually caused by faulty patient selection or technical errors. If the crossover bypass remains open for 6–8 weeks, it can be expected to remain open long-term. After several years, the greater saphenous vein will show varicose changes; however, immediately after surgery the venous pressure will normalize quickly and remain normal in spite of these later changes. During later pregnancy, the bypass causes no problems; the lumen dilates, but reassumes its normal diameter in the postpartum period.

4. Complications

Because the patient is fully heparinized during surgery and because reversal of heparinization is not desirable, the risk of bleeding is increased. The hematoma can lead to compression of the bypass and subsequently to thrombosis. Therefore, meticulous hemostasis is mandatory.

5. Postoperative Treatment

Ligation of the fistula is usually done 3 months postoperatively. Afterward, venography should be performed. Prior to ligation of the fistula, exact visualization of the bypass is not possible because of the dilution of the contrast material. This can be circumvented only by digital subtraction angiography. Anticoagulation and compression therapy should be continued after occlusion of the fistula; 6 months after the operation, anticoagulation can be discontinued. Whether continuous compression therapy is necessary can be determined by venous dynamometry.

PTFE grafts in the Palma operation. In the last few years, favorable results using alloplastic grafts have been reported with increasing frequency in the literature. Here, ring-reinforced PTFE is clearly the material of choice. Though we are able to report long-term follow-up over 14 years with the Palma operation, we do not have any information on the fate of alloplastic material over 10–15 years or during pregnancy. However, the preliminary results are encouraging.

V. "High Palma" Procedure

1. Introduction

A special form of this procedure is the "high Palma" operation as described by Vollmar, which consists of connecting the two external iliac veins [9]. This procedure is limited to the treatment of permanent occlusion or extreme stenosis of the common iliac vein. It can be done directly after thrombectomy or secondarily, applying the principles of the normal Palma operation (Fig. 27.4.13).

2. Positioning, Exposure, and Surgical Technique

The procedure is performed with the patient in a supine position and under general anesthesia. At a distance of 2 cm cephalad from the inguinal ligament, the external iliac vein is exposed from both sides preperitoneally through an oblique skin incision. Using a long clamp, a tunnel is created for the graft, between the rectus abdominis muscles and the peritoneum, above the apex of the bladder. The anastomosis of the PTFE graft (10–12 mm diameter) is done with 5–0 Prolene following oval excisions of the venous wall on both sides.

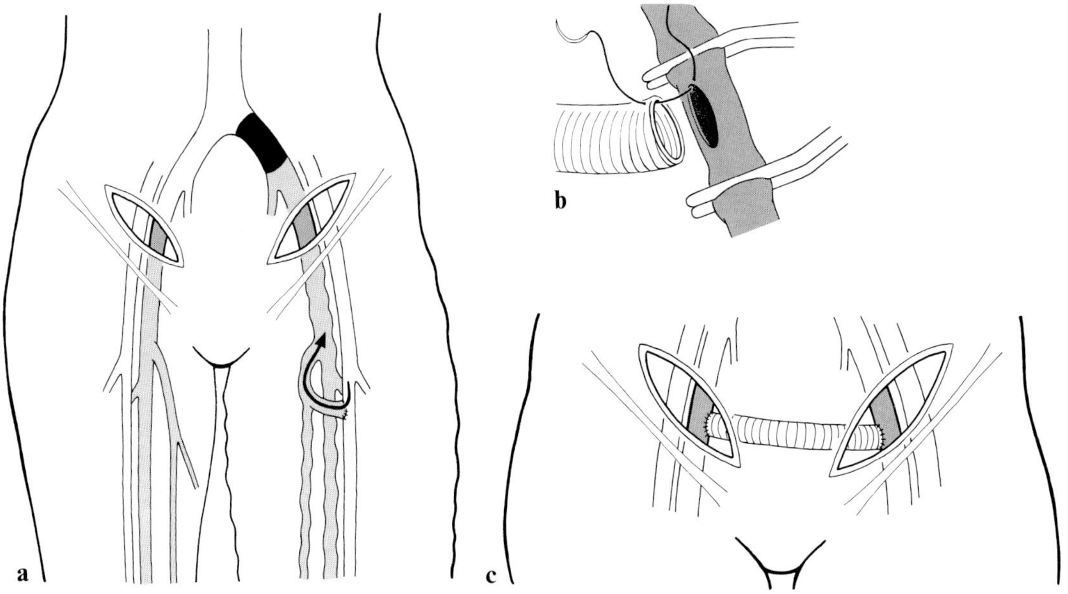

Fig. 27.4.13a–c. The high Palma operation. **a** Incision above the inguinal ligament. Both external iliac veins are exposed. **b** A ring-reinforced PTFE prosthesis (10–12 mm diameter) is anastomosed on the left side and brought preperitoneally to the contralateral side. **c** Right-sided anastomosis. A shunt at the groin level improves retrograde flow (see p. 723)

REFERENCES

1. Cockett B (1976) The pathology and surgery of the veins of the lower limb. Churchill Livingstone, Edinburgh
2. Gottlob R, May R (1985) Venenklappen. Urban & Schwarzenberg, München
3. Kubik S, May R (1979) Das Verspannungssytem der Venen in der Subinguinalregion. In: Die Leiste. Huber, Bern
4. May R (1979) In: Surgery of the veins of the leg and pelvis. Thieme, Stuttgart
5. May R (1984) Die Licht-Reflexions-Rheographie – LRR. Perimed
6. May R, Kriessmann A (1978) In: Periphere Venendruckmessung. Thieme, Stuttgart
7. May R, Weber J (1981) In: Pelvic and abdominal veins. Excerpta Medica
8. May R, Partsch H, Staubesand J (1981) Venae perforantes. Urban & Schwarzenberg, München
9. Vollmar J (1960) Der Hohe Palma. VASA 9:62

27.5 Pulmonary Embolism

W. Klinner and B. Reichart

CONTENTS

A. Surgical Anatomy

In order to perform pulmonary embolectomy and caval interruption, knowledge of the four following anatomic regions is necessary:

1. The anterior femoral region. For ligation of the superficial femoral vein, an oblique right- or left-sided incision below the inguinal ligament is performed. The same access is used in case of an emergency; the extracorporeal circulation is then connected to the femoral artery and vein.

2. Lateral cervical region. For insertion of a caval filter, the right internal jugular vein is exposed.

3. The caval suture filter, plication of the vena cava and use of a cava clip require exposure of the inferior vena cava through a median laparotomy or a right subcostal incision.

4. The embolectomy itself makes a direct approach necessary to the heart via a median sternotomy and a consecutive longitudinal opening of the pericardium.

1: For exposure of the common femoral artery and vein and their bifurcations the skin of the thigh is incised longitudinally, beginning slightly below the inguinal ligament and 1 cm lateral to where the pulse of the femoral artery is felt. This approach avoids lymphatic fistulas (see p. 392). Following incision of Scarpa's fascia, the common femoral artery and its bifurcation into the deep and superficial branch are dissected. The common femoral vein is located medial and posterior to arterial structures, as are the deep femoral and superficial femoral branches. Attention should be given to the small veins located behind the superficial femoral artery which cross the deep femoral branch. These vessels should be doubly ligated and transected, or troublesome bleeding may occur.

2: The internal right jugular vein is located behind the sternocleidomastoid muscle and enters the thorax behind the clavicle. At this point, the right brachial and innominate veins merge in order to form the superior vena cava.

After the platysma has been incised, the internal jugular vein is exposed, either by working through the fibres of the sternocleidomastoid muscle or following lateral incision. The omohyoid muscle crosses the internal jugular vein obliquely at its midpoint. After the muscle has been severed, the vein is dissected fully. It has a diameter of approximately 1–2 cm, which changes with respiration (danger of air embolism); the medial thyroid vein is the only side branch.

The vagal nerve and the common carotid artery are found posterior and medial to the internal jugular vein.

3: The abdominal part of the inferior vena cava is located in the right retroperitoneum somewhat posterior to the abdominal aorta. It may be approached through a right lateral flank incision or through a median laparotomy. If the transabdominal approach is chosen, the inferior vena cava is covered in its cranial part by the duodenum. The ligament of Treitz is then incised in order to create a better view of the vessel itself and of both renal veins. At the level of the attempted interruption – below the renals, at the level of the third lumbar vertebra – 2 to 3 lumbar side-branches are usually encountered. Care must be taken with these branches when the vein is encircled with an instrument, since bleeding from them may be very troublesome, especially when approaching the cava from a right lateral position in an obese patient with limited exposure.

The right ovarian or testicular veins empty into the cava from an anterior direction near the right renal vein. The left-sided structures merge into the homolateral renal vein. (These vein branches can only be reached via a transperitoneal approach.)

On the right side, the psoas muscle borders the inferior vena cava, which is crossed from lateral to medial by the ureter. The sympathetic trunk lies between the psoas muscle and the vena cava and above the lumbar veins.

4: For pulmonary embolectomy, a median sternotomy is preferred. After the pericardium has been opened lengthwise from the diaphragm to the innominate vein, one faces the right ventricular wall, the right atrium, the ascending aorta, the pulmonary trunk, and both venae cavae. The anterior intraventricular branch of the left coronary artery marks the border with the left ventricle. The level of the pulmonary valve is shown by the conal branch of the right coronary artery. The trunk leads in a cranioposterior direction to its bifurcation.

B. Pulmonary Embolectomy

Fulminant pulmonary emboli still pose a serious threat to a patient's life, even though their pathology and physiology have been understood for more than a century. LAENNEC described "pulmonary apoplexy" as early as 1819 [13]. In 1858, VIRCHOW [29] recognized the triad of venostasis, injury to the vein, and hypercoagulability as prerequisites for thrombosis of the deep pelvic veins. This triad, named after him, still forms the pathogenetic basis, although it seems that venostasis is the most important factor.

I. Indication for Surgical Intervention After Fulminant Pulmonary Embolism

The optimal therapy for pulmonary embolism still remains controversial. In 1908, TRENDELENBURG [26] recommended surgical treatment, although he never performed this intervention in a clinical situation. The first successful clinical embolectomy, the extraction of an embolus from the trunk of the pulmonary artery, was performed by KIRSCHNER [12] in 1924. VOSS-SCHULTE [30] reported in 1965 on 43 interventions performed between 1957 and 1963, in 7 of which the patient survived long-term. The study revealed a high operative mortality if performed without the support of extracorporeal circulation, a technique that was introduced by SHARP [22] and COOLEY [4] in the early sixties.

After BAUER [3], BARRITT and JORDAN [2] described heparin as a major principle of therapy for pulmonary emboli, the pendulum seems to have swung more and more in the direction of conservative treatment. If the patient survives the acute event for longer than 2 h and remains hemodynamically stable, the prognosis on anticoagulation alone is excellent.

Nowadays, surgical embolectomy seems to be justified only if the patient remains hypotensive despite intensive pharmacological support with catecholamines, vasodilators, and heparin. According to SASAHARA [20], embolectomy is indicated only when the systolic blood pressure remains below 90 mmHg for 1 h, the urinary output measures less than 20 ml/h, and the arterial oxygen tension stays at 60 mmHg.

If sudden cardiac arrest occurs, minimal circulation is maintained by means of cardiac massage; the patient is quickly intubated and ventilated. If the pupils remain small and react to light again, the diagnosis of pulmonary embolus and the indication for emergency embolectomy is based on the history (which includes previous surgery, delivery, and extended bed rest) and clinical findings alone. The classic signs of a large-sized pulmonary embolus are dyspnea, crushing chest pain, tachycardia, hypotension, and venous inflow obstruction; right ventricular strain patterns are seen on the electrocardiogram.

If the condition of the patient allows further diagnostic measures, i.e., pulmonary scan and pulmonary arteriography, these should be undertaken to delineate the extent of pulmonary embolization. If more than half of both lungs are involved, surgery is indicated, especially if catecholamines are necessary to maintain hemodynamic stability.

II. Surgical Techniques

1. Embolectomy in Inflow Occlusion (see also Vol. VI/1 of the Surgical Handbook, p. 561)

A median sternotomy using an oscillating or an electric saw opens the thorax (Fig. 27.5.1a). The pericardium is then incised longitudinally. The right atrium appears engorged; contractions of the right ventricle are impeded. With the aid of a large right-angled clamp, the inferior and superior vena cava are taped. A stay suture (4–0 polypropylene) is placed in the anterior wall of the pulmonary artery trunk, 1 cm above the valvular annulus; another, 4–5 cm more cranially. An assistant then pulls the two sutures anteriorly. The surgeon partially occludes the pulmonary artery trunk with a Satinsky clamp; the arteriotomy is made. The time is noted, and both venae cavae are snared. Within 5 s after the heart has emptied, the clamp on the pulmonary artery trunk is removed. A suction device is now inserted into the pulmonary artery trunk and all its branches.

At the same time, the anaesthetist repeatedly inflates the lungs in order to express peripheral thrombi, which can then be removed by suction.

Fresh and soft thrombi are sucked up and disappear in the drainage without being detected visually by the surgeon.

The heart continues to beat during these manipulations, and a minimal circulation is usually maintained. However, after 90–120 s the intervention must be discontinued. The anaesthetist immediately expands the lungs, thus filling the distal parts of the pulmonary artery system. At the same time, the snare around the superior vena cava is loosened and blood fills the right ventricle. The assistant then pulls again on both sutures within the pulmonary artery wall, facilitating the placement of the Satinsky clamp. Finally, the snare on the inferior vena cava is loosened. Usually, forceful contractions of the heart and an increase in blood pressure occur instantaneously.

The procedure may be repeated once or twice if it is uncertain whether all emboli have been extracted. Small peripheral emboli can, in addition, be removed by manual compression of the lung. This measure necessitates the opening of the pleural cavities and subsequent drainage.

Closure of the pulmonary artery incision is done with a double running suture of 4–0 or 5–0 polypropylene.

The chest is closed, leaving the pericardium open. Two chest drains are left, one behind the heart and one behind the sternum. The latter is closed with 5–7 single wire loops. Subcutaneous tissue and skin are closed separately.

2. Embolectomy with the Help of Extracorporeal Circulation

If an extracorporeal bypass machine is available, it should always be used (Fig. 27.5.1b). This will ensure that the surgeon is not pressed for time, and that support of the right ventricle after embolectomy is possible. The thorax is again opened through a median sternotomy. After heparin has been given, the aorta and the inferior and superior venae cavae are cannulated, and extracorporeal circulation commences. The pulmonary artery trunk is opened. A search for emboli in the branches of the pulmonary artery can now be made without time constraints. A curved suction device (Fig. 27.5.1c) has proven to be superior to pliable catheters.

The pulmonary artery is closed using 4– or 5–0 polypropylene. The moment stable hemodynamics are achieved, the extracorporeal circulation is stopped and the cannulae removed; protamin is given and the chest closed as already described.

3. Embolectomy During Resuscitation Measures

The patient is placed on the operating table in a supine position; both inguinal regions are prepared and draped while the cardiopulmonary bypass is being readied. Heparin is given.

Following a longitudinal incision in the groin area, the common femoral artery is dissected, together with its bifurcation into the superficial and deep branches. The vessels are encircled with umbilical tapes. Following occlusion of the femoral artery proximally and distally, a transverse arteriotomy is made and an appropriate cannula inserted and fixed in place. The arterial tubing of the cardiopulmonary bypass is connected. A fine purse-string suture is placed in the common femoral vein, which is then occluded distally and cannulated with the largest catheter. Care must be taken to advance the cannula into the inferior vena cava. The venous tubing is then connected to the heart-lung machine.

During this time cardiac massage must be continued. After extracorporeal circulation and cooling have begun (an esophageal temperature of 30°

a
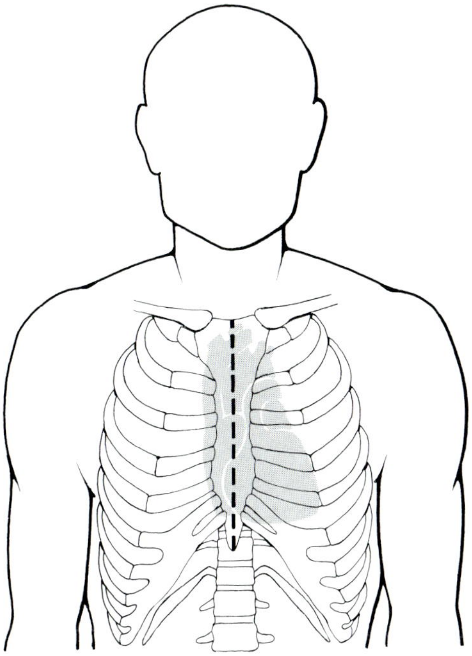

b
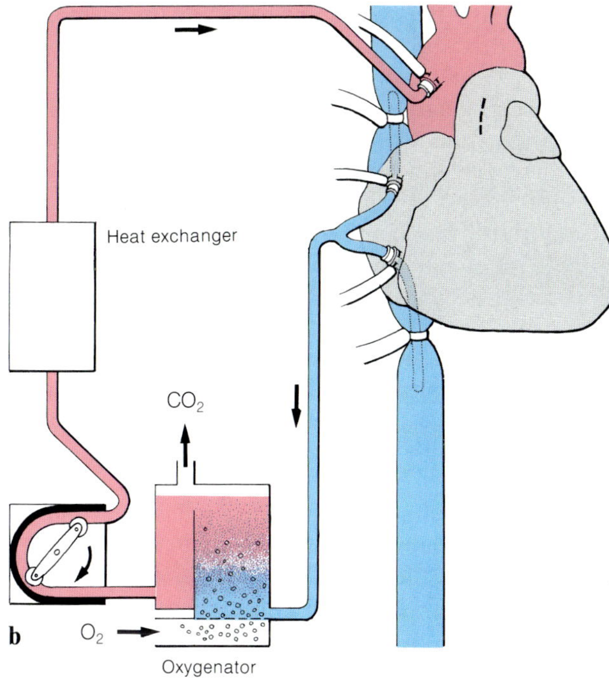

c
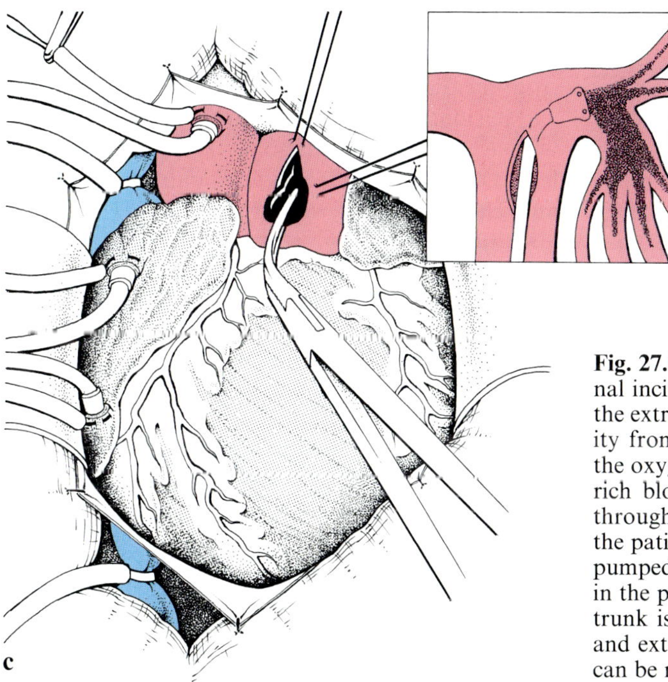

Fig. 27.5.1. a Opening of the thorax through a longitudinal incision (*broken line*). **b** Schematic representation of the extracorporeal circulation; the blood drains by gravity from both venae cavae and is first passed through the oxygenator (shown as a bubble device). The oxygen-rich blood is then moved by means of a roller pump through a heat exchanger, which makes it possible for the patient's body to be cooled and rewarmed. It is then pumped into the ascending aorta (*broken line*, incision in the pulmonary artery trunk). **c** The pulmonary artery trunk is opened. An embolus is grasped with a forceps and extracted. The inset shows how peripheral thrombi can be removed by means of a suction device

is aimed at), the thorax is opened in the fashion already described. Cooling, however, should not be carried out if aortic insufficiency is present.

If ventricular fibrillation is encountered, defibrillation should be attempted. After cannulating the superior and inferior vena cava, the cannula from the femoral vein may be removed.

On full bypass, a longitudinal incision is made in the pulmonary artery trunk, and the operation proceeds as described in Section B 11.2. The surgeon has now enough time to search for emboli in all branches of the pulmonary artery.

When no more emboli are found, the pulmonary artery is closed while the lungs are expanded; a double running suture of 4–0 or 5–0 polypropylene is utilized.

Operative mortality following pulmonary embolectomy remains high at between 20% and 90%, depending on the underlying conditions. At our hospital, 11 of 23 patients who underwent embolectomy survived long-term (=47.8%). The best results are reported by TSCHIRKOV and co-workers from Frankfurt [27]. After adopting the principles of SASAHARA for their patient selection, the operative mortality dropped from 43% to 23%.

Patients who survive pulmonary embolectomy can expect normal pulmonary function [24].

4. Catheter Embolectomy According to GREENFIELD

GREENFIELD and co-workers [7] have described a method in which embolectomy is done without thoracotomy. The long catheter is introduced into the pulmonary artery via the common femoral vein, the iliac vein, the right atrium, and the ventricle. The tip of the catheter is provided with a suction device, which is directed by means of a steering mechanism into the branch of the pulmonary artery where one suspects the embolus. When the embolus comes into contact with the suction device (the approach can be controlled by means of contrast medium), a vacuum is created at the proximal end of the catheter, thereby fixing the embolus by suction and allowing it to be removed via the femoral vein. GREENFIELD and co-workers have treated 15 patients using this technique and were able to remove the embolus in 13 cases. Three patients died, constituting a mortality of 20% [9].

5. Surgical Treatment of Chronic Pulmonary Emboli

In a patient who survives pulmonary embolism, the natural outcome is lysis and reconstitution of the vascular bed. In rare cases, however, this process does not take place. Since the work of LJUNGDAHL [14], it has been known that pulmonary emboli, which do not lyse, are transformed into tight fibrous tissue. Blocking or stenosis result and can be the cause of pulmonary hypertension and, ultimately, cor pulmonale. Clinically, these patients show severe resting dyspnea owing to chronically low arterial oxygen content.

Surgical therapy consists in desobliteration of the pulmonary artery. For this procedure, the patients must be connected to cardiopulmonary bypass as already described. An incision is usually made in a pulmonary artery branch. Then, using a dissector, a plane is developed between the wall of the pulmonary artery and the organized thrombus; the removal of the thrombus is aided in part by gentle traction. If it cannot be extracted completely, however, further incisions into the periphery of the pulmonary artery may be necessary. The operation is successful when blood flow returns from the distal part of the vessel.

Incisions in the pulmonary artery are closed with a continuous suture of 4–0 or 5–0 polypropylene. Disconnection from cardiopulmonary bypass and closure of the wound follow the technique already described.

In rare terminal cases with cor pulmonale, heart-lung transplantation may be justified.

C. Partial or Total Interruption of the Inferior Vena Cava

I. Indications

Surgical and medical prophylaxis of pulmonary embolism, which is mostly caused by deep vein thrombosis of the legs or of the pelvis, continue to be controversial.

In 1934, the principle of creating a surgical blockade between the thrombus and the pulmonary artery was first described by HOMANS [10] who recommended ligation of the common femoral vein distal to the major saphenous vein branch. This surgical procedure, however, was associated with a high recurrence rate of pulmonary emboli of up to 24%. As a result, OCHSNER and DEBAKEY [17] recommended total ligation of the inferior vena cava below the renals.

The prophylactic treatment with low dose i.v. heparin, introduced by SHARNOFF [21] in 1960, tries to counteract the pathophysiologic processes at an even earlier stage; heparin in low dosage activates the plasma inhibitors of factor X. This treatment was modified in 1971 by KAKKAR [11] who described the more convenient technique of subcutaneous injections. Since then, surgical methods of preventing pulmonary embolism – whether by ligation of the inferior vena cava or with some modification using filters or clips – are indicated only under special conditions, particularly because they are associated with significant postoperative complications, e.g., extremity edema. However, under anticoagulant therapy, there remains a 5%–25% risk of a pulmonary embolism. If pulmonary embolism has already occurred, the chance of a second episode is 4%–20%.

Nowadays, surgical interventions are still recommended when anticoagulant therapy is unsuccessful or even contraindicated, as in cases of stroke, trauma of the central nervous system, malignant hypertension or gastrointestinal bleeding. Multiple small emboli may cause pulmonary hypertension and secondary cor pulmonale. In these rare cases, the inferior vena cava should be ligated, but a filter or clip should not be used. For similar reasons, caval interruption is indicated in patients who already have pulmonary hypertension and present with signs of a threatening thromboembolism. Septic pulmonary emboli, in spite of adequate antibiotic treatment, are also an indication for caval interruption to prevent the development of pulmonary abscesses.

The opinion that the vena cava should always be blocked following an embolectomy is still controversial. According to MILLER and co-workers [15] – and our own personal experience – this prophylactic intervention is not necessary; instead, anticoagulant therapy is begun immediately after the operation and maintained for 6 months, first with heparin, then with coumarin derivatives.

II. Choice of Procedure

Of particular importance are the general condition and age of the patient, as well as any concomitant diseases. Existing heart failure necessitates choosing the quickest and the least traumatizing intervention. The magnitude of the operative trauma increases in the following order: ligation of the superficial femoral vein, positioning of a caval filter according to MOBIN-UDDIN [16] or KIMRAY-GREENFIELD [8], fixation of a caval clip according to ADAMS-DE WEESE [1] and finally – the most extensive procedure, which may be reserved for cases of septic emboli, vascular anomalies, and microemboli – total ligation of the cava using a transperitoneal approach following median laparotomy [18].

The intraluminal caval filter and the Adams-De Weese clip, which effect a partial occlusion of the vein, offer protection against bigger emboli, more than 4 mm in diameter. If smaller emboli occur only occasionally, they hardly ever cause death. One should, however, keep in mind that, following partial interruption of the vena cava, total blocking often occurs as a result of the entrapment of additional emboli, and through secondary thrombosis. Nevertheless, the primary choice of procedure nowadays will preferably be one involving partial interruption.

III. Surgical Techniques

1. Ligation of the Superficial Femoral Vein

This can be done under local anesthesia. The patient is in a supine, slightly reversed Trendelenburg position, with the upper body elevated 10° to create a positive venous pressure in the femoral vein. The incision starts at the inguinal ligament and is extended longitudinally somewhat lateral and anterior to the common femoral artery, down to the junction of the deep and superficial femoral veins. The superficial femoral vein is doubly encircled with nonabsorbable 4–0 sutures, ligated, and transected. Fresh thrombi are removed prior to this maneuver from proximal and distal with a Fogarty catheter. If the catheter cannot be passed distally, the thrombi are expressed by an Esmarch bandage, starting from the foot (see p. 722).

The ligation of the superficial femoral vein is nowadays only rarely indicated, for example, in seriously ill patients when a caval umbrella filter

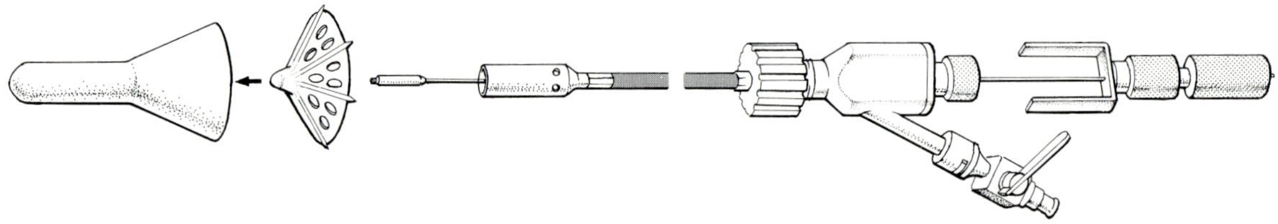

Fig. 27.5.2. Assembly of the introducer set of a Mobin-Uddin umbrella filter: There is a handle on the right-hand side which may be attached to a wire in a fixed position. The wire runs through the carrier catheter (*shown broken*) and extends it. The tip of the wire is equipped with a thin metal cone with threads on which the umbrella filter is mounted. On the left-hand side is the loading cone

is not available. Furthermore, in spite of this operation, pulmonary emboli can occur, originating from the "healthy" leg.

2. Vena Cava Umbrella According to MOBIN-UDDIN and KIM-RAY-GREENFIELD

Both filters are positioned by the same technique. The umbrella-shaped filter is attached to a catheter in the closed position and introduced into the inferior vena cava via the internal jugular vein, superior vena cava, and right atrium. The Kim-Ray-Greenfield filter can also be inserted via the common femoral and iliac vein. However, a different introducer set is needed for this route. The Mobin-Uddin filter can only be placed via the internal jugular vein.

The apparatus for introducing the Mobin-Uddin filter consists of a yellow carrier catheter, with the loading cone located on the tip. This cone contains the folded umbrella-shaped filter. A handle to allow the discharge of the umbrella is attached to the end of a wire that runs the length of the catheter and extends beyond the loading cone. The cylindrical metal tip of the wire, 1 mm in diameter, is equipped with threads. The umbrella, with a perforated covering, is 28 mm in diameter and has six spokes; it is loosely screwed onto the threads. The tips of the spokes extend 2 mm beyond the edge of the umbrella (Fig. 27.5.2).

a

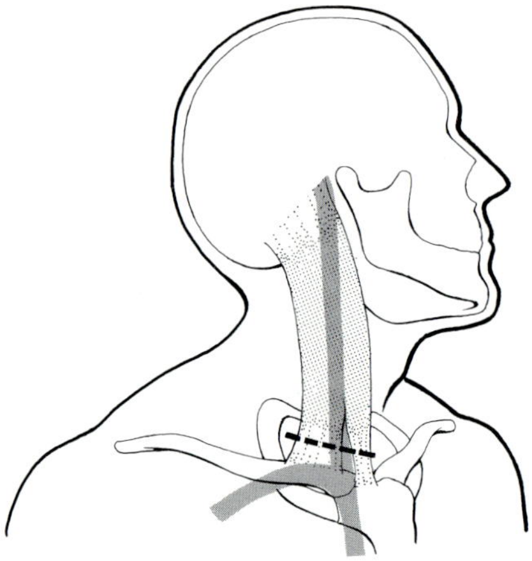

b

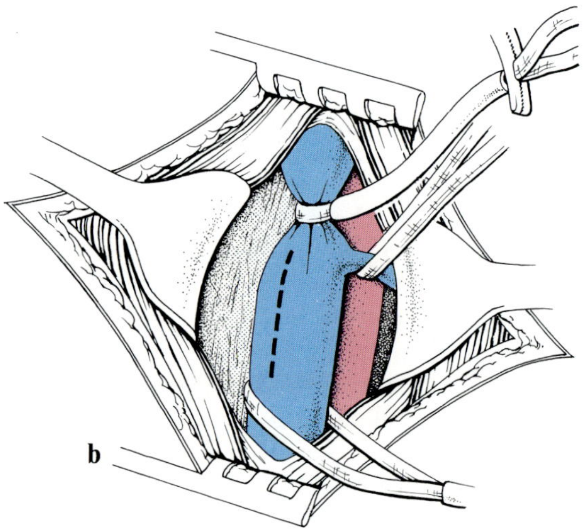

c

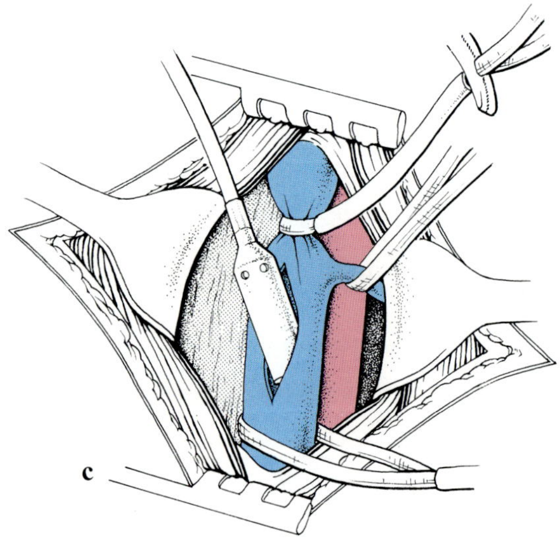

Fig. 27.5.3. a Insertion of a Mobin-Uddin umbrella filter into the inferior vena cava through the right internal jugular vein (*broken line*, skin incision). b Surgical anatomy: The internal jugular vein is dissected, doubly encircled and the tapes fitted with tourniquets. The large venous branch from the thyroid vein is also encircled. To the right one sees the common carotid artery (*broken line* indicates the planned incision into the internal jugular vein). c Insertion of the loading cone containing the umbrella; the proximal tourniquet around the internal jugular vein is pulled tight

The actual procedure is carried out under local anaesthesia, if necessary at the bedside. The patient is in a supine position, the head turned towards the left. For cosmetic reasons, the skin incision may be done transversely over the head of the sternocleidomastoid muscle 1–2 cm above the clavicle (Fig. 27.5.3a); longitudinal incisions between the clavicular and the sternal muscle insertion will, however, facilitate the venous access.

After the platysma has been transected, the two heads of the sternocleidomastoid muscle are separated bluntly in the direction of the fibres. The jugular vein is then located beneath the fascia. The vessel is dissected over a distance of approximately 4 cm and encircled proximally and distally with umbilical tape (Fig. 27.5.3b). The medial thyroid vein is divided between ligatures; if necessary, the omohyoid muscle is divided in a similar way for adequate exposure. The filter can now be introduced into the venous system: first, the internal jugular vein is occluded proximally and distally with umbilical tapes fitted with tourniquets; the vessel is then incised longitudinally. The proximal tape is loosened, allowing the loading cone with the folded Mobin-Uddin umbrella to be introduced into the lumen of the vessel (Fig. 27.5.3c). Under fluoroscopic control, the loading cone is positioned over the lower margin of the third lumbar vertebra. This point is always below the renal veins and above the iliac bifurcation (Fig. 27.5.4). In addition a cavogram, which may be produced via a side-connection of the Mobin-Uddin catheter, can provide an exact localization. This measure is especially recommended when anomalies of the inferior vena cava are suspected.

The folded umbrella is then discharged from the loading cone under fluoroscopic control and pulled gently proximally in order to allow the spokes to become engaged with the venous wall. During this maneuver, the caval filter should not tilt; if it does, one should assume that the spokes are to some extent freely movable. If unscrewed under these circumstances the umbrella could embolize into the right heart and finally into the lung. If it is not possible to fix an umbrella safely, it

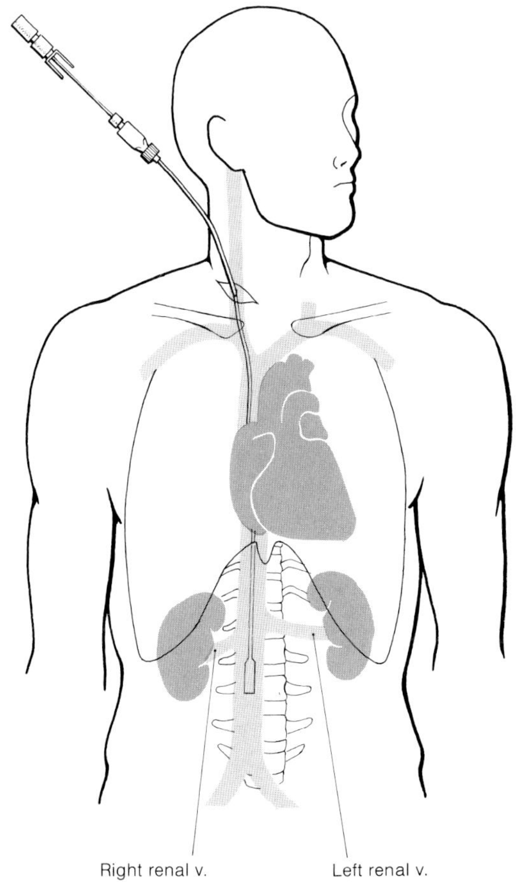

Fig. 27.5.4. Positioning of the Mobin-Uddin inferior vena cava umbrella; the correct position of the carrier catheter is shown schematically. The loading cone must be positioned below the renal veins

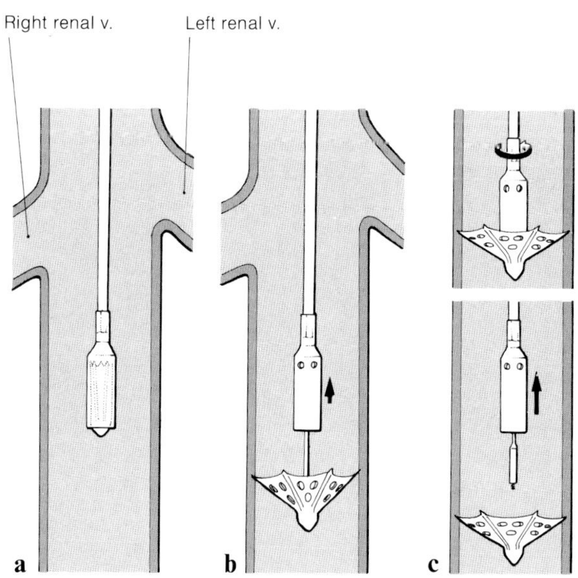

Fig. 27.5.5a–c. After the correct position below the renal veins has been ascertained (**a**) the umbrella is discharged with the aid of the wire and pulled back gently in order to allow the spokes to contact the venous wall (**b**); thereafter, the carrier catheter is removed by rotating the wire counterclockwise, thereby unscrewing it from the fixed Mobin-Uddin umbrella (**c**)

should be removed through an "emergency exit" via the iliac and femoral veins.

If the caval filter is in a satisfactory position, the wire is detached and removed (Fig. 27.5.5a–c).

The description of the positioning of the caval filter appears more complicated and dangerous than it is in reality. Incorrect placement of the filter proximal to the renal vein or in one of the iliac veins can be avoided if the proper technique is applied. Retroperitoneal hematoma – another complication – may occur when the sharp spokes of the umbrella perforate the vena cava; this can be avoided if heparin is discontinued 1 h prior to the procedure.

Umbrella filters establish a partial blockade of the inferior vena cava, thus providing protection against significant emboli while at the same time avoiding the risks of extremity edema associated with ligation. However, this theoretical concept cannot always be realized: The holes in the umbrella material cause turbulence in the venous blood flow which can ultimately lead to thrombosis of the entire surface of the filter – the incidence being 67% for all sizes of umbrella. A lower occlusion rate can be expected with newer models, coated with heparin.

Another device, the Kim-Ray-Greenfield caval filter, has been commercially available for some time (Fig. 27.5.6). It seems to have certain advantages compared with the Mobin-Uddin umbrella: The filter consists of six fine steel wires, welded together to form a tip. The separate ends of the wires are bent like fish hooks and penetrate very gently into the venous wall. In contrast to the Mobin-Uddin umbrella, the tip of the Kim-Ray-Greenfield filter points towards the heart. Because of its conical shape, thrombi form in the centre first, thus leaving the outer parts of the filter unobstructed; clinical investigations prove a patency rate of 97%.

The technique of implantation is analogous to that described for the Mobin-Uddin umbrella. Here too, a carrier catheter is equipped with a metal loading cone at the patient's end, into which the folded wire cage fits. At the surgeon's end there is, once again, an adjustable handle on a wire that runs through the catheter to extend it; the wire ends in a metal pin. During loading, the metal pin is pulled towards the bottom of the loading cone by means of the wire. The filter is then pushed as far as possible into the cone by hand and then fully inserted by means of a loading stick. In order to prevent non-opening of the filter, one must make sure that the fine wires do not become entangled during this procedure.

As with the Mobin-Uddin umbrella, precise positioning at the lower margin of the third lumbar vertebra is verified by fluoroscopy; the filter is then discharged by pushing the metal pin out of the loading cone.

A Kim-Ray-Greenfield filter may be introduced via the common femoral vein as well. This can be advantageous if the indication for a caval interruption is made during venography of the legs or during a thrombectomy procedure of the iliac or femoral veins. In these cases, a different introducer set with an oval piston in order to unfold the filter is necessary.

3. Positioning of a Vena Cava Clip According to ADAMS-DEWEESE (Suture Filter According to DEWEESE, Plication of the Inferior Vena Cava According to Spencer)

Ligation of the inferior vena cava leads to extremity edema in a high percentage of cases. As a consequence several partial interruption techniques have been developed in the past. Common to all of them is the subdivision of the large lumen of the inferior vena cava into several smaller compartments in order to trap fatal emboli on their way to the

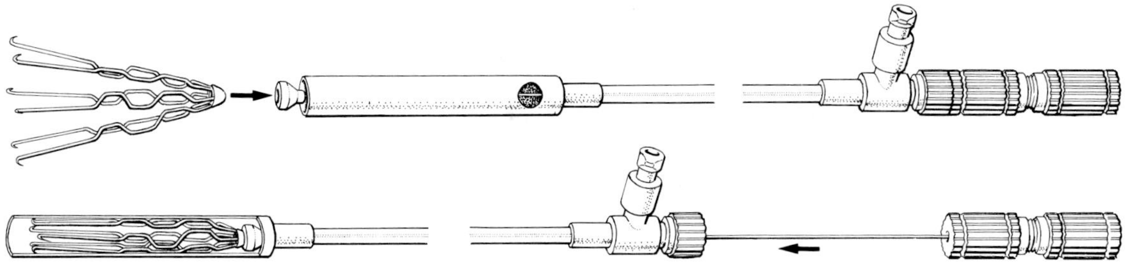

Fig. 27.5.6. Kim-Ray-Greenfield filter, including the insertion apparatus. The *drawing below* shows the folded filter within the loading cone. The two *arrows* indicate the loading move (*above*) and discharge move (*below*)

lungs, while otherwise preserving the caval blood flow. For all techniques, access to the inferior vena cava is necessary.

The DeWeese suture grid is constructed by repeatedly transfixing the vessel with sutures placed 2–3 mm apart ([5]; Fig. 27.5.7).

The method of SPENCER [25] seems to be simpler. Here, the vena cava is plicated by means of two mattress sutures placed 4–5 mm apart, thereby dividing the vessel into three compartments (Fig. 27.5.8).

The Adams-DeWeese clip represents an even simpler application of this principle [1]. This Teflon clip consists of two branches, both 35 mm in length. One branch is smooth, while the other has 3 teeth like a comb. When the clip is closed, it creates four compartments, each 4 mm in diameter (Fig. 27.5.9a, b).

The inferior vena cava is approached through an incision in the right flank similar to that used for a lumbar sympathectomy. After general endotracheal anesthesia has been induced, the patient is brought to a left lateral position. A cushion is positioned underneath the left kidney area; the left leg is flexed, the right leg extended. The skin incision follows a curve two finger breadths below the margin of the right 12th rib. The layers of the abdominal external/internal oblique and transverse muscles are separated in the direction of the fibres. The peritoneum is dissected bluntly from the surrounding fat and connecting tissue. During

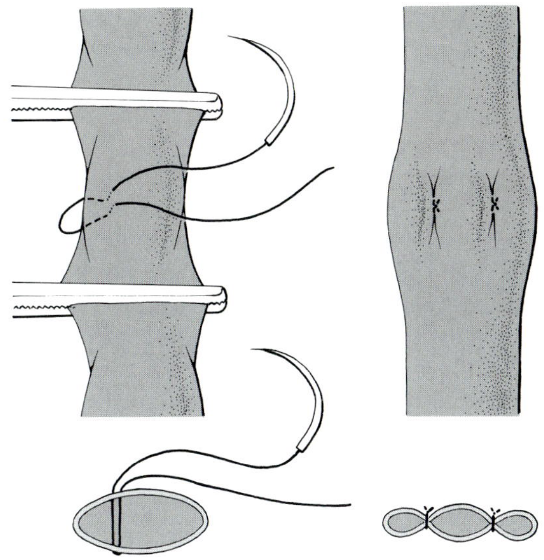

Fig. 27.5.8. Partial interruption of the vena cava according to SPENCER [25]. Two mattress sutures are placed through the vena cava 4–5 mm apart

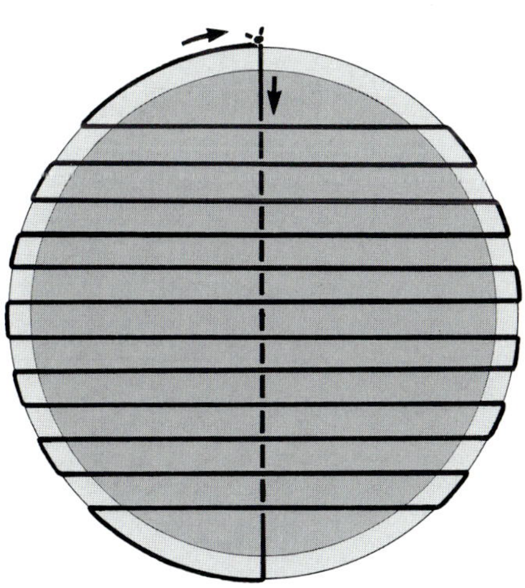

Fig. 27.5.7. Suture filter developed by DEWEESE [5]. A nonabsorbable suture is repeatedly passed through the vena cava transversely at intervals of 2–3 mm. The suture is tied in the middle of the anterior circumference

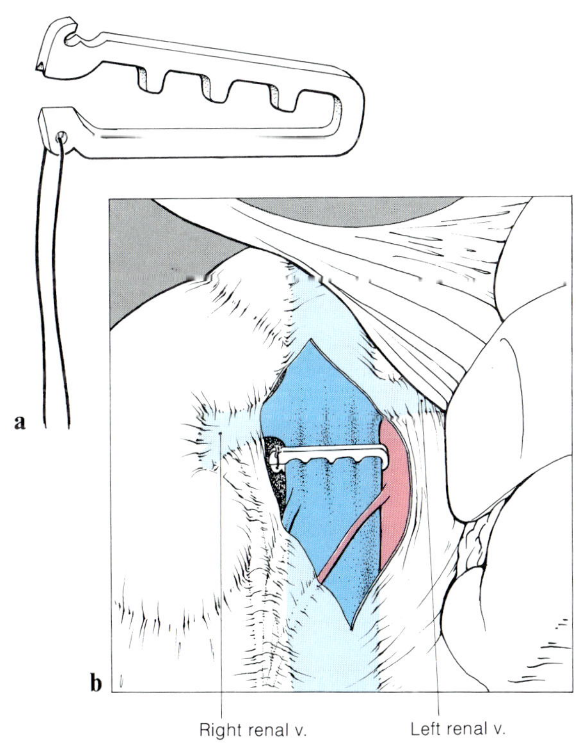

Fig. 27.5.9. a Caval clip as developed by ADAM-DE WEESE [1]. **b** Adam-DeWeese clip in the closed position. The vena cava can be approached retroperitoneally as well as transperitoneally (as shown in this case)

this procedure, the right psoas muscle can be palpated. The peritoneal sac is then held back, preferably using a large Harrington retractor. The vena cava appears medial to the psoas muscle. One should free the vein only where necessary in order to avoid undue injury to the lumbar veins. The vena cava is finally lifted gently with a vascular forceps and encircled with a large right-angled clamp. (During this maneuver one should bear in mind that there may be thrombi within the vessel. If this is the case, they can be removed after opening the cava.) The Adam-DeWeese clip is then guided with its smooth branch behind the inferior vena cava; it is closed by tying the two branches together (Fig. 27.4.9b).

The abdominal incision is sutured in layers; a drain is usually not necessary.

The clip operation carries a risk of between 1% and 9% in comparison with 3% for umbrella filter procedures [18]. Reports differ concerning the caval patency rate; bilateral edema of the legs indicates complete occlusion of the inferior vena cava at the level of the clip. In order to avoid this complication, anticoagulation treatment for a few months is recommended. If edema of the leg does occur, however, one must start immediate and effective treatment. Elastic bandages should be applied, starting from the feet up to the thigh. This makes early walking possible. While the patient is lying in bed the legs should be elevated by 15°–20°. In the later, postoperative phase grade II compression stockings should be worn until the swelling has completely subsided.

4. Ligation of the Inferior Vena Cava

Interruption by ligation is the most radical but also the safest palliative procedure. It is indicated for repeat microemboli that are too small to be intercepted by any of the techniques described above and is the only procedure that should be used for the prevention of septic emboli. One possible approach for ligation is through the right flank incision just described. However, the transabdominal access is preferable for two reasons:

Firstly, additional procedures, such as removal of septic foci in the region of the pelvis, may be necessary.

Secondly, in female patients, the ovarian veins may also be ligated in order to increase the effectiveness of the palliation. It is known that both ovarian veins can increase in size remarkably after ligation of the inferior vena cava and become the source of fatal pulmonary emboli.

After induction of general endotracheal anesthesia, the procedure is performed through a long midline incision, extending from the xiphoid to one handbreadth below the umbilicus. Then, a self-retaining retractor, for example of the Kirschner type, is inserted. Jejunum and ileum are covered with moist pads and retracted towards the right, thereby permitting a view of the duodenum, the abdominal aorta, and the inferior mesenteric vein. The ligament of Treitz is transected at the left border of the duodenum and the peritoneum incised over the abdominal aorta. The anterior surface of the aorta is exposed only in order to ascertain the position of the left renal vein. The aorta is then encircled with an umbilical tape and retracted slightly to the left. The inferior vena cava is identified on the right side of the aorta and dissected as much as necessary. A right-angled clamp is passed twice around the vessel, which is then doubly ligated using non-absorbable suture material. Finally, in females, the ovarian veins are occluded. The right vein empties at the anterior surface into the inferior vena cava, close to the right renal vein; the left drains directly into the homolateral renal vessel. In order to facilitate ligation, the inferior mesenteric vein may be transected between ligatures.

The abdomen is closed in layers, drains are unnecessary.

Ligation of the vena cava may also be achieved through a right subcostal incision. The liver is retracted cranially and the hepato-colic ligament transected. The duodenum is mobilized by the Kocher maneuver; the inferior vena cava will then be found in the middle of the operative field.

Since the approach just described is more complicated and riskier than the other, it should be used only as an alternative.

Ligation of the cava has been controversial from the start. There have always been enthusiastic advocates [18] as well as detractors [19]. Reports of a high operative mortality of up to 40% have been published; VERAT and co-workers [28] attributed a decreased p.o. exercise tolerance to the diminished venous return from the lower extremities.

More recently, however, the introduction of new techniques, such as the previously described intraluminal filter procedure for very sick patients, has contributed to greater rigour in patient selection for caval ligation and consequently to a lowering of the operative mortality. DONALDSON [6] reports a total operative mortality of 21%, SILVER

[23], of 15%. Ligation of the vena cava also carries a high morbidity: venostasis is reported in 10%–50% of cases. The clinical picture consists of edema of the legs, dermatitis, varicose veins, and chronic ulcers. OCHSNER [18], however, states that morbidity can be reduced by the early application of elastic bandages to the upper and lower leg while the patient is still in the operating room (for further therapeutic measures see p. 732). The prescription of heparin or coumarin derivatives does not seem to be necessary.

REFERENCES

1. Adams JT, DeWeese JA (1966) Partial interruption of the inferior vena cava with a new plastic clip. Surg Gynecol Obstet 123:1087
2. Barrit DW, Jordan SC (1960) Anticoagulant drugs in the treatment of pulmonary embolism. A controlled trial. Lancet 1:1309
3. Bauer G (1959) The introduction of heparin therapy in cases of early thrombosis. Circulation 19:108
4. Cooley DA, Beall AC, Alexander JK (1961) Acute massive pulmonary embolism. Successful surgical treatment using temporary cardiopulmonary bypass. JAMA 177:283
5. DeWeese MS, Hunter DC (1963) A vena cava filter for the prevention of pulmonary embolism. Arch Surg 86:181
6. Donaldson MC, Wirthlin LS, Donaldson GA (1979) Thirty-vein experience with surgical interruption of the inferior cava for prevention of pulmonary embolism. Ann Surg 191:367
7. Greenfield LJ, Bruce TA, Nichols NB (1971) Transvenous pulmonary embolectomy by catheter device. Ann Surg 174:881
8. Greenfield LJ, McCurdy JR, Brown PP, Elking RC (1977) A new intracaval filter permitting continued flow and resolution of emboli. Ann Surg 185:692
9. Greenfield LJ, Zocco JJ (1979) Intraluminal management of acute massive pulmonary thromboembolism. J Thorac Cardiovasc Surg 77:402
10. Homans J (1934) Thrombosis of the deep veins of the lower leg causing pulmonary embolism. N Engl J Med 211:993
11. Kakkar VV, Field ES, Nicolaides AN, Flute PT, Wessler S, Yin ET (1971) Low doses of heparin in prevention of deep-vein thrombosis. Lancet 2:669
12. Kirschner M (1924) Ein durch die Trendelenburg'sche Operation geheilter Fall von Embolie der A. pulmonalis. Langenbecks Arch Klin Chir 133:312
13. Laennec RTH (1819) De l'auscultation médiate. Brossen et Chaude, Paris
14. Ljungdahl M (1928) Gibt es eine chronische Embolisierung der Lungenarterie? Dtsch Arch Klin Med 160:1
15. Miller GAH, Hall RJC, Paneth M (1977) Pulmonary embolectomy, heparin and streptokinase: their place in the treatment of acute massive pulmonary embolism. Am Heart J 93:568
16. Mobin-Uddin K, Bolooki H, Jude JR (1969) A new simplified method of caval interruption for prevention of pulmonary embolism. Circulation [Suppl III] 39/40:111–149
17. Ochsner A, De Bakey M (1943) Intravenous clotting and its sequelae. Surgery 14:679
18. Ochsner A, Ochsner JL, Sanders HS (1970) Prevention of pulmonary embolism by caval ligation. Ann Surg 17:923
19. Piccone VA, Vidal E, Yarnoz M, Glass P, LeVeen HH (1970) The late results of caval ligation. Surgery 68:980
20. Sasahara AA (1967) Pulmonary vascular responses to thromboembolism. Mod Conc Cardiovasc Dis 36:55
21. Sharnoff JG (1966) Results in the prophylaxis of postoperative thromboembolism. Surg Gynecol Obstet 123:303
22. Sharp EH (1962) Pulmonary embolectomy: successful removal of a massive pulmonary embolus with the support of cardiopulmonary bypass. A case report. Ann Surg 156:1
23. Silver D, Sabiston DC (1975) The rate of vena caval interruption in the management of pulmonary embolism. Surgery 77:1
24. Soyer R, Brunet AP, Redonnet M, Borg JY, Hubscher C, Letac B (1982) Follow up of surgically treated patients with massive pulmonary embolism – with reference to 12 operated patients. Thorac Cardiovasc Surg 30:103
25. Spencer FC, Jude J, Rienhoff WF, Stonesifer G (1965) Plication of the inferior vena cava for pulmonary embolism. Ann Surg 161:788
26. Trendelenburg F (1980) Über die operative Behandlung der Embolie der Lungenarterie. Langenbecks Arch Klin Chir 86:686
27. Tschirkov A, Krause E, Elert O, Satter P (1978) Surgical management of massive pulmonary embolism. J Thorac Cardiovasc Surg 75:730
28. Verat MA, Fowler NO, Adolph RJ (1970) Cardiac output response to exercise in patients with inferior vena cava ligation. Circulation 42:445
29. Virchow R (1858) Die Cellularpathologie in ihrer Begründung auf physiologische und pathologische Gewebslehre. Hirschwald, Berlin
30. Voss-Schulte K, Stiller H, Isenreich FE (1965) Emergency embolectomy by the transsternal approach in acute pulmonary embolism. Surgery 58:317

28 Surgery for Portal Hypertension

R. Häring and A. Hirner

CONTENTS

A. Anatomy and Pathophysiology

The portal system drains all of the venous blood from the gastrointestinal tract and in part from the esophagus, spleen, and pancreas and transports it to the liver. Four large veins contribute to the portal vein (Fig. 28.1): the superior coronary vein of the stomach, the superior mesenteric vein, the splenic vein, and the inferior mesenteric vein. The portal vein itself, the splenic vein, the superior mesenteric vein, and rarely the coronary vein are of importance for the surgery of portal hypertension. An exact knowledge of the anatomic relationship of these large veins is, therefore, indispensable. The *portal vein* runs in the hepatoduodenal ligament (Fig. 28.2). Anteriorly, it is accompanied by the hepatic artery and the common bile duct. If cirrhosis of the liver is present, one usually finds enlarged and engorged lymph nodes caudal to the portal vein, which can make the dissection of the vessel more difficult. Immediately before entering the liver parenchyma, the portal vein divides into two large branches that lead to the right and left hepatic lobe. Occasionally, the right hepatic artery, originating from the superior mesenteric artery, runs caudal to the portal vein. Many variations are possible (one must be careful of accidental injuries during dissection).

The foramen of Winslow separates the portal vein from the infrahepatic portion of the inferior vena cava.

The *coronary vein* of the stomach is located at the lesser curvature, runs caudal to the left gastric artery, and joins the portal vein behind the head of the pancreas. In the presence of portal hypertension, it can assume a rather large diameter. It is one of the most important collaterals to the esophageal veins.

The *superior mesenteric vein* is located to the right of the superior mesenteric artery. Both vessels cross over the fourth portion of the duodenum. Behind the head of the pancreas the superior mesenteric vein and the splenic vein join nearly at a right angle to form the portal vein.

The *splenic vein* is formed by the confluence of several large branches emerging from the hilus of the spleen; behind the pancreas it flows into the portal vein after being joined by the inferior mesenteric vein and numerous small veins from the pancreas. These small pancreatic branches are easily torn during dissection for a splenorenal shunt.

The *inferior mesenteric vein* drains the blood from the left colon. It runs in the infraduodenal

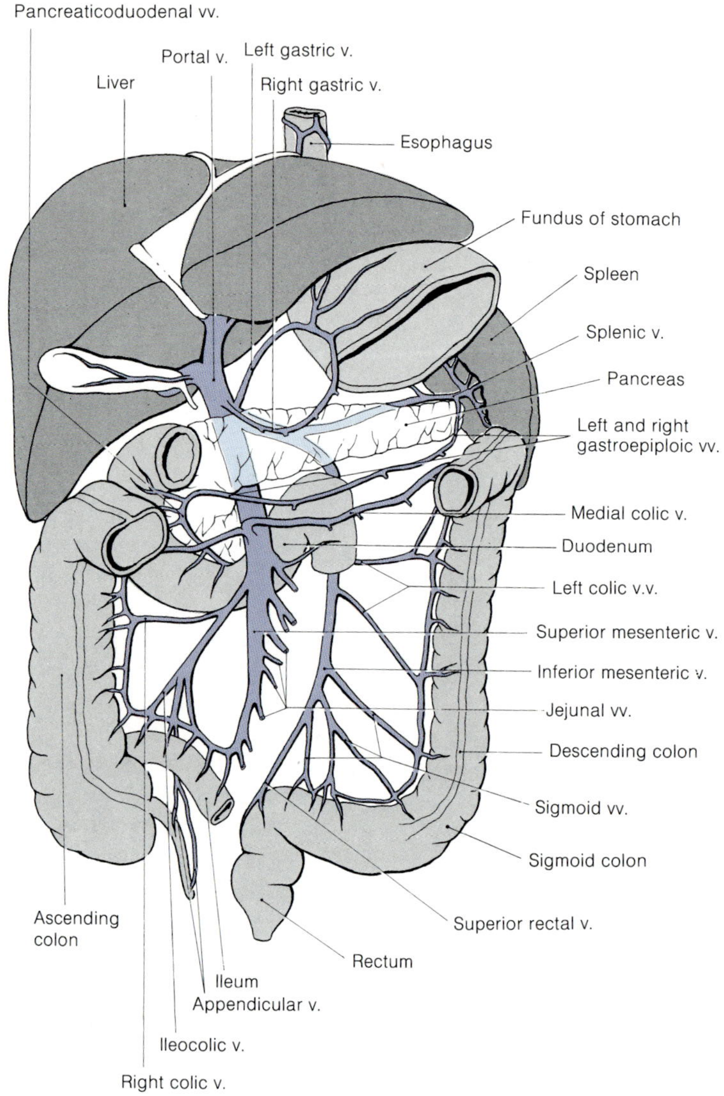

Fig. 28.1. Anatomy of the portal circulation with the main venous trunks: superior mesenteric vein, splenic vein, inferior mesenteric vein, and left gastric vein

fold beneath the transverse mesocolon and the pancreas and finally joins the splenic vein. The exact location of this junction is not constant; the inferior mesenteric vein occasionally joins the superior mesenteric vein as well.

Forms of Portal Hypertension

One can distinguish between hypertension caused by *increased resistance* and hypertension caused by *increased volume*. If it is caused by increased resistance, one can distinguish between prehepatic, intrahepatic, and posthepatic block.

1. The *prehepatic block* is caused by a thrombosis in the portal circulation. This can be located exclusively in the splenic vein (peripheral prehepatic block; Fig. 28.2a) or centrally in the portal vein itself (Fig. 28.2b). Therefore, one can distinguish a segmental from a general portal hypertension. An isolated thrombosis of the splenic vein frequently leads to bleeding from fundal varices; if the main portal vein is thrombosed, ascites or hypersplenism dominate the clinical picture.

2. An *intrahepatic block* can be either pre- or postsinusoidal (Fig. 28.2c). The presinusoidal form is caused by bilharziosis and is of no importance in Europe, where the postsinusoidal form, observed in cirrhosis of the liver, is most important. In 95% of all patients with portal hypertension, cirrhosis of the liver will be the cause; this

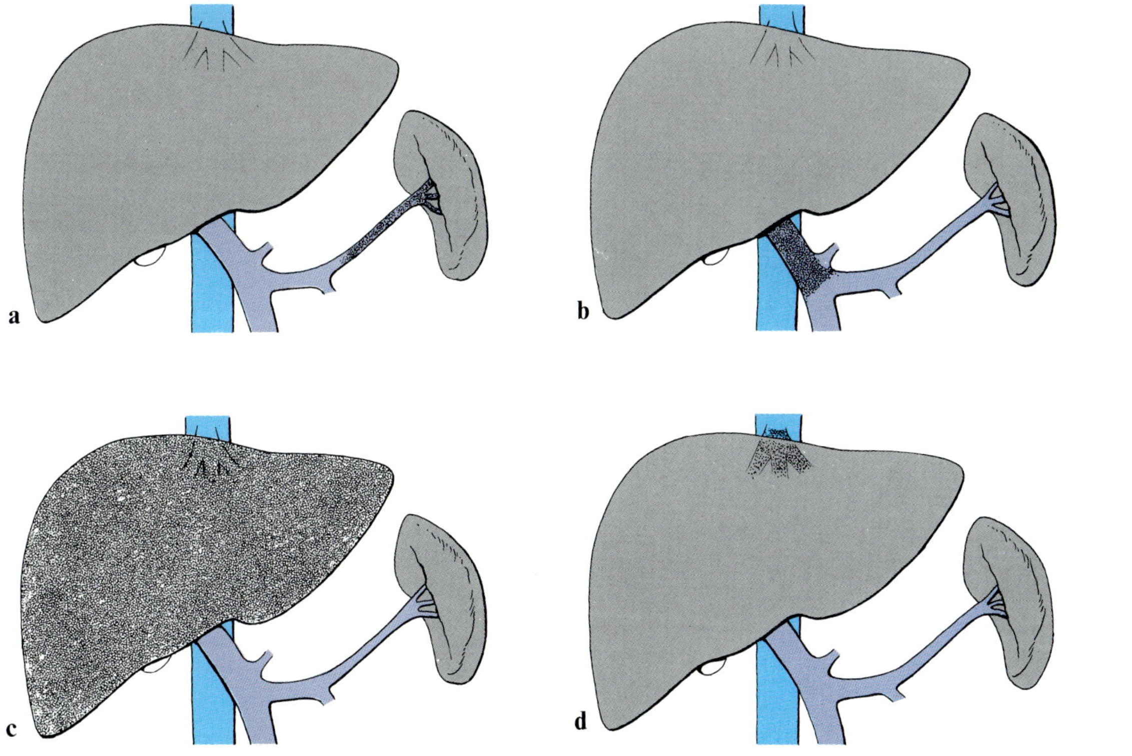

Fig. 28.2a–d. Different forms of obstruction in portal hypertension. **a** Peripheral prehepatic block with thrombosis of the splenic vein. **b** Central prehepatic block with thrombosis of the portal vein. **c** Postsinusoidal intrahepatic block with liver cirrhosis (most common form). **d** Posthepatic block (Budd-Chiari syndrome) with occlusion of the liver veins

can be alcoholic, posthepatic, or biliary in nature. Not infrequently, one finds a combination of pre- and intrahepatic block.

3. The *posthepatic block* is very rare (Fig. 28.2d). It is known as Budd-Chiari syndrome or, when small intrahepatic veins are obliterated, as "venous occlusive disease" (VOD). Essentially, what is involved here is the obstruction of hepatic venous drainage owing to the occlusion of the inferior vena cava by a tumor or to thrombosis of the hepatic veins (endophlebitis hepatica, allergic vasculitis, cytostatic chemotherapy).

4. Portal hypertension secondary to *increased volume* or *hyperkinetic* hypertension is caused by arterioportal fistulas, usually traumatic or iatrogenic in origin. They occur, e.g., after splenectomy, cholecystectomy, or gynecologic procedures. As a consequence of the arterialization, there is a significant rise in pressure in the portal system [15].

Common to all forms of block is the development of a collateral circulation to the caval system (Fig. 28.3). As a result, the diseased liver undergoes *hemodynamic changes* that are of significance for surgical therapy:

1. The hepatic artery can compensate for a reduction in portal flow up to a certain point. In a healthy person, the artery contributes one-third of the total perfusion of the liver, while in a cirrhotic patient it accounts for approximately 60%–80% of the total – in other words, double the normal volume.

2. The ability of the hepatic artery to compensate is limited to a maximal flow of 1200 ml/min.

3. In 9% of all patients with cirrhosis a reversal of flow in the portal vein occurs. This means that arterial blood is shunted away from the hepatocytes through a presinusoidal arterioportal connection into the portal vein. Thus, in every case of advanced intrahepatic block caused by cirrhosis, a hyperkinetic component is present.

For the clinical picture, the most important pathophysiologic sequela of *portal hypertension* are the following:

1. Bleeding from the esophageal and fundal varices,

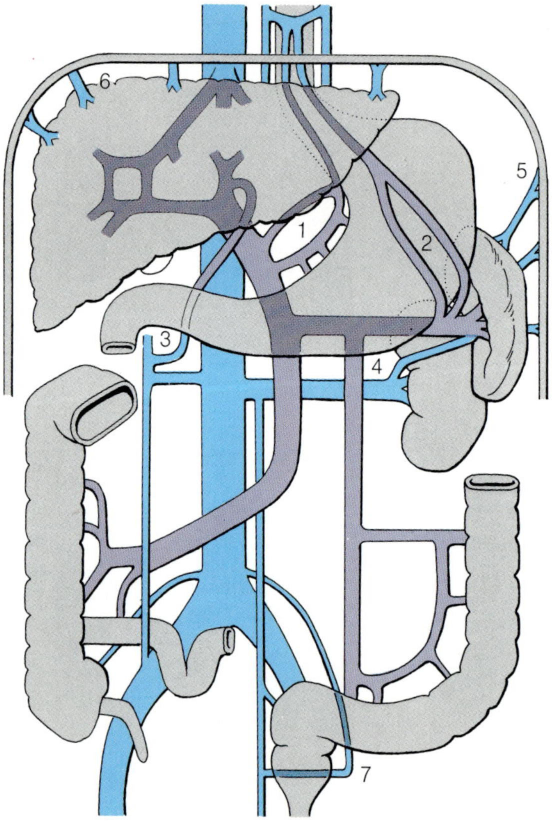

Fig. 28.3. Collateral circulation in portal hypertension. (*1*) Gastroesophageal anastomosis via the left gastric vein. (*2*) Anastomosis via the short gastric veins. (*3*) Vascular connections between the left branch of the portal vein and umbilical vein, the paraumbilical veins, and the epigastric veins. (*4*) Anastomosis between spleen and left renal vein. (*5*) Collateral vessels between the splenic capsule and the diaphragmatic veins. (*6*) Collateral connections between the intrahepatic branches of the portal vein and the diaphragmatic veins. (*7*) Retroperitoneal collateral vessels connecting to the paravertebral plexus of the vena cava

2. Ascites that is refractory to conservative therapy,
3. Encephalopathy caused by the collateral circulation, as well as parenchymal dysfunction,
4. Hypersplenism with anemia, thrombocytopenia, and leukopenia.

On the basis of the pathophysiology, *surgical treatment* of portal hypertension has the following goals:

1. Expedient control of bleeding from esophageal varices,
2. Lowering of portal hypertension to prevent recurrent bleeding,
3. Reduction of ascites that resist conservative therapy,
4. Control of hypersplenism.

B. Treatment of Esophageal Variceal Hemorrhage

Bleeding from esophageal or fundal varices is a dramatic event and carries a high mortality. Because the underlying disease, namely, cirrhosis with portal hypertension, is so complex, standardized therapy is not possible; *treatment must be individualized.*

The controversies of surgeons regarding the proper approach to the management of this or that disease are never more heated than in the case of portal hypertension. This emotionalism is due in large part to a feeling of uncertainty and helplessness in the face of very difficult problems. In the following chapter, we will try to develop an approach which in our experience has proven successful in most situations.

I. Nonsurgical Emergency Measures

Table 28.1 summarizes the nonsurgical emergency measures that have proven effective in our own hospital in cases of variceal bleeding. In this grave situation it is essential that the necessary measures be synchronized: treatment of shock, diagnostic interventions, nonsurgical hemostasis, and prevention of hepatic coma. Frequently the bleeding can be controlled temporarily by balloon tamponade, using either the Sengstaken-Blakemore or the Linton-Nachlas model. Total hemostasis can then be achieved through portal decompression utilizing the emergency shunt technique.

During the last few years, *sclerotherapy* has been advocated for esophageal varices [6, 9, 24, 28]. However, only surgical decompression of the portal system can prevent recurrent bleeding. Therefore, it is our opinion that in the treatment of portal hypertension sclerotherapy and other nonsurgical methods (tamponade, antihypertensive drug therapy) should not be viewed as an alternative to surgery but rather as an *adjuvant form of therapy* for the temporary control of variceal bleeding.

Table 28.1. Approach to massive bleeding from esophageal and fundal varices

Simultaneous measures!

Emergency treatment:

1. Treatment of shock
Volume substitution (plasma expanders and fresh blood)
Hemodynamic monitoring (blood pressure, pulse, central venous pressure, urine output)
Laboratory investigation: Hb, hematocrit, determination of blood group, liver function tests, evaluation of the clotting system

2. Hemostasis
Balloon tamponade
Replacement of coagulation factors
Heparin therapy in cases of intravascular coagulation
Endoscopic sclerotherapy of varices

3. Prophylaxis of hepatic coma
Nasogastric suction and irrigation enemas
Sterilization of the bowel (neomycin, lactulose)

Diagnostic measures:
Endoscopy
Angiography (portography)

Definitive measures:
Emergency or early shunt, portacaval, rarely mesocaval (Drapanas) or Warren shunt

Table 28.2. Child classification

	Points		
	1	2	3
Total bilirubin (mol/l)	<34	−51	>51
Albumin (g/l)	>35	−30	<30
Ascites	mild	moderate	massive
Neurologic symptoms	none	mild	marked
General condition	good	reduced	poor

A: 5–7 B: 8–10 C: 11–15

II. Diagnostic Measures

The indication for a portasystemic shunt, and the prognosis as well, must be based on thoroughgoing diagnostic procedures that address the following points:

1. The presence of bleeding or nonbleeding esophageal varices, and the cause of the portal hypertension.
2. The functional status of the liver parenchyma.
3. The hemodynamic situation, especially estimation of arterial and venous perfusion of the liver. How extensive the diagnostic procedures can be will of course depend on the urgency of operative intervention.

With respect to (*1*): The history and physical examination should provide the first clues as to whether portal hypertension may be present; this is especially true where the patient presents with cirrhosis of the liver. Esophageal varices can be demonstrated roentgenographically; however, *esophagogastroscopy* is the diagnostic method of choice during acute bleeding, as it enables one to rule out other causes of hemorrhage.

Direct splenoportography, using the Seldinger technique, is essential for the planning of a shunt operation; it provides information about the cause of portal hypertension, localization and extension of collateral circulation, abnormalities of the arterial system, hepatofugal flow, and finally, the presence of liver cell carcinoma.

With respect to (*2*): Evaluation of *hepatic function* includes synthesis, detoxification, and excretion. It is difficult to predict what the functional reserves of a cirrhotic liver with decreased perfusion will be following a portacaval shunt. Preoperative laboratory evaluation is of limited prognostic value. On the basis of our own statistically based studies we believe that the only reliable factors on which to base the prognosis are the prothrombin time and the creatinine and fibrinogen levels. It is surely better to group the patients according to Child's *classification* [7] (Table 28.2). A good, but very involved test of the parenchymal function of the liver is the *amidopyrine exhalation test*, which, together with Child's classification, allows a good estimate of liver function [16]. *Encephalopathy* plays a crucial role. It not only occurs following a portasystemic shunt operation but is often already present preoperatively. No valid clinical definition of encephalopathy exists. Psychometric testing, EEG, and determination of the blood ammonia, however, allow early detection of this problem [18].

With respect to (*3*): *Hemodynamic* investigations aid in the selection of patients for an elective portasystemic shunt. It is important to arrive at a judgment as to how much the hepatic artery and the portal vein each contribute to the hepatic flow, a relationship that is greatly altered in cirrhotic patients. In order to assess the compensatory capability of the hepatic artery, the portal vein can be totally occluded by means of a *balloon catheter*, thus simulating the conditions that will exist following construction of a portasystemic shunt. But such techniques, being very complicated, are unsuited to emergency situations. Their importance is therefore limited to cases where surgery is elective. The following methods are available: sequential liver-spleen scan [3], catheterization of the umbilical vein with occlusion of the portal vein [33], indocyanin clearance [5], cineangiodensitometry [26], transumbilical shunt simulation, and measurement of lactate extraction [17].

In acute situations, one should limit diagnostic measures to clinical evaluation, endoscopy, determination of liver enzymes, and indirect splenoportography.

III. Indications for Portasystemic Shunts

In addition to general considerations, the matters of the timing of the operation and the type of shunt are crucial factors in the indication. With respect to the timing, we differentiate:

- An *emergency shunt* for the treatment of massive variceal hemorrhage which does not respond to conservative measures,
- An *early shunt* (also called a delayed emergency shunt) within 24–48 h after bleeding has started,
- An *elective shunt*, done at least 2 weeks after variceal bleeding, and subject to strict patient selection.

The choice of *shunt* is based on the following considerations:

- Cause of the portal hypertension: pre-, intra-, or posthepatic block,
- The individual situation, i.e., acute bleeding, previous gallbladder surgery (adhesions),
- General condition and hepatic function of the patient, with special attention to the stages according to Child, the presence of encephalopathy, etc.,
- Liver perfusion, with special attention to the relative contributions of the portal vein and the hepatic artery (sequential liver scan) and to any stenosis of the celiac trunk.

One differentiates between *complete* and *incomplete shunts*, i.e., between shunts that divert all of the portal blood flow away from the liver, thereby diminishing the perfusion of the organ, and shunts that do not interfere with the perfusion of the liver but lead to a selective lowering of the pressure in the areas prone to bleeding, namely the esophagus and stomach.

Complete shunts include: The portacaval end-to-side or side-to-side anastomosis, the central splenorenal anastomosis as described by Linton [21], the central side-to-side splenorenal anastomosis described by Cooley [8], and the mesocaval anastomosis of Drapanas [10].

Incomplete shunts include: The distal end-to-side splenorenal anastomosis as described by Warren [32] and the coronary-caval technique developed by Meursing [23]. The last method can be used only in rare cases and requires significant enlargement of the coronary vein.

The *portacaval anastomosis* with simultaneous *pressure- and flow-adapted arterialization* [1, 22] of the intrahepatic portal circulation represents a special type.

In light of these considerations, the various types of shunt and the conditions under which they are indicated can be summarized as follows:

1. Portacaval Anastomosis, End-to-Side (Fig. 28.4a)

Indications: Emergency and early shunt during active hemorrhage, elective in patients with reduced portal circulation and good liver function.

Contraindications: Poor liver function, encephalopathy, hepatic coma, stenosis of the celiac trunk, thrombosis of the portal or splenic vein.

Advantages: Simple short operation, fast reduction of portal pressure, low incidence of shunt thrombosis (below 3%).

Disadvantages: Reduction in hepatic perfusion as a result of the complete diversion of portal flow, high rate of encephalopathy.

Fig. 28.4a–h. Modifications of portasystemic anastomosis. **a** Classic portacaval anastomosis end-to-side. **b** Portacaval anastomosis side-to-side. **c** Distal splenorenal anastomosis (Linton). **d** Mesocaval anastomosis, so called H-shunt (Drapanas) with interposition of a prosthesis. **e** Splenorenal anastomosis side-to-side (Cooley). **f** Central splenorenal anastomosis end-to-side (Warren). **g** Coronary-caval anastomosis (Meursing). **h** Portacaval anastomosis end-to-side with pressure- and flow-adapted arterialization (Matzander). Interposition of a vein or alloplastic material between the central stump of the portal vein and the common iliac artery ▷

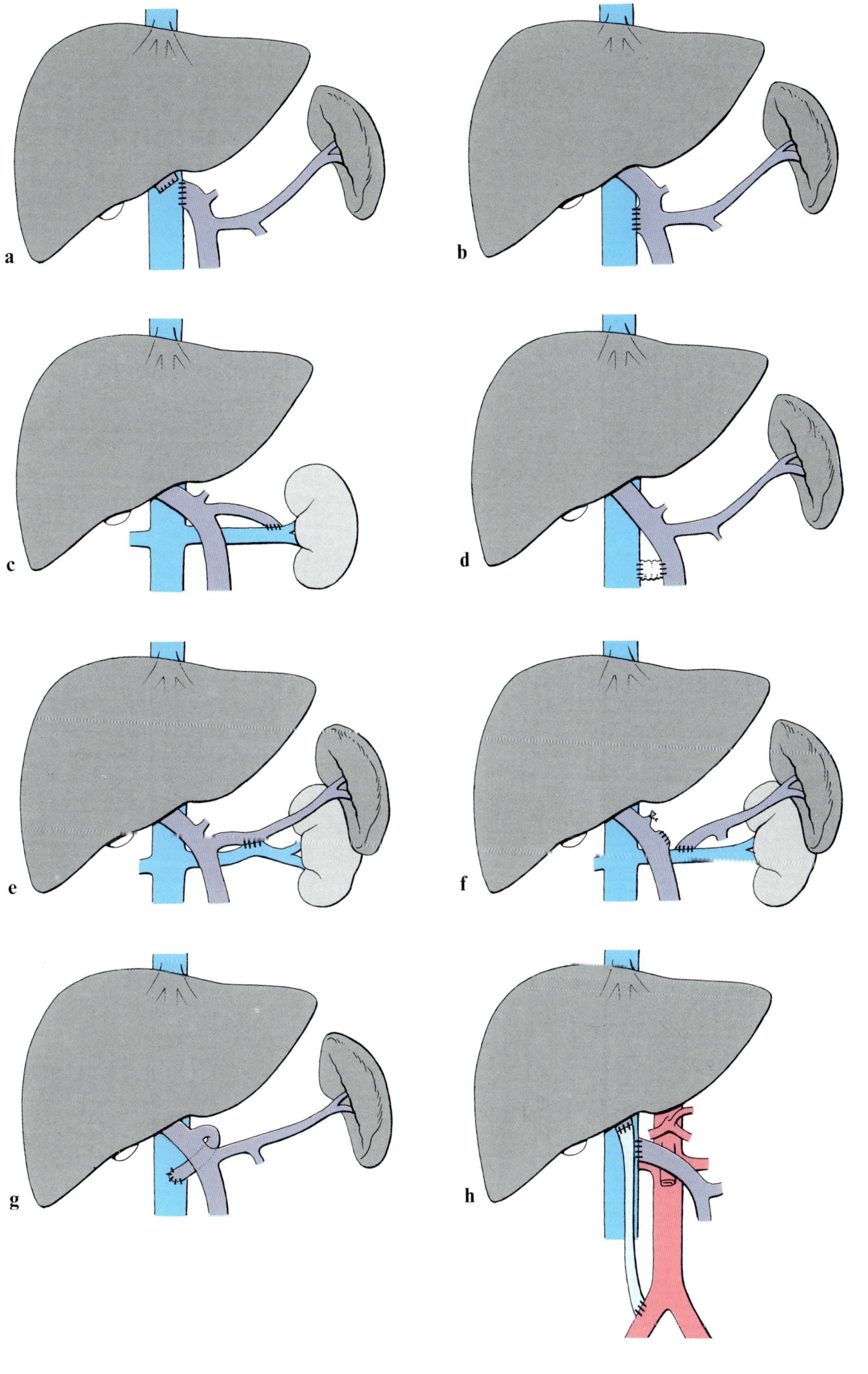
a
b
c
d
e
f
g
h

2. Portacaval Anastomosis, Side-to-Side (Fig. 28.4b)

The only clear-cut indication is the Budd-Chiari syndrome. The extremely congested liver is decompressed through diversion of the portal, and also in part the arterial flow (hepatofugal flow via presinusoidal arterioportal shunts).

A side-to-side anastomosis is functionally a complete shunt as is the end-to-side anastomosis; however, it is technically more demanding.

3. Central Splenorenal Anastomosis (LINTON) (Fig. 28.4c)

Indication: As an elective procedure following variceal bleeding, where a splenomegaly with hypersplenism is present (splenectomy). Central thrombosis of the portal vein.

Advantages: None.

Disadvantages: Extensive and technically demanding procedure involving splenectomy and extensive mobilization of the pancreatic tail. High rate of thrombosis.

4. Mesocaval Anastomosis, H-shunt (DRAPANAS) (Fig. 28.4d)

Indications: Portal vein thrombosis, prior surgical procedures in the region of the liver (highly vascular adhesions).

Contraindications: Thrombosis of the mesenteric vein.

Advantages: None that are significant, since it represents a complete shunt.

Disadvantages: Danger of kinking of the prosthesis, high rate of thrombosis.

5. Splenorenal Anastomosis, Side-to-Side (COOLEY) (Fig. 28.4e)

Indications: Thrombosis of the portal vein, previous operations of the gallbladder or liver; can also be used as an emergency shunt.

Contraindications: Thrombosis of the splenic vein and small diameter of the splenic vein.

Advantages: Because splenectomy is not required, there is a lower operative risk than with the splenorenal anastomosis according to LINTON [21].

6. Distal Splenorenal Anastomosis, End-to-Side (WARREN) (Fig. 28.4f)

Indications: Largely preserved portal circulation, poor liver function, encephalopathy, stenosis of the celiac trunk, previous operation on liver and gallbladder, central portal vein thrombosis; can also be used as an emergency shunt.

Contraindications: Excessively small splenic vein diameter, previous pancreatitis.

Advantages: Incomplete shunt, maintenance of portal liver perfusion, low rate of encephalopathy.

Disadvantages: Only selective lowering of the pressure in the region of the esophagus, stomach, and spleen; can develop into a functionally complete shunt by later collateralization; high rate of shunt thrombosis.

7. Coronary-Caval Anastomosis (MEURSING) (Fig. 28.4g)

The coronary-caval anastomosis is an incomplete shunt and can be constructed only in exceptional cases, the lumen and mural characteristics of the coronary vein being normally quite unsuited to anastomosis.

Indications: Thrombosis and cavernization of the portal vein in cases of prehepatic block, marked encephalopathy, poor liver function. It should be used only in exceptional cases.

8. Portacaval Anastomosis End-to-Side with Flow- and Pressure-Adapted Arterialization (ADAMSONS, MATZANDER) (Fig. 28.4h)

Indications: Impaired liver function, encephalopathy.

Contraindications: Emergency operations for hemostasis, portal vein thrombosis, severe arteriosclerosis of the aorta and iliac artery.

Advantages: The diversion of the portal flow is compensated by arterialization, small risk of encephalopathy.

Disadvantages: Higher operative risk, damage to the liver, and marked ascites through increased pressure in the intrahepatic portal system.

IV. Appraisal of Portasystemic Shunts

In contrast to other forms of therapy, portasystemic shunts, especially portacaval anastomosis, lower the portal hypertension markedly and definitively. They control bleeding from esophageal varices and prevent rebleeding. They influence the development of ascites and hypersplenism. With complete shunts, a serious disadvantage is that the portal hepatic blood supply is totally diverted, possibly leading to encephalopathy or significant impairment of liver function. The indication, therefore, is dependent on evaluation of the liver function and the contribution of the portal vein to the liver perfusion. Postoperative follow-up and dietetic management are also essential. Under these circumstances, encephalopathy can be controlled. Pre- and postoperative psychometric testing shows that the rate of encephalopathy is not nearly as high as expected. The increase in encephalopathy postoperatively is approximately 5% [13]. Whether the operation also changes the natural course of cirrhosis and influences life expectancy has not yet been determined. The type of shunt should be individualized for each patient. One should always keep in mind the option of the incomplete shunt (Warren's splenorenal anastomosis or the coronary-caval anastomosis), or, as a supplement to the portacaval anastomosis, a pressure- and flow-adapted arterialization.

The diagnosis of arterioportal fistula is not always easy. The following symptoms should arouse suspicion: an abdominal bruit, no signs of hepatic insufficiency, history of previous operations. Fistulas between the splenic artery and vein, as well as the hepatic artery and the portal vein, are the most common.

Because of the serious clinical picture, surgery is always indicated. The approach depends on the localization. The aim of surgery is always the elimination of the fistula without ligation of major arteries (e.g., the hepatic artery).

C. Surgical Technique and Complications

Anesthesia: Hepatotoxic anesthetic agents – e.g., halothane – must never be used in portasystemic shunt operations (see Chapter 11).

I. Portacaval End-to-Side Shunt

A long right-sided subcostal incision gives good exposure (Fig. 28.5). The collateral veins in the abdominal wall should be carefully ligated to avoid postoperative bleeding. The umbilical vein in the round ligament, however, should be spared: it provides a significant portasystemic collateral connection with the veins of the abdominal wall and can therefore be an important factor in portal decompression.

Surgery is difficult when the patient is obese, the liver is enlarged, or there have been previous operations, i.e., cholecystectomy.

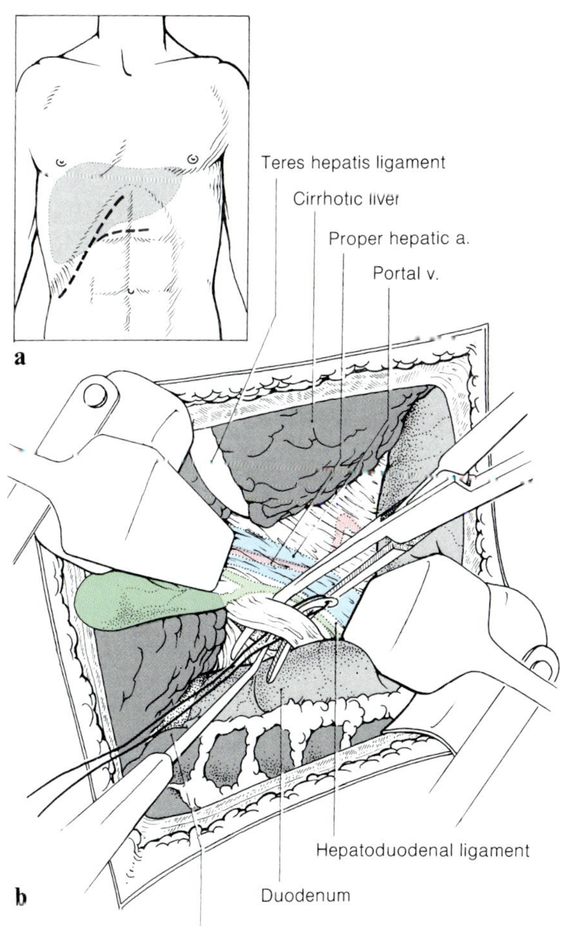

Fig. 28.5 a, b. Exposure of the portal vein. **a** Subcostal incision on the right. **b** The hepatoduodenal ligament is visualized, and the portal vein is dissected free along the lower part of the ligament. Transection of the engorged lymphatic vessels and fatty tissue in front of the portal vein

The adhesions are often highly vascularized owing to the development of portasystemic collateralization.

The operation has three stages:
1. Preparation of the portal vein and measurement of the portal pressure,
2. Dissection of the infrahepatic vena cava,
3. Performance of the portacaval anastomosis.

1. Dissection of the Portal Vein

The portal vein runs in the dorsal aspect of the hepatoduodenal ligament and is dissected from a caudal direction. It is easily palpable as an engorged vessel or, if it is thrombosed, as a firm cord. In front of the portal vein, one often encounters enlarged lymph nodes and lymphatic vessels. These are encircled with an Overholt clamp, ligated, and transected (Fig. 28.5). The biliary duct and the lymphatic tissue are then retracted ventrally with a vein retractor, allowing the blue portal vein to be seen beneath the surrounding tissue. This tissue is transected, and an Overholt clamp is placed around the vein, which is then encircled with a rubber band (Fig. 28.6a). The entire portal vein is then dissected free, from the hilus of the liver to the head of the pancreas. Small branches are divided. Occasionally, the coronary vein empties into the portal vein close to the hepatic hilus. It must be securely ligated. The pressure in the portal vein and in the vena cava is then measured with a gauge (Fig. 28.6b). The former is between 25 and 45 mmHg. During dissection of the portal vein, one frequently has the impression that it will be too short for a tension-free anastomosis with the vena cava, but this is never the case.

2. Dissection of the Inferior Vena Cava

The parietal peritoneum is opened immediately distal to the caudate lobe and lateral to the duodenum and pancreas. In this region, one frequently encounters collateral vessels, which are divided between ligatures. In the loose retroperitoneal tissue the infrahepatic vena cava can usually be freed by blunt dissection and mobilized over a distance of 5–8 cm. Occasionally, the juncture of the right renal vein with the vena cava is very high; if so, care must be taken not to injure the renal vein. However, it is not necessary to free the vena cava over its entire circumference nor to encircle it. This

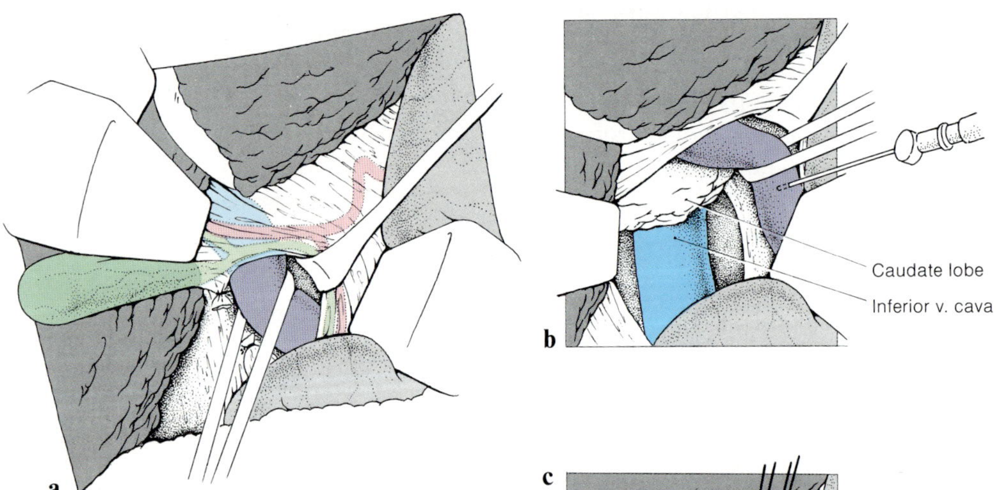

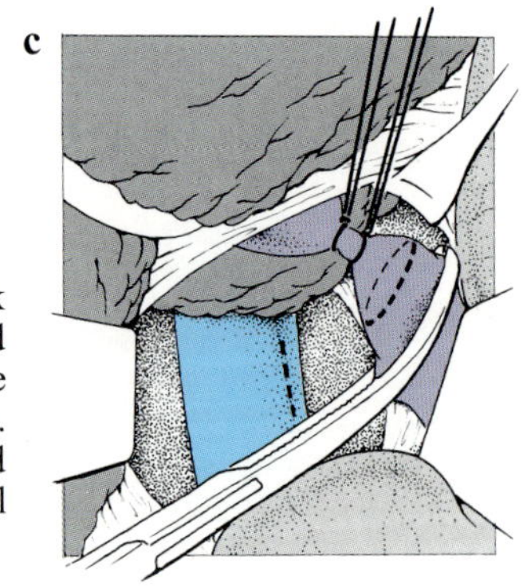

Fig. 28.6. a The portal vein is exposed with its trunk and encircled. The hepatoduodenal ligament is retracted cranially and cephalad. **b** Pressure measurement in the portal vein after puncture with a Statham apparatus. **c** The portal vein is doubly ligated toward the liver and occluded, preferably with a Glover clamp. The vessel can now be transected

would prolong the operating time and could lead to troublesome bleeding from the small side branches on the posterior wall. The dissection of the vena cava should be extended far enough cranially to expose the highest possible site for the anastomosis with the portal vein. This is done in order to prevent kinking of the portal vein.

3. Technique of Anastomosis

After both veins are dissected free, the portal vein is ligated with a no. 1 cotton thread in the hilus of the liver and additionally secured with a suture ligature. Toward the head of the pancreas, the portal vein is clamped with a curved Glover clamp and then transected close to the hepatic hilus (Fig. 28.6c). A Satinsky clamp of appropriate size is placed on the vena cava and locked. With two forceps, one approximates the portal vein to the tangentially clamped section of the vena cava to determine the site of incision. As proposed by GÜTGEMANN and SCHREIBER [11], we perform a medial convex incision on the anterior wall of the vena cava so that a lateral flap approximately 1 cm in size is produced and a large opening 2.2–2.5 cm in diameter is created (Fig. 28.7a). Corresponding to this opening, a sickle-shaped segment is excised from the anterior wall of the portal vein, so as to guarantee a wide anastomosis. One should take care to ensure that the incisional flap on the posterior aspect of the vena cava is not too short. The flap on the anterior wall of the vena cava is grasped with a stay suture and folded back laterally. The vascular clamps on the portal vein and the vena cava are then approximated, and the posterior wall is sutured continuously inside the lumen, using Ethibond or Prolene 5-0 suture and an atraumatic needle (Fig. 28.7b). One starts with a proximal and a distal corner stitch. The proximal suture is tied, and the needle is passed through the wall of the portal vein into the lumen. Now the posterior wall can be sutured from the inside of the lumen under direct vision. The distal corner stitch should be tied only after the suture of the posterior wall is half completed in order to enable the surgeon to suture the posterior margin more securely. The edges of the vessels should be transfixed obliquely in order to avoid a bulky suture line. The adventitia should not be inverted; the objective is an endothelioendothelial approximation. After the posterior wall is completed, the suture is passed to the outside at the distal corner and tied.

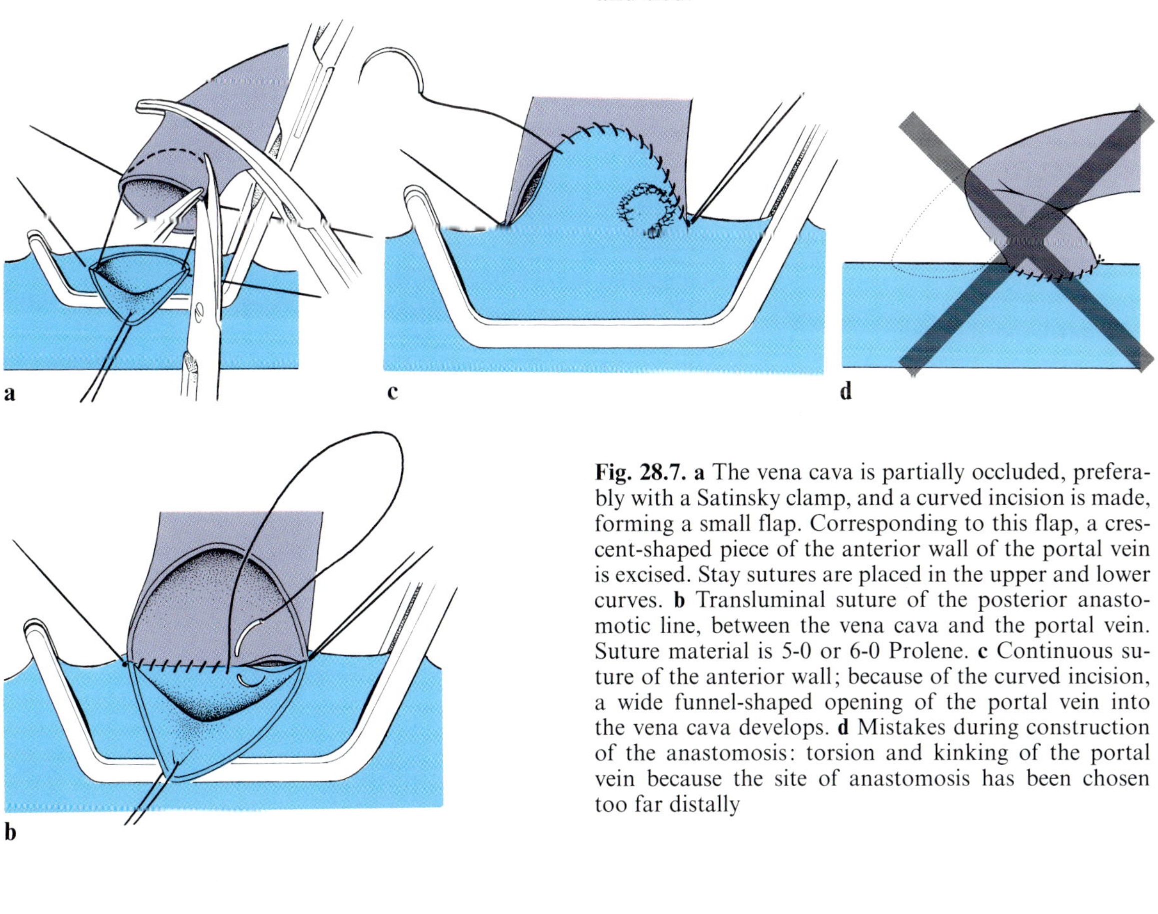

Fig. 28.7. a The vena cava is partially occluded, preferably with a Satinsky clamp, and a curved incision is made, forming a small flap. Corresponding to this flap, a crescent-shaped piece of the anterior wall of the portal vein is excised. Stay sutures are placed in the upper and lower curves. **b** Transluminal suture of the posterior anastomotic line, between the vena cava and the portal vein. Suture material is 5-0 or 6-0 Prolene. **c** Continuous suture of the anterior wall; because of the curved incision, a wide funnel-shaped opening of the portal vein into the vena cava develops. **d** Mistakes during construction of the anastomosis: torsion and kinking of the portal vein because the site of anastomosis has been chosen too far distally

Using the suture at the distal corner, the anterior wall of the anastomosis is sewn in an everting fashion, from distal to proximal (Fig. 28.7c). Prior to completion of the anastomosis, blood flow from the portal vein is checked by releasing the vascular clamp to flush out possible thrombi.

The area of the anastomosis is irrigated with normal saline solution, the suture is finished, and blood flow is restored first in the vena cava, then in the portal vein. Additional hemostatic sutures are usually not necessary.

A wedge-shaped biopsy from the liver is always taken for histologic examination. In the meantime, the portal blood has drained. To obtain the pressure gradient, the pressures in the portal vein and the vena cava are measured; the difference between them is the gradient.

Intraoperative Complications

Thrombosis of the Portal Vein. Occasionally, one will unexpectedly encounter a mural thrombus or phlebosclerotic changes of the portal vein. These changes can be so extensive that an anastomosis is impossible. Using a Fogarty catheter or a ring stripper, one should first try to remove the thrombi which did not appear during radiologic examination.

Care should be taken not to injure the wall of the vein. Postoperatively, treatment with heparin is indicated in order to prevent recurrent thrombosis (carefully watching the coagulation parameters in patients with cirrhosis). If, as happens rarely, it is impossible to perform the anastomosis, the portal vein is ligated and a splenorenal anastomosis as described by Cooley [8] or a mesocaval H-shunt is constructed.

Kinking of the Portal Vein. If the anastomosis with the vena cava is done too far distally, a distortion of the portal vein can result (Fig. 28.7d). Occasionally an enlarged caudate lobe is in the way and must be resected in order to accomplish an anastomosis without tension and kinking.

Injury to the Common Duct and the Hepatic Artery. These injuries are rare. We have never encountered such a complication. The necessary knowledge concerning abnormalities of the hepatic artery is provided by preoperative angiography. Not infrequently, the right hepatic artery arises alone from the superior mesenteric artery and runs caudad to the portal vein. Accidental transection of the artery during preparation of the portal vein would have grave consequences. Under these circumstances it is impossible to go ahead with the portacaval anastomosis.

II. Portacaval Side-to-Side Shunt

The surgical incision as well as the dissection of the portal vein and the vena cava are as described on p. 761. Because the portal vein and vena cava do not run parallel to one another, both vessels must be extensively mobilized to allow them to be approximated without tension at the site of the anastomosis. The portal vein is clamped toward the liver and toward the duodenum (Fig. 28.8a); the vena cava is partially occluded

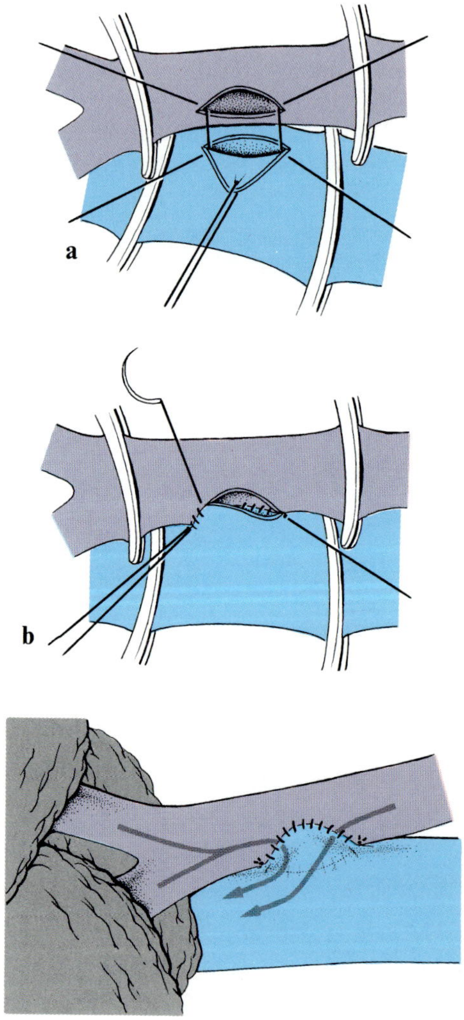

with a Satinsky clamp. A curved incision is then made caudad in the portal vein at the site where the vena cava crosses under it at an oblique angle. The vena cava is also incised in a curvilinear fashion so as to create a small flap. This incision must be made somewhat obliquely in order to prevent distortion of the anastomosis (Fig. 28.8 b). Suture material and suture technique are the same as for the end-to-side anastomosis (see p. 763) (Fig. 28.8 c).

III. Central End-to-Side Splenorenal Shunt (LINTON)

We use an extensive left-sided subcostal incision. The procedure can be divided into the following stages:

1. Splenectomy,
2. Dissection of the splenic vein,
3. Dissection of the left renal vein,
4. End-to-side anastomosis.

1. Splenectomy

Because of splenomegaly and dense vascular adhesions between the capsule, the diaphragm, and the lateral abdominal wall, the removal of the spleen can be difficult. After the lesser sac has been opened by transection of the left part of the gastrocolic ligament, the short gastric veins are divided between ligatures (Fig. 28.9). During this maneuver, an injury to the capsule of the spleen, with unnecessary blood loss, is possible. After the hilus of the spleen is exposed, one can easily identify the engorged splenic vein at the upper margin of the tail of the pancreas and, a little more cranially, the splenic artery. Both vessels are carefully dissected with scissors or an Overholt clamp and encircled. The dissection of the vein is sometimes made difficult by the fact that the very thin wall can tear, especially if phlebosclerosis is present. One must be careful here. Once the vein has been isolated over a distance of approximately 1–2 cm, the pressure is measured using a small needle and

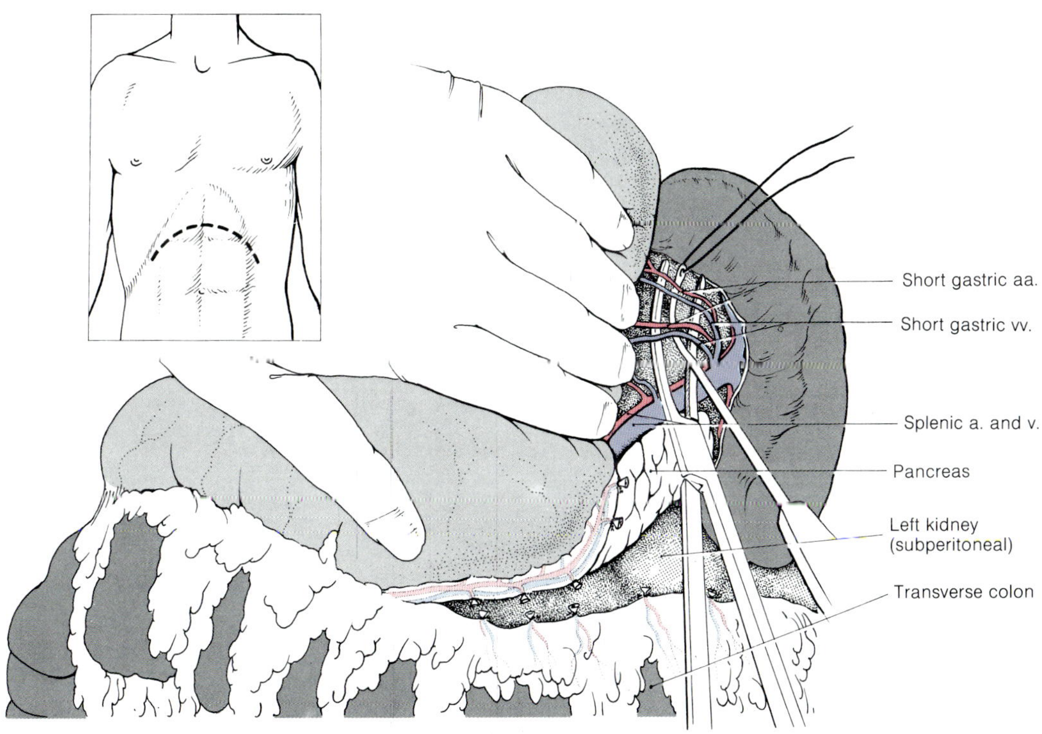

◁ **Fig. 28.8 a–c.** Portacaval side-to-side anastomosis. **a** The clamped portal and caval veins are positioned parallel to each other. Curved excision in the vena cava, creating a flap, and a crescent-shaped incision from the anterior wall of the portal vein. **b** The posterior wall of the anastomosis is complete; suture of the anterior wall is begun. **c** Completed side-to-side anastomosis

△ **Fig. 28.9.** Splenorenal anastomosis (LINTON). Opening of the abdominal cavity through a lateral subcostal incision. First, the spleen is removed. Then the lesser sac is opened, and the short gastric vessels are transected

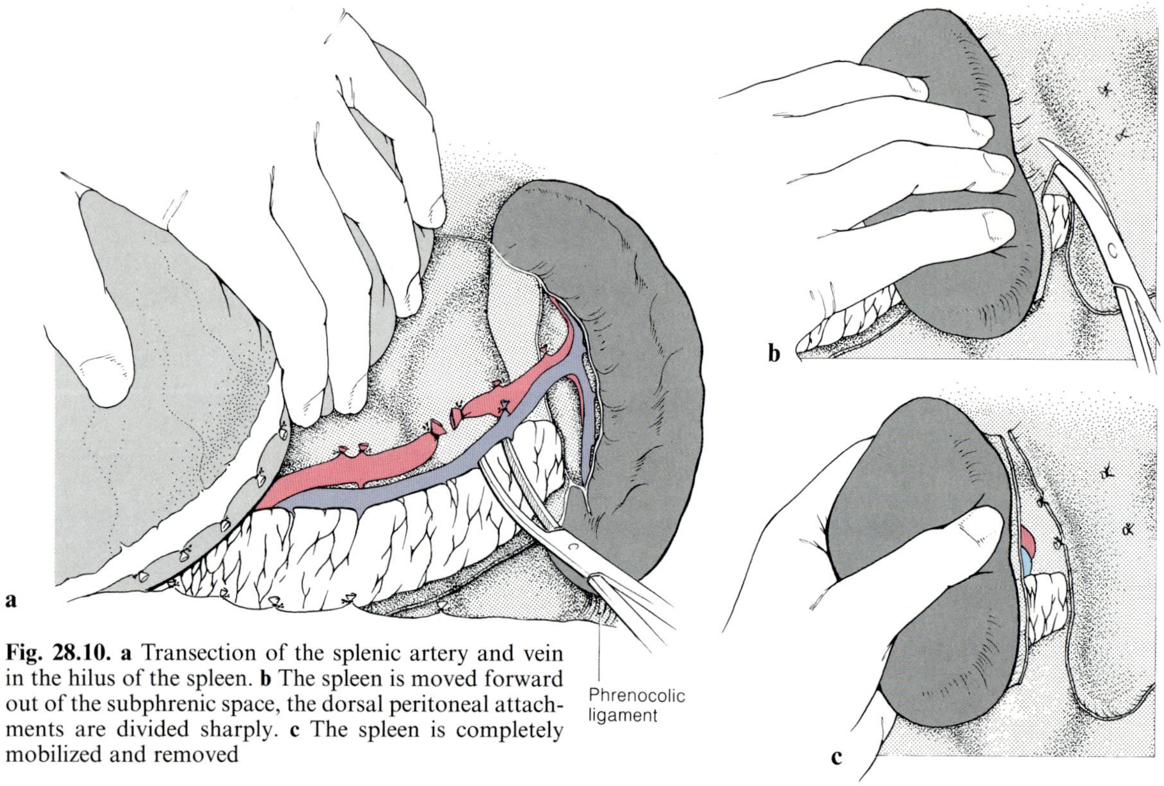

Fig. 28.10. **a** Transection of the splenic artery and vein in the hilus of the spleen. **b** The spleen is moved forward out of the subphrenic space, the dorsal peritoneal attachments are divided sharply. **c** The spleen is completely mobilized and removed

a Statham apparatus. Next, the splenic artery is divided between ligatures (Fig. 28.10a), and the splenic vein is ligated as close to the hilus as possible. Occasionally, its branches must be ligated separately. While dissecting the vessels, injury to the tail of the pancreas, which can reach into the hilus of the spleen, should be avoided at all costs. Only after the splenic vessels have been transected does one divide the splenocolic ligament, which often contains collateral vessels; any vascularized adhesions of the splenic capsule can also be transected at this time. Because of the portal hypertension, the bleeding from these adhesions can be considerable. All adhesions should be coagulated by electrocautery. The spleen is pulled medially with the left hand, a laparotomy pad is placed in the subphrenic space for tamponade, and the dorsal peritoneal attachments are incised (Fig. 28.10b). Blunt dissection continues from lateral to medial into the retroperitoneal fat. The pancreas is mobilized and reflected; occasionally collateral veins have to be ligated. Finally, the spleen can be removed (Fig. 28.10c). Because of the portal hypertension and the possibility of impaired coagulation, thoroughgoing hemostasis of the retroperitoneum is necessary.

2. Dissection of the Splenic Vein

The splenic vein is dissected from dorsal to proximal for a distance of approximately 5–6 cm, the ligature at the end of the vein being used for elevation (Fig. 28.11a). Dissection must be done very carefully because of the many very fine venous branches entering the vein from the pancreas. These are easily torn, and the resultant bleeding is troublesome. They are ligated with 3-0 cotton thread; any tears at the splenic vein are closed with 6-0 Prolene suture.

3. Dissection of the Left Renal Vein

After the splenic vein has been dissected free over the appropriate length, the pancreas is elevated and the left renal vein is dissected free from the retroperitoneum. In obese patients, the vein is occasionally difficult to identify. One should orientate oneself by the position of the kidney and by the spine, which lies medially. After the perivascular tissue is opened, the vein, which is 1 cm in diameter, can be isolated over a length of approximately 5 cm and encircled (Fig. 28.11b). Mobiliza-

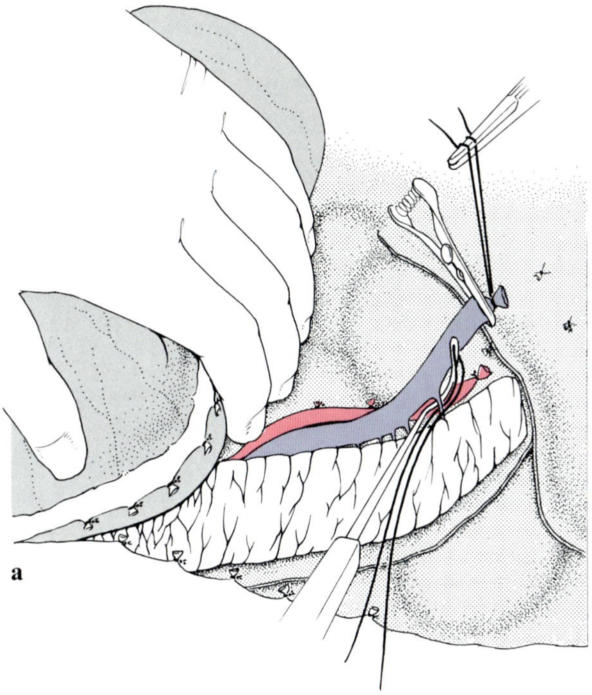

a

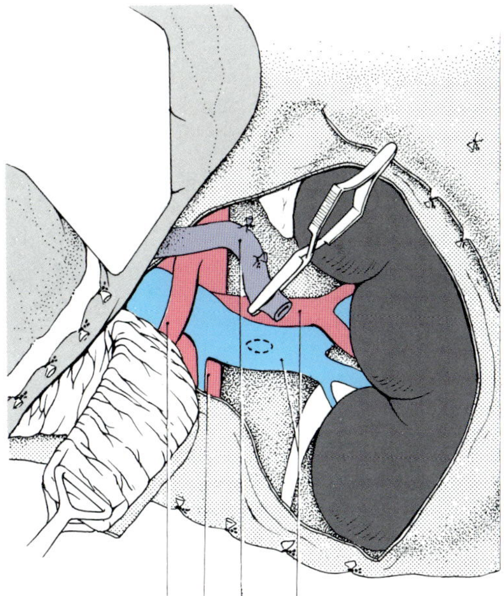

b

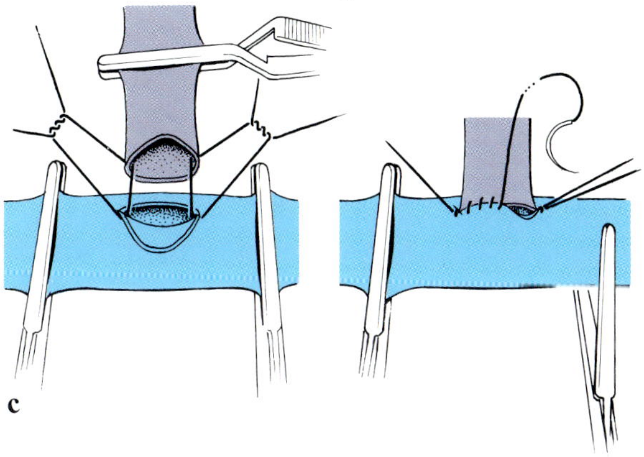

c

Fig. 28.11. a Dissection of the splenic vein. During this dissection, many tiny side branches have to be ligated. The splenic vein is mobilized over a length of approximately 1 cm. **b** The left kidney is dissected free at the hilus to expose the large renal vein which crosses the aorta. The mobilized splenic vein is occluded and approximated to the renal vein in a smooth curve. Kinking of the splenic vein must be avoided at all costs. **c** The anterior wall of the renal vein is incised in a curved fashion to create a flap, and a crescent-shaped piece is excised out of the splenic vein. Corner sutures are placed. Completion of the anterior suture line of the end-to-side anastomosis

tion occasionally requires division of the spermatic or ovarian vein between ligatures, which can be done without sequelae.

4. Anastomosis

First, one must ascertain that the splenic vein can be brought down to the renal vein without torsion, kinking, or tension. The exact position of the vein (it should be a slight arch) is of decisive importance for the function of the portasystemic shunt. The renal vein and the splenic vein are occluded with small vascular clamps. A 1.5-cm curved incision is then made in the upper circumference of the renal vein. The flap thus created should be directed caudally. It is held by a stay suture. On the anterior wall of the splenic vein a corresponding crescent-shaped piece is excised in order to create the widest possible anastomosis (Fig. 28.11c). After corner sutures with 6-0 Prolene have been placed, the posterior wall is sutured from inside the lumen, and then the anterior wall is done using an everting technique (see p. 766). It is important that the vascular clamps at the splenic vein be opened prior to completion of the anastomosis in order to flush out stagnating blood and possible thrombi. Bleeding from the suture line after the blood flow is reestablished is initially treated with compression. If this is unsuccessful, additional sutures are placed. Finally, the pressure gradient in the splenic vein is determined, a liver biopsy is done, and the splenic bed is drained. The abdomen is closed layer by layer.

a) Intraoperative Complications. If the *splenic vein is injured*, one should try a vascular suture; or, it may sometimes be necessary to dissect the vessel farther in behind the pancreas and then perform the anastomosis more medially – if necessary, with the vena cava instead of the renal vein. If this is not possible, the vein is ligated and a mesocaval anastomosis performed, as described by DRAPANAS [10].

b) Postoperative Complications. Postoperative bleeding necessitates early reintervention. An *early thrombosis* of the anastomosis is usually caused by torsion or kinking of the splenic vein. This error can only very rarely be corrected. Occlusion of the vein can result in variceal bleeding, which must be treated with a balloon tube or sclerotherapy. If surgical hemostasis is unavoidable, a portasystemic anastomosis or a venous interruption can be done. Postoperative *pancreatitis* secondary to injury of the pancreas during dissection is a serious complication and requires appropriate intensive therapy.

IV. Mesocaval or H-Shunt (DRAPANAS)

The *incision* is either a large median laparotomy or a large transverse incision in the upper abdomen. The procedure can be divided into four stages:

1. Dissection of the superior mesenteric vein,
2. Dissection of the inferior vena cava,
3. Correct positioning of the graft,
4. Completion of the anastomosis.

1. Dissection of the Superior Mesenteric Vein

The transverse colon and the greater omentum are retracted cephalad, the small bowel caudad, and the mesenteric root exposed. If the patient is obese, localization of the vein can be difficult. The following hints are helpful: to the left of the vein the superior mesenteric artery can be palpated; dorsal to the vein lies the duodenum (Fig. 28.12a). The mesenteric vein is dissected free, distal to the duodenum, over a length of 3–4 cm, and encircled.

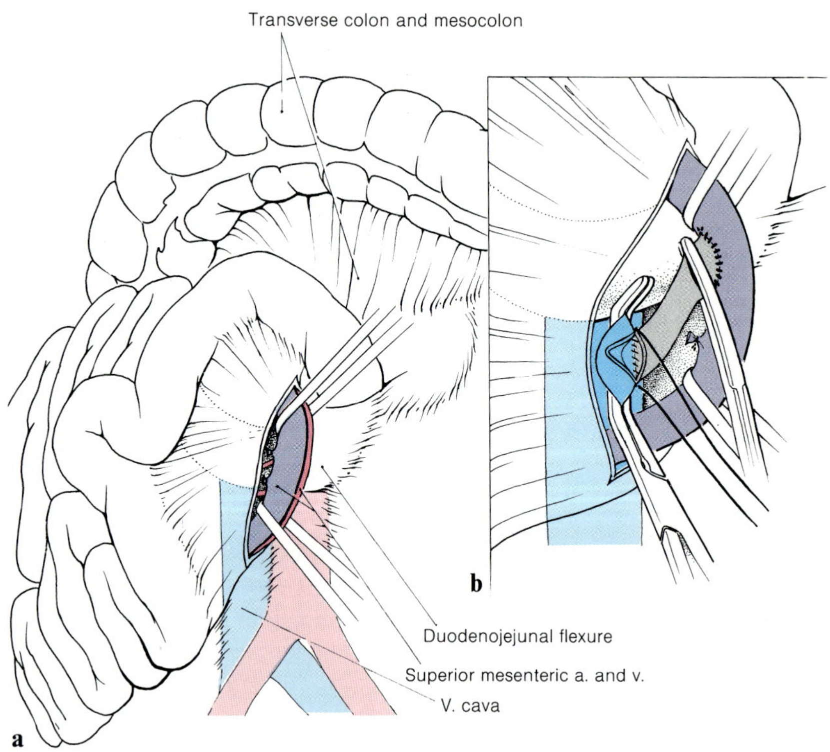

Fig. 28.12a, b. Mesocaval H-shunt (DRAPANAS). **a** The transverse colon is moved cephalad, and the small bowel is pulled to the right. The ligament of Treitz is visible; the superior mesenteric artery (left), and the superior mesenteric vein (right) cross over the duodenum. The mesenteric vein is mobilized and encircled. **b** The alloplastic vascular prosthesis is interposed between the superior mesenteric vein and the vena cava, which has been dissected free above the colon. The end-to-side anastomosis with the superior mesenteric vein is already finished, as is the posterior suture row of the anastomosis between prosthesis and vena cava

Small side branches are transected between ligatures in order to mobilize better the vein and facilitate clamping.

2. Exposure of the Inferior Vena Cava

The transverse colon is pulled caudad, and the peritoneum is incised along the lateral border of the duodenum with the same technique used during the portacaval anastomosis (see p. 762). The vena cava is dissected over a length of approximately 8–10 cm. One has to be careful not to injure the junction with the renal vein. As with the portacaval anastomosis, we do not encircle the vena cava, in order to avoid injury to the dorsal branches. The mesenteric and caval sides of the anastomosis should be placed as nearly parallel to each other as possible.

3. Tunneling of the Mesenteric Root

Prior to construction of the anastomosis, one should establish a tunnel behind the mesentery. This should be done from the right, paramedian of the superior mesenteric vein, proceeding in the direction of the exposed vena cava. During the dissection, one should be careful to avoid injury to the small mesenteric veins, as this can cause unpleasant hematomas. One should also be careful not to injure the fourth portion of the duodenum which sometimes extends rather far caudally.

4. Completion of the Vascular Anastomosis

As a vascular prosthesis, we use reinforced PTFE with a diameter of 10–12 mm. The advantages of these prostheses are wall stability and high antithrombogenicity. First, we perform the anastomosis with the mesenteric vein. For this purpose, the vessel is occluded with two clamps, and a crescent-shaped incision corresponding to the diameter of the prosthesis is made on its laterodorsal aspect, thereby creating a flap that opens out ventrally. A corresponding crescent-shaped incision is made on the anterior aspect of the prosthesis. The posterior wall of the anastomosis is then closed by continuous suture from the inside, using 6-0 Prolene suture material. When the anterior wall has also been completed, the clamps on the mesenteric vein are removed, and a Glover clamp is placed on the prosthesis, close to the anastomosis. The blood can then flow through the superior mesenteric vein again.

The graft is then brought through the previously created retromesenteric tunnel, and the vena cava is partially clamped at its ventral circumference with a Satinsky clamp. Again, a curved incision creating a small flap is made in the vena cava, and a corresponding crescent-shaped incision on the anterior aspect of the prosthesis, and both vessels are anastomosed (Fig. 28.12b). Finally, pressure is measured by puncture of the prosthesis close to the mesenteric anastomosis. The mesenteric root is reperitonealized using a 2-0 running catgut suture.

Intraoperative Complications. A tear in the superior mesenteric vein should be avoided under all circumstances because it sometimes makes the anastomosis impossible. The damaged vein must always be reconstructed, if necessary with a vein patch.

If early thrombosis of the graft occurs, reexploration should be done, and a graft thrombectomy should be attempted. If this is not possible owing to torsion or kinking, another form of portasystemic anastomosis should be tried. Postoperative bleeding, especially in the region of the mesenteric root, also requires thoroughgoing early relaparotomy and hemostasis.

V. Splenorenal/Side-to-Side Shunt (Cooley)

Large transverse incision in the upper abdomen.

In our opinion, the approach to the retropancreatic splenic vein is difficult through the lesser sac. In comparison, the transmesocolic approach is ideal. The transverse colon and the greater omentum are put under tension cranially and ventrally. The mesenteric root is pulled caudad. The ligament of Treitz and the transverse mesocolon are easily seen, and the peritoneum is incised along the duodenum. An additional incision at the base of the transverse mesocolon is made, which results in a mesocolic window as big as the palm of the hand. Now, the proximal portion of the splenic vein is dissected free. It is easily identified by orientating oneself along the course of the inferior mesenteric vein, which leads directly to the splenic vein. The vein runs behind the pancreas, which is elevated carefully with vein retractors to obtain exposure. Very careful and painstaking dissection is necessary. This can be difficult because of chronic inflammatory changes in the pancreas. A clamp is advanced beneath the vein, and the vessel is encircled. One can now divide the more or less

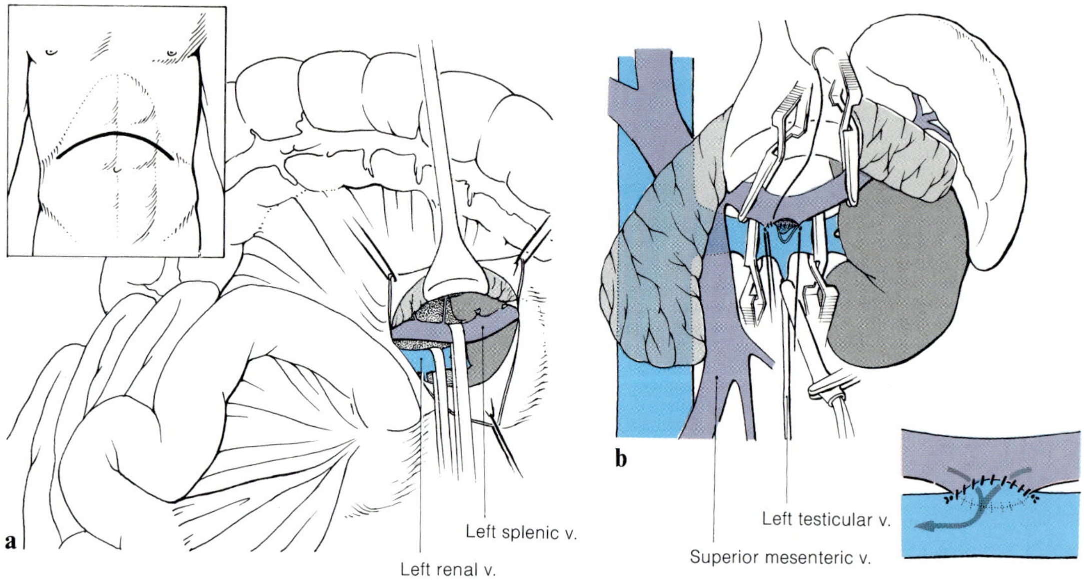

Fig. 28.13 a, b. Splenorenal anastomosis side-to-side (COOLEY). **a** Upper left: skin incision. The transverse colon is pulled cephalad, and the mesocolon is incised next to the ligament of Treitz. With this approach, the splenic vein is exposed and the lower posterior aspect of the pancreas is visible. Many very fine side branches have to be ligated and transected. The renal vein is freed and encircled. **b** Side-to-side anastomosis between splenic and renal vein. Completed anterior suture line

numerous venous branches between ligatures of 3-0 cotton (Fig. 28.13a). The splenic vein is mobilized over a length of approximately 5 cm, close to its junction with the superior mesenteric vein.

In the next step, the left renal vein is exposed, which crosses the aorta slightly caudad of the splenic vein. As a result of the portal hypertension, the renal vein is frequently covered with enlarged and engorged lymph nodes that have to be dissected away. The vessel is mobilized and encircled with tapes. The splenic vein and renal vein must be mobilized sufficiently to allow tension-free side-to-side approximation. The two vessels are then clamped with small Satinsky clamps and incised in a curved fashion over a length of 1.5 cm in order to create a wide lumen (Fig. 28.13b). For the anastomosis, we use 6-0 Prolene. The technique of anastomosis has been described in the sections on the other portasystemic anastomoses. The peritoneal window is closed with a continuous 2-0 catgut suture.

Intraoperative and Postoperative Complications. One should mention here postoperative bleeding and shunt thrombosis. The first requires early reintervention. A shunt thrombosis usually manifests itself by variceal bleeding but must nevertheless be confirmed by angiography. Initially, it should be treated conservatively. Surgical correction is done by portacaval or mesocaval anastomosis, or by venous interruption.

VI. Distal End-to-Side Splenorenal Shunt (WARREN)

The Warren shunt is the only practicable *incomplete* shunt.

Incision, exposure, and dissection for the splenorenal shunt are identical to those for the Cooley shunt (see p. 769). The differences with this approach are:

1. The end-to-side anastomosis and
2. The additional ligature of the coronary vein and the right gastroepiploic vein to interrupt the venous connections of the stomach to the portal system.

After the splenic and renal veins are mobilized and encircled with tapes, the former is ligated close to its junction with the superior mesenteric vein with a strong 1-0 cotton ligature, then clamped distally, and transected. The proximal ligature is additionally secured with a suture ligature. The

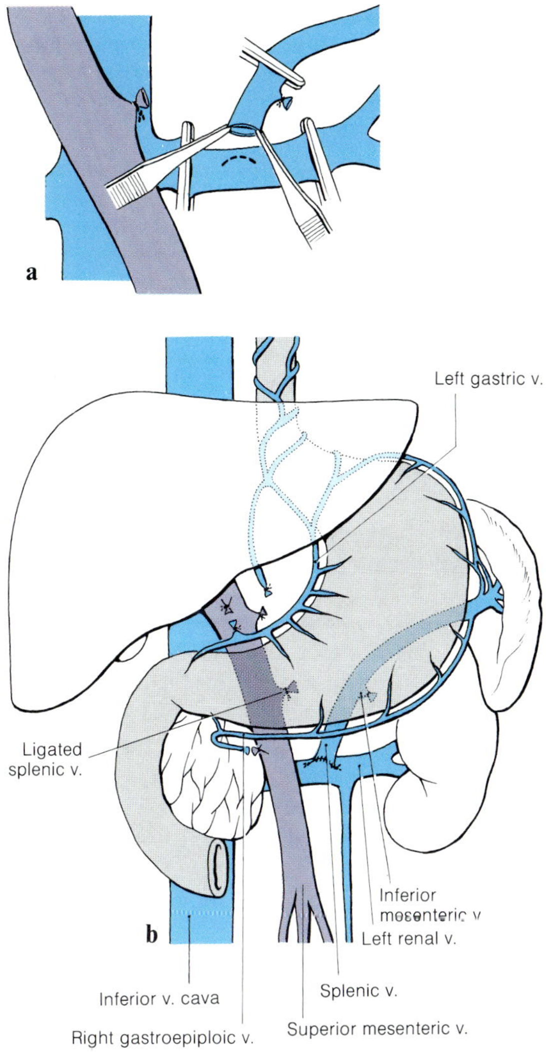

Fig. 28.14a, b. Distal end-to-side splenorenal anastomosis (WARREN). The operative approach is the same as for the Cooley anastomosis. **a** The mobilized splenic vein is ligated and transected close to its junction with the superior mesenteric vein. It is approximated in a smooth curve to the left renal vein. Kinking of the vessel should be avoided. Location of the incision at the renal vein. **b** Completion of the end-to-side anastomosis between renal and splenic vein. The left gastric vein is transected close to its junction with the portal vein. This interrupts the bloodstream from the portal vein into the veins of the stomach and esophagus. The Warren shunt selectively decompresses the portal circulation in the region of the stomach, spleen, pancreas, and esophagus (incomplete shunt). The blood supply to the liver through the portal vein is maintained

anatomic relationship of the splenic vein to the renal vein is carefully assessed to determine the correct position of the vessel and to avoid kinking and torsion (Fig. 28.14a).

After clamping, the anterior aspect of the renal vein is incised in a curvilinear fashion, so as to form a small flap directed caudally. A crescent-shaped piece of venous wall is also excised from the anterior aspect of the splenic vein. The suture is done from inside the lumen with 6-0 Prolene (Fig. 28.14b). Before finishing the anastomosis, the vascular clamps are released for a short time to flush out possible thrombi. If there is no bleeding from the anastomosis, the posterior peritoneum and the small mesocolic window are closed with a continuous suture of 2-0 catgut.

The coronary vein is now dissected free at the celiac trunk (Fig. 28.14b). It is usually engorged and is divided between ligatures. The same is done with the gastroepiploic vein, somewhat proximal to the pylorus. This finishes the operation.

Intraoperative and Postoperative Complications. The fine splenic vein can tear during operation. The leak should be closed carefully with 6-0 Prolene. If this is impossible, the vein must be ligated and another portasystemic shunt constructed (portacaval or mesocaval anastomosis).

VII. Coronary-Caval Shunt (MEURSING)

Large right-sided subcostal incision.

First, the coronary vein is identified at the lesser curvature of the stomach. It is easily found, anterior to the left gastric artery. One can now follow it to the junction of the portal vein behind the pancreas. Usually, it is covered with enlarged lymph nodes which have to be dissected very carefully. The vein should be dissected free in the direction of the cardia, and since a 10-cm segment is required, the dissection should extend beyond the angle of the stomach. At this distal site, the vein is then divided. The many side branches coming from the stomach must also be carefully dissected and divided (Fig. 28.15a).

The next step is dissection of the infrahepatic vena cava. The coronary vein is now brought underneath the hepatoduodenal ligament with the aid of a large Overholt clamp and positioned without kinking or torsion. After clamping off the vena cava, an oval segment 1–1.5 cm long is excised from the anterior wall of the vena cava, and the

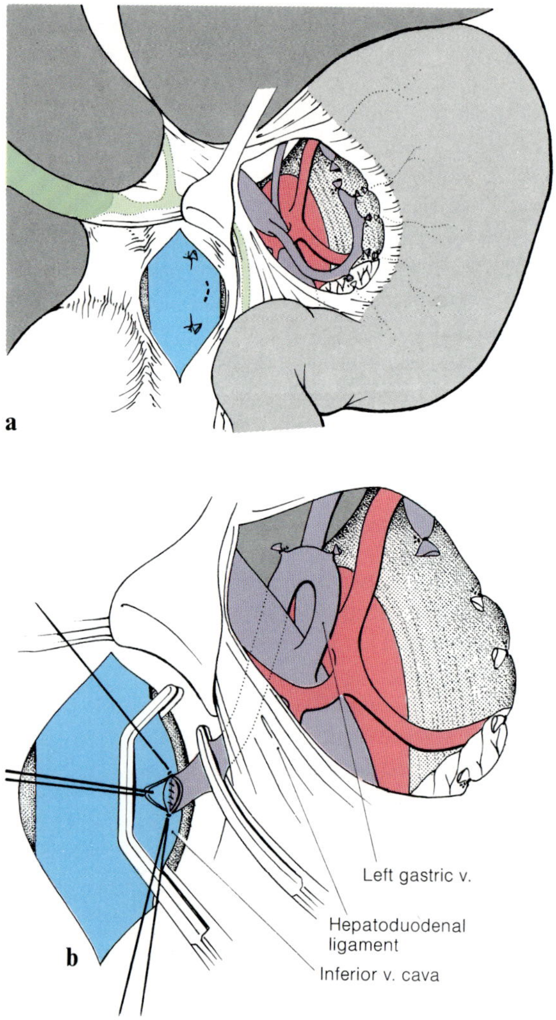

Fig. 28.15a, b. Coronary-caval anastomosis end-to-side (MEURSING). **a** The left gastric vein is dissected free at the lesser curvature of the stomach. Many small side branches to the stomach have to be ligated and transected. **b** After mobilization of the vein, it is brought behind the hepatoduodenal ligament to the infrahepatic vena cava. One should be careful to avoid kinking. End-to-side anastomosis using the technique previously described

end of the coronary vein is beveled. The anastomosis is done end-to-side with 6-0 Prolene by the usual technique (Fig. 28.17b).

Intraoperative and Postoperative Complications. If the delicate venous wall tears during dissection, the anastomosis with the vena cava can also be attempted above the hepatoduodenal ligament. Otherwise, one must ligate the vein and, if possible, construct a splenorenal anastomosis.

VIII. Portacaval End-to-Side Shunt with Flow- and Pressure-Adapted Arterialization
(ADAMSON, MATZANDER)

Large right-sided subcostal incision with extension pararectally or transrectally into the lower abdomen.

This procedure is done in three steps:
1. Portacaval anastomosis with flow measurements in order to determine whether arterialization is indicated,
2. Harvest of the greater saphenous vein, and
3. Anastomosis of the vein graft to the iliac artery distally and to the central stump of the portal vein proximally.

1. Portacaval Anastomosis, Pressure and Flow Measurement

The portacaval anastomosis is done as described on p. 762, with the exception that the central stump of the portal vein is not ligated, but occluded with a Glover clamp until the anastomosis with the greater saphenous vein graft has been completed.

Prior to division of the portal vein, exact pressure and flow measurements must be obtained. The vessel is punctured, and the free portal pressure is measured with a Statham apparatus. Then, the portal vein is occluded with a vascular clamp, and the pressure toward the liver is measured

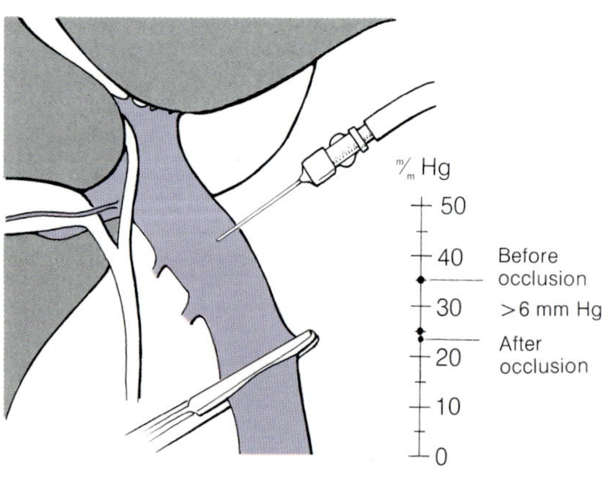

Fig. 28.16. Pressure- and flow-adapted arterialization of the liver (MATZANDER). Puncture of the dissected portal vein for measurement of the postocclusive portal pressure. Occlusion of the portal vein. The pressure is measured toward the liver. The pressure difference between free portal pressure and postocclusion pressure should be greater than 6 mmHg

(Fig. 28.16). Usually, the pressure is at least 6 mmHg lower following occlusion. This pressure gradient should be one-quarter of the free portal pressure; only in this case is arterialization indicated. If, after occlusion of the portal vein, the pressure does not fall or if it rises, one can conclude that intrahepatic arterioportal shunt connections exist and that arterialization is therefore contraindicated. The differentiation made possible by pressure measurements can be complemented by electromagnetic flow measurements, though the value of these measurements is limited in the case of veins. This information allows an individually adapted portal surgery. Arterialization makes sense if the flow is greater than 500 ml/min. At lower flow rates (300–400 ml/min) it is superfluous since no significant portal flow remains because of the advanced cirrhosis.

2. Harvest of the Greater Saphenous Vein

The distance between the stump of the portal vein and the iliac artery is approximately 15–20 cm. The venous graft must be of an appropriate length. It is removed by means of a vertical incision in the thigh below the inguinal ligament and another incision above the knee joint. A suction drain is inserted and the skin closed. The harvested vein is tested for leaks by injection with normal saline solution and preserved in heparinized saline solution until use.

3. Anastomosis of the Venous Graft

The proximal portal stump should not be too short, as there must be enough vascular wall for anastomosis with the venous graft. First, however, the right common iliac artery must be dissected free. The small bowel is covered with towels, retracted toward the left and proximally, and the iliac artery exposed. The dorsal peritoneum is incised over a length of about 8 cm, and the artery is mobilized and encircled. Care must be taken not to injure the dorsally located iliac vein. A retroperitoneal tunnel is created for the venous graft. The tunnel should run behind the mesocolon, parallel to the vena cava. It is advisable to mobilize the hepatic flexure of the colon and retract it medially and caudally.

Careful note having been taken of the direction of blood flow, the venous graft is beveled at its proximal end to match the diameter of the portal vein. The anastomosis between the portal vein stump and the saphenous vein should be performed first. This can be difficult if the liver is large and the operative field is deep in the abdomen. One starts the suture at the proximal corner of the portal vein. The suture material is double 5-0 Prolene. First the posterior wall is done in a proximal-to-caudal direction, then the anterior wall in the same manner. After the anastomosis has been completed, the vein is clamped immediately distal to the portal vein so that hemostasis of the suture line can occur. With the aid of a sponge forceps, the venous graft is then pulled down to the right common iliac artery through the retroperitoneal and retromesocolic tunnel made earlier. Torsion and kinking should be avoided at all costs (Fig. 28.17).

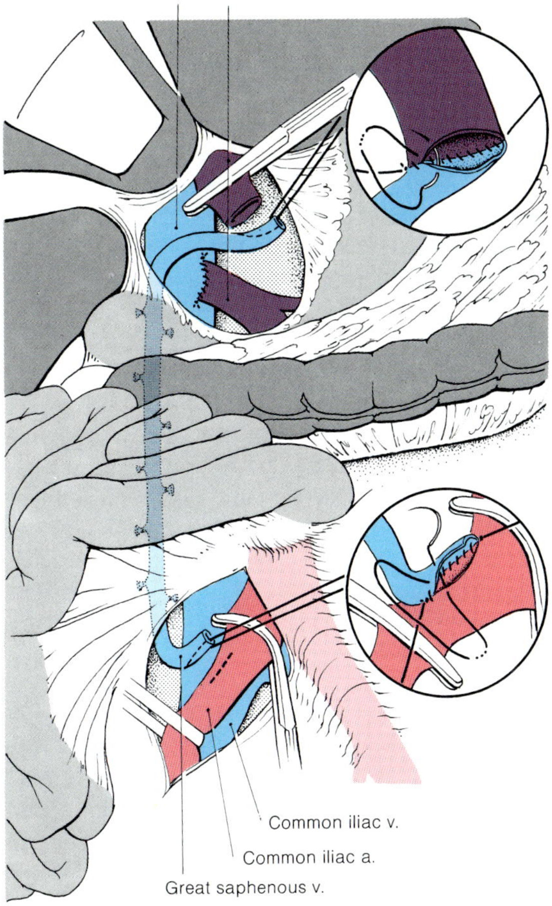

Fig. 28.17. Pressure- and flow-adapted arterialization of the liver (MATZANDER). The end-to-side anastomosis between portal vein and vena cava has already been completed. A beveled saphenous vein graft is anastomosed end-to-end to the central portal stump and is then brought through the retrocolic and retroperitoneal space to the right common iliac artery. End-to-side anastomosis between vein graft and iliac artery

The iliac artery is then clamped proximally and distally, and an oval-shaped piece of the anterior wall measuring 1–1.5 cm is excised. Heparinized saline is instilled into the artery peripherally, then the vein end is beveled for the end-to-side anastomosis, which is done from proximal to distal. Again, the suture material is double 5-0 Prolene. After the inflow and outflow have been checked, the venous graft is filled with heparinized saline solution, the suture is completed, and blood flow is restored.

Finally, the blood flow (optimally 200–300 ml/min) and the pressure in the proximal portal stump are measured. Pressures that exceed the original value by 2–3 mmHg can be tolerated; otherwise, the anastomosis or the vein graft must be banded.

Overarterialization must be avoided, because it leads postoperatively to edema, liver cell dissociation, fibrosis, and marked ascites formation. The peritoneum over the iliac artery is closed with a running catgut suture.

Intraoperative and Postoperative Complications. If the greater saphenous vein is not usable because of inadequate diameter, thrombosis, or varicose changes, or if it has already been removed, an artificial graft (PTFE graft 5 mm in diameter) can be used, though this is not as favorable. If the flow through the graft is too low, it is shortened and anastomosed directly to the aorta.

Massive postoperative ascites is usually due to overarterialization and rapidly leads to renal insufficiency. In these cases, reintervention is indicated. The transplanted vein must be banded or even ligated.

D. Venous Interruption

I. Definition

Venous interruptions are *palliative interventions* designed to arrest the blood flow to the esophagus and thereby stop variceal bleeding. They have no effect on portal hypertension itself, which remains unchanged. Therefore, they are not a real alternative to portasystemic shunts.

There are approximately 100 different kinds of venous interruptions. This large number of surgical modifications reflects not only the essential inadequacy of the procedures themselves, but also the desperation and helplessness which accompany the grim prognosis of catastrophic bleeding from esophageal varices. The in-patient mortality following venous interruption is reported between 11% and 86%.

It is impossible to describe all of the surgical techniques in detail. We therefore limit ourselves to those procedures which in our experience have proved to be the simplest and most practicable. Certainly the poor results of these procedures are to a large degree caused by the fact that a venous interruption is done only after variceal hemorrhage has recurred several times.

II. Indications and Recommended Procedures

Venous interruptions are indicated in special cases of variceal bleeding where a portasystemic shunt is not possible. They belong to the repertoire of every surgeon who deals with portal hypertension. If variceal bleeding cannot be controlled conservatively, the following are indications for venous interruption:

- Extensive prehepatic block (portal vein thrombosis without the possibility of shunt),
- Thrombosis of portasystemic shunt with postoperative variceal bleeding,
- Recurrent variceal bleeding despite an open portasystemic shunt.

We recommend the following venous interruptions:

a) Decongestion of stomach, esophagus, and diaphragm with splenectomy [14],
b) Subcardial interruption with staplers [25],
c) Esophageal interruption with staplers [19],
d) Transection of the esophagus with paraesophageal and gastric devascularization [30],
e) Abdominal resection of the cardia and fundus with splenectomy [29],
f) Thoracic esophageal transection [31].

III. Evaluation

Venous interruptions are palliative procedures that do not lower portal hypertension. During the stage of acute bleeding, they carry a higher risk than does an emergency shunt. In the literature one finds occasional reports of a lower mortality, but these reports give no information about the Child classification of the operated patients. There is also

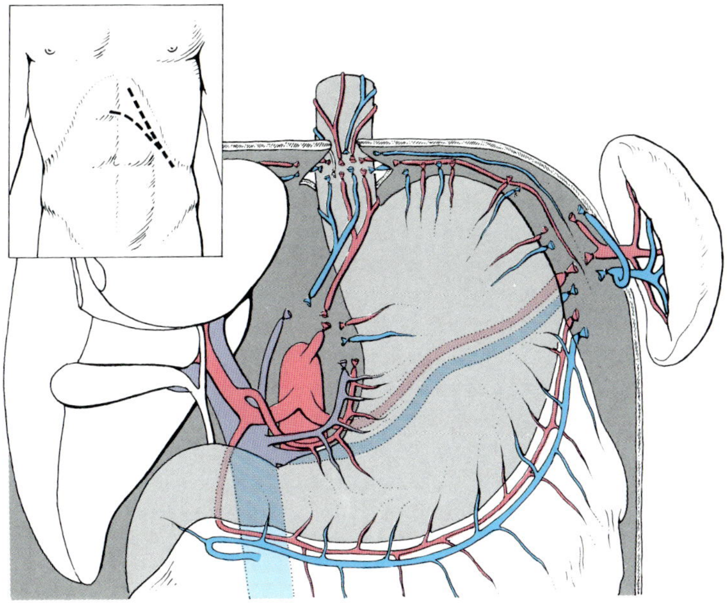

Fig. 28.18. Venous interruption (HASSAB), with decongestion of the proximal half of the stomach by stepwise skeletization of the greater and lesser curvature. Splenectomy. Furthermore, all connections between the stomach wall and the diaphragm are transected. The same is done with the periesophageal veins

a lack of detailed information on the late course following venous interruptions, especially data on recurrent bleeding and survival times. In summary, one must conclude that venous interruptions do not decrease the overall blood flow to the liver and that safe hemostasis and prevention of recurrent bleeding are questionable.

IV. Surgical Technique

For all abdominal venous interruptions, a large left-sided subcostal incision is the best approach. It allows optimal exposure of the abdominal esophagus, the upper part of the stomach, and the spleen, even when the left lobe of the liver is enlarged. In thoracic and thoracoabdominal operations, a left thoracotomy in the sixth or seventh intercostal space is recommended.

1. Decongestion of Stomach, Esophagus, and Diaphragm with Splenectomy (HASSAB) (Fig. 28.18)

After the upper abdomen has been exposed, the proximal half of the stomach, including the short gastric vessels, is skeletized. In this area, one frequently finds thick congested veins which tear easily, causing significant blood loss.

The lesser sac is now opened, and the spleen, with its artery and vein, comes into view. It is usually enlarged and adherent to the surroundings. If at all possible, the splenic vessels are isolated from an anterior direction, triply ligated with 0-1 silk, and transected. Then, the splenocolic ligament is divided; here also, large collaterals are sometimes encountered. The spleen is pulled anteriorly after the peritoneal reflection has been incised. It is dissected free, out of the subphrenic space, while the tail of the pancreas is left untouched. Careful hemostasis by means of an electrocautery and suture ligatures in the bed of the spleen is essential because of the danger of rebleeding, especially in the case of extensive adhesions. The next step is the skeletization of the lesser curvature, proceeding from the angle of the stomach proximally, during which maneuver the coronary vein and the left gastric artery are transected. Though this results in a significant reduction of blood flow to the stomach, the organ is still sufficiently supplied with blood through the right gastric artery and the right gastroepiploic artery.

Next, the peritoneum covering the esophagus is incised, and the esophagus is freed from the hiatus and encircled with a rubber band. All veins leading to the esophagus, especially those on the dorsal surface, are secured with suture ligatures and transected. The same is done with the occasionally large veins leading to the diaphragm. We have combined this procedure, first developed by Hassab, with subcardial interruption using a stapler, as described by RIENECKER [25] (see below). To avoid esophageal reflux as a result of mobilizing the esophagus and stomach, we also recommend a Nissen fundoplication, if there are no special difficulties.

2. Subcardial Venous Interruption by Stapler (Rienecker)

This is a relatively simple procedure which only interrupts the blood flow to the esophageal, not to the fundal varices. Rienecker and Danek [25] used a GIA (R) stapler which compresses the serosa-mucosa interval to 1.75 mm with four rows of staples, thereby interrupting the intramural varices. The peritoneum covering the cardia is incised, and the terminal esophagus is freed out of the hiatus and encircled with a rubber band. The lesser curvature is skeletized for a distance of 3 cm, care being taken not to injure the vagus nerves. Stay sutures are placed at the proximal and distal ends of the skeletized section of the stomach wall. The stomach wall is incised with an electric knife, the stapler is introduced, and first the anterior, then the posterior wall of the stomach is blocked with staples (Fig. 28.19a, b). The small gastrotomy is then closed in two layers and additionally covered with serosa. It is important that the staple row is close to the entrance of the esophagus; otherwise, the greater curvature and part of the fundus of the stomach will not be reached by the interruption. Technical details should be taken from the instructions supplied with the stapling instrument. The simplicity of the procedure and the short operating time are impressive.

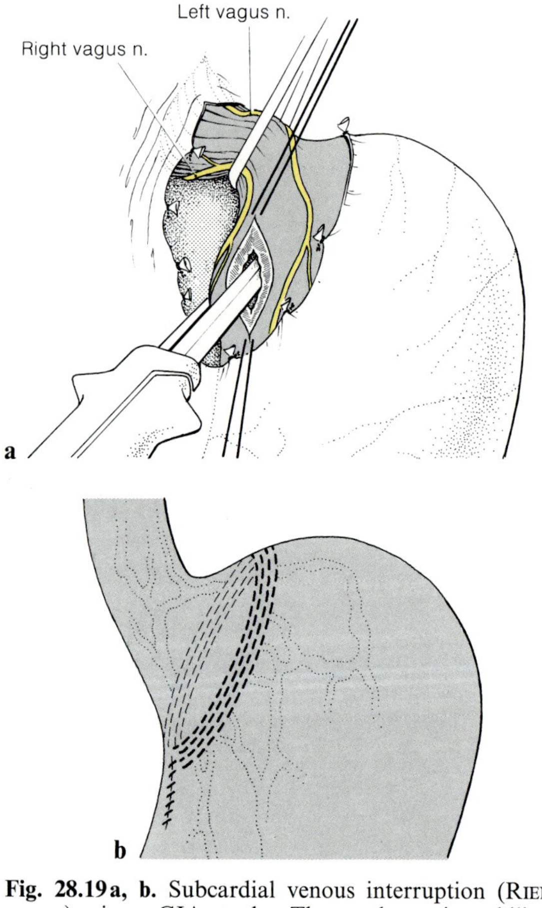

Fig. 28.19a, b. Subcardial venous interruption (Rienecker) using a GIA stapler. The esophagus is mobilized and encircled, the lesser curvature is devascularized and incised. The stapler instrument is introduced; first the posterior and then the anterior wall is blocked with four rows of staples. With this maneuver, the veins leading to the esophagus are blocked in the wall of the stomach. Closure of the gastrotomy with sutures

3. Esophageal Venous Interruption by Stapler (Kivelitz)

Years ago, Boerema developed a procedure for ligature dissection of the esophagus. The same objective can now be accomplished more simply by the use of modern stapler devices (EEA (R) stapler) developed for enteral anastomosis. The anterior wall of the stomach is opened with cautery between stay sutures. The EEA instrument is introduced through the gastrotomy into the esophagus, which has been mobilized and encircled (Fig. 28.20a). The esophagus is now ligated with 3-0 silk between the two parts of the instrument. The instrument is then closed by tightening the screw and fired (Fig. 28.20b), thereby interrupting the veins leading from the stomach to the esophagus. The gastrotomy is closed in two layers, and the staple suture is covered with the fundus of the stomach. The disadvantage of this method is that bleeding from fundal varices is not controlled.

4. Esophageal Transection and Paraesophageal Devascularization (Sugiura-Futagawa)

This procedure is done thoracoabdominally in two stages in high-risk patients.

a) Thoracic Operation. With a left thoracotomy in the sixth intercostal space, adhesions between lung and parietal pleura are removed. The inferior pulmonary ligament is incised. The lung can now be retracted cephalad. The mediastinum is opened. In the mediastinum, one finds many blood-filled

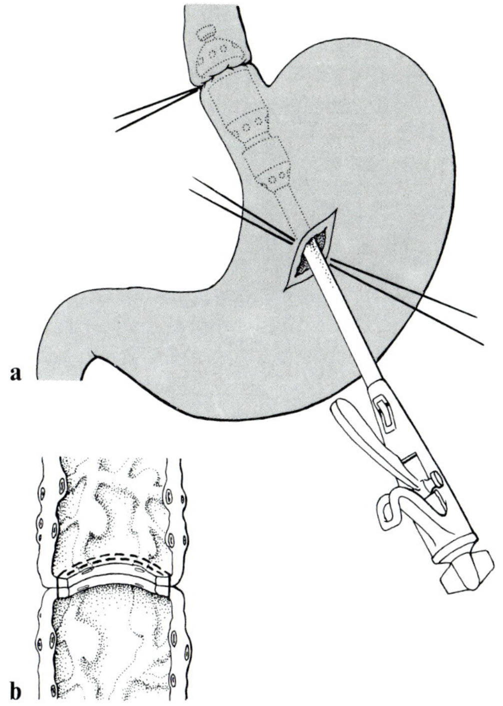

Fig. 28.20 a, b. Esophageal venous interruption (Kivelitz). **a** The abdominal esophagus is mobilized. A gastrotomy is made in the body of the stomach and the stapler instrument is advanced into the esophagus. The esophagus is ligated in a circular fashion distal to the anvil of the instrument. The instrument is fired. **b** Esophago-esophageal end-to-end anastomosis. The staple rows block the esophageal varices

paraesophageal veins running parallel to the vagus nerve and interconnecting with the esophageal venous plexus. All these shunt veins (approximately 30–50) are carefully ligated up as far as the inferior pulmonary vein (Fig. 28.21 a). Care should be taken not to injure the vagus nerves.

Now, the esophagus is mobilized, encircled, and opened after two soft clamps have been applied (Fig. 28.21 b). The muscle layer is opened longitudinally, the mucosa transversally. The varices which run in the submucosa are ligated with fine suture ligatures (Dexon (R) or Vicryl (R) 5-0 atraumatic). Afterwards, the esophagus is closed by double suture. Usually, 70–90 suture ligatures are necessary.

b) Abdominal Operation. A left subcostal incision is made. The short gastric vessels are transected between ligatures, the splenic vessels are ligated, and the spleen is removed (see p. 765). The proximal third of the greater curvature, especially the

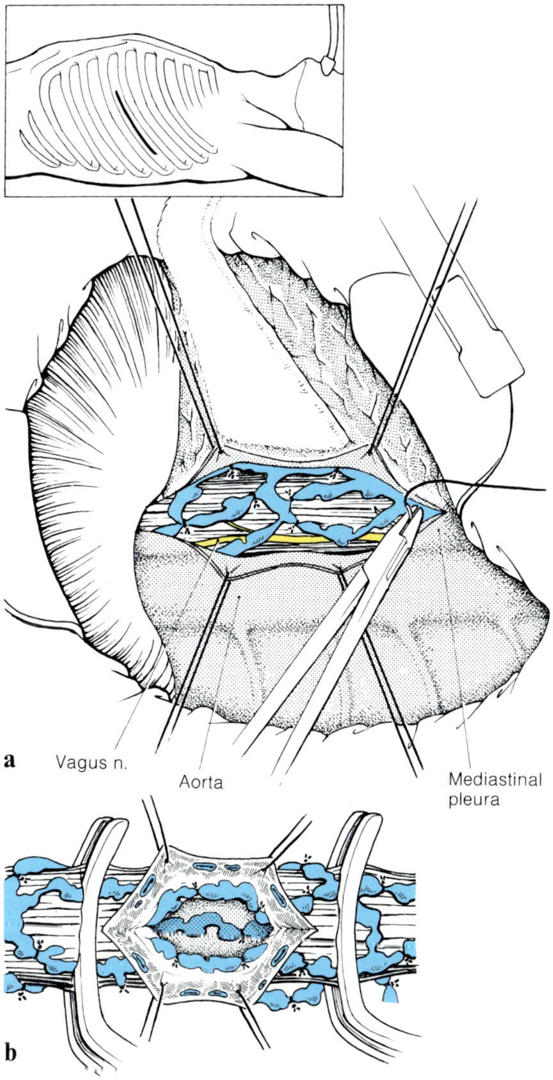

Fig. 28.21 a, b. Devascularization (Sugiura-Futagawa). **a** Opening of the left chest cavity through an intercostal incision. The lung is pushed cephalad. The mediastinal pleura is incised, and the distal esophagus is dissected free. The periesophageal veins are carefully controlled with suture ligatures. **b** The esophagus is incised after soft clamps have been placed. The intramural veins are also controlled with multiple suture ligatures

posterior wall, is carefully skeletized; then, the lesser curvature, from the angle of the stomach upward, is devascularized. A selective vagotomy and pyloroplasty is also performed. In addition, the veins leading from the diaphragm to the esophagus must be ligated and transected (Fig. 28.22). Sugiura and Futagawa [30] have operated on 276 patients using this method; only 52 of these operations came during the acute phase of bleeding.

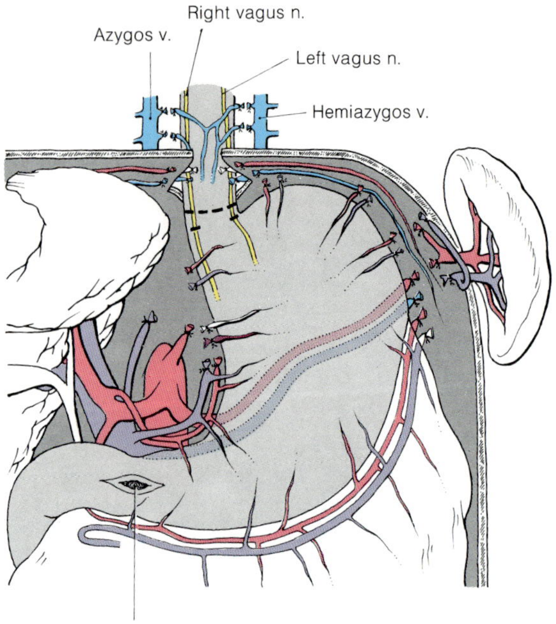

Fig. 28.22. Devascularization (SUGIURA-FUTAGAWA). Abdominal part of the operation. Devascularization of the upper half of the stomach along the greater and lesser curvature. Ligature and transection of the splenic vessels and splenectomy. Careful dissection of the phrenic veins. Vagotomy and pyloroplasty

They also recommend this procedure for elective surgery. The surgical mortality is surprisingly low, in spite of the long and extensive thoracoabdominal procedure. In emergency situations it is 11.5%.

5. Abdominal Resection of Cardia and Fundus with Splenectomy (STELZNER)

Because this is not a cancer operation requiring safety zones around the esophagus, we do not consider a thoracoabdominal approach to be necessary. Good exposure can be achieved with an extensive left-sided subcostal incision.

We start by skeletizing the fundus of the stomach, with transection of the short gastric vessels. Then, the hepatogastric ligament is divided between ligatures, and the proximal lesser curvature is carefully skeletized. Next, the esophagus is freed from the hiatus and encircled, and the left

Fig. 28.23a–c. Abdominal cardia-fundus resection with splenectomy. **a** The esophagus on the upper part of the stomach is desvascularized and mobilized. The esophagus is encircled. After a clamp has been placed, the esophagus is ligated proximal to the cardia, and the fundus of the stomach is transected with the aid of a stapling instrument. **b** End-to-side anastomosis between esophagus and stomach. The posterior wall is sutured with either continuous or interrupted sutures of fine absorbable suture material. **c** Completed end-to-side esophagogastrostomy

▽

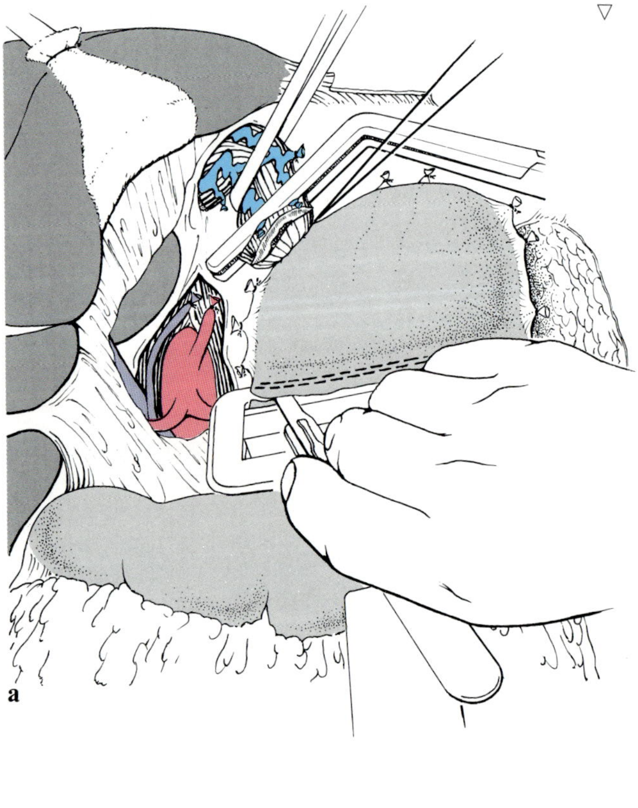

a

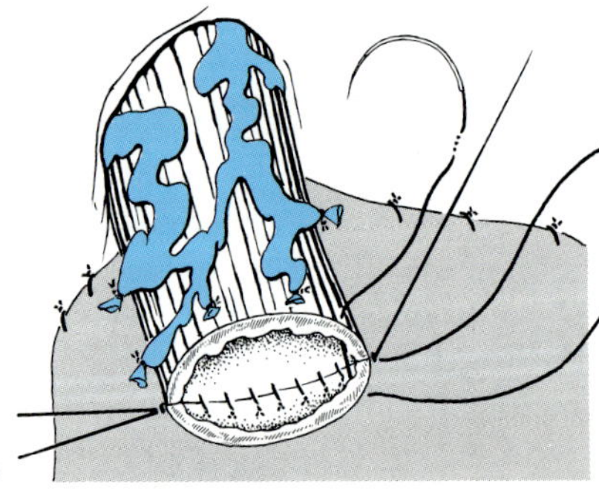

b

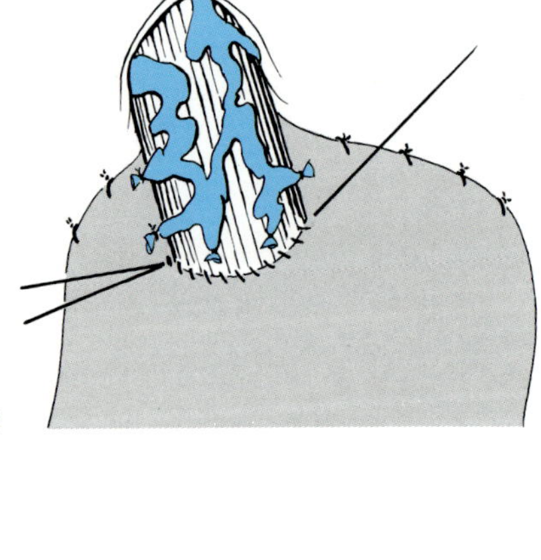

c

gastric artery and the coronary vein are ligated and transected. The esophagus is mobilized and ligated at the cardia with a heavy silk suture; then, after proximal placement of an angled clamp, the esophagus is transected (Fig. 28.23a). The stomach is then pulled distally and caudad, and a Petz apparatus is applied at the border of the skeletization. The stomach is transected between the suture rows of the Petz apparatus. The cardia, the fundus, and the small rim of the esophagus are removed.

Since the lesser sac is now open, one can expose and ligate the splenic vessels and remove the spleen (see p. 765). Careful hemostasis of the splenic bed should be observed. The suture line of the stomach is then secured with an additional running 2-0 catgut suture to obtain complete hemostasis, and the seromuscular layer is closed with interrupted 3-0 cotton sutures.

Anastomosis Between Esophagus and Corpus of the Stomach. The anastomosis is performed using a single row of all-layer sutures of absorbable material (Dexon/Vicryl 4-0) (Fig. 28.23a, b). The posterior suture row is done with mattress sutures, which allow for broad adaptation of the tissues. Since the remaining stomach is sufficiently large (unlike a cancer resection), the esophageal anastomosis can be secured in an additional fundoplication. Esophageal anastomosis can also be done with the EEA stapler. Careful hemostasis is carried out, and two drains are put in place, one in the splenic bed and one near the anastomosis. This procedure is extensive and stressful. As an emergency operation during massive hemorrhage, we think it is too risky. It should only be used as a last resort. Its advantage is that esophageal as well as fundal varices are removed. A pyloroplasty can be added but is not essential.

6. Thoracic Esophageal Transection (Walker)

The best approach is through a left thoracotomy in the sixth or seventh intercostal space. After the chest cavity is opened, the left pulmonary lobe is mobilized and pushed cranially. The mediastinal pleura is incised longitudinally, and the esophagus is freed from the mediastinum and encircled. Many vascular connections to the esophagus are encountered which have to be ligated carefully. The esophagus is mobilized over a distance of 10–12 cm and compressed proximally and distally with two soft clamps to avoid blood loss. An incision 5 cm long is made in the surface of the muscle

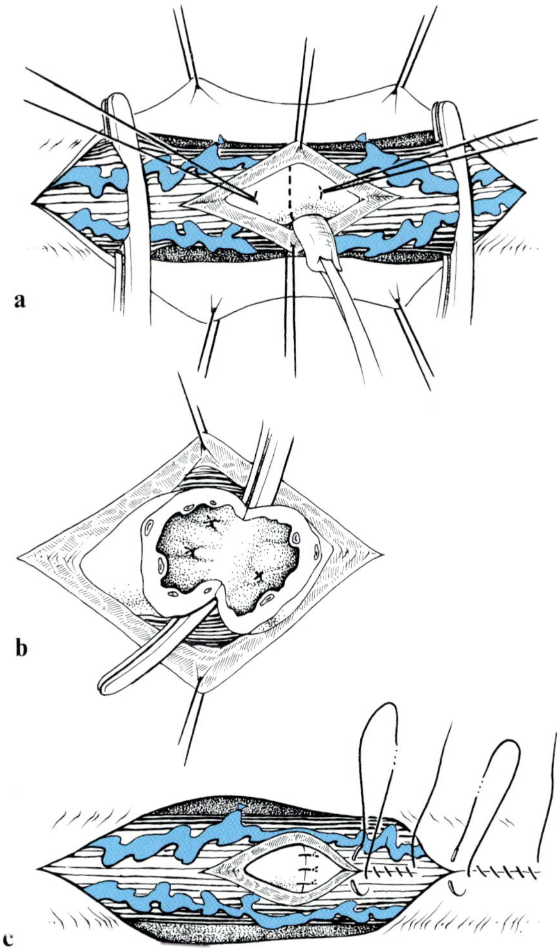

Fig. 28.24a–c. Transthoracic esophageal transection (Walker). **a** The esophagus is dissected free in its distal part after opening of the mediastinal pleura. It is grasped proximally and distally with clamps. After stay sutures have been placed, the musculature of the esophagus is opened longitudinally, and the esophageal mucosa is freed bluntly over its entire circumference. **b** The mucosal tube is transected transversally. A small posterior strip remains intact. The engorged esophageal varices are controlled with fine suture ligatures. Afterward, suture of the mucosa with interrupted absorbable sutures. **c** Closure of the musculature longitudinally with interrupted or continuous sutures

and held open with stay sutures. Now, the mucosal tube can be bluntly dissected out of the muscle bed (Fig. 28.24a). With the aid of two stay sutures, a semicircular incision is made. One can now see the varicose veins in the lumen of the esophagus. In the region of the incision, they are suture-ligated using very fine absorbable suture material (Dexon-Vicryl) 5-0. A strip of mucosa about 1 cm wide, remaining on the posterior wall, prevents retraction of the mucosa (Fig. 28.24b). The varices are now controlled one by one with suture ligatures, the mucosa is approximated with fine sutures, and the musculature is closed longitudinally using the same suture material. One should also secure the esophageal suture line with a flap of mediastinal pleura. Fundal varices cannot be controlled by this operation. This is a disadvantage.

E. Peritoneovenous Shunt in the Treatment of Refractory Ascites

Ascites not responding to conservative measures can be treated surgically. Procedures earlier used, e.g., lymphovenous anastomosis, have not stood the test of time. Today, one uses plastic valve-tube systems that transport the ascites from the abdominal cavity into the superior vena cava. LEVEEN et al. [20] first developed such a valve system in 1974.

I. Indications and Contraindications

The most important indication is ascites secondary to cirrhosis and not responsive to diuretics. Most of such patients are in the final stage of cirrhosis. A controversial indication is ascites due to peritoneal carcinosis. Contraindications are renal insufficiency, congestive heart failure, and coagulation disorders.

II. Valve Systems

The valve systems are manufactured from inert nontoxic plastic material (Silastic, Teflon); they are composed of three elements:

1. A *collector for the ascites* which is positioned in the abdominal cavity,
2. A *one-way valve* which, depending on the model, allows for the passive or active transport of the ascites and prevents retrograde flow of the blood from the vena cava into the system,
3. A *venous catheter* which is placed over the jugular vein into the superior vena cava and returns the ascites to the circulation.

The *functional principle* of the system is based on a physiologic pressure gradient between the abdominal and chest cavities. The valve opens at a pressure of 3 cm H_2O so that the ascites, which is under pressure, flows into the vena cava. The intra-abdominal pressure can be increased by the use of abdominal binders and by breathing against resistance, using a breathing bottle. The patient should breath against a resistance of 10 cm of H_2O several times daily for 15 min (Fig. 28.25).

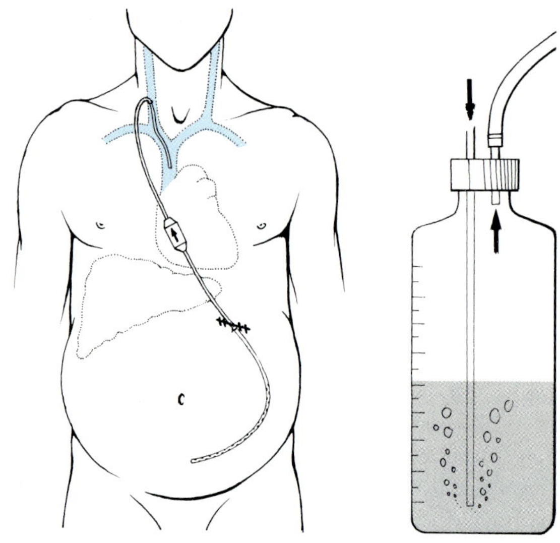

Fig. 28.25. Schematic representation of the position of a peritoneovenous shunt. The valve is located subcutaneously over the costal arch or the sternum, and the venous tubing is brought subcutaneously cephalad and inserted into the internal jugular vein. The tip of the venous tubing is positioned in the superior vena cava, close to the atrium. The figure also shows a breathing bottle by which the patient can inhale against a resistance of 15 cm H_2O. This increases the intra-abdominal pressure, and the ascites is pushed through the shunt system into the venous circulation

Four ascites valves are available. The technical principles are described in the following section.

1. LeVeen Valve

This consists of a perforated collector for the ascites and a one-way valve with a silastic tube for the vena cava, which can be shortened as needed. The valvular membrane opens when the abdominal pressure exceeds the central venous pressure by at least 10 cm H_2O. To increase this pressure gradient, the patient breathes against resistance using a breathing bottle. With this technique patient cooperation is obviously essential.

2. Storz Denver Valve

This has a flexible pump chamber with two valves. The subcutaneously implanted pump chamber can be compressed from the outside with a finger and the ascites can be pumped into the vein. The valve opens at a pressure of 1 cm H_2O and has a flow rate of 36–48 ml/min. Both valves prevent reflux into the pump chamber. It is an advantage that the ascites collector and the venous tube are marked with strips of contrast material so that precise localization by X-ray is possible during and after implantation.

3. Agishi Valve

This system uses an ascites collector with a double lumen to prevent obstruction of the collector by omentum or bowel. The membrane pump has a one-way valve which opens at a pressure of 5 mmHg and resists reflux up to a pressure of 175 mmHg. With each pump stroke, 3–6 ml ascites can be transported. A filter is located at the end of the venous catheter to prevent reflux of blood into the pump chamber and to prevent thrombosis. The loop, therefore, cannot be shortened.

4. Cordis Hakim Valve

This system is supplied in separate parts which have to be assembled intraoperatively. It has a ball valve with a closing pressure of 10–30 mm H_2O, allowing for active transport of ascites into the vein. An additional chamber is built into the system, which allows the puncture of ascites postoperatively and the irrigation of the system. Plugging by protein can thus be prevented. The ascites collector is made of semiflexible plastic and marked for fixation at the peritoneum.

III. Surgical Technique and Complications

The ascites collector should be introduced into the abdominal cavity in the left upper abdomen because in some cases a portasystemic shunt operation could become necessary later on. A 5- to 8-cm transverse incision is made in the left upper quadrant. The musculature of the rectus is pushed apart bluntly, and a purse-string suture with heavy Dexon/Vicryl is placed in the peritoneum. A stab incision is then made within the purse-string suture (Fig. 28.26a). Part of the ascites now escapes and is evacuated. The ascites collector is then introduced into the abdominal cavity and fixed in place with the purse-string suture. At the same time, the incision in the peritoneum is closed by tightening the suture (Fig. 28.26b). The *valve part* is then placed within the rectus sheath (LeVeen model) or, if one is using a pump valve (Storz Denver, Cordis Hakim), on a firm body surface (sternum, costal margin) (Fig. 28.26c). The *venous part* of the system is then introduced through the right or left jugular vein into the superior vena cava. The vein is exposed through a small supraclavicular incision lateral to the sternocleidomastoid muscle and encircled with a tape. A purse-string suture with 4-0 Prolene is placed on the anterior aspect of the vein (Fig. 28.6d). First, however, a subcutaneous tunnel is created with a forceps. After the venous tubing has been brought through this tunnel and the jugular vein has been clamped, a stab wound is made within the purse-string sutures and the vascular edges are grasped with mosquito clamps to facilitate the introduction of the plastic tube into the jugular vein and the superior vena cava. It is advanced almost to the right atrium. The purse-string suture is tightened temporarily, and the position of the catheter tip is checked by X-ray. It should not be located in the atrium, where it can cause cardiac arrhythmias. Depending on the circumstances, the tube may have to be shortened and advanced into the vein again. If the position is correct, the tube is fixed with the purse-string suture and with an additional subcutaneous suture. The tube should enter the vein in a smooth curve without kinking.

Malfunctions of the valve system can be checked in two ways:

1. After injection of radioactive technetium into the ascites-filled abdominal cavity, the transport of the tagged ascitic fluid through the valve in the external tubing can be followed scintigraphically.
2. Percutaneous injection of contrast material into the external tubing can easily detect kinking and obstruction.

In these cases, operative correction is indicated. Furthermore, *ascitic leaks* can occur where the system enters the abdominal cavity. These leaks can be controlled by suture. *Infections* leading to sepsis are serious. Mortality is high, and the shunt system must be removed in time.

A troublesome early complication is *coagulation abnormalities* with extensive bleeding along the subcutaneously embedded tubing system as well as at the site of operation. Such bleeding can be explained by disseminated intravascular coagulation already present preoperatively as the result

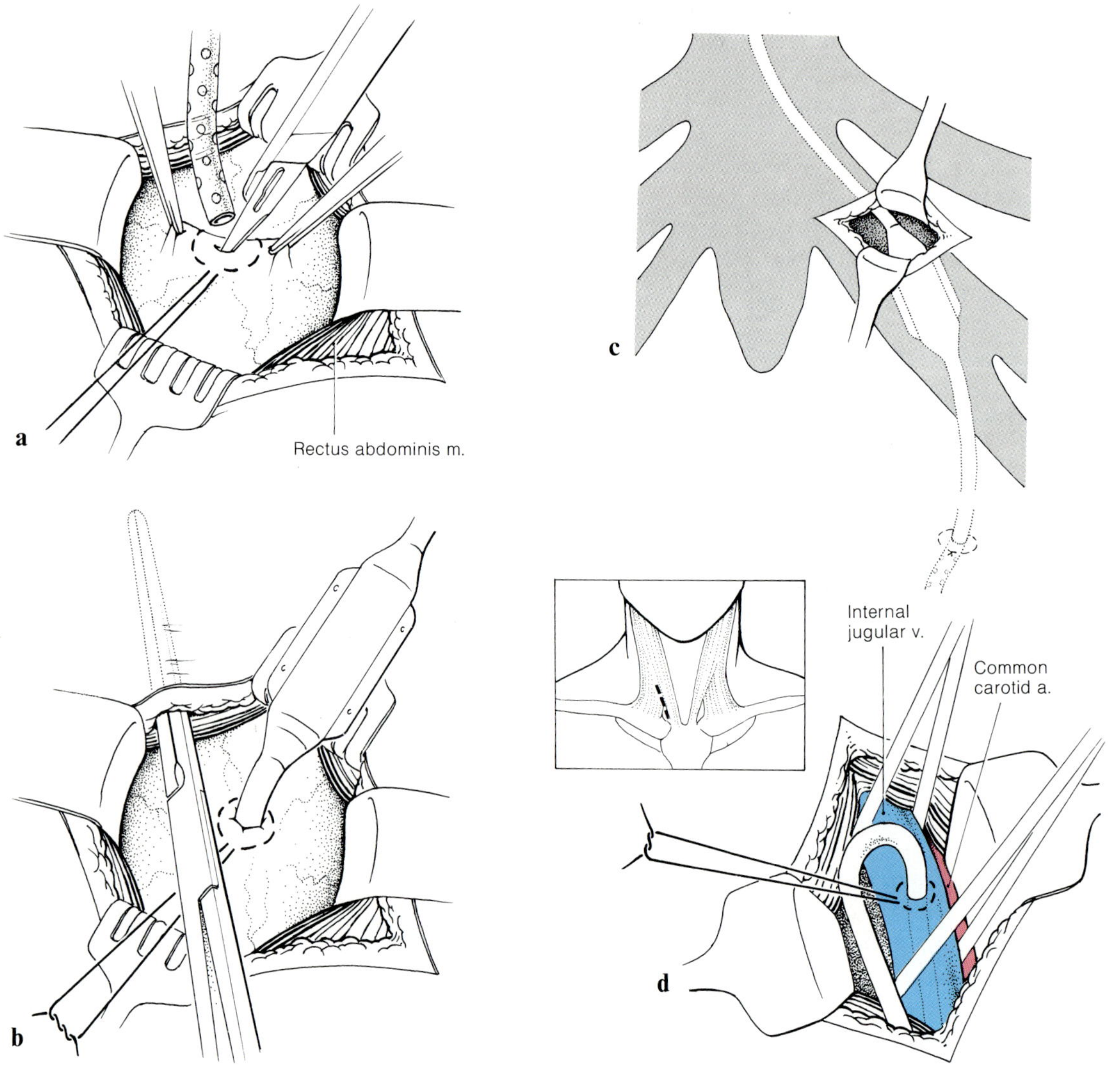

Fig. 28.26a–d. Implantation of the ascites valve. **a** After transverse incision in the right upper quadrant, the musculature of the rectus is spread apart bluntly, and a purse-string suture is placed in the posterior rectus sheath. Stab incision in the middle of the purse-string suture. The abdominal part of the tubing is inserted into the peritoneal cavity. **b** The purse-string suture closes the opening in the peritoneum. A subcutaneous tunnel is created with the aid of forceps. **c** Transverse incision over the left costal margin, close to the sternum. After a subcutaneous pocket has been created, the pump valve is placed over the costal margin. The patient is now able to compress the small balloon pump against this firm surface. **d** 5 cm incision at the lateral border of the sternocleidomastoid muscle on the right. The internal jugular vein is dissected free and encircled. Purse-string suture on the anterior wall of the jugular vein. Stab incision and introduction of the proximal part of the tubing system into the jugular vein, advancing it into the superior vena cava. One should be careful not to kink the tubing

of an impairment of the liver's ability to clear thromboplastic substances, and by intravascular coagulation caused by the continuous reinfusion of ascites. Ascitic fluid entering the blood contains tissue thromboplastin, endotoxins, products of fibrinolysis, and also clotting factors, i.e., plasminogen, antithrombin, and antithrombinogen. This complication demands the removal of the shunt system in order to eliminate ascitic flow into the bloodstream. It is necessary to try intravenous ascites reinfusion preoperatively to determine whether the fibrinogen level drops significantly, or whether products of fibrinolysis can be found in increased concentrations. The administration of vitamin K and fresh frozen plasma is essential; postoperatively the coagulation system must be checked daily.

Another complication is *congestive heart failure*, which can occur because of the increased intravascular volume. Digitalization is therefore advised.

The most common late complication is the *occlusion of the shunt system* caused by fibrin or cell elements or by a thrombosis of the jugular vein, which can extend into the superior vena cava. The occluded part of the shunt system must be exchanged.

IV. Evaluation of the Ascites Valve

If strict indications are adhered to and risk factors are excluded, the peritoneovenous shunt can effectively treat ascites that are resistant to medical management. Advantages are: minor procedure, improvement of renal function, improvement of water and electrolyte balance, simple follow-up, subjective improvement for the patient, and lower cost, as compared with high-dose diuretic therapy. We prefer the Storz-Denver system because it is less susceptible to technical complications and allows for the active transport of ascites by means of a simple maneuver that can be done by the patient.

REFERENCES

1. Adamsons RJ, Arif S, Babich A, Bult K, Lam A, Minkowitz S (1975) Arterialization of the liver in combination with a portocaval shunt in the dog. Surg Gynecol Obstet 140:594
2. Agishi T (1977) Implantable peritoneocaval shunt pump for intractable ascites. Transections 23:52
3. Biersack HJ, Thelen M, Schulz O, Knopp R, Schmidt R, Winkler C (1977) Die sequentielle Hepato-Spleno-Szintigraphie zur quantitativen Beurteilung der Leberdurchblutung. Forstschr Röntgenstr 126:47
4. Boerema I, Klopper PJ, Holscher AA (1970) Transabdominale Ligatur-Resektion des Ösophagus in Fällen von blutenden Varizen. Chirurg 41:472
5. Bradley SE, Ingelfinger FJ, Bradley GP, Curry JJ (1945) Estimation of hepatic blood flow in man. J Clin Invest 24:890
6. Brunner G (1980) Intravasale und submucöse Ösophagusvarizensklerosierung mit einem neuen flexiblen Gerät. Z Gastroenterol 18:443
7. Child CG, Turcotte JG (1964) The liver and portal hypertension. Saunders, Philadelphia
8. Cooley DA (1963) Side-to-side splenorenal anastomosis with splenic preservation for portal hypertension. Surg Gynecol Obstet 116:627
9. Denck H (1977) Die endoskopische Behandlung von Ösephagusvarizen. Chirurg 48:212
10. Drapanas Th (1972) Interposition mesocaval shunt for treatment of portal hypertension. Ann Surg 176:435
11. Gütgemann A, Schreiber HW (1962) Zur Indikation und Technik der portocavalen Anastomose. Chirurg 33:509
12. Häring R, Hirner A (1982) Blutungen aus Ösophagus, Magen und Duodenum. In: Häring R (eds) Dringliche Bauchchirurgie. Thieme, Stuttgart p 320
13. Häring R, Hirner A (1982) Der portokavale Notshunt. In: Paquet KJ, Denck H, Berchtold R (eds) Portale Hypertension. Karger, Basel, p 190
14. Hassab MA (1967) Gastro-esophageal decongestion and splenectomy and the treatment of esophageal varices in bilharzial cirrhosis: further studies with report on 355 operations. Surgery 61:169
15. Hirner A, Häring R, Bost H, Sörensen R (1978) Die hyperkinetische portale Hypertension. Chirurg 49:303
16. Hirner A, Roots I, Häring R (1982) Der Amidopyrin-Stoffwechsel als Leberfunktionstest in der experimentellen und humanen Pfortaderchirurgie (unter besonderer Berücksichtigung der Leberarterialisation). In: Weller S (ed) Chirurgisches Forum 1982 für experimentelle und klinische Forschung. Springer, Berlin Heidelberg New York, p 197
17. Hottenrott C, Böttcher W, Maul FD, Wildgrube HJ, Peter H, Förster HD, Encke A (1983) Diagnostische transumbilicale Shunt-Simulation als Indikationshilfe zum portosystemischen Shunt. Chirurg 54:149
18. Karavias Th, Häring R, Weber D (1982) Postoperative Syndrome nach portocavaler Anastomose bei Leberzirrhose. Leber Magen Darm 12:85
19. Kivelitz H, Ulrich B (1981) Klammernahtgeräte am Ösophagus. Langenbecks Arch Chir 355:455
20. LeVeen HH, Wapnik S, Grosberg S (1976) Further experience with peritoneo-venous shunt for ascites. Ann Surg 184:574
21. Linton RR, Ellis DS, Geary E (1961) Critical comparative analysis of early and late results of splenorenal and direct porto caval shunts performed in 169 patients with portal cirrhosis. Ann Surg 154:446
22. Matzander U (1981) Zusätzliche Leberarterialisation mit portokavaler End-zu-Seit Anastomose. In: Eckert P, Liehr H (eds) Akutes und chronisches Leberversagen. Intensivmedizin, Notfallmedizin, Anästhesiologie, 25th edn. Thieme, Stuttgart p 145
23. Meursing F (1913) Über eine seltene Anastomose zwischen V. portae und V. cava. Med T Geneesk 2:20, ref. Berlin Klin Wochenschr 50:643
24. Paquet KJ, Oberhammer E (1978) Sclerotherapy of esophageal varices by means of endoscopy. Endoscopy 10:7
25. Rienecker H, Danek N (1975) Operative Behandlung blutender Ösophagusvarizen durch eine subcardiale Blutsperre mittels transmuraler maschineller Klammerung. Chirurg 46:87
26. Schmidt HD (1982) Die Bestimmung der Leberdurchblutung durch die Kineangiodensitometrie. In: Paquet KJ, Denck H, Berchtold R (eds) Portale Hypertension. Karger, Basel, p 123

27. Schreiber HB (1969) Portale Hypertension. In: Baumgartl F, Kremer K, Schreiber HW (eds) Spezielle Chirurgie für die Praxis, vol II/1. Thieme, Stuttgart, p 614
28. Sohendra N, Reynders-Frederix, Doehn M, Bützow GH, Erbe W (1979) Fiberendoskopische Ösophagusvarizenverödung. Dtsch Med Wochenschr 104:161
29. Stelzner F (1967) Über die individuelle chirurgische Therapie der Blutung beim portalen Hochdruck unter Berücksichtigung der Ösophagusvarizenblutung. Bruns Beitr Klin Chir 214:86
30. Sugiura M, Futagawa S (1972) A new technique for treating esophageal varices. J Thorac Cardiovasc Surg 71:677
31. Walker M (1960) Transsection operation for portal hypertension. Thorax 15:218
32. Warren WD, Salam AA, Hutson D, Zeppa R (1974) Selective distal spleno-renal shunt. Arch Surg 108:306
33. Zöckler CE (1975) Hämodynamik der portalen Hypertension. In: Zöckler CE, Gheorghin TH (eds) Witzstrock, Baden-Baden, p 25
34. Zühlke HV, Häring R, Semsch B (1984) Der peritoneo-venöse Shunt zur Behandlung des therapieresistenten Ascites. Chirurg 55:253

29 Surgery of Lymphedema

29.1 Resectional Operations for the Treatment of Primary and Secondary Lymphedema

U. BRUNNER

CONTENTS

A. Special Prerequisites for Patient Selection and Choice of Procedure

The anatomy of the lymphatic system is described on p. 32.

Primary lymphedema of the lower extremity is characterized by reduction of the epifascial lymph collectors, especially of the ventromedial bundle. The cause of this hypoplasia has not been explained completely. Many things point to malformation. Primary lymphedema of the arm is much rarer than that of the leg and therefore less precisely characterized by lymphangiogram.

In case of *secondary lymphedema* of the lower and upper extremity, the deep or the superficial lymphatic system, or both of them, are either functionally impaired, overloaded, or have been anatomically destroyed. This may be a result of trauma, surgery, parasites, inflammatory or neoplastic processes, or a chronic venous insufficiency.

According to FÖLDI [5], in a disturbance of the lymphatic outlet of whatever origin in the extremities, the so-called lymphatic load is reduced by compensatory mechanisms. These include lymphatic as well as extralymphatic reactions. The lymphatic, regenerative functions are numerous: bypassing of defects by means of collaterals, lymphatic bypasses within the superficial or deep system itself, but also by cross connections in both directions, depending on the compartment with the lymphatic block, as well as by opening of lymphatic venous shunts. The extralymphatic reaction is the work of monocytes and macrophages, which usually support the clearance from the interstitial tissue of lymphatic substances and thereby maintain the extralymphatic protein transport. When these compensatory mechanisms fail to drain the lymphatic load, it exceeds the lymphatic transport capacity. The result is lymphostasis. Clinically, this may be evident in very circumscribed local edemas or global edema of the whole extremity. This depends on the lymphatic outlet stenoses and the possibilities for bypasses through the so-called lymph territories [7].

In the cisterna chyli, clear lymph from the lower extremity is mixed with the fatty lymph from the gut. Pathologic primary and secondary congestions in this area may result in a reflux of chylous, viscous, milky lymph back into the limb (chylous edema/chylous fistula), the abdomen (chylous ascites), the pleura (chylothorax), the pericardium (chylopericardium), the urinary bladder (chyluria), or the vagina (chylous metorrhea).

B. Indications for Resective Operations

Due to the special anatomic and pathogenetic factors involved, there is practically no regeneration of lymphatic vessels in cases of primary lymphedema, and there are also significantly fewer compensatory mechanisms, both in the pelvis and in the leg, as compared with secondary lymphedema. For both types, however, the same therapeutic principle holds true: Resectional surgery is indicated only in case of disabling symptoms.

A whole spectrum of conservative measures is available, not only as alternatives to surgery but also, from the surgical point of view, as forms of pre- and postoperative treatment [2, 5]. However, these measures will be effective only as part of an individualized treatment program, i.e., one that takes account of the special character of the swelling, specific local changes within the swelling itself, and the patient's individual circumstances. The spectrum of measures in question especially includes physiotherapy to decompress the limb and the wearing of appropriate elastic support stockings. Gymnastics especially designed for the lymphatic system as well as special hand massage have been successful. Additional measures are aimed at helping the patient understand how to live with, rather than for, the swollen limb. Diuretics are indicated only for acute swelling. Benzopyrone derivates stimulate the macrophages. These measures will not remove the lymphedema, but they may help to maintain working capacity. Improvement cannot be expected unless therapy is consistent. Only in this way is it possible to oppose the progress of the disease, which is not yet completely understood, and to protect the patient from despair.

Among the operative procedures, we fundamentally distinguish between physiologic operations and resections. The variety of procedures in current use indicates that no operative method is satisfactory in all cases. There are detailed monographs, for instance, on the leg [1] or the arm [4].

The objective of present-day physiologic methods is to drain the congested lymph through capillaries into the normal healthy body parts using pedunculated skin flaps of various thickness. Direct lymphatic venous anastomoses are an attempt to drain the peripheral lymph into the venous system. Lymph vessel transplantations (see pp. 791, 796) have the same objective but involve direct reconstructive measures within the lymphatic system. If initial evaluation reveals none of the accepted physiologic procedures to be appropriate, resectional procedures are available in cases of severe malformation. Here, the subcutaneous fatty tissue containing the lymphostatic fluid is excised. Since the lymphatic load is thereby reduced, the resection may also be acknowledged to have a physiologic component. The operative technique follows the principles of plastic surgery. Numerous modifications have been worked out in line with the basic intention. A method has been tried by Thompson, described as dermatoplasty [10], combining the idea of physiology and resection. In order to bypass obstructions within the small pelvis, Kinmonth tried an enteromesenteric shunt [6]. An evaluation of my own results and a reinspection of the literature lead me to conclude that there are currently only four methods that have any practical value.

C. Dermatoplasty According to Thompson [10]

This method aims at the drainage of the lymph in the subepidermal lymph capillaries into the muscle compartments, using a long pedicled skin flap without epithelium (Fig. 29.1.1). In order to provide a physiologic direction of lymph flow in the subepidermal plexus, the edge of the flap should be located approximately in the area of the superficial lymphatic system, normally containing the collector vessels. For instance, the prefascial lymphatic vessels of the thigh join in the direction of the collectors of the ventromedial bundle. Therefore, the incision must be chosen in such a way that the direction of normal lymph flow in the flap is toward its edge.

Typically, a dorsal full-thickness skin pedicle in the shape of a door is excised over the entire

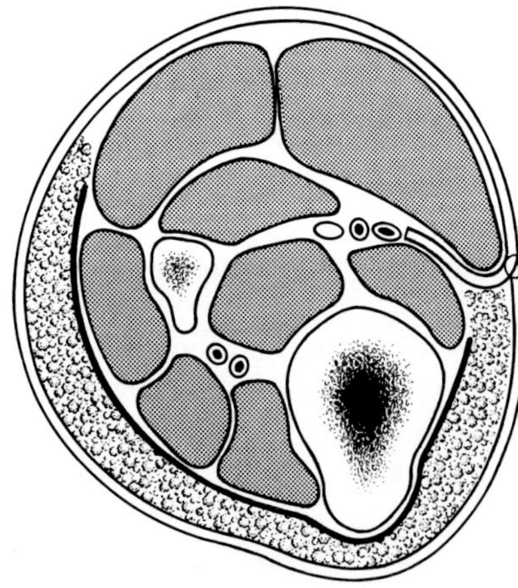

Fig. 29.1.1. Operation according to Thompson [10], partly excisional, partly for lymph drainage, creates a full-thickness skin pedicle. The compound flap is denuded of epidermis with a dermatome, is then buried between the muscles and fixed there

length of the medial side of the arm or leg, leaving enough subcutaneous capillary-containing tissue to provide nutrition. The subcutaneous tissue and the fascia underneath are excised over the entire length of the flap. Owing to excision of fatty tissue, a margin of several centimeters is left over. This margin serves as a flap providing a link to the muscle compartment. It is prepared as a skin flap by removing the epidermis with a dermatome. Then, the edge is buried between the muscles and fixed there. Finally, it is completely interiorized by closure of the skin. If the method works properly, subepidermal lymph capillaries of the skin flap will link up to the muscular and perivascular lymphatics of the deep system. The lymph draining along the skin flap should then be controlled by the muscle pump. Had the fascia not been resected, they would impair the usual regeneration of the flap.

My experience with this method has been limited mainly to operations on the leg, and I have not had good results with it. THOMPSON himself, in the final report on his results [10], held that the effectiveness of the operation was due chiefly to the extensive excision of fatty tissue and not on the improved drainage of the lymph through the buried flap.

D. Wedge Excision According to Mikulicz and Sistrunk [9]

Following successful conservative decompression of elephantiasis, performed with the ultimate purpose of hospitalizing the patient for a wedge resection, loose compound flaps remain on the shaft of the extremities as well as in the region of the joints, especially on the calf of the leg. This excess skin can be folded manually (Fig. 29.1.2), and where necessary, it can be resected in longitudinal wedges. The wedge-shaped skin incision encircles enough loose tissue to approximate the skin edge-to-edge without tension. A wedge excision is continued down to the level of the fascia, the muscles, or the ligaments (Fig. 29.1.3). Multiple suction drains and closure of the wound layer by layer with supporting sutures are recommended.

If the procedure has to be performed medially and laterally, two separate operations at different times are indicated.

The procedure is merely palliative and requires all conservative measures to assure success. Its aim is to reduce the patient's weight by massive resection and to establish the feasibility of conservative therapy with elastic stockings.

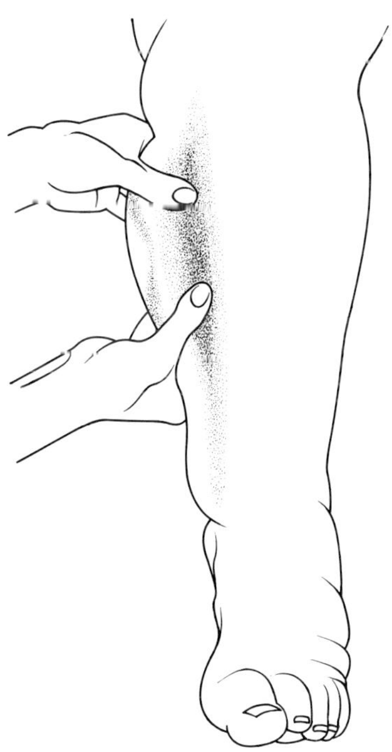

Fig. 29.1.2. Following decompression of a severe lymphedema, the excess skin becomes loose and can be folded manually

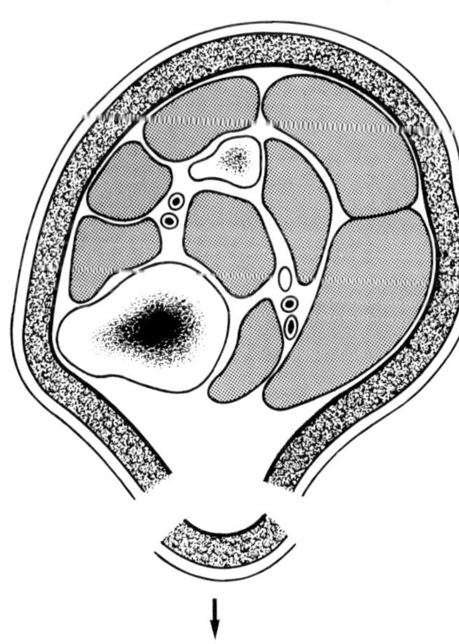

Fig. 29.1.3. Wedge excision according to MIKULICZ and SISTRUNK. The excess integument is removed in a wedge. Skin approximation without tension

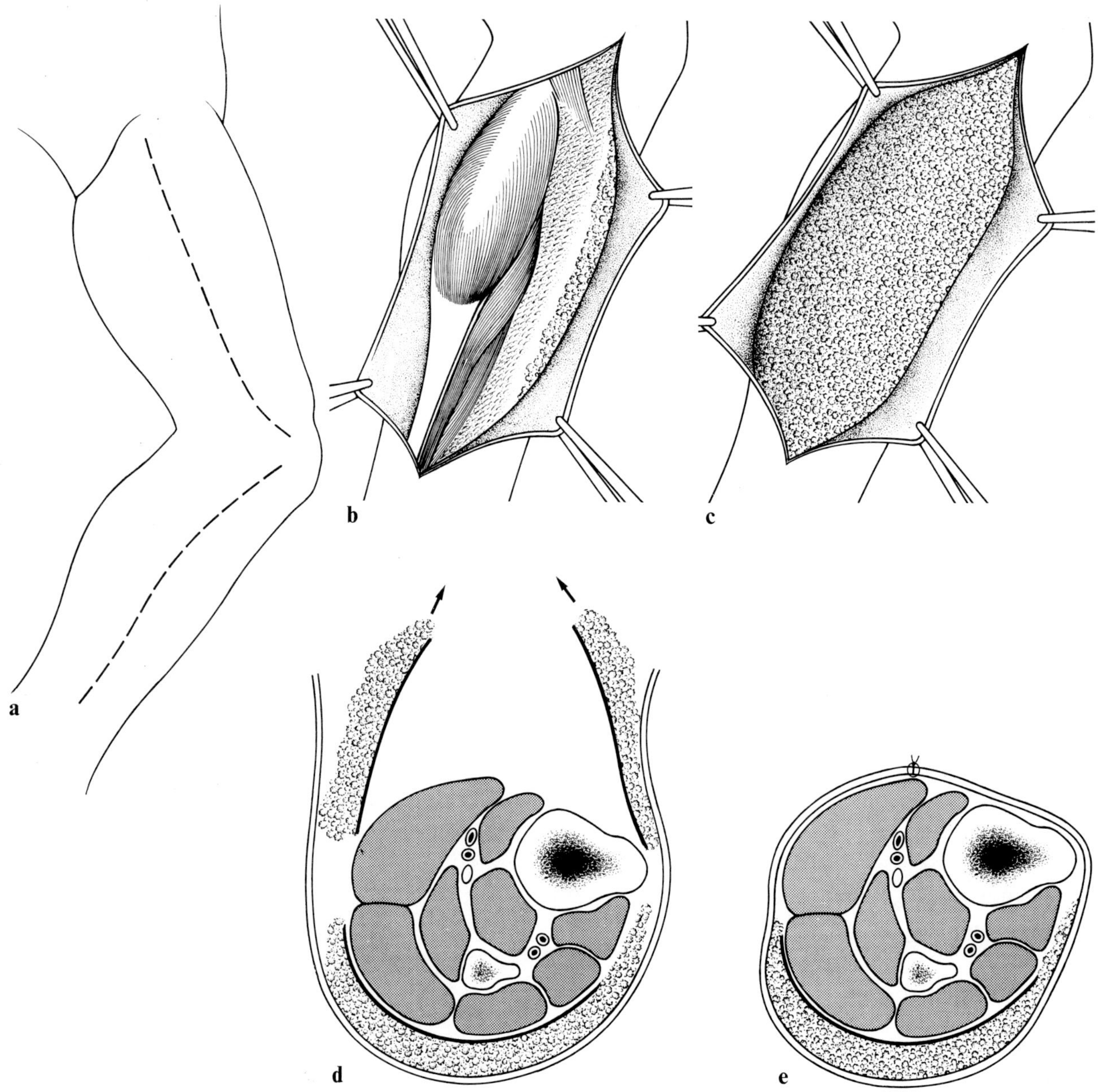

Fig. 29.1.4a–e. Extensive excision according to SERVELLE [8]. **a** Longitudinal skin incisions. **b** All subcutaneous tissue is pared off the skin with a scalpel, producing longitudinal pedicled full-thickness skin flaps that are retracted dorsally and ventrally. **c** En bloc resection of the subcutaneous fatty tissue. **d** Excision of the muscle fascia in order to provide sufficient capillary contact between the pedicled skin flap and the denuded area. **e** Closure of the skin without tension

E. Extensive Resection According to Servelle [8]

The following procedure was first described by SERVELLE in 1947. In my experience, satisfactory results were obtained, especially in younger disabled patients. The technique is shown for the medial side of the limb.

The patient is placed in a supine position. A tourniquet is applied after the leg has been suspended for at least 5 min. The tourniquet must be tightened repeatedly due to compression of the edema. Depending on the extent of the disease and the operative goal, longitudinal skin incisions are made on the medial side of the lower leg and/or the thigh (Fig. 29.1.4a). In advanced stages, the skin will have hardened or locally thickened. The incision is extended deeper to approach the fascia. Despite reduction of the edema, the subcutaneous tissue is excised carefully with a scalpel, grasping the skin only with the hand, not with forceps or clamps. In this way, longitudinal, dorsal, and ventral skin pedicles are constructed (Fig. 29.1.4b). In the second step, the fascia is denuded by en bloc resection of the fatty tissue. Depending on the situation, parts of the saphenous or sural nerve are resected (Fig. 29.1.4c). The third step is the removal of the fascia in order to provide sufficient capillary contact between the pedicled full-thickness skin graft and the denuded area (Fig. 29.1.4d). The fourth step is the release of the tourniquet followed by meticulous hemostases, which may well take 1 h. Microcoagulation should be used to protect the skin. Finally, in the fifth step, the wound is closed without tension, following placement of multiple drains of various types and excision of excess tissue (Fig. 29.1.4e).

The dressing consists of a 2-cm circular layer of hydrophilic gauze to absorb the inevitable and massive secretion during the exudative phase of the wound healing. Immediately after the operation, a circular rubber bandage providing a pressure of about 40 mmHg is applied. This rubber bandage is replaced later by an elastic textile bandage when the patient is mobilized. In a complicated postoperative course, the dressing is not changed before the 7th day.

In primary lymphedema it is often necessary to remove a hardened edematous cushion from the dorsum of the foot. In such cases, the subcutaneous fat is excised just within the layer of the peritendinous tissue of the extensor tendons, preserving their gliding ability. Pre- and retromalleolar edematous tissue is excised, preserving vascular and ligamentous structures. The placement of skin incisions depends on the local situation. On the dorsum of the foot, usually longitudinal incisions are performed. During dissection, special care must be taken to preserve the dorsalis pedis and posterior tibial arteries.

On the lateral side of the thigh and of the lower leg, the procedure is performed in similar steps. Special care is taken to preserve the fibular nerve in the region of the head of the fibula on the lateral side of the lower leg.

Postoperative complications: Seromas are treated according to general surgical procedures. Marginal necroses are removed early and covered by free skin grafts after wound debridement.

The procedure itself as well as the postoperative bandaging carry the risk of an anterior tibial compartment syndrome. This must be diagnosed and treated as early as possible; for this purpose, a regular, careful check of toe motility and peripheral pulses is essential (see p. 638).

F. Treatment of Chylous Reflux in the Leg

Chylous reflux is caused by dysfunction of the cysterna chyli. Secondary blockage and true primary lymphangiectasia with incompetent valves are the underlying diseases. The intestinal chyle no longer drains exclusively through the thoracic duct but follows the law of gravity instead. The chyle first

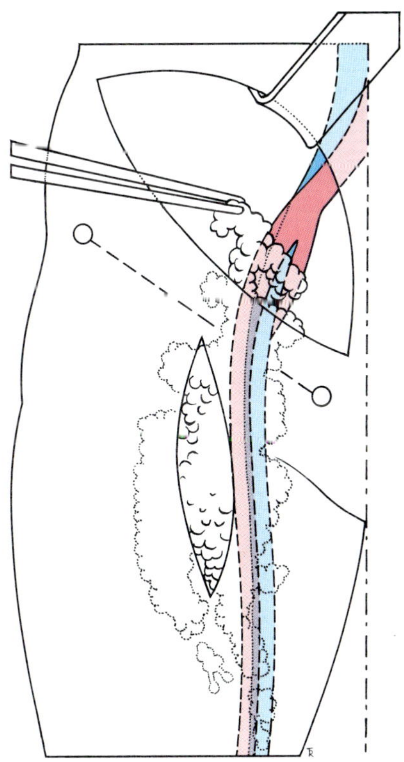

Fig. 29.1.5. Surgical treatment of chylous reflux. Removal of chyle-filled "sponges" by retroperitoneal routes at the level of the pelvis and with minimal damage to skin at the level of the leg

enters the enormous retroperitoneal lymphatic system, consisting of an enlarged pelvic lymphatic network, and from there it cascades into the periphery. The surgical treatment of choice is the ultraradical excision of the incompetent lymphatics in the retroperitoneum and in the groin (Fig. 29.1.5). This procedure is a causal treatment for chylous reflux because it is like plugging the source of the flow. Lymphedema of the leg by chylous reflux, however, is not touched. The various modifications for retroperitoneal exposure of the iliac arteries serve as the approach to the pelvis. In the leg, a more lateral longitudinal incision is beneficial, exposing the diseased lymphatic vessels subfascially with careful preservation of the skin flap. According to my observations and the literature as well, the pathology of the lymphatic vessels is quite variable. Sometimes networks of tortuous vessels, sometimes sponge-like varicose formations are found. All these pathological changes have in common that the lymphatic vessels are in close contact with arteries, veins, nerves, and muscles within the small pelvis and the groin.

With proper care being taken to preserve all of these structures, the chyle-filled lymphatics are excised as radically as possible and, if necessary, ligated and coagulated. Since the enlarged lymphatics encircle the neurovascular structures, these must be mobilized circumferentially for radical excision. One should beware of arterial spasms in young patients.

Following excision of these megalymphatics, exudation during wound healing is profuse. Suction drains placed in various layers are therefore indicated.

REFERENCES

1. Brunner U (1969) Das Lymphödem der unteren Extremitäten. Huber, Bern
2. Brunner U (1977) Manuelle Entstauung des primären Lymphödems der Beine. In: Brunner U (ed) Physikalische Therapie in Phlebologie und Lymphologie. Huber, Bern, p 46
3. Brunner U, Sonderegger A, Fleischlin C, Lang M (1984) Epidemiologie und Klinik des primären Lymphödems anhand von 500 Fällen. In: Bollinger A, Partsch H (eds) Initiale Lymphstrombahn. Thieme, Stuttgart
4. Clodius L (1977) Secondary arm lymphedema. In: Clodius L (ed) Lymphedema. Thieme, Stuttgart
5. Földi M (1983) Lymphoedema. In: Földi M, Casley-Smith J (eds) Lymphangiology. Schattauer, Stuttgart, pp 667
6. Kinmonth JB (1982) The lymphatics, 2nd edn. Arnolds, London, p 186
7. Kubik St (1980) Drainagemöglichkeiten der Lymphterritorien nach Verletzungen peripherer Kollektoren und nach Lymphadenektomie. Folia Angiol (Berl) 28:228
8. Servelle M (1947) La lymphangiectomie superficielle totale. Traitement chirurgical de l'éléphantiasis. Rev Chir (Paris) 66:294
9. Sistrunk WE (1977) Certain modifications of the Kondoleon operation for elephantiasis. Ann Surg 85:185
10. Thompson N (1965) Surgical treatment of primary and secondary lymphoedema of the extremities by lymphatic transposition. Proc Roy Soc Med 58:1026

29.2 Lymphatic-Venous and Lymph-Nodal-Venous Anastomoses

L. Nieuborg

CONTENTS

A. Indications for Lymphatic-Venous Reconstructions

I. Upper Extremity

Lymphedema following mastectomy is one of the best-known types of secondary upper-extremity lymphedema. Other types of secondary lymphedema result from axillary and/or supra/infraclavicular radiotherapy (Hodgkin's disease) and from axillary lymph node dissection for treatment or prevention of metastases in cases of malignant melanoma. Lymphedema following axillary lymph node dissection results from the removal of lymph nodes draining the lymphatics of the arm, which pass parallel to the axillary vein. Reconstruction is indicated since conservative therapy by compression is unsuccessful (absence of collateral circulation).

Exploration (early) of the lymphatic system of the arm is then required with the goal of reestablishing lymph drainage. A lymphatic-venous reconstruction is still the technique most widely used [6].

Indication for operation:

- Early secondary lymphedema without serious subcutaneous fibrosis, and an intact venous system, as demonstrated by phlebography.
- Fibrotic secondary lymphedema, when excisional surgery (subcutaneous) is considered following lymphatic-venous reconstruction (see p. 785ff.).

Contraindications:

- Partial or total venous obstruction, e.g., of the axillary vein (see lympholymphatic surgery) [1].

II. Lower Extremity

Iatrogenic lower leg lymphedema is known following gynecologic procedures (Avruel), lymph node dissection in the groin in cases of melanoma, and inguinal radiotherapy. Lymphedema may occur following vascular surgery in the groin (femoropopliteal reconstructions, operative management of vein incompetence). Secondary leg edema very soon results in serious fibrotic reactions, so that early reconstruction must be considered. Prior to exploration, however, phlebography should be performed for the purpose of documenting the deep vein branches available for the lymphatic-venous anastomosis. This is necessary because the greater saphenous vein may be absent – especially following lymph node dissection in the groin – and therefore unavailable for the anastomosis.

A lymph nodal-venous anastomosis may also be considered following abdominal lymph node dissection.

Indications for operation:

- Early secondary lymphedema, without collaterals (technetium lymph node scintigraphy)
- Late edema, where an excisional operation is being considered

Contraindications:

- Secondary lymphedema, with concomitant venous obstruction

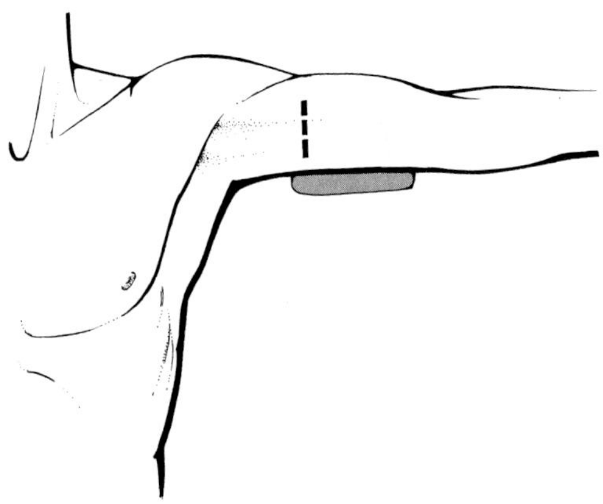

Fig. 29.2.1. Positioning of the patient for upper-arm lymph vessel exposure: transverse incision on the medial upper arm

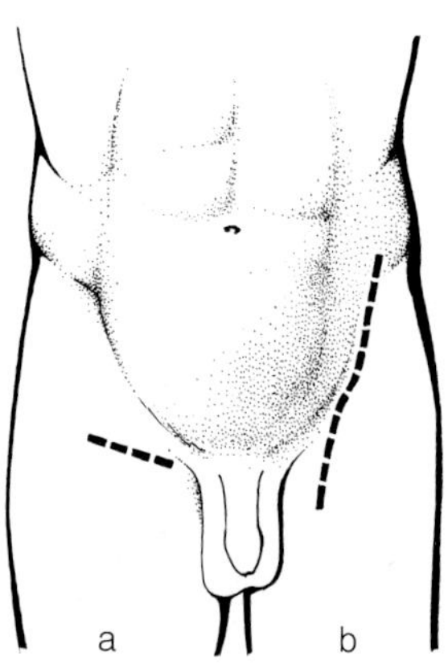

Fig. 29.2.2. Positioning of the patient for exposure of (*a*) inguinal lymphatics, (*b*) deep iliac lymphatics

B. Positioning

Reconstructive procedures on the lymphatics are performed with the patient in a supine position.

I. Arm Lymphedema

The exploration is made under intubation anesthesia or brachial plexus anesthesia. The diseased arm is placed on an arm table at a right angle to the body (Fig. 29.2.1). The elbow is slightly rotated outward. The upper arm is supported by a small cushion placed underneath it to provide good access to the lymph vessels passing subcutaneously, parallel to the brachial artery.

During the entire procedure, the surgeon sits at the medial side of the arm.

II. Leg Lymphedema

The operation is performed under epidural or intubation anesthesia. The patient is placed on an extension device or a standard operating table. In the first case, the surgeon sits between the patient's legs, which, according to our own experience, is a bad position, because the surgeon's lower arm inevitably has to be supported. When the patient is placed on a standard operating table, the soft tissue of the medial thigh is rotated outward by the placement of cushions. The surgeon sits on the ipsilateral side, at the hip joint. This positioning is also suitable for deep iliac exposure (Fig. 29.2.2).

C. Operative Approach

I. Arm Lymphedema

Exposure of the lymphatics is achieved through a transverse incision. The incision is usually placed 15 cm cranial to the medial epicondyle of the humerus, over the deep vessel sheath, and has a length of about 10 cm. The length of the skin incision depends upon the thickness of the edematous skin and subcutaneous tissue and is adapted to the local situation (Fig. 29.2.1).

It is advisable to perform the skin incision under the microscope because dilated lymph vessels are sometimes located close to the surface [5].

II. Leg Lymphedema

In the groin several incisions are possible, depending on the cause of the lymphedema.

- Following lymph node dissection of the groin: the incision is made distal to the incision of the previous operation. A transverse incision over the course of the (ligated) greater saphenous vein (15 cm) is sufficient to expose the lymphatics passing parallel to the vein.
- Following abdominal lymph node dissection of the groin: the incision is made either transversely at the level of the inguinal fold or obliquely [2] to achieve good exposure of the deep iliac lymphatics.
- Following groin irradiation: the obstructed lymphatics should be dissected distal to the irradiated area. The incision is made transversely again over a length of about 15 cm.
- Following trauma: one should never be tempted to expose the lymphatics through the previous wound. Only a few fibrotic bands will be found within the previous wound area. Also with this indication, a distal incision (transverse) should be performed.

In all the cases described, sharp dissection using a knife is possible down to the level of Scarpa's fascia. The draining lymphatics are always located below this level.

D. Technique of Dissection

I. Upper Arm Lymphatics

Following the skin incision, the entire dissection should be performed under the microscope. Usually ×10 magnification is sufficient to maintain exposure and to work atraumatically. Dissection is most quickly performed between the subcutaneous fat deposits, without division (splitting). The interstitial connective tissue bands are used to approach the microvascular structures. Each structure passing subcutaneously (nerve, vein, artery, and lymphatic) is dissected separately to preserve existing lymphatic collaterals. Small subcutaneous arteries and veins are, of course, easily recognized. Small vein branches are carefully preserved for later end-to-end anastomosis. Tapes are placed around the larger branches for a possible end-to-side procedure. Draining lymphatics can also be visualized without the aid of a dye by the small vasa vasorum located in the wall of the lymphatics. They are clearly visible against the bright contents of the lymphatics. Furthermore, the organization of the lymphatics, consisting of small pump units (lymphangiones), may be distingished following cutaneous compression.

The lymphatic valves are usually located at a distance of 3 mm from each other and are sometimes visible [2]. Usually the lymph vessel undergoes a spasm during dissection, even when the dissection is carried out according to microsurgical principles, i.e., without touching the lymphatics themselves. Papaverine (50 mg/ml) may be beneficial. A good rule to follow is to touch the lymphatics only indirectly and only to put traction on them by using the surrounding tissue. Following dissection of the dilated lymphatics and veins on the superficial fascia, the anastomosis may be performed.

II. Leg Lymphatics

The incision in the groin or in the thigh is made sharply, down to Scarpa's fascia. The fascia is then incised under the microscope. The greater saphenous vein is carefully dissected, and a tape is placed around it. If the greater saphenous vein is absent or ligated proximally (blockade in the groin), a small incision into the deep fascia should be made, followed by exposure of several branches of the deep venous system. Anatomically, the lymphatics always pass in the direct vicinity of the greater saphenous vein, mostly in three pairs. The dilated lymphatics are carefully exposed over a short distance, and tapes are placed around them. When considering a lymph nodal-venous anastomosis, a lymph node, with the afferent lymphatics, should be exposed and isolated. Following exposure of a sufficient number of lymphatics (two or three) and of the greater saphenous vein, or a comparable number of other veins, the anastomosis may be performed.

E. Anastomotic Technique

I. Lymph Nodal-Venous Anastomosis (Patch)

Among the lymph nodal-venous shunts, only the patch technique is effective. The risk that the anas-

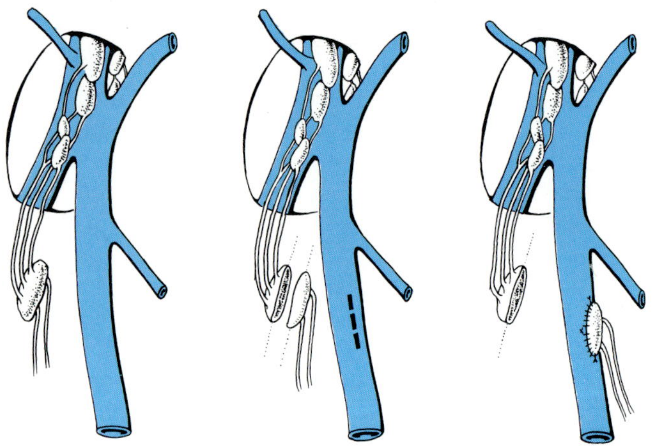

Fig. 29.2.3. Technique of lymph nodal-venous anastomosis: patch technique; suturing of the distal lymph nodal capsule (patch) to the vein, preserving the afferent lymphatics (in case of blockage in the pelvic region)

tomosis will become fibrotic is much smaller with this technique than with the conventional technique of suturing half of a lymph node into the vein.

Following dissection of an appropriate lymph node with its afferent vessels, the capsule is dissected off the underlying nodal tissue (sinus) at the entrance of the afferent lymphatics. In this manner, a rhomboid segment (window) of the capsule is removed. When inspecting the inner side, the ostia of the lymphatics should be clearly visible. The remaining nodal tissue is closed by suture ligation (if necessary, this half can also be anastomosed). Following local heparinization, the vein is cross-clamped with two vascular clamps. Between them, a venotomy is performed. The length of the venotomy is matched to the patch (about 1 cm). The patch is sutured in classic fashion using a 7-0 Prolene continuous suture. After the anastomosis has been completed, the clamps are removed. Usually, a good flow of lymph fluid in the direction of the greater saphenous vein is visible. The subcutaneous tissue and the skin are closed afterward (Fig. 29.2.3).

II. Lymphatic-Venous Anastomosis

1. End-to-End Technique

End-to-end lymphatic venous shunts usually show a longer patency than any other type. The vessels that are dissected free for the end-to-end anastomosis should be approximated without traction. Any unnecessary tension on the microsuture increases the risk of obstruction. The proximal side of the lymphatic is coagulated with bipolar electrodes; in order to avoid unnecessary damage by the clamps, the distal efferent segment is not cross-clamped during this procedure. Thus, a free flow of lymph fluid is provided. The vein is cross-clamped with a microclamp. The lumen is flushed with heparinized electrolyte solution to remove small thrombi. Prior to the anastomosis, the lumen of the lymphatic is dilated somewhat.

The end-to-end anastomosis is performed using 10-0 to 12-0 monofilament interrupted sutures. The first two sutures are placed as corner sutures, approximately 180° from each other. The wall of the lymphatic should be touched as little as possible with the microforceps in order to avoid damaging the intima. The anastomosis is completed by four additional sutures. Following removal of the clamp on the venous side, a good flow of lymph fluid should be visible within the vein. Other anastomoses are performed in the same way. Afterward, only the skin is closed to avoid compression by subcutaneous tissue in the immediate postoperative phase. For the same reason, no drains are placed (Fig. 29.2.4).

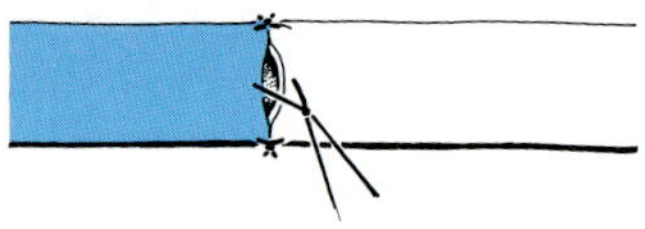

Fig. 29.2.4. Lymphatic-venous shunt. Type 1: end-to-end, with 10-0 sutures

2. End-to-Side Technique

End-to-side anastomoses are required when the vein caliber in the operative field is much greater than the diameter of the appropriate lymphatic. Following exposure and cross-clamping, a small orifice is created in the wall of the selected vein. An injection needle is best for perforating the vein wall. Through the same ostium, the vein may be flushed with heparinized solution. Proximally and distally, a suture (10-0) is placed through the ostium. Then, both sutures are passed through the lymphatic to be anastomosed and are tied. That is how the corner sutures are placed. At this moment one should carefully determine whether the anterior as well as the posterior wall of the lymphatic and the vein have erroneously been sutured together. If this is not the case, the anastomosis

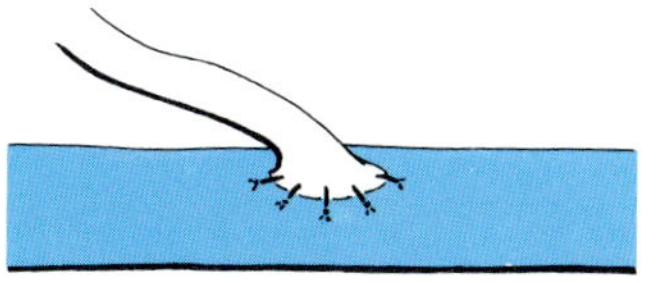

Fig. 29.2.5. Lymphatic-venous shunt. Type II: end-to-side, with 10-0 sutures

may be completed by additional sutures through the anterior and posterior wall of the lymphatic and the vein. Following completion of the anastomosis, a good flow in the direction of the vein should be visible. The other lymphatics available (donor lymphatics) may be sutured to the vein in the same way (Fig. 29.2.5). Following removal of the vein clamps, the skin is closed.

3. Pull-Through Technique

The pull-through technique is a variant of the end-to-side anastomosis. The vein is prepared in the same way. The lymphatics, however, are not sutured to the vein but inserted so that one segment is located in the lumen of the vein. The lymphatics can then be fixed by microsutures. According to some authors (JACOBS, DEGNI) the extreme end of the lymphatics functions like a valve. In routine practice, however, the risk of thrombosis is very high; consequently, this technique is suitable only in the groin, when the greater saphenous vein can be used (Fig. 29.2.6) [3, 4].

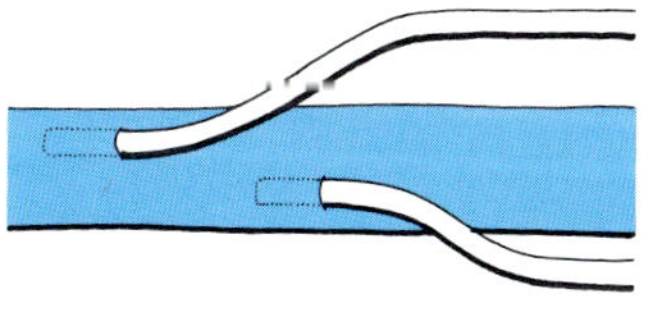

Fig. 29.2.6. Lymphatic-venous shunt. Type III: pull-through technique, fixation by single suture (DEGNI) or without suture material (JACOBS)

F. Postoperative Complications

The most serious postoperative complication following lymphatic-vein surgery is early shunt occlusion (2%–4%) which may occur by venous retrograde flow through the anastomosis.

This can be avoided by strict observation of the indication, i.e., no lymphatic-vein procedures in patients presenting with a regionally increased venous pressure from occlusion of the vein system. Postoperatively (second day), a Lymphapress apparatus may be applied (pressure 60 mmHg), for two 4-h periods per day. This provides continuous flow from the lymphatics to the veins during this critical period.

REFERENCES

1. Baumeister RGH (1987) Autologe Lymphgefäßtransplantation. In: Heberer G, van Dongen RJAM (eds) Kirschnersche allgemeine und spezielle Operationslehre, vol XI. Springer, Berlin Heidelberg New York Tokyo, p 823
2. Casley-Smith JR (1976) The functioning and interrelationships of blood capillaries and lymphatics. Experientia 32:1
3. Degni H (1974) New technique of lymphatic-venous-anastomosis for the treatment of lymphedema. VASA 3:3
4. Jacobs JWM (1981) De kunstmatige lymphaticoveneuze anastomose, een experimenteel-anatomisch onderzoek. Thesis Universiteit van Amsterdam, Mondeel Uitgeverij Amsterdam
5. Nieuborg L (1982) The role of lymphaticovenous surgery in the treatment of postmastectomy oedema. Thesis Universiteit van Amsterdam, Offsetdrukkerij Kanters BV Alblasserdam
6. O'Brien BMcC, Shafiroff BB (1976) Microlymphaticovenous and resectional surgery in obstructive lymphedema. World J Surg 3:3

29.3 Autogenous Lymph Vessel Transplantation

R.G.H. Baumeister

CONTENTS

The cause of secondary lymphedema is often a localized interruption of the lymph flow by traumatic or iatrogenic destruction of lymph collectors or lymph node groups. Restoration of passage by interposition of autogenous lymph collectors represents a true reconstruction, in contrast to excisional and draining procedures such as lymphatic-venous anastomosis [1, 2, 3, 4]. For rehabilitation, however, the extent of secondary changes caused by the lymphedema is of great importance.

A. Indications

Lymphatic grafting is a method of restoring locally blocked lymph flow. The most frequent indication is arm edema resulting from axillary lymph node removal and radiotherapy in women who have undergone a mastectomy. Blockage caused by isolated trauma or operative intervention at narrow sites of the lymph system, such as the root of the extremities and often on the inside of the knee, may also be treated by lymph vessel transplantation.

In cases of primary lymphedema, segmental atresia of the lymphatic system, like unilateral atresia in the pelvis, can be treated by means of a lymphatic crossover bypass over the symphysis.

A direct reconstruction of the destroyed lymph vessels should be attempted after an appropriate lymphatic transport deficit has been objectively diagnosed.

As a matter of routine, prior to any operative intervention, thoroughgoing conservative treatment should be tried first. If the edema improves for only a short time or recurs after the treatment has ceased, one should not delay the decision to operate because the accumulation of secondary changes may impair the result. In contrast to excision procedures, therefore, one should not wait until a massive increase of edema is noticed. Improvements in the methods for quantifying transport capacity would make it possible to select patients for reconstructive procedures before they present with the obvious clinical symptoms of lymphedema.

B. Preoperative Evaluation, Positioning, Perioperative Measures

For the most part, we deal with secondary lymphedema resulting from cancer. First of all, therefore, local recurrence or metastases must be excluded.

Preoperative scintigraphy of the edematous extremity confirms the diagnosis and allows semiquantitative determination of the reduction in transport capacity. In any case, normal lymph flow must be demonstrated in the donor leg in order to preclude the possibility of removing lymphatics in a latent edema phase. In this way, swelling following removal of lymph collectors may be avoided almost completely.

The patient is placed on the operating table, preferably on a heating cushion, and covered with a gold foil. In upper extremity edema, the arm is placed on a hand table. The head is turned to the contralateral side, thus exposing the lateral triangle of the neck.

Following closure of the wound an elastic bandage is applied to the edematous extremity as well as to the donor leg, and both limbs are elevated.

Perioperative antibiotic prophylaxis is usually performed. Postoperatively, low molecular weight Dextran is infused for 5–8 days.

C. Technique of Lymph Vessel Transplantation

I. Harvesting of Donor Lymphatics (Fig. 29.3.1)

Just prior to the procedure, Patent Blue is injected subcutaneously and intradermally in the first and second interdigital space of the donor leg. Injection of dye in the edematous extremity is carried out only in rare cases of localized edema, because usually the dye will not be transported upward in sufficient quantity to become visible.

The dissection may be carried out under a magnifying glass. Only for the final exposure of the graft ends and invisible lymphatic segments is a microscope required. For harvesting of donor lymphatics, the incision is made just medial to the femoral artery, which is palpated. Here, in the space lateral to the greater saphenous vein, the dyed lymphatics are exposed. The incision is lengthened caudally a little at a time, according to the course of the lymph collectors. The collectors are dissected until one approaches the next lymphatic isthmus, i.e., the region of the knee.

When harvesting, a small portion of fatty and connective tissue remains attached to the lymphatics to avoid exsiccation and to achieve greater mechanical stability. Only the ends to be anastomosed are cleaned of adventitial tissue. A stay suture of size 10-0 or 11-0 can be used to distingish between the anterior and posterior wall while anastomosing. Any small lymphatic end that is not to be used is ligated. The beginning of the graft is fixed by a knot to enable its passing through a Redon drain, which serves as an interim protection.

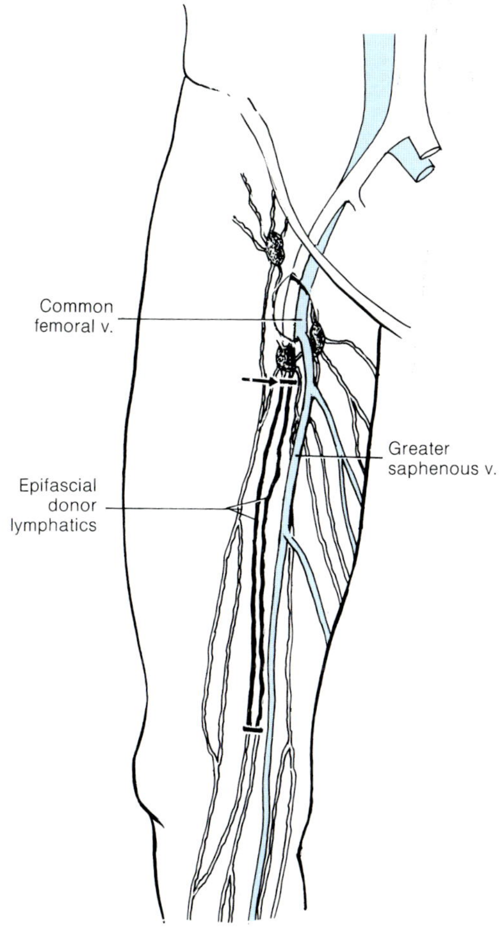

Fig. 29.3.1. Harvesting of donor lymphatics from the ventromedial bundle of the thigh, lateral to the greater saphenous vein

At the site of harvesting, two drains are placed prior to wound closure, which is done with vertical mattress sutures.

II. Lymph Vessel Transplantation in the Upper Extremity (Fig. 29.3.2)

In cases of upper extremity edema, the superficial and usually the deep lymphatics are exposed through a longitudinal incision in the proximal upper arm, over the neurovascular bundle. Additionally, the cephalic neurovascular bundle may be isolated through an incision over the cephalic vein. It is often difficult to differentiate sclerotic lymphatics from small nerves or connective tissue bands. Sometimes, diagnosis is possible only after an exploratory incision.

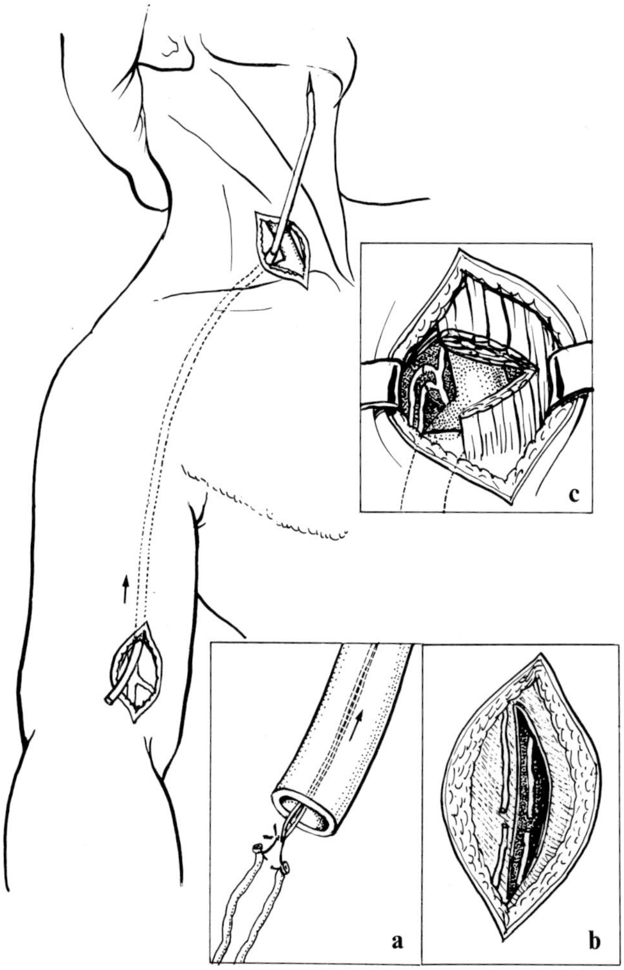

Fig. 29.3.2a–c. Incisions and tunneling of the graft bed for lymph vessel transplantation in edema following mastectomy. **a** Pulling two lymphatic grafts through the Redon tunnel. **b** An epifascial and subfascial ascending lymph vessel is dissected, and the corresponding graft ends are brought into position. **c** Cervical anastomotic site: the sternocleidomastoid muscle is incised; lympho-lymphatic end-to-end anastomosis to the deep neck collectors

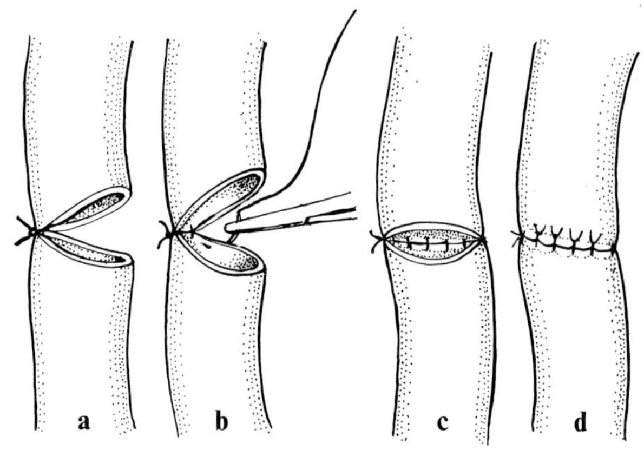

Fig. 29.3.3a–d. Schematic drawing of traction-free anastomotic technique for end-to-end lymphatic suture. **a** Corner suture. **b** Suture of the posterior wall with interrupted sutures; the lymphatic does not have to be turned by pulling on the corner suture. **c** Second corner suture. **d** Closure of the anterior wall

The dissections are carried out under the microscope. For the anastomosis, a magnification up to ×40 should be used.

In the region of the neck, the incision is made on the lateral margin of the sternocleidomastoid muscle, just above the clavicle. Severing the muscle medially, or incising the muscle, exposes the lateral wall of the internal jugular vein. In this area, the lymph collectors that are suitable for anastomosis are dissected in the fatty tissue, despite their thin walls.

The grafts are placed in the subcutaneous tissue. In order to protect them during the pull-through, a tunnel from the upper arm to the neck is created by a thick Redon drain. Care must be taken not to injure the cephalic vein; therefore, the Redon drain is passed through as far medially as possible. The collectors are then pulled through this tubing, and the Redon tubing is removed. Thus, the collectors finally course freely in the subcutaneous tissue.

Usually, end-to-end anastomoses are performed. In order to avoid lacerations of the fragile lymphatic wall, a so-called traction-free anastomotic technique is used (Fig. 29.3.3). With this procedure, the vessel does not have to be rotated by lateral stay sutures in order to bring the anterior or posterior wall around to face the surgeon.

In this special anastomotic technique, the lymphatics that are approximated for the anastomosis remain in situ throughout the entire anastomotic procedure. First, the corner suture located opposite the surgeon is tied. For the suture of the posterior wall with interrupted sutures, the lymphatic is drawn up far enough to provide sufficient space to pass the needle. After the second corner suture is knotted, the anterior wall is closed with interrupted sutures. Each of the two walls, the anterior and the posterior, requires 2–4 sutures.

Absorbable suture material is superior to nonabsorbable material. The size of the suture is from 10-0 to 12-0, the size of the needle, BV 6–8.

Cross-clamping of the lymphatics should be avoided so as not to cause additional trauma.

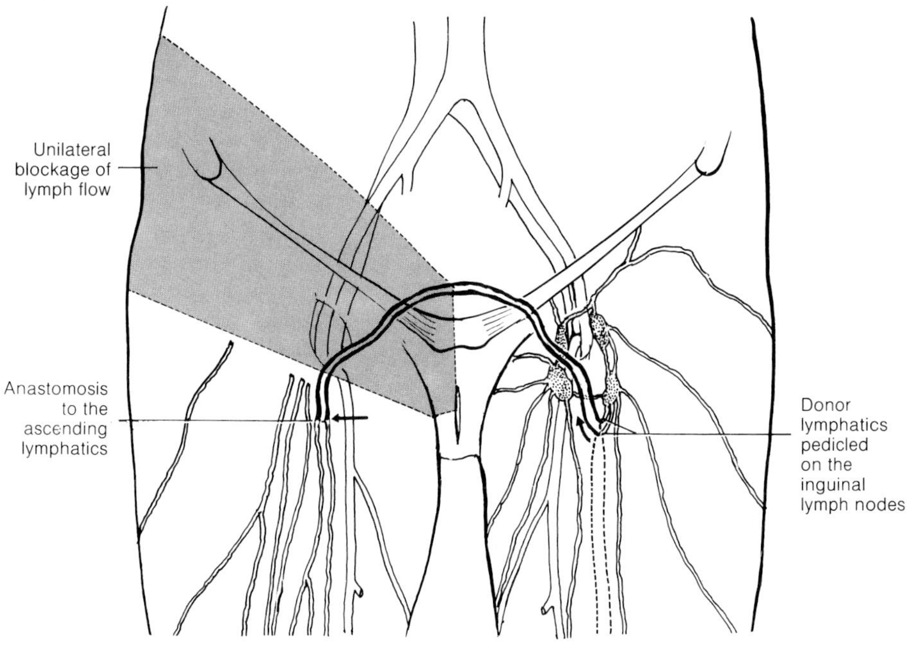

Fig. 29.3.4. Lymphatic grafting across the symphysis, pedicled on the donor side, in unilateral lymphedema of the lower extremity

III. Lymph Vessel Transplantation in the Lower Extremity (Fig. 29.3.4)

In cases of unilateral edema of the lower extremity due to blockage within the groin or the pelvis, the lymphatics of the contralateral thigh are used. They are dissected as indicated in Sect. C.I. However, they remain pedicled to the inguinal lymph nodes of the donor side. Using Redon tubing, a tunnel is created over the symphysis to an incision distal to the groin in the edematous extremity. Through this tubing the lymphatics are passed, to be finally anastomosed to the ascending lymphatics.

IV. Direct Lymphatic Reconstruction and Lymphatic Grafting

In case of fresh, regionally limited lymphedemas, resulting from local blockage of the outflow, the lymphatics distal to the site of the blockage can be exposed. They are mobilized and may, under certain circumstances, be anastomosed, without lymphatic graft interposition, to the deep or adjacent epifascial lymphatics, which lie in regions of free flow. If this is not possible, short grafts are used.

REFERENCES

1. Baumeister RGH, Seifert J, Wiebecke B, Hahn D (1981) Experimental basis and first application of clinical lymph vessel transplantation of secondary lymphedema. World J Surg 5:401
2. Baumeister RGH (1983) Mikrochirurgie des Lymphgefäßsystems. Chirurg 54:374
3. Ho LCY, Lai MF, Kennedy J (1983) Micro-lymphatic bypass in the treatment of obstructive lymphoedema of the arm: case report of a new technique. Br J Plast Surg 36:350
4. Mandl H (1981) Experimentelle Untersuchungen zur mikrochirurgischen Rekonstruktion von Lymphgefäßdefekten. Z Plast Chir 5:70

Subject Index